Clinical Orthopaedic Diagnosis

Clinical Orthopaedic Diagnosis

Fifth Edition

Sureshwar Pandey
MBBS (Hons) MS (Gen) FICS FIAMS MS (Ortho) FACFAS FACS FNAMS
Professor Emeritus, University of Ranchi
Founder and Founder Director, Charitable GNH Handicapped Children Hospital and RJS Artificial Limb Centre, Ranchi
Founder and Consultant, Ram Janam Sulakshana
Institute of Orthopaedics and Research, Ranchi, Jharkhand, India
Founder and Emeritus President and Ex-Secretary General, Indian Foot and Ankle Society [Affiliated to International Federation of Foot and Ankle Societies (IFFAS)]
Founder and Emeritus Editor, The Journal of Foot and Ankle Surgery
Visiting Professor, Universities of Tokyo, Osaka, Teikyo, Adelaide, Flinders,
Ujung Pandang, Singapore
Ex-Chairman, ASIA-CIP (IFFAS)
Founder and Chairman, Ram Janam Sulakshana Pandey Charitable
Cancer Hospital & Research and Rehabilitation Centre, Ranchi
Hon President, Asia-Pacific Society for Foot and Ankle Surgery
- Best Book Award of BOS (2000–2001) for his Book Clinical Orthopaedic Diagnosis, 2nd Edition
- Best Book Award of BOA 2002 for his Unique Books
- Best Book Award (2009–2010) for his Book—*The Clubfoot Revisited*
- Humanitarian Award of India of IOA – 2019

Anil Kumar Pandey
MBBS CORM PhD (Ortho) MAMS
Director and Consultant
Ram Janam Sulakshana Institute of Orthopaedics and Research (RJSIOR)
Associate Director and Consultant
GNH Handicapped Children Hospital and RJS Artificial Limb Centre
Executive Director and Consultant
Ram Janam Sulakshana Pandey Charitable Cancer Hospital and Research and Rehabilitation Centre
Ranchi, Jharkhand, India
Consultant—Kiran Centre for Education and Rehabilitation
Varanasi, Uttar Pradesh, India
Consultant—RAHA, Chhattisgarh, India
Reconstructive Surgeon, Rotary International Project, Government of Nigeria

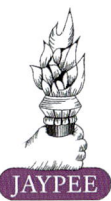

JAYPEE BROTHERS MEDICAL PUBLISHERS
The Health Sciences Publisher
New Delhi | London

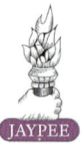

Jaypee Brothers Medical Publishers (P) Ltd

Headquarters
Jaypee Brothers Medical Publishers (P) Ltd
EMCA House, 23/23-B
Ansari Road, Daryaganj
New Delhi 110 002, India
Landline: +91-11-23272143, +91-11-23272703
+91-11-23282021, +91-11-23245672
Email: jaypee@jaypeebrothers.com

Corporate Office
Jaypee Brothers Medical Publishers (P) Ltd
4838/24, Ansari Road, Daryaganj
New Delhi 110 002, India
Phone: +91-11-43574357
Fax: +91-11-43574314
Email: jaypee@jaypeebrothers.com

Overseas Office
JP Medical Ltd.
83, Victoria Street, London
SW1H 0HW (UK)
Phone: +44 20 3170 8910
Fax: +44 (0)20 3008 6180
Email: info@jpmedpub.com

Website: www.jaypeebrothers.com
Website: www.jaypeedigital.com

© 2024, Jaypee Brothers Medical Publishers

The views and opinions expressed in this book are solely those of the original contributor(s)/author(s) and do not necessarily represent those of editor(s) or publisher of the book.

All rights reserved. No part of this publication may be reproduced, stored or transmitted in any form or by any means, electronic, mechanical, photocopying, recording or otherwise, without the prior permission in writing of the publishers.

All brand names and product names used in this book are trade names, service marks, trademarks or registered trademarks of their respective owners. The publisher is not associated with any product or vendor mentioned in this book.

Medical knowledge and practice change constantly. This book is designed to provide accurate, authoritative information about the subject matter in question. However, readers are advised to check the most current information available on procedures included and check information from the manufacturer of each product to be administered, to verify the recommended dose, formula, method and duration of administration, adverse effects and contraindications. It is the responsibility of the practitioner to take all appropriate safety precautions. Neither the publisher nor the author(s)/editor(s) assume any liability for any injury and/or damage to persons or property arising from or related to use of material in this book.

This book is sold on the understanding that the publisher is not engaged in providing professional medical services. If such advice or services are required, the services of a competent medical professional should be sought.

Every effort has been made where necessary to contact holders of copyright to obtain permission to reproduce copyright material. If any have been inadvertently overlooked, the publisher will be pleased to make the necessary arrangements at the first opportunity.

Inquiries for bulk sales may be solicited at: jaypee@jaypeebrothers.com

Clinical Orthopaedic Diagnosis

First Edition: 1995
Second Edition: 2000
  Updated Second Edition: 2002
Third Edition: 2009
Fourth Edition: 2019

Fifth Edition: **2024**

ISBN: 978-93-5465-952-2

Printed at: Samrat Offset Pvt. Ltd.

To

the fond memory of my beloved parents

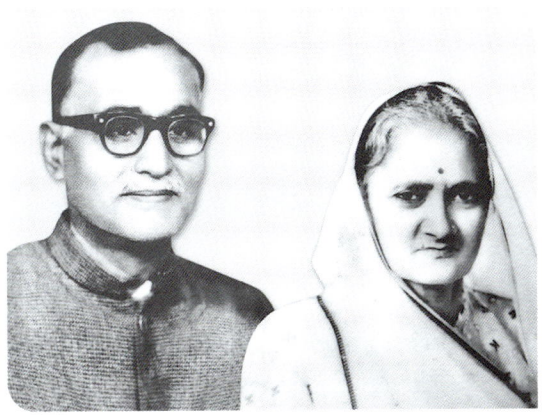

Sulakshana Pandey

and

Ramjanam Pandey

- *who were, are, and will be always with me to love, teach and guide*

- *who taught me to pursue my dreams because nothing is impossible with sincere and devoted efforts*

- *who gave me everything, but never even desired to have anything from me*

Hippocratic Oath

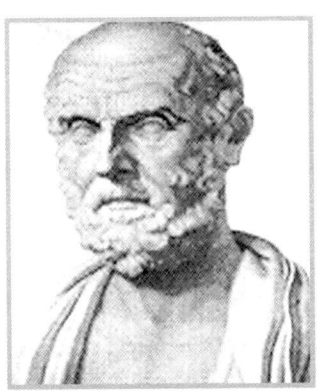

Hippocrate, a Greek physician of the 5th Century BC

I swear by Apollo Physician and Asclepius and Hygieia and Panaceia and all the Gods and Goddesses, making them my witnesses, that I will fulfil according to my ability and judgment this oath and this covenant:

To hold him who has taught me this art as equal to my parents and to live my life in partnership with him, and if he is in need of money to give him a share of mine, and to regard his offspring as equal to my brothers in male lineage and to teach them this art – if they desire to learn it – without fee and covenant; to give a share of precepts and oral instruction and all the other learning to my sons and to the sons of him who has instructed me and to pupils who have signed the covenant and have taken an oath according to the medical law, but no one else.

I will apply dietetic measures for the benefit of the sick according to my ability and judgment; I will keep them from harm and injustice.

I will neither give a deadly drug to anybody who asked for it, nor will I make a suggestion to this effect. Similarly I will not give to a woman an abortive remedy. In purity and holiness I will guard my life and my art.

I will not use the knife, not even on sufferers from stone, but will withdraw in favor of such men as are engaged in this work.

Whatever houses I may visit, I will come for the benefit of the sick, remaining free of all intentional injustice, of all mischief and in particular of sexual relations with both female and male persons, be they free or slaves.

What I may see or hear in the course of the treatment or even outside of the treatment in regard to the life of men, which on no account one must spread abroad, I will keep to myself, holding such things shameful to be spoken about.

If I fulfil this oath and do not violate it, may it be granted to me to enjoy life and art, being honored with fame among all men for all time to come; if I transgress it and swear falsely, may the opposite of all this be my lot.

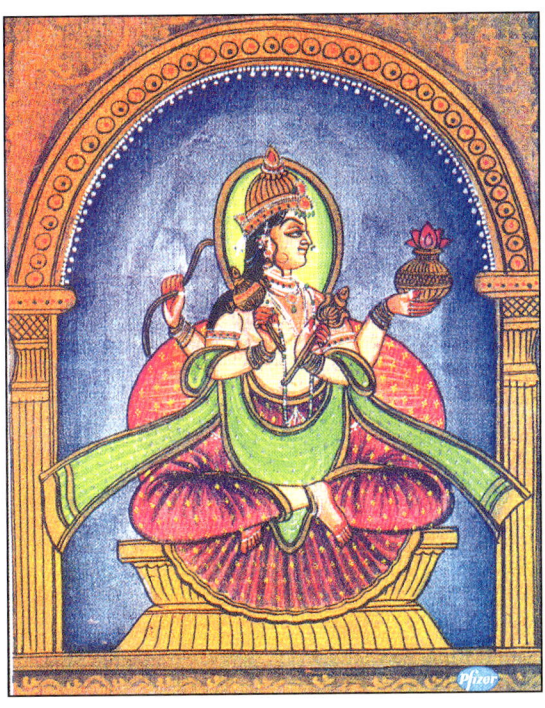

"DHANVANTARI"*
The Hindu God of Medicine

Commonly worshipped as the Hindu God of Medicine, DHANVANTARI is regarded as the original exponent of Indian medicine. DHANVANTARI has many myths and legends woven around him. He emerged with the pot of ambrosia (symbolic of medicine) in his hand from the ocean when it was churned by the contesting Gods and demons. He is viewed as the very incarnation of God VISHNU. He is said to have recovered ambrosia which had been lost, and thus obtained a share in sacrifices.

Legends make him reappear as "DIVODASA", the prince of Benaras (Kasiraja), in the family of Ayus. Dhanvantari, Divodasa and Kasiraja are names of the same person who is "the first God and who freed the other Gods from old age, disease and death", and who in his Himalayan retreat taught surgery to Susruta and other sages. DHANVANTARI appeared on earth in Benaras in the princely family of Bahuja and became known as Divodasa; he wandered about as a mendicant even during his early years.

DHANVANTARI also appears to have been an actual historical person, although his precise identity is hard to be ascertained. He taught surgery and other divisions of Ayurveda (Indian system of medicine) at the instance of Susruta, to a group of sages among whom Susruta was the foremost.

DHANVANTARI is regarded as the patron-God of all branches of medicine. While DHANVANTARI is not credited with any medical treatise of his own, in the early accounts, there is a voluminous glossary and materia medica in the nine sections known as Dhanvantari-Nighantu; it is a compilation which is probably contemporaneous with the famous Amara-kosha (A.D. 100). There are a few other works which are also ascribed to Dhanvantari.

There are numerous preparations which are ascribed to him, and many of them quite ancient.

Dhanvantari-Nighantu is considered the most ancient of the medical glossaries that are available. The original work is said to have been in three recensions; the present version which may have been based on one of them, is in six sections and deals with 373 medicinal substances; their names, synonyms, and brief description of properties being given. The work which claims to be 'like the third eye' for the practising physician, is extensively relied upon, despite several more comprehensive glossaries that have been compiled subsequently. Since there is no authentic source of information, this text can be considered more as indicative.

(By courtesy Pfizer Limited)

---

* This painting has been commissioned by Pfizer Ltd (India) based on an old painting belonging to the Late Maharaja of Mysore, Krishnaraja Wodeyar II (South India).

Foreword to the Fourth Edition

Clinical Orthopaedic Diagnosis is based upon the author's (Prof. Sureshwar Pandey) personal observations made during nearly 50 years of interaction with orthopaedic disease and patients.

With the availabilities of modern imaging modalities and investigations, there has been some reduction of the importance of clinical examinations and human-touch; however, all observations made by the modern investigative facilities are mandated to be correlated by clinical features. Clinical examination as suggested by our ancestral orthopaedic educators must include: listen, look, feel, move, measure, and compare (clinically and radiologically), all this has been documented by Prof Pandey, through the written script, tables, photographs, and drawings. The clinical approach for diagnosis is of great importance in areas of the world having constrained resources and for cost-containment in general. A sound clinical judgement helps the clinicians to ask for pertinent investigations rather than order for "MRI screening of whole spine", "scanogram of both lower limbs" in every case. Despite the development of sophisticated investigations and evolution of superspecialities during a situation of clinical and therapeutic dilemma, the clinical judgement still remains supreme.

In addition to the clinical examination methodology, relevant clinical anatomy of the region being dealt with in a chapter has been described at the beginning of each chapter. The clinical pictures and X-rays collated by Prof Pandey over the lifetime covers almost all orthopaedic diseases, deformities and traumatology. The book presents a comprehensive clinical orthopaedics, the illustrations almost present a "book-museum" of complete orthopaedics.

With continuous progress in biological science, no compendium is complete and perfect; however, Prof Pandey deserves congratulations from all students of orthopaedics and myself for his tremendous effort. Prof Pandey should continue to have a sense of accomplishment that he is leaving behind a monumental educative document for the posterity. This book is recommended to be kept in all clinics taking care of orthopaedic diseases, disorders and trauma.

SM Tuli MS PhD FAMS
Senior Consultant in Spinal Diseases and Orthopaedics
Vimhans-Primamed Hospital
Nehru Nagar, New Delhi, India
Formerly, Director, Institute of Medical Sciences, Banaras Hindu University
Professor and Head, Department of Orthopaedics
Banaras Hindu University
Varanasi, Uttar Pradesh, India
University College of Medical Sciences
New Delhi, India

Foreword to the First Edition

Professor Sureshwar Pandey has undertaken a very worthwhile project in writing a book on *Clinical Orthopaedic Diagnosis*. The importance of proper clinical examination needs no emphasis. All investigations are based on clues provided by proper and systematic clinical examination and a logical interpretation of the findings.

Unfortunately, there has been a lack of standard textbook giving a detailed and systematic approach to a methodical clinical examination of orthopaedic patients, including correct interpretation of physical signs provided by such examination. Professor Pandey has produced a textbook which embodies all the methods utilised in a systematic clinical examination of the motor skeletal system.

By providing relevant line-drawings, which are very helpful in understanding clinical features and also providing charts that include a step-by-step interpretation of the clinical findings, he has made a proper clinical approach—logical and simple.

I feel confident that the approach he has adopted in eliciting and interpreting clinical features will be most useful not only to undergraduate and postgraduate students but even to practitioners so that they can look upon this book as a guide to reduce incidents of errors in examination.

I heartily congratulate Professor Pandey on this effort.

Padmabhushan **Dr B Mukhopadhyay**
MBBS (Hons) MCh Ortho (L'Pool) FRCS (Lond) FNAMS
Emeritus Professor
University of Patna
Saidpur Road, Patna, India

Preface to the Fifth Edition

The overwhelming acceptance of the book 'CLINICAL ORTHOPAEDIC DIAGNOSIS' right from the launch of its first edition in 1995 till now — the era of its fourth edition — and launching of its present fifth edition — has definitely encouraged us to venture for this present step (the Vth Edition).

Acceptance of this book has been not only in the Indian Subcontinent, but also in several countries of the world shown by its publication as the Spanish edition. This was predicted in the Book-review of its First edition itself in the Journal of Bone and Joint Surgery (British volume 79B 1997 on page 345). Similar have been the opinions in reviews of several Journals and distinct professors and consultants. We are deeply obliged to them. We will continue to work hard to keep up their expectations.

Sureshwar Pandey
Anil Kumar Pandey

Preface to the First Edition

Orthopaedic practice demands repetitive and complex decision making. All decisions are necessarily influenced by non-scientific considerations, such as limited facilities, patients' non-compliance, and financial constraints, as well as the current limitations of orthopaedic science. Despite these impediments, we all strive towards accuracy in our decision making. Accurate clinical diagnosis forms the basis of successful management of any ailment. No doubt, the development of a sound judgement is largely a matter of experience; yet one must remember the words of Sir Astley Cooper, "Nothing is known in our profession by guess, and I do not believe that from the first dawn of medical science to the present moment a single correct idea has ever emanated from conjecture…, there is no short road to knowledge". The great Indian surgeon Sushruta has also warned against diagnosing a disease merely on speculation. He gave explicit instructions regarding exploration of the history of the disease, thorough examination (inspection, palpation, auscultation, etc.) and analysis of the symptoms and signs, before coming to a conclusion.

The immense importance of systematic clinical examination cannot be overemphasised. No one can be familiar with the clinical signs and their interpretation in a short period or just by going through the text. A rigorous apprenticeship is mandatory to learn the clinical methodology step by step, lest a snap diagnosis based on a cursory examination may prove to be disastrous. Whatsoever may be the advances in the field of investigation procedures, these must remain the supplement to and not the substitute of thorough clinical examination.

With this backdrop, an attempt has been made to further enhance the importance of 'clinical methodology' in orthopaedics. The effort has been made to create an atmosphere of positive and practical approach towards diagnosing the clinical conditions on a sound basis, so that therapy becomes easy and less complex. No patient can be examined just for one system, rather it should be the total examination of the patient. However, for the osteoarticular and neuromuscular affections, a more detailed examination than usual is necessary, such as assessment of movements, length disparities, neuromuscular status, etc.

A knowledge of clinical anatomy is quite essential for any orthopaedic student, trainee or even surgeon. To cover this, a brief description of the relevant clinical anatomy of the region dealt with was thought to be essential, and it has been given at the beginning of each chapter. Wherever it was necessary, a note on the basic physiology concerning that zone has been added. Quick and fairly clear conception of the subject can be had by going through a tabular form of description, which has been given whatever deemed to be essential. Reminder of the 'key diagnostic points' at the end of the chapters would help the clinicians come to a quick diagnosis, the trainees/residents to learn methods of elimination, and the students/examinees to quickly revise the subject.

With due apology to the stalwarts, whose names could not be included due to my ignorance, an attempt has been made at the end of the book to recall the noted works of the pioneers of orthopaedics.

The manuscript has been revised through the scrutiny of more than seven batches of postgraduate and undergraduate students in orthopaedics and the project is the result of their inspiration, encouragement and criticism. However, a lot of improvements and modifications have to be done in future editions after reviewing the frank criticisms and remarks of the readers—the real watchdogs.

I am deeply obliged to my revered teacher, Padmabhushan Prof Emeritus B Mukhopadhyay, who lit the lamp of knowledge in my mind and soul. And also to my senior and contemporary colleagues all over the country and abroad, like Emeritus Prof N Tsuyama (Tokyo), Prof SM Tuli, Prof PT Rao, Prof DP Baksi, Prof NS Laud, Dr BB Joshi, Prof RR Ganguli, Prof RC Ram, Prof SV Sharma, Prof RP Singh, Prof KM Pathi, Prof NK Agarwal, Prof K Ono (Osaka), Prof T Koshino (Yokohama), Prof B Helal (London), Prof K Bose (Singapore), Prof JM Martorell (Barcelona), Dr R Bauze (Adelaide), and others who helped me to clear my confusion at several stages. I did derive benefit, pleasure, and profit from their stimulating exchange of ideas, which I very humbly and deeply acknowledge.

My colleagues, Prof RL Rajak, Prof B Alam, Prof HN Sinha, Prof AK Mishra, Prof KP Pandey, Dr PD Singh, Dr KN Jha, Dr SS Jha, Dr RC Mishra, Dr SN Sinha, and others with whom I have been privileged to work through the years and have helped by providing healthy criticism, I am indebted to all of them.

The tiresome work of proofreading has been ably assisted by my son Dr Anil, daughter-in-law Dr Pushpa and the fleet of my very dear postgraduate students, especially Drs SP Bhagat, Awadhesh Singh and Sanjeeva Kumar, whose help cannot forget.

My family—my loving wife, sons (Dr Anil, Arun and Akhil) and their wives (Dr Pushpa, Asha and Sandhya) tolerated many of my eccentricities all through the period of preparation of this book. I cannot repay the debt. My grandchildren (Pallavi, Shivam, Vaishnavi, Shruti and Saumya) proved to be the real source of pleasure in tense moments. God bless them.

And finally, I sincerely acknowledge the help of Dr Ravi, for preparing the line drawings and Mr Ajit Kumar Shukla, for typing the manuscript.

Sureshwar Pandey

Acknowledgements

In upgrading this book to its Vth Edition, the full credit goes to tiresome efforts of the young enthusiastic doctors and pioneers of my graceful family besides my co-author Dr Anil Kumar Pandey they are: my loving wife, Dr Pushpa Pandey, Adv Arun Kumar Pandey, Smt Asha Pandey, Akhil Kumar Pandey, Smt Sandhya Pandey, Dr Kumar Sangam Shukla, Dr Pallavi Pandey Shukla, Dr Shivam, Dr Gaurav Sharma, Dr Vaishnavi, Mr Hitesh Vashistsh, Adv Shruti Pandey, Dr Mohan Tiwari, Dr Soumyanil Pandey and Dr Satyam Shrey.

I frankly admit that my driving forces are the little angles— Atharva Pranjal, Adhrit Pranjal and Yuvraj Harish.

We are extremely obliged for the untiring efforts and help rendered by our co-workers Dr Madhukar Anand, Dr Sabana Hasan, Ms Sarita Thapa, Ms Mileta Xalxo and Ms Laxmi in preparing and correcting the manuscript.

Shri Jitendar P Vij (Group Chairman), Mr Ankit Vij (Managing Director), Mr MS Maini (Group President) and the devotee team of Jaypee Bothers Medical Publishers, New Delhi, India have always been at our help with encouragement at every step, we are grateful to them.

Introductory Comments
(Based on the First Edition itself)

This textbook authored by Prof Sureshwar Pandey contains a large number of orthopaedic diseases from children to adult ones. He spent really many years to collect all these materials to complete this marvellous book. From general common diseases to even quite special rare diseases and deformities, this book is dealing with orthopaedic disorders of many kinds. One can have very clear and concise picture of orthopaedic conditions described in this book.

The readers can easily understand and refer to the contents of this book presented in simple and lucid manner, especially the detailed instructional explanations on various diseases, tests, diagnosis strategies, etc. This book is **sure to be suitable to be kept on the desk of the Outpatient Clinics to refer at every moment of questions.**

I really strongly recommend this book to undergraduate and postgraduate students and trainees who are interested in orthopaedics.

Tomohisa Koshino MD PhD
Professor and Director
Department of Orthopaedic Surgery
Yokohama City University School of Medicine and
President, University Hospital
Yokohama 236-0004, Japan

Professor Pandey's 'Clinical Orthopaedic Diagnosis' arouses scepticism against fragmentation, so-called 'subspecialities of orthopaedics'. His suggestion for a "total orthopaedist" and comprehensive knowledge of the whole musculoskeletal system as the key point to make accurate decision in any situation deserves appreciation.

"The whole art of medicine is in observation, as the old motto goes, but to educate the eye to see, the ear to hear and the finger to feel takes time" (William Osler, 1906). We really hope **this book would provide guidelines in favour of the saying, "teach him how to observe, give him plenty of facts to observe and make him proficient in his art through constant contact with diseases",** and prove precious for those who want to know.

Congratulations for your great success in publishing such an excellent textbook— "Clinical Orthopaedic Diagnosis". I am very much impressed by the fact that it covers comprehensively such a wide area of orthopaedic expertise yet implies concisely the wisdom of orthopaedics. You have presented so precious cases of wide variation...

I am very proud to have been working with such a wonderful orthopaedist and scholar.

Keiro Ono MD PhD
Ex-Professor and Chairman, Department of Orthopaedic Surgery
Osaka University Medical School, Osaka
Professor Emeritus, Osaka University Medical School
Director, Osaka Kosei-Nenkin Hospital, Osaka 553, Japan

I am indeed impressed with this book—"Clinical Orthopaedic Diagnosis" authored by Professor Sureshwar Pandey. It is a unique book on clinical methodology available today. It contains the wisdom of orthopaedics and traumatology as a whole, with an emphasis on the problems in tropical countries and developing world. Clinical methodology is quite clear supported by superb line-drawings and numerous clinical photographs.

The descriptions are simple and straightforward, but at the same time quite informative.

I am sure, those who are interested in orthopaedic surgery—students, practitioners or teachers—will find this book quite useful at all steps. **It has great potential to be accepted all over the world.**

Chairuddin Rasjad MD PhD
Professor, Department of Orthopaedic Surgery
Chairman, Department of Surgery
International Cooperation
Faculty of Medicine
Hasanuddin University
Ujung Pandang, Indonesia

Professor Sureshwar Pandey has accomplished a unique feat of collecting, analysing, and categorising the voluminous clinical material he managed to observe and treat during four decades of his active professional career. He has been a great enthusiast of proper clinical methods which are so essential for clinicians and society in general in the less privileged half of the world. A rational clinical assessment would help to employ the most appropriate and cost-effective newer modalities of investigations which are very expensive by any standards.

Most of the active orthopaedists in the Indian subcontinent deal with similar rich clinical material; however, it is to the credit of Prof Pandey to put it in a fashion to be understood by any student and practitioner of orthopaedics.

Though extensive strides have been made in the diagnostic tools in the last two decades (almost threatening to replace the humane touch by robotics); however, these serve best on the shoulders of the observations made by the clinical methods, Prof Pandey has re-emphasised for the newer generations. There is no substitute for clinical observations made by 'listening,' 'looking,' 'feeling,' 'moving,' 'measuring,' 'percussing' and 'auscultating.' Clinical methods should be a way of orthopaedics as is Yoga the way of life.

Though no compendium is complete and perfect; however, Prof Pandey deserves congratulations and gratitudes from all students of orthopaedics for his tremendous effort. I can assure Prof Pandey that he will cherish and continue to have a sense of accomplishment that he is leaving behind **a monumental document for the posterity.**

SM Tuli MS PhD FAMS
Former Director, Institute of Medical Sciences
Benaras Hindu University
Former Professor and Head, Department of Orthopaedics
Benaras Hindu University and
University of Delhi
Past President, Indian Orthopaedic Association

The Sureshwar Pandey's book **"Clinical Orthopaedic Diagnosis" is a boon to the postgraduate students and practicing orthopaedic surgeons. It has also helped me in teaching the postgraduate students.** *His collection of clinical photographs is amazing. The language is so simple that Indian students can easily understand the clinical problems in orthopaedics. Postgraduate students in my institution are using it day in and day out and have expressed great satisfaction.* **Some have stated that they have passed MS (Ortho) and DNB (Ortho) because of this book.** *I am sure this new edition will be an exciting one.*

GS Kulkarni MS MS (Ortho) FICS
Professor, Department of Orthopaedics
Director, Postgraduate Institute of Swasthiyog Pratishthan
Miraj, Maharashtra, India
Past President, Indian Orthopaedic Association

*I am glad to know "Clinical Orthopaedic Diagnosis" written by Prof Sureshwar Pandey will be published soon. The style of writing this book has got special characteristic features. Brief anatomical consideration at the beginning of the chapter, essential classification of diseases and trauma, detailed clinical tests of different diseases including those prevalent in the developing countries are the special aspects of this book. The excellent illustrations, tabular presentations of diagnostic features with keynotes at the end of each chapter will make the subject lucid to the undergraduate and postgraduate students and the practicing orthopaedic surgeons for their quick revision. The art of masterly presentation of clinical acumen of different diseases for their interpretation are important clues for **its wide acceptance to the reader.** The author deserves warm congratulation in his endeavour.*

DP Baksi MS FRCS MS (Orth) PhD (Orth) FAMS
Ex-Professor and Head
Department of Orthopaedic Surgery
NRS Medical College
Kolkata, West Bengal, India
Past President, Indian Orthopaedic Association

*It has been unique privilege for me to write my comments on the masterpiece work "Clinical Orthopaedic Diagnosis" by Prof Sureshwar Pandey. Prof Pandey, an eminent teacher in the field of orthopaedics has utilised his wide knowledge of the subject to simplify the problems of orthopaedic teaching, for which till now no other substitute was available. **It is being, and will be always appreciated by the postgraduate and undergraduate students, orthopaedic surgeons, and nonetheless the teachers.***

The text and the self-explanatory illustrations are superb and exemplary.

P Tejeswar Rao
MBBS (Hons) FRCS (Edin) FRCS (London) MCh Orth (L'Pool)
Ex-Professor and Head
Department of Orthopaedics, SCB Medical College, Cuttack
Ex-Director, Medical Education
Past President, Indian Orthopaedic Association
Cuttack, Odisha, India

*I am indeed pleased to read your new book "Clinical Orthopaedic Diagnosis". I must confess that **this is one of the concise, informative and complete principles on Clinical Orthopaedic Diagnosis.** The illustrations used in your book have clarity, the attempt to elicit clinical aids with precise analysis is noteworthy. I am certain, your book will be one of the best clinical aids for postgraduate students or young orthopaedic surgeons who can utilise it for clinical orthopaedic practice. **I am certain, the book has potential of finding worldwide acceptance.***

NS Laud
Chief, Orthopaedic Surgery and Traumatology
LTM Medical College and Hospital
Mumbai, Maharashtra, India
Past President, Indian Orthopaedic Association

Contents

CHAPTER 1 Introduction — 1
- History 3
- Documentation 7
- Examination of the Patient 10
- Examination 24
- Congenital Limb Malformations 37
- Stature Disturbances 38
- Examination of Children 39
- Assessment of Elderly 40
- Clinical Audit in Orthopaedics 41
- Evidence-based Medicine 41

CHAPTER 2 Examination of Long Bones — 43
- Blood Supply of Long Bones 44
- Methodology 45
- Key Diagnostic Points of Common Affections of Long Bones 51

CHAPTER 3 Joints — 77
- Arthritis 80
- Broadly Inflammatory Arthropathies 83
- Ankylosis of Joint 96

CHAPTER 4 Shoulder Joints — 99
- Anatomical Consideration 101
- Methodology 102

CHAPTER 5 Elbow Joints — 127
- Anatomical Considerations 129
- Ossification Around the Elbow Joint 129
- Assessment of Complications Due to Pathology in and Around the Elbow 138
- Investigations Required for Elbow Pathology 142
- Affections of Elbow 142

CHAPTER 6 Wrist Joints — 155
- Anatomical Consideration 157
- Methodology 158
- Common Swellings Around the Wrist Joint 163
- Movements 165
- Measurements 168
- Investigations Required for Wrist Pathology 168
- Key Diagnostic Points of Common Wrist Pathology 169

CHAPTER 7 Hand — 177
- Anatomical Considerations *178*
- Methodology *180*
- Movements *196*
- Gross Assessment of Movements of the Hand *196*
- Investigation *201*

CHAPTER 8 Spine — 207
- Anatomical Considerations *211*
- Applied Anatomy of Motor and Sensory Systems *214*
- Methodology *218*
- Movements *227*
- Measurements *234*
- Special Tests *235*
- Neurological Examination *240*
- Clinical Localisation of the Lesion in the Spinal Cord *255*
- Investigations for Spinal Pathology *256*
- Key Diagnostic Points of Common Spinal Pathology *258*

CHAPTER 9 Pelvis — 271
- Anatomical Considerations *273*
- Methodology *274*
- Movements *276*
- Measurements *277*
- Investigations for Pelvic Pathology *278*
- Diseases *278*

CHAPTER 10 Low Backache — 285
- Usual Causes of Backache *287*
- Investigation *293*
- Summary of Management of LBP *293*
- Prevention of Low Backache *294*

CHAPTER 11 Examination of Paralytic Patients — 297
- Anatomical Consideration *298*
- Methodology *300*
- Measurements *309*
- Movements *310*
- Neurological Examination *312*
- Key Diagnostic Points of Certain Paralytic Diseases *312*
- Proforma to Record the Muscle Power *318*
- Cerebral Palsy – Case Record *321*

CHAPTER 12 Hip — 325
- Anatomical Considerations *327*
- Methodology *328*
- Movements *333*
- Fixed Deformities of Hip *334*
- Normal Movements at Hip *337*
- Measurements *339*

- Special Tests *343*
- Investigations *348*
- Broad Assessment of Hip Functions *349*
- Key Diagnostic Points of Common Hip Pathology *351*

CHAPTER 13 Knee — 369
- Anatomical Considerations *371*
- Methodology *374*
- Movements *389*
- Measurements *392*
- Assessment of Integrity of the Quadriceps Apparatus *392*
- Physical Examination for Patellar Malalignment *394*
- Internal Derangements of Knee Joint (IDK) *395*
- Knee Instability *399*
- Investigations for Knee Pathology *403*
- Key Diagnostic Points of Common Knee Pathology *404*

CHAPTER 14 Ankle Joints — 415
- Anatomical Considerations *417*
- Methodology of Clinical Examination *418*
- Movements *422*
- Measurements *426*
- Investigations for Ankle Pathology *427*
- Neuropathic (Charcot) Arthropathy of Ankle *431*
- Osteoarthritis of Ankle *431*

CHAPTER 15 Foot — 433
- Anatomical Considerations *434*
- Deformities of the Foot *438*
- Methodology of Examination *456*
- Movements *461*
- Measurements *463*
- Investigation of a Case with Foot Pathology *464*
- Key Diagnostic Points of Common Foot Pathology *465*
- Bound Foot Deformity *485*
- Foot Involvement in Rheumatoid Arthritis *485*
- Diabetic Foot *485*

CHAPTER 16 Peripheral Nerve Injuries — 497
- Anatomical Considerations *501*
- Etiology *503*
- Methodology *505*
- Features of Different Nerve Affections of Upper Limb *505*

CHAPTER 17 Bone Tumours — 521
- Primary and Secondary Bone Tumour *522*
- Methodology *527*

CHAPTER 18 Mandible and Temporomandibular Joint — 567
- Anatomical Considerations *569*
- Methodology *569*

- Movements 571
- Investigations 571
- Key Diagnostic Points 571

CHAPTER 19 Gross Examination of Head Injury 579
- Investigations 582

CHAPTER 20 Gross Assessment of Chest Injuries 587
- Examination of Injuries of the Chest 590
- Blunt Chest Injury 595

CHAPTER 21 Gross Examination of Abdomen 597
- History 598
- Investigation 599

CHAPTER 22 How to Read X-ray Plate 601
- Reading an X-ray 602

CHAPTER 23 Advanced Diagnostic Imaging 605
- MRI 607
- Tomography 608
- Xeroradiography 608
- Endoscopy 608
- Ultrasonography 609
- Scintigraphy (Radioactive Isotope or Radionuclides Studies or Nuclear Imaging) 610
- Immunoscintigraphy 613
- Nuclear Medicine Therapies 613
- CT/CAT Scan 613
- Magnetic Resonance Imaging (MRI) 620
- Fusion Imaging 631

CHAPTER 24 Syndromes Related to Orthopaedics and Traumatology 633
- Compartment Syndrome 638
- COVID Toe Syndrome 639

CHAPTER 25 Leg Ulcers 661
- Causes of Leg Ulcers 662

Index 669

CHAPTER 1

Introduction

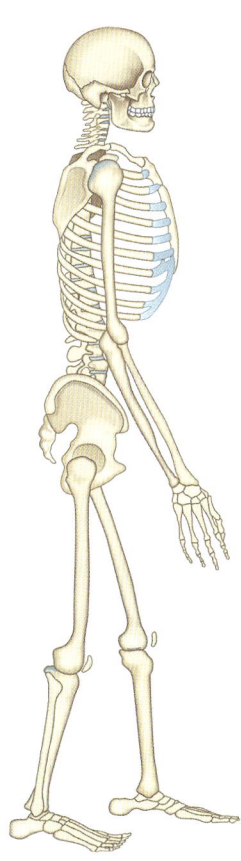

"Change is inevitable; Progress is a Choice."
—**Dean Lindsay**

"Do your little bit of good where you are, its those little bits together bring positive change in the world"

"Selfless service elicits the highest reward in life."
—**SP**

"Only way forward is to be free from narrow past"
—**Narendra Modi**

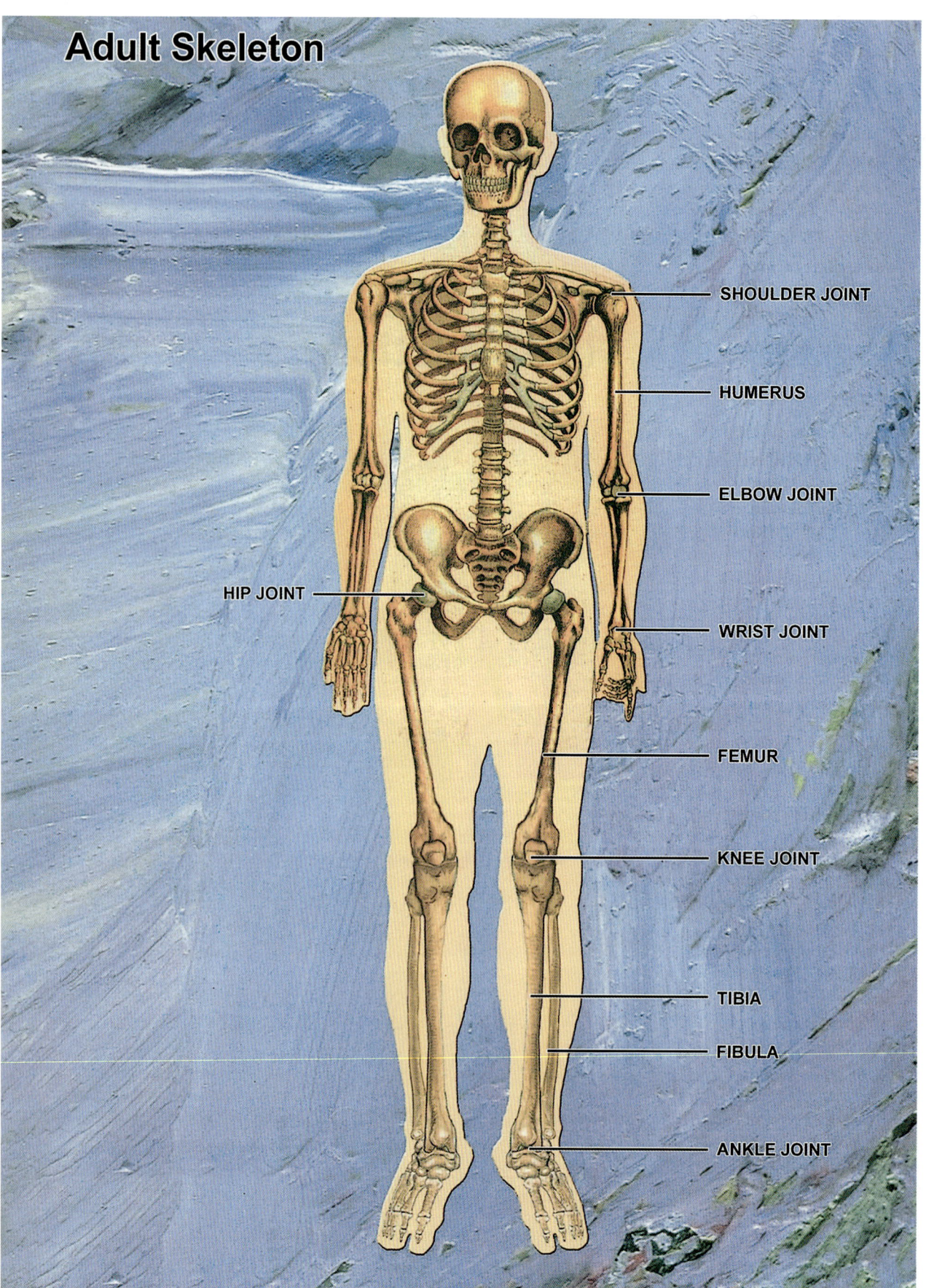

मिथ्या दृष्टा विकाराहि दुराख्यातास्तथैवच्।
तथा दुष्परिमृष्टाष्च मोहयेयुष्चिकित्सकम्।।

mithya drista vikarahi durakhyatastathawach.
tatha dusparimrstascha mohayetuchikitsakam.

Not taking a correct history and not doing a thorough examination by inspection and palpation can mislead the physician, in achieving the goal,

तस्मात् भिषक् कार्य चिकीर्षु: प्राक् कार्य समारम्भात्।
परीक्षया केवलम् परीक्ष्यं परीक्षाय कर्म समारभेत कर्त्रुम्।।

tasmat bhisak karya chikirsu praka karya samarambhat.
parikshya kevalam parikshyam parikshaya karma samarabheta kartrum.

Therefore, a practitioner keen to carry out any procedure should first of all examine and thoroughly investigate the same before venturing on the actual treatment.

(Sushruta C. 500 BC)

The word "SCIENCE" is derived from the Latin root "SCIRE" which means "to know". The original meaning of science is knowledge dealing with the material world.

"Knowledge is power".

—*Sir Francis Bacon 1597*

'The whole of science is nothing more than a refinement of everyday thinking'

—*Albert Einstein*

"Union of Science and religion alone will bring harmony and peace to the humanity".

—*Swami Vivekanand*

"I hear and I forget
I see and I remember
I do and I understand"

'*Confucious*'

The word 'patient' is derived from the Latin word 'patiens' (means sufferance). The emergence of medical practice is to relieve the suffering.

Medicare represents the essence of life experiences, the pinnacle of education and the epitome of empathy and compassion. It is a mission to heal and to comfort, and to further dignify our fellow human beings.

A 47-million-year-old fossil resembling one of the earliest ancestors of the human race has been discovered at Messal pit (important fossil site near Darmstadt, South of Frankfurt in Germany). The fossil is half of meter in length from the tip of nose to the end of tail. The fossil has been named as **"Darwinius masillae"** in honour of Charles Darwin and has also been nick-named **'Ida'**.

The first primates are believed to have evolved about 55 million years ago. It is between 40 and 50 million years ago that a division took place and humans, apes and monkeys split from other animal species—'Ida' who lived during this period is evidence of this split and proof of the common ancestry of humans, apes, and monkeys.

Aerobic respiration was thought to be ubiquitous in animals, but now it has been confirmed that this is not the case (Dorothee Huchon, a professor at Tel Aviv University in Israel). Scientists have discovered a tiny (less than 10-celled animal) parasite Henneguya salminicola that lives in salmon muscle and it does not need oxygen to produce energy needed for its survival.

■ HISTORY

Direct or indirect evidences suggest fairly acceptable developed statins of orthopaedics in ancient period, such as:

- Evidences of fractured bones healed in acceptable alignment in primitive man has been noted
- Splints made of bamboo, wood bark, reeds padded with linen have been seen on mummies
- Earliest known record about the use of crutches has been found in 2830 BC on the entrance of a portal on Hirkouf's tomb.
- Writings on the wall of the tomb of 'skar', the chief physician of one of Egypt's ruler of 5th dynasty, hint that surgery had actually been practiced in ancient Egypt (even earlier to 2000 BC). In the tomb itself 30 bronze medical instruments including scalpels, needles and a spoon were found.
- The oldest and most effective method of critical thinking has been attributed to the ancient Greek philosopher Socrates, whose credo hinges on enlightenment through questioning. It also demands exploration of the ramification of the answers to the questions, with further arguments and alternatives to consider (Editorial Jr Foot & Ankle Surg, 2020;59(2)
- History is the record of ever daily changing science and the best way is to stay connected with the latest learnings and resources in your field.

The word *'orthopaedy'* (derived from French word orthopédie and Greek word orthos+ paidion) came into existence, signifying an art of correcting deformities in children, by Nicolas Andry, a French Physician **(Figs. 1.1A and B)**, in the year 1741 who designed orthopaedic oncography in his book entitled—'L' orthopaedic Ou L'art de prevenir et corriger dans les enfants, les difformite's du corps' in 1741. English translation of the title of Andry's book published in 1743, reads '*Orthopaedia*: or the art of correcting and preventing deformities' in children ...... as may easily be put in practice by parents themselves, and all, such as one employed in educating the children. The word *'orthopaedy' comprises of two Greek words—orthos (meaning straight) + paideia (meaning rearing of children)*. However, this speciality today, is none the less, *"Orthogerontics".* Frankly speaking, unless specified, all considerations in medical practice centres around the adults and middle age (40–60 years—mediatrics),

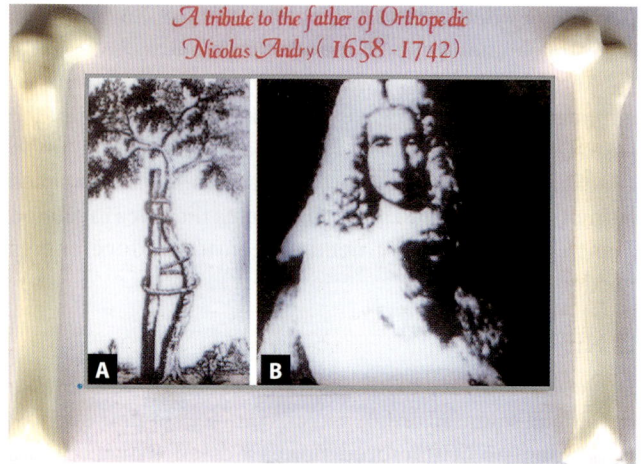

Figs. 1.1A and B: (A) Symbol of orthopaedics; (B) Nicolas Andry.

however, with constant increase in the life expectancy, the orthopaedic and trauma problems of old age (more than 60 years of age—geriatrics) are none the less, rather more, demanding. Of course, the orthopaedic problems of children (paediatrics) definitely deserve special considerations. Today, orthopaedics has grown into a multifaceted discipline and is now one of the most comprehensive specialisation in the field of medical practice, leaving too far behind the art and craft of traditional bone setters.

In order to support the curvatures of the spine, a supportive corset, made of punched iron sheet was first used by Ambroise Pare, and Gersdorff (1530) had described an iron splint for stretching contractures, still it was not until after the First World War that the principles of rehabilitation were clearly included in the arena of orthopaedics.

In the western world, *Hugh Owen Thomas (1834–1891) of Liverpool, propounded several fundamental principles of orthopaedics.* These were later put on a sound footing by his nephew, Sir Robert Jones (1857–1933), who also concerned himself with different operative techniques in this speciality. *Discoveries of anaesthesia* (Crawford Long of Athens, Georgia, 1842), ether (Mortonl), chloroform (Simpson); *antisepsis* (Joseph Lister 1867); *fundamental research on bacteria* by Louis Pasteur (1822–1895); introduction of Esmarch tourniquet in 1873 (which provided bloodless surgical field) and *X-ray* (Roentgen 1895) led to a phenomenally rapid evolution, of surgery as a whole, and orthopaedics in particular.

A probe into *ancient Indian literature* reveals that knowledge regarding the skeletal system has been mentioned in the three different systems of Atreya, Sushruta and Vagbhata. Even in the Vedic period, the craft of orthopaedic surgery was of an admirably high standard. In the oldest Aryan literature of the Rigveda, we find evidence of the use of suitable artificial limbs as substitutes for limbs accidently lost in war.

चरित्र हीं वेरिवाच्छेदि पर्णमाजा खेलस्य परितकभ्यायाम्
सद्यो जंघमाय सीं विष्णुलायै धनेहिते सस्त्रवे प्रत्यद्येत्व
ऋग्वेद १/११६/६५

In the above mentioned passage, the priest Agastya requests the clinician Ashwini to fit the artificial limb to the leg amputated in war of king Khel's wife queen Vishpala in that very night itself. Further, he requests that the limb should be strong and made up of steel but should be light like a bird's feather.

Hua Tuo (141–203 AD), in China performed many kinds of surgical operations, such as laparotomy, amputation of limb, etc. He introduced general anaesthesia to China using the Chinese herb *ma-fei-san*, along with wine as the anaesthetic.

It is interesting to note that the average human body contains enough iron to make a 3 inch nail, sulfur to kill all fleas on an average dog, carbon to make 900 pencils, potassium to fire a toy cannon, fat to make 7 bars of soap, phosphorous to make 2,200 match heads, and water to fill a ten-gallon tank — and so on. One has just to maintain this reserve.

The discovery of the structure of DNA by the 1962 Nobel laureates in medicine—Crick, Watson and Wilkin (who decoded the mystery of DNA) is not less important than Einstein's theory of relativity and Darwin's theory of evolution. This discovery solved the mystery of how the living cells divide to reproduce themselves, and further how evolutionary changes and gene mutations occur. These understandings are going to influence the high-tech medicine and management of diseases in this millennium by focussing on genetic engineering based on the structure of DNA.

Orthopaedics is the branch of medical science which concerns the investigation, preservation, development, and restoration of the form and function of the extremities, spine, and associated structures of skeletal system by medical, surgical and physical means.

Today, orthopaedics has emerged as a distinct speciality in its own right, with even different sub-branches (Cold orthopaedics, Traumatology—Accident services, Sports medicine, sub-branches for different parts of limbs, joints, spine, hip, knee, hand, foot, etc; different technologies, such as arthroscopy, arthroplasties, Ilizarov technology, etc. Rehabilitation medicine and so on). Therefore, the responsibility of an orthopaedic surgeon, in examining, investigating, diagnosing and managing the dysfunctions of the locomotor system (bones, joints, muscles and nerves), caused by congenital malformation, nutritional deficiencies, diseases, trauma, tumours and other known lesions, has also increased profoundly.

The practice of modern orthopaedics was ushered in India through the efforts of illustrious surgeons like Professors Dr MG Kini, B Mukhopadhyay, PK Duraiswamy, BN Sinha, KT Dholakia, M Natrajan, etc. In the field of rehabilitation the famous JAIPUR Foot was developed by Pandit Ram Chandra Sharma and Professor PK Sethi.

Genderwise, orthopaedics remained greatly confined to male surgeons perhaps all over world – about 5% in western countries and less than 1% in India. However, gradually numbers are increasing in the orthopaedics trainees group. Paediatric orthopaedics is attracting comparatively more younger women.

It is interesting to note that the first medical school for women was opened in Boston as The "Boston Female Medical school" founded by Samuel Gregory with just 12 students in November 1848. In 1874, the school merged with the Boston University School of Medicine, becoming one of the first co-ed medical schools.

The American Academy of Orthopedic Surgeons has defined orthopaedic surgery as "that medical speciality which embraces the investigation, presentation, development and restoration of the form and function of the extremities, the spine, and associated structures of the skeleton by medical, surgical and physical means".

Accurate clinical diagnosis forms the basis for successful management of any ailment. No doubt, the development of a sound judgement is largely a matter of experience, yet one must remember the words of *Sir Astley Cooper* (1768–1848), *"nothing is known in our profession by guess;* and I do not believe, that from the first dawn of medical science to the present moment, a single correct idea has ever emanated from conjecture. It is right therefore, that those who are studying their profession should be aware that there is no short road to knowledge; that observations on the diseased, living, examinations of the dead, and experiments upon living animals, are the only sources of true knowledge; and that inductions from these are the sole basis of legitimate theory." *The great Indian surgeon, physician and a teacher with extraordinary sharp brilliance and knowledge Sushruta (600 B.C.) (Fig. 1.2) had also warned against diagnosing a disease merely on speculation.* He, working in Varanasi, India, wrote the oldest known textbooks "Sushrusta Samhita" in sanskrit. He gave explicit description of various diseases and their management including by 300 types of surgical procedures and techniques of making incisions, probing, foreign body extraction, alkali and thermal cauterizations, tooth extractions, caesarean section and treatment of twelve types of fractures and six types of dislocations. He used 125 types of surgical instruments mostly made up jaws of animals and birds. Acharya Sushrut was born to rishi Vishwamitra and is known as the father of plastic surgery and the science of anaesthesia, even cataract surgery in detail gave explicit instructions regarding history taking, inspection, palpation, auscultation, directly by keeping the ears on chest or abdomen or indirectly by some aid, etc. An indication of the details with which the symptoms and signs were analysed can be exemplified by the *list of the types of pain which were enquired into*—i.e. whether pain was of pricking, piercing, churning, bursting, pinching, uprooting, stiffening, benumbing, indurating, contracting, or of a spasmodic nature, etc. Pain, which came on or vanished without any apparent cause, or was varied and shifting in nature was supposed to be the effects of deranged 'Vayu'.

We must express our heartfelt gratitude and salute for the great Indian geniuses of the bygone ages, who have given their unique contributions in common medical fields. Besides, Acharya *Sushruta*, the names ancient pioneers deserve special mention are Acharya *Atreya* (800 BC), whose work " Atreya Samhita" contains 46,500 verses on Ayurvedic concepts; Acharya *Charak* (600 BC), known as the father of medicine and his renowned work "Charak Samhita" is considered as encyclopedia of Ayurveda describing medicinal properties and functions of one lac herbal plants; Acharya *Patanjali* (200 BC) considered as the father of yoga – one of the six principal philosphies of India; Madhavacharya (900 or 1000 ce) is considered as an exponent of diagnosis and pathology and his authentic textual work 'Madhavanidana' describes nidana or the diagnostic process of several diseases. He elaborated on pathology, diagnosis, symptoms, conditions and causes of various diseases.

"Science is a dynamic discipline and only changes can lead to its progress"—Sir Issac Newton 1750. At the same time, science and technology are being overrated in the present civilisation and every walk of life and so in the medical field. However, the *immense importance of systematic clinical methodology* in the practice of medical science can never be ignored. There is no short cut to familiarity with clinical signs and their interpretations. A 'snap' diagnosis based on a cursory examination may be disastrous for even an experienced clinician. On the other hand, an inexperienced apprentice examining his patient, methodically step by step, will certainly give a better account of himself.

The adage "practice makes perfect" is invariably relevant in the experience, development and growth of any learner. Reznick and MacRae emphasized the wide acceptance of the Fitts and Posner 3-stage theory of motor skill acquisition, which involves "cognition, integration and automation" in sequence, being a critical part of surgical training.

There are five steps to learning: Silence, Listening, Memory, Practice, Teaching others.
—***Old Hebrew proverb***

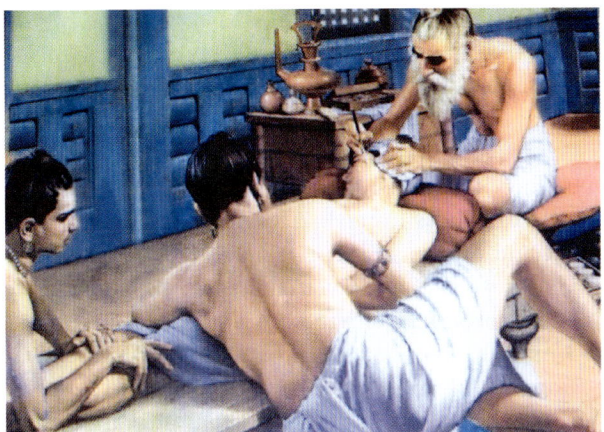

Fig. 1.2: The great ancient Hindu surgeon *Sushruta* operating upon a patient, while his trainees are holding the patient and observing the surgical procedure.

These are very true in medical education.

The *aim of the medical education* should be familiarity with the scientific principles in an approach that will allow the physician to handle logically, correctly and safely even those diseases with which he/she may not have previous experience. The only and only aim of a treating physician should be to restore the health of the patient properly, i.e., his/her ability to do what they want to do, perform the functions they wish to perform and carry out the usual activities required in everyday living. The physicians of tomorrow should be educated rather than schooled. Medical science is nowadays characterised by more and more narrow specialisation burdened by new in-depth research works. Therefore, a threat emerges that the clinicians and subsequently the medical students loose their ability to see the sick persons in their totality. This phenomenon is one of the potential sources of dehumanisation of medicine.

The development of technical approach to the medical care has gradually led to the clinician to give less and less time to the patient. Earlier, the clinician used to start the care taking with detail interrogations of the patient and/or relatives, which used to give an insight into the medical aspects of patient's past and present. Thorough physical examination was performed with great care before some tests were ordered. Though a little time consuming, such procedure promoted a holistic approach to the sick. Unfortunately, there is a gradual reversal in that trend. Clinicians are cutting down their time spent in initial conversation and primary physical examination. The cult of numbers (uncritical acceptance of quantitative laboratory determinations) has almost replaced the cute clinical observation, the friendly attitude and psychic comfort of the former days.

A clinician should not order a laboratory test/any investigation, unless he/she knows why it is being ordered and what will be done if test comes back abnormal?

Prof Peter Mortimer has astutely opined that "Dermatology is arguably the most clinical of all medical specialities because it relies less on investigation and more on good old fashioned observation and interpretation of symptoms and signs for diagnosis".

Actually, the computer addiction is prevailing over many clinicians, medical teachers and also the medical students all over the globe. The *abilities and competence of the computers are being overestimated.* However, a computer, though most helpful and serviceable in medical education and practice, cannot replace a thinking clinician with searching eyes and probing brain and the practical examination by sensitive hand and fingers. His/her associative reasoning can-not be restricted to a software programme.

In a quest of achieving the accuracy and exactness, *computer-assisted orthopaedic surgery* (CAOS) is being introduced. The principle of CAOS is simple. A digital image is produced which serves as a map for each particular procedure. That image is made available to surgeons to guide them through the operation. The accuracy can be achieved to the fraction of a millimetre or degree. Thus, surgery can be compared to an instrumental landing of an aircraft. The CAOS is being aimed to benefit the patient in having less morbidity with a better functional outcome and greater longevity for implants. However, the machines, manpower, money and methods involved in this procedure are very expensive, operational time becomes longer, and it is premature to assess and authenticate the overall benefit to the patients.

Moderately open surgery (MOS) and video-assisted endoscopic *minimum invasive surgery (MIS)* are proving to lessen the operative blood loss, operative exposure, the hospital stay and postoperative pain, but at the same time are hiking the cost of surgery and learning curve. Only good surgical training, judgement, technique and skill will be cost-effective.

Fluoro-navigation is a new surgical technique in orthopaedic trauma surgery. Fluoroscopy-based navigation system consists of a system platform, a C-arm fluoroscope adapted for use with a navigation system, and equipment for optoelectronic position detection called tracker. The system platform with an infrared camera is used for tracking and positioning the fluoroscopy (Zhou et al. 2016).

Gradually '*robotic surgery*' is also creeping in the field of orthopaedic management procedures. While the 3-D robotic procedure magnifies and makes the operating field more visible to the surgeon, it reduces pain, blood loss, scarring and post-surgery complications.

Even though, the use of robotic surgery is currently limited, mainly due to equipment, setup costs and learning curve, no wonder the future robots will facilitate surgery by anastomosing minute vessels, laser welding nerves and tendons, and performing delicate dissection discriminating fibrous scar from healthy tissue.

Robotic surgery was introduced with an aim to achieve higher speed and higher accuracy (as required in neurosurgery) or repetitive tasks (like resecting a prostate gland with a wire loop resectoscope). However, the aim of achieving the higher accuracy has been achieved, but promise of higher speed or reduced surgical time has not been satisfactorily fulfilled because of the lengthier setting up times required for robotic procedure.

The evolution and practice of microvascular surgery (consisting of the use of magnification, especially designed instruments and sutures to accurately identify, properly dissect and thoroughly repair the minute structures like blood vessels, nerves, fine structures, of eye and ear, etc.) has enhanced several surgical procedures. Its use has been immensely utilized in the surgical field of limb salvage anastomosis of amputated limb parts in accidents and limb reconstruction. The first vascular anastomosis was performed by JB Murphy in 1897 (Tamai S 2009)

The concept of modern joint replacement has been introduced as a panacea to relieve the intractable pain, to restore the functions of the affected stiff (ankylosed) joints, and to achieve/restore the overall functions of joints as much as possible. In this direction, Sir John Charnley should be credited for introducing the basics of modern hip arthroplasty, which provided millions to lead a nearly normal life.

Modern total knee arthroplasty evolved with total condylar prosthesis (with all polyethylene single piece tibial component) in 1974.

With ever increasing advancements in the metalergy of bone-fixators, and joint replacements, the present basic surgical steel alloys using cobalt-chrome–titanium and bone cement are biocompatible.

Today, in an era of rapid industrialisation and mechanisation, orthopaedics occupies an important place in the field of medical sciences. The examination and management of an osteoarticular problem, very much involve assessment of the patient as a whole. However, two factors, quite often missed, must get their place while examining an orthopaedic patient. Overall the surgeon and clinical judgement will continue to play the pivoted role in total care of the patient.

1. Proper documentation of case records, which has got immense value in this branch of reconstructive surgery, and increasing medicolegal considerations.
2. History taking and clinical examination should be rehabilitation oriented.

The Arbeitsgemeinschaft für Ostesynthese fragen (AO) group was formed in Biel Switzerland on November 6, 1958. The AO group consisting of high-powered technology, metallurgical excellence and a high level of technical skill in optimally clean and aseptic operating environment (based on the introduction of antiseptic surgery between 1860 and 1870 by Lord Lester) has led to a total change in the concept of managing the fractures by combining the principles of rigid fixation, compression and early mobilization [possible by proper anaesthesia – initiated by Morton (ether) and Simpson (chloroform)]. Fresh frozen cadaver labs dissection is increasingly becoming an integral part of any surgical training program, but for the declining availability of cadavers.

Amputation has been the most ancient of surgical procedures and today it is one of the most advanced specialised surgical procedures with simultaneous development of almost thinking–prosthesis. Today the specialised prosthesis allows the young persons to resume recreational activities and sports like dancing, running, golfing, skeing, hiking, swimming and other competitive sports.

Remember nothing is 100%, except God.

■ DOCUMENTATION

Accurate representation of the clinical findings, supplemented with sketches, graphs, photographs, X-rays, cine-films, writing tests, foot prints, topographical representation and moulds go a long way in helping the clinician in diagnosing the disease, planning of its treatment, declaring the prognosis and assessing the results of follow-up.

An *orthopaedic problem in a patient may arise from any of the following:*

- Congenital, infective, traumatic, and developmental malformations **(Figs. 1.3 to 1.27)**.
  Siamese twins are the extreme forms of congenital malformations. They are classified according to the most prominent site of conjunction: thorax (thoracopagus, **Figs. 1.4A and B**), abdomen (omphalopagus), sacrum (pyopagus), pelvis (ischiopagus), skull (cephalopagus), back, or even more than one sites (cephalothoracopagus) **(Figs. 1.3A and B)**, omphalopagus (fused at abdomen, **Fig. 1.4C**).
- Affections of bones.
- Affections of joints **(Figs. 1.26 and 1.27)**
- Affections of soft tissues around and controlling the joints, e.g.—skin [burn contracture **(Figs. 1.28 and 29)**], subcutaneous tissue [Dupuytren's contracture **(Fig. 1.30)**], muscles, tendons.
- Affections of nervous system **(Fig. 1.31)**.

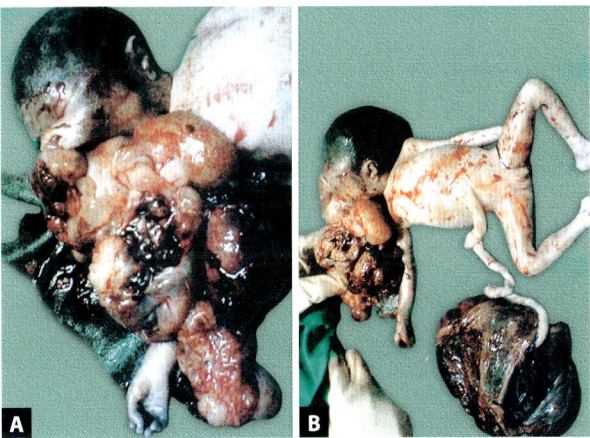

Figs. 1.3A and B: Craniopagus.
(*Courtesy:* Dr Pushpa Pandey and Dr Pallavi Pandey)

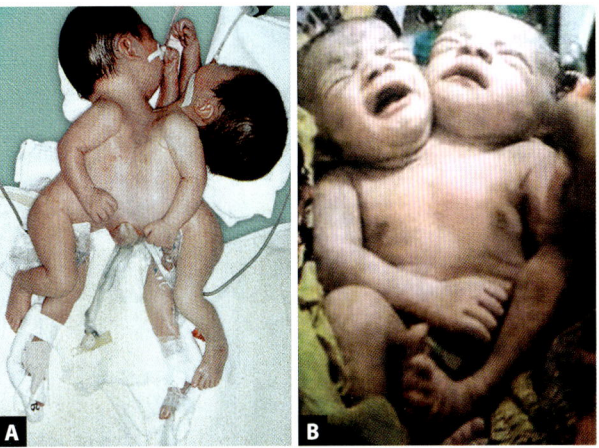

Figs. 1.4A and B: Thoracopagus—only one heart for both: A parasitic twin with four arms, four legs, heart on right side, liver on left side.
Source: Dr. Lecia Bushak, Uganda—Source of picture Asianet-Pakistan/shutterstock.com—supplied by Ms Shabana

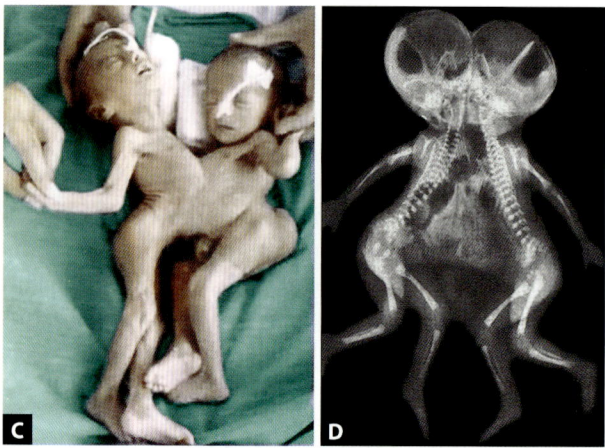

Figs. 1.4C and D: (C) Omphalopagus (fused at abdomen) and (D) Cephalothoracopagus.

Source: Herman Klapproth and Eastman Kodak in the book authored by Mae M Bookmiller (Photo supplied by Madhukar Anand)

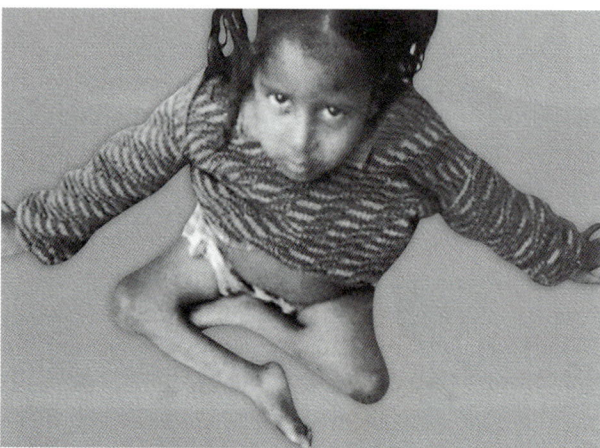

Fig. 1.7: Congenital contracture of hip, knee, ankle and foot.

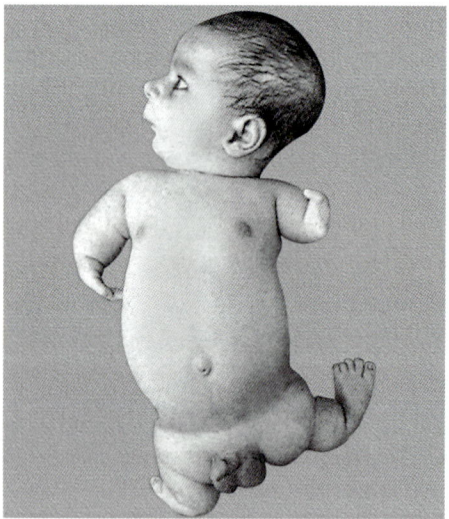

Fig. 1.5: Congenital malformation of all the four limbs—rudimentary limbs.

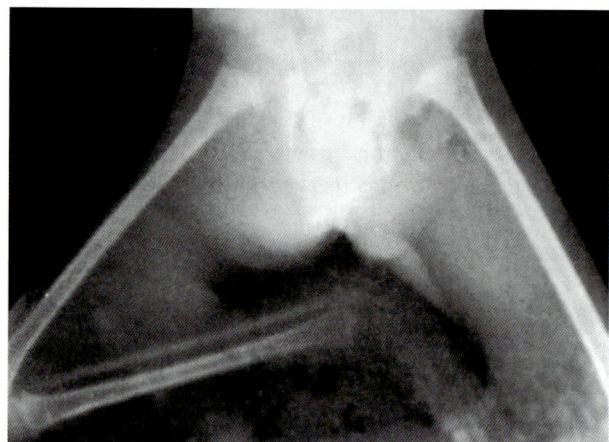

Fig. 1.8: X-ray of same child **(Fig. 1.7)**.

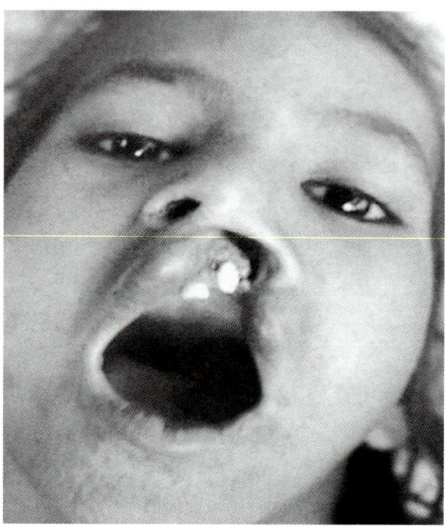

Fig. 1.6: Congenital cleft lip and palate.

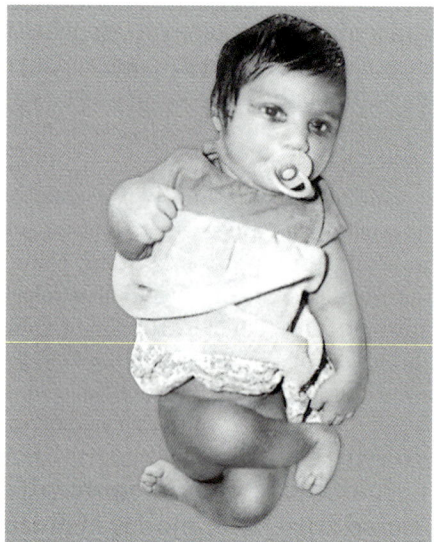

Fig. 1.9: Arthrogryposis multiplex congenita. Note bilateral club hand, left club foot, right congenital vertical talus, bilateral flexion contracture of knee joint, wide perineum indicating bilateral CDH and congenital constriction band at right lower leg.

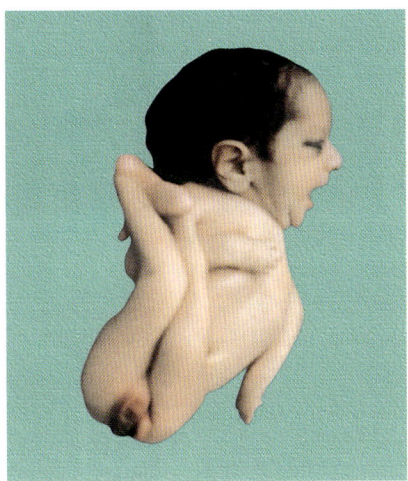

Fig. 1.10: Arthrogryposis multiplex congenita.

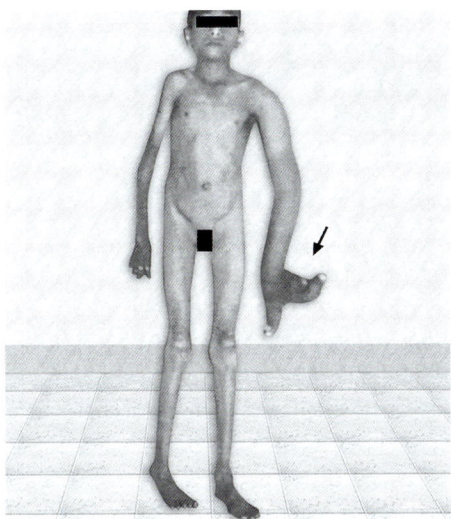

Fig. 1.11: Congenital hemihypertrophy (hyperplasia) of left upper limb.

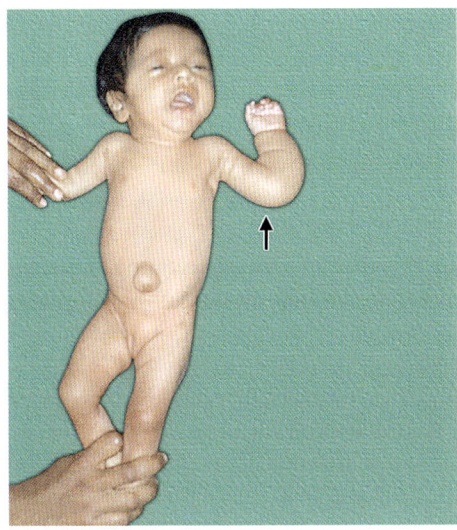

Fig. 1.12: Congenital lymphoedema of left upper limb.

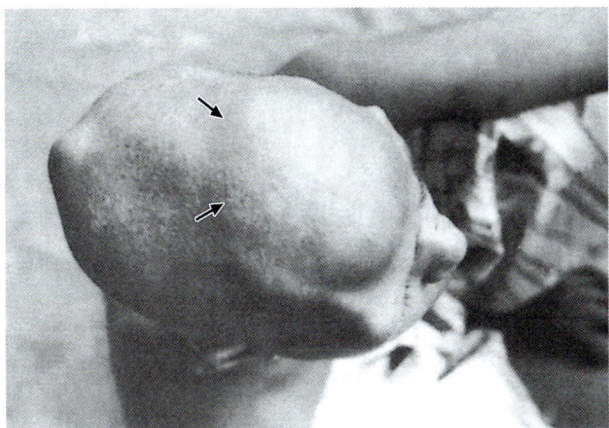

Fig. 1.13: Pott's puffy tumour in a boy aged 16 years. Percival Pott described this condition in 1700, which is osteomyelitis of skull associated with subperiosteal swelling and oedema of scalp.

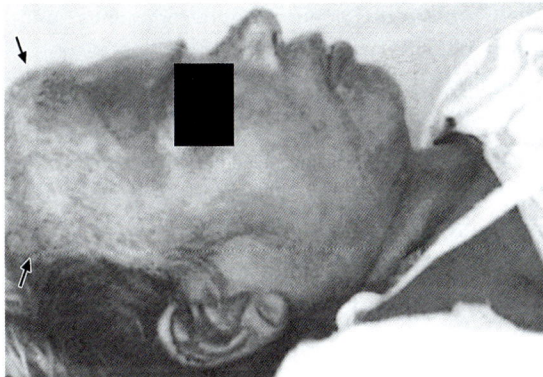

Fig. 1.14: Pott's puffy tumour in a lady aged 46 years.

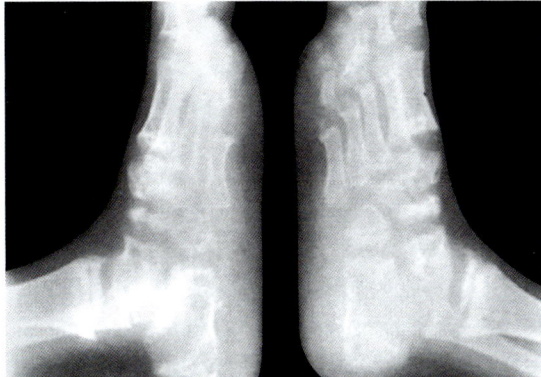

Fig. 1.15: Typical X-ray of multiple epiphysitis.

- Vascular affection of limbs [Buerger's phenomenon; Volkmann's ischaemic contracture **(Fig. 1.30)**, etc.].
- Postural abnormalities **(Fig. 1.32)**, e.g. (1) **Pisa syndrome**—a dystonic syndrome characterised by lateral flexion of the trunk associated with slight rotation due to high dose of chlorpromazine, given for neuroepileptics. There may be associated tardive dyskinesia; (2) Tortipelvis (L. tortus = twisted + pelvis = basin) meaning thereby muscular spasms in children distorting the spine and hip.

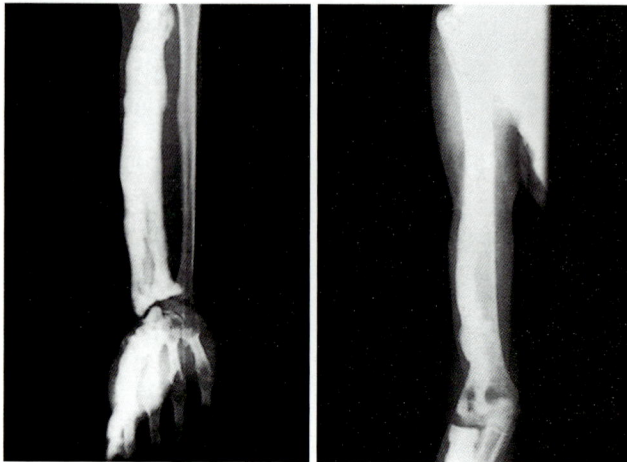

Fig. 1.16: Melorheostosis (candle bone disease). It is a rare benign disorder of unknown etiology and of insidious onset, occurring equally in male and female. There is longitudinal cortical and medullary hyperostosis of one or more contiguous bones. This disease was first described by Leri and Joanny in 1922. It is a nonhereditary dysplasia of the bone. The combination of new bone formation and resorption of the original cortex appears unique. In above X-ray pictures, note that affections are mainly of radius, lateral half of humerus and hand. The peculiar streaked sclerosis of bone resembling candle driplings. It is oftenly associated with congenital neurofibromatosis.

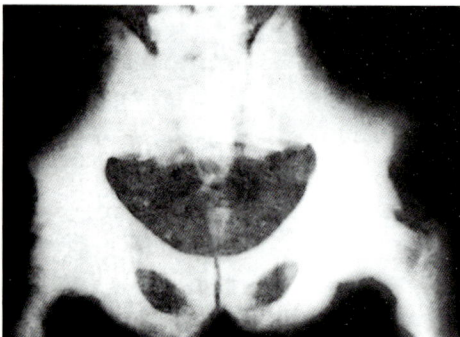

Fig. 1.17: Marble bone disease (osteopetrosis) Osteopetrosis [(osteo(=bone)+petros (=stone)] a greek word is a group of rare, heritable disorders of skeleton – a trait that can be inherited in an autosomal dominant, autosomal recessive or X-linked manner. It varies in presentation and severity ranging from neonatal onset with life-threatening complications (like bone marrow failure) to incidental findings on x-rays (like osteopoikilosis). It is caused by the failure of osteoclast development or function and mutations. Osteopoikilosis is autosomal dominant pattern in which there are multiple symmetrical circular sclerotic opacities in ischium and pubic bones. It is benign asymptomatic condition. Albers-Schonberg disease is autosomal dominant. Osteopetrosis presents in late childhood with radiologically "sandwich vertebrae".

The complications are fractures, scoliosis, osteomyelitis, osteoarthritis, hearing, and visual loss.

■ EXAMINATION OF THE PATIENT

Medical knowledge alone is not enough to meet the patient's expectations from us. Fellow feeling, friendly intentions, moral support, relief from fear, human attitude towards the patient, as well as physician's efficiency, all these are essential.

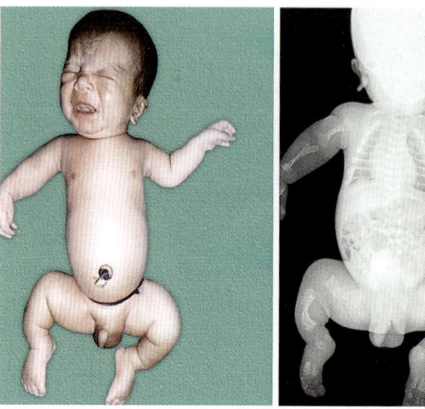

Fig. 1.18A: Osteogenesis imperfecta with multiple fractures (mostly malunited) in a new-born boy.

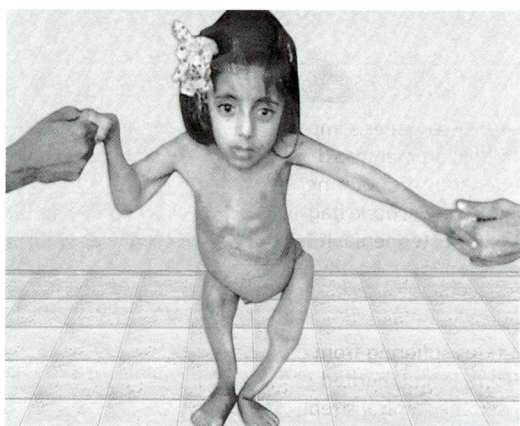

Fig. 1.18B: A girl aged 9 years with osteogenesis imperfecta with multiple deformities following multiple fractures.

The clinician must give his/her adequate time for examining the patient since as yet no computer programme has been developed to produce 'artificial intelligence' which will decrease the time needed for clinical examination and data collection.

Remember the (orthopaedic) surgeon is a doctor of medicine first and the orthopaedic surgeon the next, i.e. afterwards.

Keep anatomy of the affected part (where dead teaches the live) and physiology of the affected region (which reminds the functions) everready at the back of your mind.

Routine Hand-Hygiene

Before and after the physical examination of patient *'Routine hand-hygiene'* is essential for the safety of both, the patient and the doctor and even others. The ideal routine towards the hand-hygiene should consist of:
- Watch, bangles and jewellery should be removed
- Wash the hands and distal forearm with water and 2% chlorhexidine surgical scrub solution for 2 minutes or instant hand sanitizer
- Hands should be dried with a sterile dry towel or disposable paper towel/tissue

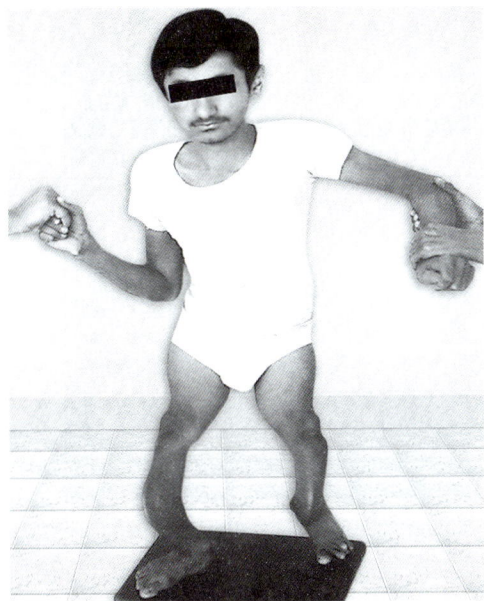

Fig. 1.19: Osteogenesis imperfecta with multiple deformities in the limbs following malunited fractures. Osteogenesis imperfecta is a heterogeneous group of heritable disorders of connective tissues. Typically there are bone fragility, recurrent fractures even with minor trauma and osteopenia. It is also known as fragilis ossium, brittle bone disease, osteopsathyrosis, Lobstein's disease, Vrolik's disease. Olaus Jacob Ekman was the first surgeon to scientifically document in 1788 his observations of bone fragility and fractures in three familial generations suffering from congenital osteomalacia. Osteogenesis imperfecta is an inherited disorder of type 1 collagen resulting in decreased mechanical strength of all bones leading to pathological fracture mainly in the first decade of life. Autosomal dominant inheritances occurs in about 60%. The bones are hard and more brittle. Blue sclerae may be seen. Joints are usually hypermobile. Skull may be deformed. The stature is usually short. Management consists of Bisphosphonate treatment (which decreases bone turnover and inhibits bone resorption) and timely corrective surgery and proper physiotherapy and occupation therapy.

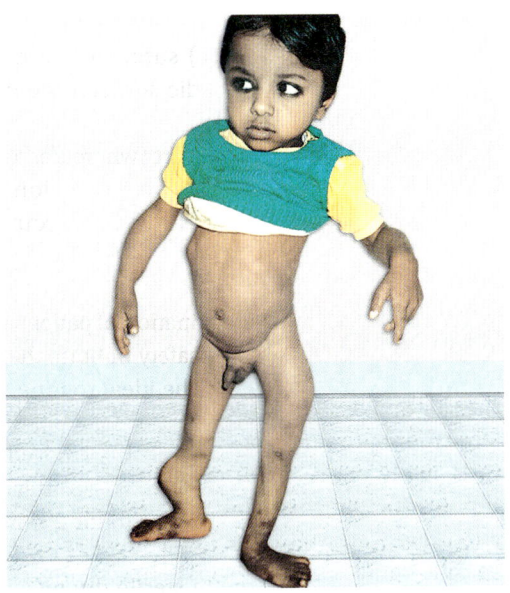

Fig. 1.20: Osteogenesis imperfecta.

- If the blood, discharge from a wound, pus or any body fluid gets unintentionally touched or is being touched without gloves in the process of examination, the above process of washing or scrubbing must be repeated before touching any other part or instrument or anything
- Subsequently, any hand rub (e.g. absolute alcohol or chlorhexidine in alcohol) should be used
- The 'hand-hygiene' should be maintained while examining each patient; while touching common objects, e.g. pen, telephone, stethoscope, etc.; putting hand in pocket, etc.

Armamentarium Necessary for Examining an Orthopaedic Patient

- A measuring tape
- Goniometer (large and small)
- A tendon reflex rubber hammer
- A pocket torch
- A pin with protected point
- Skin marker pencils and wax pencil
- A stethoscope
- A diagnostic set (tongue depressor, auroscope, ophthalmoscope)
- A plain white paper and impression ink for taking prints
- A right-angled triangle
- Camera (more important than even a stethoscope for a reconstructive surgeon)
- For neurological cases—cotton wool, tuning fork, test tubes.

Certain Factors Essential for Examining an Orthopaedic or any Patient

- Hear the patient with patience, even if he is confused, disoriented and annoying
- Reassuring the patient and gentle handling of the affected parts
- Good bedside manners
- Sympathetic appreciation of the patient's problems
- Doctor should be well-dressed, composed, and not in hurry
- As far as possible, communicate with the patient in his/her language to get the clear story and facts
- All physical complaints should be taken up seriously
- Remember that the patient is almost always right while narrating the problems
- Remember that the snap-diagnosis can be mostly wrong
- Diagnosis of Functional Neurotic Disease (FND) should always be at the last, after excluding all possible diagnosis
- You must have an insight into the patient's future rehabilitation programme
- Give importance to the need for examining the patient while standing walking, sitting, lying as a whole, and not a particular limb or system, and all vital organs of systems.
- The patient must be placed in comfortable position

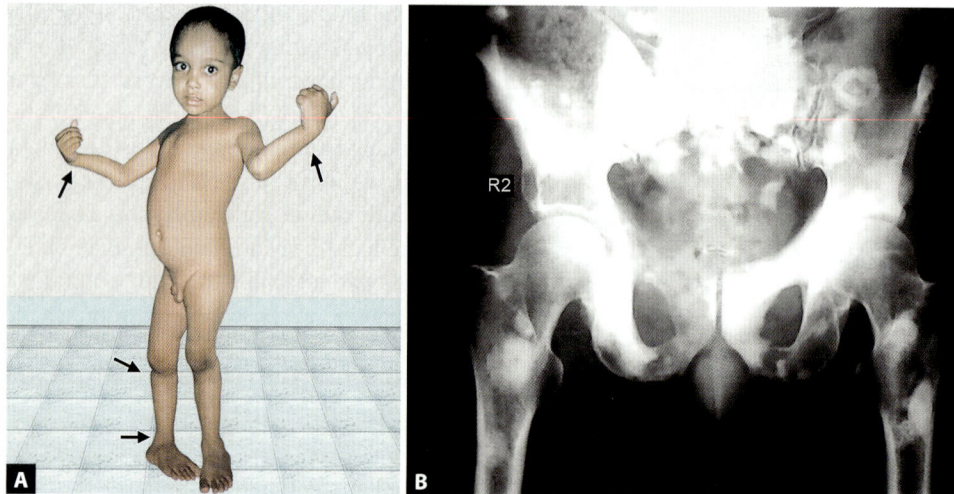

Figs. 1.21A and B: (A) Osteogenesis imperfecta. Note the malunion of forearm, tibial and femoral fractures; (B) Osteopoikilosis (osteopathia condensans disseminata; spotted bones). It is a developmental disease of skeleton in which there are rounded or elongated areas of increased density scattered throughout the entire bone, often arranged in the long axis of bone. There are deformities and secondary arthritis. There is no medical treatment of disease. Deformities and arthritis may require treatment including surgery. Prognosis to life is good.

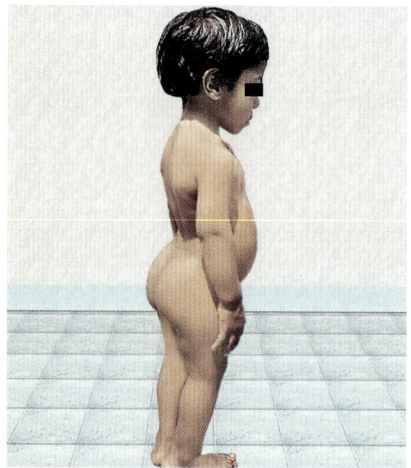

Fig. 1.22: Dwarf (rachitic).

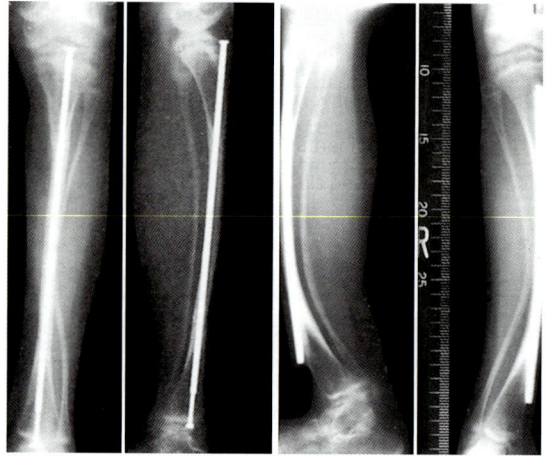

Fig. 1.23: In osteogenesis imperfecta, the fractures can be avoided by using telescoping rods.

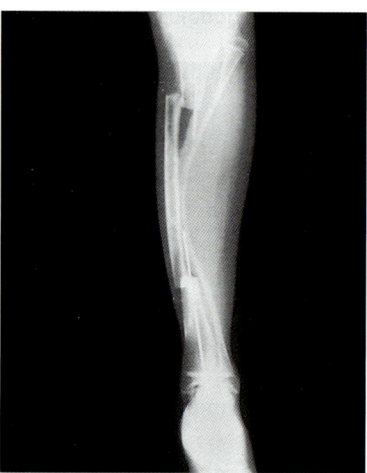

Fig. 1.24: Prophylectic telescopic rodding of the long bone can also prevent pathological fractures in osteogenesis imperfecta.

- Usually patients feel comfortable, confident and care free, when one of their relatives remain there while being examined
- The patient is to be fully exposed (except the private parts unless it is essentials) and at least the corresponding part or limb, of other side for comparison
- Do not hurt the patient during examination
- **Never examine a lady patient alone,** there must be a lady nurse and/or even the patient's own close relative by the side and in sight of the patient
- Before coming to final conclusion, remember that the **patient is always right, and doctor is always wrong unless the doctor proves that patient is not right,** which requires keen observation, thorough clinical examination, deep and detail scrutiny of patient's complaints and findings and wide application of knowledge.

The first impression, that a keen clinician gets of his patient while he/she is entering the examination room, forms the basis for his/her assessment.

At the first sight note:
- Facial expression (for stress, agony, uncared, depressed, unconcerned, anxious, hyperbola, tetanic face **(Figs. 1.33A and B)**, Mongoloid face, etc.), any facial stigma such as flattening of nasal bridge (is typical of syphilis), flattening of nose tip (characteristics of leprosy)
- Nutritional status (dehydrated, cachectic, emaciated, marasmic, hypoproteinemic, anaemic, bloated, obese, etc.) Obesity is on the rise in India. More than 30 million Indians are overweight (National Family Health Survey—NFHS).

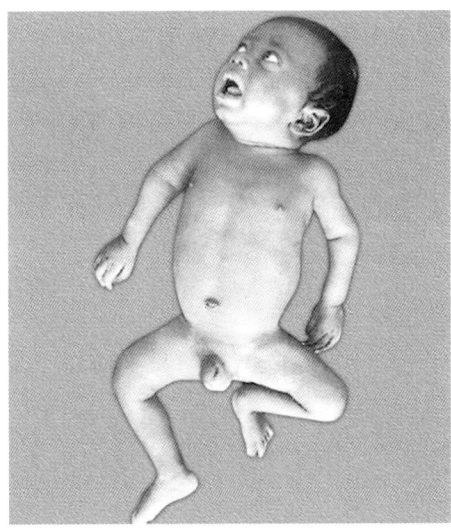

Fig. 1.26: Congenital syphilis with multiple joint affections and pseudoparesis. Congenital syphilis a rare disease (caused by Triponema pallidum bacteria) affects a child born to a mother suffering with syphilis (a highly infectious disease). Babies have delayed milestones, seizures, jaundice, anaemia, hepatosplenomegaly, deformities. (*See also* page 49 of Chapter 2 – for stigmata of syphilis).

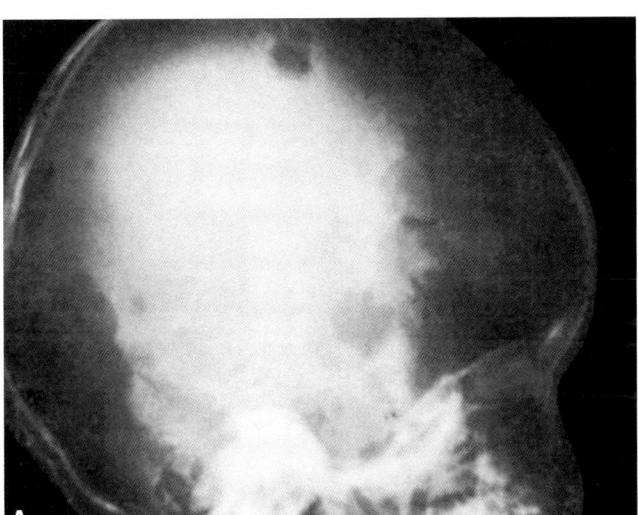

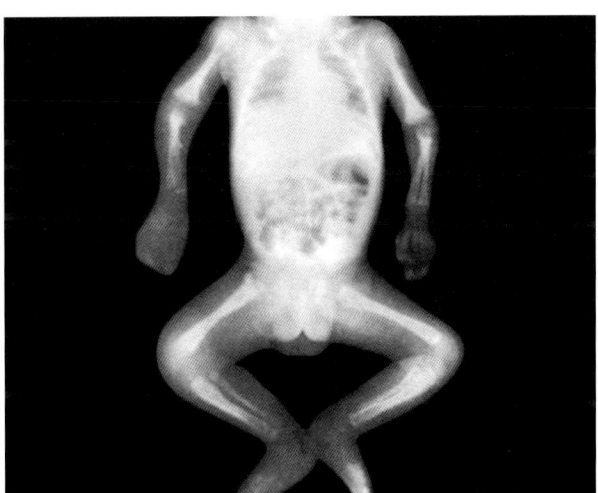

Fig. 1.27: X-ray of the child of **Figure 1.26** showing multiple metaphysitis with collection in the joints, bilaterally (in knees, hips and shoulders).

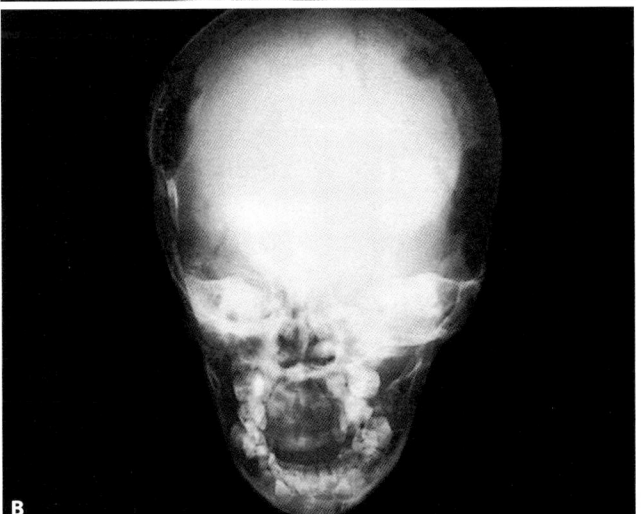

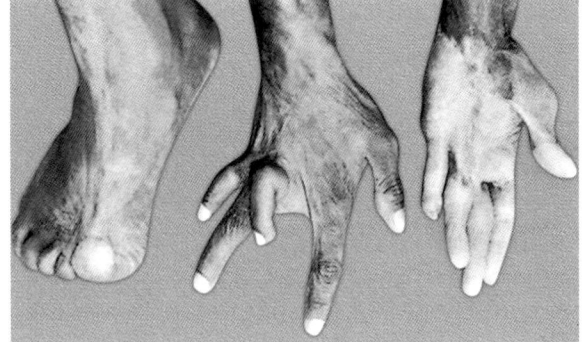

Figs. 1.25A and B: Hand-Schüller-Christian disease (a typical histiocytoses) with classic geographic skull: (A) Lateral view of skull, (B) Anteroposterior view of face and skull. Starts in early childhood. Skull and membranous bones affected; Secondary deposition of cholesterol in foam cells; Higher cholesterolaemia in most cases; Disease progress-slow; Overall benign.

Fig. 1.28: Burn contracture producing multiple problematic deformities of foot and hand.

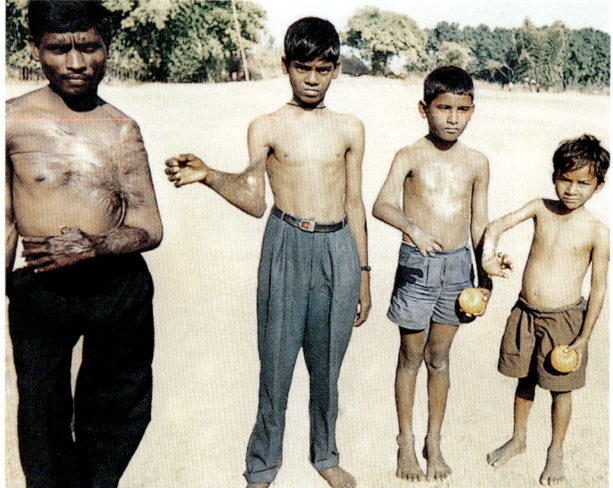

Fig. 1.29: Post-burn contracture of elbow.

In presence of vague, bizarre, unexplainable presentation (generalised pain and allied complaints):
a. Assess for the fitness of body according to the age (accelerated aging; activity assessment; stamina assessment; flexibility assessment; overall strength assessment).
b. Assess for habit/drug dependency (smoking, alcohol, drugs, narcotics, paan, paan-masala, gutka, etc.)
c. The thyroid gland secretes thyroxine (T3 & T4), which is important for development of nervous system; it promotes growth and controls body temperature.

Assess for thyroid functions, especially in ladies by thorough clinical examination, estimating T3, T4, TSH levels and other investigations if needed, e.g. fine needle aspiration cytology (FNAC) especially to know the proper nature of thyroid tissue and thyroid swelling (benign

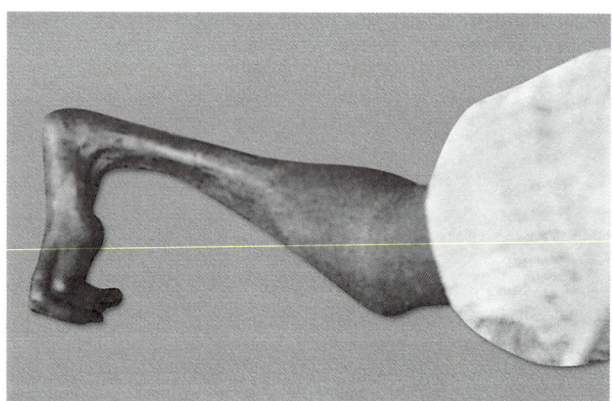

Fig. 1.30: Grotesque deformity of wrist and hand—very severe Volkmann's ischaemic contracture.

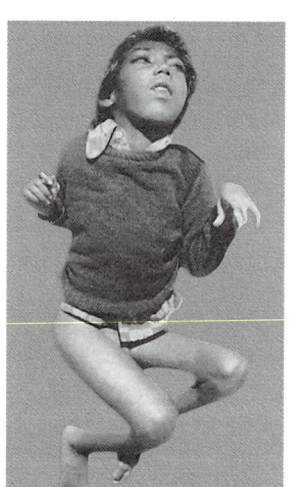

Fig. 1.31: A cerebral palsy child (spastic) with mental retardation.

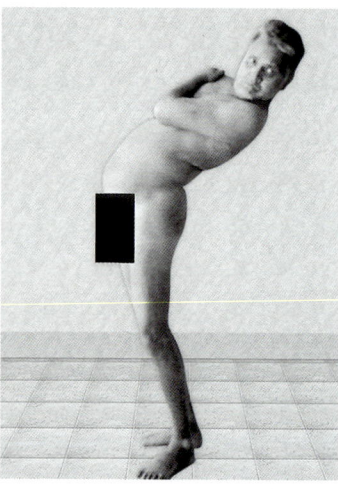

Fig. 1.32: A typical spinal deformity position due to Pisa syndrome—Refer text on page 9 of this chapter.

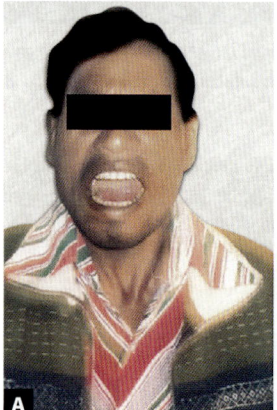
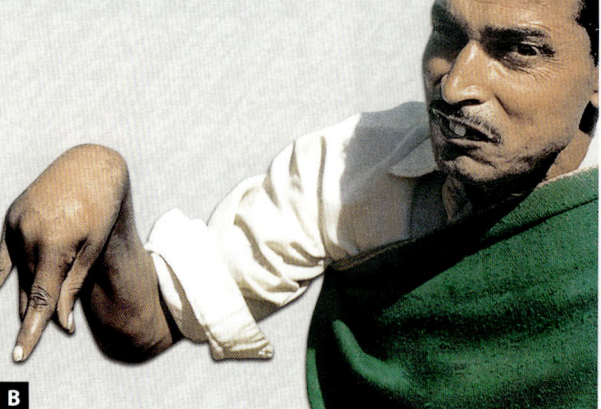
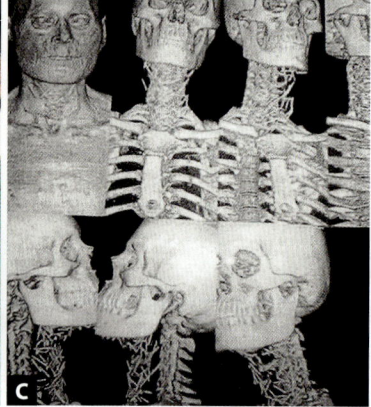

Figs. 1.33A to C: (A) Typical locking of jaw, facial expression, muscular spasm and eyes in early stage of tetanus. (B) Typical facial expression in tetanus (risus sardonicus). Note the tetanic spasm in the right hand and fingers. On the dorsum of the same hand there is reddish source-prick wound. (C) BM had 150 pins embedded in his body (throat, elbow, abdomen, ankles, etc.) without any complain nor his knowledge. It was perchance a CT finding when he consulted for pain in ankle and diabetes.
(*Source* of picture: Hindustan Times—Anonna Dutt)

or malignant); ultrasound of thyroid, which helps in defining the non-palpable nodules and the nature of swelling (cystic or solid).

Clinical features of hypothyroidism also known as "underactive thyroid" in which condition thyroid gland is not producing enough of thyroxine harmone are usually obesity; less or loss of appetite; constipation; lassitude; letharginess; increased sleep; depression, swelling of face; swelling of hands, feet, legs, thighs; generalised weakness and tiredness, dry skin, slowness of activities; increased menstrual flow; intolerance to cold; thyroid swelling, etc. These patients have low levels of T3, T4 hormones and excess of TSH (hormone).

Clinical features of hyperthyroidism an "overactive thyroid", in which too much of thyroxine harmone is produced are usually loss of weight, increased appetite, tremors in fingers, sweating, diarrhoea, sleeplessness, anxiety, exophthalmus, emotions, tension, palpitation, amenorrhoea, abortions, etc. These patients have high levels of T3, T4 hormones and low level of TSH (hormone).

Most of the thyroid dysfunctions (except advanced malignant tumours) are amenable to proper medical and/or surgical treatment.

Common Orthopaedic Complaints

- Pain
- Disability in using the limb
- Inability in using the limb
- Deformity
- Stiffness of the joints
- Swelling/abscess
- Altered gait or problems in gait
- Discharging wounds/sinus
- Limb length disparity
- Altered power and sensations
- Cramps in the calf
- Allied complaints, e.g. hyperhydrosis, tremors, muscular fasciculations.

History Taking

History of complaints forms the key step for making the diagnosis. History not only is the record of past and present sufferings but also constitutes the foundation for the future treatment, prevention and prognosis. History taking is an art of collection of data which not only gives insight into patients problems, but also provides a direction over which you are planning your examination. The importance of relevant and detailed history taking can never be overemphasised. The patient must be encouraged to tell his/her story of the problems in detail. Unless there is hyperthymesia (lacking the ability to forget anything), the patient/attendant (in case of children) may miss the continuity in expressing the problems—listen it.

Do not forget that your responsibility does not cease on getting a disease cured or a fracture united, rather management is incomplete without total rehabilitation of the patient. Therefore, history taking and examination must be rehabilitation oriented.

At first, note the patient's demographics—full name, age, sex, race, religion, occupation, topography of residence, approach road/path, surrounding and complete postal address, telephone number (including mobile), fax number, e-mail address of the patient. Carefully listen his/her story about the problem in his/her own language and words, as far as possible.

Enquire about the complaints in order of their appearance and note their duration. Each symptom should be thoroughly analysed. 'Suck each symptom dry, like a dog sucks a bone'. Sometimes patients talk irrelevant, never get irritated on them.

Chief Orthopaedic Complaints Center Around the Following

"Fortitude is the marshal of thought, the armour of will and the fort of reason."
—*Francis Bacon*

PAIN: Pain is derived from the Latin word "POENA" (meaning punishment) and was associated in early civilisation with the concepts of demons, sin, and punishment. The terminology used for pain in Ayurved is 'SHOOL'—originated from the weapon 'TRISHUL' of Lord 'SHIVA'. Pain is a more terrible lord to mankind than the death itself.

Pain is one of the four elementary sensations. It is the master symptom in medicine. Pain has been defined by the International Association for Study of Pain (IASP) as "an unpleasant sensory and emotional experience associated with actual or potential tissue damage or described in terms of such damage (except in psychological pain)". IASP has also defined "*analgesia*" as "absence of pain in response to stimulation which would normally be painful". Sensibility to pain may be normal, reduced (*hypoalgesia*), absent (*analgesia*) or increased (*hyperalgesia*). Allodynia is the perception of pain with subnormal stimuli (which normally do not produce pain), e.g. light touch, vibratory movements, etc. In simple words pain caused by stimuli that are usually not painful is called allodynia. Pain, though a prominent symptom, is a personal possessive perception which depends upon several factors like psychology of individual, environmental factors, personal will, power of tolerance, presence of different persons, place where the person is present, etc. **(Fig. 1.33C)**

Nociceptors (derived from Latin 'nocere' meaning to damage and 'capere' meaning to understand, i.e. to understand the damage) scattered in the fatty tissue around the ligaments and other tissues when pressed (e.g. by oedema) lead to perceiving of pain.

Pathophysiology of pain: Pain is a multifactorial phenomenon. Pain pathways are not hard-wired but are plastic and involve many processes that both signal and temporally increase the sensation of pain after tissue damage (e.g. after surgery). The nerve endings of A-delta mechanothermal and C-polymodal nerve fibres are the receptors for painful stimuli or nociceptors and normally they have a high threshold for activation.

The 'first pain' (sharp immediate pain) is transmitted by A-delta fibres and the prolonged unpleasant burning pain is mediated through the smaller unmyelinated C-fibres. A plethora of neurotransmitters including glutamate (most important excitatory neurotransmitters in the central nervous system) mediate transmission of the sensation of pain both in the brain and spinal cord.

Depending on the site of origin and nature, pain may classified as:

- **Nociceptive pain**—Pain produced by activation of normal nerve by noxious stimuli (mechanical, thermal, chemical). *Site of origin of pain* may be: (a) *somatic*, e.g. skin, muscles, bone, joints, (b) *visceral*—Pain in tubular structure (especially in abdominal viscera) is colic in nature, usually severe, deep pain; palpation may not reproduce pain.

  Pain in solid structure is continuous in nature, usually dull, superficially felt; and palpation always reproduces it.

- *Neurogenic pain*—Origin of pain is in nerve itself, e.g. herpetic neuralgia, diabetic neuralgia (neuritis), post-infarction pain, causalgia. It may manifest differently right from bite of small ant or a big ant or prick of paper pin or feeling of burning fire **(Fig. 1.34A)**.

  Causalgia is a clinical syndrome associated with a lesion of a peripheral nerve containing sensory fibres, first described by SW Mitchell, (the father of modern neurology) *et al* (1864). It is manifested by pain in the extremity coming spontaneously or with any stimuli, with or without change in the patient's mental state. Pain is usually of intense burning character, and may be intermittent or persistent diffused in the area of cutaneous supply of the involved nerve.

  Perhaps the only manifestation of (complains) pain in the neonate or young children is "weeping" (which may be due to hunger or fear even). Infants must not be taken as the young adults, and they should be examined with deep scrutiny.

For correct diagnosis of pain, it is better to follow 'PQRST' approach:

P = Palliative factor (what makes it less); Provocative factor (what makes it more)
Q = Quality of pain (type of pain)
R = Radiation of pain (path of reference of pain)

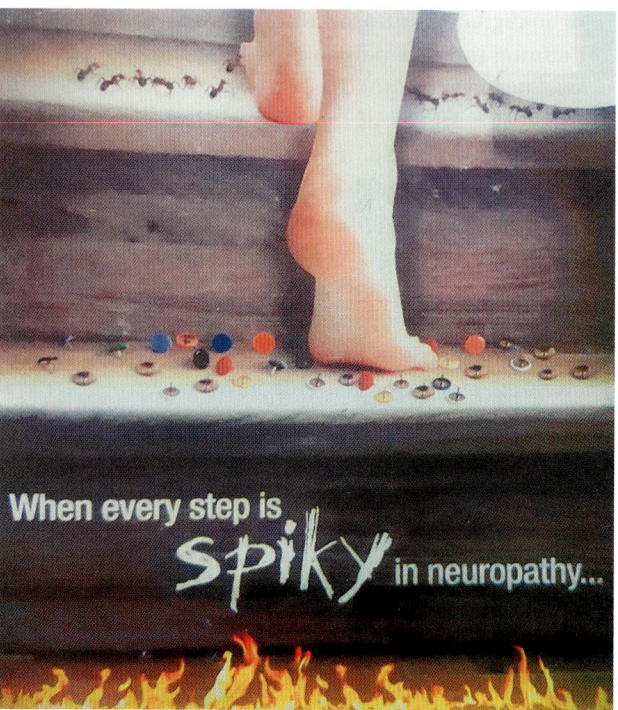

Fig. 1.34A: Neurogenic pain may manifest differently right from bite of small ant or big ant or prick of paper pins or feeling of burning fire.

S = Severity of pain
T = Timing of pain (is it all the time or intermittent, etc). With timing its *circadian* variation should be noted. Rhythms that cycle about once a day are called circadian rhythms. Those of higher or lower frequency are respectively termed *untradian* and *infradian* rhythm.

Climate pain: Few patients complain of pain only in some season; or aggravation of pain in certain climate; or after easterly wind.

- *Psychological pain*—With no organic cause various factors are responsible for origin and perpetuation of pain, e.g. mental stress, sleepless night, etc.
- *Total pain*, in which all the above three factors are responsible, e.g. pain in cancer.

  Pain in cancer patient has a dreaded psyche overlay. One of the worst aspects of cancer pain is that it is a constant reminder of the disease and death.

- *Phantom limb pain*—It was originally described by Ambroise Pare in the 17th century. It may be defined as an unpleasant sensation often painful with or without burning sensation distal to the site of a nerve injury (phantom sensation), and may result in marked physical and psychological morbidity.

Neuropathy Stages and Neuropathic Pain Causing Psychological Disturbance on Transparent (1.34B)

Chronic widespread pain (CWP): About 10% of adult population complain of CWP. The incidence is higher in

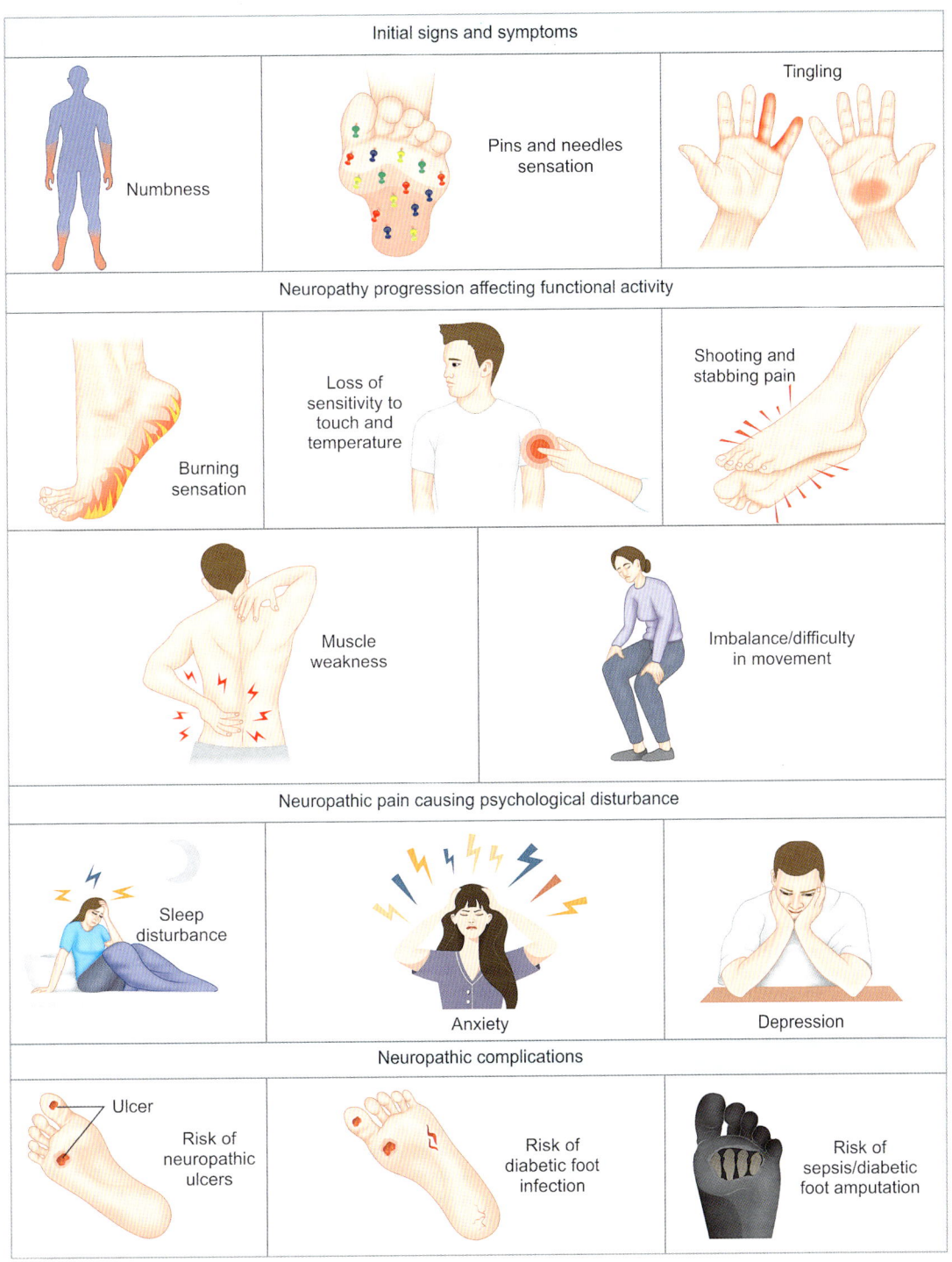

Fig. 1.34B: Stages of neuropathy.

women and generally increases with age. Usually, there is no constant correlation between CWP and tenderness. CWP is likely to be associated with depression or other symptoms of psychological distress. Once established, CWP is likely to persist or recur, especially if associated with other somatic symptoms in older age.

It is difficult to measure pain on a mathematical scale, however approximate assessment can be done in adult—*"non-verbal pain scale"* in the following way **(Fig. 1.35 and Table 1.1).** For rough assessment of ways, *"universal pain assessment tool"* Chart should be followed **(Fig. 1.35).**

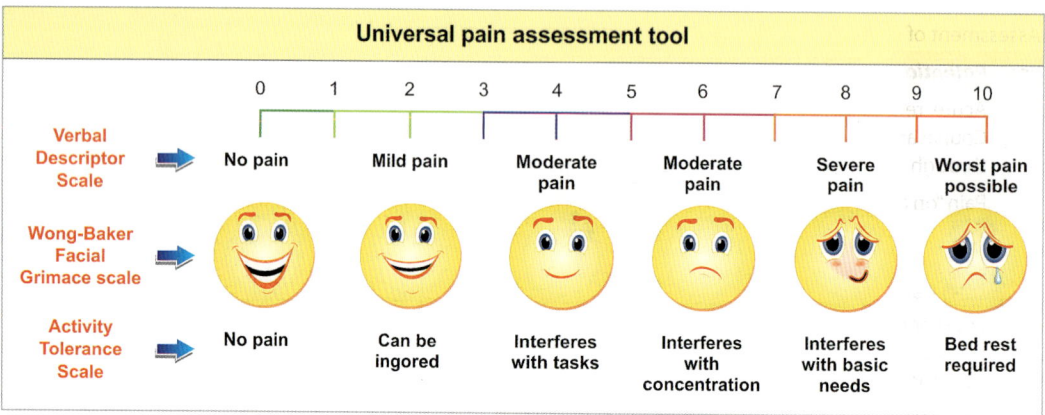

Fig. 1.35: Universal pain assessment tool.

TABLE 1.1: Nonverbal pain scale.

Parameters*	Category 0	Category 1	Category 2
Face	No particular expression or smile	Occasional grimace, tearing, frowning, wrinkled forehead	Frequent grimace, tearing, frowning, wrinkled forehead
Activity (Movement)	Lying quietly, normal position	Seeking attention through movement or slow cautious movement	Restless, excessive activity and/or withdrawal reflexes
Physiology (Vital signs)	Stable vital signs	Change in any of the following: • Systolic blood pressure >20 mmHg • Heart rate >20/minute	Change in any of the following: • Systolic blood pressure >30 mmHg • Heart rate >25/minute
Guarding	Lying quietly, no positioning of hands over areas of body	Splinting areas of the body, tense	Rigid, stiff
Respiratory	Baseline respiratory rate/SpO$_2$-pulse oximetry, compliant with ventilator	Respiratory rate >10 above baseline or 5% decreased SpO$_2$, mild asynchrony with ventilator	Respiratory rate >20 above baseline or 10% decreased SpO$_2$, severe asynchrony with ventilator

*Each of the 5 parameters is scored 0–2, which results in a total score between 0 and 10. Document total score by adding numbers from each of the 5 parameters. Scores of 0–2 indicate no pain, 3–6 moderate pain, and 7–10 severe pain

Note: The above pain scale is from Strong Memorial Hospital University of Rochester Medical Centre, 2004 (provided by Indus Citadal Aurobindo Biotech Ltd)

Assess the characteristics of pain as written in **Table 1.2**.

Certain Sitewise Reference of Pain

The speed of reference of pain in the human body is about 250 feet in one second.
- From cervical region to shoulder, arm and even up to fingertips (brachalgia or cervicobrachial neuralgia)
- From supraclavicular region to arm, forearm, fingers
- From shoulder to arm, forearm, hand and fingers
- From wrist to thumb, index finger (mainly from front of wrist)
- From upper mid dorsal spine to side of chest (girdle pain)
- From lower dorsal spine to abdominal wall
- From upper-mid lumbar region to loin, groin, upper medial aspect of thigh
- From lower lumbar region to lumbosacral region to along sciatic roots—*sciatica*
- From sacroiliac joint to back of thigh and knee
- From hip to anteromedial aspect of thigh and knee
- From thigh to knee according to the aspect of thigh involved
- From knee to shin of tibia.

Congenital insensitivity to pain and anhidrosis (CIPA): It is an autosomal recessive trait, with several defects of the gene NTRK 1 (neurotrophic tyrosine kinage), characterised by disturbance in pain and temperature perception due to involvement of the autonomic and sensory nervous system. Congenital insensitivity to pain is a difficult problem to control and treat. Congenital absence of pain is called as *analgia*.

Exact measurement of pain is rather impossible at the present stage, however, pain threshold can be assessed by *dolorimeter,* e.g. by providing a ratio of finger tenderness on the affected/unaffected hand in complex regional pain syndrome (CRPS).

Usually, it is not possible to pin-point the site of origin of pain with just a casual examination. However, the methodical examination usually leads to the approximate or even exact site of origin of pain.

Superficial sites (like skin and subcutaneous plane) as origin of pain are mostly quite obvious. Muscle pain is

TABLE 1.2: Assessment of characteristics of pain.

Characteristics	Potential elements
Temporal	Acute, recurrent or chronic; Onset and duration Course and daily variation, including break-through pain*
Intensity	Pain "on average" Pain "at its worst" Pain "at its least" Pain "right now"
Topography	Focal or multifocal Focal or referred Superficial or deep
Quality	Any descriptor (e.g. aching, throbbing, stabbing, churning or burning) Familiar or unfamiliar
Exacerbating/ relieving factors	Volitional (incident pain) or non-volitional

*Breakthrough, episodic, incidental and transient are few of the terms commonly used to refer to pain flare that can occur as a symptomatic overlay to baseline persistent pain.
Breakthrough pain has three subtypes:
1. Incident pain: Pain with activity or movement (most common)
2. Idiopathic pain: Pain with no known cause
3. End-of-dose pain: Pain appearing before a scheduled dose of around-the-clock analgesic medication.

carried on somatic sensory neurons and is usually well-localised. Squeezing the affected muscle increases the pain. The exact cause of chronic myofascial pain is not discernible in most of the cases, but, probably, it represents alterations in the peripheral or central pain circuits. Reference of pain to and from muscles and regional structures is common.

Pain due to pathology in bone is mostly constant, well-localised, worst at night and gets augumented by movement of the affected part and/or weight bearing in a case of lower limb weight-bearing bones. Bone pain may be referred to the nearby joint. Bone pain may occur due to inflammation, injury, infarction, increased intraosseous pressure, stretching of periosteum, or combined causes.

Somatic afferent nerves carry the pain fibres and the pain is well-localised, especially when periosteum and endosteum are involved.

Neuropathic pain may manifest continuous or intermittent. It may manifest differently and to different magnitude.

Complex regional pain syndrome (CRPS): *Also see* in the chapter on "Syndromes" on Page 639.

Drs Mitchell, Moorehouse and Keen described CRPS 125 years ago.

CRPS previously known as reflex sympathetic dystrophy (RSD) comprises of abnormal pain, swelling, vasomotor disturbances, contracture and osteoporosis. Exact cause is not known. Hand and foot are mainly affected, although knee, elbow, shoulder and even hip (in pregnancy) may also be affected. On the whole, CRPS is often unrecognised and poorly understood.

Usually, CRPS starts by a month after precipitating trauma, by which time direct effects of injury mostly subside, and a new diffuse unpleasant neuropathic pain arises. Spontaneous or burning pain, *hyperalgesia* (increased sensitivity to a noxious stimulus), *allodynia* (pain provoked by innocuous stimuli, e.g. gentle touch) and *hyperpathia* (the temporal and spatial summation of allodynia) are common feature. Pain is unremitting, however, sleep is usually not affected.

- *Concerning pain:* Note its site, depth of severity (ignorable—trivial; not ignorable as it interferes in activities—moderate; constant even in rest—severe; tossing and incapacitating—very severe), mode of onset, character, diurnal variation, path and site of radiation, relation with activities and rest, relieving/aggravating factors. *Reference of pain can be due to* same source of sensory supply or cortical confusion between embryologically related areas
- *Deformity:* Mode of onset, progressive or static, any earlier attempt for correction, disabilities due to deformity
- *Disability* or *Inability* in using the limb, with clear description
- *Limitation of movement:* How it started, whether progressive or static; any massage done and, how it hampers the activities
- *Swelling:* Site, how it started, associated with pain or painless, size, increasing gradually or rapidly, any decrease in the size if ever, any similar or other type of swelling elsewhere
- *Discharging wound:* How it started, type, colour and nature of discharge, intermittent or continuous, painful or painless, any history of indigenous applications or cauterization and any history of bony spicules in the discharge
- *Constitutional features:* Like fever, anorexia, constipation, headache, urinary trouble, eye trouble, night sweating
- *Cramps:* Cramps and cramp-like complaint in both calves are not uncommon. There can be several causes, which may be specific or nonspecific. **Claudication** [(the word derived from Latin 'Claudicatio' = to limp) the Roman emperor Claudius (10 BC to AD 54)—walked with limp probably due to polio] should be differentiated from the cramps. Claudication may be due to neurological (e.g. **spinal stenotic syndrome**) or vascular causes (e.g. **Buerger's phenomenon**), and they can be confused with each other. In rare cases, both causes may co-exist presenting with superimposed features. The neurogenic and vascular claudications can be differentiated as in **Table 1.3**.

In claudication (vascular e.g. Buerger's phenomenon; neurogenic, e.g. spinal stenotic syndrome), the patient feels gradually ensuing catch in both calf muscles after some walking. The walking distance, before the symptoms start appearing, gradually decreases. The claudication of spinal origin usually disappears after sitting or bending forward in chair, while that of vascular

TABLE 1.3: Difference between neurogenic and vascular claudication.

Neurogenic claudication	Vascular claudication
• Claudication is in the calf muscles due to pressure on or affection of cauda equina (spinal nerve roots). Patient after exerting/walking for sometime develops neurogenic pain and paraesthesia along the lower limb (mainly the calves, but may be in buttocks as well)	• Claudication in the calf muscles due to narrowing of the vascular tree (earlier spasmodic, but gradually organic narrowing due to atheromatous deposits and fibrosis). Pain may be also in thigh
• Spinal canal stenosis is most common cause	• Buerger's disease is the most common cause
• Persons beyond 40 years of age are usually affected	• Young and middle age groups are usually affected
• Males are more affected	• Mostly in males
• Patient complains of pain usually, in both calves/legs; catch and tightness in muscles; difficulty in walking; paraesthesia	• Patient complains of gradually increasing pain and fatigue and burning sensation, usually to start with in one leg, but later on in both after some walking
• Pain character—numbness, aching—proximal to distal	• Pain character—cramping—distal to proximal
• Burning is not associated with pain	• Burning is usually an accompanying symptom
• Movements of back—Limited	• Movements of back—Normal
• Pain is aggravated by extension of back	• Pain is aggravated by continuation of walking
• There is no particular time or walking-distance for initiation of the claudication. Rather distance of walking before precipitating of symptoms may remain same	• Claudication always starts after walking some distance, which gradually decreases (the length of distance) with the advancement of pathology
• Claudication pain is relieved only by bending forward or sitting, not only by resting where standing. Rather as soon as patient stands from sitting posture, the pain is initiated	• Claudication pain gets relieved after rest for sometime. Pain is not relieved after stooping
• Going uphill reduces the pain	• On going uphill pain is not reduced, rather it may increase
• Cycling reduces the pain	• Cycling does not reduce the pain, rather it may increase
• Peripheral vascular pulsation normal (according to the age)	• Peripheral vascular pulsation (dorsalis pedis pulsation upwards) is decreased, or even may not be felt
• Skin—normal	• Skin—loss of hair; shiny
• There may be neurological deficit features (muscular weakness, wasting, sensory or visceral affection)	• No neurological deficit
• Atrophy—occasional	• Atrophy—uncommon
• Usually there is no trophic changes	• Trophic changes do develop
• Gangrene does not develop	• Gangrene develops in advanced cases
• X-ray, CT scan, MRI helps in confirming the diagnosis	• Doppler flowmetry is helpful to assess the status of the peripheral circulation
• Management mainly consists of surgical decompression of the spinal stenosis. Non-operative management like limitation of activities, spinal exercises, neurotropic vitamins, orthotics have limited role	• In early stages, management mainly consists of antiplatelet, antiatherogenic, vasodilator drugs (medical sympathectomy). If no response—surgical sympathectomy. For gangrene—amputation

origin requires rest from walking for relief. Neurogenic claudication is defined as the onset of lower extremity pain, paraesthesia or weakness on walking.

In cramps (the muscle cramps are common in about 60% of the adult population), the patient feels a sudden painful catch in the calf muscles with or without the contracted muscles forming a hard ball *(systremma)*, which almost disappears within a few seconds, either following local massage or rest or itself, leaving behind a dull aching pain lasting for few hours to a day or two. Constipation, overexertion and walking without habit can precipitate cramps in the calf. Calcium deficiency and advanced pregnancy can also induce these cramps.

However, symptoms like cramps may also be seen in lumbar spinal canal stenosis, vague ankylosing spondylitis, cirrhosis, thyrotoxicosis, poly-inserinitis, metabolic diseases, e.g. hyponatraemia (as in heat stroke) and hypomagnesaemia, myopathies, aesthenia, hemodialysis, and depressive syndromes in adults. Chronic leg compartment syndrome and stress fractures should be differentiated from intermittent claudication.

- Any other complaints, even unrelated to orthopaedics, should be noted chronologically. Usually there are more than one presenting complaints, which may appear one after another or simultaneously. Note the sequence of their appearance.

Raynaud's Phenomenon

Raynaud's phenomenon usually occurs in ladies and in upper limbs. It is a self-limited reversible vasospastic disorder characterised by transient stress-induced (e.g. cold temperature) ischaemia of digits, nose-tip, and/or ears. Due to vasospastic alterations in blood flow a triphasic colour response is usually noted. The initial colour is white/pale (ischaemic pallor), the blue (congestive cyanosis) and finally red (reactive hyperaemia).

Management: Stop smoking (if smoker); keep hands and body warm—repeated soaking in warm water; vasodilators (calcium channel blockers, e.g. nifedipine); angiotensin II receptor antagonists; topical nitroglycerine ointment. In severe cases, intravenous prostacycline and its analogue are helpful.

Buerger's Disease (Thromboangiitis Obliterans: TO)

Buerger's disease also called thromboangiitis obliterans is an inflammatory obliterative nonatheromatous vascular disease which most commonly affects small and medium-sized arteries, veins and nerves typically in young smoker males (18–50 years). Initial manifestation is ischaemia or claudication of both legs (and sometimes hands) which begins distally and progresses proximally. Pedal-leg claudication, dysesthesias, sensitivity to cold—ultimately ending in gangrene and ulceration. It should be differentiated from atherosclerosis, embolic autoimmune disease, diabetes neuropathy affection of foot, hypercoagulable state. Confirmation is by arteriogram.

Management: Stop smoking (if smoker), trial of calcium channel blockers, foot care, sympathectomy, treatment of the ulcer (if present) and ultimately amputation.

Hyperhidrosis (Excessive Sweating)

Normally, sweating occurs when ambient temperature is greater than 32.5°C and during exercises. In hyperhydrosis there is excessive and uncontrollable sweating induced by sympathetic hyperactivity. It occurs typically in young people involving palmar, plantar or axillary areas, etc. where eccrine glands are most dense. The eccrine glands are innervated by cholinergic fibres from sympathetic nervous system and shows exaggerated response to mental stimuli. Secondary hyperhydrosis may occur in hyperthyroidism, obesity, menopause and condition involving autonomic deregulation, e.g. in cardiovascular accident patients and paraplegics. Botulinum toxin type A injection has been found to address this problem at palmar, axillary, facial and other sites with overactive eccrine glands.

Causes of Generalised Sweating

1. During shock, vasovagal attack, anxiety, excruciating pain, motion sickness.
2. In systemic diseases, e.g. rickets, infantile scurvy, hyperthyroidism, pink disease, tuberculosis (night sweating).
3. Drugs, e.g. alcohol, salicylates, pilocarpine.
4. Occasionally, during menstruation.

Localised Hyperhidrosis

Localised hyperhidrosis occurs due to:
1. Injury to spinal cord or nerve.
2. Brain tumours.
3. Post-encephalitic Parkinsonism.

Few Common Sites of Hyperhidrosis

Site	Cause
Palms and Soles	May be normal Psychoneurosis Rheumatoid arthritis
Sweating at tip of nose	Granulosis rubra nasi
Generalised with small vesicles on the skin and trunk	Miliaria or sudamiel
Lesions in crops on any part of body with perspiration.	Miliaria papulosa or rubra (prickly heat)

Tremor (Latin—Tremor, Tremere, Shake, Tremble; Greek—Tremein, Tremble)

Tremor may be defined as involuntary shaking of the body or limbs (regular or irregular; rapid or slow; fine or coarse) with an oscillatory character. Involuntary rhythmic movements occur due to alternating contractions of opposite groups of muscles.

Tremor may be grouped under following headings:

- *Physiological,* e.g. due to fear, emotion, weakness, anxiety, alcoholism, fever, nervousness and cold climate.
  The tremor of anxiety is usually fine and rapid but it may be coarse and irregular.
- *Benign essential tremor:* It occurs as a familial disorder as the coarse distant tremor, usually exaggerated in awkward postures, e.g. when the patient holds his outstretched fingers pointing to each other in front of his nose. Though it is usually relieved to some extent during movement, but it is present both at rest and movements.
- *Senile tremors* are similar to benign essential tremor.
- *Parkinsonian tremor:* In Parkinsonism, tremor is usually the initial presentation for which patients seek advice. It first involves the fingers and spreads to proximal portion of arm, and gradually it may extend to the tongue, lips and legs. The tremor is rapid, rhythmic, and alternating tremor, mainly in flexion/extension, but often with rhythmic rotatory component between finger and thumb (**pill-rolling tremor**). It is often associated with features of extrapyramidal disease, such as hypokinesia, cogwheel rigidity, postural abnormality, gait disorder (festinant

- *Cerebellar tremor:* It usually occurs in elderly persons, in whom the tremor occurs only during movements (intention tremor). Such tremors increase when the limb approaches a target and gets relieved when the affected limb is supported and relaxed.
- *In thyrotoxicosis,* tremor is always rapid.
- *Hysterical tremor* usually involves a limb or whole body and is characteristically worsened by examiner's attempt to control it.
- Tremors of hand may be even *congenital.*
- *Tremors may also occur in multiple sclerosis, uraemia, hepatic failure, mercurial poisoning,* etc.

Muscular Fasciculations

These are *spontaneous contractions of groups of muscle fibres.* They originate from abnormal generator sites in the peripheral nervous system. They vary in distribution and frequency and most commonly occur in motor neurone disease (anterior horn cell disease), however may also occur in fatigued normal subjects.

Many patients complain of generalised weakness and vague pain in body, joints or limbs. Usually, the cause is systemic, such as generalised weakness or fatigue, anaemia, hypothyroidism, hypoproteinaemia, cardiopulmonary disease, chronic infection, hyperthyroidism, depression, poor physical condition, malignancy, etc.

History of Present Illness

Let the patient narrate the story of his ailments in his own words from the beginning to the present condition. Pick up the salient points. Dilate on each point with relevant leading questions. Any history of injury or febrile attacks must be explored through leading questions. Treatment received and medicines taken for the present complaints should be noted in detail.

Broadly orthopaedic problems fall in two major groups—injury related or noninjury related.
- *In Case of Injury*—Enquire about its mode and nature, and if associated with any abnormal sounds, the amount of impact, the portion of body hurt, immediate effects of injury, delayed effects of injury, could he/she stand and walk or was carried (then mode of carriage), did the injury affect mobility/activities.

High velocity injuries are getting more and more common and usually produce multiple injuries with or without injury to vital organs. Hence enquire with leading questions about the general effects of polytrauma [e.g. shock, haemorrhage, electric shock, burn **(Figs. 1.41A and B)**, etc.] and about level of consciousness at the time of trauma and later on.

Modes of injury
- Direct hit (contact injury)
- Indirect injuries
  - Rotational strains (e.g. fracture neck femur)
  - Violent muscle pulls (e.g. fracture of patella)
  - Compression injuries (e.g. compression fracture of vertebra).

In Case of Fall—Height of fall, surface on which fallen, level of consciousness after falling, if he could stand up or walk or even take weight on the affected side or not following the injury, immediate posture after injury, any manipulation at the site of injury by himself or any one else.

After the injury
- Mode of transportation to home or hospital
- Attempts by bone setters or quacks and/or any other treatment given.
- *Fever*—Onset, any associated rigor, range of temperature, continuous or intermittent, if only at particular time, e.g. in the evening, sweating, response to treatment, accompanying symptoms.

Enquire about appetite, polyuria, loss of weight.

History of Past Illness

Any earlier injury; history of earlier infections, specially tuberculosis, syphilis, leprosy, pyogenic; average duration of bleeding after any cut; any particular treatment received. History about TORCH profile (To = toxoplasmosis, R = rubella, C = cytomegalovirus, H = herpes virus), which can be detected with ELISA test.

The *incidence of bone and joint tuberculosis* is on increase over the past decade in several regions of the world, may be due to the spread of human immunodeficiency virus (HIV) infection. Diagnosis of osteoarticular tuberculosis is becoming frequently difficult due to polymorphism of the disease, bizarre manifestations, and the weak specificity of the clinical features and more emergence and increase in the incidence of drug resistant tuberculosis. Hence, wherever is any doubt, histological examination (besides other investigations) is essential to confirm the diagnosis.

Personal History

Occupation, any tobacco/drug habit, personal hygiene, hobby, sensitivity or allergy to any drug or object.

Occupation should be verified and noted clearly. Several conditions, especially in upper limb have been attributed to manual activities, which require force, repetition, overuse or the use of an awkward posture alone or in combination, e.g. carpal tunnel syndrome, lateral or medial epicondylitis, **de-Quervain's disease**, **Dupuytren's disease,** ganglia and carpometacarpal arthritis in the thumb. The blame was so deep that the de-Quervain's disease was called **Washerwoman's strain,** because there was discomfort during wringing out clothes or turning a mangle. However, except for a very few conditions, mixed or even opposite conclusions have been drawn about the occupation as the causative factor for such conditions. Exacerbation of the symptoms should be distinguished from the causation of the underlying condition, especially keeping in view the legal aspects and compensation factor involved in several works and manual activities.

The term **'repetitive strain injury'** used to generally describe the conditions noted above has now been replaced by *'work-related upper-limb disorder'* (WRULD). More recognised WRULD are cramp of the hand and forearm, which can occur after 'repetitive work'; traumatic inflammation of the tendons of the hand and forearm or of the associated tendon sheaths can occur in those involved in manual labour or whose occupation demand frequent or repeated movements of the hand or wrist; carpal tunnel syndrome occurs more in hand-held vibrating tool users and so on.

Without blaming a single factor, the incidence of above mentioned non-traumatic soft tissue musculoskeletal disorders may be a synergy between genetics, physiology and lifestyle factors (intrinsic) in addition to biomechanics and workplace (extrinsic) risk factors.

In case of females, enquire about marital status, number of children, any gynaecological complaints.

In relevant cases, enquiry must be made about the factors which can lead to the dust and fibre generated diseases like silicosis, asbestosis, coal workers pneumoconiosis.

Family History

Any familial incidence related to the recent complaints, tuberculous infection in family, any hereditary disorder **(Figs. 1.36 to 39)**.

Social History

- Economic background, status of living, approach road/path/way to house
- Topographical surroundings
- Barriers in and around home
- Education in the family.

History of present illness is more or less analysis of relevant points. The onset of the symptoms can provide clue to the origin of the disease, e.g. Congenital (present since birth); Developmental (defect in developmental period of childhood and adolescence); Infective/Inflammatory (associated with constitutional features); Metabolic (nutritional and/or economic deficit); Endocrinal (evidences of hormonal imbalance); Traumatic (history of injury); Neoplastic (painless or painful, gradually or rapidly increasing, swelling or ulcer—benign or malignant); Degenerative (in older age groups, or chronic or old pathologies); Idiopathic (causes not known); by indirect questions assessment for HIV.

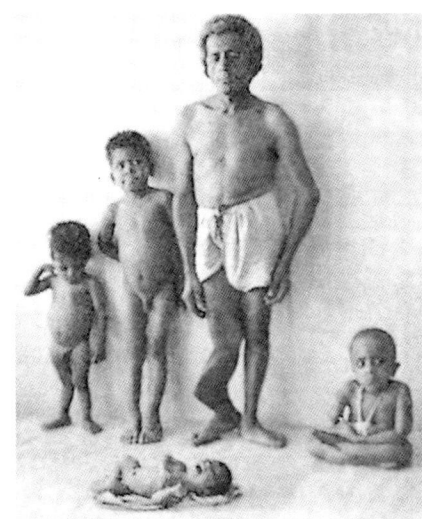

Fig. 1.36: A family of five, all having deformities of the limbs due to osteogenesis imperfecta—hereditary familial disorder characterized by fragility of bone, blue sclera, deafness, laxity of joint and secondary dwarfism. The basic pathology is failure of formation of osteoblast. The long bones become shorter and thinner with thin cortex and medullary cavity – they have tendency to bend and fracture with minimal trauma; however, they heal readily with abundant callus. The overall bone is osteoporotic. There is no specific treatment.

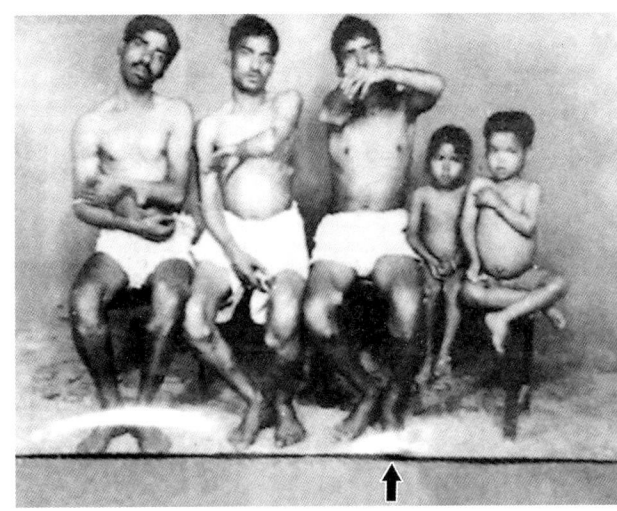

Fig. 1.37: Group photograph of available family members showing multiple exostosis, familial incidence had been followed up to four generations. Third brother in this group consulted for his foot lesion (exostosis in 1st web, **Fig. 1.38**).

History of past illness: Trauma, tuberculosis, syphilis, gonorrhoea, bleeding diasthesis.

Personal history: Addiction, immunization, allergy or sensitivity to drugs, education, hobby.

In case of females: Any gynaecological disorder, number of children.

Family history and social status: Social status, hereditary disorder, economic status, infectious disease.

EXAMINATION
- General examination
- Regional examination
- Local examination.

General Examination
Start the examination of the patient with the idea that you are examining the patient as a whole NOT a system nor a limb only. Start with the assessment of level of assess consciousness, level of intelligence, and level of appreciating power. Wherever needed (like unconciousness, head injury, poisoning, stroke, etc.) the level of consciousness should be assessed by Glasgow coma scale.
- Look, intelligence, built, any special posture, cyanosis, oedema, pulse, temperature, blood pressure, jaundice, lymph glands, nail conditions (the appearance of nails can serve as a barometer of a patient's general health).
- *Attitude*—While entering the examination room, note the first impression and posture (general, regional, local) **(Figs. 1.31 and 1.32)**. To maintain a particular posture the concerned bones remain in tone with extra power **(Fig. 1.40)**.
- *Attitude of standing and height* (in cms)
  - with full weight
  - with partial weight
  - with support.

If patient can stand, also perform Trendelenburg's test.

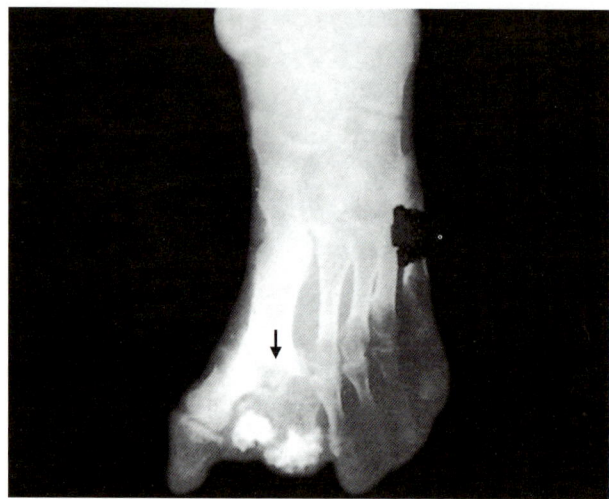

Fig. 1.38: X-ray of the foot of the third brother in the family of **Figure 1.37**. Note the disabling exostosis from the first metatarsal.

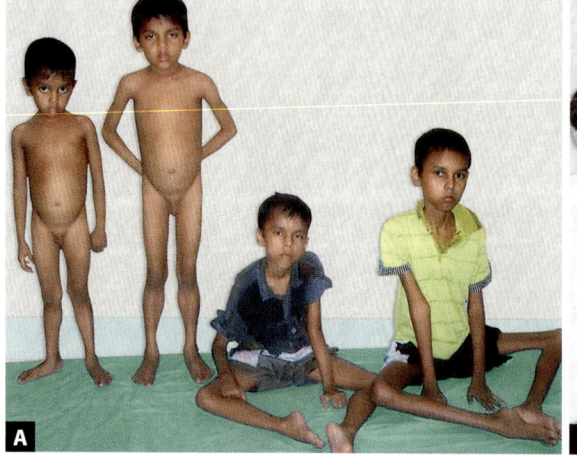
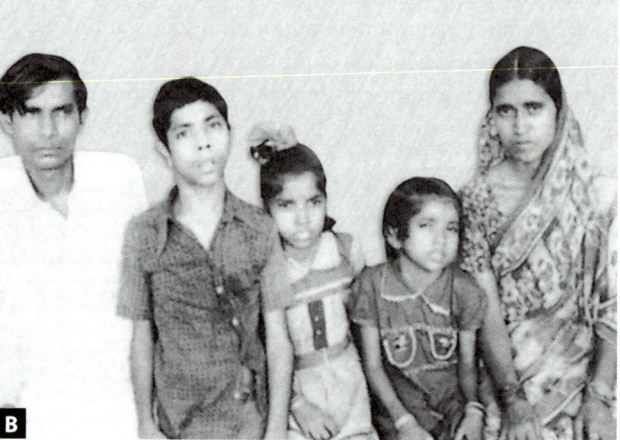

Figs. 1.39A and B: (A) Four own brothers suffering form myopathy; (B) A family of five—all suffering from myopathy.

History and Record Chart

Name	Age	Sex	Race	Religion	Occupation	Registration No.
	Marital status and family					Complete postal
	Photographic records with dates					address:
						Telephone:
Complaints	— Pain					Fax:
	— Deformity					E-mail:
	— Disability					Any other information
	— Disparity of limb length					
	— Swelling					
	— Any other.					

Body Mass Index (BMI), kg/m^2

	|← Weight (lb) →|																			
	120	130	140	150	160	170	180	190	200	210	220	230	240	250	260	270	280	290	300	310	320
4'10"	25	27	29	31	34	36	38	40	42	44	46	48	50	52	54	57	59	61	63	65	67
4'11"	24	26	28	30	32	34	36	38	40	43	45	47	49	51	53	55	57	59	61	63	65
5'0"	23	25	27	29	31	33	35	37	39	41	43	45	47	49	51	53	55	57	59	61	63
5'1"	23	25	27	28	30	32	34	36	38	40	42	44	45	47	49	51	53	55	57	59	61
5'2"	22	24	26	27	29	31	33	35	37	38	40	42	44	46	48		51	53	55	57	59
5'3"	21	23	25	27	28	30	32	34	36	37	39	41	43	44	46	48	50	51	53	55	57
5'4"	21	22	24	26	28	29	31	33	34	36	38	40	41	43	45	46	48	50	52	53	55
5'5"	20	22	23	25	27	28	30	32	33	35	37	38	40	42	43	45	47	48	50	52	53
5'6"	19	21	23	24	26	27	29	31	32	34	36	37	39	40	42	44	45	47	49	50	52
5'7"	19	20	22	24	25	27	28	30	31	33	35	37	38	39	41	43	44	46	47	49	50
5'8"	18	20	21	23	24	26	27	29	30	32	34	35	37	38	40	41	43	44	46	47	49
5'9"	18	19	21	22	24	25	27	28	30	31	33	34	36	37	38	40	41	43	44	46	47
5'10"	17	19	20	22	23	24	26	27	29	30	32	33	35	36	37	39	40	43	43	45	46
5'11"	17	18	20	21	22	24	25	27	28	29	31	32	34	35	36	38	39	41	42	43	45
6'0"	16	18	19	20	22	23	24	26	27	29	30	31	33	34	35	37	38	39	41	42	43
6'1"	16	17	19	20	21	22	24	25	26	28	29	30	32	33	34	36	37	38	40	41	42
6'2"	15	17	18	19	21	22	23	24	26	27	28	30	31	32	33	35	36	37	39	40	41

Normal · Obese · Morbid obese

Conversion factors:
Weight in lbs/2.2 = Weight in kilograms (kg)
Height in inches × 0.0254 = height in meters (m)
1 foot = 12 inches

- *Weight:* Body weight should be taken with bare minimum clothings and in erect standing position in kilograms.

Since *obesity* has been the cause and predisposing factors for several diseases, including cancers (like brain cancer, multiple myeloma, oesophageal cancer, post menopausal breast cancer, cancers of thyroid, gall bladder, stomach, liver, pancreas, kidney, ovaries, uterus, and colon.) its assessment is essential.

More than 30 million Indians are overweight and obesity continues to rise (National Family Health Survey). Further, obesity is on the rise in India. Prevalence of obesity is 12.6% in women and 9.3% in men in India. It is becoming a worldwide epidemic. WHO reported 500 million of world population being obese. Obesity is a great risk factor for osteoarthritis. It is associated with increased morbidity and mortality. Cohen et al (2013) have observed that trunk fat is associated with poor bone quality, decreased trabecular bone volume, decreased, stiffness, greater cortical porosity, and decreased bone formation in premenopausal women with a normal

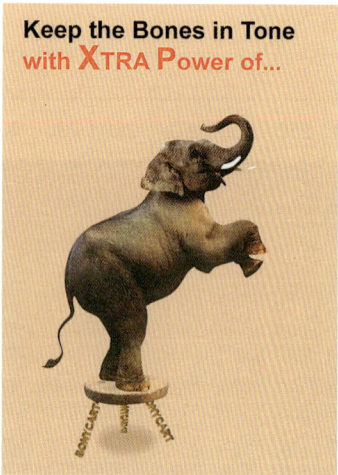

Fig. 1.40: Elephant standing on stool.

bone mineral density. The relative bone strength decreases with increasing fat mass and this relationship is strengthened with increasing age. Overweight and obesity are generally associated with a higher morbidity and mortality. However, Modig K et al have published their registry-based cohort study concluding that the overall increased risk of death associated with a high body mass index (BMI) has been found to decline with increasing age. This phenomenon has been called the "*obesity paradox.*"

The WHO (1997) and National Institute of Health (NIH 1998) have endorsed the Body Mass Index *(BMI) as a measure of obesity*. BMI, expressed as weight in kilograms divided by the square of height in meters (kg/m^2), has been adopted as the preferred method of expressing body weight, especially from obesity point of view, since BMI correlates greatly with most laboratory measures of the body fat. According to assessment of BMI, *under-weight* (BMI <18.5 kg/m^2); *normal range weight* (BMI 18.5–24.9 kg/m^2); and *over-weight* (BMI >25 kg/m^2) 25.0–29.9 mg/kg^2, or obese CBMI, e'' 30 mg/kg^2 have been defined. *Obesity* has been *classified into three classes:* Class I: 30.0–34.9 kg/m^2, Class II: 35.0–39 kg/m^2; and Class III: >40 kg/m^2. The risk of morbidity and mortality is increased in BMI range 25.0–29.0 kg/m^2, moderate in class I, severe in Class II, and very severe in class III groups.

Body Mass Index (BMI): Body Mass Index (BMI) 18 to 19 is considered normal in the case of most adolescents. Anything more indicates risk of becoming overweight as they get older.

The crux of obesity management are diet therapy (eat small, frequent meals = fruits, walnuts, almonds, sandwiches; avoid fried food and aerated drinks, drink 8–10 glasses of water every day), augmented physical activities, behaviour modifications, changing of lifestyle and pharmacotherapy [anorectic drugs—e.g. appetite suppressants, noradrenergic agents (acting on opposite centre), serotonergic agents (acting on hypothalamus to decrease satiety), adrenergic/serotonergic agents, etc.].

Proper sleep is also helpful in achieving a balanced body. Eight hours sleep in the right is thought to be ideal (which, perhaps people of Finland, only enjoy) however, seven hours of good sleep to the night may be taken as balanced one.

- *Gait*
  - Limp or lurch
  - Specific gait—recognised patterns of gait (*also see* Pages 243–246):
    - waddling
    - high stepping
    - hemiplegic (spastic)
    - ataxic
    - scissor
    - festinant
    - lathyriatic
    - stamping
    - knock knee, etc.

Systemic Examination

- Skull and face—Contour, swelling, decubitus ulcer, and any stigmata (of syphilis, rickets, etc.).
- Neck—Lymph nodes, venous engorgement, any swelling.
- Cardiovascular system—Pulse, blood pressure, heart.
- Respiratory system—Thoracic cage, rib contour, chest expansion, abnormal shape of chest (flat, barrel, pigeon), rib hump, rachitic rosary (Harrison's sulcus, scorbutic rosary).
- Abdomen—Liver, spleen, kidney, any lump, iliac fossae, any abnormal finding.
- Central nervous system:
  - Higher mental functions
  - Cranial nerves
  - Motor system: Power, bulk, tone, reflexes, coordination, involuntary movements
  - Sensory system.
- Genitourinary system.
- Endocrinal functions.

Regional Examination

The examination of the part complained of only, does not complete the examination, because sometimes the symptoms felt in one part have their origin in another region—proximal or even distal. For example, pain in the leg is often caused by a lesion in the spine, pain in the knee may have its origin in the hip, a pain or tingling and numbness in hand may have its origin in the cervical spine, pain in forearm or even arm may have its origin in wrist region (e.g. in carpal tunnel syndrome). Hence, the necessity of regional examination.

- For lower limb problems, examine lumbar region to tip of toes

- For upper limb problems, examine cervical region to tips of fingers
- For trunk problems, examine thoracic, lumbar, and abdominal regions, besides spine (and the supply region if spinal cord is involved)
- Also examine the regional lymph nodes.

Local Examination

Inspection (Look for)

For proper observation the patient and the part to be examined should be viewed in coronal, transverse, and sagittal planes, while the patient is in perfect erect position, if possible. The centre of gravity lies just anterior to the second sacral segment where all (coronal, transverse and sagittal) planes converge. Look for:

- Posture of the patient and position of part/limb—attitude.
- Inspect from different sides.
- Normal anatomical points
  - Bony
  - Soft tissue.
- Skin:
  - Colour
  - Texture
  - Elasticity/stretchability
  - Erythematous changes
  - Puckering
  - Cafe-au-lait spots
  - Tattoo marks
  - 'Pachh'/vaccination scar
  - Superficial cuts or scars (linear scar with/without suture mark—usually operative scar; irregular scar—injury; broad, adherent puckered scar—old suppuration)
  - Warts or callosities.
- *Muscle condition:*
  - Swelling
  - Wasting
  - Spasm
  - Contracture
  - Fasciculations.
- *Vascular:*
  - Venous prominence
  - Pulsation
  - Varicosities.
- Abnormal findings, e.g. swelling, sinus, ulcer.

In case of ulcer(s), note the followings: site, size, shape, surface, floor, base, margin (edge), relation to deeper tissues, surrounding tissues, discharge on the surface [especially ICHOR (a thin watery discharge from an ulcer or unhealthy wound) which usually denotes chronicity and deeper involvement], pigmentation, regional lymph nodes.

Broadly, the *ulcers are classified as* (i) non-specific, (ii) specific, (iii) malignant **(Table 1.4)**.

Examination of Any Sinus

A *sinus* (Latin = a hollow; a bay or gulf) is a *blind ending, usually lined by granulation tissue track opening onto the skin or mucous membrane* [cf. *Fistula* (Latin = a pipe or tube) is *a tunnel connecting two epithelial or endothelial surfaces*]. Sinus may be (1) *congenital* (arising from the remnants of embryonic ducts that persist instead of being obliterated or (2) *acquired* (usually secondary to the presence of foreign body or necrotic material.

Note:

- Number, site, relation with deeper tissues, relation with skin, margin, discharge—intermittent/continuous, colour and type of discharge, relation with pain, possible source, discharge of any bony spicule—diagnostic of chronic pyogenic osteomyelitis, nature of scar (if healed)

TABLE 1.4: Ulcers (ulcer may be defined as discontinuity of epithelial surface).

Non-specific ulcer	Specific ulcer	Malignant ulcer
• Varicose ulcer (ulcer developing on underlying varicose veins)	• Tuberculous (undermined edge), pigmented surrounding; serous, sero-sanguinous or sanguineous discharge	• Carcinomatous (everted edge)

Trophic ulcer
  [trophe (Greek) = nutrition]
  (ulcers developing due to impairment of nutrition which depends upon properly intact vascular and nerve supply) e.g.
  – Ischaemic ulcer,
  – Diabetic ulcer,
  – Ulcers developing in spina bifida, tabes dorsalis, leprosy, peripheral nerve injury—due to anaesthetic skin, and are called neuropathic/perforating ulcer
	• Pyogenic (sloping edge)
	• Syphilitic (usually punctated)
	• Actinomycotic (multiple ulcer with sulphur granules)
		• Rodent ulcer (basal cell carcinoma usually occurring on upper face
		• Marjolin ulcer (carcinoma developing on scar)

• Tropical ulcer		

- Sinus tract—feel of tract, traceability of tract to parent site, tract fixed to bone or mobile. Probing should be avoided.

Causes of persistence of sinus: Persistence of infection; presence of dead tissue within, e.g. bony sequestrum; presence of any foreign body, e.g. bullet, metallic foreign body, pieces of cloth, etc; persistence of cavity within the bone; epithelialisation/endothelialisation of sinus track; puckering of soft tissues around the tract; intractable infection, e.g. fungal infection; malignant changes in the tract; diabetes; general debility; prolonged use of corticoids; persistent discharge, e.g. of urine, cerebrospinal fluid, faeces, etc. after irradiation.

Sinuses must be differentiated from fistulae which are abnormal communications between two epithelium lined surfaces.

Palpation

- *Superficial (touch)*: Skin condition; temperature; sensation; superficial tenderness; anatomical points—bony, soft tissue; induration (oedema)—regional/local; arterial pulsation; crepitus (may be due to entrapped gas, e.g. in surgical emphysema, gas gangrene; fracture; tenosynovitis).
- *Deep Palpation (feel)*: Deep tenderness—It should be avoided in presence of any inflammation (clinically diagnosed by noting the cluster of symptoms and signs of *calor* (heat due to vasodilatation), *dolor* (pain), *rubor* (redness due to vasodilatation), *tumor/tumour* (swelling mainly due to oedema, exudate) and *functio-lessa* (less or loss of function). Deep palpation should be done by direct pressure, indirect twist, and deep thrust. *Tenderness of a bone, joint or soft tissue can be classified into four grades according to the reaction* (facial and verbal) *of the patient* during examination for tenderness.

  Grade I — The patient says that part is painful on pressure.
  Grade II — The patient winces.
  Grade III — The patient winces and withdraws the affected part.
  Grade IV — The patient repeatedly avoids allowing the part to be touched.

While palpating (mainly for the soft tissues) the "*tendor point*" and "*trigger point*" can be differentiated as follows:

Parameters	Tendor point	Trigger point
Tenderness	Focal	Focal
Referred pain	No	Yes
Distribution	Widespread	Regional
Usual cause	Inflammation/fibromyalgia	Myofascial pain/neurofibromatous lesion
Presence of abnormal tissue	No	Possible

Deep palpation of the bone: Bone should be palpated for surface, alignment, deep tenderness, abnormal prominence, disturbed relationship of the normal bony landmarks, any crepitus (fracture).

Palpate the girth of bone for **Thickening** (there is increase in almost all surfaces of bone which are usually irregular and anatomical configuration is distorted). Bone is thickened usually due to deposit from outside, e.g. in chronic osteomyelitis); **Broadening** (breadth of the bone increases, surfaces of the bone almost regular, anatomical configurations are usually identifiable. Broadening occurs from within, e.g. in rickets); **Expansion of bone** (bony surfaces are expanded, surfaces are usually nodular or bluntly irregular, all dimensions of bone in the affected zone are increased, e.g. in giant cell tumour).

Deep palpation of a joint: Palpate for:
- Synovial thickening—The normal synovium is not palpable, while thickened synovium feels soft/boggy/doughy; feel for any tenderness.
  To palpate a joint for synovium an optimum pressure to balance your thumb-nail (about 4 kg/cm^2) should be adequate.
  Many times, it becomes difficult to ascertain the origin of pain—whether from intra-articular or extra-articular structures. However, stressing a joint is easily accomplished by gentle passive range of motion of the joint by the examiner. In contrast, pain occurring while the patient performing active range of motion against a joint held rigid by the examiner is usually due to pathology in the surrounding tendons. Further, by selective direct palpation of periarticular structure (such as skin, subcutaneous tissue, tendons, etc.) one can ascertain the origin of pain to a fair extent.
- Joint line—A slit all around in between the articular ends—feel for any tenderness, any abnormal mass.
- Fluid in the joint—Yielding/cystic/fluctuant/tense feel.
- Articular ends—For any tenderness, roughness, crepitus.
- Adjoining bones—For any thickening, expansion, crepitus, irregularity, tenderness.
- Abarticular (at a distance from or not involving a joint) structures and tissues.

  Crepitus is an audible and/or palpable 'grating' sensation felt during joint movements. Crepitus may be *fine* or *coarse*. The *fine crepitus* of inflamed synovium is of uniform intensity and perceptible only with a stethoscope. The *coarse crepitus* is of variable intensity, can be detected easily and transmitted from damaged cartilage and/or bone. It can be elicited by gently compressing a joint throughout its range of motion.

Palpation of fossae (if any)

Palpation of muscles: Girth, feel, tone tenderness and pliability of muscles.

Examination of any swelling should be in detail: skin over the swelling, site, size, margin, extent, surface, any veinous prominence, hyperaesthesia on the surface, shape, vascularity, tenderness, consistency (cystic, very soft, soft, doughy, firm, hard, stony hard), fixity (to superficial structures—subcutaneous tissues, skin; to deeper structures), deeper relations, mobility, fluctuation test, transillumination test (if cystic).

Examination of nodules:
- The regional lymph nodes should be examined according to the affected region, such as cervical chain of lymph nodes; submandibular lymph nodes; supratrochlear lymph nodes; axillary group of lymph nodes, para-aortic group; inguinal group, popliteal group of lymph nodes. Lymph glands should be examined for size, extent of enlargement, surface, tenderness, adhesions (matting), mobility, consistency, relation to superficial and deeper structure.
- Other nodular enlargements—In several diseases, there are painless nodules in relation to subcutaneous tissue, tendons, joint capsules, ligaments, adjoining connective tissue, such as—in rheumatoid arthritis subcutaneous nodules develop usually over bony prominences in the periosteum or the deeper layers of skin. In rheumatic fever, mobile subcutaneous nodules develop usually over bony prominences or tendons. In hypercholesterolemia, nodular swellings develop over fingers/toes/upper eyelid.

Springing

To elicit pain at the site of lesion by intermittently compressing the distant part of the parallel bones, e.g. in fracture of the neck of radius pain can be elicited by compressing the lower forearm.

Transmitted movement: In case of fractures, feel for transmitted movements across the fracture site which will not be felt, if there is displaced fracture. However, in impacted or incomplete fractures movements can be transmitted across the fracture site.

Percussion (tap)

Specially over the bone in suspected crack fracture or some deep pathology; over the joints if suspected deep pathology like gout; over the spinous processes to elicit tenderness in spine.

Auscultation (hear)

- If needed, e.g. for systolic bruit (haemangioma)
- May be of value in localising crepitations, snaps, mild friction rubs in joints.

Measurements

- Linear measurements
- Circumferential measurements.

Linear measurements

- Apparent measurement
- True measurement.

Apparent measurement (mostly useful in lower limbs)
- Make the limbs parallel to each other and to the trunk
- Handle the unaffected limb to make the limbs parallel (without touching the affected limb)
- Measure from any fixed central point to the most distal sharp bony point of the long limb bone.

Therefore, in the lower limb, measure from:
- Manubrium sterni or xiphisternum or umbilicus } to the tip of medial malleolus
- In the upper limb—from vertebra prominence (C_7) to tip of radial styloid process.

True measurement
- Reveal the concealed deformity by handling the affected limb
- Limbs to be kept in identical position after revealing the concealed deformity
- Measurement is ipsilateral and then comparison with the other side is done.

Lower limb
- Total length—from anterior superior iliac spine to medial malleolus
- Segmental length
  - Anterior superior iliac spine to mid-medial knee joint line (thigh length)
  - Mid-medial knee joint line to tip of medial malleolus (leg length)
  - The components of thigh length are measured as follows:
    - Infratrochanteric—tip of greater trochanter to knee joint line
    - Supratrochanteric—indirect measurement, e.g. through Bryant's triangle.

Upper limb
- Total length—from acromion angle to radial styloid process tip
- Segmental length
  - From acromial angle to lateral epicondylar tip (arm length).
  - From lateral epicondylar tip to radial styloid process tip (forearm length).

Circumferential measurements

- At affected point—for any swelling
- At fixed distances, proximal and distal, from the affected part—
  - For muscular wasting (atrophy)
  - For muscular hypertrophy
- For disorganised joint.

Across Measurements (for cross check-up of measurements)
In identical position of the limbs:
- From left anterior superior iliac spine to right medial malleolus tip

- From right anterior superior iliac spine to left medial malleolus tip.

Note the overall posture of the patient—posture accompanies movement like a shadow.

Movements

Ascertain first that the patient is not having '*abulia*' (loss or impairment of the ability to perform voluntary actions or to make decisions).

Ask to perform—Active movement—performed by patients without any assistance; performed by others—or even by the help of patient's opposite limb—passive movement.

Always compare with the opposite joint. In general, the range of movements at any joint, is more in females than males. First look for and acertain about *ankylosis* or *stiffness of the joint*. Also identify any hypermobility of joint. The easily measurable criteria are hyperextension of knee and elbow more than 10° with concomitant fifth finger metacarpophalangeal hyperextension and thumb-forearm apposition (Beighton and Horan 1969).

Ankylosis (no apparent movement in a joint)
Types of Ankylosis
- Bony (True)
  - No movement even on using force
  - No pain in the joint on trying to move it even by using force.
  - Bony trabeculation across the joint in X-ray.
- Fibrous (False)
  - Slight yield or jog of movement on using force
  - Pain in joint on trying to move by using force
  - Joint line visible in X-ray.

Stiffness in the joint (i.e. joint in which complete movements cannot be obtained—either active or passive): Limitation of movements can be:
- In all directions—due to arthritis
- Not in all directions—due to synovitis and/or spasm of muscles.
- Fixed movement in one or more direction—due to fixed deformity.

Limitations of movements are painful in active arthritis (due to stretching of or pressure on the inflamed capsule and/or rubbing of exposed subchondral bone) and painless in healed ones (due to short fibres fibrous bondage).

Milder form of joint stiffness (arthrofibrosis) mainly due to intra-articular surgery or injury (mainly in the knee joint) disrupts the kinematics of the joint and may lead to degenerative changes.

Types of joint stiffness (Table 1.5)
- Extra-articular, e.g. due to burn contracture, myositis ossificans, post-infective contracture of periarticular tissues, congenital contracture, e.g. quadriceps contracture, arthrogryposis multiplex congenita, etc.

TABLE 1.5: Types of joint stiffness.

Extra-articular	Intra-articular
• Obvious evidences of extra-articular tightness or adhesion like scars, subcutaneous fixity, musculotendinous contracture, sinus tract in vicinity	• No obvious scar, adhesion, sinus or contracted tissues
• Joint line is usually nontender, except when any inflammatory process lies over the joint line	• Joint line tender
• Painless range of free movements active and/or passive	• Possible movements are usually painful, especially at the extremes
• On X-ray—joint space sharply defined and clearly visible; articular ends nearly normal	• Joint margins fluffy, joint space reduced. Articulating bony ends usually osteoporosed with or without evidences of underlying pathology
• Dealing with the contracted extra-articular tissues, releases the stiffness	• Dealing with the extra-articular tissues does not release the stiffness
• Manipulation under general anaesthesia is not helpful in mobilising the joint	• Manipulation may mobilise the joint • Arthroscopic arthrolysis may improve stiffness • Arthroplasties of different types are usually required for mobilising the joint

- Intra-articular, e.g. due to septic arthritis, tuberculous arthritis, intra-articular fractures, etc.

If there is no ankylosis, assess the movements in various planes:
- Sagittal plane—flexion/extension
- Coronal plane—abduction/adduction
- Rotational plane—external/internal; supination/pronation.

The range of movement of a joint should be measured by the *goniometer* (the term goniometry is derived from Greek words—Gonio = angle + Metron = measurement). Measurement by goniometer is better than the clinical observational methods. For more accurate measurements mechanical or electronic inclinometers have been suggested (Lea and Gurhardt 1995).

For each movement:
- Fix the 'neutral zero position' which is extension for most joints rather than 180° to avoid confusion
- Mark lag of movement (usually extensor lag)
- Assess angle of fixity of any movement (e.g. fixed flexion deformity)
- Range of active movement
- Range of passive movement
- Range of utility or activity = Free active movement
- Range of possibility = Free active movement + Free passive movement.

- Any pain during the movement—If painful focus is in the vicinity of the joint (not in the joint), patient will still be reluctant to initiate active movement. Taking the patient in confidence, passive movement can be demonstrated to variable range, in such cases
- Limitation of terminal range
- Achievement of 'critical arc'
- Achievement of ADL (activities of daily living)
- Any abnormal movement (e.g. hypermobility in neuropathic joint, e.g. *Charcot's joint*)
- Any abnormal sound during the movement (heard/felt). In normal joints, movements are smooth and gliding without any palpable or audible friction or noise. Chronic inflammations, roughened surfaces of cartilage (e.g. in osteoarthritis), cartilage injuries, loose bodies in joints are often associated with audible/palpable friction, clicks or crepitations (grating sounds) on movement of joints. However, few persons have apparently normal joints which crackle or pop on certain movements
- Assess the power of controlling muscles.

Active movement of a joint—Movement produced by patient himself, without any assistance. Active movements of joint can be restrained by muscular contraction.

Passive movement—Movement produced at a joint either by help of patient's other limb and/or examiner or anyone else. Passive movements of joint are restrained by the ligaments attached to the bones on either side of the joint.

Fixed deformity: It is a fixed position of a joint from where the limb cannot be brought back to neutral position, but further movement in the same axis (direction) may be possible.

Normally, active and passive ranges are equal.

Passive range is more than active in:
- Paralysed joint
- Lax/Torn
  - Capsule
  - Ligament
  - Tendon
  - Muscle.
- Subchondral/condylar fracture.
  Test for any laxity or tear of the aforesaid components.

Critical arc: For any joint, the minimum range of active movement, which is necessary for the important functions of that joint.

ADL (Activities of Daily Living): The bare minimum necessary for daily living, like—eating, clothing, cleaning the private parts and minimum necessary mobility.

Understanding about the muscle action: In producing the movement, a single muscle cannot be all effective, rather the movement produced will be the ultimate outcome of the actions of several muscles acting in different capacities individually or in groups.

Muscles can be—
- *Agonists:* Chief muscle (prime movers) to produce particular action
- *Synergists:* (syn = with) Acting with the agonists they augment the effort
- *Antagonists:* Their action is against that of the agonists. By neurological reflex, they go for relaxation to make the action of agonists effective
- *Fixators:* They stabilise the fulcrum, while the agonists produce controlled desired action, e.g. in abducting the arm the deltoid contraction becomes more effective when the muscles attached from shoulder girdle to trunk act as fixator.

Power of controlling muscles **(Table 1.6)**: The assessment should be accurate from prognostic point of view. According to Medical Research Council (MRC) scale, muscle power is grouped under five grades. We feel that each grade is further divisible into 4 quadrants; depending upon lag of completion of full range, the deficit can be assessed, as, e.g.

'2- - -', '2- -', '2-', '2'.

Special tests: (Pertaining to individual joints) Diagnostic tests must have the following qualities—sensitivity, specificity, reproducibility, predictability, accuracy, minimum hurting to the patient.

TABLE 1.6: Grading of muscle power.

MRC scale		Suggested subgrouping (Pandey's)
'0'—	Not even flicker of contraction	'0'
'1'—	Flicker of contraction	'1'
'2'—	Contraction of muscles with no assistance and gravity eliminated, but moving the joint to full range	Depending upon lag of completion of full range 2- - -, 2- -, 2-, 2
'3'—	Contraction of muscles against gravity but with no resistance, moving the joint to full range	Depending upon extent of lag of completion of full range 3- - -, 3- -, 3-, 3
'4'—	Contraction of muscles against gravity and with moderate resistance, moving the joint to full range	Depending upon extent of lag of completion of full range 4- - -, 4- -, 4-, 4
'5'—	Normal	Depending upon extent of lag of completion of full range 5- - -, 5- -, 5-, 5. (While '5' is normal, the rest are subnormal in that order).

Heel Walking/Toe Walking

Children should walk with normal heel strike by the age of three years. If the patient can walk, quick inferences can be drawn by making him/her walk on heels and toes alternately. If the child is having persistent toe walking beyond the age of three years it is abnormal.

If he can walk swiftly in both positions without any complaints—probably there is no serious affection in the lower limbs including its neuromuscular control.

Erect posture along with integrity of the hip, knee, ankle and foot are essential for painless, quick, heel/toe walking.

Any limb-length disparity will obviously affect these walking and any inequality will be apparent.

If patient cannot walk swiftly, there are two broad probabilities:

If there is inability/difficulty in walking on heels, it may be due to:
- *Weakness* of muscles and/or abnormal joint condition:
  - Weakness of dorsiflexors of ankle; stiffness of the ankle joint.
  - Probable weakness in quadriceps femoris and erector spinae
  - Unstable hip.
- *Pain*—This may be felt due to any of the following pathologies:
  - Pain in back of thigh, knee and leg—due to sciatic stretch
  - Pain in sacroiliac region, in hip region (affection of the joint line, e.g. trauma, tuberculosis)
  - Back of the knee, e.g. in cases of trauma— posterior cruciate lesion, condylar fracture/crush of tibia (upper end)
  - Pain at ankle—In any traumatic, inflammatory, degenerative or neoplastic condition
  - Pain at heel—Any cause of painful heel syndrome (discussed in chapter on Foot, Pages 469–471).

If there is inability/difficulty in walking on toes, it may be due to:
- *Weakness* of muscles and/or abnormal joint condition:
  - Weakness of plantarflexors; stiffness of ankle (except where in equinus); genu recurvatum; unstable hip.
- *Pain*—Pain in the forefoot—trauma, metatarsalgia, inflammatory lesion.
  Usually pain in ankle is not complained of in early affections because the gravity line falls forwards.
  - If pain is in knee region—in case of trauma—probably anterior cruciate involvement, involvement of anterior horn of semilunar cartilage, affection of the quadriceps apparatus.

Peripheral Circulation

Impaired peripheral arterial circulation may produce symptoms in a limb, especially in lower limb. So a thorough examination should be done to assess the state of circulation, which is done by examination of the colour and temperature of skin, the texture of skin and nails and by palpating for arterial pulsation, which must always be compared with opposite side.

Peripheral nerves (e.g. lateral popliteal nerve, ulnar nerve, etc.) should be checked for the following:
- Tenderness
- Thickening
- Beading
- Irritability
- Detail muscle power and sensory charting of the supply zone of concerned nerve.

Observe about any change/disturbance in synchronous activities; even the finer activities like sneezing - an interesting fact - it is impossible to sneeze with your eyes open.

Investigations

For confirming the clinical suspicion, certain investigations are needed. One must not have a 'shortgun approach' in ordering the investigation (all around investigations), rather it must be an 'arrow head' targeted approach to order the really just needed investigations.

All results of laboratory investigations must be correlated with the clinical findings. Clinicians and patients are mostly, rather always, interested in less invasive, less costly and faster diagnostic tests. However, while ordering such tests, physicians must ensure that they are maximum reliable and are not liable to commit errors. The old standard trusted tests/investigations are usually gold standard diagnostics. However, new tests/investigations are being added/loaded— they must be adopted only when their efficacy and utility have been properly judged and their accuracy has been well tried. Investigations may be grouped under following heads:
- General investigations
- Special investigations
- Electrical investigations
- Radiological and allied investigations.

General Investigations
- Routine haemogram
- Erythrocyte sedimentation rate (ESR)
- C-reactive protein (CRP)—A significant reduction in the CRP level after initial treatment is a good indicator of a favourable clinical outcome
- Routine urine examination
- Stool examination
- Grouping and cross-matching of blood
- HIV test
- Test for hepatitis B
- **Assessment for diabetes (Table 1.7).**

Diabetes is a metabolic disorder in which there is too little or no production of insulin in body or body does not respond

TABLE 1.7: Assessment for diabetes and allied complications.

Name of the test	Purpose
Fasting blood glucose, post-prandial blood glucose reflect acute changes in blood glucose	To assess the current blood glucose level
Glycosylated haemoglobin HB A1C (Glucose Memory Test), i.e. assessment of glucose or glucose phosphate moieties bound to the amino terminal value of one or both beta chains	To monitor blood glucose/sugar control for the last 2–3 months
Assessment of fructosamine	For assessment of diabetic control
Routine urinalysis. Morning and post-prandial sample	To assess the presence of sugar in urine and overall status of renal function
Urine micro alb/spot	To detect even a minute quantity of albumin in urine
Blood urea	To assess the kidney function
Serum creatinine	To assess the kidney function
Fasting lipids and lipid profile	To assess cholesterol
SGOT/Serum proteins	To assess liver functions
ECG, ECHO, TMT	Diabetics are more liable to have heart problems, which can be detected by these (investigations) tests
X-ray chest	To detect any lung and (chronic) cardiac pathology
Ultrasonographic scan of abdomen	To assess the abdominal organs
ABI/Biothesiometry	To assess the blood flow and nerve sensation in the feet

NB: The level of HB1C, which comprises 3–6% of the total haemoglobin in healthy individual, is proportionate to the average glucose concentration and the lifespan of RBC in circulation. Hence, in haemolytic anaemia the HB1C has lower value due to shorter lifespan of RBC and in polycythemia or post-splenectomy HB1C value increases due to longer lifespan of RBC.

Medications other than metformin should be avoided when an older patient's HbA1C is less than 7.5 per cent, because the risk of hypoglycaemia is larger and the potential benefits of treatment are smaller for older persons with diabetes.

The interrelation between diabetes and bone physiology and pathology is very complex. In type 1 diabetes the bone mineral density remains constantly low. In type 2 diabetes it remains similar or higher than the nondiabetes. However, in both types of diabetes the bone fragility appears to be more for given density.

to available insulin in body. Type 2 diabetes mellitus (T2DM) is rapidly increasing in India. The prevalence is about 8.8% (Diabetes Atlas).

Worldwide, diabetes mellitus has reached epidemic proportions and is increasing due to population growth, aging, consequences of industrialization, urbanization, increasing prevalence of obesity and limited physical activity. India, said to be the diabetes capital of the world is expected to have 57 million diabetic patients by the year 2025 (Shankar et al. 2005). About 5 in 100 patients with diabetes mellitus will develop peripheral neuropathy, out of which 8.5 per 1000 is likely to suffer from charcot neuroarthropathy. (Galli et al. 2018).

Erythrocyte sedimentation rate (ESR) is a measurement of the distance in millimeters that RBCs fall within a specific tube (Westergreen or Wintrobe) over 1 hour and 2 hours—and the average of two hours fall is calculated. It is an indirect measurement of alteration in acute phase reactants (a heterogeneous group of proteins which are synthesized in liver in response to inflammation) and quantitative immunoglobulins.

C-reactive Protein (CRP) is a pentameric non-specific acute phase protein comprised of five identical non-covalently linked 23KD subunits arranged in cyclic symmetry in a single plane. CRP is produced as an acute-phase reactant by the liver in response to interleukin 16 and other cytokines. It is present in trace concentration in the plasma of all humans. Elevation in the level occurs within 4 hours of tissue injury/insult with peak within 24–72 hours. It falls rapidly in the absence of inflammatory stimuli. It is measured by immunoassay or nephelometry. CRP test, though costly, is more specific as compared to ESR (which is inexpensive, easy to perform and is affected by multiple variables).

CRP disappears when inflammatory process is suppressed by steroids or salicylates. This test is used to monitor recovery from infection. It is most useful as an indicator of activity in rheumatoid disease like rheumatoid arthritis and rheumatic fever.

Special Investigations

- *Serum biochemistry*, e.g. sugar, urea, calcium, phosphorus, alkaline phosphatase (particularly alkaline phosphatase isoenzyme determination by electrophoresis which differentiate alkaline phosphatase of osteoblastic origin from alkaline phosphatase from other sources), acid phosphatase, fluorine, creatinine, serum and urine amylase and lipase for chronic pancreatitis.
- *Serology*—Washerman's reaction (WR)—presently not necessarily recommended, Kahn, VDRL, Rheumatoid factor (Rose Wallar test).
- Human Immunodeficiency Virus (HIV)—AIDS was first diagnosed is 1981 in patients with immunodeficiencies of known causes. After that its cause—infection by HIV—a human RNA retrovirus was identified in two strains as HIV1 and HIV2. The human RNA retrovirus produces reverse transcriptase, which converts RNA to DNA and incorporates into the host chromosomes. The virus produces deregulation and destruction of the 'T' lymphocytes and thus an immunodeficient state. There are four clinical stages of HIV infections (1) acute primary HIV infection, (2) chronic asymptomatic HIV infection,

(3) symptomatic HIV infection, and (4) advanced HIV-associated opportunistic disease or AIDS. Most of the patients develop antibodies for HIV within 6 months of initial infection.

The orthopaedic/trauma surgeons/dentists do treat HIV patients in causality, emergency, out-patient department, clinics and operation theatre, and thus they are theoretically and even practically exposed for acquiring the infection in any stage. The magnitude of risk of disease transmission due to puncture during operation broadly depends upon frequency of punctures and number of HIV positive patients handled.

To diagnose the HIV infection a serological test—the **enzyme-linked immunosorbent assay (ELISA)**—has been developed to detect the HIV antibodies, of course it indicates a past infection. If the test is reactive and remains reactive, it should be confirmed by "Western blot test".

- *Guthrie test*—(Robert Guthrie—American bacteriologist and physician described this test): It is done to assess the possibility of detecting developmental, genetic and metabolic rare disorders in newborn babies. It is a spot test done by soaking the pre-printed collection cards (Guthrie cards) in blood obtained by pricking one of the heels of the newborn.
- Immunohistochemistry is a process in which cell-specific antigens/proteins on the cell surface are identified using antibodies, the tagging of which is identified using a color reaction, radiostope or immunofluorescence.
- *Arthrocentesis*—Aspiration of any collection and its examination—physical, chemical, cytological, serological, culture and sensitivity, inoculation test. Arthrocentesis should be avoided if cellulitis is overlying a swollen joint, in bleeding diatheses (haemophilia, anticoagulation therapy, thrombocytopenia).
- *Foot print*, Ichnogram (imprint of the soles of the feet taken in standing position), hand print.
- *Arthroscopy* (Diagnostic/therapeutic—knee, shoulder, ankle, elbow, wrist, hip and even IP joints).
  Arthroscopy: The word 'arthroscopy' comprises of two Greek words: 'arthro (= joint) + skopeir (to look). The term literally means 'to look within the joint'. Japanese physician Dr Takagi was the first to perform arthroscopy with a cystoscope in 1918. Nowadays, arthroscopy is being widely used to diagnose and variably deal the pathology (mainly traumatic) affecting the interior of the joints. It is particularly useful for the knee, followed by shoulder. However, its use is being extended to other joints like ankle, wrist, elbow, hip, spine and even interphalangeal joint.
- *Biopsy:*
  - FNAC (Fine needle aspiration cytology)
  - Needle biopsy
  - Aspiration biopsy
  - Core biopsy
  - Endoscopic/arthroscopic biopsy
  - CT-aided biopsy
  - USG-aided biopsy
  - Open biopsy
  - Excisional biopsy.

Electrical Investigations

- Electrocardiography (ECG)
- Electroencephalography (EEG)
- Electromyography (EMG)
- Strength duration curve
- Nerve conduction test
- Electrophoresis.

Radiological and Allied Investigations

One should remember that *imaging procedures may only give a "shadow of truth" and "truth" can only be nearly accomplished by thorough clinical examination.*

The utilization of medical imaging continues to rise. Associating the degree of radiation exposure with the risk of carcinogenesis is being discussed for long and perhaps this risk is silently increasing. This risk can be reduced by the clinicians by using nonradiographic assessments or reduce exposure by specifying exact areas of interest or deploying alternate modalities such as ultrasound or MRI.

- *Plain radiography; xeroradiography: Xero = dry*, thus xeroradiography does not involve the wet process of developing and fixing the film (using the photoconductive behaviour of a selenium plate and by photoelectric process, the conventional X-ray exposure is recorded as positive image)
  - Routine projections
    - Anteroposterior/posteroanterior view
    - Lateral view
    - Oblique view (internal oblique and external oblique, i.e. opposite rotational oblique)
  - Special projections
    - Axial view
    - Stress radiography.

Plane film radiograph will not show an osseous erosion until approximately 40% decrease in bone density has occurred.

- *Contrast radiography*
  - *Air contrast radiography*
  - *Radio-opaque dye contrast radiography* [water soluble (metrazimide), oil soluble]
  - *Myelography*
  - *Radiculography*
  - *Discography.*

Carried out for the patients with low back pain, discography is a safe, accurate, reproducible, objective diagnostic tool when tested for volume, pressure, fluoroscopic changes and pain provocation. The process involves the injection of water-soluble nonionic contrast dye into a disc in an effort to relate a radiographic image with the patient's pain.

- *Arthrography*—X-ray of joint after injecting contrast dye
- *Sinography*—X-ray of sinus tract after injecting contrast dye
- *Venography:* After applying a fine tourniquet just above the malleoli a nonionic contrast medium is injected to outline the veins
- *Plathysmography* assesses changes in volume of a limb or digit over the cardiac cycle
- *Arteriography*—In arteriography a radio-opaque solution is injected into the arterial tree, generally by a retrograde percutaneous method involving the femoral artery (occasionally brachial or axillary artery)
- *Cystography* is done by injecting the contrast medium through a catheter introduced into the bladder. The micturating cystogram is done to look for the presence of vesicoureteric reflex
- *Lymphangiography* is used to demonstrate the nature of lymphatic abnormalities and to diagnose lymphoedema. Pedal lymphangiogram is done by injecting blue dye subcutaneously between the toes to outline the lymphatic vessels
- *Duplex imaging*—A duplex scanner uses B mode ultrasound to provide an image of vessels
- *Doppler flowmetry*—To assess the status of the peripheral circulation, a continuous wave ultrasound signal is beamed at an artery and the reflected beam is picked up by a receiver
- *Laser Doppler flowmetry*—For direct measurement of the circulatory disorders in chronic compartment syndrome (CCS)
- *Doppler ultrasonography*—A doppler flow probe is used to exclude arterial disease, and to determine the patency of a vein. A bidirectional flow probe is used to detect venous reflex
- *Bone densitometers*—To assess the bone mineral density (BMD)—the single best method to diagnose osteoporosis and to assess the future risk of osteoporotic fractures. Of many types of densitometers, two commonly used are:
  - *Ultrasound densitometer*—nonionising, safe and cheap, but not that precise
  - *Dual energy X-ray absorptiometry* (DEXA)—it is accurate, precise and reproducible with 'Gold standard results', but is costly.

- *Tomography* (stratigraphy; planigraphy; Tomos = cut or section)—X-ray taken after being focussed at a desired depth blurring all the structures above or below, and anterior or posterior of the area of interest.
- *Stereoscopic*—bi-dimensional picture studies
- *Cine-radiography*
- 3D C-arm CT
- *MPR and SSD—Multiplanar reconstruction* (MPR) and surface shade display (SSD) combined together provides 3D images and virtually brings the advantages of CT. It is especially useful in operation theatre, and is extremely suited to minimally invasive surgery (MIS). It is very useful in spine and trauma surgeries, and helps in choosing the right implant
- PET – Positron emission tomography (PET) picks up metabolic activity and has tremendous potential - both in initial evaluation and in monitoring response to treatment as well as infection.
- *Scintigraphy* (**Radioactive isotope studies or radionuclide studies** or **nuclear imaging**)**.** A three phase study aiming to show the vascular, soft tissue and bone uptake is performed using TC-99 m MDP. It is sensitive for detecting osseous abnormalities, but should be correlated with plain radiograph or other techniques, since it is nonspecific
- *Granulocyte scintigraphy* is a sophisticated investigation to diagnose osteomyelitis especially in acute stage, of course it is not that useful
- *Ultrasonic scanning*, and high resolution ultrasonography
- *Computer assisted X-ray tomography*
- *Computerised tomography* and intrathecal low osmolarity contrast media studies
- Plain tomography is being replaced by computerized axial tomography with coronal and axial reformations. These are of much value in assessing the complex fractures, such as pelvic injuries, acetabular injuries, pilon fractures, fractures around knee, shoulder injuries, etc.
- *Nuclear Magnetic Resonance Imaging (NMRI)* or Magnetic Resonance Imaging *(MRI)*—In order to avoid using the word nuclear, which induces fear, the changed terminology is MRI, also kinematic MRI where required.
- *Spinal cord monitoring*—Recording of somatosensory evoked potentials (SEP)
- *Neurosensory testing (NST)* with the pressure specific sensory device (PSSD) is a state-of-the-art non-invasive painless and accurate diagnostic instrument by which one can carefully evaluate the degree of neuropathy starting at its very early onset, especially in diabetic neuropathy, Hansen's neuropathy, etc.
- Meterecom (a 3D skeletal analyser)—A precise, computer-based, non-invasive, 3-dimensional digitizer designed to access bony landmarks, at any point on the body for various patient's positions
- *Roentgen-Stereophotogrammetric Analysis* (RSA) allows the accurate three-dimensional measurement of relative

implant movement and in certain circumstances, measurement of wear. The accuracy of RSA can be up to the detection of 0.1–0.8 mm for translation movement and 1–2° for rotation at the 99% significance level
- *MSI* (Roser Boldlex 1995): The combination of technique of MRI and magnetoencephalographic recording (MEG) is being known as *magnetic source imaging (MSI)*. This indicates a functional description rather than only anatomical detail
- *Study of genome*—Virtually, *every human ailment*, except perhaps modern trauma *has some genetic basis*. A Genome is all the DNA in an organism including its genes. Genes carry information for making all the proteins required by all organisms. DNA is made up of four similar chemicals (called bases and abbreviated as A, T, C and G) that are repeated millions or billions of times, throughout a genome. The human genome has 3 billion pairs of bases. The sequencing of these three billion base pairs is likely to be as fundamental to medical science in next few hundred years as the periodic table was to chemistry in the last. Understanding the genetic make up will help greatly in the field of gene-therapy both for cure and prevention.

Next step in the *Genomic* is *Proteomics* (isolation and identification of proteins from normal versus perturbed cells).

In the next decade, genetic tests will routinely predict individual susceptibility to disease. It was expected that by 2020 gene therapy should become a common treatment at least for a small set of conditions. By 2050 many potential diseases will be cured at the molecular level before they arise.

Clinical Diagnosis

Basically clinical diagnosis is based on sound knowledge of anatomy, physiology, and pathology; a specific history and detail clinical examination. To come nearest to the (final clinical) provisional diagnosis, always keep in mind that patient has been always right and the clinician remains always wrong, unless the clinician proves that the patient was not right in his/her expression. In the process of making a diagnosis at the end of careful listening and analysing the history, guess the diagnosis; after thorough clinical examination make a provisional clinical diagnosis, which should be nearly confirmed by the relevant investigations. But the final confirmation of diagnosis should be made only after histopathological examination wherever possible and indicated (medicolegal aspect).

Thorough clinical examination leads to more or less accurate clinical diagnosis. However, in certain situations, this may not be possible. In such conditions, provisional diagnosis with immediate differential diagnosis should be mentioned. The most probable provisional diagnosis should be reached by the process of elimination, starting from the common to rare conditions.

In expressing the diagnosis of the disease, it is essential to make it a complete expression under the following headings:
- Duration
- Anatomical site affected
- Causative pathology with its stage of advancement
- Any obvious complication
- Any particular treatment given
- Affection of the patient's routine life, specially the activities of daily living (ADL), e.g.:
  - 5 months old, untreated, advanced tuberculous arthritis of right hip joint with discharging sinus, and patient not able to perform ADL.
    or
  - 7 weeks old conservatively managed traumatic ununited fracture of neck of left femur with 2 cm of supratrochanteric shortening and patient not able to perform ADL.

Management

"In imparting management adhere on two core principles: one from humanities the other from medicine: "Do unto others as you would have them do unto you" AND "first, do no harm."

In clinical practice, the word management comprises understanding of broad outline of main etiological factors, principal pathology, diagnosis, planned investigations and treatment.

It is very important to spend the time and energy to reach to the best possible decision. *"The decision is more important than the incision"* (Rang M 1990). The reasonably correct diagnosis and plan of management are reached only by repeat examination, repeat examination and repeat examination....

Place yourself (or your near and dear one) in place of your patient and decide what best you will like to be done for you (or your near and dear) and do the same for your patients.

Evolution of fracture-fixation and placement (1860 to 1870s) of metallic or allied implant started after the advent of antiseptic surgery (between 1860s and 1870s) by Lord Lister. In fact, Lister himself was one of the first to successfully fix a fractured patella using a silver wire.

Congenital anomalies (birth defects) are structural and functional abnormalities present since birth, caused by various factors such as micronutrient malnutrition, single gene defects, etc. (WHO/CDC/ICBDSR-2014). On broader considerations, causes of birth defects can be classified into three groups: Genetic, environmental, and complex. Congenital anomalies affect 1–2% of neonates, and of these 10% are in upper limb. (Lamb 1982). Genetics is science of inheritance. Now gene splicing by genetic engineering has become possible. Mapping of human genome will be possible completely very soon.

Causes of birth defect (Czeizel AE. 2005)

Genetic causes (25%)	Environmental causes (15%)	Complex causes (60%)
• Women giving birth after 35 years of age. • High rate of consanguineous marriages	• Infectious disease such as rubella • Maternal diseases such as diabetes mellitus or diseases with high fever • Teratogenic drugs, alcohol and smoking • Environmental pollutants	• Gene-environmental interaction • Polygenic liability is triggered by environmental 'risk' factors

Source: Adapted from Czeizel AE. Birth defects are preventable. Int J Med Sci. 2005;2(3):91-92.

High prevalence of birth defects is reported worldwide, with an alarming prevalence of 6 to 7% in India with very limited chance of complete recovery. Prevention is the only medical solution for avoiding congenital anomalies (Czeizel AE 2005). Neural tube defects like spina bifida and anencephaly can be prevented up to 70% with appropriate folic acid supplementation (at least 400 mcg daily) during entire reproductive age of a woman (quoted in Pfizer Limited– Booklet – quoting UA experts list top preventable birth defects). Other measures like rubella vaccination can prevent mild birth defects such as congenital dislocation of hip.

■ CONGENITAL LIMB MALFORMATIONS

(Based on CME lecture by Prof HKT Raza)

Congenital anomalies of the limbs can be considered under two broad headings:

- *Congenital limb malformations*, such as clubfeet, polydactyly, syndactyly.
- *Anomalies due to failure* of formation of certain parts of body which have been named as congenital limb reduction anomalies or congenital skeletal limb deficiencies.

"Thalidomide tragedy" in 1961–62 (when there was a high incidence of phocomelic children born to mothers who had taken thalidomide for morning sickness) aroused interests in this group of anomalies.

Effects of any indigenous medicine **(Fig. 1.42)**.

Classification of Congenital Anomalies

(Based on as proposed by Swanson AB 1976—and adopted by the International Federation of Societies for Surgery of the Hand)

- *Failure of formation* (Congenital skeletal limb deficiencies or congenital limb reduction anomalies)
  - Transverse arrest, e.g. absence of all fingers; amputation through carpus, forearm or arm
  - Longitudinal arrest, which may be pre-axial or para-axial, e.g. absence of radius and thumb; absence of tibia and medial ray of foot.
- *Failure of differentiation* (Separation of parts)
  - Soft tissue involvement
  - Skeletal involvement e.g. simple or complex syndactyly.
- *Duplication* (Polydactyly)
- *Overgrowth* (Macrodactyly)
- *Undergrowth* (Brachydactyly)
- *Constriction ring syndrome*
- *Generalised abnormalities and syndromes* (Limb anomalies as a part of syndromes).

According to Frantz and O'Rahilly classification which is simple, though it does not account complex anomalies like syndactylism, fused joints (etc.):

- *Terminal defects:* Involves the distal rays + proximal segments like forearm or leg, in which there may be

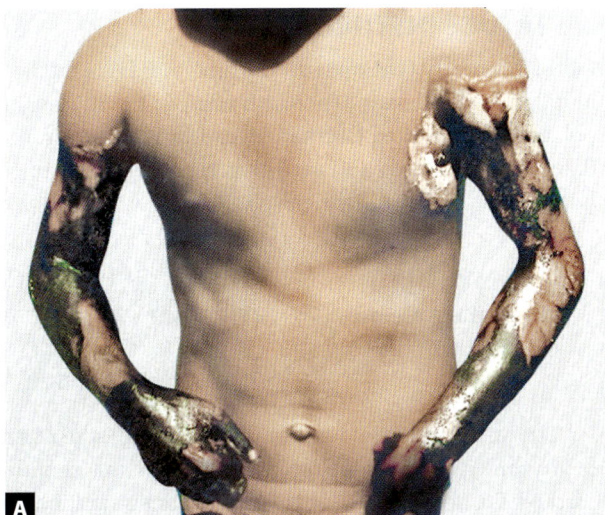
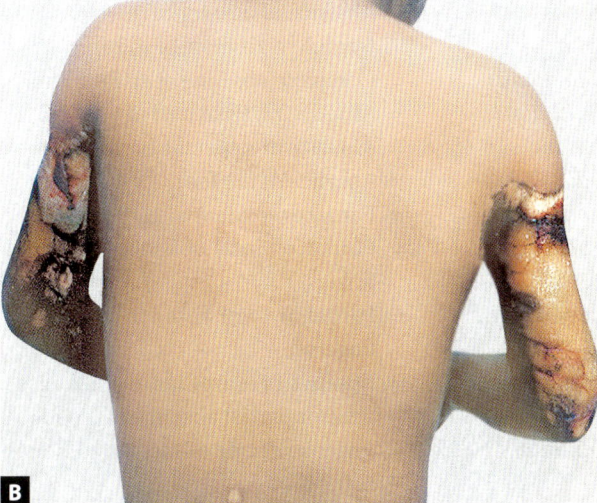

Figs. 1.41A and B: Typical bilateral symmetrical electrical burn in upper limbs. For such cases management in even best burn units leave behind various legacies.

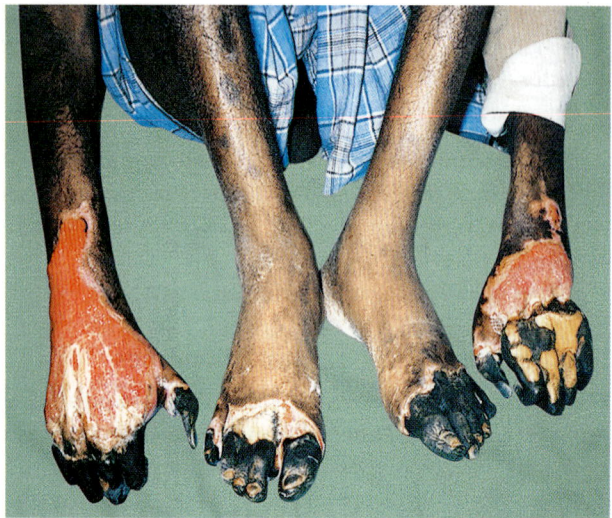

Fig. 1.42: Bilateral almost symmetrical gangrene of both hands and feet due to toxicity of an indigenous medicine.

transverse defects (absence of all fingers, amputation through carpus forearm or arm) OR longitudinal defects which may be pre-axial or para-axial (absence of radius with thumb or absence of tibia with medial rays of foot).
- *Intercalary defects (intermediate segment is missing):*
  - There may be transverse defect alone phocomelia (e.g. distal part of radius and ulna are absent). Complete phocomelia, e.g. radius, ulna and humerus are absent; tibia, fibula with hypoplasia or aplasia of femur.
  - Longitudinal, e.g. absence of radius or ulna or fibula or tibia alone.

Descriptive Terms Usually Used While Describing Congenital Anomalies

Acheiria (achiria)	= Absence of hand
Acheriopodia	= Absence of hands and feet
Adatylia (adactyly)	= Absence of fingers/toes
Agenesis	= Absence of development
Amelia	= Complete absence of a limb
Amelia totalis	= Complete absence of all four limbs
Amputation	= Absence of distal part of a limb
Aphalangia	= Absence of a specific bone or bones
Apodia	= Absence of the foot
Ectrocheiria	= Partial or total missing of hand
Ectrodactyly	= Partial or total absence of digits/fingers
Ectromelia	= Partial or total absence of hand or fingers
Ectrophalangia	= Absence of one or more phalanges
Ectropodia	= Total or partial absence of the foot
Hemimilia	= Absence of one of the paired bones of the limbs
Hypophalangia	= Less than normal number of phalanges
Intercalary deficiency	= While proximal and distal portions of limb are intact, the middle portion is missing
Longitudinal deficiency	= Absence of the limb extending parallel to the long axis (may be pre-axial, post-axial or central)
Meromelia	= Partial absence of a limb
Oligodactyly	= Absence of few fingers
Paraxial deficiency	= Only the pre-axial or post-axial portion of the limb is affected
Peromelia	= Hemimelia, especially the ending in stump
Phocomelia	= In its complete form, the arm and forearm are absent in the upper limb and the thigh and leg are absent in the lower limb (the hands and feet sprout directly from the trunk). The deficiencies may be proximal (arms and thighs missing) or distal (forearms and legs missing)
Post-axial	= Pertaining to the ulnar side of the upper limb, and the fibular side of the lower limb
Pre-axial	= Pertaining to the radial side of the upper limb, and the tibial side of the lower limb
Terminal deficiency	= Absence of limb with all portions in line with and distal to defect involved
Transverse deficiency	= Entire width of the limb is affected.

Because of immense power adaptability for functions, the persons with the terminal transverse defects should be better managed with fitting with suitable prosthesis.

■ STATURE DISTURBANCES

(After Mercer's Orthopaedic Surgery. (Eds). Dutchie RB and Bentley – Edward Arnold 8th edition, 1983) Most of the persons with stature disturbances can carry out their routine daily physical needs and activities, accepting their physical handicaps. However, the psychological problems persist with them.

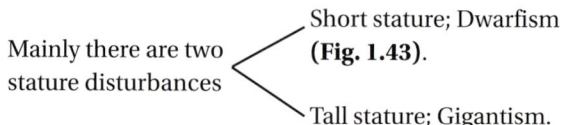

Mainly there are two stature disturbances
- Short stature; Dwarfism **(Fig. 1.43)**.
- Tall stature; Gigantism.

The anterior lobe of pituitary gland controls the activities of thyroid gland, the adrenal cortex and the sex glands through its secretion of thyrotropic, adrenocorticotropic, and gonadotropic secretions. Besides other factors, these contribute in achieving/affecting the stature.

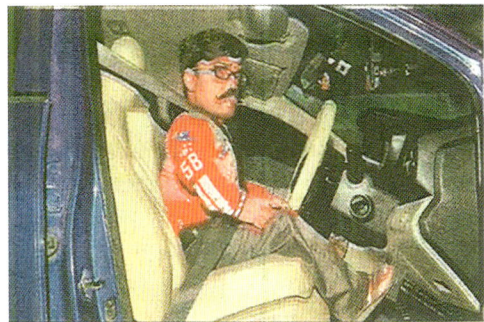

Fig. 1.43: Hindustan Times December 06, 2021. Dwarf GS 42 years old of three feet height – Perhaps 1st Indian dwarf to obtain official COD V driving license. He modified his car mechanism to lift the seat and other equipment for his height.

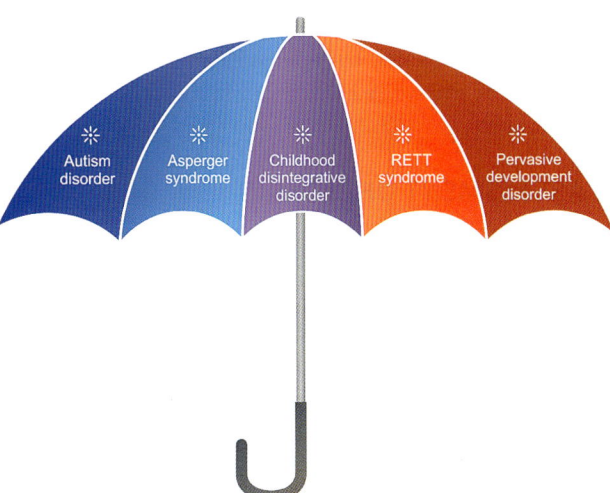

Fig. 1.44: Five types of autism under the umbrella of autism spectrum disorder.

The term dwarf is applied to an individual whose physical dimensions are considerably below those peculiar to his/her race, whereas the term short stature usually implies only a unexpected decrease in height. The congenital hypothyroidism (cretinism) and hypopituitarism (usually occur due to compression or destruction of gland) produce dwarfism.

When growth–both longitudinal as well as accretion (increase by a gradual build up of layers) – is increased proportional to that of normal during adolescence, and when the epiphysis continue to grow and fail to close, the syndrome of tall stature or *gigantism* develops. The common causes are hyperpituitarism, cerebral gigantism, arachnodactyly, Marfan's syndrome, homocystinuria, chromosomal abnormalitism of the xxy/xyy types, and the constitutional or familial type in otherwise healthy individual.

However, if a person with disturbed stature desires to obtain something/some job, which is not coherent with his/her physical dimensions, it becomes problematic – such as a dwarf desiring for owing a car and driving it. However by exploiting one's hidden talents one can achieve his/her persistent desire, even though it is not consistent with his/her physical dimensions. This can be examplified by the achievements of a dwarf (with height of about three feet) who could own a car and ride it **(Fig. 1.43)**.

▌ EXAMINATION OF CHILDREN

"If a child cries when you examine it, then it's probably your fault."

—**John Apley**

"All too often children are examined but not looked at."

—***Aicardi 1998***

The above sweeping statement may not be all correct, but the basic philosophy is right. It is always paying to spend some time trying to gain their confidence. Younger children are always comfortable in mother's lap. Some toys and toffees will help you to make familiar with child. While in mother's lap, watch the expression, general built and behaviour and obvious abnormalities, movements of the limbs, etc. before touching the child.

The clinician should not be over-eager to look at the 'test results' and bias the mind but should observe the quality of activities and behaviours of the child patiently. The qualitative approach takes experience and practice that comes only with time.

The clinician/orthopaedic surgeon should have working knowledge of developmental and behavioural milestones and the infants and children (including the pre-school children and school-going ones) should be assessed categorically. Children with *autism* manifest limitations in social interaction from the very beginning, which gradually affects their social communication skills. This leads to **'autism spectrum' (Fig. 1.44)**. Parents may say that the child was speaking during the first two years but this is very likely 'echolalia' or meaningless repetition of words. Autism was first described in 1943 by Leo Kanner an American psychiatrist. They should be watched carefully about their physical activities, gait pattern, behaviour, communicating skills etc. Girls tend to be slightly more advanced in behaviour and communication skills.

Today in several cases, the orthopaedic surgeons do not have the time (or pose to show that have no time) for examining the child patients in detail. They cannot expect the same cooperation from the children as in adults. However, at least two common types of examinations must be performed (1) screening examination to detect disorders which may remain asymptomatic still can cause significant morbidity (such a DDH and scoliosis, etc.), (2) focused examination for the problems/complains for which the child has been brought.

While the basic methodology remains the same, one should not expect to get same degree of cooperation as in average adults. Try to derive as much information as possible in the short period when the child cooperates with. The child gets irritated by repeated examinations and gets frightened by the white coats, examining tools and serious environments.

■ ASSESSMENT OF ELDERLY

"In the end it is not the years in your life that count. It's the life in your years."
—*Abraham Lincoln*

Fasting is good for your neurons and enhances synaptic plasticity.
—*Mattson et al. 2003*

William Shakespeare termed old age as the second childhood. The degeneration of cells and weakening of neuro-receptors (neuro-responsive system) may be responsible for the child-like behaviour of old people.

By 2000 AD, the average life expectancy in India has just crossed 60 year mark and is gradually increasing (which was just around 30 in 1947), while that in USA is now more than 75 years (72 for men and 79 for women).

Heterogenous population above the age of 60 to 65 should be in the bracket of elderlies. Chronologically, they can be subgrouped as: young old (60-69), old (70-79), very old (>80). This century has proved to be the '*Century of longevity*' and a "*century of cognitive decline*". Though the maximum height of age has not increased, the average life expectancy has remarkably increased globally and thus unprecedentally increasing the numbers of elderlies in the world with all their problems. As on today, the number of centenarians is round about 1,35,000 and is likely to increase to 25,00,000 by the year 2050. With 1,15,000 in India alone, i.e. one centenarian will be in every 5,000 of population.

In Indian mythology, the achievement of '*desired death*' has been noted by several saints and kings. Saint Tulsidas lived for 126 years, Ramaniya for 120 years, Kanchi Parmacharya for 100 years and so on. Even politicians like Guljarilal Nanda and Morarji Desai touched their 100 years.

Besides the chronological count, the old age requires a broad assessment. *Comorbidity* is the hallmark of the elderlies. Multiple system involvement at a time, symptoms varying from 6 to 12 and diagnosis around 2 or 3 at a time usually characterise the clinical profile of elderly patients (Venkobe Rao 1990). Usually, there is overlay of depression and/or anxiety—a condition called '**Cothymia**' (Tyrer 2001).

The feeling of loneliness and neglected by their near-ones adds to the problems of the elderlies (at least in the Indian subcontinent).

Desiring and maintaining independence is of paramount importance in this more frail patient population. With increasing advancements in the field of medical care, technology and surgical approaches the possible operative management of diseases and trauma effects may offer a real advantage in allowing earlier motion and independence in activities of daily living without any risk of complications.

At the back of mind the elderlies apprehend—I fear of losing my independence.

Exact causes of ageing are not well established—hovering around 30 theories. However, more convincing ones are: (1) deccumulation of unrepaired DNA (free radical theory), (2) concept involving telemeres. Economics, though helpful, do not essentially influence the longevity.

There are two aspects of old age. The positive aspect visualises the old age as the period of grandeur and exquisiteness, crystallised wisdom and crystalline intelligence. On the opposite aspect, it is looked down upon as a period of dreary waste land with diseases, disabilities, dependence, depression, decay and an ailing continent. In the gradual ebbing away evening period of life, many elderlies have to unwillingly face a *host of losses—loss of status*, income, self-respect, body functions, sense organs (e.g. vision, hearing, etc.), memory, mental status, motor power, mobility (due to instability, muscle power loss, paralysis, fractures, etc.) near and dear ones, etc. The sense of wellbeing remains in a small percentage of elderly (on an average about 30%).

Worrying about these points they gradually lessen their sleeping hours. In India people sleep, on an average less than seven hours, whereas in Finland people sleep, on an average for eight hours.

"*Preventive Geriatrics*" involves the concept of 'successful ageing' by improving the health of the mass above sixty to sixty five entering into the arena of 'old age', so that they pass their final years in a state of 'engeria'—the term coined by Aristotle to qualify the state of freedom from disease, disabilities, dependance, depression and death-phobia without being burden to others, and be ready to welcome the well-earned death gracefully.

Geriatric medicine is not a new concept. At least the great Indian surgeon Sushruta classifying Ayurveda into 8 diversions has categorically described one of them as "*Old-age-medicine*".

A "healthy lifestyle" is the hallmark of "preventive geriatrics". It involves nutritious diet, avoiding smoking and alcohol, less sodium intake in diet, adequate fresh fruits and green vegetables, high complex carbohydrate, reduced saturated fat, adequate protein (non-animal source), cognitive exposure, cognitive stimulation in childhood, healthy natural environment, reduced exposure to pollution and infection, physical and intellectual activities, and none the less religious and spiritual believes and YOGA practices and meditation—are the ingredients to foster the happy journey through the evening of life. Spirituality has been observed to have definite scientific base. There is a set of neuronal circuits in the left temporal lobe (limbia system) which serves as a substrate for religeousity, spirituality and belief in God. Music initiates a magic like environment in old age by helping the old people stay calm and relaxed.

While examining an elderly person, **Alzheimer's disease** must be kept in mind. It results due to deposits of amyloidal substances and several other inflammatory proteins in the brain (*Also see* Page 634).

Physical examination processes of the elderly person are more or less the same as described in individual chapters. However, they deserve more sympathetic and respectful approach in each step of examination. Confusing pain syndromes are not uncommon in the elderly, e.g. Hip-spine syndrome—significant lumbar canal stenosis and arthritis of lower extremity joints may co-exist. This combination of radiculopathy and osteoarthritis usually produce diagnostic confusion. However, careful respectfully repeated examination taking the elderly patient in full confidence, diagnostic tests, and investigations are essential to discriminate them, since both require separate effective management.

While examining, some forms of 'Yoga' practices, commensurate to their age, physique and ailments, should be demonstrated to the elderlies, which will definitely help them to come out from the evils of senility, loneliness, depression, psychiatric morbidity and considerable impairment of quality of life (QoL).

—*Like 'Nail to Vault Yoga' (Pandey's)*

■ CLINICAL AUDIT IN ORTHOPAEDICS

Ernest Codman became known as the first true medical auditor following his work in 1912 on monitoring surgical outcomes.

Clinical audit compares current practice to the standard practice. The clinical audit is essential to assess ones performance. Audit guides us, if we are doing the things in the right way and right direction. Of course, the knowledge about the things to do and progress comes from research, and keeping oneself refreshed with the latest development.

"Be lifelong learner under the proven leaders, for changing the lives of needy"

Health Risks of being an Orthopaedic Surgeon

Besides the risks faced by any surgeon, the orthopaedic surgeons face higher ones too like due to noise, vibrations of tools, exposure to chemicals, blood borne pathogens, hazards of radiation, noises generated by drills, trapped suction tip whistles in tissue. Further updating equipments, change from pneumatic to battery powered tools, etc. keep on increasing the risks proportionately.

Training of young surgeons must be in disciplined way and as much as possible stress free. Maintaining the proper duty hours. Loaded shifts and job stressors should be avoided burnout . These can be further eased and regularised by adopting "employee social support program"effects of radiation exposures (in procedures requiring C arms fluoroscopy) may lead to dermatitis, skin cancer, cataract, thyroid gland changes, bone narrow suppression, congenital defects in offsprings, etc. Radiation can be minimized by using ALARA principles, lead apron, by avoiding horizontal fluoroscopy as far as possible:

For assessing the results of treatment of various orthopaedic diseases and injuries various parameter-based scales are being suggested, most of which are the suggesting surgeons' based and/or mechanical instruments based, where the receivers' (patients') role does not remain dominant. However, gradually, the patient-reported outcome measures are becoming widely used tools to assess the impact of injury or disease and subsequent treatment on a patient's physical and psychosocial well being from the patient's perspective.

The statement attributed to Frank Dobie – "The average PhD thesis is nothing but a transference of bones from one graveyard to another " (Quoted by Singh and Gupta 2021)

■ EVIDENCE-BASED MEDICINE

The concept of evidence-based medicine originated in the id of 19th century in Paris; however, its formal version developed in Canada in early 1990. David Sackett (1996) defined it as "the conscientious, explicit and judicious use of current best evidence in making decisions about the care of the individual patient. It means integrating individual clinical practise with the best available external clinical evidence from systematic research. With the passage of time, it is becoming clear that only result of any research is inadequate for taking an action, rather expertise and experience of the clinician is equally important for diagnosis and subsequent management.

Evidence-based medicine concerns a systematic approach of finding and analyzing the published data to form the basis for making the clinical decision.

For recommending to health professionals the evidence-based medicine has been categorised into four grades assessing on the degree of transparency and practicability as follows:

1. *High degree:* In this category Randomized Control Trials (RCTs) (the gold standard for the assessment of treatment efficacy) are without any serious limitations.
2. *Moderate degree:* RCTs are with serious limitations, i.e., further research is likely to have an impact on the confidence in the estimate effect.
3. *Low degree:* In this group, further research will have impact on the confidence and may change the estimate of effect.
4. *Very low degree:* Here any estimate effect is uncertain.

The evidence of research, clinical expertise and values of patient, combined together aim to improve the quality of clinical care of the patients. The practical adoption, realization, and true application of evidence-based medicine oriented Randomized Control Trials provide strong pillars for truthful and useful research for publication of scientific papers or even for meaningful PhD thesis, otherwise

"Do your little bit of good where you are, its those little bits together bring positive change in the world"

QUEUE comes from 'Queen's Quest'. Long back a long row of people was waiting to see the Queen. Someone made the comment Queen's Quest.

■ BIBLIOGRAPHY

1. Aicardi J. Diseases of the Nervous System in Childhood, 2nd edn, London: Mac Keith Press with Cambridge University Press; Philadelphia: JB Lippincott.
2. Andry N. Orthopaedia: or the art of correcting and preventing deformities in children. London: Millar. 1743;1:36-37.
3. Beighton P, Horan F. Orthopaedic aspects of the Ehlers Danlos syndrome. J Bone Joint Surg (Br). 1969;51:444-53.
4. Brengem CC, Mass M, Breugen SJM et al. Vascular malformations of the lower limb with osseous involvement. J Bone Joint Surg. 85-B:399-405.
5. Cohen A, Dempster DW, Recker RR, et al. Abdominal fat is associated with lower bone formation and inferior bone quality in healthy premenopausal women: a transiliac bone biopsy study. J Clin Endocrinal Metab. 2013:98;2562-72.
6. Congenital anomalies (birth defects) Available from https:/www.nhp.gov.in/disease/gynaecology-and-obstetrics/congenitalanomalies-birth-defects [Last accessed 14th February 2020]
7. Czeizel AE. Birth defects are preventable. Int. J. Med. Sci. 2005;2(3):91.
8. Diabetes Atlas, Global Fact Sheet, 8th edition. Brussels, Belgium: International Diabetes Federation; 2017.
9. Galli M, Scavone G, Vitiello R, et al. Surgical treatment for chronic Charcot neuroarthropathy. Foot (Edinb) 2018;36: 59–66.
10. Lamb DW, Wynne-Davies R, Soto L. An estimate of the population frequency of congenital malformations of the upper limb. J Hand Surg Am. 1982;7(6):557-62.
11. Lister J. On the antiseptic principle in the practice of surgery. Lancet. 1867;2:353-6.
12. Mattson MP, Duan W, Guo Z. Meal size and frequency affect neuronal plasticity and vulnerability to disease: cellular and molecular mechanisms. J Neurochem. 2003;84(3):417-31.
13. Modig K, Erdefelt A, Mellner C et al. "Obesity Paradox" holds true for patients with hip fracture. A registry-based cohort study. J Bone Joint Surg Am. 2019:101;888-95.
14. National Institute of Health: Clinical guidelines on the identification, evolution and treatment of overweight and obesity in adults. The evidence report. Obes Res. 1998; 6 (Suppl 2).
15. Pare A. The works of that famous Chirurgion Ambroise Parey—translated by T Johnson. London, R Cotes and W Du-gard. 1649.
16. Rang M. Cerebral palsy. In: Morrissy RT, editor. Lovell and Winter's pediatric orthopaedics. 3rd ed. Philadelphia: Lippincott; 1990. p 465-506
17. Raza HKT. Congenital Limb Reduction Anomalies. CME lecture IOACON 2005;1-8.
18. Roger Boldlex. A century of Medical Imaging, Paraplegia, 1995;33:685-86.
19. Sackett DL, Rosenberg WM, Gray JA, et al. Evidence-based medicine: what is it and it isn't? BMJ. 1996;312(7023): 71-2.
20. Sharma R. Birth defects in India. Hidden truth, need for urgent attention. Indian Journal of Human Genetics. 2013; 19(2):125.
21. Shyam A. Evidence-based medicine and research in Textbook of Orthopaedics & Trauma. Evidence-based medicine and research. In: Kulkarni GS, Babhulkar S. (Ed). Textbook of Orthopaedics & Trauma, 3rd edition. New Delhi: The Health Sciences Publishers; 2016; pp. 78-86.
22. Singh T, Gupta P. Can we consider scholarship of teaching learning rather than focusing only on publications for recognition of medical teachers by national medical commission? – Editorial: Annals of the Medical Sciences (India). 2021;57(1):1-2.
23. Tamai S. History of microsurgery. Plast Reconstr Surg. 2009;124(6 suppl):e282-94.
24. UA experts list top preventable birth defects. Available from https://www.pharmacy.arizona.edu/news/2011/ua-experts-list-top-preventable-birth-defects [Last accessed 15 February 2020]
25. World Health Organization. Obesity: Preventing and managing the global epidemic report of WHO consultation on obesity. Geneva. 1998.
26. WHO/CDC/ICBDSR. Birth defects surveillance: atlas of selected congenital anomalies: World Health Organization; 2014.
27. Zhou KH, Luo CF, Chen N, Hu CF, Pan FG. Minimally invasive surgery under fluoro-navigation for anterior pelvic ring fractures. Ind Jr Orth. 2016;50:250-5.

CHAPTER 2

Examination of Long Bones

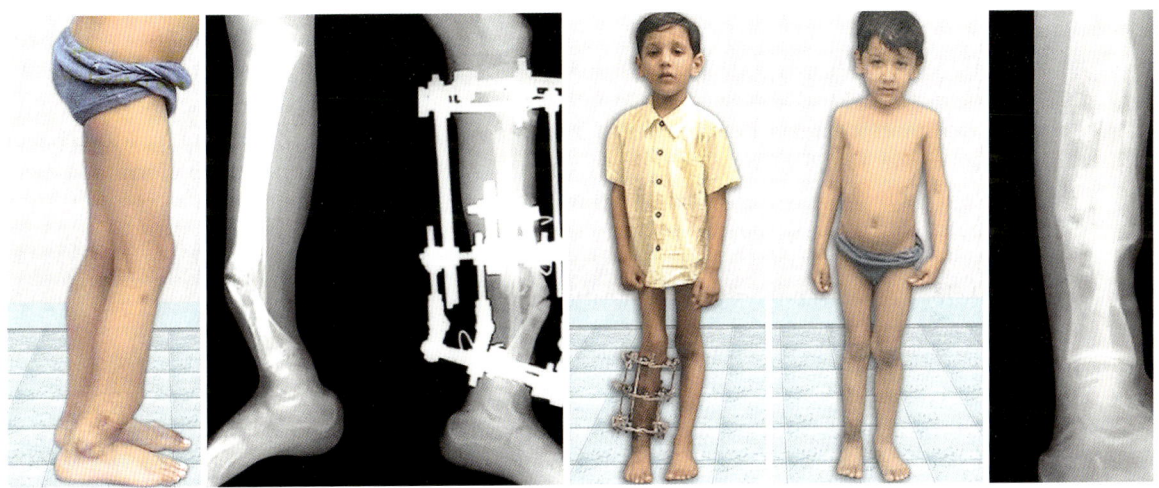

"We may learn wisdom: First, by reflection, the noblest; Second, by imitation, the easiest; and Third, by experience, the bitterest."

—*Confucius*

"The origin of all science is in the desire to know causes".
—Klilliam Hazlitt 1829

■ INTRODUCTION

Except when it is acutely affected, e.g. fracture or acute inflammatory lesions, the affections of the shaft remain unheeded for varying periods. The movements of the adjoining joints are not affected in the majority of shaft affections. Therefore, the patient has comparatively less disability. Of course, in all shaft affections, the examination of the adjoining joints is essential. The shaft of the short long bones, e.g. metacarpals, metatarsals and phalanges will be examined as discussed in the chapter of Hand and Foot.

Anatomical Consideration

The long bone, before fusion of its growing epiphyses, can be descriptively divided into:
- *Diaphysis:* The central portion of shaft up to the metaphysis at both ends
- *Metaphysis:* (The flared transitional zone between the diaphysis and epiphysis). Metaphysis are the ends of diaphysis proximal to the epiphyseal growth plates on each side. It is difficult to draw an exact line of demarcation between diaphysis and metaphysis. The structure of the bone is much more compact in diaphysis than in the metaphyseal region. At the metaphysis, the cortical layer of bone is very thin. However, the metaphyseal region contains mostly highly vascular cancellous or spongy new bone
- *Epiphyseal growth plate:* Epiphyseal growth cartilage or plate lies transversely between metaphysis and epiphysis, and is responsible for longitudinal growth of the bone
- *Epiphysis*: The ends of the long bones are the epiphysis (between growth plate and articular cartilage). In infancy, most of the bulk of the epiphysis is cartilaginous, having a central area of ossification. With the advancement of age, the bony bulk of the epiphysis increases
- *Articular cartilage*: The epiphysis is capped with a layer of hyaline cartilage at its extreme ends. This smooth gliding shiny surface is bathed all the time with the synovial fluid for facilitating the movements of the joints.

A typical long bone is cylindrical with expanded ends. The *periosteum,*—a tough, thin connective tissue layer, is more and more closely adherent as we go from the centre to the ends. It covers the entire bone except the articular cartilage, and attachments of tendons, ligaments and joint capsule. In infants and children, the periosteum is thick, more vascular and cellular and is on the whole comparatively loosely attached. With increasing age it becomes thinner, less vascular, less cellular and more firmly attached.

Periosteal blood vessels lie on the outer face of periosteum anastomosing with the adjacent muscular blood vessels.

Nerve supply of the periosteum is mainly vasomotor and run along the periosteal blood vessels.

The periosteum is a fibrocellular structure having two layers—*outer fibrous* (dense collagen fibrous tissue and fibroblast like cells) and *inner cambium* (vascular) layer. In the inner cambium layer osteoblasts, having very potent osteogenic activities, are interspersed here and there. They are responsible for the circumferential growth of the long bones.

▌BLOOD SUPPLY OF LONG BONES (FIG. 2.1)

Taking all together the volume of blood supply of the long bones account for 5–10% of the cardiac output.

The long bones have three main sources of blood supply:
1. Nutrient system
2. Periosteal system
3. Metaphyseal system

Nutrient System

The nutrient artery usually perforates the shaft of a long bone in its middle third. After piercing the cortical layer at a definite place for each bone, it divides into ascending and descending branches. These branches travel along the Haversian canal, forming anastomosis at different levels all around and ultimately form anastomotic rings in the metaphyseal area.

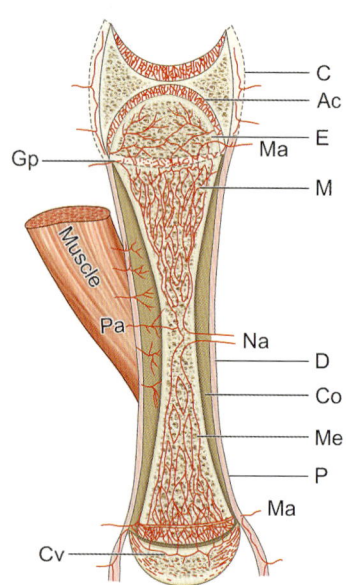

Fig. 2.1: Different parts of long bone and its blood supply. (C: capsule; AC: articular cartilage; GP: growth plate; Ma: metaphyseal artery; M: metaphysis; Na: nutrient artery; D: diaphysis; Co: cortex; Me: medulla; P: periosteum; Pa: periosteal artery; Cv: circulus vasculosus)

Periosteal System

The periosteum receives blood supply from the adjoining soft tissues especially the muscles, which send tiny perforating branches almost to their attachment to the bones. These small branches ultimately anastomose with the branches of the nutrient system and are responsible for supplying about outer two-thirds of the bony wall.

Metaphyseal System

Direct branches from the articular blood vessels or the adjoining muscular blood vessels form an anastomotic leashing, almost all around the metaphyseal surface. From this circular arterial system, multiple perforating branches enter the metaphysis. They heavily interlace among each other as well as with the ends of the nutrient system.

Short bones are supplied by numerous periosteal blood vessels. A rib is supplied by a nutrient artery and periosteal vessels.

Veins

Variable sinusoidal networks are formed in the regions of epiphysis, metaphysis and diaphysis. These in turn drain into venous channel leaving the bone through all its surfaces which are not covered by articular cartilage. Valveless nutrient veins accompany the nutrient arteries.

Lymphatics

Lymphatic vessels are found accompanying the periosteal vascular plexuses but their presence within the bone substance has never been convincingly demonstrated.

Nerves

They are distributed freely within the layer of the periosteum. Finally myelinated and non-myelinated nerve fibres accompany the nutrient vessels into the interior of the bone and even into the perivascular spaces of the *Haversian* canals. Articular ends of the long bone are very rich in nerve supply.

Most of the part of the shaft of a long bone is protected by several layers of soft tissues, i.e. muscular, fascial, fibrofatty, subcutaneous and cutaneous layers. However, all the layers may not be complete all around all over in all bones, e.g. in tibia. Therefore, examination of the shaft of a long bone mandatorily implies the examination of soft tissues, neurovascular bundles and the bony axis. The long bone supports the central core axis of the limbs, and it also provides surface for attachment of different muscles.

The marrow of long bones are mostly red, specially at the ends, therefore, the haemopoietic activity is also subserved by the long bones. The long bone also acts like a long lever for effective functional mobility at the adjoining joint fulcrum.

■ METHODOLOGY

History Taking
(As in the Chapter 1 on Introduction)

General Examination

General, systemic and cursory regional examination must precede the local examination of the shaft (As in the Chapter 1 on Introduction).

Local Examination

Local examination includes the following:
- Inspection
- Palpation
- Percussion
- Squeezing
- Measurement
- Auscultation.

Examination of the shaft is not complete till the adjoining joints are thoroughly examined.

Inspection—Prerequisites

- The part to be examined or even the entire limb must be adequately exposed for examination
- The corresponding part of the opposite limb must be examined for comparison
- Both limbs must be kept in identical position (position the unaffected limb in the same posture, in which the affected limb has been kept comfortably by the patient).

Look for

A. The position, shape, thickening or thinning of the part
B. Skin surface regarding its look, texture, colour, creases, varicose veins, vascularity, presence of scar, sinus, obvious pulsation through skin. Any abnormal swelling must be examined as per the examination of the swelling anywhere in body (shape, surface, vascularity/any prominent vein on surface, mobility, consistency, relationship to deeper structures and surrounding structures, fixity, etc.) (*see* **Figs. 2.54B and C, 2.55 to 2.57**); lymphoedema (**Figs. 2.56A to D**); elephantiasis (**Figs. 2.57 to 2.59**).
- Look at the long bone from diaphysis to epiphyseal ends and compare its symmetry with the opposite side. There may be angulation or bowing [congenital (**Figs. 2.5 to 2.11**) traumatic, syphilitic—sabre tibia (**Fig. 2.12**), degenerative collapse, Paget's disease, etc.]. Look at metaphyseal area for any broadening (if bilateral—usually rickets, if unilateral—usually traumatic or neoplastic)
- Epiphyseal area may be thickened or there may be swelling.
- With a suspicion of rickets or syphilis always look for their stigmata.

Stigmata of rickets

Basic pathogenesis in rickets (also in osteomalacia) is failure in deposition of calcium and phosphorous salt in osteoid tissue. Bones become soft and porotic. Bone bends easily under pressure and even by body weight. Epiphyseal line is normally 2 mm thick regularly defined cartilage but in rickets it becomes wide as irregular band **(Figs. 2.2A to C)**. Metaphyseal part becomes irregular and broad due to excessive proliferation of epiphyseal growth plate cells with cupping effect at wrist epiphysis and ankles.

- Children below 7-8 years coming from low socio-economic group are usually affected
- Child has flabby look and remains dull
- Child remains irritable
- Child remains restless during sleep
- Child does not take part in playing
- Delayed walking – Develops abnormal gait – waddling gait.
- Stunted growth
- Develops secondary anaemia
- Has poor muscle tone: protuberant abdomen (pot-belly); separation of rectus muscles.
- Has irregular bowels
- Flabby skin and subcutaneous tissue
- Rachitic rosary – rosary like swelling at costochondral junction due to hypertrophy of cartilage cells (not tender)
- Harrison sulcus – a horizontal depression at a few cms above lower costal margin caused by pull of attached diaphragm of softened ribs **(Fig. 2.4)**.
- *Pectus carintum:* In this condition sternum sticks out more than usual.
- Barrel shaped/pigeon chest – Anteroposterior dimension of chest is greater than the transverse, with angled manubrium sterni **(Fig. 2.5G)**.
- Pectus excavatum **(Fig. 2.5H)** (also called Funnel condition sternum sinks into the chest.
- Prominent parietal region ⎫ These altogether present
- Flattening of occiput and vertex ⎬ enlarged squared appearance of head –
- Frontal bossing ⎭ caput quadratum.
- Open fontanelles
- Craniotabes (crackling cranial bones due to thinning and softening of bone at places.
- Rachitic dwarfism (specially in renal rickets) **(Figs. 2.2A to C)**

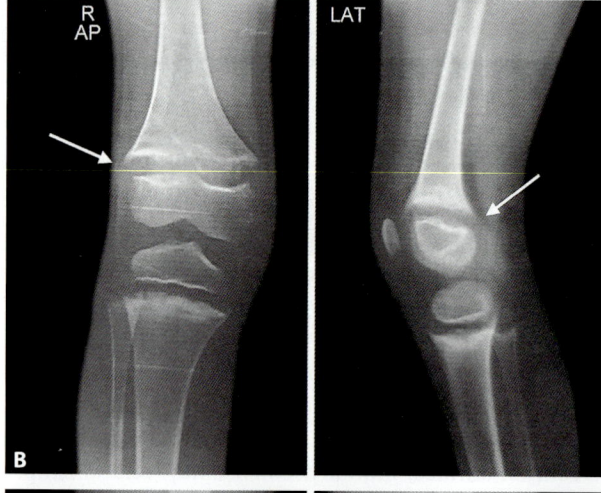
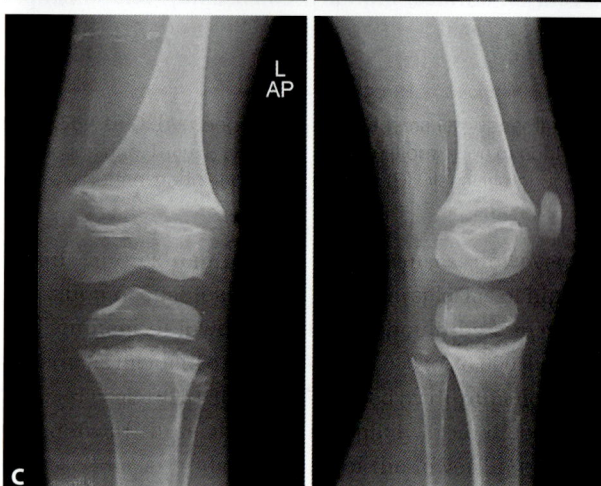

Figs. 2.2A to C: X-ray of renal rickets.

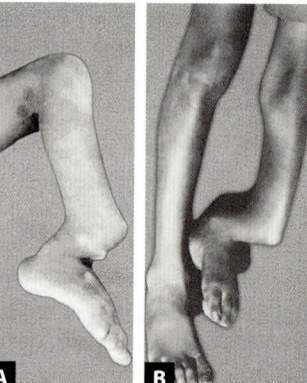
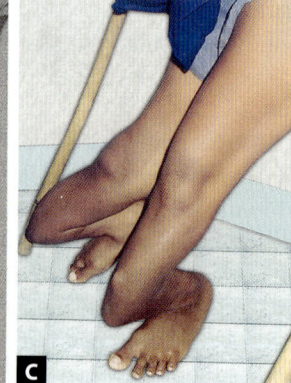

Figs. 2.3A to C: Congenital pseudoarthrosis (often associated with neurofibromatosis) of tibia with gross angulation (A and B) is most frequently encountered, but this pseudoarthrosis may occur in any long bone (e.g. forearm bones—usually only ulna or radius; femur). Bilateral pseudoarthrosis of tibia is extremely rare (C).

Examination of Long Bones

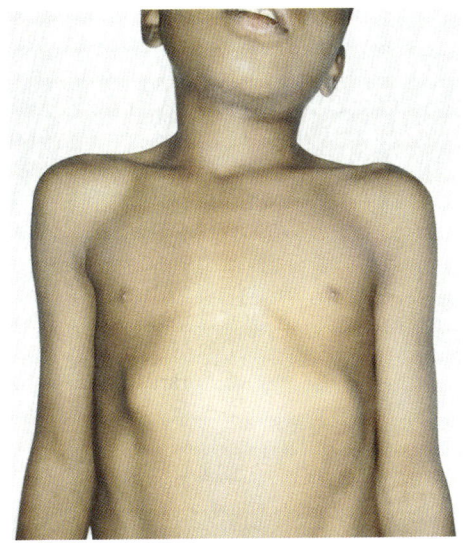

- Broadening in wrist and ankle regions (double malleoli)
- Coxa-vara, anterolateral bowing of Femur, genuvalgum varum, anterolateral bowing of lower third of tibia with Flattening of tibia and secondary adapting changing in the foot (for genu valgum varum or bowing, wind swept deformity (**2.13 to 2.15**).
- In renal rickets there is renal dysfunction due to glomerular or tubular disease, is associated with parathyroid hyperplasia—leads to less deposition of calcium in bone. There are dwarfism, pseudo rickets and osteitis fibrosa cystica (Refer **Figs. 12.83, 13.13**)
- Fluorosis may be confused with rickets.

Laboratory Findings
- Serum alkaline phosphate level is increased
- Serum phosphate level is reduced

Fig. 2.4: Harrison's sulcus and rachitic rosary.

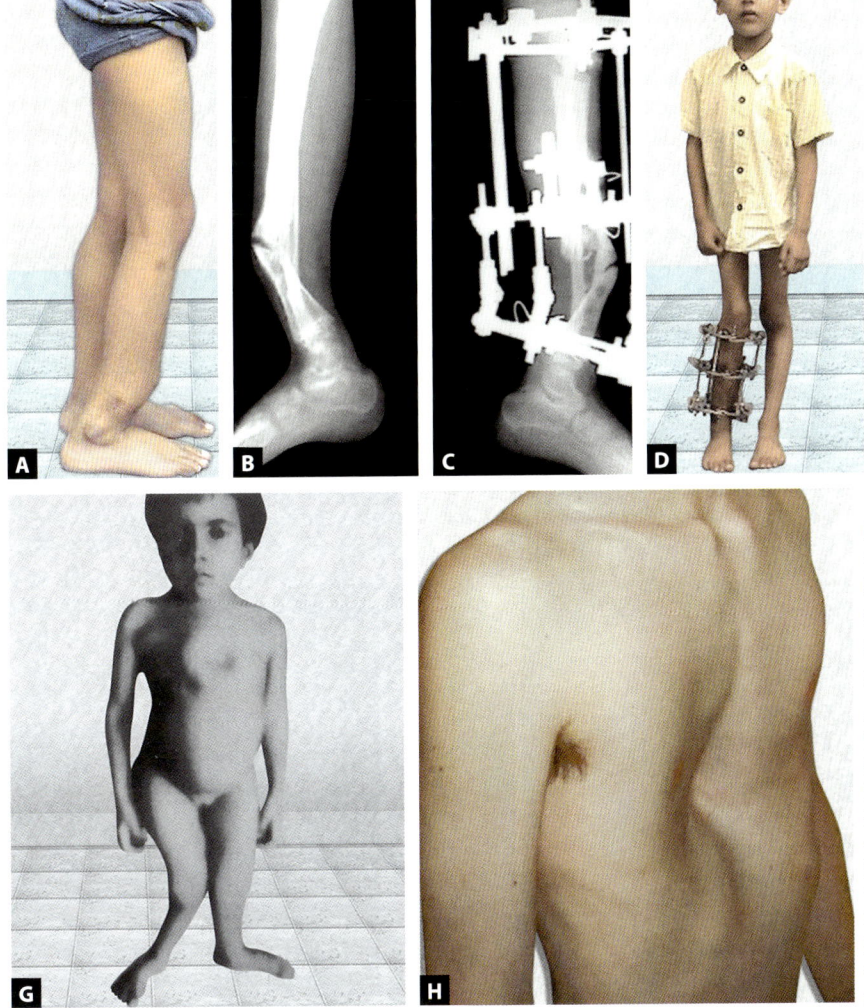
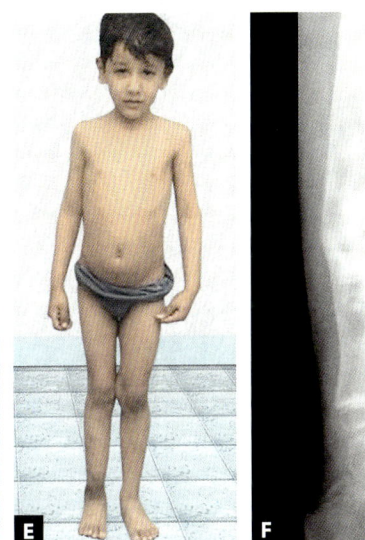

Figs. 2.5A to H: Congenital pseudoarthrosis tibia—managed by Ilizarov apparatus. Treatment by Ilizarov apparatus appears comparatively practical and effective.

Courtesy: Dr RA Agrawal, Dr Mohan Tiwary.

Source: Wikipedia.

Advantages of Ilizarov apparatus: It can be used for:
I—Immobilization
L—Limb lengthening
I—Infection control
Z—zig-zag (deformity) correction
A—Adaptable to most of the bones
R—Reliable apparatus
O—Overall good results
V—Versatile in use

In managing osteomyelitis, Ilizarov's concept was—osteomyelitis, infection burns in the fire of regeneration.

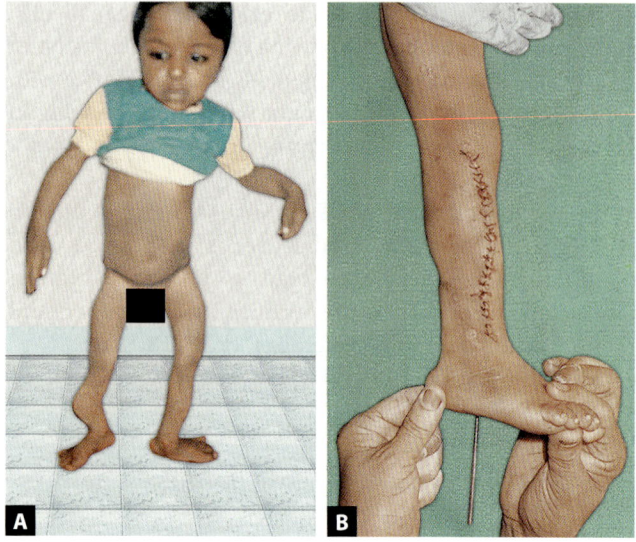

Figs. 2.6A and B: (A) Congenital pseudoarthrosis of tibia; (B) Operated pseudoarthrosis—immediate postoperative picture.

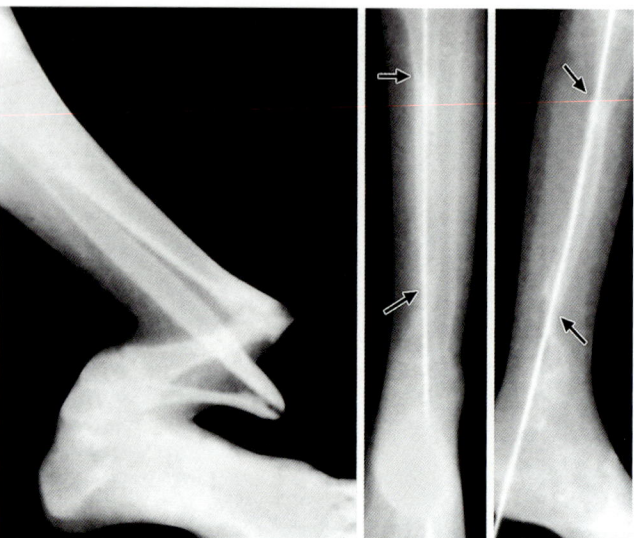

Fig. 2.7: X-ray picture of congenital pseudoarthrosis of lower third of leg bones (common site)—Pre- and post-correction radiographs.

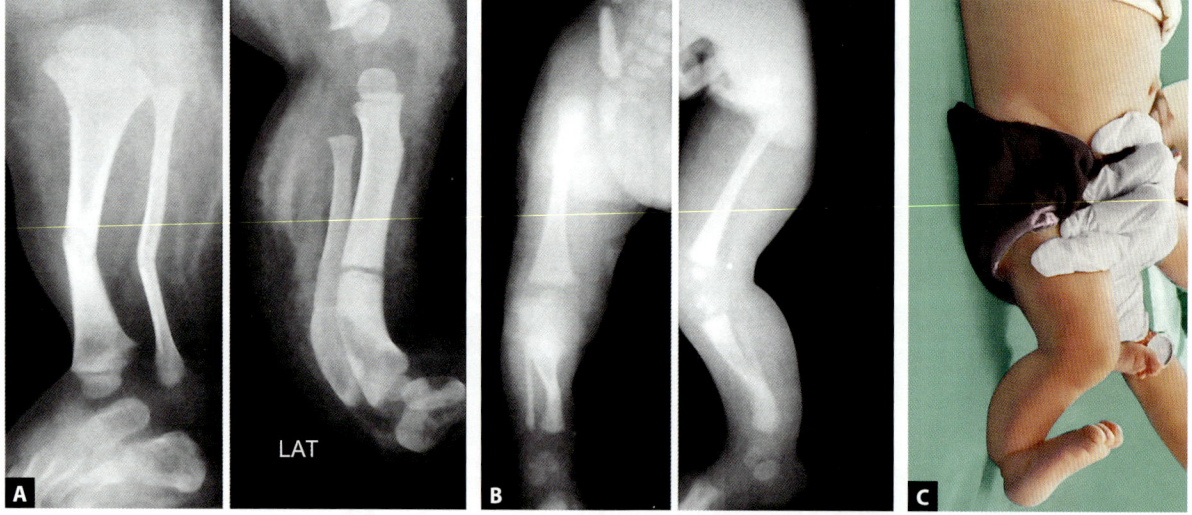

Figs. 2.8A to C: (A) Congenital fracture leg bones leading to pseudoarthrosis; (B and C) Posterior bowing of leg (tibia) – One should not hurry to operative correction – it may end in pseudoarthrosis.

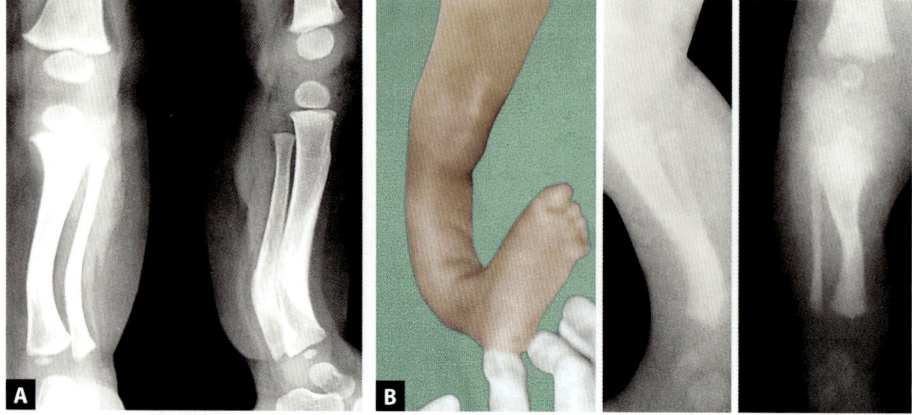

Figs. 2.9A and B: (A) X-ray picture showing posterior bowing of leg bone. Resist-temptation of operative correction, wait and watch; (B) Congenital posterior bowing of tibia.

Examination of Long Bones

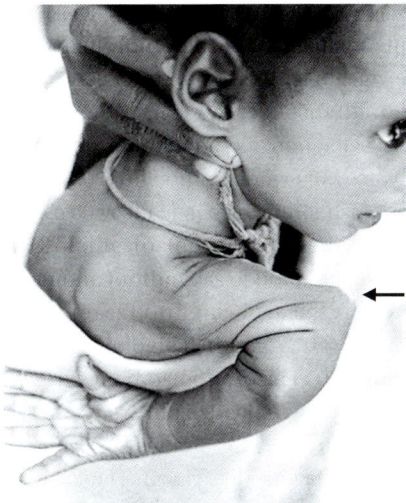

Fig. 2.10: Congenital **pseudoarthrosis** of humerus.

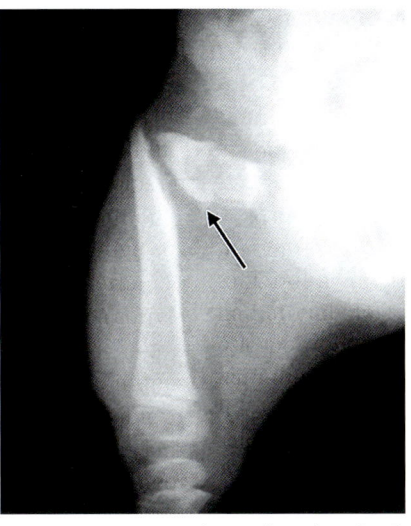

Fig. 2.11: Congenital **pseudoarthrosis** of femur (unusual site).

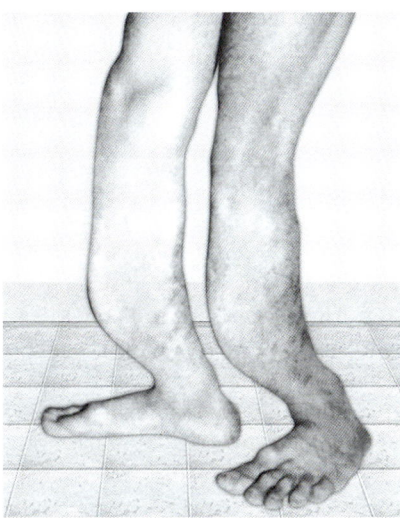

Fig. 2.12: Sabre tibiae (due to syphilis).

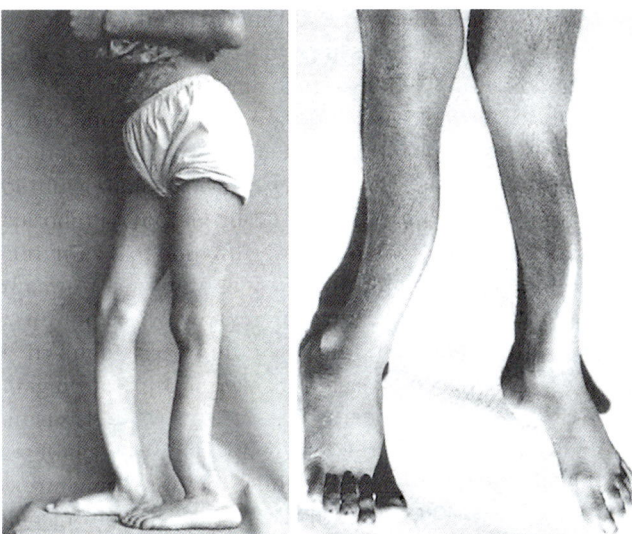

Fig. 2.13: Rachitic bilateral bow leg. Note the bowing in the lower third with side-to-side flattening of tibia.

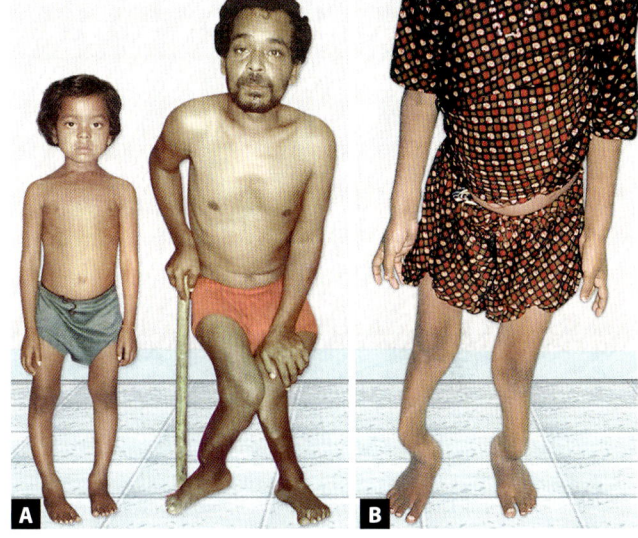

Figs. 2.14A and B: (A) Father – bilateral genu valgum and daughter – bowing of right leg having deformities in lower limbs due to **fluorosis**; (B) Rachitic bowing of both tibiae. Note the widening at both wrists.

- Serum calcium level is usually normal, but may be reduced
- Urinary calcium level is reduced.
- Delayed closure of fontanelle, craniotabes Crackling cranial bone due to thinning and softening of bone at places frontal bossing, flattening of occiput and vertex – present enlarged, squared appearance of head–caput quadratum
- Delayed eruption of teeth, decaying of teeth
- Protuberant abdomen, hepatomegaly
- Broadening in wrist region and ankle (double malleoli)
- Coxa-vara, anterolateral bowing of femur, genu valgum or varum, anterolateral bowing of lower third of tibia with flattening of tibia and secondary adaptive changes in the foot (for genu valgum, varum or bowing wind swept deformity) **(Figs. 2.13 to 2.15)**. In renal rickets there is renal dysfunction due to glomerular or tubular disease, is associated with parathyroid hyperplasia–leads to less deposition of calcium in bone. There is dwarfism, pseudorickets and osteitis fibrosa cystica.
- Rachitic dwarfism (specially in renal rickets) **(Refer Figs. 12.83 and 13.13)**.
- Flurosis may be confused with rickets.

Stigmata of syphilis

Syphilis a highly infectious disease caused by Treponema pallidum bacteria is nowadays becoming rare disease due

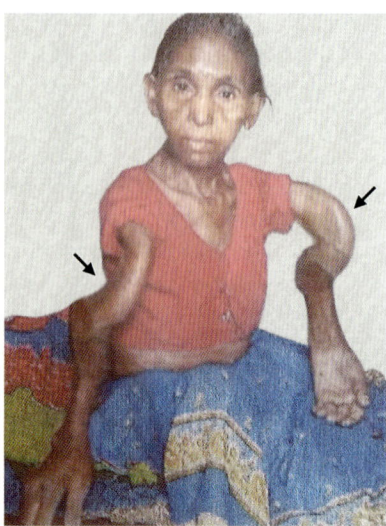

Fig. 2.14C: Note the acutely curved arms due to **fluorosis** (*Source of photo:* Hindustan Times).

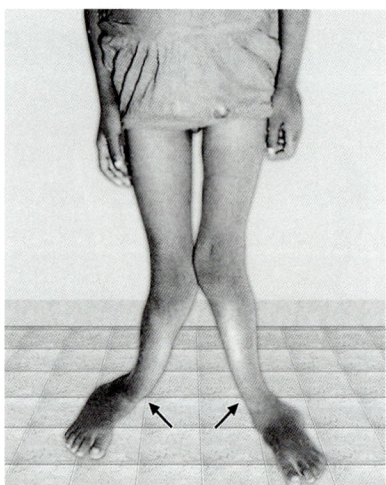

Fig. 2.15: Rachitic bilateral genu valgum with anterior bowing in the lower third junctional zone and secondary pes planus.

to awareness about this disease and its mode of spread and availability of higher antibiotics. Congenital syphilis occurs when a child is born to a mother with syphilis. In established certain stigmata develop.

- Alopecia
- Frontal bossing
- Depressed nasal bridge, perforation of nasal septum (cf. flattening of nose-tip in leprosy)
- Hutchinson's teeth ⎫
- Keratitis   ⎬ Hutchinson's triad
- Auditory nerve deafness ⎭
- Snuffles
- Enlarged lymph nodes—occipital and epitrochlear
- High arching palate, perforation of palate, mucous patches
- Gumma of testis
- Condylomatas [anal region **(Fig. 9.1B)**, mouth]
- Sabre tibia **(Fig. 2.12)**

- Clutton's joint (symptomless symmetrical synovitis with boggy fluid distension usually in childhood due to congenital syphilis) **(Fig. 3.9)**
- Charcot's joint (*see* **Figs. 12.75, 13.48B and 13.49**)

Fluorosis is an endemic osteosclerotic disease resulting from excessive ingestion of fluorides in drinking water Fluoride content in normal water is less than 1 ppm.

Fluorosis is a cosmetic condition that affects the teeth. It is caused by overexposure of fluoride during the first eight years of life, during which most of the permanent teeth are being formed. Teeth of those affected by fluorosis may appear mildly discoloured. Patient can develop white spots and brown stains. Pitting or mottling of enamel can happen in severe cases.

Deformities of limbs may develop like rickets **(Figs. 2.14A and 2.14C)**

Fluoride occurs in natural water. Where natural levels exceed 2 parts per million, The Centers for Disease Control and Prevention (CDC) recommends for changing the source of drinking water for the children. Fluoride containing products should be kept out of reach of children.

Children who consume more amount of fluoride in a short period can have, vomiting, pain abdomen, diarrhea.

Fluorine directly stimulates osteoblastic activity. Fluorapatite crystals are laid down in bone. Excessive calcium gets deposited in bone and soft tissue.

In skeletal fluorosis patients complain of pain and stiffness in back and joints.

Palpation

Confirm the findings of inspection.

Superficial palpation (touch): Temperature, hyperaesthesia, hypoaesthesia, anaesthesia, texture of skin (smooth, rough, etc.), superficial crepitation, superficial tenderness to be noted.

Deep palpation (feel): Feel the muscles, deeper soft tissues and normal bony shaft after displacing longitudinal muscle fibres to the sides wherever possible. Note any abnormality like crepitus, abnormal swelling, fixity of the soft tissues, irregularity of the bone, etc. Crepitus may be an important finding while examining the shaft of a long bone (confirms fracture, if with history of injury; confirms pathological fracture in expansile lesion of the bone, e.g. giant cell tumour). However, it should not be attempted only for the sake of confirming fracture in clinical examination. After all, crepitus results from rattling of the bony fringes at the fractured ends. This crackling is going to break the thin fragile fringes and thereby, reduce the possibility of locking of the fragments following reduction. If it is done for diagnosing an expansile lesion (giant cell tumour), the thin expanded fragile cortical shell sustains micro-fractures, thereby allowing leakage of the underlying contents and dissemination of the pathological tissues hitherto confined within the bony cortical shell. In the course of gentle examination or gentle handling of the limbs, if crepitus or abnormal mobility are felt, they will be a welcome finding. However, one must not attempt to demonstrate these clinical signs in acute lesions.

If the general curvature of the shaft is not identical with the opposite side this should be clearly noted. Note the site of abnormal contour, the direction of bulge, and the change in curvature. Palpate surface of curvatures as far as practicable as if examining a bony lump. Whenever possible, any abnormal vascular finding should be noted (pulsation, thrill, compressibility, pulsatile swelling, ballooning and varicosities). Palpate the soft tissues, layer by layer all along. Any abnormal tender spot should be thoroughly scrutinized. At times, nodular or oblong firm soft tissue swellings are felt at varying depths which are usually tender on direct pressure (most likely neurofibroma). In case of neoplasm, its status, as regards benign or malignant, should be decided clinically as described in the Chapter 17, Bone Tumours.

Percussion (Tap)

Percussion of a long bone usually subserves more or less the function of squeezing. However, tenderness in the shin of tibia or other subcutaneous bone is well demonstrated by this method.

Squeezing

Periosteal tear and haematoma, a very minor crack fracture or a deep-seated painful bony lesion may not be accurately diagnosed by the routine method of examination. In such cases, squeezing of the palpable portion of the shaft of the bone may provide a clue. By squeezing, pressure stress is generated on the surface of the bone which travels along the long-axis of the bone. The moment the wave encounters the discontinued area, the subperiosteal nerve endings are triggered by the vibratory waves and the patient complains of pain at the site.

Measurement

Linear measurement of the shaft includes total and segmental length measurement of the limb (as described in the concerned chapter). Limb-length equality is significant from cosmetic and functional points of view. Lower limb length discrepancy affects the gait, increases energy expenditure, and may lead to backache, scoliosis and decreased spinal mobility. 0.5–2 cm of limb length discrepancy usually remain asymptomatic, however, the discrepancy of more than 2.5 cm needs care.

The circumferential measurement of the shaft must be done at the symmetrical levels of the shaft (e.g. mid shaft levels) for muscular wasting or increase in girth. Besides, the girth at the level of any abnormal swelling must be compared to that of the unaffected limb.

Inequality in the limb length especially in the lower limbs, needs equalization—smaller ones (about 2.5 cm) by compensatory footwears, and bigger ones by surgical procedures as and when needed. These differ in growing age and adults. During the growing age, it is helpful if the remaining extent of growth can be predicted. Two techniques are mostly used for predicting the growth-remaining:
- *Green-Anderson growth-remaining chart:* For utilising this charting properly, one will have to estimate the percentage of growth inhibition for the concerned patient by taking two measurements at the interval of at least 3 months. The difference of growth between the normal limb and the affected limb is multiplied by 100 and the result is divided by the growth of the normal limb
- The above *Green-Anderson's chart has been simplified by Moseley* by mathematically manipulating the original data to allow it to fit on a straight line graph, which is easier to appear and visually graphic.

Auscultation

This clinical ritual sometimes is much informative, e.g. hearing for a systolic bruit in a highly vascular swelling of the long bones.

Investigation

- Beside the routine haemogram and urine analysis, X-rays are very important. This should be taken preferably in three planes, i.e. anteroposterior, lateral and oblique. If possible, X-ray of the corresponding part of the shaft of other limb must be included in same plate for comparison. This helps in detecting the minor changes in the texture, girth and curvature of the bones. In the X-ray, the entire shaft must be exposed specially where inflammatory and neoplastic lesions are suspected. The skip lesions in the same shaft have been noted in several cases
- Orthotomography—It is done to detect any suspicious lesion, which cannot be detected by ordinary X-rays, e.g. osteoid osteoma
- Radioisotope-scanning
- Computerised axial tomography
- Magnetic resonance imaging (MRI)
- For confirmation of any lesion histopathological examination may be necessary. Of course before this, other investigations including radioscanning must be completed. Histopathological examination can be done by either aspiration biopsy or open biopsy. The latter is more authentic.

KEY DIAGNOSTIC POINTS OF COMMON AFFECTIONS OF LONG BONES

Congenital Anomalies of Lower Extremity (*see* Figs. 2.49, 2.50, 2.59)

Important congenital anomalies of lower limb are:
- *Limb length discrepancies:* Limb length discrepancy of more than 2.5 cm is significant since it may lead

to awkward gait, back pain, hip and knee pain, compensatory scoliosis, decreased spinal mobility, increases energy expenditure in walking due to excessive vertical rise and fall of pelvis, cosmetic concern. Limb length discrepancy may also be due to acquired causes, such as following trauma; infection (chronic osteomyelitis—infective focus just beneath the growth plate irritates the growth plate leading to lengthening, whereas damage of growth plate and sequestrating out of a portion of bone lead to shortening); paralytic condition (e.g. poliomyelitis cerebral palsy); juvenile rheumatoid arthritis, tumours and tumorous like conditions (which stimulates asymmetrical growth).

- *Congenital recurvatum* (hyperextension of knee) and congenital dislocation of knee is divided into 3 grades according to severity.
  - Congenital hyperextension
  - Congenital hyperextension with anterior subluxation of tibia on femur
  - Congenital hyperextension with anterior dislocation of knee.

  The basic pathology is the contracture of anterior capsule of knee and quadriceps apparatus. Associated pathologies are intra-articular adhesions and hypoplasia or absence of patella.

- *Congenital dislocation of patella* (Fixed lateral dislocation of patella)—It is often bilateral and familial. Milder forms are usually missed in X-ray up to the age of about 4 years because of lack of ossification in patella. However, MRI and ultrasound can delineate the cartilaginous patella. Severe cases associated with flexion contracture of knee, can be detected soon after birth. It may be a part of **arthrogryposis multiplex congenita** (AGMC) and **Down syndrome**. Congenital dislocation of patella may be confused with habitual dislocation of patella (obligatory dislocation of patella) which the patient can reproduce voluntarily by flexing the knee. Of course, the basic pathology of both (congenital and habitual dislocations) remains the same, i.e. contracture of quadriceps mechanism. In congenital dislocation, the vastus lateralis may be absent or severely contracted. Patella remains small and shapeless. The medial side capsule of knee is stretched. The patellar tendon is attached more laterally. Usually, there is genu valgum and external rotation of tibia on femur.

- *Congenital constriction ring* of leg and thigh (Streeter's syndrome) (*see* Chapter 24—Syndromes Related to Orthopaedics and Trauma, Page 622).

- *Congenital pseudoarthrosis of tibia and fibula.* Congenital pseudoarthrosis is a special type of non-union which may remain occult or manifest at birth. Its exact cause is not known, however, neurofibromatosis may remain associated in good number of cases.

- *Congenital pseudoarthrosis of fibula* may precede or accompany the pseudoarthrosis of tibia. Pseudoarthrosis of fibula manifest in several grades, such as: (1) bowing of fibula without pseudoarthrosis, (2) pseudoarthrosis of fibula without ankle deformity, (3) with ankle deformity, (4) fibular pseudoarthrosis with latent pseudarthrosis of tibia. Treatment is complex with almost same uncertainty as that of tibial pseudoarthrosis. Primary aim should be to prevent ankle deformity such as by tibiofibular synostosis.

- *Congenital pseudoarthrosis of tibia* is a rare condition (incidence about one in 2,50,000 live birth). Association of neurofibromatosis is in quite large number of cases (50-90%). Boyd classified pseudoarthrosis of tibia into six types: (1) Pseudoarthrosis tibia (PT) with anterior bowing and defect in tibia manifesting at birth, (2) PT with anterior bowing and an hourglass constriction of tibia, the tibia remains at high risk of fracture by the age of 2 years. The tibia is tapered, rounded, sclerotic with obliterated medullary canal. This type is most common and has poorest prognosis of healing. (3) PT develops in congenital cyst at about junction of middle and distal third. Anterior bowing develops preceding or following the fracture. Prognosis is good after operative treatment. (4) PT develops in sclerotic zone. Medullary cavity is partially or completely obliterated. Incomplete fracture becomes complete and fails to unite and PT develops. If treated in incomplete stage of fracture, the prognosis is good. (5) PT develops with dysplastic fibula. Gradually PT of both tibia and fibula develops and then prognosis becomes poorer. (6) PT develops as an intraosseous neurofibroma or schwannoma. It is rarest form. Its prognosis depends upon the aggressiveness and management of primary osseous lesion.

  Management of pseudoarthrosis, with main stress or bone grafting and intramedullary fixations, remains variably uncertain. Use of recombinant human bone morphogenetic protein (rhBMP) is an adjunct to treatment. Treatment by Ilizarov apparatus may be effective **(Figs. 2.5A to H)**.

- *Congenital angular deformities of leg*—Congenital angular deformities of leg are primarily of two types—in one type, the angulation of leg is anteriorly, which is usually associated with or may lead to congenital pseudoarthrosis; in other type there is posterior bowing of leg, which tend to improve with the growth of the child. Both types may be associated with variable medial or lateral angulation. Variable shortening of the affected limb is usual accompaniment. In a distinct syndrome, the anterior bowing of tibia is associated with duplication of great toe along with shortening of tibia, clinodactyly and anomalous maturation of metacarpals and carpals.

- *Congenital deficiencies of the long bones—*
  - Proximal femoral focal deficiency

TABLE 2.1: Characteristics of osteomyelitis in different age groups.

Infancy	Childhood	Adult
• 1 year (0–1 Year) • Usually secondary to umbilical infection	• Maximum incidence (1–17 Years) • Haematogenous from any septic focus	• 17 years onwards • Usually open fractures • Haematogenous

Organisms:
• Staphylococci
  H. influenzae
  Streptococci
  Pneumococci
	• Staphylococci
	  Streptococci
	  Pneumococci
	  Salmonella and others
	  In sickle cell anaemia, *Salmonella* group more common
		• Staphylococci, Pseudomonas, bacillus *Proteus*, and others. In heroin addicts *Pseudomonas aeruginosa* is predominant organism, besides *Staphylococcus aureus* and gram-negative bacilli

• Constitutional features less marked	• Rare infecting organism *Staphylococcus lugdunensis* for acute osteomyelitis • More marked	• Moderately marked
• Site—Usually intra-articular metaphysis and epiphysis	• Metaphyseal Primary epiphyseal osteomyelitis is extremely rare	• Usually diaphyseal
• Local temperature—very little/insignificant/or even not raised	• Always raised	• Mild to moderately raised
• Pus not under pressure	• Pus under tension	• Less pus (located in medullary, cavity)
• Veil like periosteum is easily perforated by pus	• Sub-periosteal pus collection persists for some time elevating periosteum for longer and wider distance before bursting	• Adherent periosteum does not allow wider spread of pus
• Diffuse local oedema manifest quite early—even whole limb may be swollen	• Pitting oedema more or less localised to area of affection (pus collection)	• Pitting oedema localised to area of deeper pus collection
• Joint affection frequent because infection can easily penetrate along the communicating blood vessels through epiphyseal growth plate	• Joint affection less frequent except at sites where metaphysis is intracapsular	• Indirect joint affection in late cases due to muscular adhesions
• Sequestrum formation much less	• Very common	• Smaller/thin sequestra, except in open fractures (where bigger sequestrum). Sequestrum if formed, gets extruded, or incorporated or has to be extracted
Complications • Dissolution of intra-articular cartilage • Unstable joint	• Extensive diaphyseal affection • Pathological fracture • Persistant sinus	• Flares • Persistant sinus • Pathological fractures
• Marked shortening (due to dissolution of epiphysis, gross damage of growth plate, or diaphyseal sequestration • Angular deformities more common • Chronic conversion much less	• Limb length disparity—lengthening more common (due to increased vascularity near growth plate) • If joint involvement—epiphyseal separation • Chronic conversion much common	• Shortening and/or deformities due to malunited pathological fractures • Chronicity more common • Malignancy—epithelioma in sinus Sarcoma in bone • Amyloidosis

- Tibial hemimelia: It is a rare congenital disorder with longitudinal deficiency of tibia and relatively intact fibula. Historically Otto was the first to describe it in 1841. It has been variously classified and treatment is mainly surgical with varying results.
- Fibular hemimelia.

Osteomyelitis (Table 2.1)

Cellulitis is soft tissue infection involving the skin and subcutaneous tissues, clinically diagnosed by soft tissue swelling, erythema, warm affected area, ill-defined margin separating it from the adjacent uninvolved skin. Cellulitis on MRI shows thickening of subcutaneous tissues ill-defined increased signal intensity of superficial soft tissue on T2-weighted sequences and corresponding low signal intensity on T1-weighted sequences.

Broadly 'osteomyelitis' is inflammation of bone, but it comprises of two words—osteitis (inflammation of bone) + myelitis (inflammation of marrow). It affects the cortex, marrow, periosteum and even the surrounding soft tissue. Inflammation may be defined as the reaction of vascularised living tissue to local tissue injury or insult by different stimuli. Osteomyelitis sets in when adequate number of sufficiently virulent organism overcomes the host's natural defence mechanisms, beside some local factors, such as relative absence of phagocytic cells in the metaphysis of bones in children, where haematogenous osteomyelitis is more common. Haematogenous osteomyelitis is the generic name for infection of bone and narrow by the circulating organism in the blood from distant source. The body's main defence mechanisms are (1) Neutrophil response; (2) Humoral immunity; (3) Cell-mediated immunity; (4) Reticuloendothelial cells. Deficient production and/or function of any (or combination) of above predisposes the host to infection. *Osteomyelitis may be acute, subacute, and chronic* depending upon the period of infection, the virulence and dose of infective organism and the immune system, age, general nature and condition of the host.

In acute osteomyelitis the symptoms and signs of systemic infection dominate. In subacute osteomyelitis there are no obvious signs of systemic involvement, though local signs are there. Chronic osteomyelitis dominantly present with recurrent infections and discharging sinuses.

Acute Haematogenous Osteomyelitis (Figs. 2.16A to C)

(= infection of bone and marrow by circulating organisms in the blood from a distant source in the body)

- Its incidence is gradually decreasing due to improvement in standard of health, hygiene, nutrition and living
- In preantibiotic era the morbidity and mortality following osteomyelitis was fairly high
- Usually occurs in childhood, and more in males
- Vague history of insignificant trauma, followed by pain
- Constitutional features—high temperature (around 39°C) persisting for few days, patient looks ill and toxic.
- Affected part (metaphyseal region) swollen, warm, distended, erythematous; *pitting oedema (indicates deep pus collection, e.g. sub-periosteal abscess).*
- *Posttraumatic osteomyelitis* develops when infection follows through an open wound
- Soft tissue infection in overlying or neighboring area may lead to *contiguous osteomyelitis*
- Clinical features base on pathophysiological evolution of acute haematogenous osteomyelitis as summarised in three stages (Treuta 1968): Stage I—a boil in the bone manifesting as constant severe pain, swelling, local tenderness; Stage II—features of established inflammation with increase in above clinical features. Inflammation is mediated through several soluble factors including a group of secreted polypeptides known as cytokines. Inflammatory cytokines are different for acute inflammation and chronic inflammation. In inflammation, redness (rubor) and heat (calor) are due to increased vascularity, swelling (tumour) is due to increased inflammatory fluid and white blood cell, pain (dolor) is due to released chemical compounds and pressure on nerves in the vicinity of inflammation and less of function (functio laesa) is mainly due to pain and mechanical interferences (such as swelling); Stage III—subperiosteal abscess stage (clinical features as noted above)
- Neighbouring joint mildly swollen, however fair range of passive movement can be demonstrated. But patient does not want to move his limb due to pain
- Regional lymph nodes enlarged, soft and tender
- When asked for, he/she can point to the site of maximum pain, which is also very tender, i.e. this is the point of focus in the metaphysis

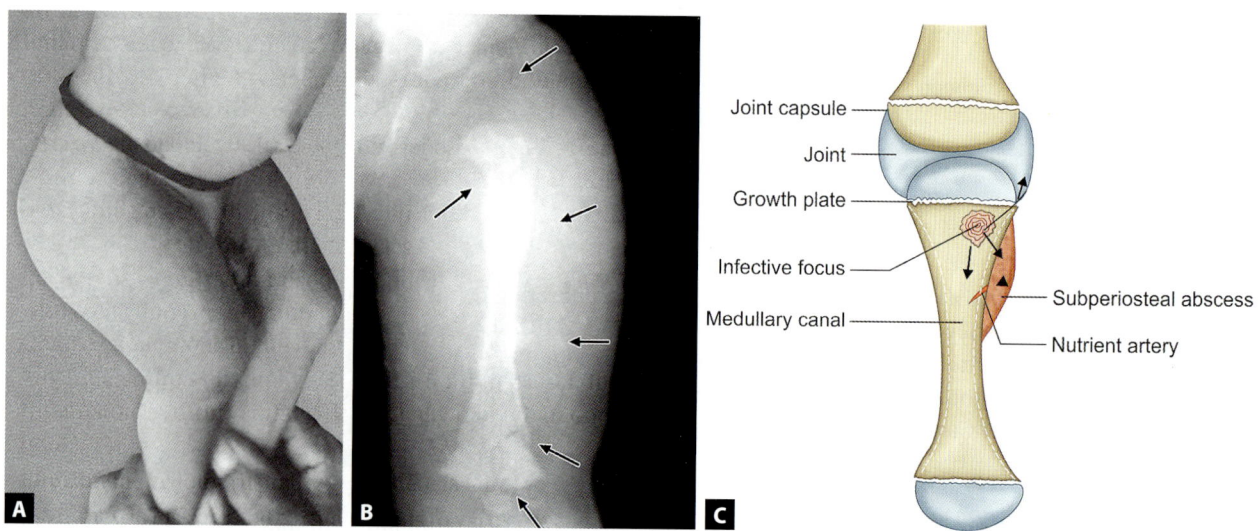

Figs. 2.16A to C: (A) Acute haematogenous osteomyelitis of right femur in 25 days old infant; (B) Osteomyelitis of femur with septic arthritis hip with huge abscess in 35 days old child; (C) Path of travelling of pus from the infective focus in metaphysis.

- Bacterial pyomyositis (infection of skeletal muscle by staphylococci or other organisms) is common in tropics, which can be easily confused with acute osteomyelitis, especially in adults.
- Adult osteomyelitis is an infection of bone in which > 90% of cases are the result of contiguous spread from nearby skin due to trauma, surgery or diabetic ulceration. Osteomyelitis may be a comorbidity with cellulitis.
- Vertebral osteomyelitis is the common presentation of hematogenous osteomyelitis in adults, more in males, and it may be confused with tuberculous disease. CT or MRI show the pathological anatomy more clearly. In MRI bright signed is seen on T_2 – weighted images and a low – intensity image on T_1 weighted image.

Investigations
- *Total and differential count of WBC*
  - Polymorphonuclear leucocytosis, usually below 15,000/mm^3
  - Blood ESR raised
  - C-reactive protein raised.
  - Serum procalcitonin at a cut–cuff of 0.4 ng/mL is a sensitive and specific marker in the diagnosis of septic arthritis and acute osteomyelitis.

The level of neutrophil CD64 expression is better predictor of local musculoskeletal infection than the CRP, ESR and WBC count.

CD64 is one of the Fc receptor for IgG commonly known as F receptor 1 (FcγRI). It plays a role in antibody-dependent cytotoxicity, the clearance of immune complexes and the phagocytosis of targets opsonised with IgG and mediates the release of pro-inflammatory cytokines (Tanaka et al. 2009).
- *X-ray:* May be non-contributory till 10–12 days.
  - *Within 48 hours:*
    - Loss of normal delineation between the subcutaneous and muscular shadows (*Glenn* 1948)
    - Linear transverse lines extending from muscle outwards.
  - *10–12 days:*
    - Localised rarefaction at the site of origin of the disease (earlier in infancy) due to hyperaemia
    - Early subperiosteal new bone formation
  - *12–20 days:*
    - Soft tissues present almost homogeneous look
    - Surrounding bone also rarefied due to increased vascularity
    - Increasing subperiosteal reactionary longitudinal bone laying
  - *21 days onwards:*
    - Definite features of periostitis and bone destruction. 30–50% of the bone matrix must be lost to show a lytic lesion on X-ray.

- Blood culture may be positive in 30 to 50% of cases, however, a negative culture does not exclude the diagnosis of acute pyogenic bone and joint infection.
- Culture of the aspirate and/or scraped tissue indicates the causative organism (also true for subacute and chronic osteomyelitis)
- Special investigation
  - *Radioisotope studies* (radionuclide scanning) for hot spots. It is a useful technique for diagnosis of osteomyelitis. Most commonly used radioisotopes are technetium-99m (^{99m}Tc) phosphate, gallium 67 (^{67}Ga) citrate and indium-111(^{111}In)-labeled leucocytes. The most commonly used is ^{99m}Tc phosphate which can detect osteomyelitis within 48 hours of clinical onset of infection. The bone scan with ^{99}Tc phosphate is done in three phases (flow phase, intermediate equilibrium phase, and delayed phase). In osteomyelitis, there is an increased uptake in all three phases. However, ^{99m}Tc phosphate bone scans are unreliable in neonates (<6 weeks old) and are usually negative in good number (>60%) of these neonates. Radionuclide scan is useful in patients who have metallic implants in their body in whom CT and MRI are rather contraindicated for fear of producing artifacts:
- *CT scanning* is helpful in identifying sequestrum or subchondral bony plate destruction. In acute osteomyelitis CT detects intraosseous gas, osteolysis, soft tissue masses and foreign bodies
- In ultrasonography, an abscess cavity and any joint effusion can be localised
- *MRI* is important investigation to rule out cartilaginous epiphyseal infection. MRI detects the intramedullary changes much earlier, however, the changes are non-specific since anything which causes oedema or hyperaemia can produce the signal changes similar to that of osteomyelitis. The typical findings of osteomyelitis in MRI are the decrease in the normally high marrow signal on T1-weighted images and a normal on increased marrow signal intensity on MRI sensitivity is 92% and specificity 86% in the detection of osteomyelitis (Klein DA et al, 2020) T2- weight images with marrow enhancement after gadolinium administration. STIR (Short Tau Inversion Recovery) signals have a high negative predictive value for osteomyelitis of almost 100%.

Subacute Osteomyelitis
- The second half of the 20th century saw truly, the remarkable advances in the therapy of bacterial

infections, still it is not uncommon to see the cases of subacute or chronic osteomyelitis
- For convenience acute osteomyelitis presenting beyond 3 weeks may be known as subacute one, however, pathology may start *de-novo* as subacute presentation. Due to indolent course, the diagnosis of primary subacute osteomyelitis is usually variably delayed
- The pathogenic organisms of primary subacute osteomyelitis are usually *Staphylococcus aureus* and *Staphylococcus epidermids*
- Constitutional features present but less marked
- Patient can move the affected part slightly
- Part swollen (but not so much as in acute osteomyelitis)
- Local temperature mild to moderately raised, local tenderness and appearance of bony thickening
- Neighbouring joint is less swollen but with terminal painful limitation of the movements (due to the fact that the controlling muscles which were oedematous at the beginning now start developing adhesions)
- Regional lymph nodes enlarged but less tender
- WBC count is usually not/or mildly raised
- ESR is raised in about 50% of cases
- From the bone aspirate or biopsy material pathogenic bacteria can be identified in only 50-60% of cases.
- The combination of normal ESR and CRP is reliable for predicting the absence of infection (also in the case of chronic osteomyelitis)

X-ray (see Fig. 2.17A):
- Soft tissue shadow starts getting smaller
- Localised rarefaction irregularly spreads in the medullary cavity and/or towards cortex
- Periosteal longitudinal bone laying well-marked
- In extensive diaphyseal affections, there may be indication of early pathological fracture.

Primary subacute osteomyelitis in children is rare. The diagnosis is mostly delayed due to slow onset of disease, intermittent pain, lack of typical constitutional features and subtle radiological changes. However, MRI can provide precise informations about the location and extent of infection. In MRI, the gadolinium-enhanced imaging is the most sensitive. It also helps in proper planning of the treatment. Fortunately, primary subacute osteomyelitis in children does not follow an aggressive course and if early detected, mostly it is amenable to non-operative management—with rest to the part, antibiotics and supportive therapy. Differential diagnosis should be effect of trauma, eosinophilic granuloma, tuberculosis, fungal infection, osteoid osteoma, chondroblastoma, Ewing's sarcoma, osteosarcoma, etc.

Chronic Osteomyelitis (Figs. 2.17B and 2.62)
- Chronic osteomyelitis is a dreaded sequel to acute haematogenous osteomyelitis
- Prolonged history

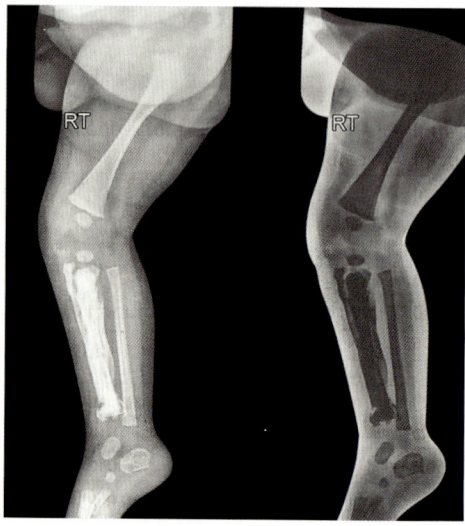

Fig. 2.17A: Subacute osteomyelitis affecting whole right tibia.

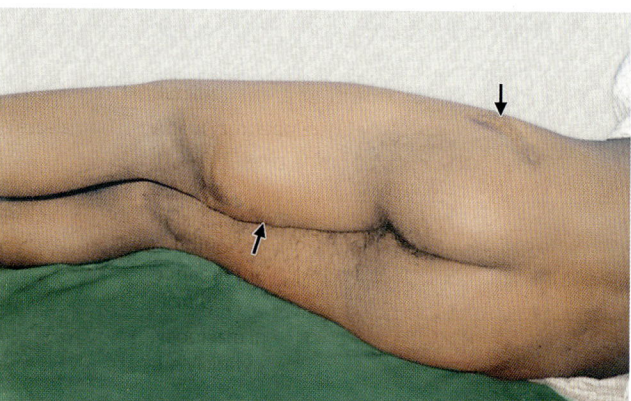

Fig. 2.17B: Chronic osteomyelitis of left trochanteric region—relapsed after 60 years. Note the earlier operative scar healed by second intention; also note the huge collection of pus on the back of thigh.

Recurrence of pain occurs quite often due to:
- Dull pain in the night due to low grade lurking infection
- Pain on minor hurt (usually not cared for) due to underlying subdued infection; or an adhered subcutaneous tissue on the bone (e.g. on tibia)
- Flare of infection—pain recurs with/without constitutional features
- Secondary infections are common.
- No constitutional features except when there is flare
- Discharging or healed sinuses, usually fixed to the bone
- Cultures from sinus tract and deeper bony lesions may differ. Usually S. aureus is the most common isolate in chronic osteomyelitis followed by gram - negative rods like pseudomonas which are usually resistant to many antibiotics.
- Metastatic bone infection is not uncommon.

- History of discharge of small bony spicules, is diagnostic clinical feature
- May be deformities (usually angulation) **(Figs. 2.18 to 2.22)**; neighbouring joint usually stiff or having limited movement; affected bone thickened for variable lengths; may be tender
- May be limb length disparity (usually affected bone is longer) **(Figs. 2.23 to 2.27)** [cf. other common causes of limb disparity, e.g. congenital **(Figs. 2.28 to 2.36)**, haemangioma **(Figs. 2.37 and 2.38)**, lymphangioma **(Fig. 2.39)**, and dyschondroplasia **(Figs. 2.40 to 2.42)**], following trauma
- Regional lymph glands insignificant
- Wherever possible, it is worthwhile to obtain a biopsy material from the lesion for histological and microbiological evaluation of infected bone
- Chronic osteomyelitis is difficult to cure completely.
- Adjacent joint involvement producing septic arthritis with its complications like its damage, deformation, disorganization, stiffness etc.

X-ray: Soft tissue shadow usually shrunken (due to wasting and adhesions).

- May be *sequestrum (a dead piece of bone separated from the living in the process of necrosis, by granulation tissue and/or pus)* **(Fig. 2.44A)**.

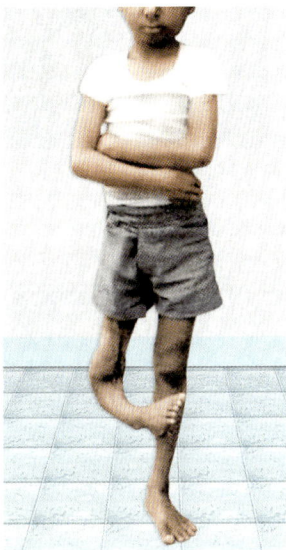

Fig. 2.18: Gross angulation and shortening of right leg due to destruction and bone loss in upper end of tibia following chronic osteomyelitis.

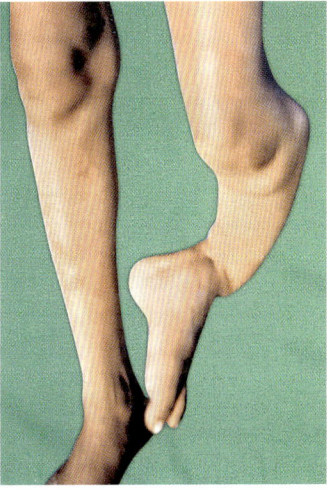

Fig. 2.20: Gross angulation and shortening of left leg following chronic osteomyelitis and destruction (sequestration) of the tibial diaphysis.

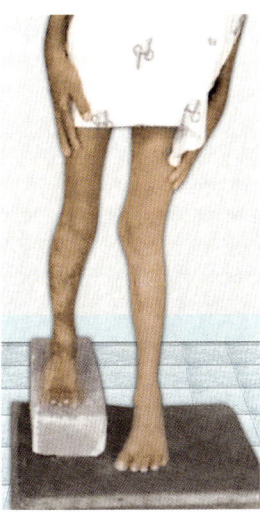

Fig. 2.19: Same patient **(Fig. 2.18)** after fibular muscle pedicle graft Tibialization of ipsilateral fibula was first suggested by Hahns in 1884 to bridge a gap of 12 cm in a 8 year old male child with a segmental loss in tibia due to chronic osteomyelitis. In his patient transposed fibula was tibialized by 75% in 8 months after surgery. tibialization of ipsilateral fibula can be done to make up the gap in tibia due to segmental extrusion in chronic infection, traffic accident, or after excision of neoplasms.

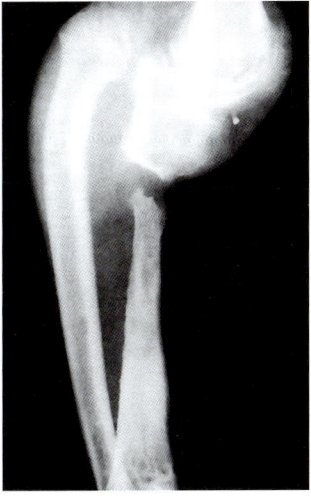

Fig. 2.21: Gross deformity and shortening following sequestrated out diaphyseal segment in pyogenic chronic osteomyelitis of tibia with overgrowth of fibula.

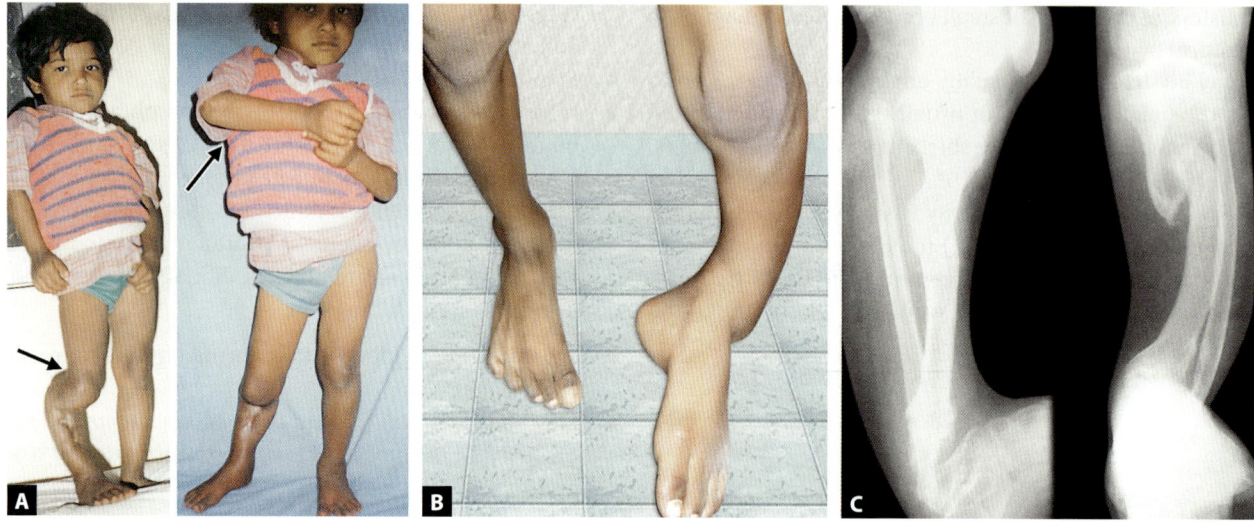

Figs. 2.22A to C: (A) Multifocal chronic pyogenic osteomyelitis in a 5 years old child; the affected right femur has lengthened; the right ulna has osteomyelitis in upper part; in right leg upper tibial diaphysis has sequestrated out and there is overgrowth of fibula; (B) Grossly malunited compound fracture of left tibia with overgrowth of fibula and subluxed fibular ends; (C) X-ray of the same patient.

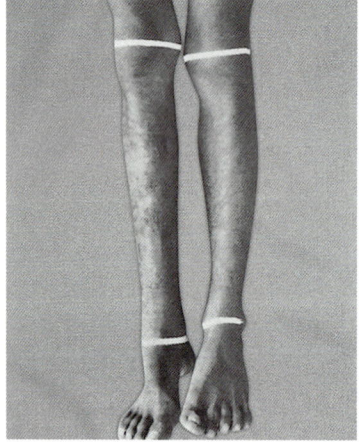

Fig. 2.23: Lengthening of right leg due to chronic osteomyelitis of right upper third of tibia.

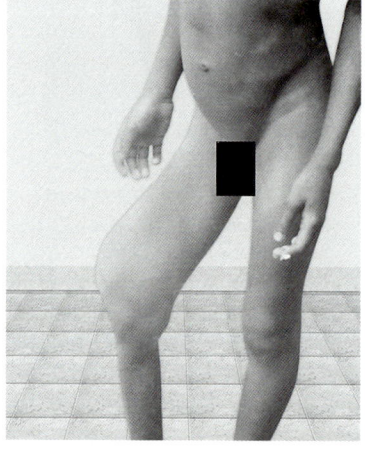

Fig. 2.24: Relapsed chronic osteomyelitis of femur with huge collection of pus. Note the lengthening of thigh.

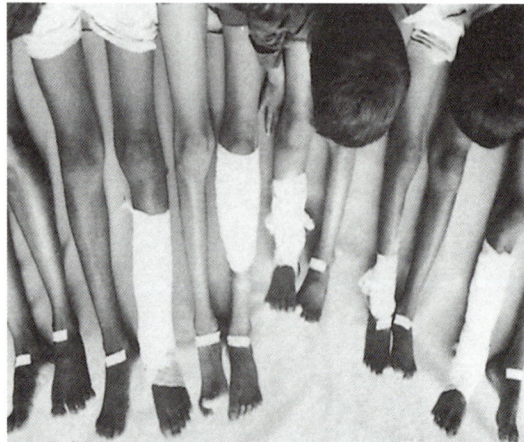

Fig. 2.25: Group photograph of patients having limb-length disparity (usually lengthening) which is common following chronic osteomyelitis.

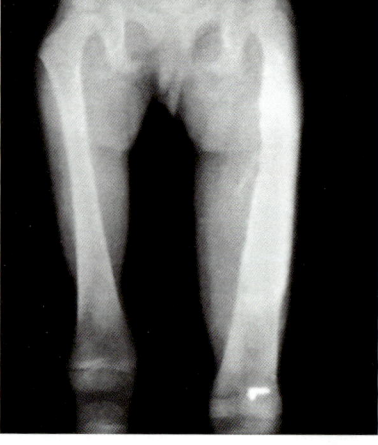

Fig. 2.26: Lengthening of left femur due to chronic osteomyelitis (diaphyseal affection extending upto almost upper metaphysis).

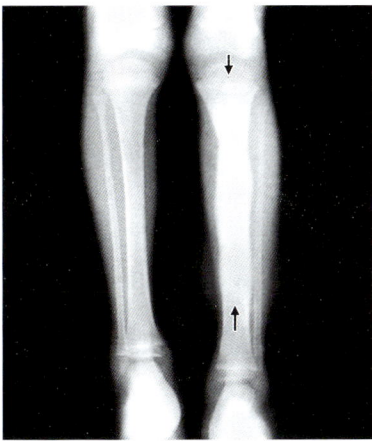

Fig. 2.27: Lengthening of left tibia due to (metaphyseal extending almost to upper growth plate) chronic osteomyelitis.

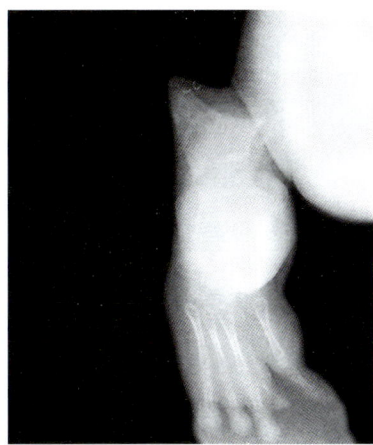

Fig. 2.28: Congenital absence of right thigh, knee, leg, ankle and hind-foot, which have been represented by a mass placed in horizontal continuity of the spider like forefoot.

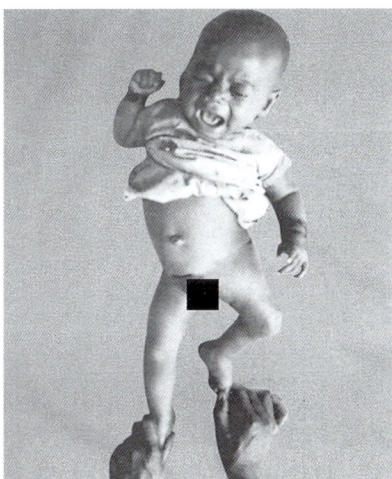

Fig. 2.29: Congenital short femur and leg bones with gross dysplasia of hip and flexion deformity of knee—all in left lower limb.

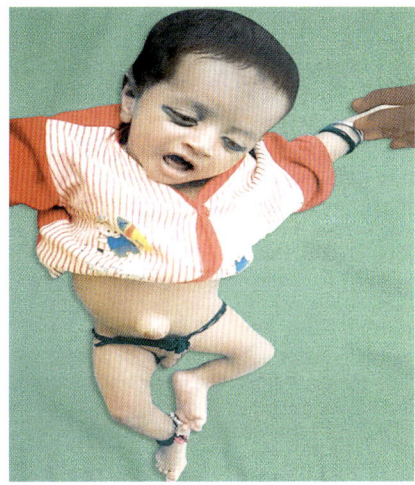

Fig. 2.30: Congenital absence of left upper femur and exomphalos.

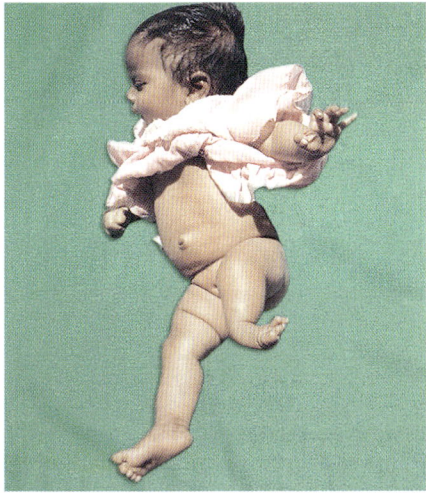

Fig. 2.31: Congenital absence of upper left femur + deficient growth of left leg + calcaneovalgus deformity of foot.

- *Sinus track denoted by irregular translucent passage* reaching up to the bone (due to *entrapped air*).
- Surrounding new bone formation—involucrum.
- Evidence of healed pathological fracture, malunion, may be nonunion
- Relics of damaged cartilaginous growth plate.

Brodies Abscess

- Usually in the upper end of the tibia, upper end of the femur **(Fig. 2.53)**, lower end of the tibia, lower end of the femur, upper end of the humerus
- Brodie abscess is a localised type of subacute or chronic osteomyelitis
- Causative organisms (like *S. aureus*) are of low virulence
- Usually in late teens or in young adults; present with chronic dull pain in the metaphyseal zone, specially after work or exertion; slight to moderate pitting oedema

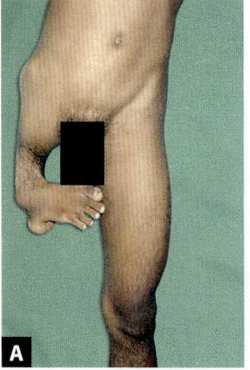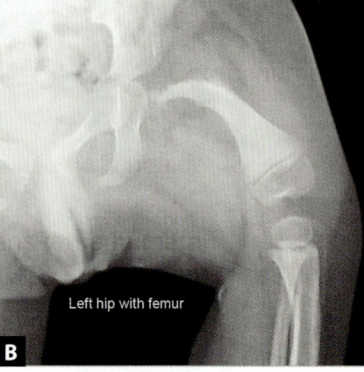

Figs. 2.32A and B: (A) Congenital short right femur and leg bones with absent knee joint; (B) Congenital deficiency of proximal femur—Aitken's type C

Patients with severe *congenital femoral deficiency* develop flexion and external rotation contractures of the limb. Femoral shortening of more than 50% of the normal side usually have instability of the hip and knee.

Proximal femoral focal deficiency (PFFD) is an uncommon congenital defect where there is dysgenesis (defective morphogenesis) of proximal portion of femur. The growth of femur is greatly hampered resulting in marked shortening of femur. No obvious genetic predisposition has been observed except probably in cases of femoral hypoplasia – unusual facies syndrome.

Aitken's four-part classification of PFFD appears systematic.
A—Hip joint is formed, femoral neck is absent, femur is short
B—Femoral head is rudimentary and significant deficiency of proximal femoral shaft; and pseudoarthrosis between femoral shaft and head
C—Femoral head is absent, acetabulum is shallow, and proximal femur is represented only by small tuft
D—Femoral head and acetabulum are absent with significant deficiency of femoral head.

Severe congenital femoral deficiency cannot be completely compensated, however, demanding procedures like that of resection, rotationplasty, femuropelvic arthrodesis followed by fitting with suitable prosthesis help much in rehabilitating the patient.

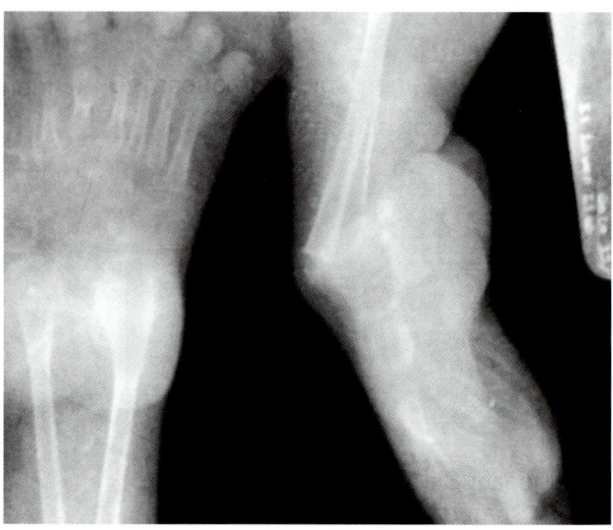

Fig. 2.35: Congenitally disorganised leg bones, ankle and foot.

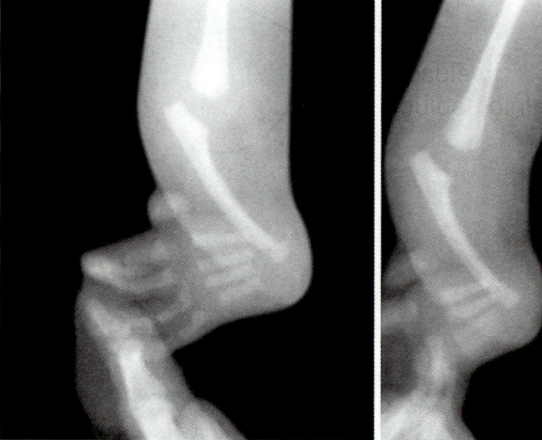

Fig. 2.36: Congenital absence of fibula with distorted development of tibia, knee, ankle and foot.

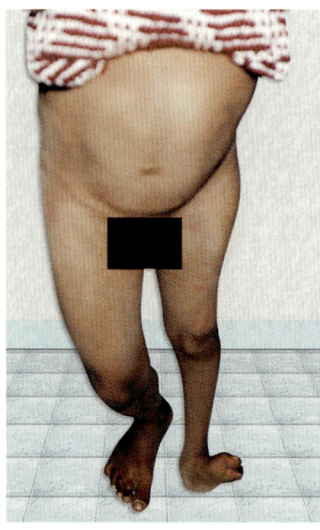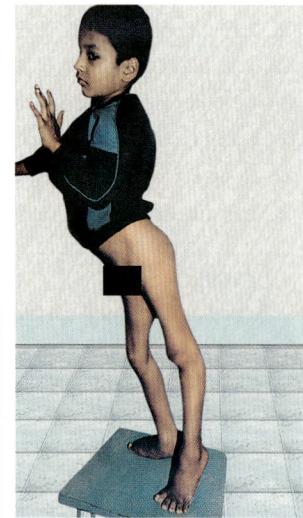

Fig. 2.33: Congenital shortening of thigh and leg bones with disorganised ankle and foot (left lower limb). The patient is compensating the shortening by flexing other side hip and knee.

Fig. 2.34: To compensate shortening of lower limb (congenital shortening of leg) that limb needs to be kept in equinus at ankle-foot and hyperextension of knee.

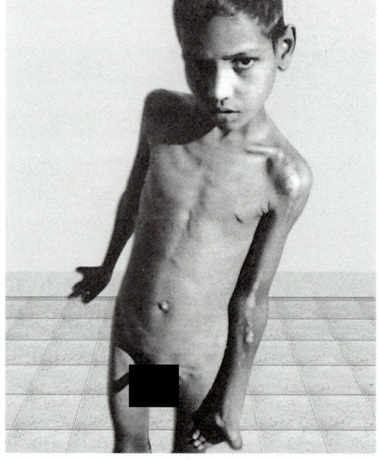

Fig. 2.37: Linear sebaceous naevus syndrome with lengthening of the left upper limb. Note the linear pattern of sebaceous naevi almost in continuity in front of shoulder, arm, elbow, wrist and thumb. There are congenital anomalies in hand along with lengthening of left upper limb.

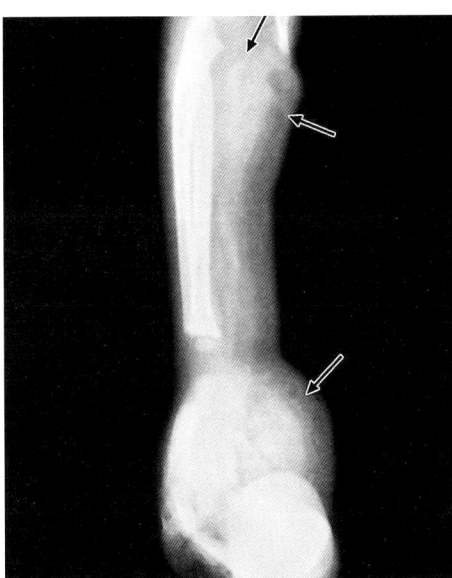

Fig. 2.38: X-ray of forearm and hand showing the swelling and the calcified mass shadow in haemangiomatous zone in front of forearm and hand. Cautions excision of pathological mass may be possible, however, functional recovery (may be) usually remains limited.

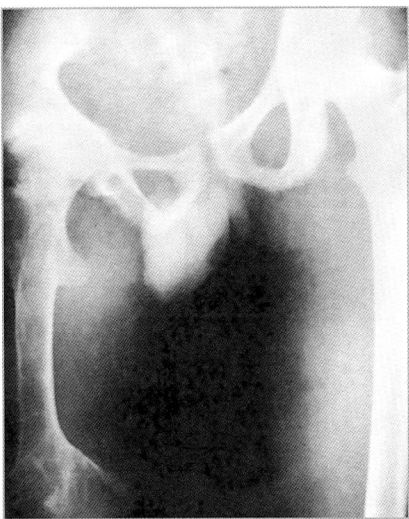

Fig. 2.40: Dyschondroplasia. Note metaphyseal enlargement, thickened shaft, shortening of bone and mottled epiphysis.

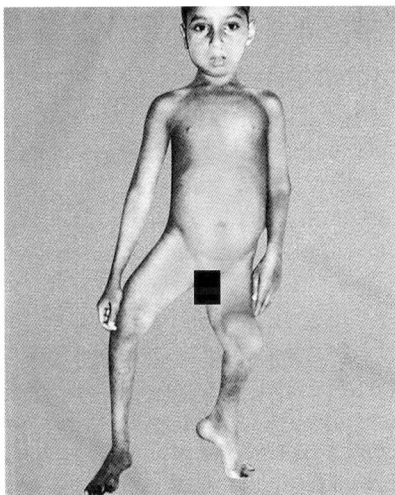

Fig. 2.41: Dyschondroplastic left femur and tibia.

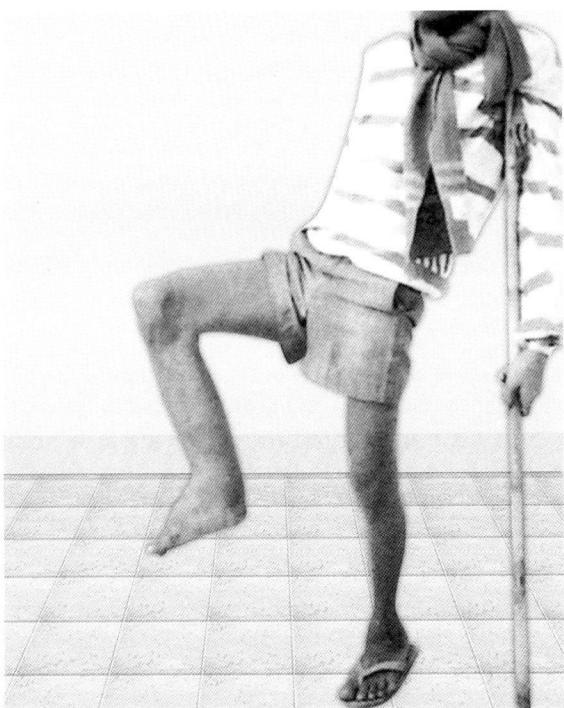

Fig. 2.39: Congenital cavernous lymphangioma with lymphoedema leading to enlargement of right lower limb (both length and breadthwise).

Lymphangioma is congenital malformation of lymphatic system and usually occurs in children before 2 years of age. On the basis of size of sinuses, histologically, it can be subclassified into cavernous lymphangioma and cystic hygroma. Cavernous lymphangioma can be effectively treated by surgical excision followed by the injection of OK-432 (an anticancer agent showing immunopotentiation—Picibanil)

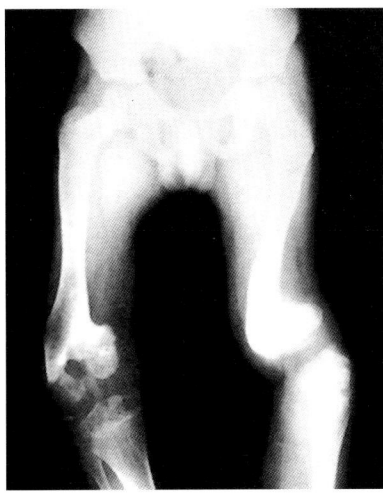

Fig. 2.42: X-ray of the same boy **(Fig. 2.39).**

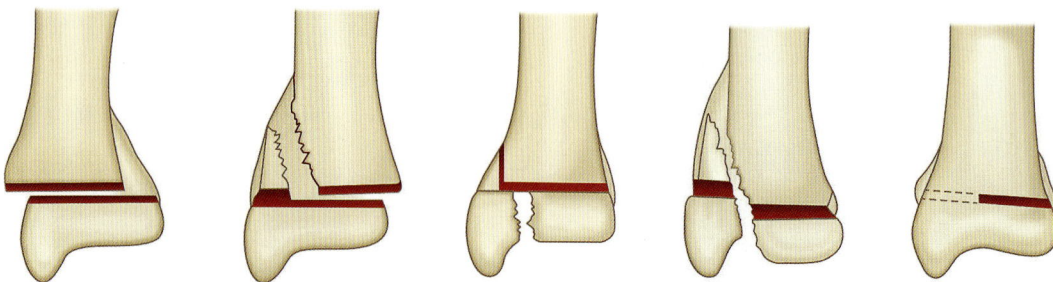

Fig. 2.43: Salter-Harris classification of physeal fracture.

- Underlying bone is tender
- Neighbouring joint usually not affected.

X-ray: Usually, there is localised area of irregular rarefaction surrounded by sclerosed zone, however, there may be varied appearance.

Excision of the affected zone usually cures it. Thorough curettage, culture from the curetted material (organism may be cultured in about 50% of cases) and the indicated antibiotics—may also be line of treatment.

Implant – related Osteomyelitis

With spurts in using the implants for treating the fractures, the incidence of implant related infection osteomyelitis is also on increase. An implant – associated infection is defined as a host – immune response to one or more microbial pathogens on an indwelling implant. Based on mode or timing of presentation of infection Coventry described (modified by Fitzgerald et al.) a three stage classification system for implant related infections: type 1. Infection occurs in immediate postoperative period caused by infected hematomas or superficial wound infections.

Type 2 infections also most probably set in at the time of surgery but its manifestations are delayed (6 to 24 months) due to small inoculum or organism of low virulence, type 3 infections are least common manifesting usually after 2 year, and infection is by haematogenous spread.

Fractures (Tables 2.2 to 2.5)

Fracture of Long Bones

Fracture is the mechanical disruption of mineralized bone along with its collagenous matrix.

Examination of closed fracture markedly differs from that of an open one. *Open fractures* are almost always diagnosed by the patient/relatives themselves. What is required is, *after relevant X-ray, war-footed management of these open fractures with the sole aim of converting them to closed type.* Fractures around the joints and intra-articular fractures present more or less with joint problems.

Fracture in Children

The long bones of children have epiphyses and physes, the latter being the weakest point in the bones of children. Their integrity and anatomy must be preserved/restored to as normal as possible to avoid growth arrest and angular deformities. The fractures may involve epiphyses and physes. Based upon the morphology of fractures as seen in X-ray Salter and Harris have classified these fractures into five types (*See* **Fig. 2.43**):

Type I: Epiphysis is completely separated from the metaphysis usually resulting from a shearing or avulsion force, and tends to occur in early childhood.

Type II: It is the most common type. The fracture plane runs transversely across the growth plate to a variable extent and then exits through the metaphysis on opposite side forming a spike (**Thurston-Holland sign**) attached to the epiphyseal plate. It usually occurs in children over 10 years of age due to shearing or avulsion force.

Type III: Starting from the intra-articular side, there is fracture through the epiphysis and the fracture runs through the physis and exits peripherally. It is less common type.

Type IV: There is more or less vertical splitting of epiphysis and physis and the splitting fracture line exits through the metaphysis, with the joint incongruity.

Type V: There is compression or crush fracture of the physis (hardly discernible in X-ray) and it produces permanent damage with inevitable growth arrest and future deformity.

Green Stick Fracture

Here there is fracture of the mineralized bone leaving the collagenous matrix intact.

It is an incomplete fracture in which only one cortex is broken with the fractured ends telescoped within each other, while the opposite cortex usually bends in the same direction, as occurs in an attempt of breaking a green bamboo stick. Infants and children are brought with bowed affected part, which is swollen and tender at the fracture site, however, limb can be used to a fairly good extent. Since, the fracture is always incomplete and impacted, there is no abnormal movement at the fracture site.

Features of a Fracture

- History of optimum indirect or direct violence
- Immediate or delayed appearance of ecchymosis

TABLE 2.2: Classification of fractures (Considering broad etiological factors).

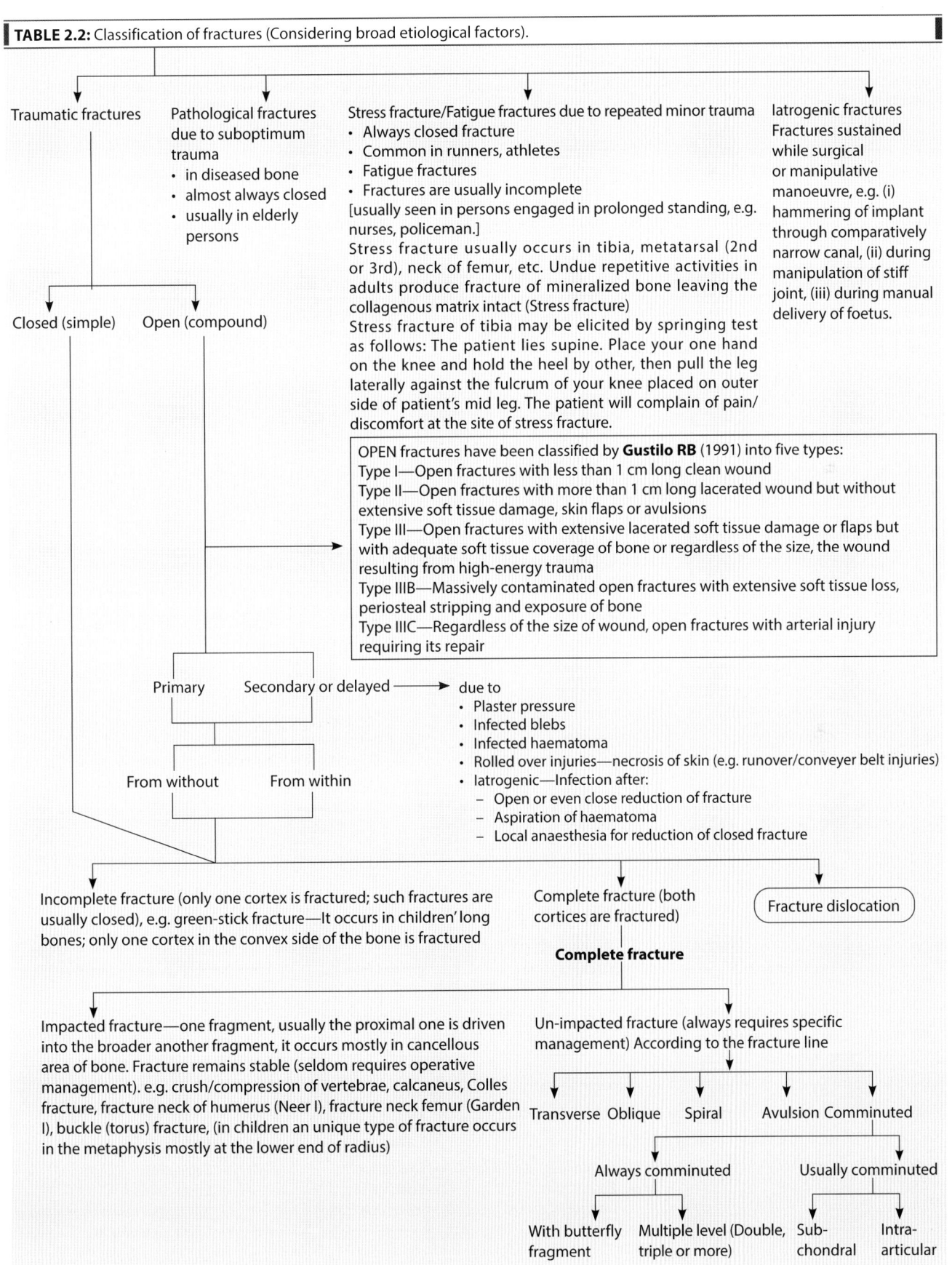

Contd...

Contd...

Displacements of Fractures: (Distal fragment is always to be considered for describing displacements in relation to the proximal fragment)

(i) Shifts—Upward (overlap), downward (distraction)
(ii) Tilts/Angulation—(consider convex side) mainly the valgus, varus, anterior or posterior angulation,
(iii) Rotation/twist—external/internal
Translation:
- Sidewards (lateral and medial)
- Forwards/backwards

NB: Ping-pong fracture—a depressed fracture of skull resembling the indentation that can be produced with fingers pressing firmly on a ping pong ball.

TABLE 2.3: Working time table for different stages of uncomplicated fracture healing—in weeks (Based on Perkins G.).

Child, Upper limb, long bone, Spiral fracture	Ensheathing callus (gluing) 5–6 days (3/4th week)	Clinical union 1½ (weeks)	Consolidation 3 (weeks)	Radiological union 6 (weeks)

For each of the following, multiply by 2
- Adult
- Lower limb long bone fracture
- Transverse fracture

TABLE 2.4: Salient features of different stages of fracture healing.

	Ensheathing callus	**Clinical union**	**Consolidation**	**Radiological union**
Symptoms	• Pain +++	• Pain +	• No pain	• No pain on any stress
	• Swelling +++	• Swelling ++	• Swelling +	• Swelling ±
	• Cannot bear any stress	• Can bear gravitational stress but not angulatory one	• Can bear up to angulation stress	
	• Two ends at fracture move separately	• Two ends at fracture move as one	• Two ends at fracture move as one	
Signs	• Warm	• Slight warm	• Local temperature normal	
	• Firm fusiform swelling—due to organising haematoma and soft tissue swelling over and around the fractured ends, fracture ends can be felt in displaced fracture	• Fracture ends not felt		
		• Surface regular		
		• Firm or hard swelling	• Swelling less and hard	• Hard, more or less uniform
	• Tenderness +++	• Tenderness +	• No tenderness	• Non-tender slightly fusiform swelling
	• Surface at fracture site smooth except at the spiky ends	• Fracture ends not felt	• Surface regular	
		• Surface regular		
X-ray	• Fracture line clearly visible	• Fracture line visible	• Fracture line may be visible	• Fracture line not visible
	• Hazy soft tissue swelling	• Callus	• Callus	• Callus
		– Exo callus	• Exo callus	• Exo callus –
		– Endo callus	• Endo callus	• Endo callus ±
		– Interstitial callus	• Interstitial callus	• Interstitial callus converted to trabecular bone
				• Medullary continuity ±

TABLE 2.5: Complicated status of fractures.

	Delayed union	Ununited fracture (Rarely it can include delayed union, but left to as such it usually proceeds to non-union)	Non-union — Fibrous union	Non-union — Pseudoarthrosis
1	2	3	4	5
1. Pain	+	+	None/slight	None
2. Swelling	+	±	+	None
3. Local temperature	± ↑	± ↑	Normal	Normal
4. Movement at fracture site	May yield on stress	Present	Slight movement on stress (Patient may not be aware of)	Painless hypermobility (patient complains of it)
5. Angulation	May bear	Cannot bear any stress	Slight yield on angulation stress	No need to test—being hypermobile, e.g. "double elbow" (Refer Fig. 5.7)
6. Tenderness at fracture end	Tender	Tender	Not tender	Not tender
7. Surrounding muscles	Wasting +	Wasting + (or slightly)	Wasting ±	Marked wasting
8. Functional affection	Varying	Fully affected	Not much	Markedly affected
9. Optimum period	Optimum period for stages of clinical union and consolidation delayed	Optimum period crossed (but not to the limit of nonunion) for clinical union still there is stress-mobility at fracture site	24–36 weeks (on average)	24–36 weeks or more (on average)
10. Bondage of fracture ends	Organising callus (but delayed)	Fibrous tissue	Dense fibrous tissue	A cavity forms in fibrous tissue lined by pseudosynovial tissue
11. X-ray	Callus not sufficient; Fracture line visible	Callus none or irrelevant Fracture line clearly visible Ends rarefied Medullary canal open	Callus: • atrophic type—no callus • Oligotrophic-slight, irrelevant callus • hypertrophic—elephantoid callus at the fracture ends Fracture ends may not be sclerosed Medullary cavity may not be closed	Callus none; fracture ends rounded and sclerosed (as if there was no fracture) Medullary canal closed
12. Suggestion	Prolonged immobilisation; Osteoinduction; Phemister's graft	Osteoinduction Open reduction— • internal fixation • bone graft • replacement arthroplasty	Osteoinduction Phemister's graft May require open reduction and internal and or external fixation	Open reduction, freshening of sclerosed ends Internal fixation/external fixation, e.g. Ilizarov's method Bone grafting ±

- Immediate feeling of pain; may be some rattling noise during the fracture; difficulty or inability in using that limb; gradually increasing swelling; deformities according to displacements, angulation and rotations
- Localised persistent bony tenderness; squeezing of proximal and distal end of fractured bone leads to pain at the site of fracture. To elicit tenderness, press through healthy tissue (pressure on contused soft tissue may be misleading)
- *Crepitus:* If one gets crepitus during casual examination, it should be noted, but do not attempt to demonstrate it
- Irregular bony ends (with or without gap) may be felt
- Abnormal mobility at the suspected fracture site; however in impacted fractures (e.g. **Colles fracture**, fracture upper end of humerus, Garden type I fracture of neck of femur), where one fracture end is partially or completely telescoped within another end, there will be

no mobility at the fracture site and patient can invariably use the limb, of course, with variable pain
- May even present with early complications of fractures, e.g. wrist drop in fracture shaft humerus; skin necrosis in dislocation of the ankle; effect of partial cessation of blood supply—early features of ischaemic changes (as given in Chapter Elbow)—**Volkmann's ischaemia**.

Juxta-articular and Intra-articular Fractures
- They may be associated ligamentous injury of the joint (especially the intra-articular ones)
- Presentation mainly concerns with adjoining or affected joints
- The affected bony ends may be widened and tender
- Joint movements are painfully restricted
- The concerned joint is swollen and tender
- Deformities are due to angulation and subchondral collapse of bones
- In the knee joint, stress tests must be done to recognise, the possible internal derangements of the knee joint
- In *battered baby syndrome*, the fractures are usually juxta-articular with/without intra-articular communication **(Fig. 2.43A)**.

Pathological Fractures (Figs. 2.44 to 2.46)
- History of minor trauma (suboptimal for that age and bone). The bone is inherently weak due to some local destructive lesion or generalised bone weakening.

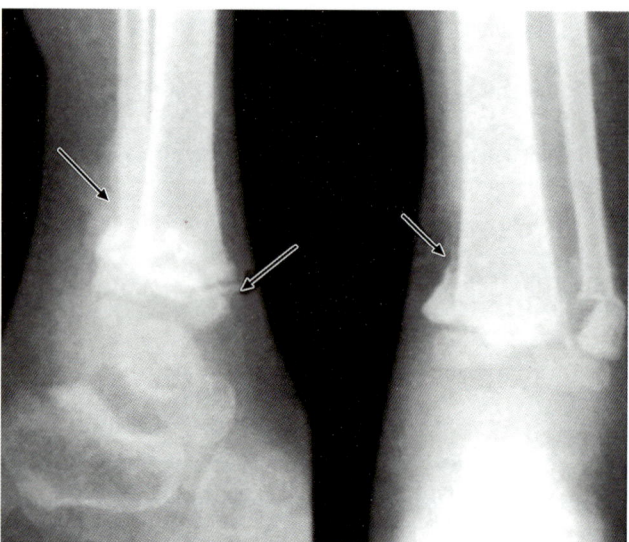

Fig. 2.43A: Multiple injuries of twisting strain produced in same ankle—battered baby.

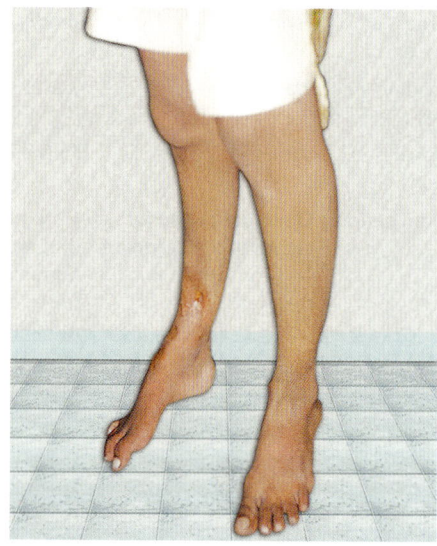

Fig. 2.45: Osteomyelitis lower end of tibia producing shortening and posterior bowing deformity—due to malunited pathological fracture.

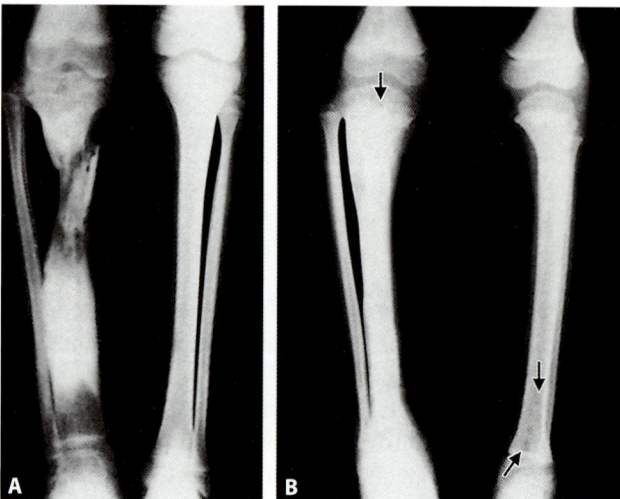

Figs. 2.44A and B: (A) Extensive osteomyelitis of right tibia with pathological fractures and sequestrating out necrosed segment. It is bound to end up in a shorter leg. (B) Shortening of right tibia due to chronic osteomyelitis with affection of growth epiphysis.

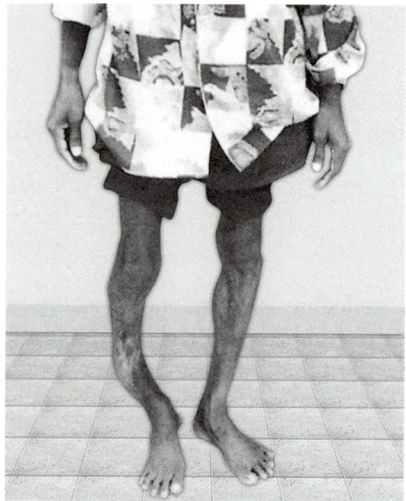

Fig. 2.46: Malunited pathological fracture in osteomyelitis with marked bowing and shortening of leg.

- May be history of earlier local pathological lesion with persistent or occasional pain at the site, with or without swelling.
- Enquire for general debilitating conditions like diabetes mellitus, tabes dorsalis, alcoholism, malnutrition and prolonged hypoproteinaemia, prolonged morbidity, osteomalacia, Paget's disease, malignancy, osteogenesis imperfecta **(Figs. 1.18A to 1.21B and 2.45)**.
- **Osteogenesis imperfecta** is a disease of mesenchymal tissue with defective or deficient collagen in bone, skin, sclerae and dentin. Clinically, multiple fractures in osteoporosed bones with bowing of long bones, blue sclerae, dentinogenesis imperfecta form the *diagnostic triad*. There is no specific laboratory test to confirm the diagnosis. It has been broadly classified as (a) *Osteogenesis imperfecta congenita* in which there are multiple wormian bones around the base of skull, evidence of multiple fractures, bowing of long bones, short extremities and generalized osteoporosis; (b) *Osteogenesis imperfecta tarda*, which may be of type 1—where there is bowing of long bones, OR, type 2—it is of milder type without bowing. Healing of fractures is usually achieved, however, great care is required in handling, supporting and bracing in the initial stage. The bisphosphonates has been used to reduce osteoclast-mediated bone resorption. Telescoping medullary rod (or expandable rods) with small flanges at proximal and distal ends has been used to prevent fractures of long bones in their entire length with simultaneously coping with the growing long bone **(Refer Fig. 1.23)**.
- After maturity the selected deformities of long bones may be corrected by osteotomy (ies) to improve the function and look as far as possible
- **Osteoporosis**—a systemic bone disease, progressing with the population longevity, and characterised by low bone mass and microarchitectural deterioration of bone tissue with a consequent increase in bone fragility and susceptibility to fracture; gradual dorso-lumbar and lumbar kyphosis and loss in height.

Complications of Fractures

Whenever a fracture is diagnosed one must look for its possible complications.

(i) Early Complications (0–2 weeks)

- *General*: Haemorrhage, *shock*, acute respiratory distress syndrome (ARDS), *fat embolism*, crush syndrome, thromboembolism, fracture fever; infection, *tetanus*, gas gangrene **(Figs. 2.48A and B)** in open fractures
- *Necrotising fasciitis:* It is a progressive rapidly spreading inflammatory infection (due to aerobic, anaerobic or mixed flora) located in the deep fascia with secondary

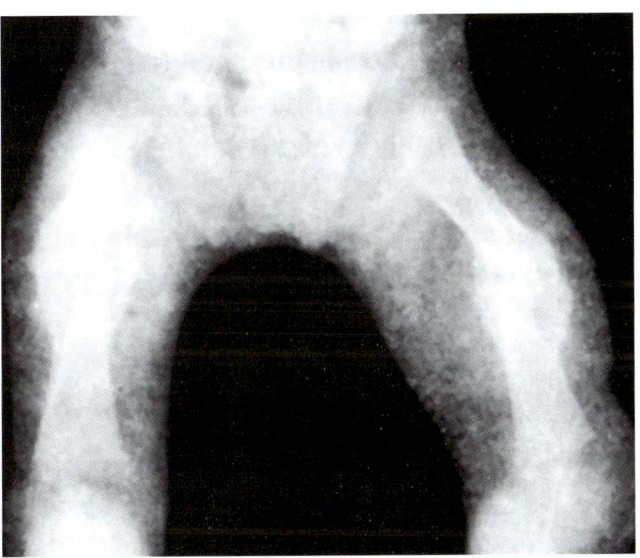

Fig. 2.47: Osteogenesis imperfecta with multiple fractures of femoral shaft. *See also* **Figs. 1.18A, 1.18B, 1.19, 1.20.**

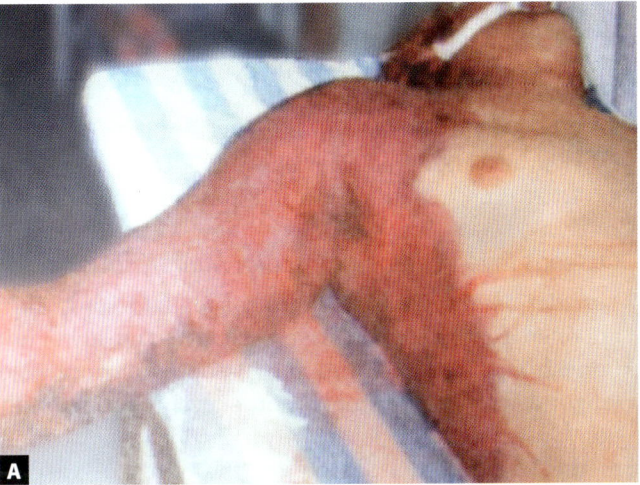
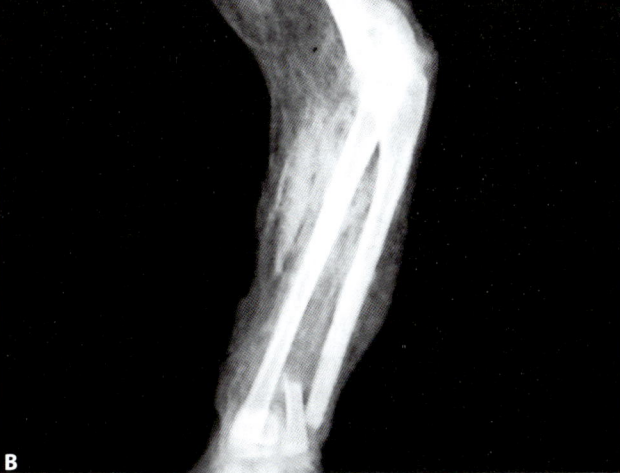

Figs. 2.48A and B: (A) Acute gas gangrene (*Courtesy:* Dr Rajgopal Shenoy K); (B) Extensive linear gas along muscles and soft tissue planes—in gas gangrene.

necrosis of the subcutaneous tissues. It also presents, radiologically, in almost similar fashion due to presence of air in subcutaneous plane. Though the clinical picture may vary, but the infection usually progresses rapidly along the deep fascia plane and unless attended promptly, high morbidity and mortality is usual outcome

- *Local*
  - Compounding (primary) at the site
  - Affections of peripheral nerves. (In spinal injuries—damage of spinal cord)
  - Affections of main blood vessels (partial—leading to ischaemia; complete—leading to gangrene)
  - Torn/ruptured tendon
  - Blister formation
  - Acute Volkmann's ischaemia.

(ii) Intermediate Complications (2–12 weeks)

- *General*: Deep vein thrombosis, pulmonary embolism; tetanus; *decubitus complications* (renal failure, pressure sore, chest infection)
- *Local: compartmental syndrome:* Setting of the features of ischaemic changes in hand or foot; development of different deformities and stiffness of adjoining joints
- *Secondary compounding of the fracture* due to plaster pressure, infected blebs, rolled over injury (e.g. run-over, conveyer belt injuries), iatrogenic (infection after open reduction, aspiration of fracture haematoma, local anaesthesia for reduction of closed fracture)
- *Myositis ossificans*: Basically, it is a subperiosteal calcification, though it has been thought to occur in muscles. Usually, injuries around elbow and hips, are associated with myositis ossificans or heterotopic ossification. Other established risk factors for heterotopic ossification include head injury (CNS injury); severe burn; personal factors, such as gender, age, and probably genetics.
  - *In early stage:* Area of impending myositis (usually cubital fossae, anteroinferomedial aspect of groin, around the shoulder, etc.) feels indurated and resistant, warm and slightly tender, with limitation of movements at the affected joint
    - *X-ray*: Fluffy to irregularly calcified radio-opaque area with no definite margin and no trabecular pattern of bone (usually seen after 3 weeks).
  - *In late cases:* Area neither tender nor warm, localised plaque like bony mass may be felt after 6 weeks. Though movements improve but are still limited
    - *X-ray*: Localised, regular, condensed radio-opaque shadow with sclerosed, circumscribed margin and usually not related to site.
- *Nerve affection*: e.g. *lateral popliteal nerve palsy* (due to pressure by splint or bed)
- *Plaster disease:* (Stiffness of joints, wasting of muscles, skin changes, pressure point sores).

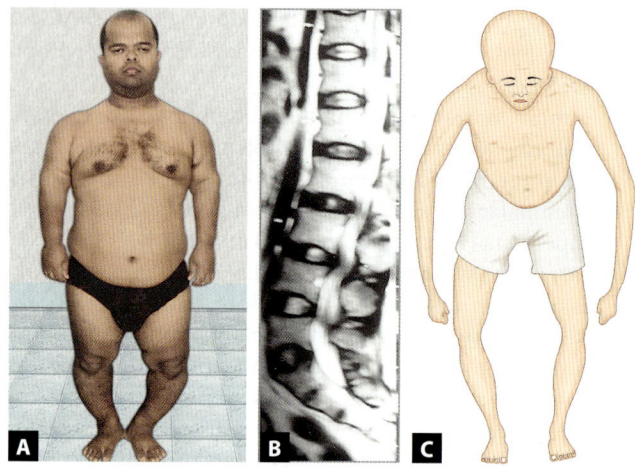

Figs. 2.49A to C: Achondroplasia: (A) Patient presented with the features of lumbar canal stenosis; confirmed by MRI (B); outline of a patient of Paget's disease (C).

(iii) Late Complications (after 12 weeks)

- *General complications*: Accidental neurosis; depressive psychosis; tetanus
- *Local complications*:
  - Malunion
  - Delayed union
  - Non-union
  - Sudeck's osteoneurodystrophy
  - Avascular necrosis of bone
  - Post-traumatic degenerative arthrosis
  - Friction tendinitis
  - Tendon rupture
  - Growth disturbances
  - Delayed nerve complication (e.g. carpal tunnel syndrome, tardy ulnar palsy)
  - Stiffness of the joint, which may even be ankylosed.

Interposition of soft tissue in between the fractured fragments is a potent cause of delayed and non-union. It should be suspected when:

- There is no sensation of crepitus while manipulating the fracture
- When there is wide gap in between the fragments—clinically and/or radiologically
- There is no, or hardly any, callus formation (in X-ray).

Osseous Involvement in Vascular Malformations

Vascular malformations are rare congenital lesions which are often associated with skeletal changes (mostly in long bones), such as bony and soft tissue hypertrophy, leg length discrepancy, compression effects (denting on the bony cortex), sclerotic changes, rarefaction, etc. According to the International Society for the Study of Vascular anomalies, vascular anomalies have been classified into either *vascular tumours* (mostly haemangiomas) or *vascular*

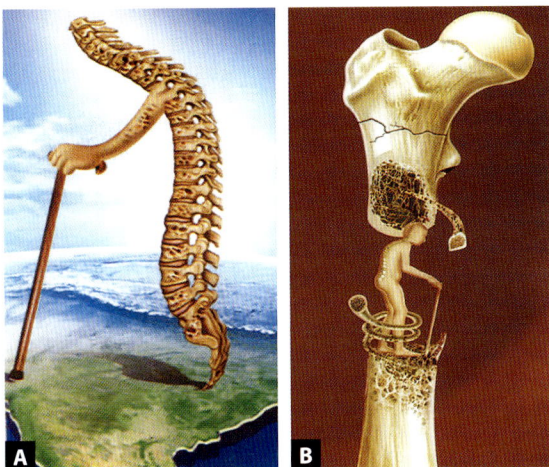

Figs. 2.50A and B: (A) Spinal posture and disability due to osteoporosis; (B) Osteoporosis leading to pathological fracture, spinal deformity and disabilities represented by a person (standing in between the pathological fractured bone-ends) with dorsal kyphosis and walking stick in right hand. Note the osteoporosis texture of femur.

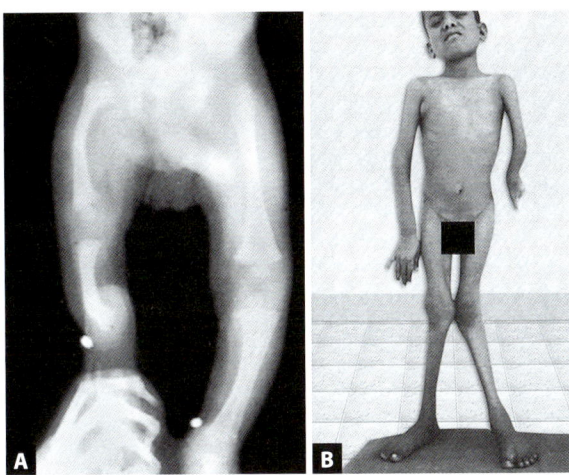

Figs. 2.52A and B: (A) Congenital shortening and bowing of ipsilateral femur and tibia and absence of fibula; (B) Congenital shortening of arm, forearm, and hand with ankylosed joints (elbow, wrist, fingers and thumb) and marked genu valgum with comparatively long legs.

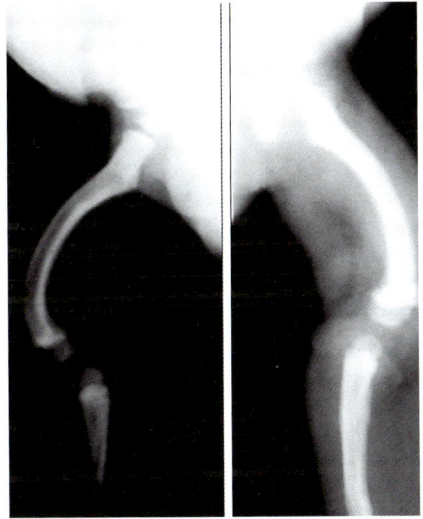

Fig. 2.51: Congenital anterolateral bowing of femur.

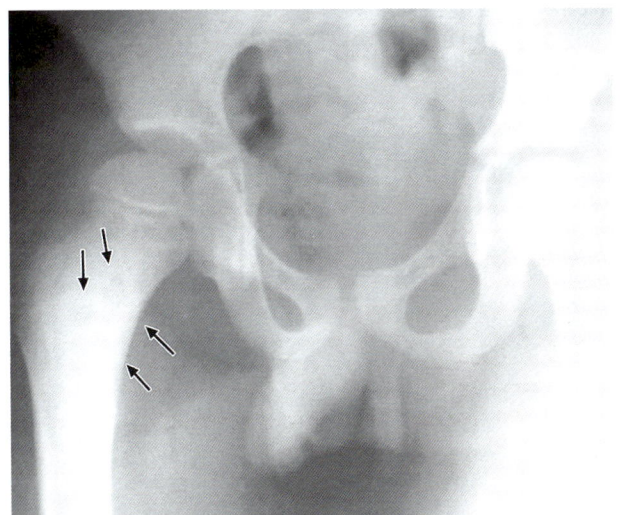

Fig. 2.53: Brodie's abscess in upper end of femur and cervicotrochanteric region.

malformations. Haemangiomas are characterised by endothelial proliferation, a phase of rapid postnatal growth followed by slow evolution, which is almost complete by 10 years of age. These should be managed by non-operative modes except when there is recalcitrant ulceration or bleeding or functional problems (e.g. dyspnoea, obstruction of the upper eyelid, etc.).

Vascular malformations are rare and are congenital caused by a defect during vascular embryogenesis. These can be either high flow lesions (arteriovenous malformations) which usually manifest clearly by 6 years of age or low flow lesions (venous malformations) which are often visible early in life either as a small blue patch or a soft blue mass usually manifesting clearly by the age of 1 year.

Skeletal changes are commonly associated with vascular malformations while they are rarely seen in conjunction with haemangiomas. Anatomically, vascular malformations can be either capillary, venous, lymphatic, arterial, or combination of the above.

Achondroplasia (Figs. 2.49A and B)

Achondroplasia is a congenital development disorder of unknown etiology affecting mainly the long bones–more in females. *Achondroplasia is one of the most common form of osteochondrodysplasia.* It is the most frequent form of short-limbed dwarfism caused by mutations in the $FGFR_3$ gene. It has autosomal dominant inheritance, though most cases are sporadic. The gene responsible for it was mapped to chromosome 4(4p16.3) (Velinor met. et al). These dwarfs due to achondroplasia grow to a maximum of 122 cm in boys and 117 cm in girls. Dwarfism with disproportionate shortness

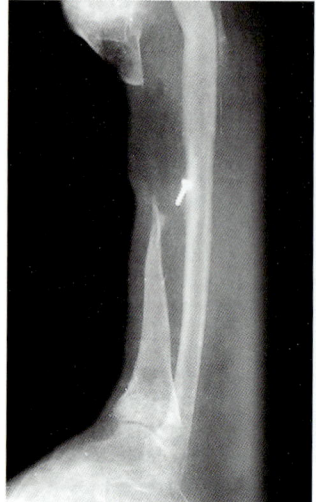 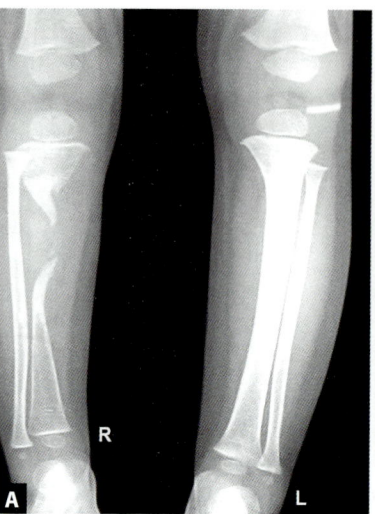 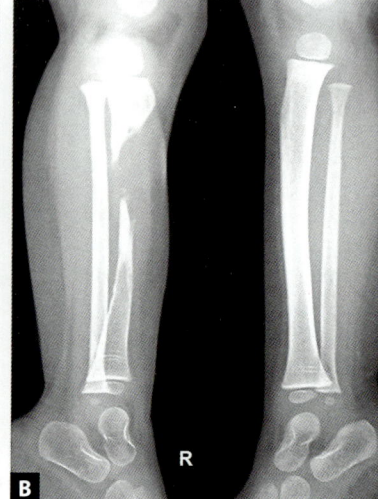 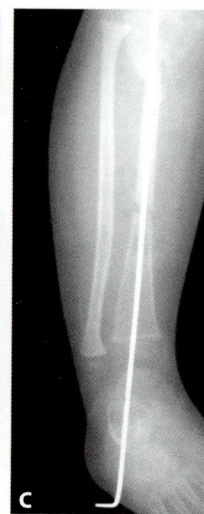

Fig. 2.54: Chronic osteomyelitis of tibia with sequestrated out upper diaphyseal portion (following operative fixation of fracture—note a left-out screw lying embedded in soft tissue) and overgrowth of fibula.

Figs. 2.55A to C: Chronic osteomyelitis of tibia with sequestrated out upper diaphyseal portion and overgrowth of fibula (A & B). Gap created due to sequestration has been made up by using a segment taken from opposite fibula as bone graft fixed with k-wire (C).

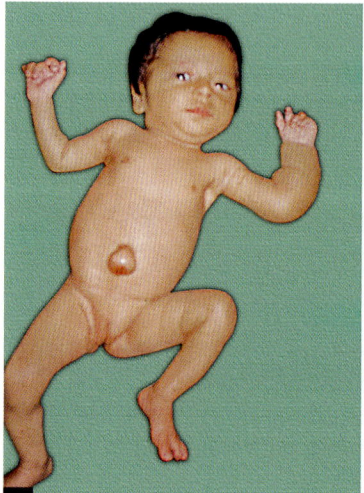 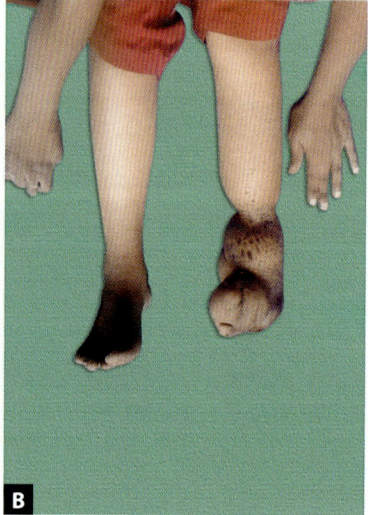 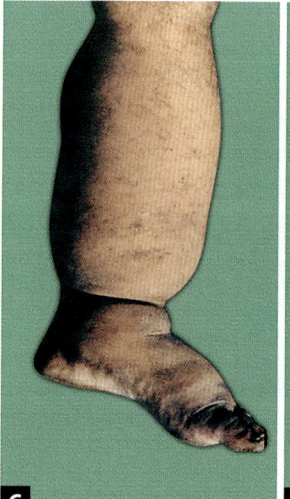 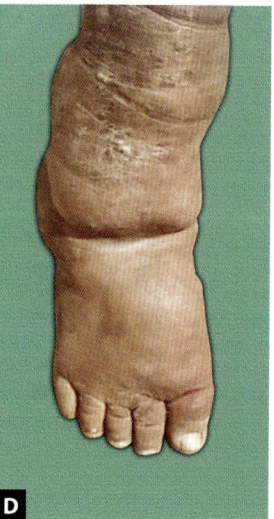

Figs. 2.56A to D: (A) Congenital lymphoedema left upper limb; (B) Congenital lymphoedema of left lower leg, ankle and foot following a constriction ring. There is also congenital malformation of right hand and fingers (syndactylism); (C) Filarial lymphoedema with elephantiasis, without fissuring, nodulation or ulceration; (D) Filarial lymphoedema with fissuring.

of trunk and extremities has many causes, however, the association of atlantoaxial instability, dysplasias of hip, and malalignment of lower extremities should be a matter of concern. Its incidence is about 1 in 26,000 to 28,000 live birth (Oridi IM et al. 1995). It is characterised by rhizomelic, short-limbed dwarfism relative macrocephaly, frontal bossing, a depressed nasal bridge, bowing of the lower limbs, short humerus, trident hands, variation in the length of the fingers, and lack of full extension of elbow, which is the earliest clinical manifestation and the most common abnormality of the upper limb (it is due to posterior bowing of the distal humerus, which if greater than 20°, leads to loss of extension of elbow).

Management is mainly surgical to correct any obvious deformity and limb lengthening is primarily done to restore proportion of spine height to lower limb height.

Paget's Disease (Osteitis Deformans) (Fig. 2.49C)

Its cause is not exactly known. Environmental, some viral (slow) infection and genetic factor have been suspected

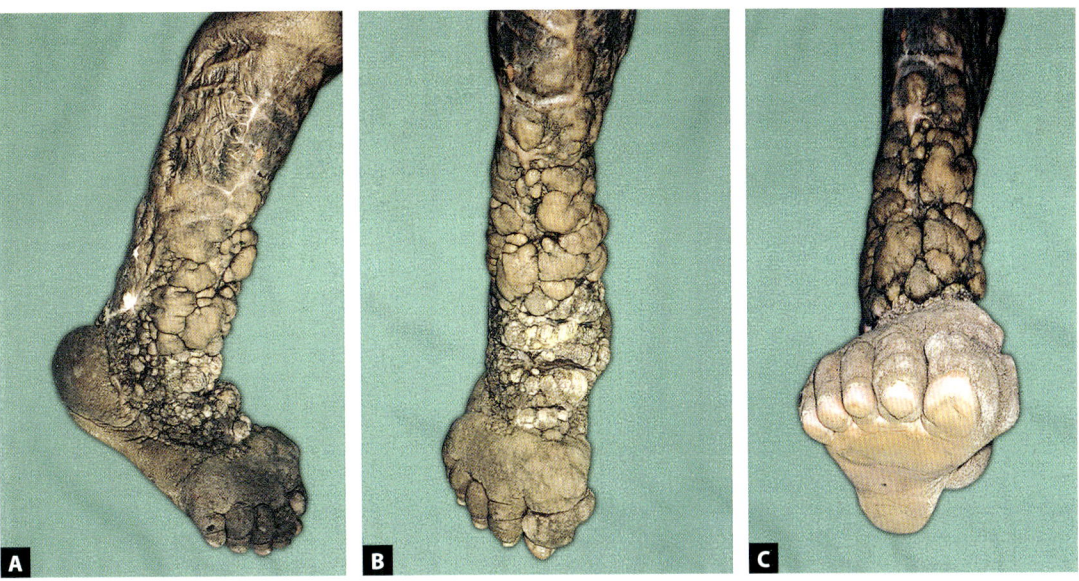

Figs. 2.57A to C: Filarial elephantiasis with deep fissures and ulcers and warty nodulations. Note that the sole and toes are normal.

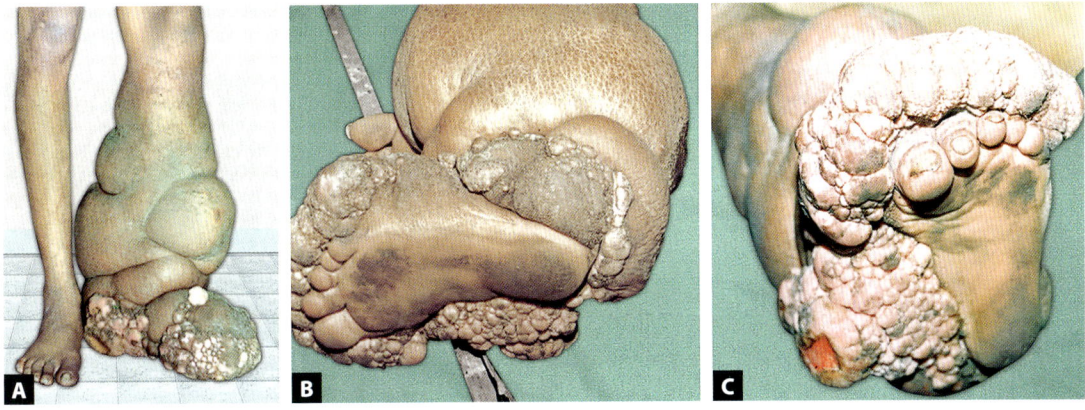

Figs. 2.58A to C: Elephantiasis with enormous swelling of the foot and ankle, with furrows, lobulations, nodules, ulcerations and warty projections. Note that the toes and sole are not affected (**tortoise foot**).
Courtesy: Dr KD Sharan.

to play some part in its causation. There is an increased resorption of bone combined with rapid growth of new bone, disordered architecture and decreased mechanical strength.

Except the bones of hands and feet, any bone may be affected. Mostly it affects several skeletal segments (polyostotic, but it may affect even 1 bone-monostatic). Paget's disease was first described by Sir James Paget (a surgeon and pathologist trained in London UK) in 1877. Paget's disease bone has been even seen in medieval skeleton (Wells c 1975). It is second most common (after osteoporosis) in United kingdom. The typical bony deformities are increased girth of calvarium, thoracic kyphosis, genu varum, and flattening of vertebrae leading to shortening of spine. Thus, the arms look disproportionately longer as compared to trunk. Most of patients remain asymptomatic throughout life. Patient may complain of dull pain in bone even at rest. Spontaneous fracture may develop in affected bone. Rarely (secondary) osteogenic sarcoma may develop.

It affects the old people of mostly the Anglo-Saxon race. The unregulated bone turnover is the main disorder. In the beginning, there is excessive osteoclastic resorption (lytic phase) followed by excessive bone formation (osteoblastic phase) with cortical and trabecular thickening.

X-ray in the lytic phase presents "blade of grass" or "flame" appearance starting at the end of bone and extending towards diaphysis in advancing inverted 'V' shaped lytic lesion. Later on, in osteoblastic phase, there is sclerosis and thickening of cortices and trabeculae. SPECT – CT improves identification of Paget's disease of bone – (Favid 2010) Scintigraphy, usually show hot spots. In MRI, the marrow signals remain normal. In biopsy, a typical mosaic pattern with wide lamellae, irregular cement lines, and fibrovascular connective tissue is seen.

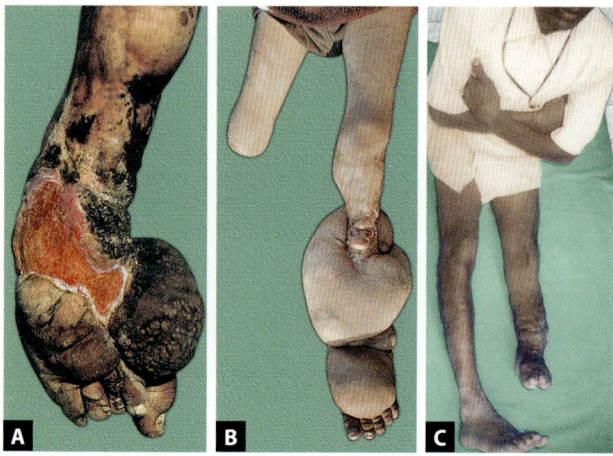

Figs. 2.59A to C: (A) Post-traumatic elephantiasis and ulcer should be treated with below – knee amputation and suitable prosthesis; (B) Post-traumatic lymphoedema of left leg and foot: right lower limb suffered traumatic amputation—A challenge case; by proper plastic surgery left lower limb can be preserved for weight bearing and aided ambulation; (C) Shortening of left lower limb leg following neglected compound crush injury in the childhood. May be lengthened by Ilizarov distraction.

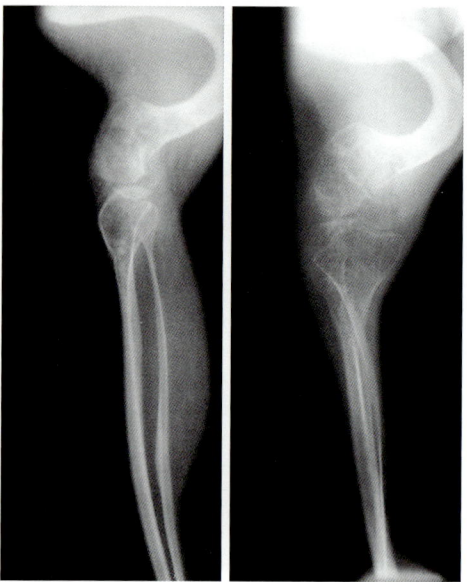

Fig. 2.61: Congenital acute bowing of femur. Operative correction is very difficult, and hardly fruitful. Patient should be encouraged to use walking aids for mobility (such as walker, or crutches).

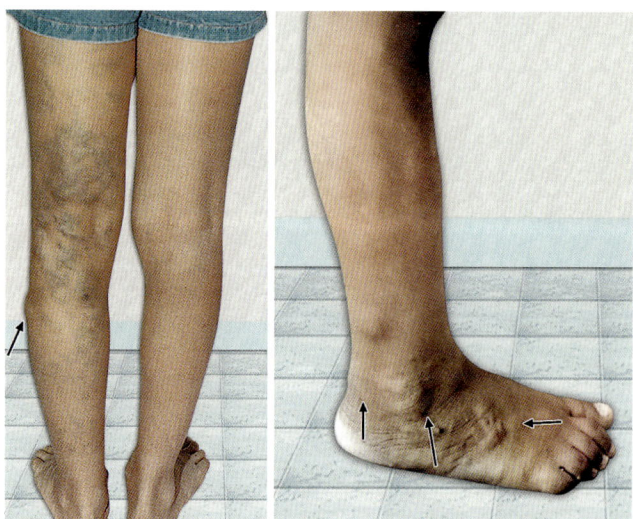

Fig. 2.60: Congenital varicose veins.

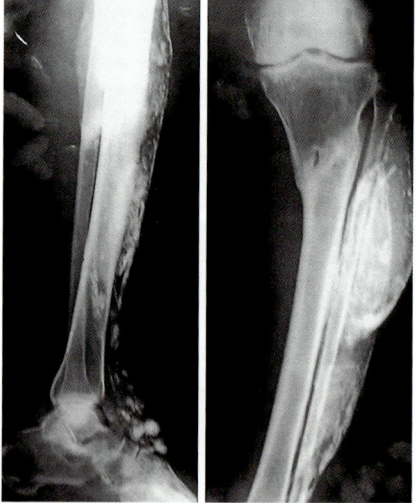

Fig. 2.62: Old traumatic infection—osteomyelitis with collection of pus and with calcified loose bodies in relation to fibula. Treatment should be excision of fibula (leaving the ends) and pathological tissues; antibiotics according to culture and chemosensitivity.

Management of main disease is by NSAIDs, calcitonin or bisphosphonates.

Osteoporosis (Figs. 2.50A and B)

It is a chronic, progressive multifactorial systemic bone disorder resulting in increased bone fragility due to low bone mass measured as bone mineral density (BMD) and microarchitectural deterioration of bone tissue. It is one of the most important and most common medical disorders affecting the post-menopausal women. Low bone mass is the main determinant of osteoporosis and *determination of bone mineral density (BMD) is the single best method for diagnosing osteoporosis* and to assess future risk of osteoporotic fractures. Bone mass is maximum up to third decade which is maintained till the age of 50. From then, resorption predominates and the bone mass starts to decrease.

Osteoporosis was first officially recognised as a disease by *WHO in 1994* and was defined as: *"Osteoporosis is a systemic disease characterised by low bone mass and microarchitectural deterioration of bone tissue leading to enhanced bone fragility and a consequent increase in fracture risk"*. In osteoporosis, there is decrease in bone density (mass per unit volume) with a normally mineralised trabecular pattern greater than would be expected for an individual of a given age and sex.

Literally *'osteoporosis'* means thin and porous bone. It is the most common metabolic bone disease in the world. In India, about 80% of women above 40 years of age and 50% of men above 60 years of age are either osteopenic or osteoporotic.

Total testosterone resulted in the most productive sex hormone for the loss of bone mass. Hence, it is important to evaluate sex hormones in males with osteoporosis for a correct and 'physiological' therapy.

Although osteoporosis is debilitating condition, it does not affect the life expectancy directly and it is preventable.

Besides several vague causes (such as poor nutrition, lack of physical activities, obesity, multiparity, etc.) intensive neo-adjuvant chemotherapy for highly malignant osteosarcoma can also affect the bone mass. Any serious disease during the period of bone accumulation (e.g. a malignant bone tumour and its treatment) may predispose patients to *methotrexate osteopathy,* which is characterised by pain in the osteoporosed bones and an increase the risk of fracture.

Most of the patients of osteoporosis have generalised aches and pain. Progressive loss of height with thoracic kyphosis *(Dowager's hump)* gradually develops. There may be indigestion associated with pot belly. The patient may have episode of acute pain in the back while at rest or during routine activities like coughing, sneezing or straining. However, *the most common clinical manifestation of osteoporosis is an increased susceptibility to fracture,* rather condition is frequently asymptomatic until this point (of fracture). Fragility fracture, for which subjects with osteoporosis are at great risk.

Riggs *classified osteoporosis into two types: Type I or postmenopausal type* tends to occur at younger age group, and are more liable to sustain fractures of vertebrae and in the wrist region; cancellous bone loss is maximum in this type I osteoporosis. *Type II or senile type osteoporosis* occurs due to age-related bone loss and is more liable to sustain fractures in hip region. In this type II, there is relative universal bone loss. [Of course nasal spray of Salmon calcitonin is being claimed to retard the rate of bone absorption and thus reducing the risk of developing osteoporotic fractures and osteoporotic pain.]

Malaysian Osteoporosis Society (2012) has suggested a classification of osteoporosis as primary and secondary quoted by Babhulkar S (2016)

Primary Osteoporosis:
- Postmenopausal osteoporosis
- Age–related osteoporosis occurs in both sexes
- Idiopathic osteoporosis is rare

Secondary osteoporosis:
- *Endocrine:* Cushing's syndrome, hypogonadism, thyrotoxicosis, hyperthyroidism
- *Drugs:* glucocorticoids, heparin, anticonvulsants (phenytoin)
- *Chronic diseases:* Renal impairment, liver cirrhosis, malabsorption/postgastrectomy, chronic inflammatory polyarthropathies (e.g. rheumatoid arthritis)
- *Others:* Nutritional, multiple myeloma, malignancy, osteogenesis imperfecta.

For diagnosing osteoporosis, earlier, X-rays were the only tool, but by the time X-ray manifestations occur, the bone had already lost 50–70% of calcium. However, *nowadays, osteoporosis can be diagnosed even in its asymptomatic stage with the help of DEXA* (Dual Energy X-ray Absorptiometry). It is a quick, non-invasive, simple, precise, reproducible, and safe (using only 1/10th dose of normal X-ray), technology. The X-ray is composed of two energy levels that are absorbed by the bones and soft tissues differently, and from these differences, the computer calculates the level of calcium in the bones. Though the whole body can be scanned, only the hip, spine and sometimes forearm, wrist being the fracture prone sites, are scanned. The bone density measurement thus obtained is compared with that of a young adult (T-score), and to a reference value of persons of similar age and sex (Z-score). Severity of osteoporosis is estimated on the basis of WHO classification using T-score. WHO has attempted to define when the condition becomes pathological in terms of the estimation of BMD using *dual energy X-ray absorptiometry* (DEXA) scanning. A BMD of less than 2.5 standard deviations below the expected value for the particular age and sex is considered diagnostic.

Radiological indices of proximal femur such as cortical thickness indices and calcar-to-canal ratio, appear reliable in diagnosis of osteoporosis with less radiation exposure and also cost effective in comparison to DEXA scan. Cortical thickness index less or equal to 0.4 ± 0.03 and calcare-to-canal ratio less than or equal to 0.5 ± 0.02 fall into osteoporotic range (Burlic et al. 2019).

Ladies (usually more than 50 years old), complain of vague pain in the bones, more in the flat bones, more in the night, and features of fracture with even trivial injuries.

In adult patients:

WHO criteria for clinical Diagnosis of Osteoporosis.	
BMD (Bone Mineral Density T- score (femoral neck)	Diagnosis
T score > - 1	Normal
-1 > T score > - 2.5	Osteopenia(low bone mass)
T score ≤ - 2.5	Osteoporosis
T score ≤ - 2.5 with existing fracture	severe osteoporosis

"Osteoporosis" is defined as bone mineral density (BMD), as demonstrated by dual photon X-ray absorptiometry (DXA) scanning, of less than 2.5 SD below the young adult mean (the T-score). Children do not achieve their adult bone density until the third decade. Osteopenia is declared when the BMD is less than 1.0 SD below the young adult mean (the T-score). The term osteopenia is not recommended in children, because fracture thresholds have not been established in children for specific Z-scores. The term recommended by the ISCD is "low bone density for age" and is defined as a bone mineral density that lies less than 2 standard deviation (SD) below the age-and-sex matched mean (the "Z-score").

Besides routine investigations concerning any bone – pathology, kidney, liver, thyroid, parathyroid function tests, specific investigation to diagnose osteoporosis are:
- Routine plane X-rays of more osteoporosis – susceptible region (like – hip, vertebrae, wrist, forearm)
- DXA (gold standard for measuring BMD)
- Quantitative ultrasound
- Quantitative compound tomography
- MRI
- Bone turnover markers (BTM)

International Osteoporosis Foundation One-Minute Osteoporosis Risk Test: If the answer is 'yes' to one or more of the following questions; it denotes risk of osteoporosis and proper assessment and BMD measurement should be done:
1. Have either of parents broken hip after minor bump or fall?
2. Have you broken a bone after a minor bump or fall?
3. For women—Did you undergo menopause before the age of 45 years?
4. For women—Have your periods stopped for 12 months or more (other than because of pregnancy)?
5. For men—Have you suffered from impotency, lack of libido or other symptoms related to testosterone levels?
6. Have you taken corticosteroid tablets for more than 3 months?
7. Have you lost more than 3 cm in height?
8. Do you drink alcohol heavily?
9. Do you smoke more than 20 cigarettes in a day?
10. Do you suffer frequently from diarrhoea (e.g. due to celiac disease or Crohn disease?)

The following may also form the predisposing factor for inducing osteoporosis:
- Rheumatoid arthritis
- Cardiovascular disease
- Type 2 diabetes
- Asthma
- Drugs—tricyclic antidepressants
- History of falls
- Chronic liver disease
- Menopausal symptoms
- Other endocrine disorders.

The WHO defined osteoporosis in adult women using T-scores as follow:
- *Normal*—A value of BMD within 1.0 standard deviation (SD) of the young adult reference mean
- *Osteopenia*—A value of BMD more than 1.0 SD but less than 2.5 SD below the young adult reference mean
- *Osteoporosis*—A value of BMD that is 2.5 SD or more below the young adult mean
- *Severe osteoporosis*—A value of BMD that is 2.5 SD or more below the young adult reference mean in the presence of one or more fragility (osteoporotic) fracture (e.g. typical osteoporotic fractures like compression of spine, Colles' fracture, femoral neck fractures).

Besides other precautions, the combination treatment with ibandronate, vitamin D3 and calcium has therapeutic advantage in the management of osteoporosis.

WHO has suggested the use of the tool called as FRAX (fracture risk assessment tool) which is a fracture risk calculator and is freely accessible on the web (www. Shef.ac.uk /FRAX). It for identifying cases at fracture – risk. It can predict absolute risk for fracture even for 10 years ahead. (quoted by Babulkar 2016). However, it has to be used very cautiously in India today, in lack of complete proper required data.

In treating osteoporosis only one form of calcium does not appear to be sufficient, it is advisable to administer 4 active forms of calcium, which supplement each other such as follow:

Calcium sulphate, which is easily absorbed in the body and fills the bone – voids which fights osteoporosis.

Calcium silicate provides strength to bones and speed up fracture healing

Calcium oxide provides bioavailable form of calcium and supports formation of healthy bone, especially in elderly people.

Calcium carbonate (as found in/by oysterpearl) act as an ideal supplement for improvement and maintenance of strong bones

OSTEOSARCOPENIA

The concept of *osteosarcopenia* is defined in relation with the patients having *osteoporosis* and *sarcopenia* (Kaji 2014, kull 2012)

Sarcopenia is an age - related disease characterized by a progressive loss of muscle mass and function. Sarcopenia has its own International Classification of Diseases in the 10th revised clinical Modification (ICD - 10 - CM) the prevalence of osteosarcopenia is not rare.

The combined effect of sarcopenia and osteoporosis presents a serious problem in the elderly, because of their propensity for falls which may lead to fragility fractures. The risk of fracture in men suffering with osteosarcopenia is increased by 3.5 fold or even more as compared to those suffering from sarcopenia and osteoporosis alone (Yu et al. 2014).

Osteoporosis was defined as a BMD 2.5 standard deviations (SDs) below the peak bone mass of a young, healthy, gender and race - matched reference population according to the WHO diagnostic classification. The relation between BMD (T-score) and SMI was used for classification of osteosarcopenia (T-score ≤ –2.5 and low SMI), and normal (high T-score and high SMI) – (Yoo JI, Hyunho K et al. 2018).

■ BIBLIOGRAPHY

1. Aitken G. Proximal femoral focal deficiency: a congenital anomaly. In Aitken GT (ed). A symposium on proximal femoral Focal Deficiency: A congenital Anomaly. Washington DC: National Academy of Sciences; 1969. p1.
2. Babhulkar S. Osteoporosis and Internal fixation in osteoporotic Bones IN Textbook of Orthopaedics & Trauma 3rd Ed. Edts: Kulkarni GS, Babhulkar S. 2016. JAYPEE Brothers.
3. Breugem CC, Maas M, Bregem SJM, Schaap GR. Vascular malformations of the lower limb with osseous involvement. J Bone Joint Surg. 2003;85-B:399-405.
4. Burlic U, Patil K. chamakeri P: Reliability of Radiological indices in comparison to Dexa scan in diagnosis of osteoporosis. IOACON 2019, Abstract Book, Kolkata. p.122.
5. Clinical guidance on Management of osteoporosis 2012. Petaling Jaya: Malaysian osteoporosis society (Persatuan osteoporosis Malaysia). Endorsed by the Malaysian health Technology Assessment section (MaH TAS); Medical Development division, Ministry of Heath Malaysia.
6. Farid K, caillat VN. Spect CT improves the identification of Paget's diseases of bone. Joint bone spine 2010;77;243–254.
7. Hempfing A, Placzek R, Gottsche T, Meiss AL. Primary subacute epiphyseal and metaphyseal osteomyelitis in children. Diagnosis and treatment guided by MRI. J Bone Joint Surg. 2003;85-B:559-64.
8. Kaji H. Interaction between muscle and bone. J Bone Metab 2014;21(1):29–40.
9. Klein DA, Lee BH, Bezhani H, Droukas DD, stoffels G. The clinical utility of MRI in evaluating for osteomyelitis in patients. Presenting with uncomplicated cellulitis. The Journal of foot & Ankle surgery. 2020;59:323–329.
10. Kull M, kallikorm R, Lember M. Impact of a new sarco – osteopenia definition on health – related quality of life in a population. based cohort in Northern Europe. J Clin Densitom. 2012;15(1):32–8.
11. Paget J. on a form of choric inflammation of bones (ostitis deformans. Med Chir Trans. 1877:60;37–64).
12. Report of a World Health Organization Study Group: Assessment of fracture risk and its application to screening for postmenopausal osteoporosis. WHO Tech Report Serg. 1994;843.
13. Riggs BL, Melton LJ III. Evidence of two distinct syndromes of involutional osteoporosis. Am J Med. 1983;75:899-901.
14. Tanaka S, Nishino J, Matsui T, et al. Neutrophil CD64 expression in the diagnosis of local musculoskeletal infection and the impact of antibiotics. J Bone Joint Surg. (Br) 2009;91-B: 1237-42.
15. Yoo JI, kim H, Ha Y – C et al. osteosarcopenia in patients with Hip fracture is related with Mortality. J korean Med sci. 2018; 33(4):e27.
16. Yu R, Leung, Wooj. Incremental predicative value of sarcopenia for incident fracture in an elderly chinese cohort: results from osteoporotic fractures in Men (MrOs) study. J Am Med Dir Assoc. 2014;15(8):551–8.

CHAPTER 3

Joints

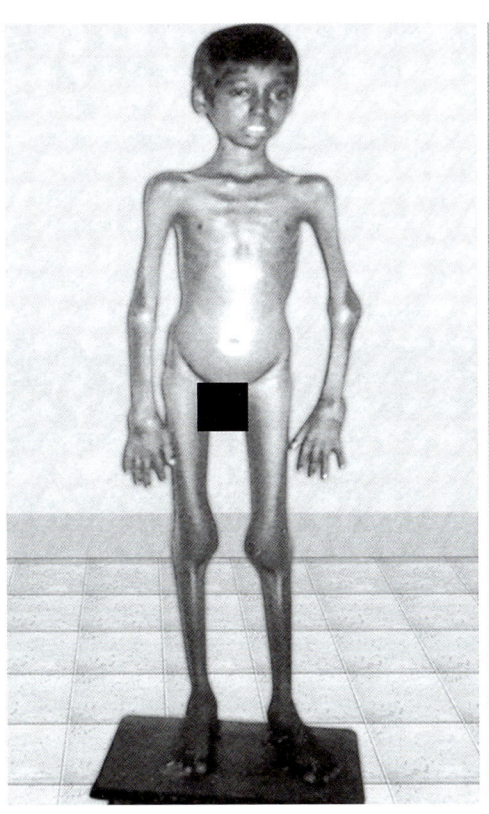
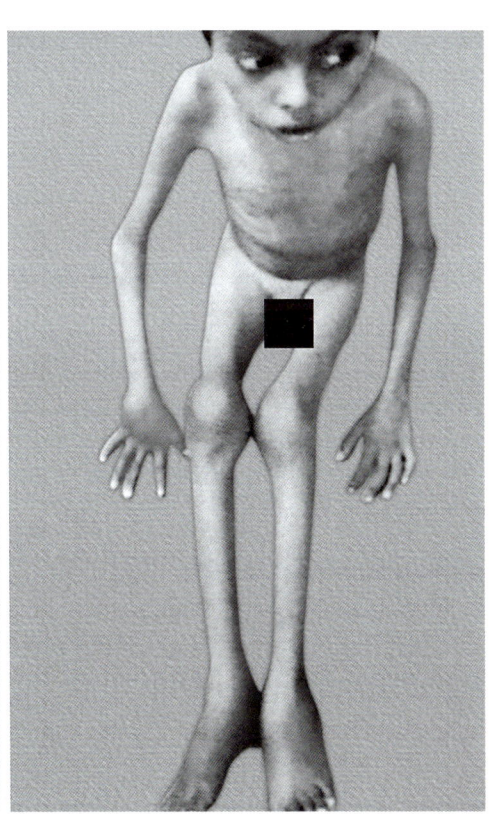

"There is no problem so great that you can't walk away from it."
—*Charles Schulz*
"Study the past if you would define the future."
—*Confucius*

"As it takes two to make a quarrel, so it takes two to make a disease, the microbes and its host."
—**Charles V Chapin 1856-1941**

The junctions between the skeletal components, where slight to free, movements occur may be defined as the '*joints*' or articulations or arthrosis or juncturae.

The joints (**Arthron**) in between the skeletal structures are essential for mobility and stability. So the jointed exoskeleton of crustaceous and insects accounts for the name of their phylum—the **Arthropodae (Flowchart 3.1)**.

Five components of musculoskeletal system are:

1. Muscles
2. Tendons
3. Ligaments
4. Cartilage
5. Bone.

All these structures contribute to the formation of a functional and mobile joint.

There are approximately 206 bones in the human skeleton that are connected by joints

Major functions of musculoskeletal system are:

- Structural support
- Purposeful motion.

Basically the *joints can be placed into two broad groups:*

1. *Synovial* or freely mobile joints (juncturae synoviales or diarthroses).
2. *Nonsynovial joints*, which can be (a) Fibrous or fixed joints (juncturae fibrosae or synarthroses), (b) Cartilaginous or slightly movable joints (juncturae cartilaginae or amphiarthroses), which may be (i) Symphyses (fibrocartilage) or (ii) Synchondroses (hyaline cartilage)

Variants of Non-Synovial Joints

- *Sutures:* e.g. in between skull bone components
- *Synchondroses:* Temporary cartilaginous junctions between the diaphyses and epiphyses in the growing age group
- *Schindylesis:* In this articulation, a rigid bone fits into a groove on a neighbouring element, e.g. junction between the vomer and the rostrum of the sphenoid bone
- *Gomphosis—(peg and socket joint):* It is a specialised form of fibrous articulation in which the teeth are fixed in the mandible and maxillae
- *Syndesmosis:* In this articulation, two bony surfaces are bound together by an interosseous ligament, where little movement is possible, e.g. in sacroiliac joint
- *Symphysis:* It is a fibrocartilaginous articulation of non-synovial type, in which there is an intervening fibrocartilaginous disc or connecting pad. A limited range of movement is possible, e.g. symphysis pubis.

Synovial Joints

Synovial joints are the most common joints of the human body and allow load bearing, low friction, wear-resistant movement between opposing bone surfaces.

The synovial joint is an organ which simultaneously ensures stability and movement. Synovial joint may be:

Synovial joints (diarthroses) are:

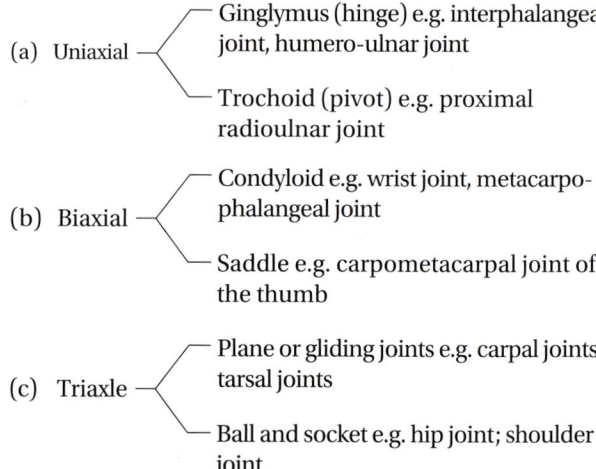

In a synovial joint, the concerned bones are linked together by a *fibrous capsule*, which mostly encloses the joint completely (except the hip joint) and *intra- or extra- capsular accessory ligaments*. The joint capsule consists of two layers.

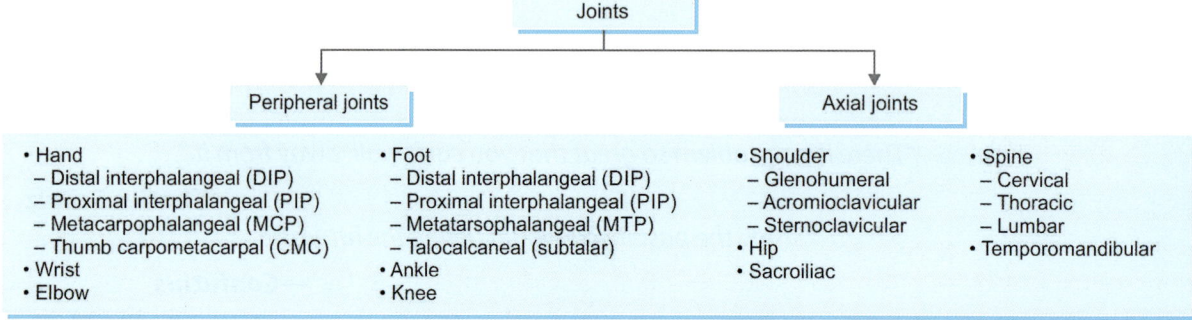

Flowchart 3.1: Classification of joints.

1. The outer layer stratum fibrosum is composed of dense fibrous tissue and completely encircles the ends of bony components. It is attached to the periosteum of articulating bones by Sharpey's fibres and is reinforced by ligaments and musculotendinous structures which cross the joint. Its vascularity is poor, but is rich in innervation by joint receptors.
2. The inner layer stratum synovium contains synoviocytes- The specialized cells that can synthesize hyaluronic acid found in synovial fluid. This layer is highly vascularized but poorly innervated and is insensitive to pain, however when subjected to heat or cold it can undergo vasodilatation or vasoconstriction. It also produces matrix collagen. It is involved in nutrition and waste product disposal of synovium.

The articulating surfaces of the bones are covered with a thin layer of *hyaline cartilage* (rarely fibrocartilage), which accounts for a very low co-efficient of friction (0.002 or less). Articular cartilage is avascular and aneural. The capsule is lined by *synovial membrane* (developed from embryonic mesenchyme), it differentiates from the mesenchymal tissue around the articular disc, clearing the articular surface by the fifth month in utero, which also covers almost all the intra-articular structures except the articulating surfaces which remain in contact and compression. The synovial membrane is rich in blood vessels and plays important role in physiology and metabolism of the joint. Normal synovium contains synovial lining cells that are 1–3 cells deep. The synovial lining cells reside in a matrix rich in type I collagen and proteoglycans. There are two main types of synovial lining cells, which can be only differentiated by electron microscopy. *Type A cells* are macrophages-like and have primarily a phagocytic functions, and *type B cells* are fibroblast-like and produce hyaluronate, which accounts for the increased viscosity of synovial fluid. This membrane secrets synovial fluid from the synovial layer of the membrane and also removes materials from the joint cavity, e.g. crystalloid, soluble dyes, etc. The synovial fluid acts like a lubricant and also provides nutrition to the articular cartilage. The **synovial fluid** (synovia means "like egg-white") is a clear or pale yellow highly viscous (fluid remains intact when slowly pulled between thumb and the index finger) glairy fluid of slightly alkaline pH (at rest). It shows viscous, elastic, and plastic components. The synovial fluid is almost similar to plasma except that it contains hyaluronic acid and a glycoprotein known as a Lubricin. It is an ultra-dialysate of blood plasma to which proteoglycans has been added by the joint tissues. Hyaluronic acid, synthesised by synovial lining cells type B, is secreted into the synovial fluid and makes it viscous.

The glycoprotein lubricin gets absorbed at articulating surfaces preventing direct surface to surface contact and thus reduces surface wear.

Physiological Characteristics

Physiological characteristics of normal synovial fluid are as follows:
- It remains in *thin film* covering surfaces of synovium and cartilage within the joint space; its pH is 7.4
- *Temperature* 32°C (peripheral joints remain cooler than core body temperature)
- Its *colour* is colourless and transparent
- *Cell count* is less than < $200/mm^3$, with 25% neutrophil; other cells are monocyte (predominant), lymphocytes, macrophages, free synovial cells
- *Protein content*—1.3–1.7 g/dL (20% of normal plasma protein)
- *Glucose content* within 20 mg/dL of the serum glucose level after 6 hours of fasting
- *String-sign* (*measurement of viscosity*) is 2.5–5 cm.

Apart from facilitating sliding of the articular surfaces, the synovial fluid also supplies nutrients and oxygen to the avascular cartilage.

In normal human knee joint, the volume of synovial fluid is +1 ml

Joints included in joint count are as follows:

The *synovial joints* may be:
- *Simple*—have only two articulating—male and female—surfaces
- *Compound*—have more than one pair of articulating surfaces, e.g. elbow joint
- *Complex*—where an articular disc or meniscus of fibrocartilage is present, e.g. knee joint.

According to the approximate shape of the synovial joints they have been classified as follows:
- *Plane joints*, in which apposing articular surfaces are fairly flat. Movements at this type of joint are sliding and translational, e.g. intercarpal joints, intermetatarsal joints
- *Hinge joints* (ginglymi) are uniaxial joints, having to-and-fro movements in one plane, e.g. elbow joint
- *Pivot (trochoid) joint* is uniaxial joint, in which rotational movements occur around a longitudinal axis running through the centre of the central bony pivot. The pivot may rotate within the ring, e.g. in proximal radioulnar joint, the radial head rotates within the annular ligament; or the ring may rotate around the pivot, e.g. the ring, formed by anterior arch of atlas and its transverse ligament, rotates around the dens of axis vertebra
- *Condylar joint* is basically an uniaxial joint but some additional rotational movements also occur, e.g. temporo-mandibular joints in which two convex knuckle-shaped male surfaces (condyles) articulate upon two concave female surfaces
- *Ellipsoid joints* are biaxial joints, in which oval convex male surfaces articulate with an elliptical concave female surface, e.g. radiocarpal joints, metacarpophalangeal joints

- *Saddle (Sellar)* joints are biaxial joints with their apposing surfaces concavo-convex, e.g. carpometacarpal joint of thumb; ankle joint; calcaneocuboid joint
- *Ball and socket joints* are multiaxial joints in which a globular head of one bone articulates with the cup like concave surface of other, e.g. hip joint, shoulder joint.
- *Osteokinematics* is movements of bone in space e.g. in flexion of forearm bones
- *Arthrokinematics* indicates the joint surface movements such as:
  - Rolling as in knee joint
  - Sliding as in proximal phalanx over metacarpal
  - Spinning as in radial head spins on capitellum

ARTHRITIS

Literally, arthritis means = the inflammation of the joint.

Arthralgia means joint pain which may be associated with other clinical features of inflammation in arthritis.

Pathologically, it includes inflammation at different levels:

Capsulitis = inflammation of capsule
Synovitis = inflammation of synovium

In progressive orthropathy, synovitis is a silent but active contributor.

Chondritis = inflammation of articular cartilage
Subchondral osteitis = inflammation of subchondral bone.

Clinically, *Synovitis* and *true arthritis* should be differentiated on their merits **(Table 3.1)**.

Presentation of Arthritis

The term 'rheuma' (first appeared in the literature in 1st century AD) refers to a "substance that flows".

The word "rheumatism" was introduced in the literature by the French physician Dr G Baillou in 1642, who emphasized that arthritis could be a systemic disorder. The 'rheumatology' is devoted to the study of rheumatic diseases and musculoskeletal disorders—which are over 120.

According to acuteness of presentation, virulence of the organisms, and resistance of the patients, *arthritis may be grouped under three headings:*

1. *Acute arthritis:*
   - Specific, e.g. pyogenic (bacterial) **(Fig. 3.1)**
   - Non-specific, e.g. allergic, haemophilic
2. *Subacute arthritis:*
   - Specific
     - Pyogenic **(Figs. 3.2 and 3.3)**
     - Tuberculous
     - Gonococcal
     - Syphilis
     - Filarial
   - Non-specific
     - Allergic
     - Villonodular synovitis

TABLE 3.1: Difference between synovitis and true arthritis.

Synovitis	True arthritis
Inflammation of synovial tissue Synovitis, if remains untreated or inadequately treated, leads to arthritis	*Inflammation* (with/without destruction) of *articular* cartilage Arthritis always *includes synovitis*
Clinical presentation: Pain, swelling, with/without variable flexion (spasmodic), cautious movements	Pain, variable swelling, spasmodic or fixed flexion and/or other deformities, limitation of movements
Good range of movements are possible after taking the patient in confidence. Only terminal movements in one or more directions may be painfully limited due to mechanical intracapsular pressure over the inflamed synovial tissue	*Movements are limited in almost all directions*. Pain starts almost from very beginning or quite early when the movements are attempted
More common in children especially in tuberculous and pyogenic synovitis. However, rheumatoid, villonodular, traumatic, and degenerative synovitis usually occur more in adults	In any age group (according to the causative factor)
X-ray findings: Joint space is usually increased due to synovial proliferation and secretion; There is no destruction of the articular cartilage, nor subchondral cystic destruction	In X-ray, the joint space is variably *reduced* depending upon the extent of destruction of the articular cartilage; subchondral and articular destructions are obvious There may be collapse of the articular surface
After proper treatment complete recovery is possible	Complete recovery is never possible and some form of legacy is bound to persist

- Post-diarrhoeal
- Haemophilic

3. *Chronic arthritis:*
   - Specific (infective)
     - Tuberculous, **(Figs. 3.4 and 3.6)**
     - Pyogenic **(Figs. 3.5A and B)**
     - Syphilis, **(Figs. 3.7 and 3.8)**
     - Hansen's disease **(Figs. 15.102 and 15.103)**
     - Actinomycosis **(Figs. 15.112 to 15.114)**
   - Crystal arthritis
     - Gout **(Figs. 9, Refer Figs. 15.100 and 15.101)**
     - Pseudogout
   - Collagen arthropathy—rheumatoid arthritis and its variants
   - Villonodular synovitis (can be treated by arthroscopic/open synovectomy; injection of 90Y or radiation)
   - Osteoarthritis
   - Haemophilic arthritis
   - Neuropathic arthropathy usually results from:

Joints

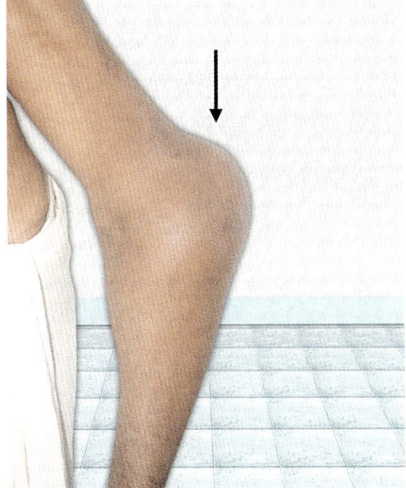

Fig. 3.1: Acute septic arthritis of elbow.

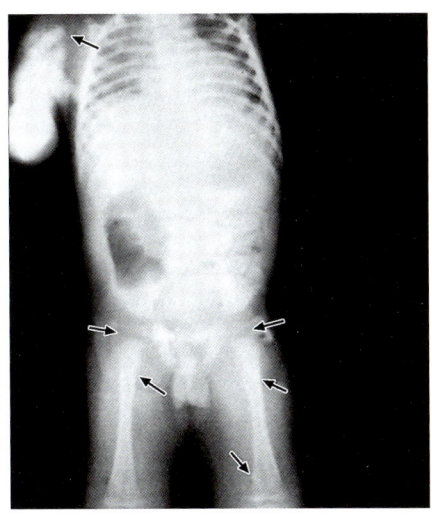

Fig. 3.2: Multifocal pyogenic arthritis (both hips and right shoulder). Note the associated congenital malformations of right upper limb.

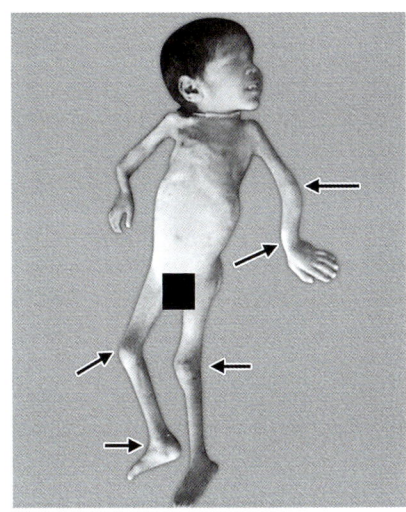

Fig. 3.3: Multifocal pyogenic arthritis in a marasmic child.

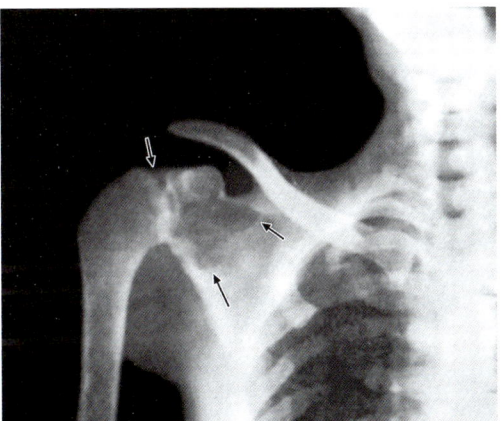

Fig. 3.4: *Tuberculous caeca* of right shoulder with a destructive cystic lesions in adjoining scapula and humeral head. Joint space is reduced.

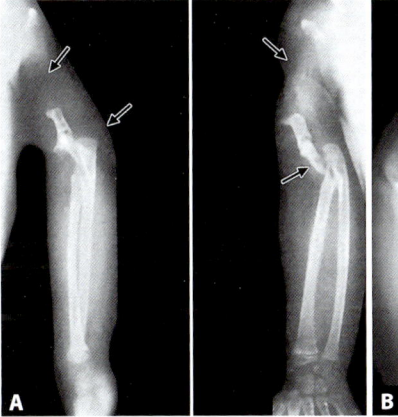

Figs. 3.5A and B: (A) Chronic (old)—Pyogenic arthritis of shoulder and elbow with extensive osteomyelitis of humerus which has sequestrated out; (B) Septic arthritis of right hip with pathological dislocation and osteomyelitis of upper part of femur, femoral neck and head. Septic arthritis is more common in children.

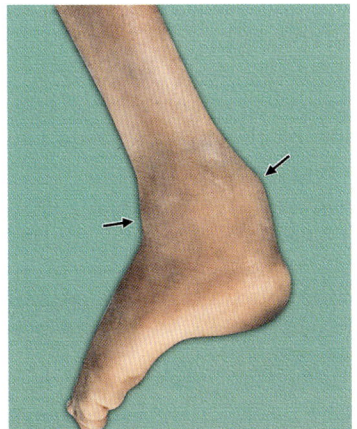

Fig. 3.6: Tuberculous arthritis of ankle-swelling of the ankle joint is due to the collection of infected fluid and caries material and tuberculous synovial thickening.

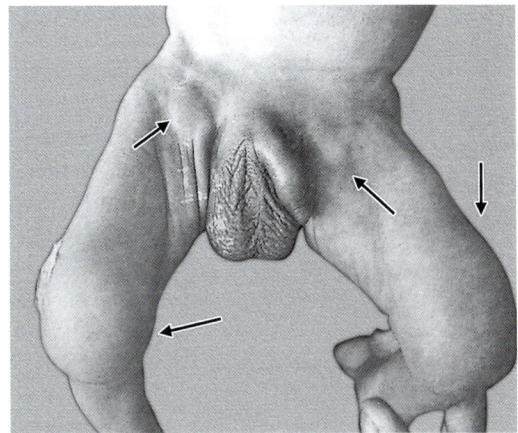

Fig. 3.7: Congenital syphilis (affection of joints and lymph glands) (Fig. 13.81).

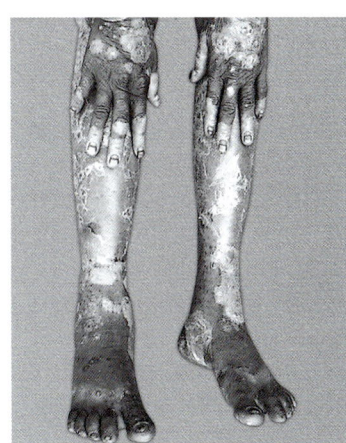

Fig. 3.8: Late pinta with mixed overlap lesions of dyschromia, hypochromia, and achromia. Areas with complete loss of melanin mimic vitiligo.

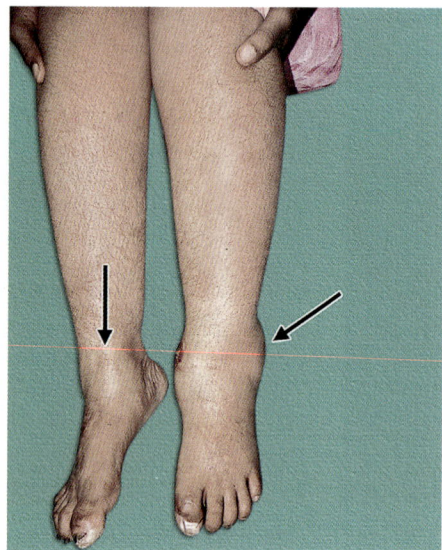

Fig. 3.9: Gouty arthritis of ankles L>R. Note the affection of (Rt) 1st metatarsophalangeal joint with reddish look.

- Neuromuscular disorders, e.g. syringomyelia
- Chronic infection, e.g. syphilis, Hansen's disease **(Refer Figs. 15.102 to 15.103, 15.104)**
- Chronic alcoholism
- Diabetes
- Vanishing bone disease (Gorham disease) may also manifest as neuropathic arthropathy **(Refer Figs. 17.87 to 17.89)**.

According to broad-based etiology, the arthritis may be considered as:
- Idiopathic (most of osteoarthritis)
- Inflammatory (collagen arthropathy—ankylosing spondylitis, psoriatic arthritis, Reiter's syndrome, post-diarrhoeal, etc.)
- Infective (septic arthritis, syphilitic, tuberculous, viral)
- Metabolic (crystal arthritis—gout, pseudogout; ochronosis; scurvy, etc.)
- Endocrinal (acromegaly, hypothyroidism, hyperthyroidism)
- Vascular (haemophilic, osteonecrotic)
- Neoplastic (benign—pigmented villonodular synovitis, systemic vasculitis; malignant—metastatic involvement of joint, primary involvement, e.g. in synovioma, chondrosarcoma.

According to the number of joints involved, the arthritis may be prefixed as:
- Monoarticular (arthritis), i.e. only one joint involvement
- Polyarticular (polyarthritis), i.e. several joints involved, either simultaneously or sequentially—it includes oligoarthritis (usually 2–4 larger joints are asymmetrically involved) and classical polyarthritis in which more than 4 joints are involved, usually symmetrically including the small joints of hands and feet.

TABLE 3.2: Following conditions are usually seen in monoarticular arthritis and polyarticular arthritis.

Monoarticular arthritis	Polyarticular arthritis
Septic: • Bacterial • Mycobacterial • Fungal • Lyme disease	*With acute polyarticular symptoms:* • Gonococcal • Meningococcal • Lyme disease • Acute rheumatic fever • Bacterial endocarditis • Viral, e.g. rubella, hepatitis B & C • Parvovirus, Epstein-Barr, HIV
Traumatic: • Following fracture • Following internal derangement • Following haemoarthrosis	*With chronic polyarticular symptoms:* a. Inflammatory – Rheumatoid arthritis – Polyarticular juvenile rheumatoid arthritis – Systemic lupus erythematosis – Polymyositis – Reiter's syndrome – Psoriatic arthritis – Polyarticular gout – Sarcoid arthritis – Polymyalgia rheumatica
Crystal deposition diseases: • Gout • Pseudogout—Calcium pyrophosphate dihydrate deposition • Hydroxyapatite deposition • Calcium oxalate deposition • Palindromic rheumatism	
Miscellaneous: • Osteoarthritis • Juvenile rheumatoid arthritis • Coagulopathy • Aseptic necrosis of bone • Foreign body synovitis • Pigmented villonodular synovitis • Synovioma	b. Non-inflammatory – Osteoarthritis – Calcium pyrophosphate deposition (CPPD disease) – Polyarticular gout – Fibromyalgia – Benign hypermobility syndrome – Haemochromatosis

Disorders involving the joints are a varied group of diseases. Mainly various types of arthritis—primary degenerative conditions; infective arthritis; and immunoinflammatory conditions, e.g. rheumatoid arthritis; and seronegative-spondyloarthropathy (SSA). In these groups. following conditions are usually seen **(Table 3.2)**:

The *expression about pain in multiple joints* are usually as:
- *Polyarthritis which denotes definite inflammation of more than 4 joints* demonstrable by physical examination (as swelling, tenderness, warmth, limitation of movements due to pain). The acute polyarticular disease and chronic inflammatory diseases usually present with polyarthritis
- *Polyarthralgia denotes pain in more than 4 joints without demonstrable inflammation by* physical examination. SLE, *polymyalgia* rheumatoid, vasculitis, systemic sclerosis usually present with polyarthralgia
- *Diffuse aches and pains* are hardly localised and manifest as vaguely originating in joints, bones, muscles, tendons, etc. Physical examination does not reveal any inflammatory change in the joint. Fibromyalgia, SLE, polymyositis, hypothyroidism, polymyalgia rheumatica usually present with vague aches and pains.

In polyarthritis, the joints are usually involved in three characteristic temporal patterns:
- *Migratory pattern:* Certain joints are affected for few days and then features remit in them only to reappear in other joints, e.g. in rheumatic fever, gonococcal arthritis—early phase of Lyme disease
- *Additive pattern:* Initially, few joints are involved, and while the symptoms persist in them, other joints are also involved, e.g. in rheumatoid arthritis, SLE, etc.
- *Intermittent pattern:* In this pattern, repetitive attack of acute/subacute polyarthritis occur with complete remission in between the attacks.

BROADLY INFLAMMATORY ARTHROPATHIES

(Including immunoinflammatory conditions)
- Rheumatoid arthritis
- Rheumatic fever
- Juvenile rheumatoid arthritis
- Collagen vascular:
  - Systemic lupus erythematosus (SLE)
  - Scleroderma
  - Polymyositis (dermatomyositis)
  - Mixed connective tissue disease
  - Polyarteritis nodosa
- Psoriatic arthritis
- Reiter's syndrome
- Polymyalgia rheumatica
- Gonococcal arthritis
- Crystal arthritis—Gout; Pseudogout
- Miscellaneous
  - Tuberculous
  - Peripheral arthritis of inflammatory bowel disease
  - SABE (subacute bacterial endocarditis)
  - Viral arthritis
  - Amyloid arthropathy.

Salient Features of Inflammatory Polyarthritic Conditions

Rheumatoid Arthritis (Deforming Symmetrical Distal Polyarthritis)

The earliest known appearance of rheumatoid arthritis was noted in skeletal remains of American Indians from 4500 BC, found in Tennessee. A high prevalence of arthritis is still found among North American Indians in Tennessee (3.5–5.3%).

According to the WHO Indian Rural Study, about 5.5 million Indians are likely to be suffering from rheumatoid arthritis.

Rheumatoid arthritis is a chronic relapsing immuno-inflammatory multisystem disease, known for its highly variable course and the patients remain at high risk of developing progressive joint destruction and even premature death. Patients are of all ethnic group and the disease is prevalent in 0.5–1.5% of the general population worldwide. The patients have both joint-related symptoms (chronic inflammatory polyarthritis characterized by pain, swelling, stiffness and deformities involving multiple joints usually in symmetrical pattern) as well as general malaise and lassitude and their physical and psychosocial function may deteriorate rapidly. However, the disease course varies considerably. The exact cause is not known. A blend of environmental factors, and genetic factors and even host factor, is not sufficient to explain all about the disease.

The five item criteria (age, weight, inflammation, immobility and overuse of corticoids) give more significant indications to clinically suspect and rather diagnose the patients of rheumatoid arthritis and the induced osteoporosis.

Extracellular vesicles (EVS) which are released from cells and are found in all types of body fluid have been found to have potential roles in inflammatory arthritis including rheumatoid arthritis. EVS have been shown to exert both pro and anti inflammatory effects. EVS may show a new way to deliver and target therapeutic agents in rheumatoid arthritis in better way.

Salient features
- *Ladies in thirties* are mainly affected (Female:male — 2.5:1), however, disease sets in earlier age in India. Peak age of onset is between 35–50 years
- *Several joints* (3 or more than 3) *are affected*—mainly the small joints of hands and feet (but distal interphalangeal joints are not affected). Usually, symmetrical joints are affected. To assess the hand disability, grip-strength and pinch measurements are the most related parameters
- *Morning stiffness* of the joints (specially the fingers and wrists). The time that patients of polyarthritis take to "limber up" from "morning stiffness" in the morning can roughly differentiate the inflammatory arthritis (where it lasts for more than one hour) from the non-inflammatory arthritis (it takes less than 15 minutes, e.g. in osteoarthritis)
- *Pain stays for hours, more in the morning;* increases with activities and massage
- May be *low-grade fever*
- Secondary weakness in the limbs
- Some muscle wasting (but less than tuberculosis)
- Fatigue, limited mobility, and feeling of inability to do even simple everyday tasks lead to mood variations and even variable depression
- *Swelling in and around the joint*; locally warm; joint tenderness; synovial thickening; deformities according to the joint affected and the neglect
- Patients of rheumatoid arthritis have the risk of having early onset of cervical spine affections mainly due to: C corticoid use, S = seropositive RA, P = Peripheral joint destruction, I = involvement of cervical nerve (paraesthesia, weakness, pain in neck) N = nodules—rheumatoid nodules, E = established disease for more than 10 years *(C Spine)*

- This systemic inflammatory disorder is caused by lymphoproliferative disease within synovium, which results in cartilaginous destruction, periarticular erosions and attenuation of ligaments and tendons
- The deformities (such as swan neck deformity, boutonniere deformity, z-deformity in thumb, ulnar deviation of fingers piano key ulnar head. etc.) develop in the fingers with the damaged joints even by the normal actions of extrinsic flexors and extensors, tightness of intrinsic muscles, displacement of the lateral bands of the extensor hood, rupture of central slip or of the long flexor or extensor tendons. The disfiguring deformities of hand affect the functions of hand and thereafter socialization of the patients
- The ankle is usually mildly affected, like cystic swellings around the malleoli. In foot the forefoot is much more affected (like hallux valgus, toe deformities), than hind foot (like subtalar joint affection)
- *Rheumatoid nodules* are found in about 25% patients. They present as painless firm nodules usually on extensor surface of forearm olecranon, occiput, fingers and rarely in heart, lung, vocal cords. They have characteristic histology of a central area of fibrinoid necrosis surrounded by a zone of palisades of elongated histiocytes and a peripheral layer of cellular connective tissue
- May be associated systemic diseases
- Cardiovascular system affected in about 15% of cases
- *Extra-articular manifestations* are seen less frequently in Indian patients.

The *synovium is the primary site for inflammatory process in rheumatoid arthritis*. Inflammatory infiltrate consists of mononuclear cells, primary CD_4 + (helper) T lymphocytes, activated macrophages and plasma cells. The synovial cells proliferate and the inflamed synovium becomes oedematous and boggy and develops villous projections. This *proliferative synovium (known as pannus)* can invade bone and cartilage leading to destruction of joint. The symmetric erosive synovitis is the characteristic, and in some cases extra-articular involvements can also occur. Gradual articular cartilage and bone destruction occurs following growth of inflamed synovial tissue over the articular surface. Extensive bone erosion seen as marginal joint erosions in X-ray denotes poor prognosis.

These pathological processes involve cell-cell inter-actions between lymphocytes, monocytes/macrophages, and type A and B synoviocytes. These cell interactions produce matrix metalloproteinases, cathepsins, and mast cell proteinases, which cause cartilage and bone destruction. Osteoclast formation from cells of macrophage/monocyte lineage at the cartilage-pannus junction is associated with destruction of bone matrix.

An increase in receptor activator of NF-Kb (RANKL) in the inflamed joint of RA patients, produced by infiltrating activated T cells and macrophages, is probably responsible for *joint erosions*. Rather, RANKL is thought to be central mediator of osteoclast development in RA and other bone loss pathologies. Hence, highest level of RANKL protein expression are seen during active disease. On this basis, it is being identified that osteoprotegerin OPG/RANKL/RANK pathways would be important future therapeutic targets to treat joint destruction in RA (Crotti TN et al. 2003).

Anti-RA33 antibody assay—85% specific for rheumatoid arthritis.

Early rheumatoid arthritis exhibit elevated Autoantibody Titres against mildly oxidized LDL [Arthritis Res Ther 2007, 9(1)].

Serum interleukin-1β level remain significantly associated with the presence of erosions at the onset of rheumatoid arthritis. [Clin Exp Rheumatoid 2007; 25(5):684-689].

Persons, who are to later develop rheumatoid arthritis, usually have significantly increased levels of several cytokines, cytokine-related factors and chemokines representing the adaptive immune system (Th 1, Th 2, and Treg cell-related factors). After the onset of disease the involvement and activation of the immune system becomes more general and widespread.

[Source: Arthritis and Rheumatoid, vol 62, Issue 2, Pages 383-391. www.sciencedaily.com/releases/2010/01/100128091736.htm]

Anti-cyclic-citrullinated-peptide (Anti-CCP) antibodies hold promise for early and more accurate detection of rheumatoid arthritis before the disease advances for irreversible damage. The anti-CCP antibodies are detected by using a solid phase enzyme immunoassay with an analytic sensitivity of 1.0 u/mL No cross reactivity to other auto antigen is found; sensitivity of the method is 68%. Positive results occur in 60–80% of rheumatoid arthritis patients and specificity is 92%. The positive predictive value of Anti-CCP for rheumatoid arthritis is far greater than Rheumatoid factor.

Using ELISA technology—Reference range:
- <=0.90—Negative
- 0.91–1.10—Equivocal
- >1.11—Positive.

In the process of detecting early biomarkers of rheumatized arthritis using miRNA expression profiling in whole blood it has been observed that miRNA-24 values were significantly lower in patients of rheumatoid arthritis when compared with healthy controls. The miRNA-125a-5p were significantly higher in patient of rheumatoid arthritis compared to healthy controls. The miRNA-132 values were significantly lower in patients with rheumatoid arthritis when compared to healthy controls. (Manimaran et al. 2010).

Clinical Diagnosis

For clinical diagnosis, criteria laid down by the American College of Rheumatology in 1987 appears more parallel in

which four out of seven laid down criteria should be there for more than 6 weeks. Criteria are:
- Early morning stiffness
- Arthritis of 3 to 4 joints
- Small joints of hand and foot should be involved
- Arthritis should be symmetrical
- Presence of rheumatoid nodules
- Positive RE test
- In X-ray peri articular osteopenia and erosion of articular surfaces.

Clinical uses
- For diagnosing early rheumatoid arthritis (usually after 3-6 months of symptoms)
- Prediction of severity of disease—early rheumatoid arthritis patients with anti-CCP positivity may develop a more erosive form of the disease as compared with anti-CCP negative patients
- To differentiate elderly-onset rheumatoid arthritis from polymyalgia rheumatica and erosive SLE.

X-ray findings
- In *early stage* periarticular soft tissue swelling
- Later on periarticular osteoporosis
- Joint erosion occur within first 2 years, though cartilage damage manifest at a much earlier stage
- Pencilling of cortex.

X-ray findings in rheumatoid arthritis can be conveniently *remembered* as:

A = Alignment abnormal
B = Bone—Periarticular soft tissue swelling later on osteoporosis
C = Cartilage destruction uniform—symmetric loss of joint space
D = Deformities are usually symmetrical and are mainly in hands and feet
E = Erosions are mainly marginal
F = Fusion (in advanced stage)—joints (mainly wrist, elbow, ankle) undergo fibrous ankylosis
S = Swelling around joints; subluxation of joints due to ligamentous laxity and destruction.

Pathogenic stages of rheumatoid arthritis
Stage 1 - No radiological bone/cartilage erosion
Stage 2 - Osteopaenia with/without subchondral bone or cartilage destruction
Stage 3 - Obvious destruction of bone and cartilage
Stage 4 - End-stage disease with fibrosis or ankylosis

With progress of disease:
- Reduction of joint space, but the bony margins are sharply delineable
- Destruction of articular cartilage, then of subchondral bone (much less than tuberculosis)
- Subluxation of joint due to ligamentous laxity and destruction
- Secondary osteoarthritic changes.

Aspiration of joint: Fluid is serous and cloudy; On clinical viscosity test, the fluid breaks into droplets easily and becomes watery.

Joint fluid contains 2,000–50,000 cells/mm with 40–80% polymorphs.

Total haemolytic complement (C/H50) is not depressed.

Management: Rheumatoid arthritis is a progressive disease, and *it must be treated early, aggressively and effectively to prevent joint damage and morbidity.*

Outline of Management

There is *no known exact cause nor cure for rheumatoid arthritis.* Probably, the disease is triggered by activation of T lymphocytes in genetically predisposed individuals with defined HLA class II haplotypes. Optimal management requires early diagnosis and timely use of the agents that can slow down the progression of disease and reduce the functional disabilities.

The American College of Rheumatology in the 2015 Annual meeting endorses the treat-to-target approach for rheumatoid arthritis, in which clinicians set specific goals of low disease activity or remission.

Therapeutic goals for drug therapy in rheumatoid arthritis:
- Short-term suppression of inflammatory changes to reduce pain and improve mobility by basic drugs like aspirin and NSAIDs
- Long-term suppression of inflammatory changes to preserve the joint structures and to lessen the morbidity by DMARDs.

The following groups of drugs are:
- *Non-steroidal anti-inflammatory drugs* (NSAIDs), e.g. Aspirin, ibuprofen, ketoprofen, mefenamic acid, indomethacin, naproxen, diclofenac, piroxicam, meloxicam, coxib groups, lornoxicam, etc.
- *Disease modifying anti-rheumatic drugs* (DMARDs) have revolutionised the management of rheumatoid arthritis: Drugs are hydroxychloroquin, chloroquin, auranofin, oral gold, sulphasalazine, injectable gold salts, D-pencillamine, methotrexate, cyclophosphamide, azathioprine, cyclosporine. These drugs appear to have helped in decreasing dramatically the rheumatic hand deformities
- *Corticosteroids*—Orally or intra/periarticularly or tissue infiltration
- *Biological response modifier* (BRM), e.g. Monoclonal antibodies (Murine, Chimeric, Humanized); Anti-cytokine; Anti-lymphocyte therapy; Anti-adhesion molecules.
- In a phase 3 trial, baricitinib [$(C_{16}H_{17}N_7O_{25})$ is an oral JAK1 and JAK2 inhibitor] monotherapy is more effective than methotrexate monotherapy and more effective than the combination of methotrexate and baricitinib

(Laird Hrrison 2015). Filgotinib (is a highly selective JAK1 inhibitor) appears to be safe and effective for rheumatoid arthritis patients who have an adequate response to methotrexate therapy (Pam Harrison 2015).

Usually, the following drugs are used along with other therapeutic measures:

- *Drugs:* Aspirin (methyl salicylate); NSAIDs; Gold or D-penicillamine; methotrexate; sulphasalazine; chloroquine; steroids—intra/periarticular and/or systemic
- Current guidelines recommend treatment with non-steroidal anti-inflammatory drugs (NSAIDs) or conventional synthetic disease modifying antirheumatic drug (csDMRD) therapy with or without concomitant glucocorticoid therapy as the first line of treatment (Smolen et al. 2014)
- A second substantial development has arisen from the advent of "strategically smart" approaches (Smolen et al. 2016). Together these developments have improved the prognosis of patients of rheumatoid arthritis significantly leading to reduction in joint damage, functional disability, comorbidity and mortality (McInnes et al. 2017).
- Rest to the inflamed part in functional position
- *Reduction of joint stress*
- *Guarded physiotherapy* (guarded isometric non-weight-bearing/non-stressed isometric exercises to maintain tone of the muscles); hydrotherapy; heat therapy including hot shower/bath; mud therapy. Sometimes ice application provides better analgesia
- Supportive/corrective *orthotics*
- *TENS*—Transcutaneous electrical nerve stimulation reduces pain after acute stage, especially backache
- *Surgery:*
  - Synovectomy (open or even careful arthroscopically) with/without joint debridement (after 6 months of drug therapy and when the synovium is affected) can effectively relieve pain for a long period with improvement in the range of flexion and function
  - Joint replacement—partial or total
  - Arthrodesis
- Rehabilitation
- Reduction of weight—weight gain threatens remissions in rheumatoid arthritis
- Psychological management
- About 15–20% of patients deteriorate despite best of treatment
- When patient becomes apprehensive about falls, which definitely reduces the quality of life, using a cane or walker or holding rails is more desirable and should be recommended.

Poor prognostic points in rheumatoid arthritis: Older age; female sex; gradual onset; rheumatoid nodules; high rheumatoid factor titre; high titre of serum cartilage oligomeric matrix protein (COMP); elevated acute phase reactants; MHC class II allele; HLA DR-4; juxta-articular bone erosion.

Epidemiologie studies have shown 1.5–2.0 times increased risk of cardiovascular morbidity and mortality in patients of rheumatoid arthritis. The increased risk is not only the traditional risk factors, but also rheumatoid arthritis severity or acute systemic inflammation (Meissner et al. 2016)

Noted variants of rheumatoid arthritis

- Felty's syndrome is triad of rheumatoid arthritis, splenomegaly and leucopenia generally a neutropenia ($<2000/mmm^3$) or thrombocytopaenia (*see* Page 644)
- Palindromic rheumatism, in which multiple afebrile attacks of monoarthritis or oligoarthritis occurs, however, the problems last only for 2–3 days and do not leave any residual effects
- Secondary Sjogren syndrome (*see* Page 633)
- Vasculitis may be associated with rheumatoid arthritis, in which skin and lung are involved
- Juvenile idiopathic arthritis.

Collagen Vascular Conditions

Systemic Lupus Erythematosus (SLE)

Nondeforming Symmetrical Distal Polyarthritis

- *Investigations:* Routine blood tests, ASO titres, C-reactive protein, ECG, echocardiogram, X-rays of joints
- Oral contraceptive pill may precipitate relapse
- SLE is the prototype of a systemic autoimmune disorder in which immune complexes or cytotoxic antibodies give rise to tissue damage often resulting in end organ damage failure or even death
- More common in female
- Systemic joint involvements
- Mucosal lesions
- Rashes
- Systemic reaction
- Brain or visceral organ involved
- Hair loss
- Leucopaenia
- Serological test for syphilis falsely positive
- X-ray non-contributory, no erosion.

Lab findings

- Aspiration—non-inflammatory joint fluid with good viscosity and mucin clot; Total WBC count 1000–2000 WBC/mm, cells are mostly small lymphocytes
- Serum C/H50 mostly depressed
- Anti-nuclear antibody titre elevated
- Anti-native-human DAN antibody titre increased.

Scleroderma

- Tight tough skin
- Raynaud's phenomenon
- Resorption of digits
- Constipation
- Lung, heart, kidney involvement

- Symmetrical kidney contractures
- Little/no synovial thickening
- Positive ANA with speckled or nuclear pattern
- X-ray—calcinosis circumscripta.

Polymyositis (Dermatomyositis)
- Proximal muscle weakness—mainly the pelvic and pectoral girdle muscles
- Muscular tenderness
- Skin changes
- Typical nail and knuckle pad erythema
- Symmetrical joint involvement
- Elevated CPK (creatine phosphokinase)
- EMG shows combined evidence of myopathic and denervation pattern.

Mixed Connective Tissue Disease
- Swollen hands
- Raynaud's phenomenon
- Tight skin
- Symmetrical joint and tendon involvement
- X-ray—may be joint erosion
- Positive ANA-speckled pattern
- Anti-ribonucleoprotein antibody increased
- Good response to corticoid therapy.

Polyarteritis Nodosa
- Symmetrical involvement
- Diverse clinical picture of systemic disease
- Diagnosis is usually histologically.

Rheumatic Fever (Migratory Polyarthritis)
- Children and young adults (0–35 years) are affected, mostly in developing countries
- Persistent sore throat
- Disease is delayed inflammatory reaction following infection with specific Lancefield groups of group A *Streptococci*
- Classically, 1-4 weeks after streptococcal pharyngitis, malaise, fatigue, fever, anorexia develop followed by painful tender warm swelling (inflammatory) in a single big joint. Sterile turbid fluid appear in the joint. Inflammatory changes subside spontaneously in few days only to reappear in another joint—thus a migratory polyarthritis
- Rashes and other skin lesions may appear
- Tissues affected are heart/pericardial involvement, joints, skin and central nervous system
- Elevated antistreptolysin O titres
- Carditis may develop. Valvular disease may develop as a long-term complication
- Joint involvements respond dramatically to aspirin
- There is no residual joint deformity
- Oral contraceptive pill may precipitate relapse
- *Investigations:* Routine blood tests, ASO titres, C-reactive protein, ECG, echocardiogram, X-rays of joints.

Spondyloarthropathies

Spondyloarthropathies (SPA) are a group of inter-related chronic inflammatory rheumatic diseases that primarily include: Ankylosing spondylitis, Reiter's syndrome, reactive arthritis, arthritis associated with psoriasis and inflammatory bowel disease and a form of juvenile chronic arthritis, undifferentiated SPA, juvenile onset of ankylosing spondylitis.

Common characteristics of SPA are:
- Typical pattern of arthritis, usually in lower limbs as asymmetric arthritis
- Radiographic sacroiliitis
- No manifestation of rheumatoid nodules or any other extra-articular features of rheumatoid arthritis
- Presence of HLA-B27
- Extra-articular features, such as anterior uveitis, aortic valve aggregation
- Rheumatoid factor not positive.

Rheumatoid factor (RF) is the general term used to describe an auto-antibody directed against antigenic determinants on the Fe fragment of immunoglobulin G. RF positivity is associated with more severe disease, with extra-articular manifestations including subcutaneous nodules and with increased mortality. However, a positive RF without clinical evidence of rheumatoid arthritis (RA) does not suggest RA. Also, all patients with positive rheumatoid factor do not have rheumatoid arthritis.

Juvenile Rheumatoid Arthritis (Fig. 3.10)
- It is a group of disorders which overlap with the adult disease, i.e. rheumatoid arthritis
- Usually in 2–15 years of age–less than 18 years of age Juvenile idiopathic arthritis is the most common type of arthritis affecting children.
- Symmetric joint involvement
- Backache
- Rashes
- Fever
- RA Factor—negative
- X-ray—periostitis, erosion in late cases
- Recur in adults
- HLA-B27 antigen present in 90%.

American college of Rheumatology criteria of JRA: onset, 16 years; Arthritis at least in one or more joint; Duration of disease at least 6 weeks or longer; other form of juvenile arthritis excluded.

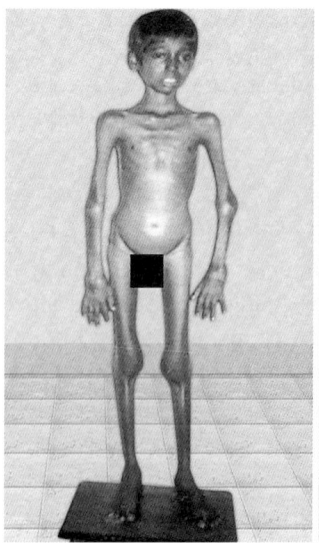 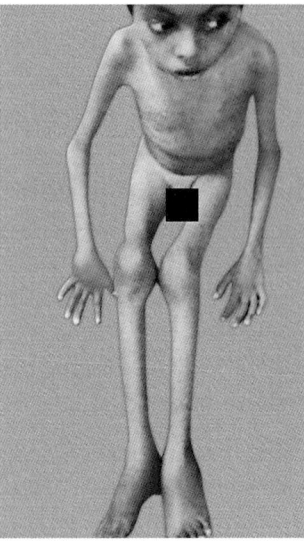

Fig. 3.10: Juvenile rheumatoid arthritis.

Still's Disease

Still's disease, described in 1897 by George F Still, a pathologist, is a variant of juvenile rheumatoid arthritis characterised by seronegative chronic polyarthritis in association with a systemic inflammatory illness. It can also occur in young adult, with prodromal sore throat, and other symptoms like severe arthralgia, myalgia, malaise, weight loss and fever.

Psoriatic Arthritis

- Asymmetric boggy joint and tendon swelling
- May be skin or nail changes prior or post to arthritis
- Distal interphalangeal joints predominantly involved
- X-ray—periostitis and erosion
- RA factor—negative
- Aspirated joint fluid—inflammatory changes with polymorph preponderance
- C/H50 mostly not depressed
- Polyarthritis accompanies psoriasis, in 5–50% of cases with genetic predisposition almost equal in both sexes.

Reiter's Syndrome

As originally described in 1916, *Reiter's syndrome* (now considered to be a form of reactive arthritis) is a *clinical triad of urethritis, conjunctivitis and arthritis* following infectious dysentery, however, only about 35% of cases present with above triad.
- Young males much more affected
- Associated urethritis, iritis, conjunctivitis
- Keratosis blennorrhagia
- Asymmetric joints affection mostly in lower extremity
- Balanitis circinata
- Painful ulcers in mucous membrane
- Loss of weight; generalised weakness
- C/H50 increased in serum and joint fluid with 3–5 Reiter's cells (phagocytosed polymorphs)
- Joint fluid shows 5,000–30,000 leucocytes/mm^3
- Prepondering macrophages in joint fluid.

Enteropathic Arthritis

Bowel diseases (e.g. ulcerative colitis, Crohn's disease) associated with inflammatory arthritis—Both ulcerative colitis and Crohn's disease related arthritis affect knee and ankle predominantly. However, upper extremity and small joint involvement are more common in ulcerative colitis than in Crohn's disease.

Gonococcal Arthritis

Gonococcal arthritis; caused by N. Gonorrhea, is a sexually transmitted disease (may be associated with HIV infection) common in men (complaining acute pain during urination). Affected man complains of yellowish or bloody discharge, and pain during urination and intercourse. Arthritis manifest 4-6 weeks after acute infection affecting tendons, small joints of hands, wrist, knee, elbow, ankle to be treated by support of joints and antibiotics.
- Migratory arthritis/tenosynovitis (settles fully in one or more joints)
- Either sex affected
- Primary focus in urethra, female genitourinary tract, rectum or oropharynx
- Skin lesion—vesicles mostly in genitalia
- On smear examination gram-negative diplococci isolated
- Positive culture from primary site, blood, joint fluid but not from vesicular fluid.

Reactive Arthritis

Reactive arthritis is a sterile inflammatory synovitis due to an infection by organisms which infect mucosal surfaces, especially urogenital or enteric infections (e.g. *Chlamydia trachomatis*, urea plasma urealyticum, *Salmonella typhimurium, Shigella flexneri*, etc). Urogenitally infected subjects are usually sexually active males, whereas enterogenic reactive arthritis exhibit equal sex distribution (*Also see* Reiter's syndrome in the chapter on 'Syndromes related to Orthopaedics and Traumatology).

The *clinical features of reactive arthritis* are similar to those found in spondyloarthropathies. The patients usually manifest extra-articular affections, such as skin, eye, enthesopathy, etc. Most of the patients recover fully, however, there may be recurrences.

HLA-B27 a human antigen encoded on the short arm of chromosome 6 as part of the major histocompatibility complex (MHC) is a MHC class I molecule. There is strong association between the presence of HLA B27 antigens and an increased incidence of ankylosing spondylitis as well as several other diseases, such as Reiter's syndrome, anterior uveitis, psoriatic arthritis, *Salmonella* or *Yersinia* arthritic infection and arthropathies associated with inflammatory bowel disorders. These diseases are collectively termed as *seronegative spondyloarthropathies.* A HLA-B27 positive patient is more likely to exhibit spondyloarthropathies than on HLA B27 negative. The alleles of HLA B27 associated with ankylosing spondylitis are B2702, B2703, B2704, B2705, B2707 and B2708.

Polymyalgia Rheumatica

Polymyalgia rheumatica is an inflammatory syndrome of unknown aetiology and it usually affects the older persons characterised by pain and stiffness in the shoulder and/or pelvic girdle. It responds quickly to glucocorticoid therapy (prednisolone 10–15 mg daily).

Clinical features of polymyalgia rheumatica can be summarised in SECRET
S = Stiffness and pain
E = Elderly individual (more than 50 years)
C = Constitutional symptoms; effects mostly the Caucasians
R = Rheumatism—arteritis
E = ESR raised (markedly elevated)
T = Temporal arthritis

- Symmetric pelvis or pectoral girdle affection, but no loss of strength
- Morning stiffness of long duration
- Easy fatigue is prominently manifested
- Loss of weight
- Joints involved: shoulder, sternoclavicular, knees, etc.
- Alpha 2 and gamma globulin elevated
- Anaemia
- Serum CPK (Creatine phosphokinase)—normal
- Prednisolone even in low dose (10–20 mg) relieves well.

Crystal Synovitis Arthritis

Gout (see Fig. 3.9)

- Gout, word is derived from Latin word "gutta" which means "drop", was introduced in 13th century AD. Earlier it was believed that acute attack of disease happens due to dropping of poison in the field. Thomas Sydenham classically described this diseases in 1983. It is more common in caucasian.
- Gout may be primary or idiopathic in 90% of cases, where there is no obvious cause and secondary in 10% which occurs in acquired disorders with prolonged hyperuricaemia.
- Crystal synovitis results from the deposition of certain crystals in and around the joints, such as monosodium urate monohydrate urate monohydrate crystals (in gout); calcium pyrophosphate dihydrate (CPPD) and hydroxyapatite (HA). Crystal synovitis is seen in mainly three conditions—Gout, Seudogout, CPPs.
- Gout is a common inflammatory joint disease worldwide with its incidence gradually increasing especially in elderly population of western countries. It is rather a collective name for several disorders that is characterised by the formation and deposition of monosodium urate (MSUr) crystals.
- *Pathogenesis of gout:* Following uric acid overproduction or underexcretion due to genetic (e.g. in primary gout) or acquired (e.g. in secondary gout) causes, it accumulates in tissues and extracellular fluid. With supersaturation of fluid with uric acid its crystals form in the tissues. When the crystals shed in the joint fluid, the polymorphonuclear neutrophils phagocytose them and produce acute inflammation (Choi et al. 2005)
- Mostly hereditary disease (occurs in family)
- Gout usually does not occur in premenopausal women
- Gout usually does not affect the joints close to spine
- Men are at greater risk than women. Usually males in forties or more are affected but incidence difference between males and females decrease with increasing age
- Risk Factors–Seafood, meat, alcohol, obesity, hypertension
- Disturbed electrolyte balance proceeds acute attack
- Onset is usually acute. The initial attack, usually occurs in late night or small hours of morning with severe burning pain, tingling, warmth in joint which rapidly swells and becomes excruciatingly tender. The overlying skin becomes red (inflammatory). There may be constitutional features (like headache, malaise, fever)
- Adrenal cortex activity; adequate corticosteroid activity counteracts gouty attack
- Joints affected: Pain in big toe (metatarsophalangeal joint), mid-foot, ankle, elbow, knee, shoulder, hand joints, wrist
- Nervous tissue is not affected (invaded) except compression of digital nerve
- The acute joint inflammation, that is characteristic of gouty arthritis is caused by the deposition of monosodium urate crystals due to hyperuricaemia (>7 mg/dL in men and >6 mg/dL in premenopausal women). Joints are swollen, warm, tender with inflamed look; movements are painfully limited
- Uric acid (discovered by Scheele in 1774) is the end result of purine metabolism
- Tophi (First described by Galen in 3rd century AD) **(Figs. 15.100, 15.101)** may be present in chronic cases in big toes, thumb, pinna of ear, Achilles tendon
- In late cases deformities may develop
- Serum uric acid is raised
- Blood ESR is raised
- Renal complications of gout are nephrolithiasis, acute gouty nephropathy, chronic gouty nephropathy

- Gouty patients are usually hypertensive and have impaired renal function, examination and investigation of renal and cardiovascular systems are essential

The presentation of gout can be divide into four stages:

Stage 1 – Asymptomatic hyperuricated-No clinical feature; few patients may develop urinary, calculi.

Stage 2 – Acute gouty arthritis –typical clinical presentation usually in men affecting smaller joints, attacks resolve in few days to few weeks.

Stage 3 – Intercritical gout the patient remains asymptomatic in between attacks of gouty arthritis, urate crystals get deposited usually in previously affected joints.

Stage 4 – About 50% of patients who have suffered from gout for 10 years or more develop nodules or tophi contains uric acid crystals.

Prognosis of properly managed gout is excellent with normal life span.

X-ray: Soft tissue swelling; subchondral variable irregular-sized cystic appearances; chalky white deposits of urates; joint space reduced; destruction of adjoining bones; deformities develop

- Decreased urinary 17-ketosteroids—reduction below 3 mg/24 hours is a constant finding in gout
- **Synovial fluid** contains WBC (10–60,000/mm^3 with predominating polymorph. It contains *monosodium urate monohydrate crystals* seen by compensated polarized light microscope (or sometime by ordinary light microscopy) as negatively birefringent needle-shaped rods.
- Gout can be diagnosed with almost absolute certainty by polarization microscopy.

Outline of management
- *Rest*
  - General for few days
  - Local support, e.g. elevation on pillow. (physical strain, trauma, surgery, mental stress, over eating may precipitate or exaggerate the acute attacks)
- *Drugs*
  - In acute cases:
    - Colchicine (0.6 mg tablet even up to 6–8 tablets on the first day depending on severity; thence one tablet twice daily for few months
    - Indomethacin—50 mg QID to 25 mg TID
  - In chronic cases:
    - Colchicine 0.6 mg BID for 9–12 months
    - Xanthine oxidase inhibitor, e.g. allopurinol 100–200 mg daily
    - Uricosuric agents (if uric acid remains increased), e.g. probenecid 0.5–2 g/day.

Urate-lowering agents, such as allopurinol (standard dose 300 mg/day) and uricosuric agents to reduce and maintain the serum urate level below 5.0–6.0 mg/dL.

Febuxostat, a new non-purine selective and potent inhibitor of xanthine oxidase/xanthine dehydrogenase is reported to be useful alternative for allopurinol. Its anti-hyperuricaemic efficacy is at 80–120 mg/day; it is well-tolerated even for longer period even up to 6 months. Treatment-related adverse effects are mild to moderate like headache, nausea, gastrointestinal upset.

Pseudogout: Calcium Pyrophosphate Dihydrate Crystal Deposition Disease

Same elderly age group as gout; Onset less acute than gout; Knees are more commonly affected. Other joints affected in neorates are metacarpophalangeal, wrist, elbow, shoulder, hip, knee

- Mental stress, over physical activities, surgery may precipitate the acute attack
- May be flexion contracture
- *X-ray:* Chondrocalcinosis (calcium deposit in cartilage, ligaments, meniscus, joint capsule) is common (cf. *chondrocalcinosis* is also common in hyperparathyroidism, hemosiderosis, hemochromatosis, hypophosphatasia, hypomagnesemia, hypothyroidism, neuropathic joints, gout, in elderlies).
- Clinical similarity to gout promoted the name pseudogout for this "crystally induced arthropathy"
- Other changes may be like those in gouty arthritis.

Synovial fluid contains calcium pyrophosphate dihydrate crystals, (Calcium pyrophosphate dihydrate, shed from articular cartilage, crystalizes within the joint as small rhomboidal, weakly positive birefringent crystals which trigger the inflammation) which are weekly positive birefringent but have a different extinction angle compared to the urate crystals—usually rhomboid or rectangular in shape.

The WBC count in this synovial fluid is 5–60,000/mm^3 with polymorphs predominating.

Outline of management
- Colchicin may give quick relief
- Indomethacin as in gout
- Intra-articular corticosteroids after aspirating the fluid, if any.

Calcium pyrophosphate deposition (CPPD), an illness manifested by swollen joints are often misdiagnosed as gouty arthritis. CPPD is sometimes referred as pseudogout and about 25% of patients of CPPD present with swelling of the first metacarpal. For acute CPPD management should be ice or cool pack, rest, aspiration of joint and intra-articular corticosteroids injection.

For chronic (CPPD) calcium pyrophosphate crystal inflammatory arthritis, oral NSAIDs, colchicine, a low dose corticosteroid, methotrexate and hydroxychloroquine should be useful. Allopurinol, Febuxostat (40 mg/80 mg claimed to be more effective for hyper uricemia and gout at inhibiting xanthine oxidase activity and reducing urate levels, and noticable less cardiovascular risk.

Prophylaxis against frequent recurrent acute calcium pyrophosphate crystal arthritis can be achieved with low dose of colchine or low dose of oral NSAIDs.

Miscellaneous Joint Inflammation

Peripheral arthritis of inflammatory bowel disease, tuberculosis, SABE (sub-acute bacterial endocarditis), viral arthritis.

Acute Septic Arthritis (Bacterial Septic Arthritis) (Flowchart 3.2)

- Acute onset with high fever (with/without rigor and fluctuations)
- Septic Arthritis is more common than osteomyelitis
- More common in children: the ratio in adults to children is 1:15
- The most common causative organism of septic arthritis in children is *Staphylococcus aureus* followed by A *Streptococcus, Enterobacter, Haemophilus influenzae*. Young male ill-nourished and under developed children are more affected. Sickle-cell haemoglobinopathy, respiratory distress syndrome and umbilical artery catheterisation increase the susceptibility
- Acute septic arthritis of childhood is a potentially devastation disease that may cause permanent disability or even death clinically. They are brought with fever, swelling of joint and feature of pseudo paralysis child cress more on touching or moving the joint. Hip is the most common joint affected followed by knee, elbow and shoulder.
- Vague or insignificant history of injury
- *Clinical evidences* of local severe inflammatory changes including hyperaesthesia, and painful limitation of movements, hot abscess (in patients of low resistance abscess may not be hot/warm)
- Acute septic arthritis is serious specially in children and that too of the hip joint. Pathological dislocation of hip occurs predominantly in children and it is rare in adults
- The ratio of septic arthritis in adults to children is 1:1.5 approximately
- *X-ray:*
  - Enlarged soft tissue shadow
  - Joint space may be increased (due to collection in the joint)
  - There may be fuzzy appearance across the joint
- *Blood examination:* High leucocytosis with polymorphs predominance; Blood ESR—raised
- *Serial CRP-high*; High platelet count
- *Blood culture* may be positive for the infective organism (usually *Staphylococcus aureus* in about 65%, Beta-haemolytic streptococci, gram-negative bacilli, *Streptococcus pneumoniae*, polymicrobial). *Staphylococcus aureus* preferentially localises to joints (a collagen adhesion factor, under the influence of a 'cna gene', has been found to be an important virulence factor which contribute to joint localization)
- *Joint aspiration:* purulent joint fluid with yellow, yellow-whitish flakes; turbid fluid; on clinical viscosity test—very watery; total count of WBC—increased usually more than 15,000 with predominating polymorphs; synovial glucose very low (less than 60% of the concurrent serum glucose); synovial culture usually reveal the causative

Flowchart 3.2: Evaluation of a hot swollen joint.

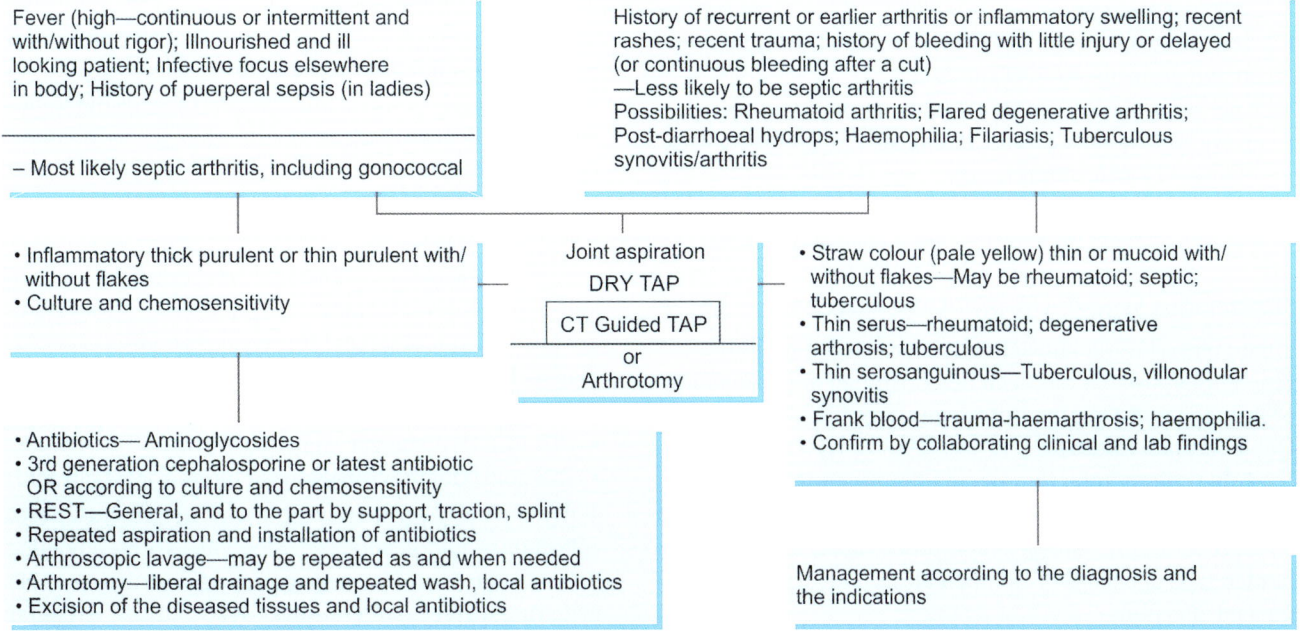

organism, however, culture may be negative in good number of patients
- *"Pseudoseptic" arthritis* should be differentiated with the patient of poorly controlled rheumatoid arthritis, who presents with one or more inflamed joints with very high synovial fluid leucocyte count— (>1,00,000 cells/mm^3). The aspirated fluid cultures are negative. The patients respond to high dose of corticosteroids rather than antibiotics.
- Fungal septic arthritis is a rare disease caused by *Aspergillus* species and it occurs mostly in immunocompromised patients. *Aspergillus* and TB coinfection can also occur in immunocompromised patient (Golmia et al. 2011).

Ultrasound is most sensitive tool for detecting even small effusion collection in the joint, specially hip. Non-echo-free effusion from clotted haemorrhagic collections are characteristic of septic arthritis.

In MRI, significant findings in septic arthritis are signal intensity alterations of the bone marrow, and signal intensity alterations and contrast enhancement of the adjacent soft tissues.

Transient synovitis mimic septic arthritis, however, in it the MRI findings are an effusion in the contralateral (asymptomatic) joint and the absence of signal intensity abnormalities of the bone marrow.

Complications of septic arthritis: damage of articular cartilage, growth plate, damage of blood supply, dislocation of joint, joints instability, limb length disparity, deformity of limb.

Outline of management
- General rest; hydration; nourishment
- Rest to the part
- Repeated aspirations, joint lavage, intra-articular antibiotics
- Systemic broad range antibiotics according to culture and chemosensitivity
- Arthrotomy—drainage, lavage, removal of necrosed materials, installation of antibiotics.
- The sequelae of septic arthritis in neonates can be prevented by early diagnosis and early intervention with emergency arthrotomy lavage.
- Strict adherence to guidelines for antibiotics administration to avoid multi drug resistance organisms.

Tuberculous Synovitis/Arthritis (see Figs. 3.4 and 3.6)

Tuberculosis has remained in symbiosis with mankind since time immemorial. It has been demonstrated in the remains of iron age and Egyptian mummies (Samhitas Wikipedia-Quoted by Jain AK2016).

Tuberculous infection occurs by inhalation or ingestion of *Mycobacterium tuberculosis or Mycobacterium bovis*. Most of the osteoarticular tuberculosis is caused by human type of bacilli. Of all tuberculosis patients 1-3% have skeletal affection.

Because of proper prophylactic measures and effective chemotherapy tuberculosis was being considered to be almost controlled specially in developed countries. However, an increase in the number of cases is excepted transglobally due to the emergence of multiresistant strains of bacteria and HIV infection. The highest rate of new cases is in Southeast Asia, but the highest rates of infection and mortality are in sub-Saharan Africa (WHO). The government of India plans to eradicate tuberculosis by 2025.

Of all the patients suffering from tuberculosis nearly 1-3% have involved of the skeletal systems (Tuli SM 2016). Vertebral tuberculosis is the most common form of skeletal tuberculosis. Any osteoarticular tuberculosis lesion results by haematogenous spread from a primary focus in soft tissue lesion such as lung, lymph gland, gastro-intestinal region, kidney etc.

- Subacute onset to chronic onset
- May be vague history of trauma
- May be history of primary focus in the body, e.g. lung, lymph gland, abdominal viscera
- History of chronic immunodeficiency
- History of chronic drugs
- Alcoholics
- Clinically evident tuberculosis is a reflection of reduced immunity of the patient
- Complains of pain, swelling, deformities, limitations of movements, stiffness of the joint, cold abscess, sinuses
- Warm tender swollen joint
- Movements restricted (due to muscular spasm, destruction of the articular cartilage, still later due to ankylosis
- Cold abscess in the dependant part of the joint (usually), or at distant places due to tracking of the pus along the path of the least resistance
- Sinuses—typical of tuberculous nature (usually)—multiple, undermined margins; pigmented surroundings; serous, serosanguinous or sanguinous discharge)
- Aspiration of the swollen joint: serous or serosanguinous fluid which may contain yellowish-white flakes; predominant polymorph leucocytosis
- Blood ESR raised; differential leucocytes— lymphocyte count is increased
- Culture may show acid-fast bacillus (about 65%). Sputum and gastric cultures of patient of pulmonary involvement are positive in more than 50%, which is confirmatory for diagnosis
- Firm supportive tests for tuberculosis are:
  - TB PCR (Polymerase chain Reaction)
  - TB gold (Quantiferon essay for interferon μ (gamma))
- *X-ray:* Initially joint space may be increased due to collection of fluid; generalised osteoporosis of the adjoining bones; reduction of joint space due to destruction of the articular surface; subchondral destruction—irregular

cystic spaces; tuberculous sequestra; collapse; cold abscess, if present, casts soft tissue shadow.

The accurate diagnosis of osteoarticular tuberculosis is complex and difficult. However, according to WHO guidelines the diagnosis of extrapulmonary tuberculosis can be made on the basis of strong clinical suspicion and firm support of imaging pictures with therapeutic clinical response.

Outline of management

Essentially and practically osteo-articular tuberculosis is more a medical disease with specific indications of surgical intervention mainly where excision of the diseased and damaged tissues is indicated and subsequently for restoring the joint and joint-functions.
- General rest
- Local rest (by plaster/splint support; traction)
- Chemotherapy (antituberculous drugs). The antitubercular drugs have been available since 1948–1951.

Chemotherapy of tuberculosis has been now well standardized and notified and accepted but for the emergence of drug-resistance tuberculosis. Bacilli demonstrating resistance to a single antitubercular agent are termed Mono drug resistance. Resistance to both isoniazid and rifampicin is termed as MDR and extensively drug-resistance tuberculosis (XDR-TB) is defined as resistance to INH and rifampicin along with resistance to any fluoroquinolone and at least one injectable second line antituberculosis drug. Bacteria demonstrating resistance to all known antitubercular drugs are termed as total drug resistance (Jain et al. 2018).
- Orthosis in the convalescing stage (non-weight bearing for the lower limb)
- If cold abscess—repeated aspiration through non-dependant zone and installing of streptomycin; if no satisfactory response—excision of the cold abscess along with/without excision of the source and the tract.

Surgery for the tuberculous joint: When non-operative management is not satisfactory OR in complicated cases:
- Arthrotomy, lavage, and synovectomy
- Excision of the diseased tissue
- Arthrodesis in second stage (i.e. after excision in first stage) OR in one stage itself as excision arthrodesis
- Arthroplasty—Excisional arthroplasty, e.g. in hip joint, elbow and shoulder joints.

Replacement arthroplasty only when the treated joint has remained continuously healed for at least 3 years.

Prophylaxis against tuberculosis is strongly recommended at least for special risk persons like household contacts, nurses, medical students and all those who are liable to be in contacts with active cases or fomites. The protection afforded by BCG (Bacilli Calmatte Guerin) in control of tuberculosis is around 80% (Tuli SM 1916).

A positive Mantoux test (allergic inflammatory response to an antigen) is present in a patient of tuberculosis of some standing (1–3 months – Tuli SM 1916). If it is negative in a known previously negative person, it is diagnostic.

Osteoarthritis (Degenerative Arthritis; Non-Nodal Non-Erosive Degenerative Joint Disease; Osteoarthrosis) (also see Fig. 13.82)

Loosely speaking '*arthritis*' denotes rheumatoid arthritis in younger age groups, and osteoarthritis in elderly age group. John Spender originally coined the word "*Osteoarthritis*" which is a misnomer (Parish 1963). It is a degenerative joint disease (or osteoarthrosis). It is non-inflammatory polyarthritis of large joints. Altman et al. (1986) told that osteoarthritis is not a single disease rather it is "a heterogeneous group of conditions that led to joint symptoms and signs." Joint osteoarthritis is an irreversible condition characterized mainly by degeneration of articular cartilage. Symptoms include joint pain, of deterioration function and ultimate physical disability.

Worldwide osteoarthritis is the most common joint disorder affecting 9.6% of males and 18% females aged >60 years. With the continued increase in elderly population, osteoarthritis is gradually becoming a major medical, financial and social problem.

Osteoarthritis or *osteoarthrosis is an idiopathic slowly progressive disease of arthrodial joints occurring late in life,* though earlier was thought to be an idiopathic disease is now recognised to be multifactorial resulting from the interaction of a variety of systemic and local factors including age, genetic predisposition, obesity, trauma and mechanical properties of the synovial joint. Low dietary Magnesium intake has been found to be associated with osteoarthritis more studied in DA knee. Hypomagnesia is linked to increase circulating cytokine level which may lead to bone resorption that worsens DA and predisposes to osteoporosis.

Osteoarthritis is a common disease with multiple predisposing factors and it can affect almost every joint in the human body. In the lower extremity knee, hip and ankle are affected in that order.

Basically *osteoarthritis is of two types—primary or idiopathic* type and *secondary type.*
- Primary osteoarthritis is always in elderly people—about 70% of women and 60% of men above the age of 40–60 years are usually affected
- Secondary osteoarthritis can occur in earlier age as well (e.g. post-traumatic; healed infections of the joint; old Perthes disease or otherwise osteonecrosis of the bone involved in the joint, etc.).

The pathodynamics consists of "morphologic, biochemical, molecular and biomechanical changes of both cells and matrix leading to softening, fibrillation, ulceration and loss of articular cartilage, sclerosis and eburnation of subchondral bone, osteophytes and subchondral cysts (Keuttner and Goldberg 1995). Cartilage destruction due to biomechanical and biochemical factors is at the core of arthritis. Joint capsule is little affected. Adhesions are usually not formed.

Cytokines and growth factors probably play a substantial role in the pathophysiology of the disorder. Interleukin-1 and tumor necrosis factor beta may activate enzymes involved in proteolytic digestion of cartilage. Collagenolytic enzymes are supposed to contribute to the breakdown of cartilage. When catabolism exceeds cartilage synthesis osteoarthritis develops

- This is a disease of articular cartilage with degradation of the proteoglycan matrix leading to fissuring, thinning and loss of articular cartilage and secondary thickening of subchondral bone. The bony margins proliferate to form lippings, spurs and exostoses.
- *Clinically,* there are recurrent episodes of pain, synovitis with effusion, stiffness and progressive limitation of movements
- Pain mainly after rest and fairly relieved after mild to moderate activities (severe activities usually increase the pain)
- Pain in the knee may be due to osteoarthritis of hip joint as well. However, pain (usually grion pain) with internal rotation and flexion of hip may be referred to the knee.
- Circadian rhythmic variation in pain, stiffness, and dexterity is often seen in osteoarthritis (and also in rheumatoid arthritis). It has implications in organising activities of daily living and timing the drug administration
- Variable asymmetric joints may be involved at a time
- Knee and hip osteoarthritis cause greatest disability followed by the osteoarthritis of hand (mainly thumb root joint)
- Distal interphalangeal joints are affected (cf. rheumatoid arthritis where these joints are not affected)
- Enlargement of distal and proximal interphalangeal joints of fingers is frequently seen (Heberden and Bouchard nodes, respectively)
- Overweight people (BMI >25 kg/m^2)—obese people (obese women > obese men in ratio of 3:1) are at high risk of developing osteoarthritis of knee, hip and hand
- May be disuse atrophy of the muscles
- Local temperature not raised except when there is flare with collections in the joint
- Coarse crepitations in the joint
- Morning stiffness (usually less than 15 minutes—cf. in rheumatoid arthritis stiffness last usually more than one hour)
- Effusion in the joint (usually when there is flare)
- Asymmetric loss of knee cartilage leads to varus or valgus deformity
- Range of the movements are reduced specially in the terminal range (more in flexion)
- Deformities of the joints—mainly it is angular deformity, specially in direct weight-bearing joints, e.g. in knee and ankle
- Joint movements are restricted
- Contractures may develop
- Ankylosis of joint usually do not develop
- *X-ray:*
  - In osteoarthritis weight bearing X-rays are more helpful–typically four views X-rays should be taken: Bilateral weight-bearing posteroanterior, Lateral, 45 degrees of flexion posteroanterior (Rosenberg) and 20 degrees of flexion patellofemoral (Laurin) views Posteroanterior flexion weight-bearing view is more useful for defecting osteoarthritis.
  - Joint space gradually narrows down
  - Subchondral sclerosis
  - Subcortical cysts
  - Marginal osteophytes (and eburnations)
  - Collapse of joint
- On aspiration of the joint (when there is effusion):
  - Fluid is usually clear and straw colour/serous
  - Clinical viscosity test—fluid remains intact when slowly rubbed and pulled between thumb and the index finger, i.e. viscosity is high or good as in normal cases
    - Glucose content is normal
    - Cell count is 2000/mm^3 (cf. normal is 200/mm^3) with more of monocytes.

Outline of management
- Drugs—NSAIDs (Non-steroidal anti-inflammatory drugs)
- Aligning the weight transmission in lower limbs by the alteration of the shoe heel; providing inserts; bracing
- Limited supports (to maintain the functions simultaneously)
- Postural adjustments, e.g. sitting, standing, sleeping postures; chair adjustments
- Intra-articular steroids and allied injections
- *Surgery:*
  - Arthroscopic lavage; arthroscopic/open joint lavage and cleaning
  - Osteotomy (e.g. high tibial osteotomy for knee and McMurray's osteotomy for the hip)
  - Joint replacement (e.g. total hip and knee replacements). Total knee arthroplasty is being taken as gold standard for knee osteoarthritis.
  - Arthrodesis of the joint (more suitable in manual workers and labourers and failed TKR.)
  - Possible measures in future: gene therapy; bone-marrow transplantation for stem cells.

Clinical differentiation between rheumatoid arthritis and osteoarthritis is presented in **Table 3.3.**

TABLE 3.3: Clinical differentiation between rheumatoid arthritis and osteoarthritis.

	Rheumatoid arthritis	Osteoarthritis
Geographical distribution	Most Common in temperate climate	Can occur anywhere
Race	More in white population	No such predilection
Familial tendency	Often history of rheumatoid arthritis or other collagen arthropathy in family	No such family history in most of the cases
Past history	May be history of rheumatic fever, tonsillitis, sore-throat, sinusitis	May be history of postural defects/mechanics or trauma
Age	Usually in 20's or 30's may be 40's	Usually in 40's, 50's, 60's
Sex	Females are more affected	Both sexes almost equally affected, of course obese woman more often
Onset of disease	Usually insidious	Always insidious—may be intermittent flare
General condition	Usually looking ill, anaemic, undernourished. May be slight febrile	Mostly well-nourished, more common in obese
Involvement of joints	Multiple joints usually symmetrically involved; small joints of hands (proximal interphalangeal joints) and feet	Usually big weight bearing joints (knees, hips, ankle), distal interphalangeal joints
Morning stiffness	Usually lasts for more than one hour	Usually lasts for less than 15 minutes
Appearance of joints	Early—periarticular swelling, fusiform fingers	In early stage—may be variably swollen In advanced stage—variable deformity like varus collapses flexion deformation, etc. of knee etc.
	Late—variable deformities of fingers, ulnar deviation of wrists; other affected joints also variably deformed Stiffness of joints	Early—slight swelling of joint Late—more swelling of Joint, variable limitation of movements; Heberden's node in fingers
Wasting of muscles	Marked wasting in late cases	Nothing significant
Skin changes	Skin atrophy and glossy, redness of thenar and hypothenar eminences, cold and clammy skin	Nothing significant
Subcutaneous nodules	May be psoriasis Present in about 20%	May be psoriasis Not present

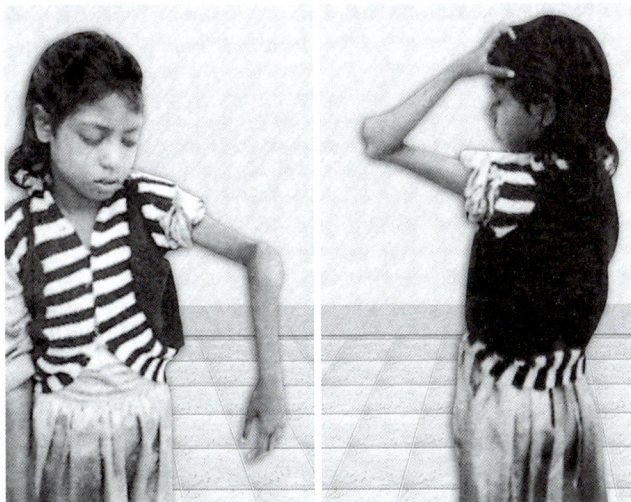

Fig. 3.11: Post-variolar arthritis of left elbow.

Viral Arthritis (Fig. 3.11)

Viral arthritis usually occurs during the viral prodrome. Arthralgia with/without rash are the presenting feature. Hepatitis virus (Hepatitis A or B), Rubella virus, mumps virus can lead to arthritis. Mumps virus may cause migratory polyarthritis, which usually involves big joints with variable symptoms. However, symptoms usually resolve in about 2 weeks.

- History of preceding or concomitant systemic viral illness
- Mixed clinical picture of viral and septic infections
- Aspirated joint fluid can show inflammatory changes with polymorphs preponderance
- Culture of virus from the joint fluid.

Post-variolar arthritis manifests as disorganised variably stiff joints (usually bilateral; elbow is a common site). Though smallpox has been eradicated, but its legacies would be seen for few more decades, specially in tropical and allied countries.

Chikungunya

Chikungunya is a self-limiting illness caused by chikungunya virus of gene alphavirus. The disease spreads by the bite of *Culex* and *Aedes* mosquitoes.

Clinical features: Patient complains of severe headache, chills and rigors, nausea and vomiting and fever more than

40°C, severe pain in different joints. Due to excruciating pain in joints, patient assumes the posture of being bent up—this bending up posture refers to name the virus as 'chikungunya'—the Makonde word which means cone which bends up. Chikungunya fever was first reported in 1952 from Makonde plateaus (along the border between Tanzania and Mozambique). Management is mainly symptomatic and rest.

Dysenteric Arthropathy

- Sterile seronegative synovitis/arthritis as a complication of intestinal infection with *Shigella* or *Salmonella* or cases of *Yersinia*
- Clinical manifestations of asymmetric polyarthritis or arthralgia, following weeks of definite diarrhoeal illness, abdominal pain
- Knee, ankle, and wrist are commonly affected
- Diagnosis is by stool examination and agglutination tests
- Usually, it clears in weeks or months with management of intestinal infections.

Poncet's Disease or Tubercular Rheumatism

- Poncet (1897) described cases of polyarthritis occurring in patients suffering from tuberculosis
- Polyarthralgia may be associated with tuberculosis (usually extra-articular tuberculosis), however this association may be controversial
- The joint aspirate is watery or straw-coloured fluid whose culture is (mostly) negative
- Symptoms may subside with NSAIDs and physiotherapy, however, anti-tubercular drugs may be given for 6 months.

■ ANKYLOSIS OF JOINT

Ankylosis of a joint means fixity of the joint, in any position depending upon the pathology and posture (cf. *arthrodesis* is a planned operative fusion of a joint in possible functional position).

Aims of Examining an Ankylosed Joint (Tables 3.4 and 3.5)

- To know the possible cause
- To know the type of ankylosis
- To evaluate the capability of the joint in presence of the ankylosis or incapacitating effects of the ankylosis
- To plan the treatment
- Stretchability of the ankylosed joint:
  - Yield of skin
  - Yield of subcutaneous tissue
  - Yield of blood vessels
  - Yield of tendons
- To predict the prognosis
- To assess the effects of ankylosis on the adjoining joints and posture.

TABLE 3.4: Causes of ankylosis.

Extra-articular		Intra-articular	
		Soft tissue	Bony
Skin	• Contracture	• Capsular contractures	• Intra-articular fracture
	• Congenital	• Synovitis	• Infective conditions, e.g. pyogenic, tuberculosis
	• Postburn	• Intra-articular ligamentous affections	• Collagen arthropathy
Subcutaneous tissue	• Dupuytren's contracture		• Degenerative changes
	• Fibrosis		• Neoplasm
Muscles	• Fibrosis		
	• Myositis		
	• Neoplasm		
Tendon	• Fibrosis		
	• Neoplasm, e.g. xanthoma		
	• Bursitis		
Vessels	• Aneurysm, e.g. in popliteal fossa		
Bone	• Inflammatory condition of bones in the vicinity		
	• Neoplasm in the vicinity		

TABLE 3.5: Types of ankylosis.

True or bony	False or fibrous
• No yield even on stress	• Yield on stress
• No pain even on stress	• Pain on stress
• Marked atrophy of the surrounding soft tissues specially muscles	• Comparatively less atrophy of the surrounding soft tissues
• Causes of ankylosis usually intra-articular	• Mixed causes (intra-or/extra-articular or both)
• Radiological findings	• No trabeculations across the joint
– Trabeculations across the joint	• Joint line always present
– No joint line left	• Detail assessment
• Management	• Planned physiotherapy
– Detail assessment specially related to functional loss	• Analgesic
– If adjustments possible, rehabilitation in original or changed job	• Reassurance
– If treatment required	• Management of primary cause
– Operation:	• Operation:
♦ Excisional arthroplasty	• Total joint replacement
♦ Total joint replacement	• Excisional arthroplasty
♦ Planned arthrodesis	• Planned arthrodesis

Tumoral Calcinosis

First report of tumoral calcinosis was by Duret in 1899 (Synonym: calcium tumour; calcifying bursitis; calcifying collagenolysis; kikuyu bursa). Inclav was the first to introduce the term "tumoral calcinosis". Exact cause is not known. May be inborn error of phosphorus metabolism and mechanical trauma or repeated minor injuries. The disease is probably a result of metaplasia of connective tissue cells. The disease has a genetic background. It occurs in younger patients, affects multiple joints and has a familial tendency. Lateral aspect of hips and buttocks are more likely to be affected. The disease has a benign clinical course with slowly growing masses. On X-ray nature of crystals are lobular (cf. in pseudogout crystals are more delicate and granular). There are no bony abnormalities. The calcium deposits are characteristically periarticular. On microscopy, macrophages, multinucleated giant cells and chronic inflammatory cells lining the fibrous bands are seen.

Complications are rare—may be ulceration in overlying skin, secondary infection and fistula. Surgical excision is the main treatment. Recurrence may occur, which will require repeated excision.

Musculoskeletal Manifestations in HIV (Table 3.6)

TABLE 3.6: Joint, bone and muscles related manifestations in HIV*.

Rheumatic manifestations associated with HIV:	Diffuse infiltrative lymphocytosis syndrome (DILS) 5%
Articular: • Arthralgia (45%) • Reiter's syndrome • Psoriatic arthritis • Undifferentiated spondyloarthropathy • HIV-associated arthritis • Painful articular syndrome (10%)	*Vasculitis* *Infective:* • Septic arthritis • Osteomyelitis • Pyomyositis
Muscular: • Myalgia • Polymyositis • Myopathy (i.e. HIV-wasting, zidovudine-induced nemaline rod)	*Others:* • Soft-tissue rheumatism (e.g. tendinitis, bursitis) • Fibromyalgia (30%) • Avascular necrosis (due to protease inhibitors) • Gout

*Adapted from Espinoza LR: Retrovirus-associated rheumatic syndrome. In: McCarty DJ, Koopman (Eds). Arthritis and Allied Conditions, 13th edn. Philadelphia, Lea and Febiger, 2001, 2670-2683.

BIBLIOGRAPHY

1. Alexander Y. Hui, William J, McCarty, Koichi M, et al. (2012). A systems biology approach to synovial joint lubrication in health, injury, and disease. WIREs syst Bid Med. 2012;4: 15-17.
2. Altman R, Asch E, Bloch D, et al. Development of criteria for the classification and reporting of osteoarthritis: classification of osteoarthritis of the knee. Arthritis Rheum. 1986;29: 1039-49.
3. Choi HK, Mount DB, Reginato AM. Pathogenesis of gout. Ann Intern Med. 2005;143:499-516.
4. Crotti TN, Smith MD, Weedon H, et al. Receptor activator NF-kB ligand (RANKL) expression in synovial tissue from patients with rheumatoid arthritis, spondyloarthropathy, osteoarthritis, and from normal patients. Ann of Rheumatic Diseases. 2003;1:9-16.
5. Golmia R, Bello T, Marra A, et al. Aspergillus fumigatus joint infection: A review. Semin Arthritis Rheum. 2011;40: 580-4.
6. Jain AK et al. Drug-resistant spinal Tuberculosis–quoted– Multidrug and extensively drug-resistant TB (M/XDR-TB) global report on surveillance and response. 2010 Indian J Orthop. 2018:52(2);100-7.
7. Khanna NB. Therapeutic spectrum of rheumatoid arthritis. The Archives of Bones and Muscles. 2001:(1)2:29-36.
8. McInnes IB, Porter D, Sieberts. Choosing new targets for Rheumatoid Arthritis Therapeutics: Too Interesting to Fail. Arthritis Rheumatol, 2017;69-6:1131-34.
9. Meissner Y, Zink A, Keknow J, et al. Impact of disease activity and treatment of comorbidities on the risk of myocardial infarction in rheumatoid arthritis. Arthritis Res Ther. 2016; 18:183.
10. Samhita S. Wikipedia, The free encyclopaedia—Available from: http://www.en:Wikipedia.ORg/wiki/Sushruta_ Samhita [Last assessed on 2015 Nov 02]—Quoted by Jain AK. Tuberculosis of spine: Research evidence to treatment guidelines. Ind Jr Orth. 2016;50:3-9.
11. Smolen JS, Aletaha D, McInnes IB. Rheumatoid arthritis. Lancet. 2016;388:2023-38.
12. Smolen JS, Landewe R, Breedvedd FC et al. EULAR recommendations for the management of rheumatoid arthritis with synthetic and biological disease-modifying antirheumatic drugs 2013 update: Ann Rheum Dis. 2014;73: 492-509.
13. West SG. Rheumatology Secrets, 2nd Edn. Indian Reprint New Delhi: Elsevier. 2004.
14. World Health Organization. Disease outbreak: Chikungunya and Dengue in the South West Indian Ocean, 17 March 2006, Geneva, WHO.

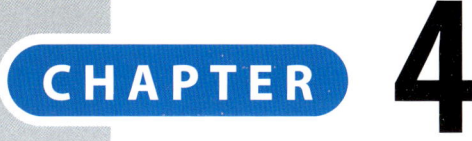

Shoulder Joints

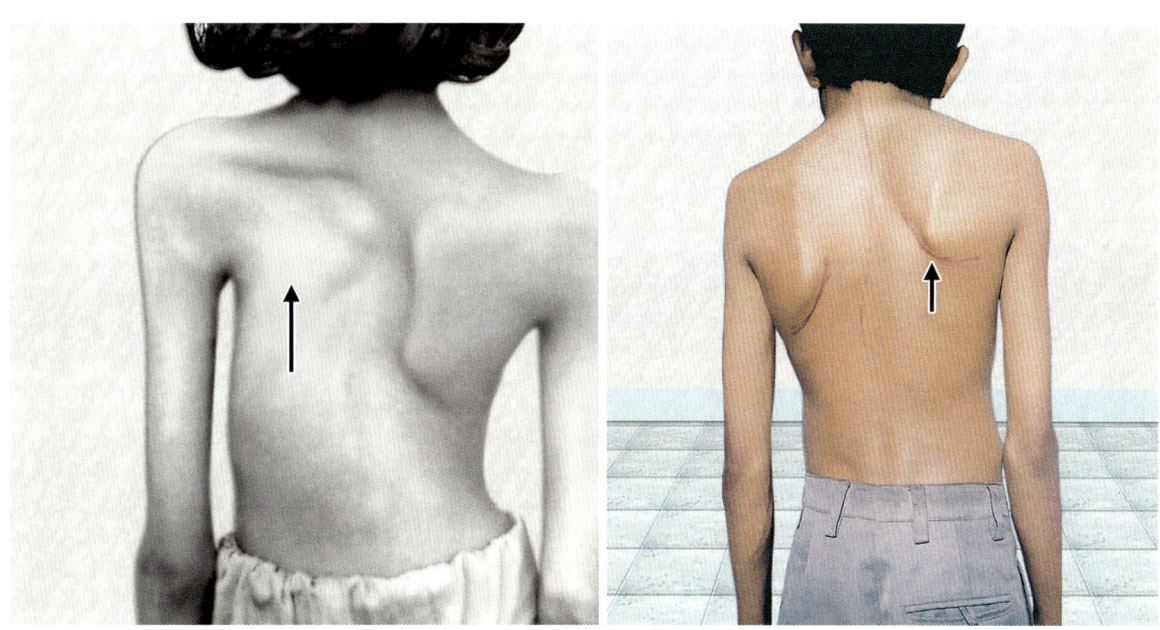

"A person who won't read has no advantage over one who can't read."
—*Mark Twain*
"Life always begins with one step outside of your comfort zone."
—*Roy T Bennett*

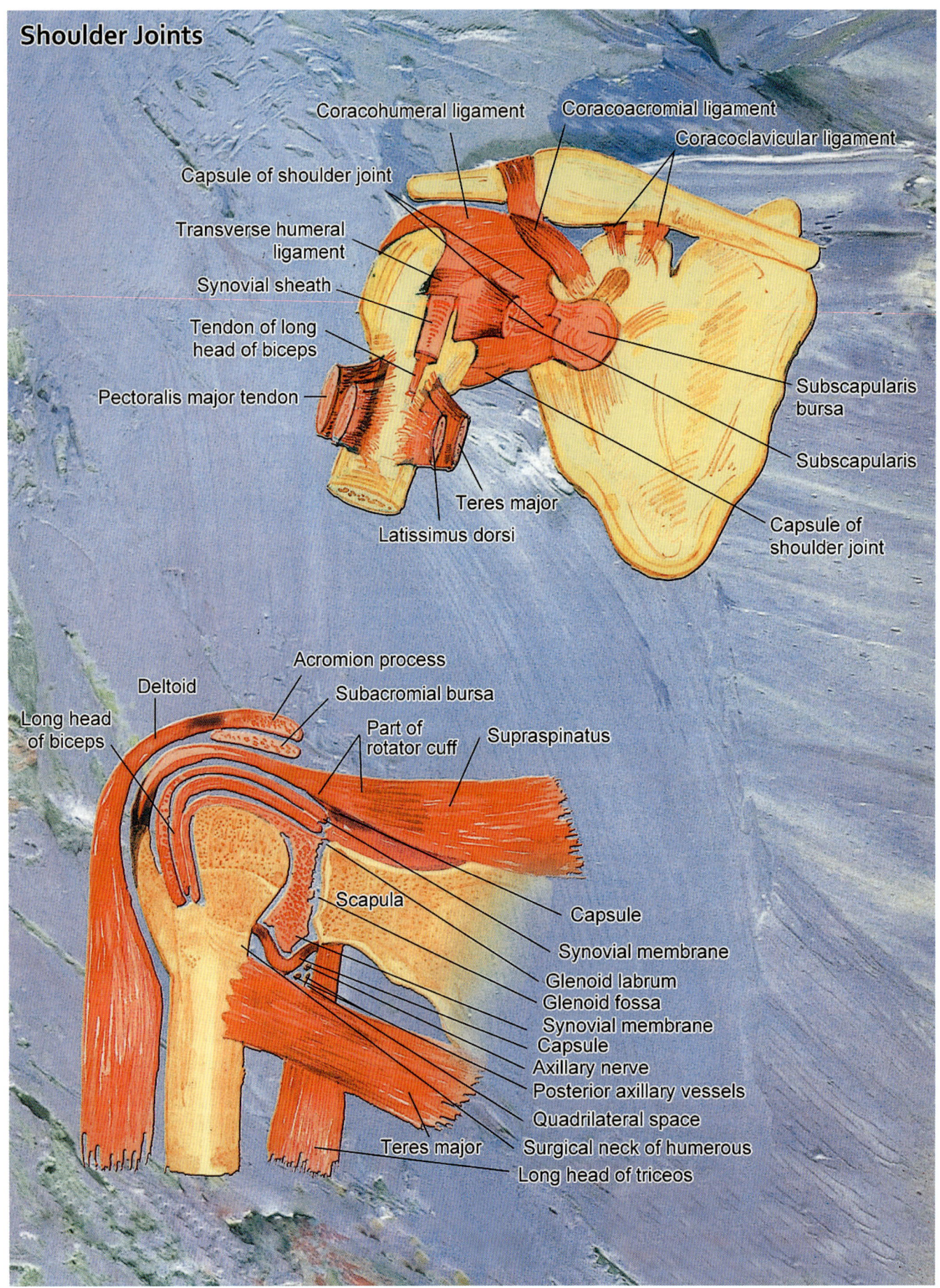

INTRODUCTION

In the process of evolution from quadrupeds to bipeds, the forelimbs developed into upper limbs. In quadrupeds, they serve the purpose of weight bearing and attack. In bipeds, their responsibilities are mainly concentrated on subserving fine functions, holding an object, attack and defence. The main axis of the upper limb also changed with some rotational element at the root joints, i.e. at forequarter girdle. Therefore, the long axis of the upper limb in human beings is neither set parallel nor at right angles, but oblique to the trunk.

ANATOMICAL CONSIDERATION

The upper limb more or less hangs from the body. The only skeletal connection from the trunk to the upper limb is via the acromioclavicular joint, the strut of clavicle and the sternoclavicular joint. It, therefore, assumes the responsibility of a shock absorber, preventing a thrust from the upper limb from being transmitted to the trunk. For a clinician, the word 'shoulder' should include the shoulder girdle as a whole, since an affection anywhere in the shoulder girdle has to affect the shoulder functions. The shoulder girdle broadly comprises of bones (humerus, scapula, clavicle, sternum), joints (glenohumeral, acromioclavicular, sternoclavicular and scapulothoracic), their ligamentous connections, and the overlying muscle, tendons and bursae.

The shoulder joint has greatest range of movements of any joint in the body and hence has the highest rate of dislocations.

The *movements at shoulder* is the sum total of movements at different joints of the shoulder girdle (i.e. *glenohumeral articulation, scapulothoracic gliding, acromioclavicular and sternoclavicular joints*). In most of the affections of cervical spine, the shoulder region may be involved. Rather, at times, the complaints lie only in the shoulder for a pathology in the cervical spine. Therefore, it is imperative to examine fully the cervical and cervicodorsal regions for shoulder complaints. The *rotator cuff* consists of musculotendinous attachments to the greater tuberosity (teres minor, supraspinatus and infraspinatus), lesser tuberosity (subscapularis) and adjoining capsule of the shoulder joint. The dynamic interplay of the rotator cuff and deltoid muscle is essential for smooth functioning of shoulder. The rotator cuff acts as horizontal stabilisers and steerer holding the humeral head in the glenoid during the abduction of shoulder.

Directly or indirectly the shoulder helps in placing the hand in the best position for different activities of daily living.

The skeletal anatomy of the *glenohumeral joint* comprises two retroverted non-constrained articular surfaces. The glenoid articular surface is pear-shaped because of the anterior incisura acetabuli. Its mean transverse diameter is 24 ± 3.3 mm; mean superoinferior diameter is 35 ± 4.1 mm; mean posterior version is $2.0 \pm 4.2°$ (-7 to -12); and mean radius of curvature is 36.6 ± 7.4 mm (Mallon et al. 1992).

The glenoid labrum is a circumferential rim of fibrocartilaginous structure attached to the margin of glenoid fossa. Functionally, it increases the concavity of relatively flat bony glenoid and serves as stable attachment site for the biceps origin, glenohumeral ligaments and capsule. Thus, it becomes a critical static stabilizer of the shoulder. It is prone to injury with traumatic or recurrent subluxation/dislocation of shoulder.

The *proximal end of humerus has a cartilaginous surface which is tilted 45° upwards and about 20° posteriorly with reference to distal intercondylar line.* The humeral retroversion is $26.9 \pm 12.22°$ on the right and 21.2 ± 11.02 on the left (Mallon et al. 1992).

The glenohumeral joint is not a ball and socket joint like hip joint, rather it is "ball on a dish" articulation. Unlike hip joint where femoral head is well contained in acetabulum, in shoulder joint, the humeral head has much greater freedom of motion on the relatively flat glenoid—anatomically deepened by the fibrocartilaginous labrum forming a peripheral rim for the glenoid that increases both the surface area and its concavity.

The *glenohumeral joint is superiorly protected by osseous ligamentous arches formed by the coracoid process, coracoacromial ligaments, and the under surface of the acromial process.* The subacromial bursa lying between the capsule and the arches virtually protect the humeral head from impingement against the acromial process and is liable to undergo degenerative inflammation quite often.

The *vascular supply of the humeral head* plays a major role in the outcome of trauma or diseases. The arterial arcuate circulates within the humeral head and receive its blood supply from four major sources—The metaphyseal artery, the branch of anterior circumflex artery in the bicipital groove, arteries from the rotator cuff, and the medial branch of the posterior circumflex artery. Hence, a fracture through the anatomical neck will lead to complete devascularisation of the head fragment carrying the articular surface.

The non-specific inflammation and adhesions affecting the capsule, the rotator cuff, subacromial bursa and the surrounding ligaments, manifest more or less in the same way, ultimately resulting in frozen shoulder. The coracohumeral ligament, mainly meant for acting as checkrein against extreme external rotation of humeral head, gets variably contracted in rotator cuff syndrome/frozen shoulder thus earlier limiting the external rotation.

The clavicle subserves its strut action through strong coracoclavicular ligaments (trapezoid and conoid parts) which helps in suspending and stabilising the arm in its allocation. Hence, any rupture of this ligament, associated with injury of acromioclavicular ligament causes subluxation/dislocation of the joint.

Long head of biceps originates from supraglenoid tubercle, invaginating through the synovium and passes in the bicipital groove, strapping the head of the humerus firmly in the glenoid cavity in all its movements. This makes this tendon vulnerable to degenerative inflammation, attrition and even varying ruptures. The biceps tendon is valuable surgical landmark separating the lesser tuberosity from the greater tuberosity and therefore is of help in identifying the various fragments with their attached cuff tendons.

The *power transmission from scapula to humerus* is through the glenohumeral groups of muscles which directly cross the joint namely teres major, deltoid (has three functionally dependent portions—anterior, middle and posterior) and the rotator cuff (consists of musculotendinous units of subscapularis (forms anterior cuff and inserts in lesser tuberosity), supraspinatus, infraspinatus, and teres minor (these three form posterior cuff and insert on three facets of greater tuberosity—the biceps and its tendinous long head may also be considered as part of the rotator cuff). The rotator cuff is a primary dynamic stabiliser of shoulder and also provides some power in motion. It acts primarily to maintain the mid-range stability of glenohumeral joint during movements.

The shoulder remains stable by the help of its dynamic and static stabilizers. Dynamic stabilisers are the rotator cuff, the tendon of long head of biceps, and the scapular muscles which help in controlling the shoulder through the midrange of motion. The static stabilisers exert control at the extremes of motion. They include the glenoid fossa, glenoid labrum (which increase the stability by deepening the relatively shallow, almost plate like, articular surface of glenoid fossa), glenohumeral joint capsule and the glenohumeral ligaments (which are thickening of the capsule that individually limit motion depending on the position of the arm). The scapulothoracic articulation also contributes to glenohumeral instability. Several clinical examination procedures are involved in assessing the function and integrity of shoulder but there is hardly anyone for definitely identifying the instability.

The shoulder is notorious for undergoing stiffness, not only following its own pathology, but also following the pathology situated centripetally or centrifugally, e.g. in cervical spondylosis or shoulder hand syndrome (Steinbrocher et al. 1943).

The *axillary nerve*, which supplies deltoid and teres minor muscles, is tensed in internal rotation and relaxed in external rotation of shoulder. It is at risk in the fractures of the proximal humerus.

Vascular lesions are infrequent in fractures of proximal humerus, and are mostly venous (rarely arterial).

■ METHODOLOGY

Different clinical conditions affecting the shoulder do produce almost similar clinical presentations, such as in impingement syndromes, rotator cuff tears, bicipital tendinitis, adhesive capsulitis, calcific tendinitis, nerve entrapment syndromes, etc.

The comprehensive clinical examination of shoulder should include cervical spine examination, thoracic inlet examination, neurological examination of upper extremity, shoulder girdle examination, examination of shoulder joint proper, acromioclavicular joint, sternoclavicular joint, the scapulothoracic articulation and muscles stabilising the scapula during active shoulder motion, the long head of biceps, the subacromial bursa and the rotator cuff. The main aim of examining the shoulder should focus on identifying the structure involved in pathology (traumatic or disease) and the stability of shoulder.

History Taking

The usual complaints concerning shoulder are: (i) Limitation of movements, (ii) pain in the region of shoulder joint, (iii) inability/weakness to lift the limb, (iv) swelling in the region of shoulder joint, and (v) wound or sinus in the region of shoulder joint.

Injuries of shoulder joints are usually the result of indirect violence. Of course, falling on the shoulder point can also produce various injuries. The actual mode of sustaining the injury should be noted, e.g. (i) fall on outstretched hand or point of shoulder or on point of elbow, (ii) direct hit from any direction at shoulder, (iii) hyperabduction strain of the shoulder.

Pain

Besides enquiring about the nature, site, relation with activities, diurnal variation of pain, always ask about its radiation, especially from or to the cervical region, arm, forearm, or hand. Note the actual direction and point of radiation. Pain in the shoulder region may be referred from the affections of the viscera. Referred shoulder pain may be also from thoracic contents, such as cardiac origin angina pectoris (to one or both shoulders), aortic aneurysm; pleural origin—pleuritis (usually of central part of diaphragm); lung origin—pneumonia, Pancoast syndrome (e.g. Pancoast carcinoma of apical part of lung); Diaphragm origin—subdiaphragmatic, supradiaphragmatic and diaphragmatic pathology (e.g. gallbladder, liver and pancreatic pathologies). Referred pain from spleen pathology is to the left shoulder only. Referred pain from gallbladder and liver is to the right shoulder.

General and Systemic Examinations

As in Chapter 1 "Introduction".

Regional Examination

For the shoulder affections, examination from the cervical and cervicodorsal spine to the tip of the finger is essential. If any pathology is detected in this range, that part should be examined thoroughly. The regional lymph nodes (the supraclavicular and axillary groups) should also be examined.

Local Examination

Prerequisites

(i) Patient must be examined standing on the floor or sitting on a stool, (ii) neck to the tip of fingers must be exposed fully from all sides, (iii) opposite shoulder must be examined for comparison, (iv) the limb should be kept freely hanging by the side of chest in anatomical position, i.e. elbow extended and forearm supinated as far as practicable. Limb length disparity and the portion where the disparity lies can be easily seen in this posture (*see* **Fig. 4.2A**).

Attitude

Attitude of the patient in relation to the shoulder is sometimes typical depending upon underlying pathology (*see* **Figs. 4.1 to 4.6**). The position of the neck, the shoulder point and the supported or unsupported upper limb should be noted. Many a times the attitude itself is diagnostic, e.g. patient with *fracture clavicle* inclines his neck to the affected side and supports the elbow in opposite hand keeping the arm by the side of the chest. Patient with *anterior dislocation of shoulder* loses the contour of shoulder, develops flattening of deltoid bulge, drooping of axillary fold and keeps the elbow away from the chest (**Fig. 4.1**). In luxatio erecta, the arm is kept widely abducted and sometimes internally rotated. In *Erb's palsy*, the child keeps the arm abducted and internally rotated, elbow extended, forearm pronated, wrist partially flexed, thumb in palm and fingers semiflexed, i.e. position of the *policeman receiving tip* (Refer **Figs. 16.4 to 16.6**).

Contracture of the deltoid muscle may develop secondary to congenital fibrosis (**Figs. 4.2, 4.3 and 4.46**), intramuscular injection or trauma leading to fibrosis of the muscle. Abduction contracture of shoulder and winging of scapula due to the deltoid contracture should be differentiated from abduction contracture of shoulder due to other causes, e.g. brachial plexus palsy (it usually involves the infraspinatus and teres minor muscles and abnormal

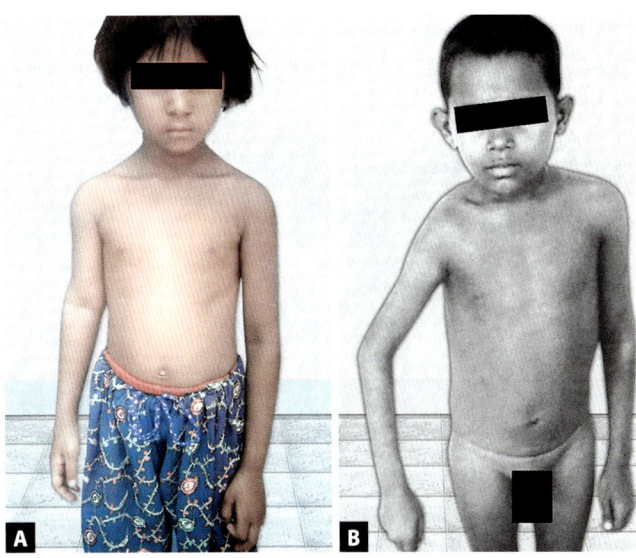

Figs. 4.2A and B: (A) Note that the right upper limb is shorter (congenital) than the left and arm portion is mainly short; (B) Fixed abduction deformity of shoulder due to congenital contracture of intermediate fibres of deltoid.

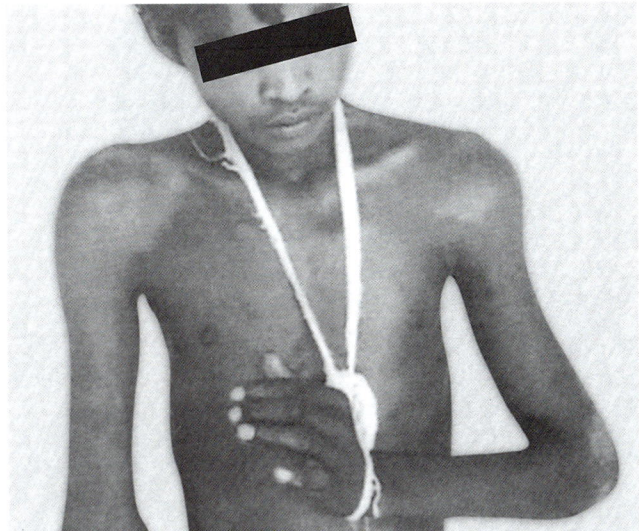

Fig. 4.1: The typical attitude of anterior dislocation of shoulder.

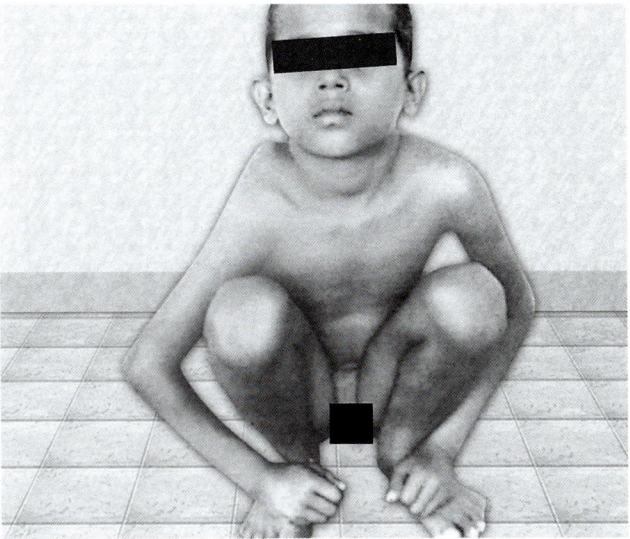

Fig. 4.3: Same patient (**Fig. 4.2B**) in sitting posture. Note the projecting scapular acromion process on deltoid contracture side.

involuntary movement—dyskinesia—is a prominent feature); prescapular space occupying lesion, e.g. abscess **(Figs. 4.4 and 4.5)**, osteochondroma, deltoid muscle tumours (*see* **Figs. 4.49 to 4.51**); septic arthritis of shoulder (*see* **Figs. 4.53 and 4.54**).

In *Klippel-Feil syndrome (congenital webbed neck)*, hairline lies almost on shoulder level **(Fig. 4.6)** with/without high-placed scapula **(Figs. 4.6 and 4.7)**. In *Sprengel's shoulder* Sprengel (1891) and Kolliker (1891) described the first cases in the Lagenbecks (Archiv Für Klinische Chirurge in 1891, however Kolliker applied Sprengel's name to this clinical condition. The first description of the deformity was by Eulenberg which was published in 1868 in Germany – (After Patwardhan S 2016) (most common congenital malformation of shoulder girdle)—*congenital elevation of scapula,* upper border of which may lie well above the shoulder, scapula is usually hypoplastic and misshaped. The inferior angle is medially rotate causing the glenoid to face inferiorly. There is asymmetry in shoulder contour and restriction of shoulder and cervical spine movements. Eulenberg described this condition first in 1863 as 'hochgradige dislocation der scapula', but Sprengel illustrated this condition in 1891, hence his name is associated. Some associated anomalies are almost always present like absent or fused ribs asymmetric chest wall, Klippel-Feil syndrome **(Fig. 4.6)**, Congenital scoliosis **(Fig. 4.9B)** Cervical rib, spine bifida. The cosmesis and function of the shoulder can be fairly improved by surgery, such as Mear's procedure (2001) in which scapular osteotomy, partial excision of scapula and release of the long head of triceps are done **(Figs. 4.8 and 4.9)**. In deltoid contracture, there is fixed abduction deformity at the shoulder (*see* **Figs. 4.2 and 4.3**).

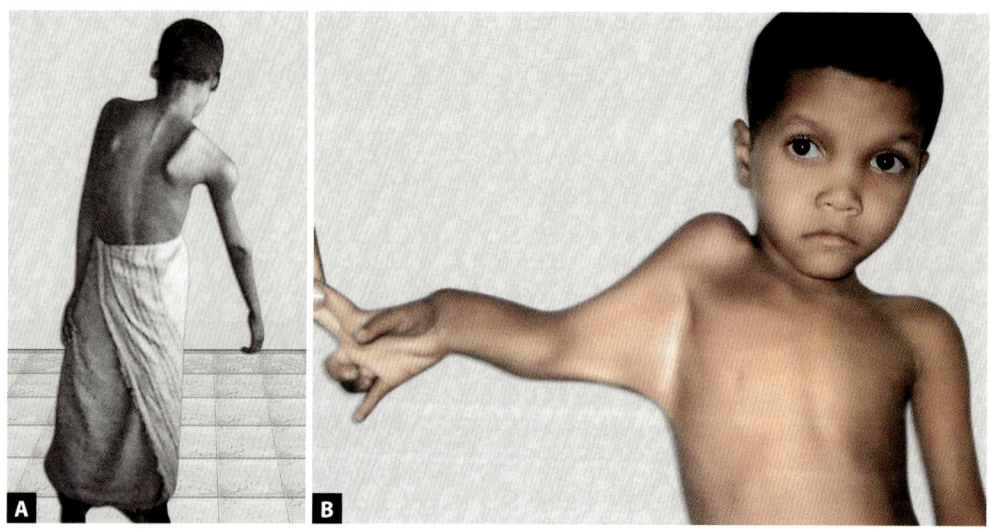

Figs. 4.4A and B: (A) Fixed abduction deformity of shoulder due to 7 weeks old prescapular abscess which is also encroaching upon the posterolateral aspect of shoulder; (B) Congenital webbed axilla—management by plastic surgery (release and reconstruction of web).

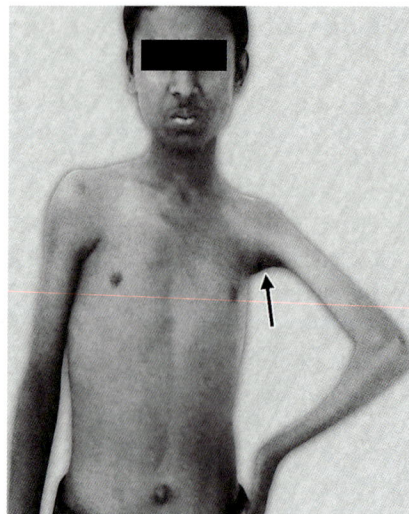

Fig. 4.5: Fixed abduction deformity of shoulder due to axillary abscess.

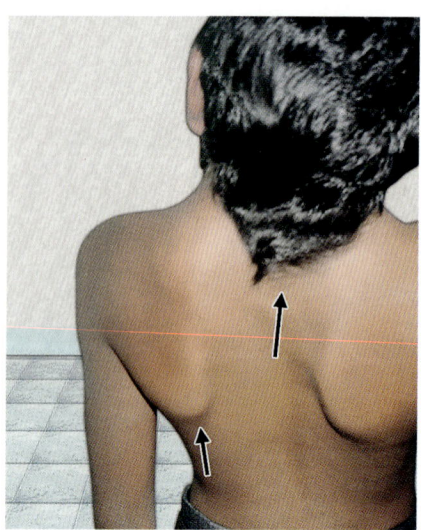

Fig. 4.6: Klippel-Feil syndrome. Note the level of hair-line, and congenital elevation of left scapula.

In gross congenital malformations, examination should be done on the lines pertinent to that particular case (*see* **Figs. 4.10 and 4.55**).

Inspection

Inspect from the front, side, back and the top simultaneously comparing with the opposite side. Note the condition of skin, its vascularity, presence of any swelling **(Figs. 4.11, 4.45B)**, abnormal pulsation, wasting, fasciculation, etc.

From the front: Relation of the two clavicles from the sternoclavicular to acromioclavicular joints, anterior deltoid bulge, supraclavicular fossae, infraclavicular fossae, pectoral bulge, anterior axillary line and folds, contour of the shoulder and approximation of the elbow to the chest.

From the sides: The deltoid bulge and the side of the arm.

From the top: Acromioclavicular elevation and angle of acromion, the bulge of the shoulder.

From the back: Right from midspinal line, medial border of scapula and scapular prominence, scapular (supra- and infraspinatus) fossae, level of inferior angle of scapula, posterior deltoid bulge, posterior axillary line and folds. Any abnormality in comparison to the other side must be noted **(Figs. 4.8 and 4.9)**.

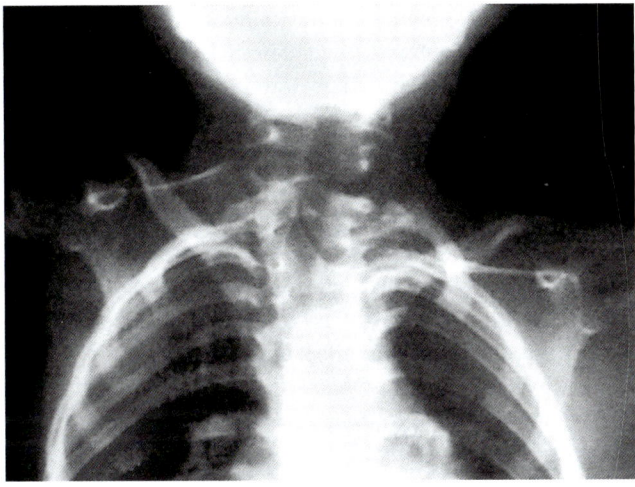

Figs. 4.7: X-ray of the same patient (Fig. 4.6) of Klippel-Feil syndrome.

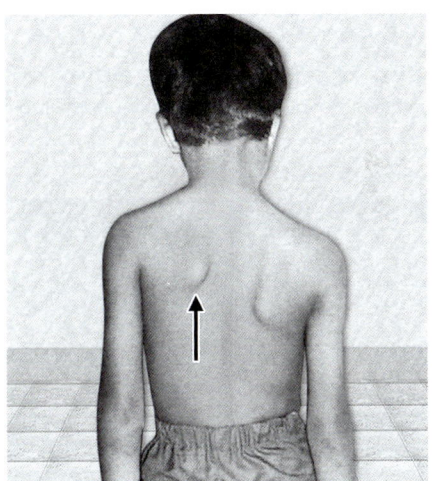

Figs. 4.8: Sprengel's shoulder on left.

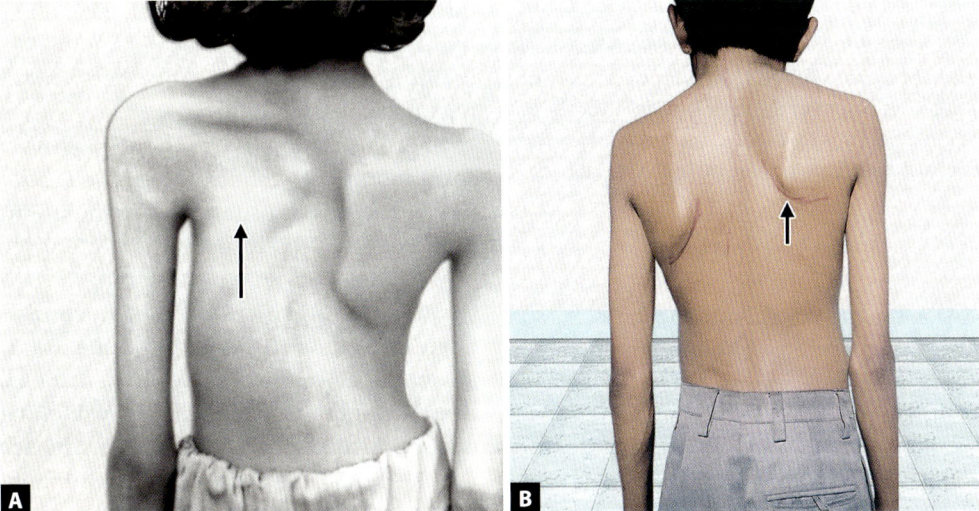

Figs. 4.9A and B: (A) Congenital absence (or rudimentary development) of infraspinous portion of high ridden left scapula with mild thoracic scoliosis; (B) Sprengel's shoulder on right with mild scoliosis. Sprengel's shoulder is the most frequent congenital shoulder deformity caused by arrest in caudal migration of scapula during embryonic development. Patient has cosmetic and functional problems. Various treatment like muscle release procedures with relocation of scapula; excision of superior angle of scapula, excision of omovertebral mass with partial scapulectomy. Mears procedure consisting of partial resection of scapula and release of long head of triceps with part of teres minor has usually produced better results.

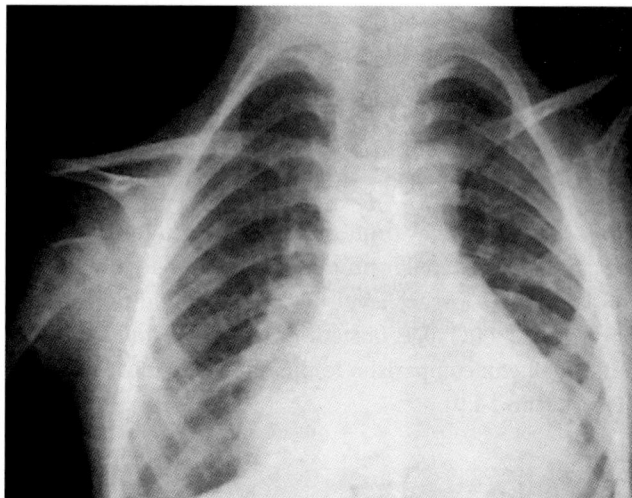

Fig. 4.10: Gross congenital malformations in the cervical regions and absence of more or less both upper limbs.

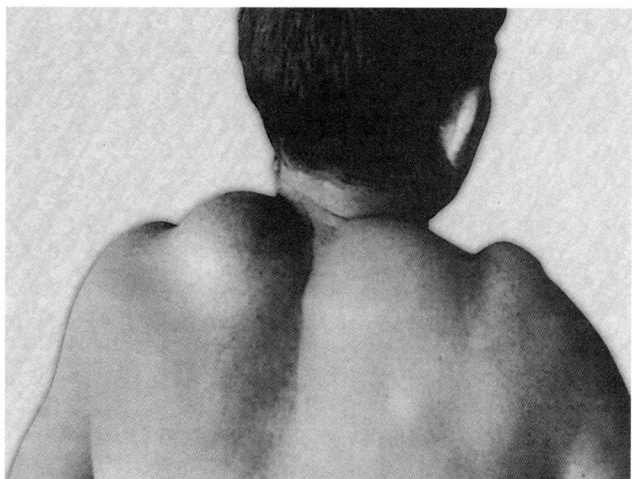

Fig. 4.11: Note the abnormal rounded swelling over the right shoulder and on both sides of root of the neck and also over the left shoulder top—pseudolipoma due to repeated friction trauma in one who carries bamboo stick with hanging load on both sides (Bhar).

Palpation

(a) Superficial—(As in the chapter on Introduction)
(b) Deep—Besides the common points as noted in the chapter on 'Introduction' *locate and palpate the following*, and note any abnormality. The main bony landmarks of the normal shoulder—the tip of coracoid, the greater tuberosity of humeral head and the acromion—form a right angle at the greater tuberosity. Palpate (i) clavicle from sternoclavicular to acromioclavicular joint, (ii) tip of the coracoid process, (iii) angle of acromion, (iv) the body and angles of scapula, (v) hollowness of the base of axilla, (vi) hollowness or fullness of infraclavicular fossae, (vii) palpate the supraclavicular region for pulsation or any other abnormality of the subclavian artery and upper medial aspect of the arm for the brachial artery, (viii) palpate the different groups of lymph glands in axillary and supraclavicular regions, (ix) in acute traumatic cases palpate for any dislocated articulating end or displaced bony fragment, and in late ones for any myositis or myositic mass, (x) the ipsilateral chest and breast (specially in ladies) should be palpated for any pathology. Sometimes the carcinoma of breast, specially that of axillary tail of Spence (or allied affection) manifest as stiffness and pain in shoulder region.

Tenderness of the shoulder joint is mainly elicited at two regions; just lateral to the coracoid process anteriorly, and just below and behind the acromial angle posteriorly. In bicipital tendinitis, tenderness is along the biceps tendon on the anterosuperior slope of the shoulder bulge. Tenderness over the region of glenoid, head of humerus, tuberosities and upper humeral shaft should be noted separately.

A *cystic* (the word cyst is derived from the Greek word meaning bladder) *swelling around the shoulder* should be confirmed by the usual methods of demonstration. Collection in the shoulder joint is usually localised anteriorly, posteriorly or inferomedially. However, when the collection increases, cross-fluctuation (anteroposteriorly) can be demonstrated. A cystic hygroma, having typical compressibility and very clear transillumination, may manifest anteriorly.

In doubtful cases of *fasciculation,* tapping over or squeezing the deltoid muscles can be useful in initiating the bout.

Since the muscular padding is very thick almost all around, on palpation one gets very little clue about the fracture ends unless they are quite obvious. One should not attempt to elicit crepitus and abnormal mobility. Most of the fractures around the shoulder are generally impacted and require hardly any interference. Overenthusiastic attempts at demonstrating crepitus and abnormal movements may disimpact the fractured ends.

If on inspection, the roundness of the shoulder is lost, search for *abnormal position of the head of the humerus*. In dislocations, it usually lies in the infraclavicular fossa (anterior), and rarely just posteroinferior to the acromion or its spinous process (posterior) or the subglenoid region (inferior). In fresh cases of dislocations, the finding of depressed contour should be enough to diagnose it. Any attempt to move the shoulder, to note the movement of the head under the palpating fingers, will initiate endless pain and spasm. In the paralytic shoulder, the deltoid mass thins out, the head of the humerus stands prominent much below the acromial process, thereby having a 'step' in between the acromion and the head of the humerus in which the finger can be well insinuated **(Figs. 4.12 and 11.32)**. Atrophy of the deltoid, abnormal mobility of the shoulder (mainly passive) and the *'step sign' are diagnostic of paralytic subluxation or dislocation.*

Movements (Normal Movements of Shoulder, Table 4.1)

Let the patient stand with his upper limbs hanging by the side of the chest in anatomical position, i.e. shoulder adducted, elbow extended and forearm supinated. Elicit the movements (active and passive) and note the results under the standard headings as given in the chapter on 'Introduction'. If the active movement is restricted, possible passive range of movement can be tested by holding the patient's hand by examiner's one hand, while his 90° flexed elbow is supported by the examiner's other hand.

Measurements

- Linear
- Circumferential.

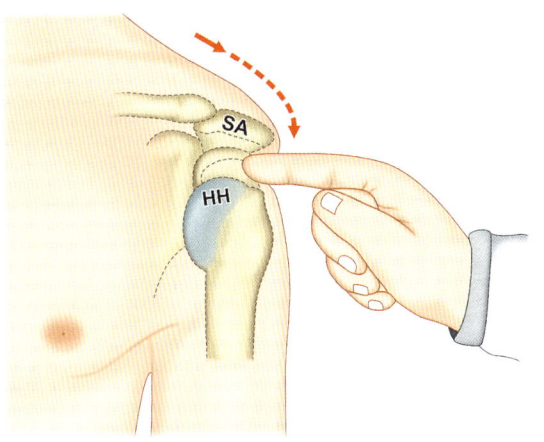

Fig. 4.12: Paralytic subluxation—step sign.

TABLE 4.1: Movements at shoulder.

Movement	Range	Prime movers	Assisted by	Root control	Limiting factors	Remarks
1	2	3	4	5	6	7
Flexion Patient stands with arm hanging by the side, elbow extended and forearm supinated. Ask him to take hand towards the mid-line	0°–135°	Pectoralis major, pectoralis minor, anterior fibres of deltoid, coracobrachialis	Biceps brachii	C5	Nothing specific except tension of posterior capsule	In extreme flexion internal rotation supervenes
Extension Diametrically opposite to that of flexion	0°–55°	Latissimus dorsi	Posterior fibres of deltoid, teres major	C5, 6	Tension of shoulder flexor muscles. Contact of greater tuberosity of humerus with the acromion	
Abduction Extended elbow moving away from body. The glenohumeral and scapulothoracic components of abduction can be tested as follows. Stand behind the patient and hold the inferior angle of scapula firmly in between thumb and index finger of one hand. While doing abduction, so long as the movement is at glenohumeral joint, scapula will not resist. The moment scapulothoracic gliding starts, resistance is felt by the holding hand. Note the extent of each component (Normal: 90°+ 90°)	0°– almost 180°	While subscapularis muscle steadies the humeral head in glenoid socket, initiation is by supraspinatus (15°–30°), by middle fibres of deltoid up to 90°, deltoid straps around the humeral head on the glenoid, making the glenohumeral component into one unit. Beyond 90°, the locked scapulohumeral component glides over the chest wall till the extended elbow goes overhead. In this gliding mechanism, muscles involved are serratus anterior, trapezius, latissimus dorsi. The seat of this movement for all practical considerations; the initial 90° of abduction		C6 Accessory nerve	Up to 90°— none. Beyond 90°—at terminal stage by contact of the arm against the side of the head	(i) In extreme abduction, external rotation of the shoulder supervenes (ii) In terminal stage, some gliding movements occur at the sternoclavicular and acromioclavicular joints. (iii) **Painful arc** syndrome (pain in arc of 60°–120°) occurs in supraspinatus tendinitis, subacromial bursitis, partial supra-spinatus tear, calcific deposits in subacromial bursa and rotator cuff, crack/ fracture of greater tuberosity

Contd...

Contd...

Movement	Range	Prime movers	Assisted by	Root control	Limiting factors	Remarks
1	2	3	4	5	6	7
		is at glenohumeral joint, then gliding of locked scapulohumeral components over the posterolateral aspects of chest is supplemented by gliding movements of the clavicle at acromioclavicular and sternoclavicular joints. However, detailed work has shown that there may be involvement of the scapula or even the clavicle right from the beginning of abduction (Turek, SL 1954)				
Adduction						
Diametrically opposite to abduction	180°–0°	Pectoralis major, latissimus dorsi, teres major	Gravity	C5, 6	Contact of arm with chest wall	
External rotation						
While arm is by the side of the chest, elbow flexed at 90° and forearm supinated, move the extended hand outwards	0°–70° to 90°	Teres minor, infraspinatus, posterior fibres of deltoid		C5	1. Tension on internal rotators 2. Tension of upper portion of capsular ligament and coracohumeral ligament	Never try to demonstrate the rotational movement in extended position of elbow as rotational elements of forearm will be superadded
Internal rotation						
While the position as above, move the extended hand towards the mid-body plane	0°–80° to 90°	Subscapularis, pectoralis major, teres major, latissimus dorsi	Anterior fibres of deltoid	C5, 6, 7, 8	1. Tension of external rotators 2. Tension of upper portion of capsular ligament	
Circumduction						
With the upper limb extended at the elbow and wrist, complete a circle starting from the adducted position of the arm	360°	Combination of all of the above		C5, 6 Accessory nerve		If any of the above movements is affected, true circumduction will not be possible

Linear Measurements

- Apparent measurements
- True measurements.

Segmental measurements should also be done.

Apparent measurements: Apparent measurement is not of much value as in the lower limbs. However, it can give some idea.

Method: With the affected upper limb in a position as kept comfortably by the patient, the opposite upper limb is put parallel to it. Measure from the tip of the seventh cervical spine to the tip of the radial styloid on both sides while the trunk is aligned to the limbs.

True measurements: Prerequisites—Limbs must be kept in identical position at each joint, i.e. shoulder, elbow and wrist. Palpate and mark the angle of acromion (pass a finger laterally on the spine of scapula, at the extreme outer end posteriorly, an angle is formed known as the *angle of acromion*), lateral epicondyle of the humerus and tip of the styloid process of radius.

Total linear measurement of the upper limbs is done by measuring from the angle of acromion to the tip of radial styloid process **(Fig. 4.13)**.

Segmental measurements are for arm and forearm components. For the arm, measure from acromial angle to the tip of the lateral epicondyle and for the forearm, from the lateral epicondylar tip to the tip of the radial styloid process. If the lateral epicondylar tip is not discernible (e.g. in comminuted fractures, congenital absence, iatrogenic) identical fixed bony points can be taken for comparative measurement (e.g. medial epicondylar tips, radial head, olecranon tips).

Circumferential Measurements

Besides noting the wasting at the mid-arm level, or at equidistant from the acromial angles, circumferential measurements should also be done around the shoulder joint, i.e. across the base of axilla to the top of the shoulder. For all practical purposes, any increase in this measurement indicates an increase in the girth of the shoulder joint and *vice versa*.

The anterior and posterior axillary folds should be measured and compared with the other side **(Fig. 4.14)**.

Method: Abduct the shoulder as far as practicable up to 90°. Keep the opposite shoulder in the same position. Axillary folds stand prominent. Measure from the junction of the axillary folds with the arm to their junction with the trunk (both anterior and posterior folds).

Special Tests

Hamilton Ruler Test (Figs. 15A and B)

In a normal shoulder, a straight ruler cannot touch the acromial process and lateral epicondyle of humerus at the same time **(Fig. 4.15A)** because of the prominence of the deltoid bulge, which is supported by the head of humerus. If the support is lost, the ruler can touch both the points (e.g. in dislocation of the shoulder, congenital absence or iatrogenic excision of the head of humerus; complete paralytic atrophy of the deltoid, as in polio paralysis; dissolution of humeral head in septic arthritis) **(Fig. 4.15B)**.

Callaway's Test

The girth from axillary base to shoulder top is symmetrical and same on both sides. If the head of humerus occupies an abnormal position, e.g. in dislocation, the girth increases on the affected side.

(Fallacies—axillary abscess, huge lymphadenopathy, collection in the shoulder joint).

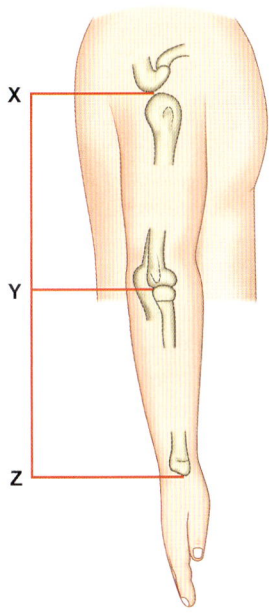

Fig. 4.13: True measurement of upper limb XY—arm length; YZ—Forearm length; XZ—total linear measurement of upper limb.

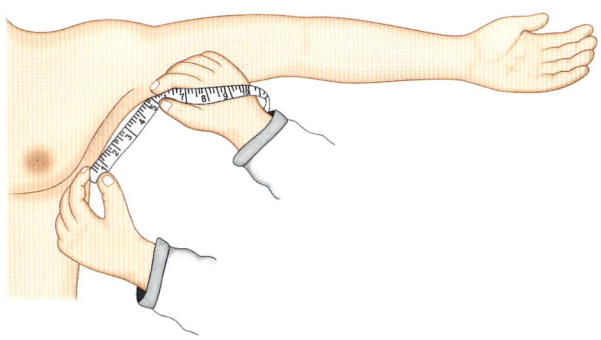

Fig. 4.14: Measurement of axillary folds.

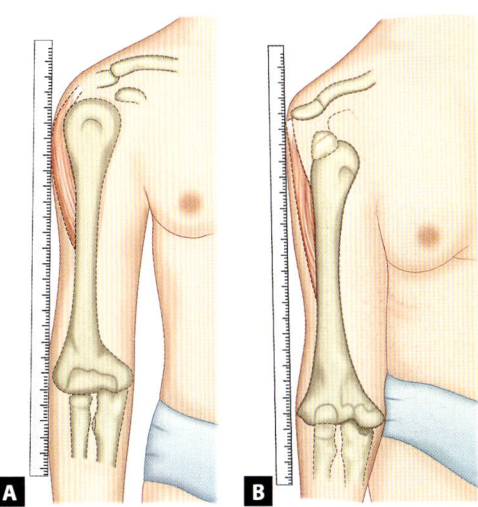

Figs. 4.15A and B: Hamilton ruler test.

Duga's Test (Fig. 4.16)

Normally after full flexion at the shoulder, the elbow can be brought to near about the midbody plane and the hand to the opposite shoulder top. In dislocation of the shoulder joint, the full flexion of the shoulder cannot be achieved, the elbow, therefore, cannot be brought to the midbody plane and thus the hand cannot be taken to the opposite shoulder.

Bryant's Sign

In anterior subcoracoid dislocation of the shoulder, the anterior axillary fold looks elongated and seems to be at a lower level.

Test for Integrity of the Brachial Plexus

Test for integrity of the brachial plexus is essential as it may be variably damaged in anterior dislocation of shoulder.

Erb's palsy (upper brachial palsy)—look for the typical attitude and posture of hand—*policeman tip position* and test for the muscle supplied by C5,6.

(*See* Chapter 16 on Peripheral Nerve Injuries).

Test for Integrity of the Axillary Nerve

It is manifested by loss of deltoid action, i.e. abduction of shoulder (though initiation of abduction is possible by the intact supraspinatus muscle) and sensory loss over the 'regimental badge' area at upper outer aspect of the arm.

(*See* Chapter 16 on Peripheral Nerve Injuries).

Radial Nerve

Manifested by wrist drop (Refer **Figs. 16.19 and 16.20**).

Test for Thoracic Inlet Syndrome

This syndrome comprises the pathologies in which there is compression of the subclavian artery and/or lower roots of the brachial plexus, e.g. scalenus anticus syndrome (nerve compression by scalenus anticus muscle), costoclavicular syndrome [nerve compression (in between) by first rib and clavicle], subclavian aneurysm, cervical ribs, Pancoast tumour, exuberant callus in fracture clavicle, etc. (*See* Chapter 8 on Spine), complex regional pain syndrome, shoulder hand syndrome.

Tests for Bicipital Tenosynovitis (Bicipital tendinitis)

- *Yergason's manoeuvre:* Patient flexes the elbow and then supinates the forearm against resistance. The resulting forceful contraction of biceps effects distal movement of the tendon and causes pain in the bicipital groove
- The elbow is flexed 90° and examiner's three fingers are firmly placed along the anterosuperior slope of the deltoid bulge (line of bicipital groove); ask the patient to alternately rotate the shoulder externally and internally. Patient will complain of pain when the inflamed tenosynovitis will pass under the pressing fingers
- *Speed's test:* The patient complains of pain in the bicipital groove with resisted elevation of the arm, while the elbow and forearm are fully extended forward.

Test for Complete Rupture of Supraspinatus

It is difficult to categorically distinguish pure supraspinatus and other rotator cuff ruptures from any pathology of the subacromial region. However, in complete rupture, a gap may be felt beneath the acromion, which will be tender. Patient cannot initiate active abduction at the shoulder (glenohumeral joint), but once the arm is passively abducted to about 90°, he can sustain and further actively abduct the shoulder due to deltoid action.

Incomplete rupture of the supraspinatus and other rotator cuff muscles can be diagnosed by infiltrating local anaesthetic in the affected area, which abolishes the pain and spasm, allowing the patient to abduct the shoulder from the very beginning.

Test for Complete Tear of Rotator Cuff

The *rotator cuff* consists of the tendons of supraspinatus, infraspinatus and teres minor. The most important *function of rotator cuff* is to stabilise the humeral head against the glenoid as the arm is elevated. The rotator cuff along with deltoid allows elevation of the arm overhead. If the stabilising function of rotator cuff is compromised (as in full thickness tear of rotator cuff), the unopposed pull of deltoid displaces the humeral head upward towards the acromion. Elevation is generally limited to 30°–40°.

The average thickness of the normal tendon of the rotator cuff is 10–12 mm. It may be torn in its complete or partial thickness (not rare), of course in most situations, it is difficult to clinically differentiate between the two. At times partial tear can be more painful than the full thickness tears. Nocturnal pain is the most irritating symptom and is the principal

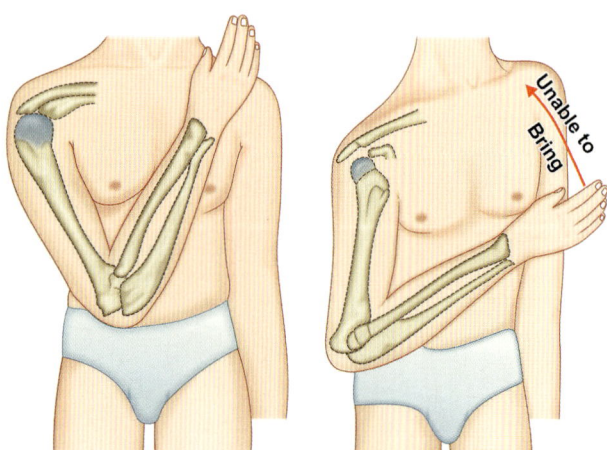

Fig. 4.16: Duga's test.

problem in both partial and full thickness tears. Partial thickness rotator cuff tear is a common pathology among shoulder disorder in people over 50 years of age.

The *clinical features of rotator cuff disease* (tears) are nonspecific. Fukuda et al. (1996) categorised them into two groups:
1. *Those caused mainly by the inflammation* of subacromial bursa (bursitis) and tendon (tendinitis)—symptoms are various types of pain, signs of fluid, a painful arc, an impingement sign, a positive procaine test and contracture—these features are usually reversible with non-operative management.
2. *Those caused due to torn tendon* (mostly degenerative tears). Clinical features are: Pain (usually nocturnal—both in partial and complete tears). Positive arm-drop sign, crepitus, weakness of muscles and atrophy of supra- and infraspinatus. These features usually do not reverse with conservative treatment alone.

Arm-drop-sign—Stabilising the scapula with one hand, the examiner passively abducts the patient's affected shoulder to 90° and asks him to sustain it. In case of complete tear, the patient cannot sustain the abducted arm and it drops by the side of the trunk.

Clinically diagnosed rotator cuff tears can be further assessed and confirmed by arthrogram and MRI.

Treatment of the various local injection of autologous platelet-rich plasma into shoulder joint appears to be more effective in reducing the pain and improving the functional result.

Test for Detecting Subacromial Impingement of the Rotator Cuff

Painful arc syndrome (Fig. 4.17)—Patient is asked to abduct his/her internally rotated arm over his/her head. In case of impingement of rotator cuff in between the humeral head and the acromion, he/she starts getting pain at about 60° of abduction, which continues till about 120°, and then disappears.

Calcifying Tendinitis of Rotator Cuff is a common degenerative disorder of unknown etiology mostly seen in aging people and in persons with occupation demanding prolonged use of arms in internal rotation and slight abduction (such as typists). Reactive calcification of varying size occurs in rotator cuff, which undergoes spontaneous resorption in course of time with subsequent healing of the tender. It rarely ossifies.

Neer's Impingement Test (Sign)

Jarjavay first described the 'subacromical bursitis' in 1867. Neer in 1972; described impingement syndrome characterised by a ridge of proliferative spurs and excrescences on the under surface of the anterior process of acromion, probably caused by repeated impingement of

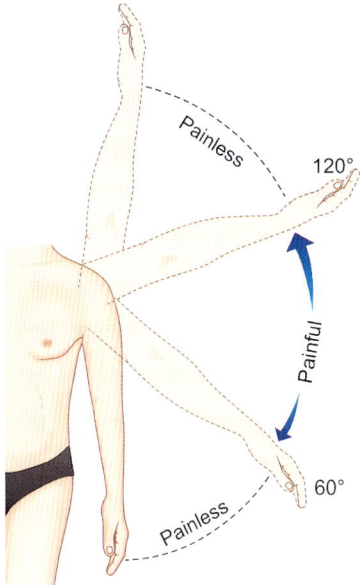

Fig. 4.17: Painful arc syndrome.

the rotator cuff and the humeral head with traction of the coracoacromial ligament.

Neer's impingement test is done to differentiate impingement syndrome (mainly subacromial pathology) from 'frozen shoulder' arthritis. Here the clinician prevents scapular rotation with one hand, while with the other hand he raises the affected arm in forced forward flexion and abduction, thus causing the greater tuberosity to impinge against the acromion. Pain is produced in all the above conditions. Neer impingent test (sign) is positive, if the pain is elicited in the mid arc of motion. If the pain is primarily the result of impingement, it can be reduced or eliminated by injecting 10 mL of 1% lignocaine beneath the anterior acromion.

Test for Anterior Shoulder Instability

The best signs for anterior shoulder instability are the apprehension and relocation signs.

Apprehension (sign) test: It is performed to detect any instability of the shoulder (e.g. in recurrent subluxation/dislocation of shoulder). The patient lies supine keeping his/her shoulder muscles relaxed. The suspected shoulder is gradually abducted to 90° and then gently externally rotated pressing the shoulder along the long axis of the arm. In case of instability, the patient becomes gradually apprehensive and tries to resist any further movement by his other hand and making the shoulder stiff. This is a positive apprehension sign.

The *relocation test* is done with the patient in the same position as during the apprehension test except that a posteriorly directed force is applied to the humeral head while continuous maximum external rotation of this shoulder is maintained. This force relocates the joint and thus in a patient with anterior instability, the apprehension and pain resolve.

This test is useful is differentiating anterior instability from primary impingement.

Test for Detecting Coracoiditis

The repeated acute or chronic work by arm (and shoulder) may lead to inflammation of the attachment region of short head of biceps and coracobrachialis muscles at the tip of the coracoid process. There may be history of injury in the coracoid process tip region.

When the patient is asked to adduct and externally rotate the humerus, the pain is reproduced in the shoulder region, if there is coracoiditis.

Another test: the patient is asked to perform supination of the forearm with flexed elbow and flexed shoulder against resistance OR do adduction of the flexed shoulder—in both situations pain is reproduced in shoulder.

Jobe Test

Jobe described this *supraspinatus test* in 1983 to test the integrity of the muscle. The patient is asked to place the shoulder in 90° of abduction, 30° of forward flexion and internal rotation so that the thumb is pointing towards the floor. The muscle is tested, i.e. patient is asked to initiate abduction against resistance put by the examiner—there will be weakness and insufficiency in supraspinatus if there is tear or pain associated with rotator cuff impingement.

Investigations Required for Shoulder Pathology

Besides the routine X-ray, haematological investigations and urine analysis, some special investigations may also be required, according to indications.

X-ray

It is of great importance in any shoulder affection. It is always useful to take a comparative X-ray of the opposite shoulder. The shoulder girdle must be fully exposed along with a minimum of the upper one-third of the arm. In suspected referred pain around the shoulder, X-ray of cervical spine is necessary.

The X-rays should be taken at least in two planes, preferably at right angles to each other.

Anteroposterior X-ray—Patient lies supine with the arm adducted. The plate is kept behind the shoulder and beam is focussed from the front at the shoulder level. With any suspicion of subluxation/dislocation at the acromioclavicular joint, anteroposterior X-ray should be taken, while the patient stands, keeping his upper limbs hanging by the side of his chest, with some equal weight tied to his hands. Standing position X-ray should also be taken in case of paralysed shoulder.

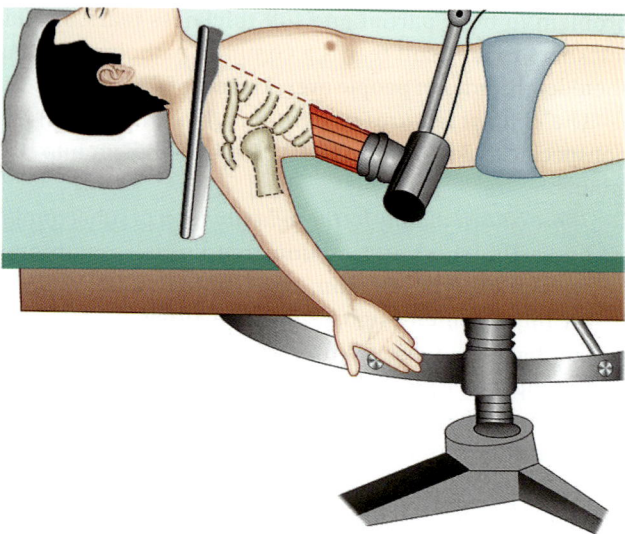

Fig. 4.18: Positioning for lateral axillary view.

Anteroposterior view in neutral position: A true anteroposterior X-ray of the glenohumeral joint (i.e. Grashey view) helps in clear delineation of the articular cartilage of the glenoid and the humeral head.
- The anteroposterior X-ray in internal rotation is useful for detecting the *Hill-Sachs lesions*
- The anteroposterior X-ray in external rotation provides good view of the greater tuberosity and proximal humeral physis in skeletally immature patients.

Lateral axillary (transaxillary) view: The shoulder is abducted to about 90° and the plate is kept on the shoulder top. The X-ray is shot through the base of the axilla **(Fig. 4.18)**.

Axillary lateral view shows the clear anatomy of glenoid rim, acromion, coracoid, and proximal humerus. The supraspinatus outlet view is a lateral view of scapula with the X-ray tube tilted 10° caudad. It helps in evaluation of rotator cuff disease.

Special Anteroposterior Projection

This special X-ray projection demonstrates the *Hill-Sachs lesion* (a humeral head impaction fracture) in recurrent dislocation of the shoulder **(Fig. 4.19)**.

While shoulder is abducted about 30° and internally rotated about 60°–90°, the plate is placed behind the shoulder and the beam is shot from the front at the shoulder level. In certain recurrent anterior dislocations, a radiological step can be delineated on the posterosuperolateral aspect of the head of the humerus (Hill-Sachs lesion or Broca lesion) presumably due to repeated compression (impingement) over the posterosuperior surface of head by impaction against the anterior margin of the glenoid, though it may also be congenital defect. A similar defect may be seen on the anteromedial sector of the head in recurrent posterior dislocation of the shoulder.

Three-dimensional CT scan and MRI are useful in demonstrating respectively the bony and soft tissue lesions (due to trauma or disease) which are not discernible in plain X-ray. MRI is specially helpful in detecting the subtle rotator cuff tears.

Aspiration of the Joint

Whenever collection is suspected, aspiration should be done through anterior approach and the aspirate should be submitted to physical, biochemical, cytological, culture and chemosensitivity examinations.

Arthroscopy

This investigation is being utilised to locate *Bankart's lesion* (the anterior margin of the glenoid cavity and capsule, with or without the glenoid labrum get torn off, presumably in the first traumatic dislocation, the non-healing of which has been blamed for recurrence), any foreign body, loose bodies, to study the condition of synovium and articular surfaces.

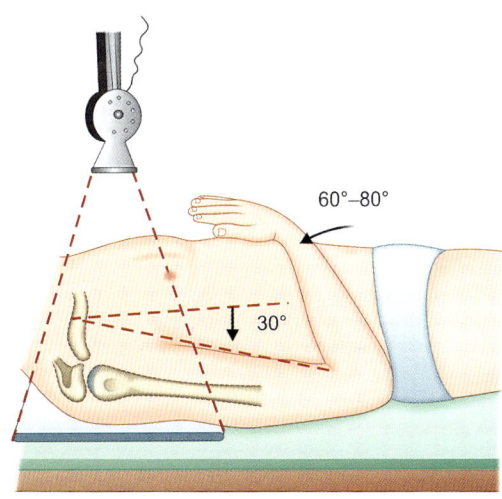

Fig. 4.19: Positioning for X-ray to demonstrate Hill-Sachs lesion.

Arthrography

Either utilising air or contrast dye, this investigation is useful for delineating the joint space, any filling defect, any leak of contrast medium into the surroundings (e.g. in complete rupture of supraspinatus, Bankart's lesion).

Arthrotomy

This step is seldom required for diagnostic purposes.

Key Diagnostic Points of Common Shoulder Affections (Table 4.2)

Traumatic Conditions

- *Traumatic Dislocation* **(Figs. 4.20 to 4.27) (Flowchart 4.1)**
  - Young adult with comparatively good muscle built
  - History of comparatively severe injury
  - Loss of normal contour of the shoulder
  - Abnormal attitude of the upper limb, e.g. elbow held away from the side of the chest, loss of shoulder bulge
  - Globular bony swelling at abnormal sites around the shoulder joint, according to the type of dislocation **(Fig. 4.20)**
  - Axillary girth increases
  - Anterior axillary fold lowers down
  - Ipsilateral hand cannot be brought to the contralateral shoulder
  - Look for possible neurovascular damage (axillary nerve, brachial plexus)
    (Fallacies—In (i) Fracture dislocation, (ii) Paralytic dislocation, where all above features may not be positive).
    In dislocation of shoulder joint, there is pseudo-lengthening (apparent lengthening) of the arm, and it appears as if the arm is originating at the lower level from the trunk when compared to other side
  - Rarely avascular necrosis of humeral head may occur as a late complication (*see* **Fig. 4.28**)
- *Recurrent Dislocation of Shoulder Joint*
  - Recurrent anterior dislocation is more common while posterior is rare
  - Subjects are usually young adults with good musculature

TABLE 4.2: Common affections of shoulder.

Traumatic	Paralytic	Degenerative and infective lesions
• Fracture surgical neck of humerus • Anterior dislocation of shoulder • Avulsion fracture of greater tuberosity • Fracture outer end of clavicle • Subluxation/dislocation of acromioclavicular joint • Fracture neck of scapula	• Poliomyelitis • Brachial plexus palsy • Motor neuron disease	• Periarthritis/adhesive capsulitis/frozen shoulder • Subacromial bursitis/calcification • Bicipital tendovaginitis • Tuberculosis shoulder • Septic arthritis

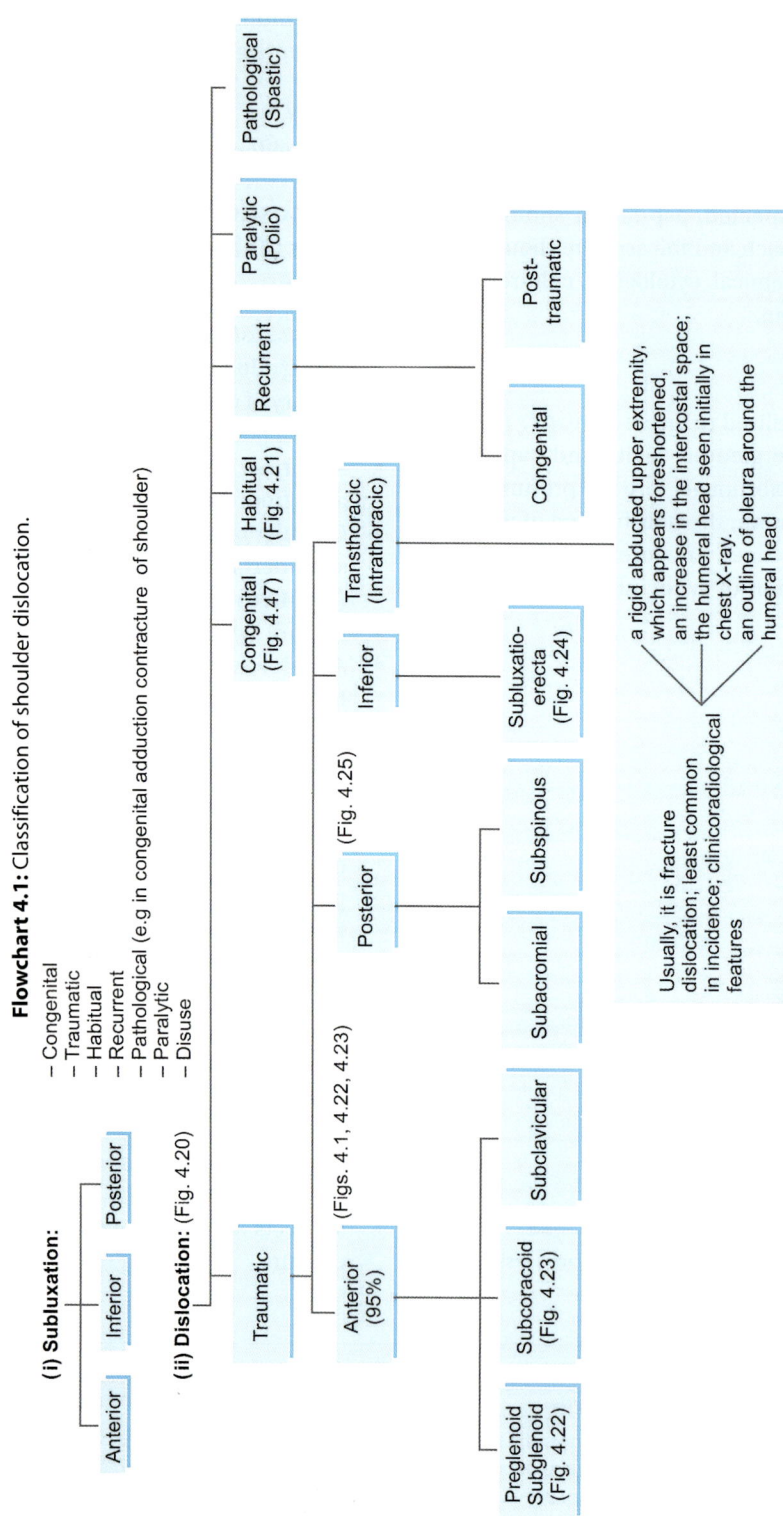

Flowchart 4.1: Classification of shoulder dislocation.

- History of recurrence even without significant trauma.
- No confirmatory clinical signs, however, subject may get apprehensive about dislocation with the limb put in a particular provocative position. While the shoulder is held in maximum external rotation and 90° or more abducted position and extension, the humeral head is pushed forward from behind. The patient becomes apprehensive and complains of pain in shoulder, and/or a sense of impending subluxation (*apprehension test*). By reducing or relocating the humeral head back into its normal position by manual pressure on the humeral head, the patient feels relieved of the apprehension symptoms (*relocation test*)
- A special X-ray may demonstrate Hill-Sachs lesion (anterior dislocation)
- Arthroscopy may demonstrate Bankart's lesion in anterior dislocation and reverse lesion in posterior recurrent dislocation.
  - *Fractures around the Shoulder:* Most of the fractures can be accurately diagnosed only after taking the X-ray
    - The most common fracture here is of the surgical neck of the humerus **(Fig. 4.29)**.
      - Elderly persons
      - History of fall on outstretched hand
      - Pain in shoulder region
      - In impacted fracture, fair/good range of passive shoulder movements

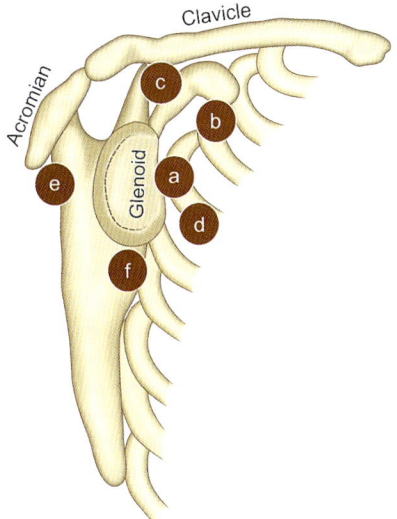

Fig. 4.20: Types of dislocation of shoulder—Circle represents the position of dislocated humeral head. a = preglenoid, b = subcoracoid, c = subclavicular, d = intrathoracic, e = subspinous, f = infraglenoid (subluxatio erecta).

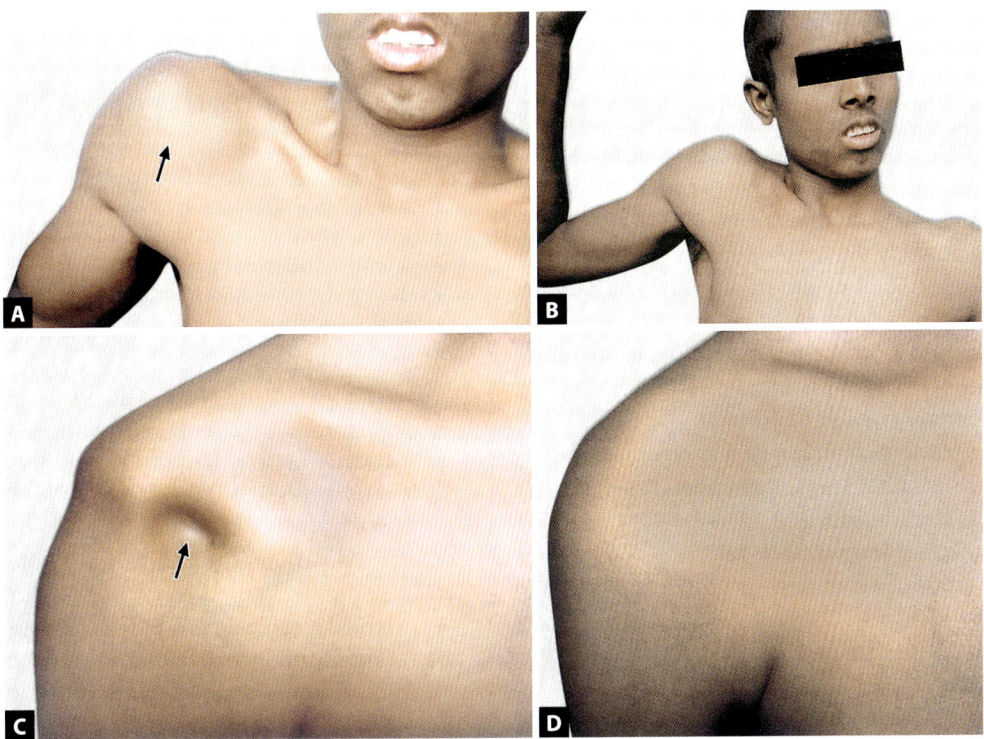

Figs. 4.21A to D: Habitual dislocation shoulder. Note the infraclavicular bulge produced due to dislocated humeral head (A); autoreduction at his will (B); voluntary inferior dislocation (C); autoreduction at his will (D).

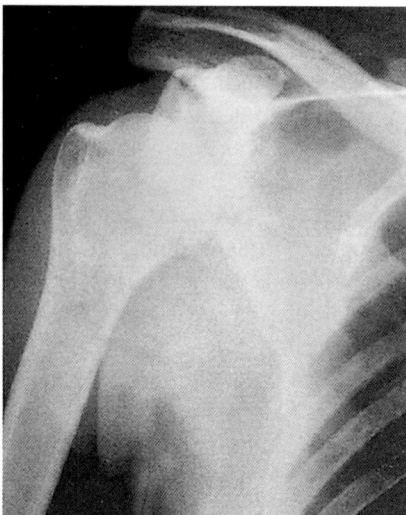

Fig. 4.22: Preglenoid dislocation of shoulder.

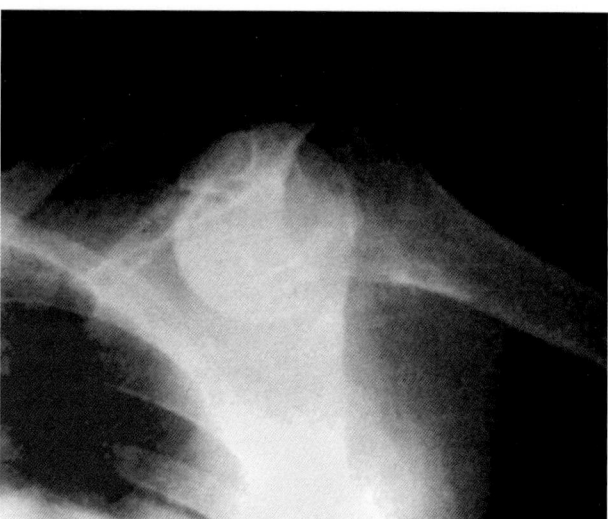

Fig. 4.23: Subcoracoid dislocation of shoulder.

- In unimpacted fractures, movements at the fracture site itself can be felt
- Ecchymosis in arm.
- *Dislocation of acromioclavicular joint* **(Fig. 4.30)**
  - Usually due to fall on shoulder joint, resulting in either subluxation (coracoclavicular ligament intact) or dislocation (coracoclavicular ligament torn). Indirect thrust violence from outside while the shoulder is kept abducted above 90°
  - In *subluxation*—outer end of clavicle, which just projects under the skin, is tender, clavicle is stable
  - In dislocation—outer end of the clavicle obviously ridden up, tender and the clavicle is unstable
  - X-ray is confirmatory.
- *Sternoclavicular dislocation* **(Figs. 4.31 to 4.34)**
  - Comparatively uncommon injury produced due to fall on shoulder point or outstretched hand; or direct hit from the front
  - Sternal end of clavicle may subluxate/dislocate forwards or backwards with upward shift
  - Local tender swelling at the joint
  - Rarely, clavicular end can be demonstrated mobile due to unstability **(Figs. 4.31 and 4.32)**
  - X-ray is confirmatory.
- *Fracture clavicle* **(Figs. 4.35 to 4.37)**
  - One of the most common fractures in children and adults
  - Due to fall on outstretched hand and by direct hit
  - Typical attitude
  - Fracture of middle two-third of clavicle is common **(Figs. 4.35 and 4.36)**; may be of outer end (Fig. 4.37) (confused with acromioclavicular subluxation/dislocation); may be of inner end (confused with sternoclavicular subluxation/dislocation)
  - Common displacement of clavicular-shaft fracture—medial fragment displaced and tilted upwards (due to pull of sternomastoid), and lateral fragment displaced downwards by the weight of the arm
  - Locally fracture end felt as an irregular end, which is tender; in late cases as a bony swelling at the fracture site (exuberant callus)
  - X-ray confirmatory.

Nontraumatic Conditions

- *Pyogenic Arthritis* **(Figs. 4.38, 4.39, 4.53, 4.54)**
  - Acute onset with constitutional features
  - Inflammatory swelling all around
  - Pitting oedema
  - All movements restricted and severely painful
  - Lymph nodes enlarged
  - Polymorphonuclear leucocytosis
  - Aspiration of pus—On culture causative organism usually grows.
- *Tuberculous Arthritis* **(Figs. 4.40 and 4.41)**
  - Rare forming 1-2 % of skeletal tuberculosis
  - Chronic history (in adults usually confused with periarthritis shoulder). More or less constant pain, more on activities
  - Disease originates in heads of humerus, glenoid of scapula
  - Marked atrophy of muscles all around the shoulder
  - Marked tenderness all around joint line, even on the adjoining bone (in periarthritis/frozen shoulder adjoining bone not that tender; flexion, and adduction movements are free). Tenderness of the head can be easily elicited through the axilla
  - Movements painfully restricted in all directions (in periarthritis, flexion and adduction not limited)

Shoulder Joints

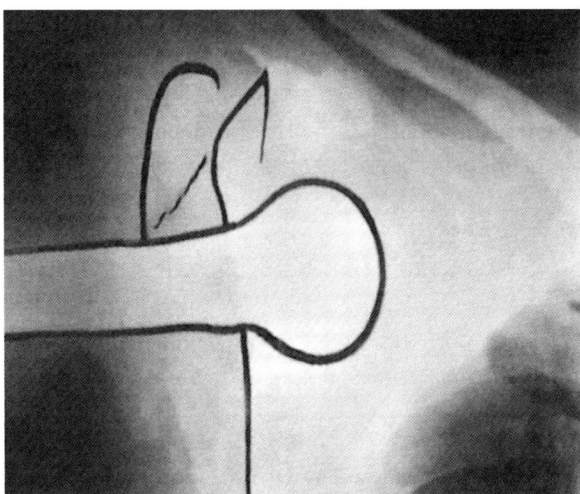

Fig. 4.24: Subluxatio erecta.

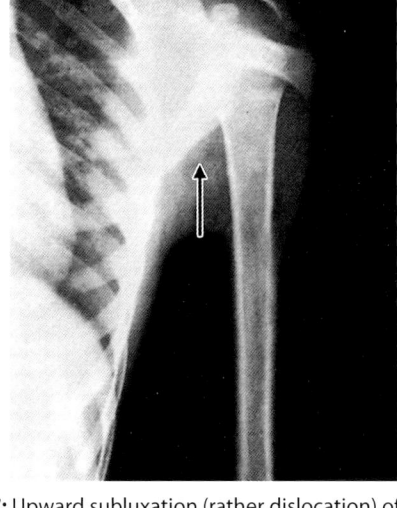

Fig. 4.27: Upward subluxation (rather dislocation) of shoulder.

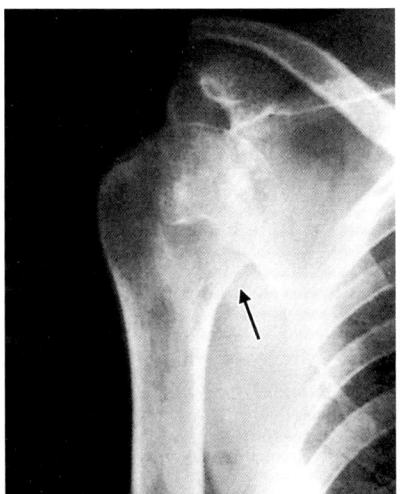

Fig. 4.25: Posterior dislocation of shoulder.

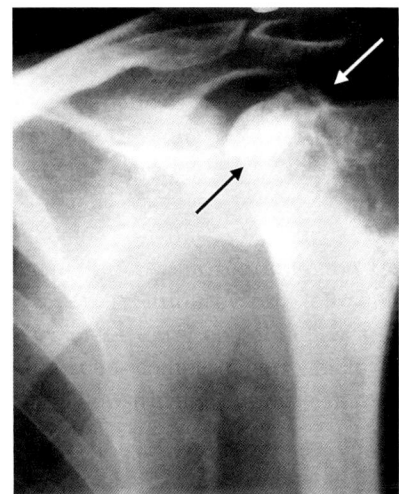

Fig. 4.28: Avascular necrosis of humeral head.

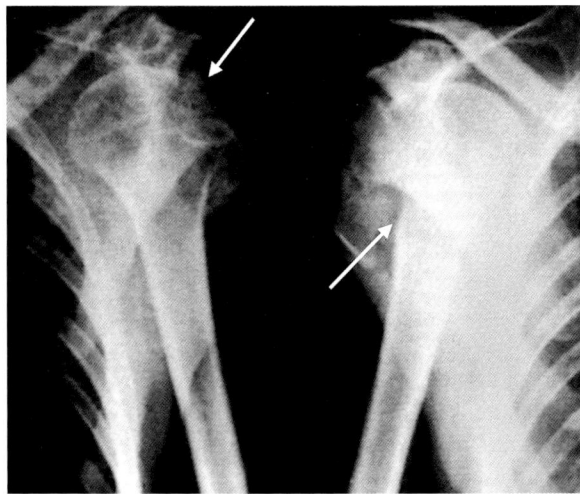

Fig. 4.26: Fracture dislocation of shoulder—bilateral.

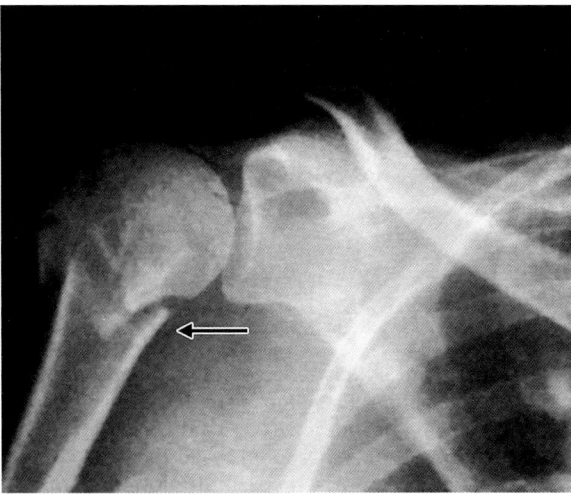

Fig. 4.29: Fracture of surgical neck of humerus.

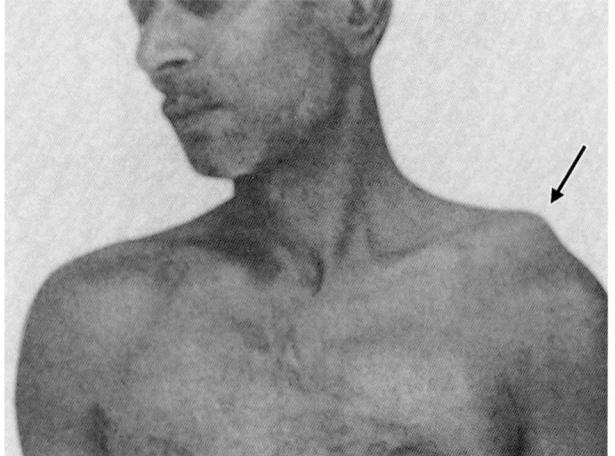

Fig. 4.30: Left acromioclavicular dislocation.

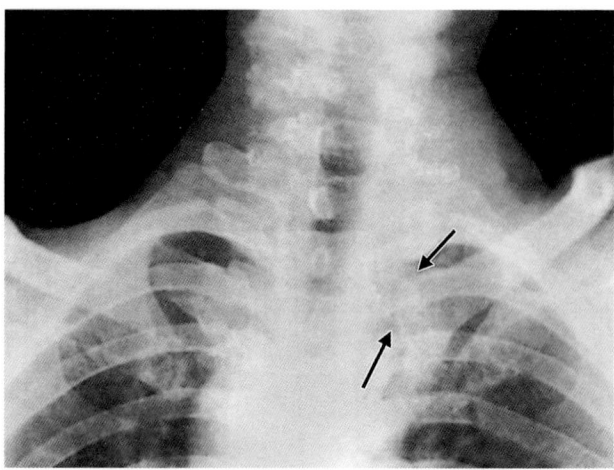

Fig. 4.33: Subluxated sternoclavicular joint.

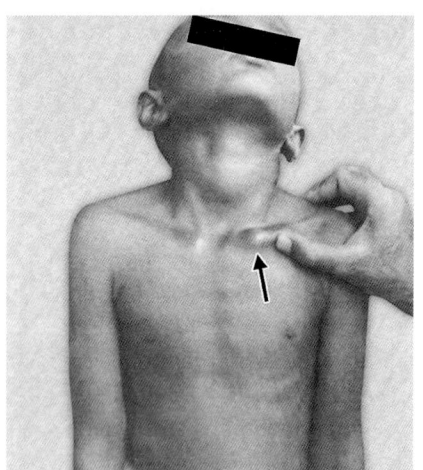

Fig. 4.31: Sternal end of clavicle can be pushed up.

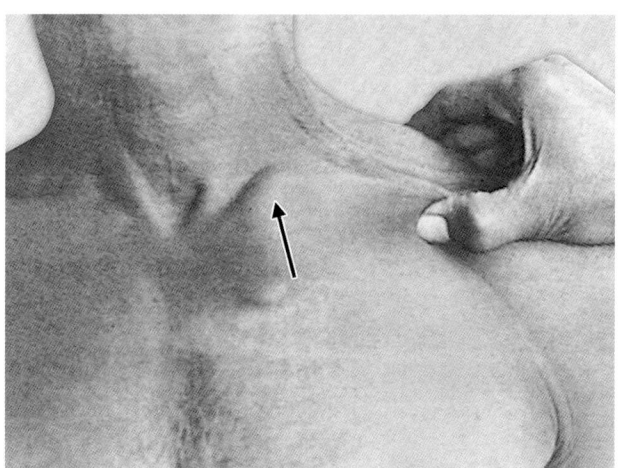

Fig. 4.34: Dislocated sternal end of clavicle can be pushed up.

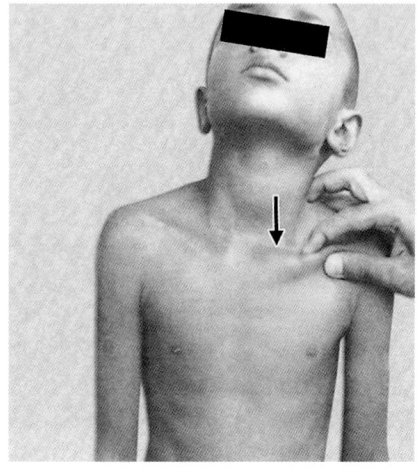

Fig. 4.32: Sternal end of clavicle can be pushed down.

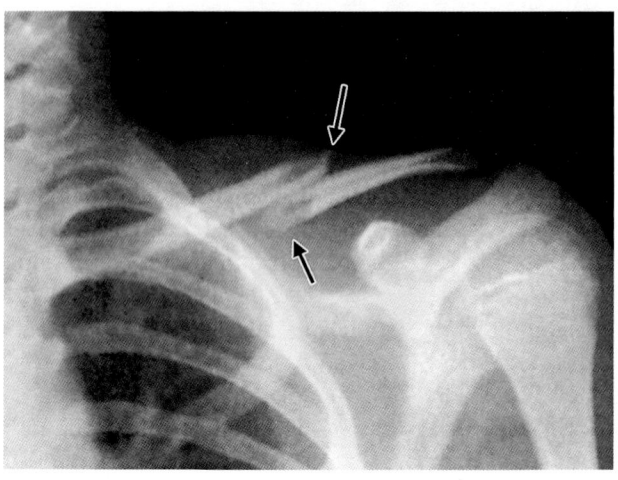

Fig. 4.35: Fracture clavicle with typical displacement.

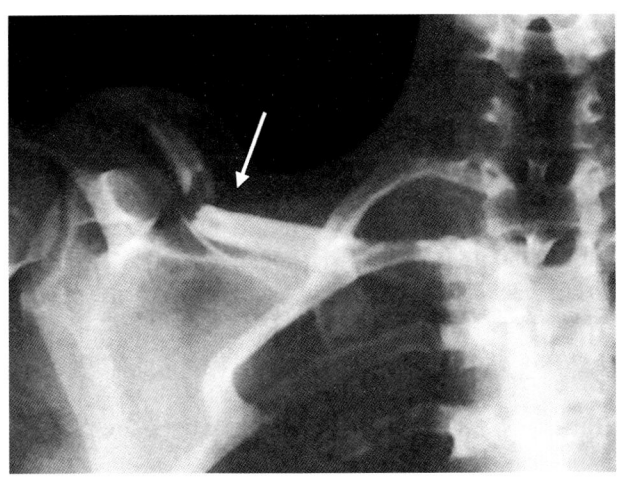

Fig. 4.36: Fracture clavicle with atypical displacement (medial fragment is displaced down).

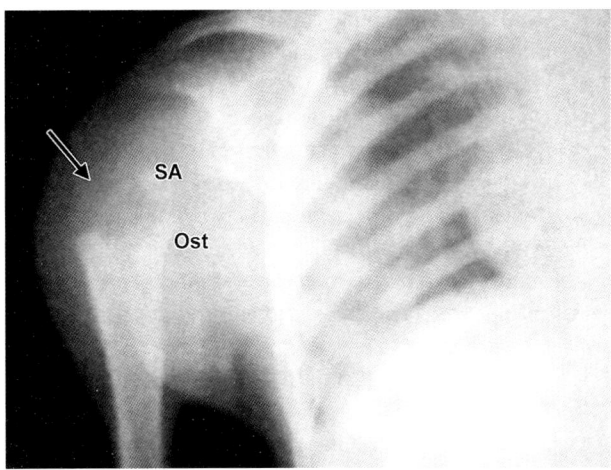

Fig. 4.39: Septic arthritis of the shoulder and subacute osteomyelitis of upper region of humerus in an infant.

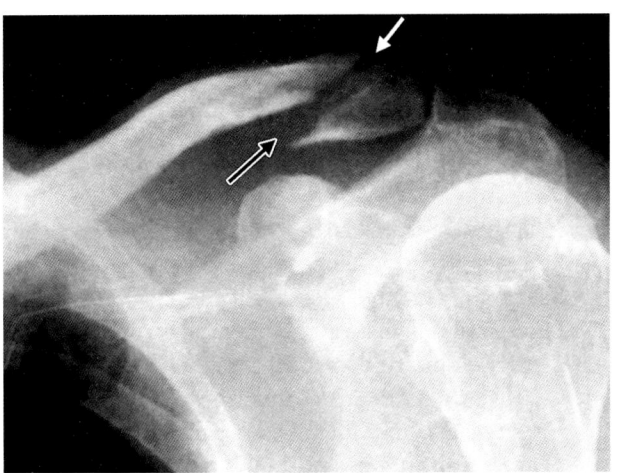

Fig. 4.37: Fracture outer end of clavicle.

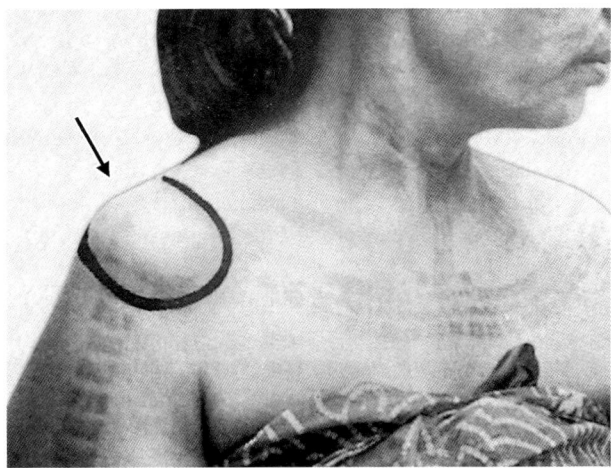

Fig. 4.40: Tuberculosis of shoulder joint with cold abscess.

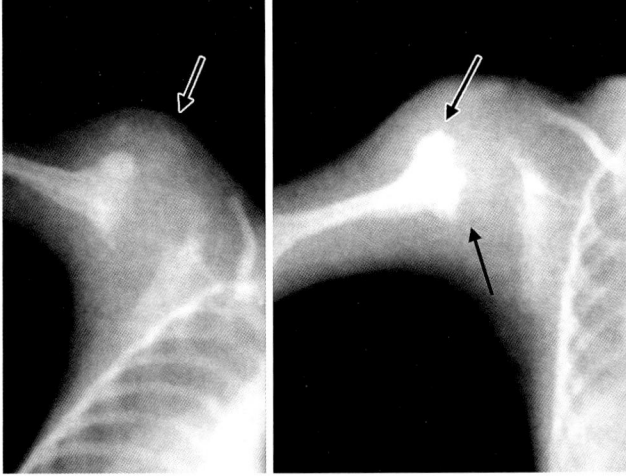

Fig. 4.38: Primary septic arthritis of shoulder with osteomyelitis of upper part of humerus in an infant.

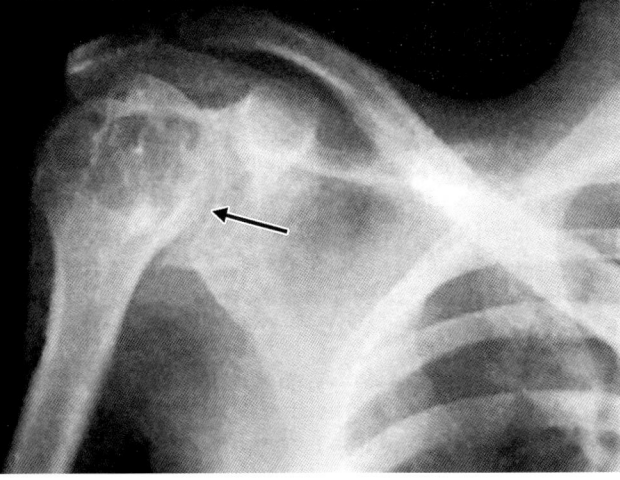

Fig. 4.41: X-ray of the same patient **(Fig. 4.40)**.

- Cold abscess, usually not accompanied (shoulder tuberculosis is commonly of dry atrophic form also known as *caries sicca*)
- Lymph glands may be enlarged
- *Radiologically:* Typical features of a tuberculous lesion (joint space reduced; generalised rarefaction; irregular bony destruction; irregular bony collapse, etc.).

■ *Periarthritis/Freezing Shoulder/Frozen Shoulder:* E Codman coined the term *"Frozen shoulder" in 1934 and described it as a condition difficult to define, difficult to treat and difficult to explain from the point of pathology.* It comes on slowly with pain over the deltoid insertion, inability to sleep, painful incomplete elevation and external rotation of shoulder, the restriction of both active and passive movements with a normal radiograph. Earlier S Duplay used the term "periarthritis scapulohumeral" to describe the condition in 1872. Later, J Neviaser used the term "adhesive capsulitis" in 1945 reflecting the findings at surgery and at postmortem.

The descriptive terminology in the ongoing pathology may be used as periarthritis → freezing shoulder (adhesive capsulitis) → frozen shoulder → thawing phase.

Primary frozen shoulder is characterized by the disabling pain and global stiffness of shoulder; leading to significant functional disability.

The incidence of this problem is about 2.5% in general population of 35–50 years of age with females predominating over the males.

It is usually unilateral. Both shoulders may be affected in about 10–20% of cases (mainly diabetics).

The primary pathology in adhesive capsulitis is within the glenohumeral joint capsule. The exact pathology is unclear, however condition is largely believed to be a chronic inflammatory process, involving the rotator cuff and joint capsule, which leads to shortening of the usually loose tendinous cuff and progressive loss of motion.

Adhesive capsulitis is the initial manifestation of an ongoing pathology which usually culminates in frozen shoulder. The term 'adhesive capsulitis' was coined by Neviaser (1945) to describe a thickened and contracted joint capsule which appeared to be drawn tightly around the humeral head with relatively reduced or absent synovial fluid and chronic inflammatory changes in the subsynovial layer of the capsule. External rotation, terminal internal rotation and terminal abduction are painfully restricted.

Significant glenohumeral joint pathology can usually be excluded if passive external rotation of the shoulder is pain free.

Freezing shoulder: Severe pain is the most common presenting symptom of the freezing or synovitis phase of adhesive capsulitis due to synovitis. There is painful restriction of rotational movements and abduction but shoulder can be abducted more than 90° (glenohumeral joint not completely frozen).

Frozen shoulder: Glenohumeral movements are frozen. Rotational and abduction movements are markedly painfully restricted. Less than 90° of abduction is possible by scapulothoracic gliding (glenohumeral joint completely frozen).

The aetiopathogenesis of this condition is not exactly known. Almost all cases are self-limiting, of course in variable period (4 months to 2 years or even more).

Clinically, three symptom-related phases can be defined. However, it is difficult to draw dividing lines.

1. *Initial phase* (Periarthritis and freezing process)—Insidious onset of pain, which gradually increases in intensity (few weeks to 9 months) with gradual restriction of active and passive movements (freezing process), as noted above.
2. *Second phase* (The stiffness of shoulder is established and with it the intensity of pain starts decreasing in 4–9 months—Frozen shoulder (glenohumeral movements frozen, scapulothoracic gliding movements possible to variable extent).
3. Finally in the 'thawing phase', the resolution starts, gradually returning the shoulder to almost normalcy in 6–24 (or more) months.
   - No specific aetiology of primary frozen shoulder has been identified
   - May be history of insignificant injury following which the symptoms develop
   - Diabetics are more prone, which leads to think about this condition to be an 'algoneurodystrophic process'. Other endocrine disorders like hypothyroidism, triglyceridemia and corticotropin deficiency have been associated with adhesive capsulitis
   - Dupuytren's contracture and thyroid dysfunction may have high prevalence of frozen shoulder
   - Severe pain at rest (usually at night). Pain usually starts on getting out (arising) of bed in morning or after inactivity, which usually diminished or clears after exercises and activities
   - On right-sided shoulder complaints, the right lower chest and upper abdominal pathologies must be excluded. On left-sided shoulder complaints, cardiovascular system must be examined thoroughly.
     - Mild-to-moderate wasting of supraspinatus, infraspinatus and deltoid
     - Tenderness at anterior and/or posterior shoulder joint line
     - Gradual limitation of abduction and external rotation (when markedly advanced—frozen shoulder)
     - Small nodules may be palpated on the surface on trapezius or adjoining muscles. Pressure on the nodule may initiate pain with or without radiation to the neck and/or upper arm.

- Flexion and adduction are usually free, even in advanced cases. (cf. in tuberculous affection all movements are restricted and painful).
  - In late cases, rarefaction in surrounding bones, more of tuberosities.
- In elderly and even in adults, X-rays of shoulder must be taken to eliminate any hidden pathology [e.g. early giant cell tumour (GCT), secondary carcinoma, etc.].

Pathological findings: Macroscopically, there is contracture of coracohumeral ligament. Microscopically in the capsular contracture, there are inflammatory and fibrotic changes (with dense matrix of type I and type II collagen).

Adhesive capsulitis (manifested by simultaneous loss of both active and passive range of motion) *and rotator cuff pathology*-induced condition can be *broadly differentiated as follows:*
1. *Lag sign*—The patient is asked to elevate the affected arm. If there is lack of terminal range, supporting the patient's elbow elevate the arm and note the passive range (lag of range as compared to normal side). Similarly, the patient's active external rotation of shoulder with arms keeping at the sides of chest is compared with the patient's passive range of motion.
   The presence of the lag sign, external rotation weakness or pain with restricted external rotation suggests pathology in the rotator cuff.
2. *Capsular irritation sign*—It may differentiate between early adhesive capsulitis from primary rotator cuff disease. The patient keeps the arm by the side. Gently externally rotate the arm beyond the normal range, which will stretch the anterior capsule. This will be painful in presence of synovitis or capsular irritation—characteristic of adhesive capsulitis. The distinction between painful passive stretch of anterior capsule and painful restricted active external rotation helps in distinguishing the adhesive capsulitis and primary rotator cuff impingement or disease.

Management: Reconciliation; exercises; cold/heat therapy; intra-articular steroid injection (into the proper glenohumeral joint) plus exercises; suprascapular nerve block; hydrodistension (intra-articular distension with or without steroids hydrodistension and steroid injection have pain relief and improved joint mobility for long term); manipulation under anaesthesia (MUA); in conservatively failed cases—surgery—arthroscopically (release is performed using a radiofrequency hook through the anterior portal with standard posterior portal used for visualization) or open release of anteroinferior capsular structure with/without MUA. Suprascapular nerve block is used more frequently by anaesthetists and rheumatologists in the treatment of frozen shoulder (Mortada M 2017).

- *Supraspinatus Tendinitis/Subacromial Bursitis/Shoulder Impingement Syndrome/Painful Arc Syndrome:* It is a multifactorial disorder with continuum of degenerative, inflammatory processes and attrition of the structures in the subacromial space, i.e. SITS—Supraspinatus, infraspinatus, teres minor, subscapular muscles; subdeltoid bursae; capsule and biceps tendon. Impingement usually occurs following weakness or destruction of the rotator cuff muscles (SITS muscles) which are stabilizer of the humeral head against the shallow glenoid fossa.

If arm can be fully painlessly abducted, palm can be taken fully behind the neck and dorsum of hand can be taken to about opposite infrascapular region that shoulder is almost normal. However, if there is pain only in 60°–120° abduction of shoulder, there is possibility of partial rupture of supraspinatus tendon, supraspinatus tendinitis or subacromial bursitis. These three conditions produce similar clinical features. Pain throughout the range of abduction indicates synovitis or arthritis. During abduction of arm, the supraspinatus tendon and its insertion on the greater tuberosity of humerus must pass beneath the acromion. The function of subacromial bursa is to decrease the friction or impingement under acromion. However, repetitive forceful motion produces mechanical irritation and thence inflammation of the tendon and bursa.

Hawkin's test: It is done to test for impingement, in which pain is produced by abducting the shoulder to 90° and flexing the elbow by 90° and then shoulder is internally rotated. In this manoeuvre, the greater tuberosity is moved to the under surface of the acromion producing the pain.

Neer's test also produces pain on full flexion in abduction of shoulder.
- Typical history of pain at the shoulder in a certain arc of abduction movement (60°–120°) (*see* **Fig. 4.17**)
- Tenderness below the subacromial area and over the greater tuberosity
- X-ray may reveal abnormal subacromial calcification (**Figs. 4.42 and 4.43**) due to deposition of crystals of calcium pyrophosphate dihydrate (CPPD). Calcification in tendons is relatively common with CPPD crystal deposition, specially in rotator cuff, tendo Achilles, gastrocnemius and quadriceps, etc.). Calcific tendinitis, specially of shoulder is recently commonly being treated by *extracorporeal shock-wave lithotripsy*. However, long-term clinical follow-up studies is essential to watch for the possible complication of avascular osteonecrosis of the humeral head due to possible damage of the blood supply of the head.
- *Bicipital Tendinitis:* Biceps instability and biceps tendinitis are common disorders of the long head of biceps. Mechanical impingement of the biceps tendon against the coracoacromial arch (like rotator cuff impingement) is, probably, the cause of biceps tendon degeneration. There is inflammation in the tendon sheath of biceps usually, where it emerges anteriorly from the capsule of the shoulder joint. The overuse can also produce this inflammation.

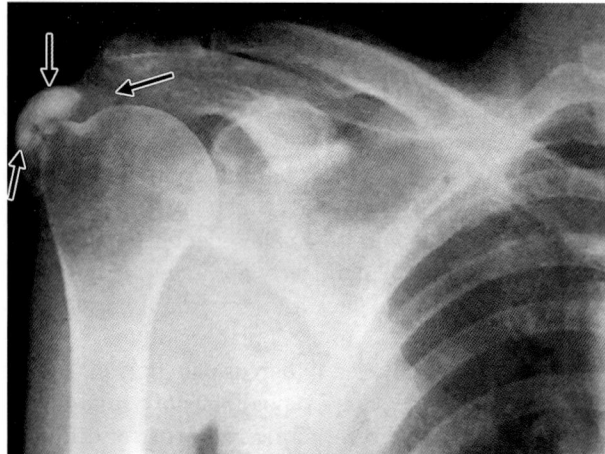

Fig. 4.42: Calcified subacromial bursa.

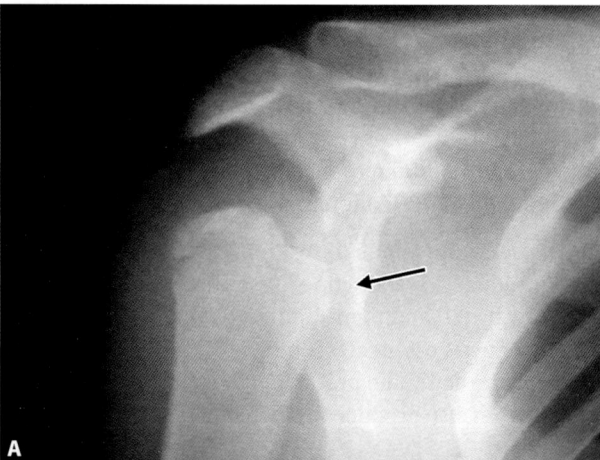

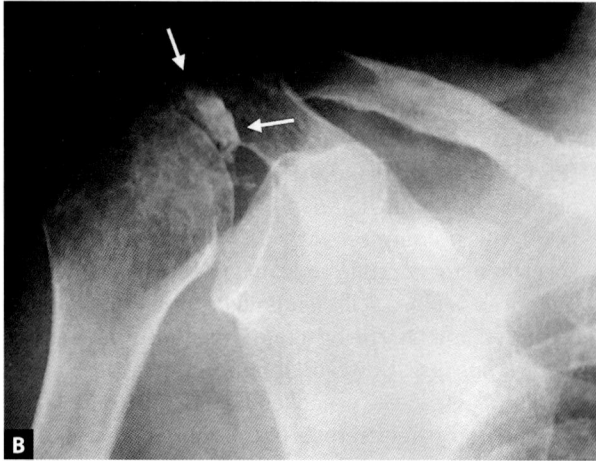

Figs. 4.43A and B: (A) Avascular necrosis of humeral head, which may be a cause of chronic pain in shoulder; (B) Calcified subacromial bursa.

abduction of shoulder and flexion at elbow simultaneously. Maximum tenderness on anterolateral slope of shoulder (along the bicipital tendon). *Yergason's sign is present*—while the elbow is flexed by 90° with pronated forearm, ask the patient to supinate forearm against resistance, patient will complain of pain in the anteromedial aspect of shoulder, i.e. bicipital groove—indicating inflammation along the long head of biceps.

When less than 25% of the overall tendon is involved, degeneration can be reversible even by non-operative management. However, if more than 25% of the tendon is involved in degeneration (fraying, tearing, tendon subluxation) surgical treatment is indicated in the form of debridement, tenodesis or tenotomy.

Tenodesis is better for biceps muscle health and action and should be preferred in younger, active and non-bulky patients.

Recently, lesions/injuries of the superior labrum—SLAP *(superior labral anterior and posterior)* have been recognised as a significant cause of shoulder pain (Synder et al. 1990) and can be confused with the lesions of long head of biceps. It usually occurs due to acute shoulder traction or compression or repetitive overhead activity (throwing or overhead movements). *Active compression test* is usually positive. In this test, the arm is kept in 20° adduction and 90° of forward elevation and the examiner applies downward force on the forearm while the hand is pronated and supinated—the patient will complain of pain and weakness, which is compared with the normal side. In SLAP lesion pain is worst in the pronated position—which is positive test.

O'Brien Test: The patient keeps arm in 900 of forward flexion and adduction at the shoulder and is asked to flex his arm against resistance. In positive O'Brien Test the arm will drop down due to pain at shoulder joint.

MR arthrography is superior to plain MRI for diagnosing SLAP lesions. Preferred management is by surgery, mild cases by debridement, and severe cases by repair or excision.

- *Fibrous Dysplasia* **(Fig. 4.44)**
  - The term fibrous dysplasia was coined by Lichtenstein in 1938
  - In young adolescent, more in males
  - Trivial injury producing pain in the upper arm or shoulder region
  - May be earlier history of off and on pain
  - X-ray reveals multicystic or monocystic expansion of the upper humeral end beneath the growth cartilage with/without pathological fracture. Patient may present with fracture through the lesion.
- *Sternoclavicular Tuberculosis*
  - It is not common condition and presents vaguely with complains of pain mild fullness, mild rise of local temperature, mild inflammatory look, tenderness in the sternoclavicular joint line, pain in the joint region on passively moving the clavicle, active extreme range of shoulder movements produces pain in the

Ultrasound may corelate the clinical site of tenderness with the involved pathology. MRI delineates the biceps tendon in its groove, the surrounding osteophytes and any associated rotator cuff pathology.

Patient complains of pain in the region of insertion of the pectoralis major on the humerus and may shoot down along the arm; and/or in anterolateral region of shoulder in

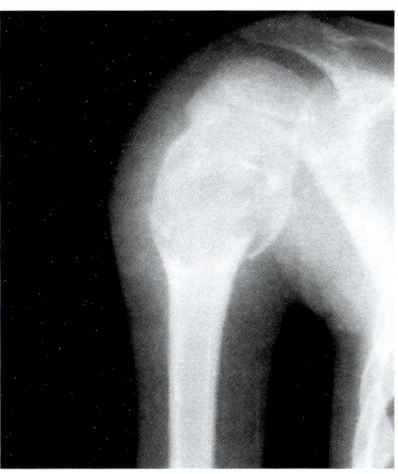

Fig. 4.44: Unicameral bone cyst with pathological fracture (Latin: Unus = one; camera = vault)—mimicking fibrous dysplasia.

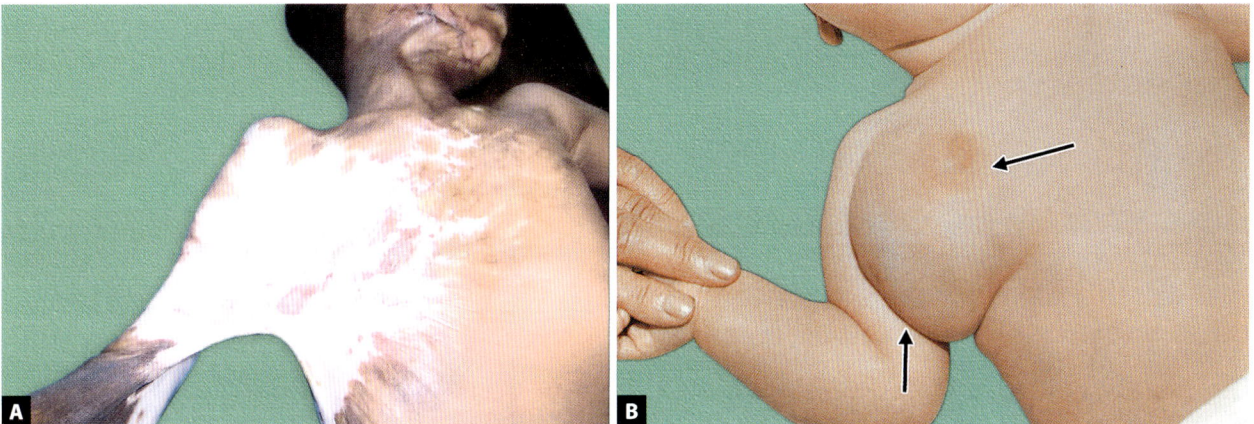

Figs. 4.45A and B: (A) Post-burn contractural adduction deformity of shoulder with gross limitation of abduction of shoulder; (B) Congenital lymphoedema.

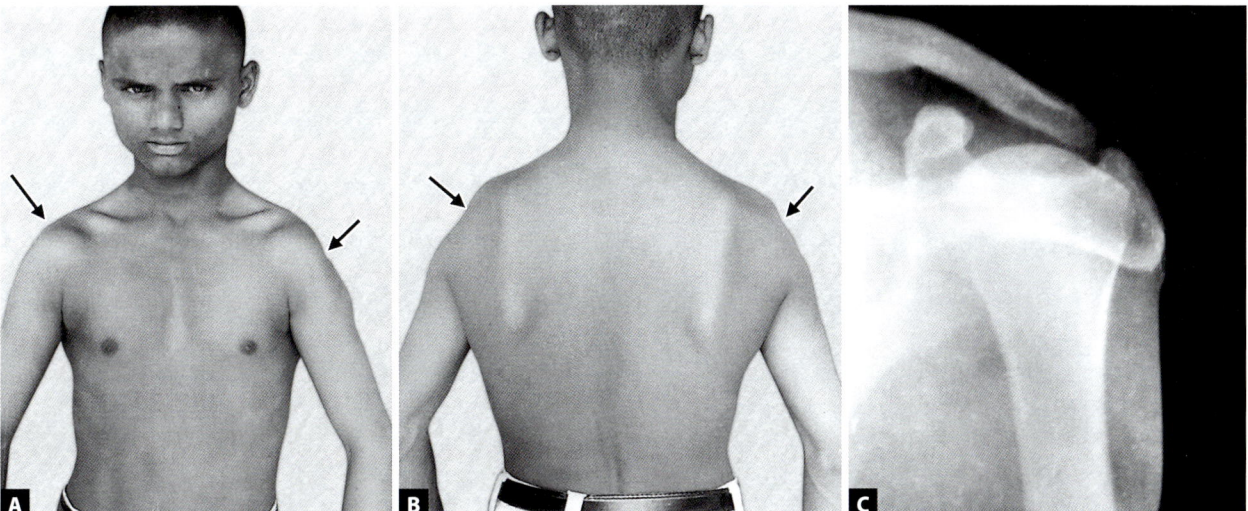

Figs. 4.46A to C: Bilateral congenital contracture of deltoid muscles: A—photo from front, B—photo from back, C—X-ray picture of left shoulder.

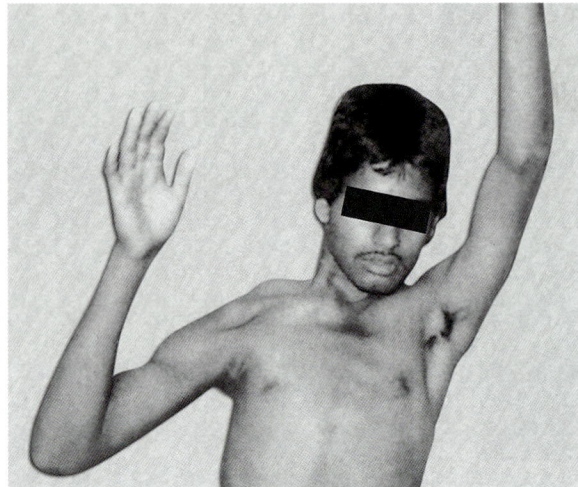

Fig. 4.47: Fixed abduction deformity of right shoulder due to congenital dislocation of shoulder.

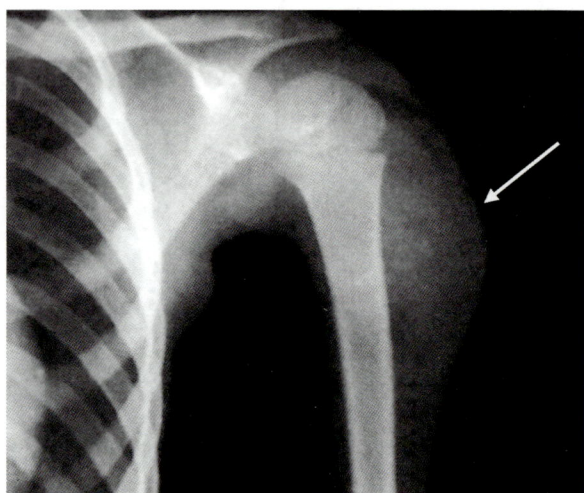

Fig. 4.50: X-ray of same patient (Fig. 49). Note the shadow of haemangiomatous mass in deltoid muscle.

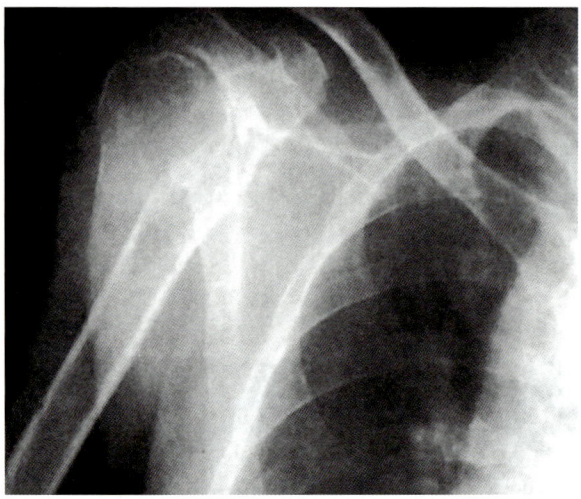

Fig. 4.48: Fixed abduction deformity of shoulder due to neglected fracture subluxation/dislocation of shoulder.

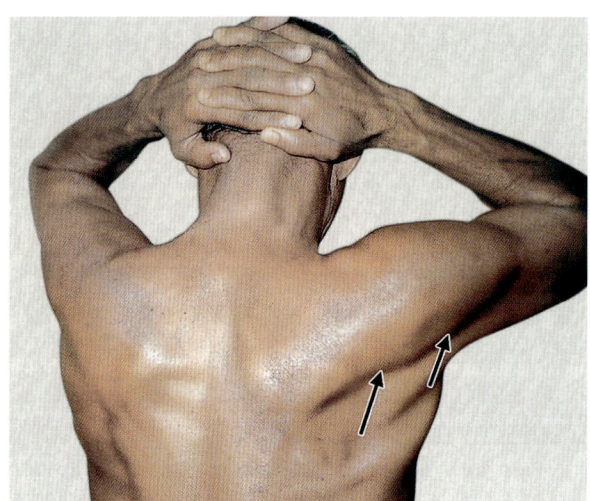

Figs. 4.51: Haemangiomatous mass in right deltoid muscle.

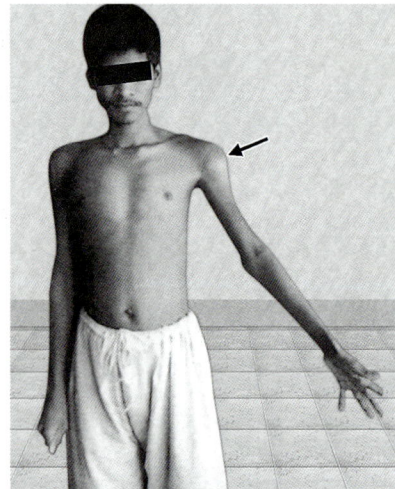

Figs. 4.49: Fixed abduction deformity of shoulder due to haemangioma in deltoid muscle.

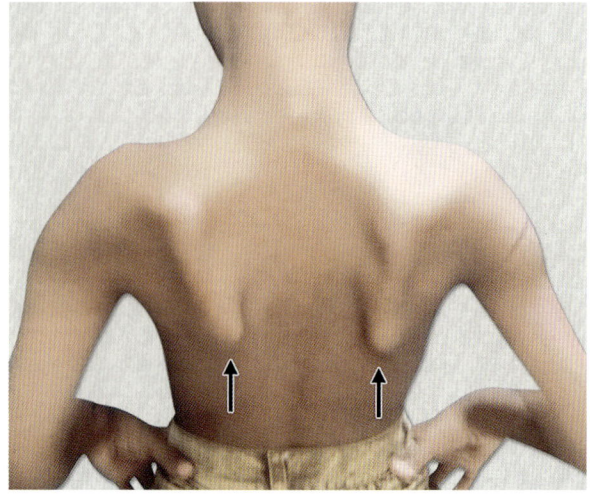

Figs. 4.52: Winging of both scapulae (*Also see* Figure 11.36).

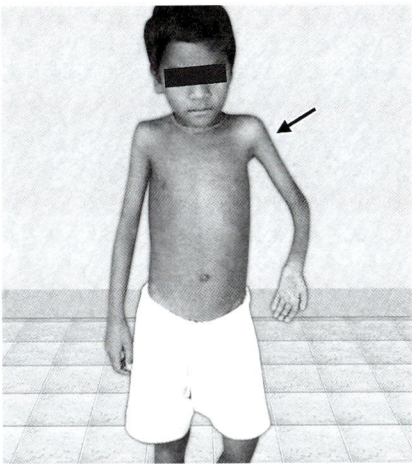

Fig. 4.53: Fixed abduction contracture of shoulder due to neglected chronic septic arthritis of shoulder.

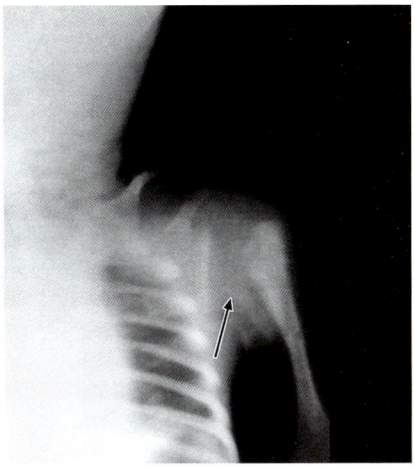

Fig. 4.54: Septic arthritis shoulder with osteomyetis of upper region of humerus in a neonate.

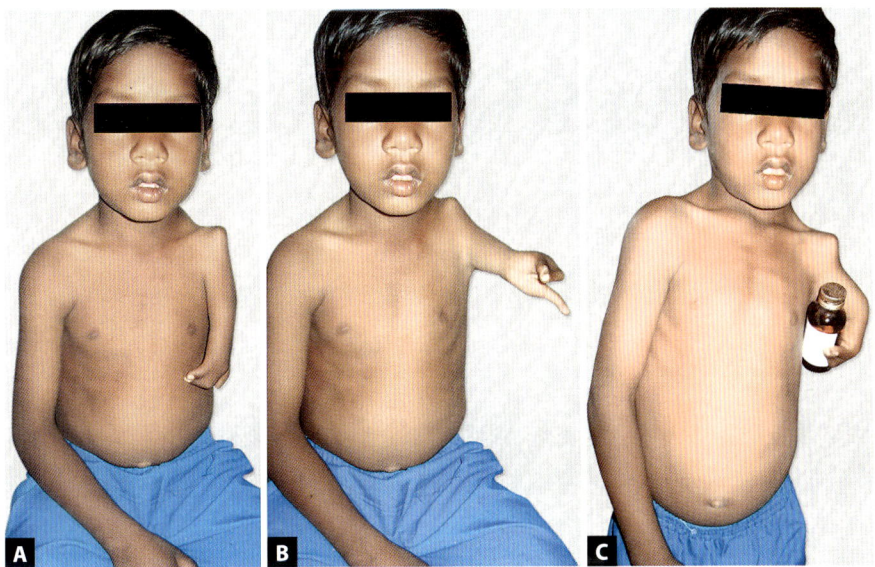

Figs. 4.55A to C: Congenital deficits in arm, elbow, forearm, wrist, hand and fingers. However, he can use left upper limb for ADL and necessary works. He should not be subjected to any surgery.

joint region. X-ray is not that contributory unless clear picture of both sides are exposed. With a high index of suspicion focused MRI is helpful. Variable confirmation may be achieved with tuberculosis oriented pathological investigations and biopsy (needle biopsy or open biopsy). Early commencement of antituberculous treatment is helpful.

■ BIBLIOGRAPHY

1. Bulgen DY, Hazleman BL. Immunoglobulin-A, HLA-B27 and Frozen shoulder. Lancet. 1981;2:76.
2. Chambler AFW, Carr AJ. The role of surgery in frozen shoulder. J-Bone Joint Surg. 2003;85-B:789-95.
3. De Palma AF, Gallery C, Bennet C. Anatomy and degenerative lesions of the shoulder joint. Ann Acad Orthop Surg Instr Course lecte Ann Arbor. Edwards, 1949;6.
4. Fukuda H. The management of partial thickness tears of the rotator cuff. J Bone Joint Surg. 2003;85-B:3-11.
5. Jobe F, Giangarra CE, Kvitne RJ, et al. Anterior capsulolabral reconstruction of the shoulder in athletes in overheand sports. Am J Sport Med. 1991;19(5):428-34.
6. Mears DC. Partial resection of scapula and release of long head of triceps for management of Sprengel's deformity. J Pediatr Orthop. 2001;21:242-5.
7. Montada M. Treatment of frozen shoulder in diabetic patients: using suprascapular nerve block, 8th International Conference of Orthopedic Surgeons and Rheumatology, Rome, Italy 2017 (March 22–23), published in Finecure Medica p 36.
8. Simpson NS, Schwappach JR, Toby EB. Fracture-dislocation of the humerus with intrathoracic displacement of the humeral head. J Bone Joint Surg. 1998;80A:889-91.
9. Sprengel OK. Die angeborene verschiebung des schulterblattes nach oben. Archive fur rlinische chirurgic, BERLIN. 1891;42:545-9.
10. Synder SJ, Karel RP, Del Pizzo W, et al. SLAP lesions of the shoulder. Arthroscopy. 1990;6:274-9.
11. Turek SL. The painful and stiff shoulder. J Int Coll Surg. 1954;22:695.

CHAPTER 5

Elbow Joints

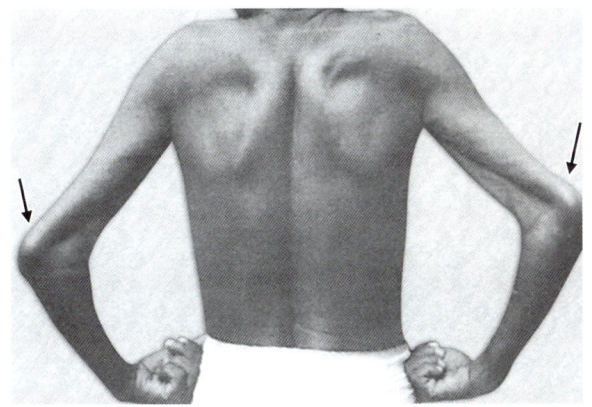
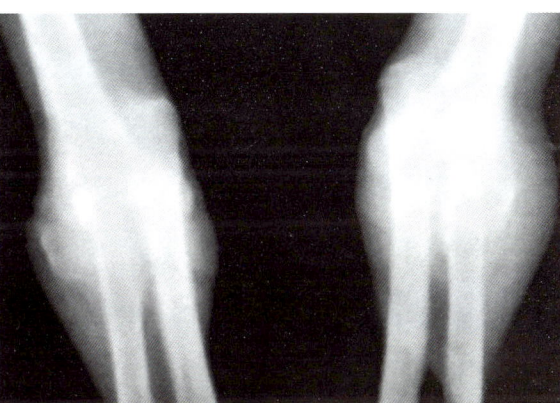

"Self awareness can help us head in the direction of everlasting peace, love and happiness."
—*Mihir Paul*

*"To live peacefully replace suspicion with trust; manage differences
with dialogue and build your future with cooperation."*
—*SP*

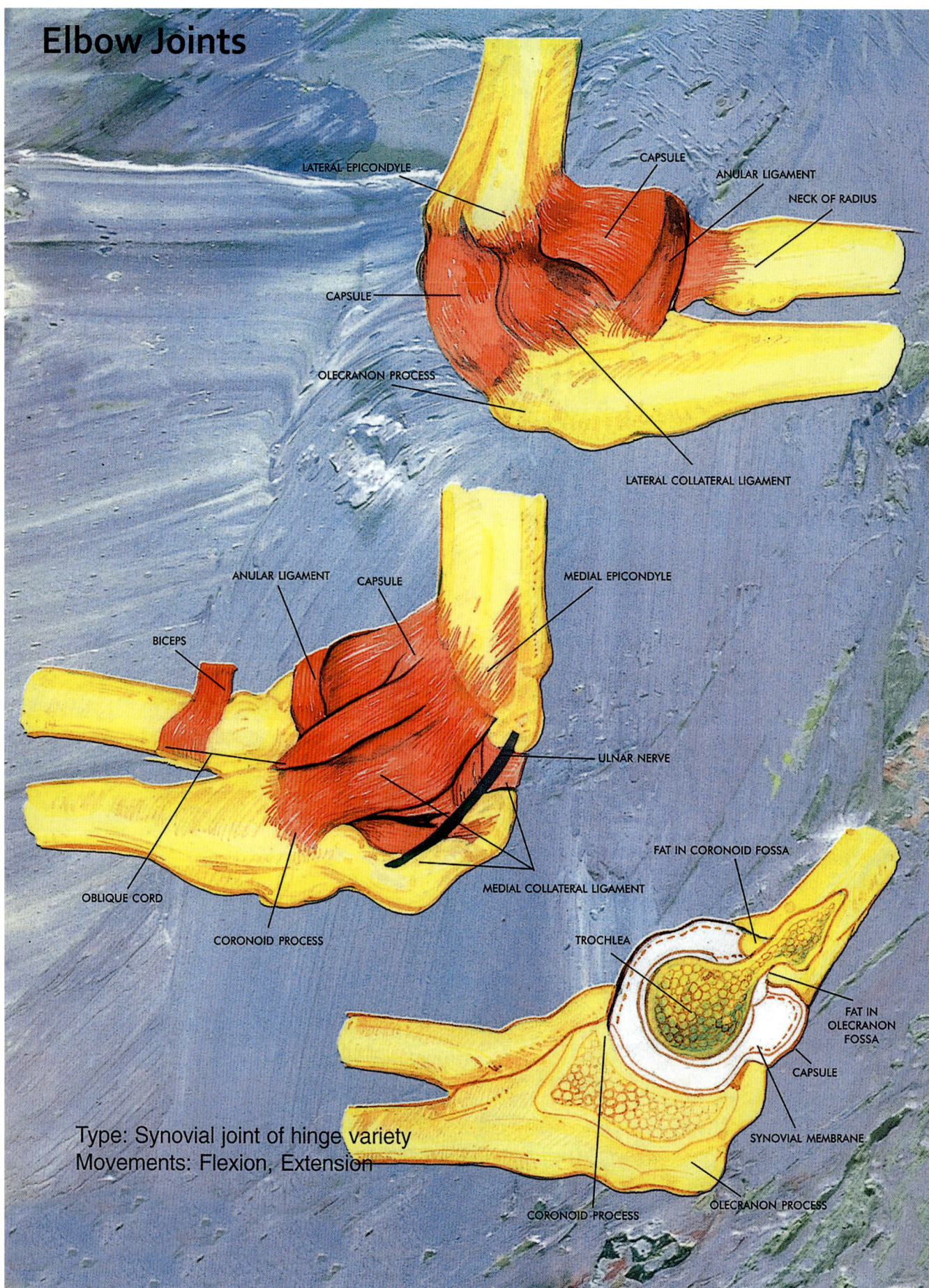

INTRODUCTION

The elbow joint (a hinge joint), is perhaps the main joint responsible for communicating the actions of the hand to the trunk. It is a compound joint having ulnohumeral and radiohumeral components. The elbow joint comprises of two articulations—the hinged ulnohumeral and radiohumeral components. The main articulation is in between the semilunar trochlear notch of the ulnar olecranon process embracing and moving around the transverse drum of the spool-shaped trochlea of the distal humerus, the trochlea forms the medial two-thirds of the lower humeral articular surface. The rounded convex capitular portion, which forms lateral third of lower humeral articular surface and on which the shallow concave top of the radial head pivots and glides, forms the humeroradial joint—a passive articulation. The radial head rotates in the annular ligament during pronation and supination of the forearm. The upper radioulnar joint communicates with the elbow joint proper. The synovial reflections of these joints are also intercommunicating.

The stability of elbow joint is maintained by three factors: (1) highly congruent joint geometry, (2) capsuloligamentous integrity, (3) intact balancing musculature—mainly the biceps, triceps, brachialis and anconeus.

ANATOMICAL CONSIDERATIONS

- The *trochlear notch* keeps its grip on the lower trochlear articular end almost throughout the full range of elbow movements. In the fully pronated position of the forearm, the trochlear notch assumes a wrenching grip over the trochlear portion of humerus and thus for all practical purposes the joint is locked. The main thrust is thereby directly transmitted in a straight line from the ulna to the lower end of the humerus
- The medial lip of the spool-shaped *trochlea* is more prominent and extends more distally (5–6 mm) than its lateral lip. This forms an oblique axis at the ulnohumeral joint, which results in the normal valgus angulation at the elbow—the carrying angle (10–15°, more in females)
- The *lower articular end of humerus* is placed about 40° tilted forwards in relation to the long axis of the humeral shaft
- The functional efficiency of elbow movements markedly improves in collaboration with the actions at the radioulnar joint
- Due to causes not well known, the elbow is very *notorious for developing post-traumatic myositis ossificans* (with or without any history of massage)
- In front of the elbow and a little above its level the *brachial artery* is very much vulnerable, and can undergo spasmodic contraction following exogenic or endogenic stimuli. Therefore, Volkmann's ischaemia (which if not promptly managed) followed by ischaemic contracture is more likely to develop, following injuries in this region
- The *three important peripheral nerves of the upper limb* lie in close relation to the elbow joint. Of these, the *ulnar nerve* theoretically appears to be in a more vulnerable position, being placed in close association with the back of the medial epicondyle and then passing through a tight fibro-osseus tunnel. The *median nerve*, like the brachial artery, lies just in front and above the elbow level and is vulnerable in any injury, especially in supracondylar fracture. The *radial nerve,* lying closely related to the lateral supracondylar ridge, and the anterior capsule of the elbow is also likely to suffer in elbow injuries. *In order of frequency, the median nerve (indicated mainly by pointing index and sensory loss in index finger), the radial nerve (indicated by wrist drop) and the ulnar nerve (indicated by clawing tendency and sensory deficit in the little finger and half of the ring finger)* are affected in injuries around the elbow. The injuries—supracondylar fractures, Monteggia fracture dislocations, baby car fracture dislocations, elbow dislocations, fracture neck of radius, fracture medial epicondyle of humerus—are likely to affect the nerves, in that order
- The radial head, the lateral epicondyle and the tip of the olecranon forms a triangle over the posterolateral aspect of the joint. This space is occupied by the anconeus muscle overlying the joint capsule. With fluid collection in the joint, this **'anconeus triangle'** bulges out
- The fascial compartments in front of the elbow are comparatively tight, therefore, any swelling in this region is likely to jeopardise the neurovascular bundles quite early
- If viewed from the back, the 90° flexed elbow presents three bony prominences of an inverted equilateral triangle, the two basal points of which are the medial and lateral epicondyles of humerus, and the tip of olecranon process forms the apex. In fully extended position of elbow, these three bony points fall in a straight transverse line **(Figs. 5.1A to C)**.

OSSIFICATION AROUND THE ELBOW JOINT (FIG. 5.2)

Methodology

History Taking

Besides detailed history taking as in general chapter, special attention must be paid to the following points: In cases of traumatic conditions—mode of injury; history of massage; number of attempts of manipulative reduction; history pertaining to impending features of Volkmann's ischaemia, *history for haemophilia*

Pain and affection of motion due to any cause, is poorly tolerated and leads to variable functional impairment.

General and Systemic Examinations

(As in the chapter on Introduction).

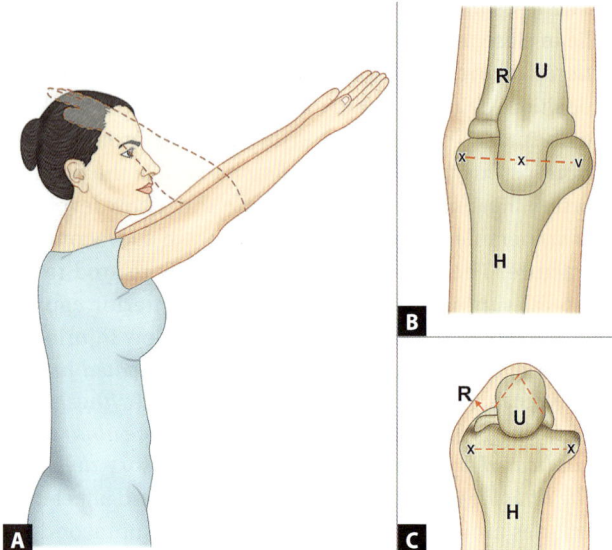

Figs. 5.1A to C: (A) Position of the elbow in which the relation of the three bony points should be ascertained, (B) Relation of the three bony points in extension, (C) Relation of the three bony points in 90° flexion. (H: humerus; U: ulna; R: radius)

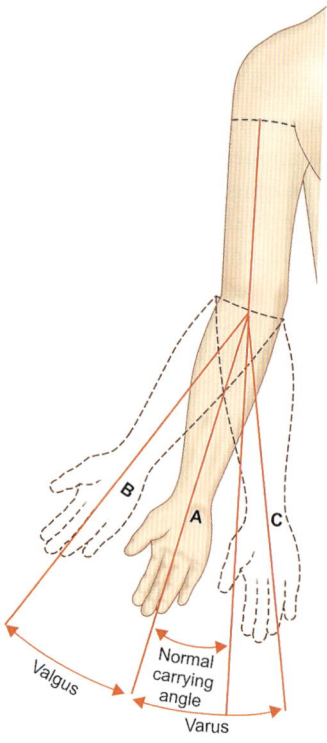

Figs. 5.3A to C: (A) Normal carrying angle; (B) Cubitus valgus; (C) Cubitus varus.

- The position of the shoulder, forearm and the hand of the normal side must be in identical position with that of affected one, preferably, with the arm lying by the side of the chest.

Attitude: Note the attitude of the elbow and presence of any contracture **(Fig. 5.52)**. The carrying angle of the elbow should be marked in supine and extended position of the forearm. The *angle formed in between the extended long axis of the arm and the long axis of the forearm at the central point of the extended elbow axis is the **carrying angle*** **(Fig. 5.3A)**. It varies between 15° and 20° if measured from inner side, i.e. about 170° if measured from outer sides of extended arm and forearm. The carrying angle is comparatively more in females to prevent forearm rubbing against the sides of pelvic region (which is wider in the females) while walking with extended elbow. It varies from 10° to 20° (more in females than in males). A difference of more than 10° between the carrying angles of right and left elbows is also abnormal. Exaggeration of this carrying angle (i.e. if outer angle is less than 165°) is called *cubitus valgus* **(Fig. 5.3B)**. Reduction, neutralisation or reversal of carrying angle is *cubitus varus* (i.e. outer angle is more than 175°) **(Figs. 5.3C to 5.5)**. In cubitus varus in children, the *Baumann's angle* in AP view X-ray of the extended elbow (the angle created between the physeal line of the lateral condyle and the long axis of the humerus) is increased as compared to the opposite normal side. In most of the pathologies in and around the elbow, there is varying degrees of flexion deformity at the elbow. In an old,

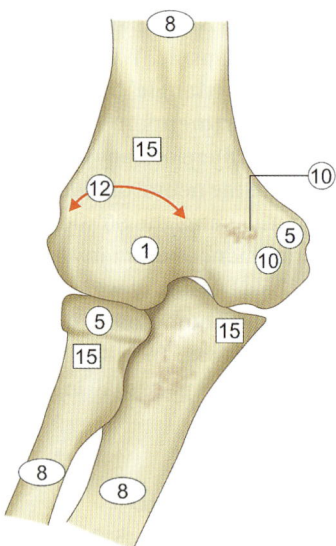

Fig. 5.2: Ossification around elbow: Oval circle denotes primary ossification centre in weeks (IUL), complete round circle denotes secondary ossification centre in years, square denotes fusion of epiphysis in years.

Regional Examination

As usual for the upper limbs (from the cervical spine to the fingertips).

Local Examination

Prerequisites
- Both the elbows must be examined in identical position
- The patient should either stand or sit on a stool

unreduced posterior dislocation of the elbow, the joint is flexed to about 45°, the triceps tendon stands prominent and the olecranon tip projects prominently (*see* **Fig. 5.37**).

Inspection: Assessment should be done in symmetrical position (in case of deformity the normal elbow should be kept in identical position to that of deformed one) from the back, the front and from the sides. Fixed bony and soft tissue points should be looked at. *Biceps is flexor of elbow, shoulder, and supinator of forearm:*

From the front: Biceps bulge (**Fig. 5.6** note rupture of biceps which can occur due to injury or overuse), cubital fossa, upper forearm bulge, biceps tendon prominence, superficial veins, any fixed flexion deformity (**Figs. 5.7 and 5.8**).

From the back: Triceps muscle bulge and tendon, olecranon process, callosity or any other swelling on the point of the elbow (e.g. in *student's elbow/bursa*, **Figs. 5.5B and 5.9**), paraolecranon depression, anconeus triangle, upper end of the ulna, back of the medial and lateral epicondylar tips represented by depression on the surface.

The triceps is a pennate muscle with three heads (lateral, long, medial). It occupies the posterior compartment, it is inserted on to the olecranon through triceps expansion. The main function of triceps is to extend the forearm at the ulnohumeral joint. Rupture of triceps tendon, traumatic or degenerative is rare, commonly occurs due to its sudden contraction (like in weight lifting, fall on outstretched hand or direct blow).

From the outer side: The lateral epicondylar prominence, bulge of the brachioradialis and long extensors of the wrist, or any abnormality.

From the inner side: The medial epicondylar prominence, supracondylar depressions and the bulge of the common flexors.

Any abnormality, like swelling (**Fig. 5.10**), sinuses, scars on any aspect should be noted clearly, as dealt within the chapter on Introduction.

Palpation

Superficial palpation: Besides palpating as discussed in the Chapter 1 Introduction, specially feel for any local rise of temperature and any superficial tenderness.

Deep palpation: Confirm the findings of inspection. Special points besides the general considerations are: the muscles around the elbow should be palpated for texture, bulk and pliability. In delayed traumatic cases, specially palpate for the presence of firm to hard bony plaques in the muscle mass

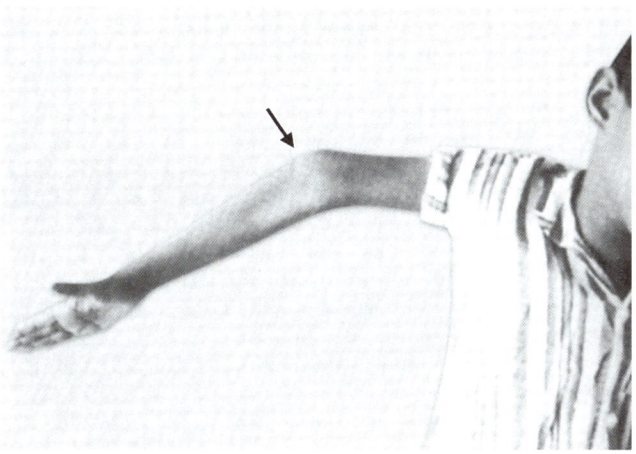

Fig. 5.4: Photograph showing marked cubitus varus deformity following malunited supracondylar fracture. In prone position of forearm this deformity looks further exaggerated. Painless movement of elbow are usually preserved. Deformity can be corrected by supracondylar osteotomy of humerus.

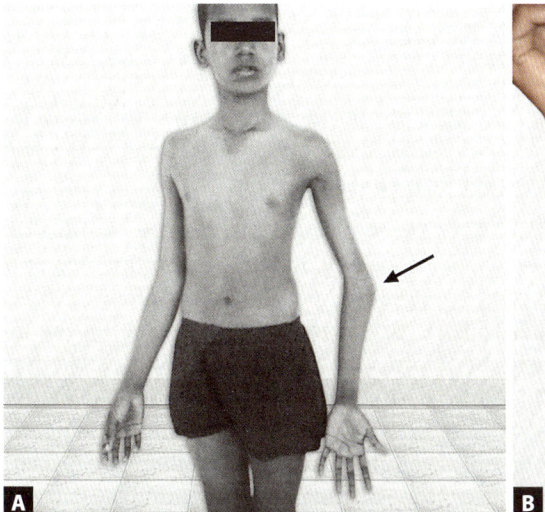
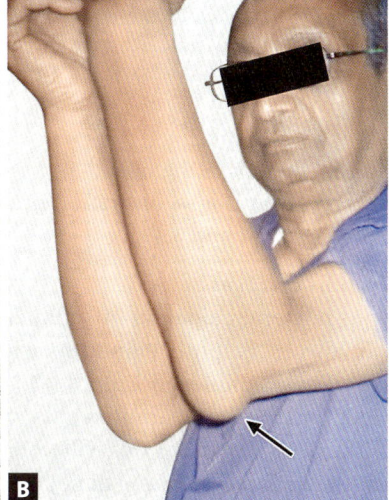

Figs. 5.5A and B: (A) Cubitus varus deformity. Exact deformity should be assessed in supine position of forearm, and corrected by osteotomy it required. (B) Inflamed olecranon bursa (student's elbow)—should be treated by aspiration, antibiotic according to culture of aspirate and at last excision if required.

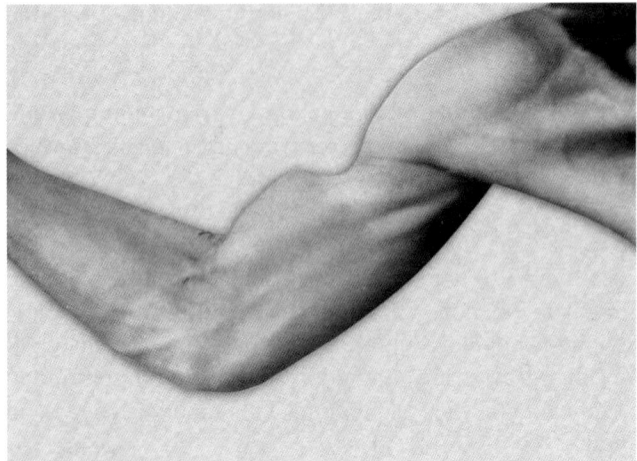

Fig. 5.6: Normal biceps bulge interrupted due to its tear; note that in performing active flexion of the elbow, the torn biceps mass stands markedly prominent—Popeye Muscle – Popeye Sign.

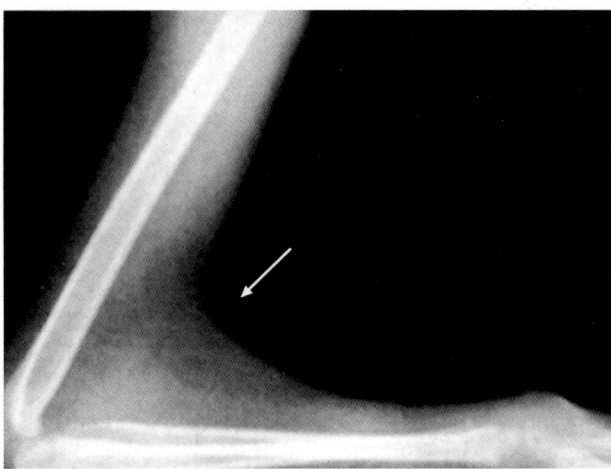

Fig. 5.8: Congenital flexion contracture of elbow, leading to fixed flexion deformity— even after excisional or replacement arthroplasty, the functional result is poor mainly due to ill-developed muscles around the elbow.

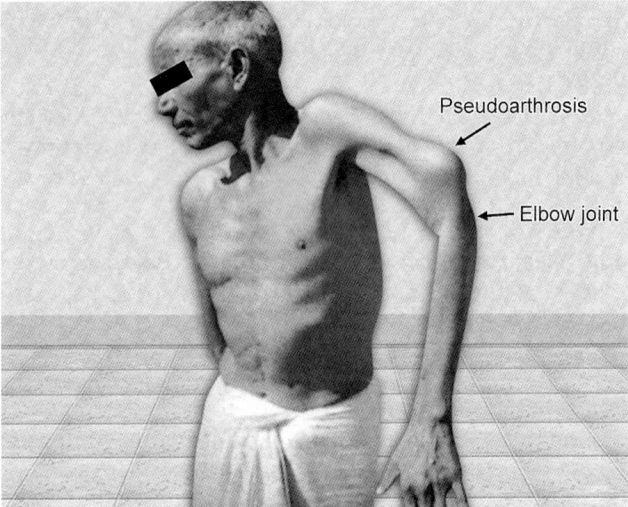

Fig. 5.7: Photograph showing abnormal angulation above the elbow joint in attempt of flexing the elbow **(double elbow)** produced due to pseudoarthrosis following fracture of lower humeral shaft—it shoulder be managed by excision of pseudoarthrosis and proper osteosynthesis and bone graft (if appears necessary).

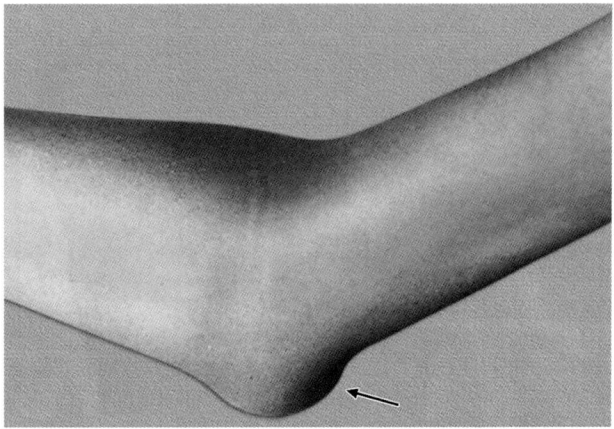

Fig. 5.9: Olecranon bursitis—should be managed by aspiration, antibiotics (according to culture of aspirate), and at last excision of the bursa.

(myositis ossificans). Feel the tips of the lateral and medial epicondyles, the supracondylar ridges, olecranon process, and head of the radius **(Figs. 5.11 and 5.12)**.

Palpation of supracondylar ridges

Method: Simultaneous bilateral palpation in symmetrical position of limbs is always helpful. Palpation will be convenient with the elbow semiflexed (about 45°) and the forearm supinated or even semisupinated as far as possible **(Fig. 5.11)**. The two epicondylar tips will stand out prominently. Hold the lower forearm in one hand, and use the thumb and middle finger of the opposite hand to palpate the epicondylar tips. Proceed vertically upwards from the epicondyles along the shaft of humerus in the midplane of the arm—the sharp bony supracondylar ridges are felt on the two sides (note any abnormality, like tenderness, irregularity, and thickening, etc.).

Three-point relationship: Confirm the normal relation of the epicondylar tips to the olecranon tip. Normally, in 90° flexed position of the elbow, they form more or less an isosceles triangle ***(see* Fig. 5.1)**, the interepicondylar line forms the base. If it is not possible to put the elbow in the desired position of palpation, palpation should be done in whatever position is possible. Comparison should be done with the elbow of the other side placed in similar postures, for assessing and comparing the correlation.

Fallacies in the three-point relationship: Fracture of the either epicondyle, fracture olecranon, excision arthroplasty of elbow may affect the relationship.

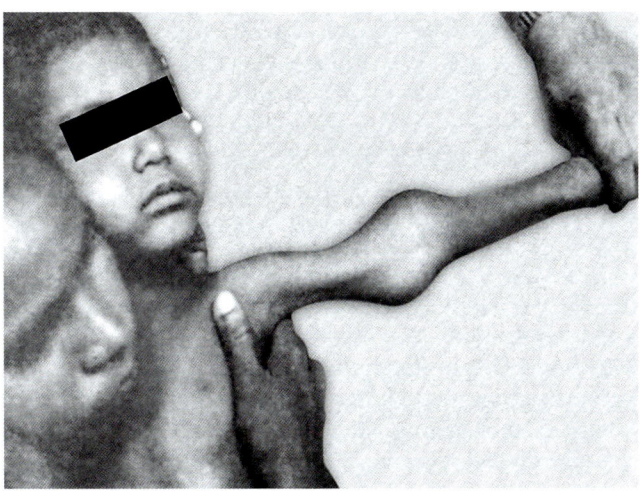

Fig. 5.10: Photograph of a patient of villonodular synovitis of elbow showing huge synovial swelling—should be managed by cautions synovectomy.

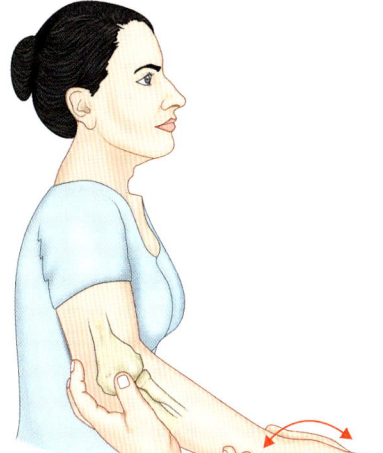

Fig. 5.12: Palpating the radiohumeral joint line and head of the radius.

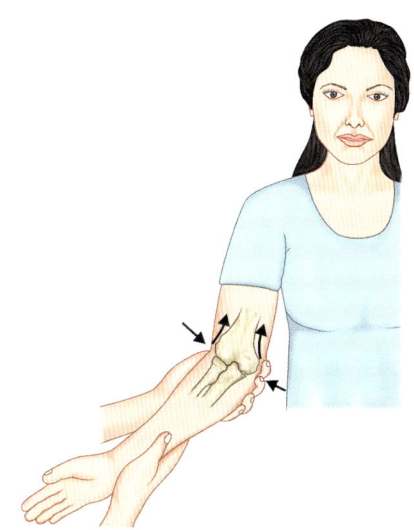

Fig. 5.11: Localisation of the epicondylar tips and palpating the supracondylar ridges.

Palpation of epicondylar region: Feel for bony tenderness, e.g. for lateral epicondylitis (tennis elbow) or medial epicondylitis (golfer's elbow or pitcher's elbow or Baseballer's elbow or javeline thrower's elbow, Little League elbow syndrome or manifestation of chronic tension stress injuries of elbow). Hold the distal forearm in one hand, with (your right hand holding the patient's right hand) the elbow of the patient in about 35° flexion. With the thumb and middle finger of your opposite hand, press the epicondylar areas. In lateral epicondylitis, there is maximum tenderness in the anteroinferior region of the lateral epicondyle. In medial epicondylitis, maximum tenderness is in the anteroinferior region of the medial epicondyle.

Both epicondyles lie in same line or slightly posterior to the supracondylar ridges. *In case of internal rotation of the lower fragment in supracondylar fracture, the lateral epicondylar tip remains anteriorly in relation to the supracondylar ridge.*

Palpate the *ulnar nerve* behind and above the medial epicondyle (**see Figs. 5.50 and 5.51**) as far as possible and note its position, pliability, any thickening and/or beading, and tenderness.

Method: Support the lower forearm in the same position as above, using one hand. Gently roll the pulp of the middle finger of the other hand behind the medial epicondyle. The ulnar nerve can be felt like a slippery cord. Palpate the nerve as far above as possible up and down, since in Hansen's neuritis its thickening is more marked in this region.

Palpation of joint line: The prominent brachialis and biceps muscle and their musculotendinous masses prevent the palpating fingers from reaching up to the joint line from the front. From the back, the olecranon process and the comparatively broad and tight tendon of the triceps do not allow the fingers to reach up to joint proper. However, on both sides of the main triceps tendon, the uppermost part of the olecranon notch of the humerus can be partially felt. On the outer side, the humeroradial joint line is felt as a transverse slit beneath the outer margin of the rounded capitulum.

Method: Bilateral palpation is always helpful. Flex the elbow at 35°–45° for comparison. Hold the lower forearm in one hand (right hand holding patient's right forearm). The upper end of the patient's forearm is supported on the palm of the opposite hand, the thumb is placed on the outer side of the level of the elbow joint. The tip of the thumb can feel the rounded bulge of the outer margin of the capitulum. Keeping the thumb just below it, rotate the forearm. The head of the radius can be felt rotating. *Just above the head of radius, a transverse slit can be felt* (**see Fig. 5.12**). For all practical purposes, this represents clinical palpation of the elbow joint. Since the elbow is a composite joint, tenderness in this region indicates tenderness in the elbow joint as well. However, when there is a synovial bulge (*see* **Fig. 5.10**), the joint is grossly affected and it is difficult to palpate the joint line. Palpation *along the interepicondylar line anteriorly* will also demonstrate the *elbow joint tenderness.*

Fluid in the joint: Swelling of the elbow can be also due to any haemarthrosis or any pathological collection. On the whole it is difficult to clinically find out little or even moderate collections. However, *fullness* specially posterolaterally in the *anconeus triangle,* if it is not boggy in feel, is in all probability due to fluid in the joint. In such situations, the elbow is kept in semiflexed position, because in this position the joint capacity is maximum. Positive cross-fluctuation between the medial paraolecranon swelling and the posterolateral swelling indicates fluid in the joint. In huge collection, *a tense bulge may be palpated in the cubital fossa.*

A collection in the triceps bursa should be differentiated from any collection in the joint. In 45° flexed position of the elbow the bursal collection will stand as two identical sacculations on both sides of the triceps. Try to elicit cross-fluctuation, keeping both index fingers on both sides of the triceps. In triceps bursitis, it is positive.

Palpate the *supratrochlear lymph glands* on the medial side of the elbow. Also palpate the *axillary group of glands* which drain this area.

Movements (Table 5.1)

Movements should be tested at *humeroulnar, humeroradial,* and *superior radioulnar joints.* Besides assessing the flexion and extension movements occurring at the proper elbow joint (a hinge joint), movements occurring at the forearm joints should also be examined. These joints are true *(synovial upper and lower radioulnar joints)* and false (working through interosseous membrane) effecting rotational movements of the forearm.

At proper elbow joint (the humeroulnar hinge joint) the movements occur from the *zero position of full extension to terminal flexion* (vide the **Table 5.1** on movements).

Method of Assessing the Movements

Compare the movements on both sides. Though movements can be tested by making the patient sit or stand, it will be better to make him/her sit on a stool **(Fig. 5.13)**. Let the patient lean over a table with arm fully supported over the table from shoulder to elbow (there should be no gap in

TABLE 5.1: Normal movements of elbow and forearm.						
Movements	*Axis*	*Range of motion*	*Prime movers*	*Nerve supply*	*Assisted by*	*Limiting factors*
Flexion	At elbow joint—a line joining the two epicondylar tips	0° to 145°–160°	1. Biceps brachii 2. Brachialis	C-5, 6 (Musculo cutaneous nerve)	Brachioradialis	1. Contact of front of upper part of forearm with front of arm 2. Engagement of coronoid process of ulna into coronoid fossa of humerus
Extension (Reversal of flexion) Hyperextension	-do-	145°–160° of flexion to 0°–10°	Triceps	Radial (C-7, 8)	1. Anconeus 2. Gravity	1. Locking of olecranon process into olecranon fossa 2. Tension of anterior capsule of elbow (along with its reinforcement) 3. Tension of flexor group of muscles of the forearm
Supination	At radioulnar joints— a line passing through centre of head of radius to ulnar attachment of triangular disc	0° to 90°	1. Biceps brachii 2. Supinator	Musculocutaneous (C-5, 6) Radial (C-6)	Brachioradialis	1. Tension of pronators 2. Tension of anterior radioulnar ligament and ulnar collateral ligament of the wrist 3. Tension of lowest fibres of interosseous membrane and the oblique cords
Pronation	-do-	-do-	1. Pronator teres 2. Pronator quadratus	Median (C-8, T1)	Brachioradialis	1. Tension on dorsal radiocarpal ligament 2. Tension of dorsal radioulnar ligament 3. Tension of ulnar collateral ligament 4. Tension of lowest fibres of interosseous membrane

Elbow Joints   135

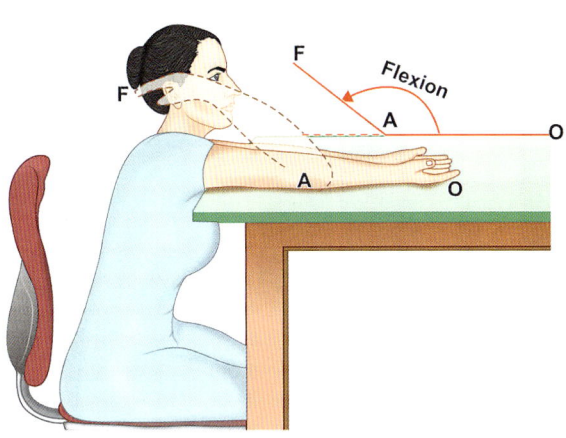

Fig. 5.13: Movements of elbow—flexion and extension.

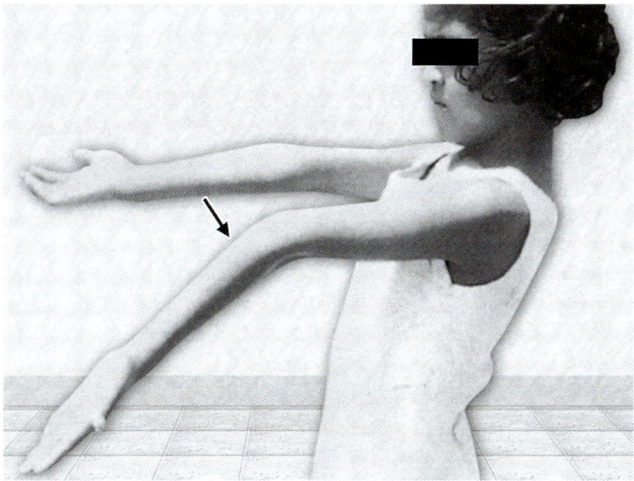

Fig. 5.15: Photograph of a girl having abnormal hyperextension at elbow—cubitus recurvatum.

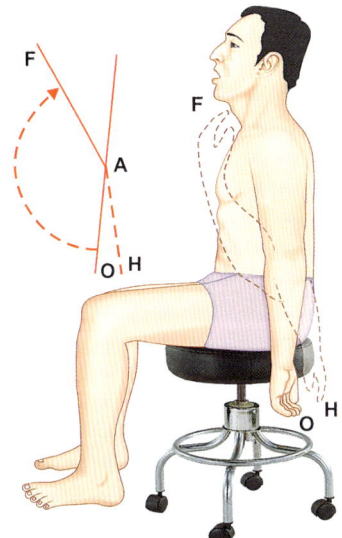

Fig. 5.14: With arms by the side (<OAF—flexion; <OAH—hyperextension); (F: flexion; O: neutral position; H: hyperextension).

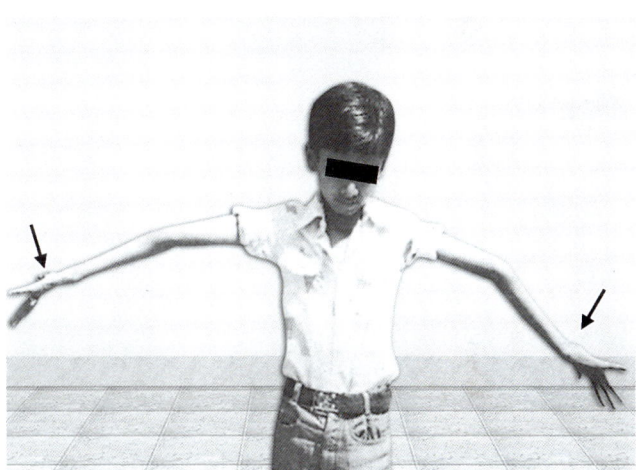

Fig. 5.16: The boy is having hyperextension of both elbows.

between table surface and back of the arm). The forearm is kept in fully supinated position with wrist extended and fingers fully opened up. View from the side, ask the patient to touch the table from the back of the hand without lifting the shoulder at all. This will demonstrate extending back to zero extension position. From this position, ask the patient to approximate the front of upper forearm to the front of lower arm as far as possible, again without lifting the shoulder—this will be flexion.

Another method: If the patient cannot lean—let the patient stand or sit on a stool **(Fig. 5.14)** and view from side. Both arms are close to the sides of the chest with the elbow point being in vertical pendulum line to that of the shoulder. Ask the patient to keep the forearm in fully supinated position and extended at elbow as far as possible. In this position, hyperextension at the elbow can also be noted. Certain individuals have fairly varying extent of laxity. In them the elbow can be hyperextended up to 15°–20° **(Figs. 5.14 to 5.16)**. From zero extension position he/she is asked to approximate the palm towards the shoulder—this will be flexion.

Rotational Movements

Let the patient stand or sit on the stool with arm vertical and by the side of the chest. The elbow is flexed as far as possible up to 90° with wrist extended and fingers opened up. Ask the patient to rotate the palm towards the sky and towards the ground **(Figs. 5.17 to 5.19)**. Movements should be measured from zero position of mid-prone either way. Note the extent of rotational movements and the discrepancy if any. Most of our daily activities are done with the forearm in pronation.

Snapping elbow: *Snapping elbow is mostly due to recurrent dislocation of ulnar nerve.* However, the medial head

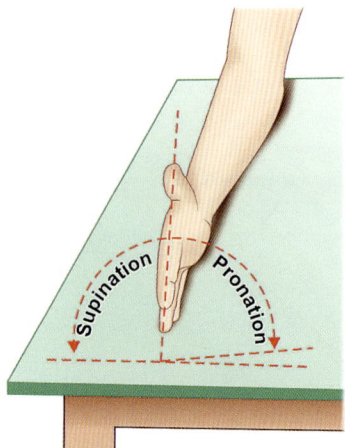

Fig. 5.17: Rotational movements of the forearm (supination and pronation).

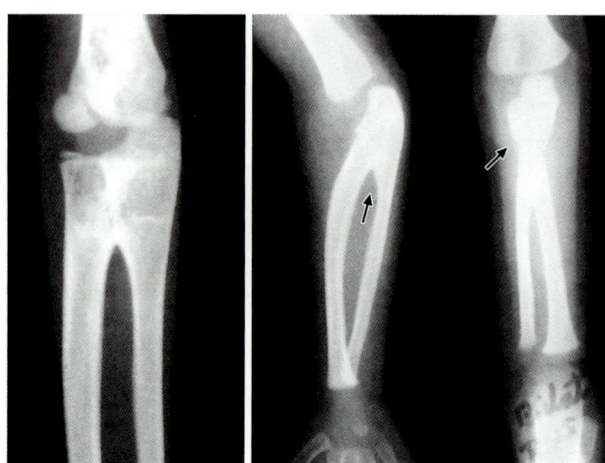

Fig. 5.19: Congenital upper radioulnar synostosis—rotational movements of forearm not possible in such cases and most of the forearms are fixed in supination. Such synostosis should be corrected by osteotomy to place the hand in a more pronation which is the functional position to carry out most of our daily activities.

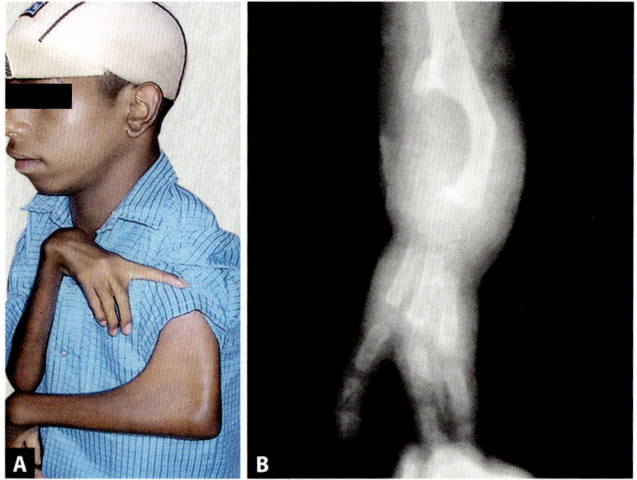

Figs. 5.18A and B: (A) Congenital webbed elbow limiting the extension of elbow. It can be released by plastic surgery—release and reconstruction; (B) Congenital absence of elbow and ulna—no question of having any rotation in forearm or any movement in elbow region.

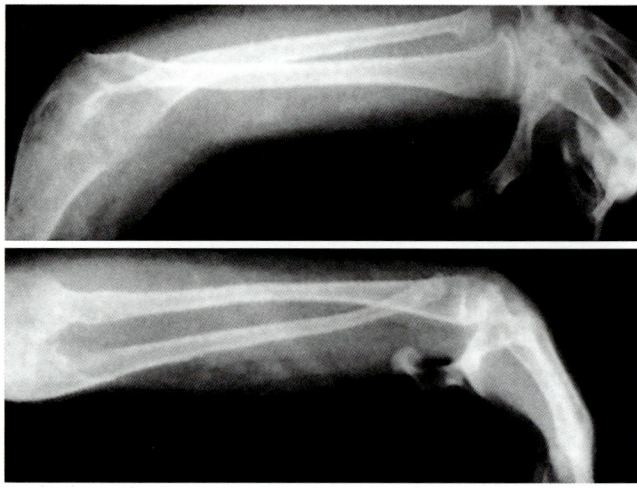

Fig. 5.20: Post-burn contracture of wrist, thumb, fingers and forearm joints and ankylosed elbow—can be managed to variable extent by excisional arthroplasty of elbow (replacement arthroplasty mostly fails due to damaged muscles; arthrodesis of wrist joint and planned physiotherapy).

of triceps muscle or tendon also may dislocate over the medial epicondyle resulting in snapping while elbow is flexed from extended position or *vice versa*. Dislocation of ulnar nerve and medial head of triceps tendon may co-exist producing the clinical finding of at least two snaps at the elbow. The condition may be asymptomatic or symptomatic (discomfort on the medial side of elbow with or without ulnar neuropathy—irritation or palsy). Snapping can be heard, seen, palpable, and reproducible.

The main cause of this condition is *anatomical variations*, e.g. shallow groove on medial epicondyle, hypermobility of ulnar nerve, abnormal configuration of the triceps (e.g. thickening of the fascial edge of medial head of triceps, accessory triceps tendon).

It should be differentiated from bicipital tendinitis, intra-articular abnormalities, medial epicondylitis, Little League elbow syndrome, recurrent dislocation of ulnar nerve itself. Non-symptomatic ones should be ignored, but symptomatic ones need operative management (exploration, dealing with the anatomical abnormality, anterior transposition of ulnar nerve).

As indicated in the Chapter 1, *note the following while assessing the movements:*

- Ankylosis (or congenital absence of joint or fusion of joint **(Figs. 5.18 and 5.19)** or congenital flexion contracture of elbow joint (*see* **Fig. 5.8**) or post-burn **(Fig. 5.20)** or post-infective ankylosis of joint, if any
- Fixation of zero position

- Lag of movement
- Fixity of movement
- Range of activity
- Range of possibility
- Limitation of terminal movement
- Pain during movement
- Achievement of critical arc (15° supination to 15° pronation)
- Abnormal movements
- Achievement of ADL (Activities of daily living)
- Abnormal sounds during movements
- Power of controlling groups of muscles.

Measurement

Linear

(i) As in shoulder joint, for arm and forearm, (ii) Locally, measure the distance between the lateral epicondyle to the olecranon tip, and medial epicondyle to the olecranon tip and compare with the corresponding measurements in the opposite elbow, kept in similar position. *In posterolateral dislocation,* the distance between the lateral epicondyle and the olecranon tip will be decreased. Similarly, *in posteromedial dislocation*, the distance between the medial epicondyle and olecranon tip will be decreased. *In supracondylar fracture,* these distances will be undisturbed. However, in comminuted supracondylar fracture, depending upon the displacement of the fragments, the measurements will be variable. One can have a rough estimation of displacements and rotation by these measurements, e.g. *if the distance between the lateral epicondyle and olecranon tip is decreased it indicates external rotation of the outer fragments and vice versa*. Similar inferences can be had from the medial measurements too. These measurements will also be useful in assessing the displacement of epicondylar fractures, specially that of the medial. *In lateral condylar fractures*, in a few second and in all the third grades, it is difficult to palpate the epicondyle. In *a medial epicondylar fracture* beyond grade I, the distance between the medial epicondyle and the olecranon tip will be correspondingly decreased. Similarly, one can assess almost accurately the localisation and types of olecranon fractures. In fresh fractures of olecranon, one may feel the gap as an aid to diagnosis but in old fractures, the amount of decrease in these aforesaid distances can be a guide to the displacements.

Circumferential

Measure the symmetrically aligned elbows (the normal limb aligned and put according to the diseased one) at the interepicondylar line and olecranon tip. For muscular girth, measure at points equidistant from the tip of olecranon, towards the arm and forearm.

Measurement of Cubitus Varus and Cubitus Valgus (*See* Figs. 5.3 to 5.5, 5.21A and B)

Both upper limbs should be symmetrically extended at the elbow and supinated at the forearm as far as possible (affected elbow will be the guide). Join the midpoint of the interepicondylar line to the midpoint of the interstyloid line at the wrist. This will be the central axis of the forearm. Join the midpoint of the interepicondylar line to the centre of a transverse line drawn outwards from the point, where the anterior fold of axilla meets the arm, to the upper outermost bulge of arm. This, for practical purposes is the central axis of the arm. Prolong this line downwards. *The angle formed in between the long axis of the arm and the forearm is the "carrying angle"* (normal 10°-15°; more in females). If this angle is more on the affected side, it denotes *cubitus valgus deformity* (**Fig. 5.21B** denotes cubitus valgus developed due to displaced unreduced fracture of lateral condyle of humerus, **Fig. 5.21A**) and the amount of increase in the carrying angle measures the extent of cubitus valgus. In *cubitus varus*, the forearm axis drifts towards, or even beyond the arm axis. Up to neutralisation of carrying angle, the normal carrying angle minus that on the affected side will be the measurement of cubitus varus. If the central axis of the forearm drifts further inwards, the cubitus varus will be measured as follows—carrying angle of the normal side + the angle subtended by the central axis of the arm with the medially drifted central axis of the forearm.

Cubitus varus deformity, the common complication of supracondylar fracture develops mainly due to uncorrected medial tilt and medial rotation of the distal fragment. The medial tilt can be confirmed as follows:

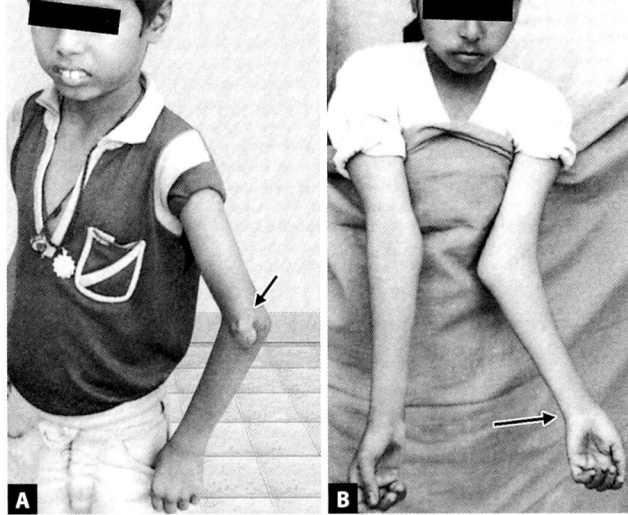

Figs. 5.21A and B: (A) Photograph of a boy having displaced unreduced fracture of the lateral condyle of humerus; (B) Typical cubitus valgus deformity following ununited fracture of lateral condyle of humerus.

Ask the patient to bring both, about 90° flexed, elbows towards the mid-line. Note the position of the medial epicondylar tips. In case of medial tilt, it will be on a higher level.

Medial rotation of the lower fragment can be *assessed as follows:*

Both arms are kept close by the side of chest with elbows flexed at about 90°. Ask the patient to externally rotate both the upper limbs at shoulder. On the affected side, the external rotation will be limited more or less by the same degree as the medial rotation.

ASSESSMENT OF COMPLICATIONS DUE TO PATHOLOGY IN AND AROUND THE ELBOW

Besides any stiffness and deformity, look especially for any vascular (e.g. compartmental syndrome—VIC) or neurological complications *(affections of peripheral nerves). If the patient can make a firm normal looking fist and open up the hand fully, all peripheral nerves are almost intact.*

Test for Impending/Threatening Volkmann's Ischaemic Contracture (*Also see* Table 5.3)

Following any injury in and around the elbow and the upper forearm, (e.g. war injuries, missile or high-velocity injuries, side sweep injury or bullet injury), any tight bandage/plaster in this area, after reducing any fracture or dislocation in this area, or after operating in this area—**Always apprehend** threatened vascular insufficiency (compartmental syndrome) and:
- Elevate the limb/part.
- Examine the patient/part again and again to note if pain, swelling, congestion, number is/are increasing.
- Release the tight bandage/plaster/or any suspicious pressing object.
- Reduce the dislocation/fracture at the earliest; remove (any) foreign body which can/likely to press on the adjacent/underlying blood vessels.
- If intercompartmental pressure is increasing-Release it surgically at the earliest-LEST precipitate the problems as in **Figures 5.22A to D** may result.

In compartment syndrome, the circulation within a closed compartment is compromised due to increase in pressure within the compartment leading to necrosis of muscles, nerves, subcutaneous tissue and even skin. When the compartment syndrome is suspected, compartment pressure should be measured by special instrument. Compartment pressure over 30 mm Hg or within 20 mm Hg of the diastolic pressure are indicative of compartment syndrome.

There are four interconnected compartments in the forearm: 1. superficial volar compartment, 2. deep volar compartment, 3. dorsal compartment, 4. compartment containing the mobile wad of Henry—brachioradialis, extensor carpi radialis longus and extensor carpi radialis brevis. The volar compartments are most commonly involved in compartment syndrome, however, dorsal and *mobile wad* compartments may also be involved along with the volar ones or in isolation.

Increased tissue pressure is the key to compartmental syndrome. Once the pressure is raised, it can compromise the local circulation by decreased perfusion pressure, arteriolar closure, and reflex vasospasm. In compartment syndrome/threatened Volkmann's ischaemia:

Look for—(i) **P**ain—Disproportionate unrelenting pain is usually the earliest feature—believe your patient if he complains of pain (moderate to severe) especially in the forearm, (ii) *Finger stretch test* or *passive muscle stretch test*—**p**assive stretching of the fingers aggravates the pain, which is progressive, it indicates that the muscle is ischaemic, (iii) **P**uffiness—swelling of the fingers, dorsum of the hand and palm, (iv) **P**allor—earlier, there is *cyanotic hue* and then increasing pallor may develop, (v) **P**alpation of the muscular compartment elicits tenderness, which is one of the specific signs of compartmental syndrome, (vi) **P**ressing the nailbed—delayed capillary refilling, (vii) **P**ulse (radial) may be feeble, to absent, (viii) **P**araesthesia—in the hand and fingers, (ix) **P**ower—ask the patient to move the fingers. Earlier pain might have been the preventing factor in moving the fingers, but later actual neurogenic paresis supervenes, (x) **P**erception of temperature—ischaemic hand and fingers are comparatively colder.

Paralysis and **p**ulselessness are the late findings. If the process has progressed to this point, the pathological changes are more likely to be irreversible **(Figs. 5.22 to 5.25)**.

Warm and red skin overlying the affected compartment suggests cellulitis or thrombophlebitis.

If the problem is not apprehended, diagnosed and managed promptly, the established ischaemic effects develop, such as various degrees of contractures paresis and allied changes, i.e. The Volkmann ischaemic contracture (described by Volkmann in 1881) in which the necrotic muscle and nerve tissue and other affected tissues are replaced by fibrous tissue.

The patient presents with flexed fingers [(with or without flexed wrist)(or flexed toes)] leading to clawing effect of the fingers or toes (intrinsic plus type). Main clinical sign is Volkmann's sign or muscle length phenomenon. Here, when wrist is further flexed, the fingers can be actively and/or passively extended. But with gradual extension of the wrist, the fingers again get flexed. This occurs because there is contraction of fibrotic muscle and tendon without any synovial adhesion in the tendon sheath. With adhesion between tendon and its sheath (as happens in tenosynovitis) the extension of tendon is prevented.

Chronic exertional compartment syndrome: It is reversible ischaemia occurring due to a non-compliant osteofascial compartment which is unresponsive to the expansion of muscle volume developing after exertional exercises due to increased blood flow and oedema and muscle hypertrophy. It is commonly seen in young adult recreational runners,

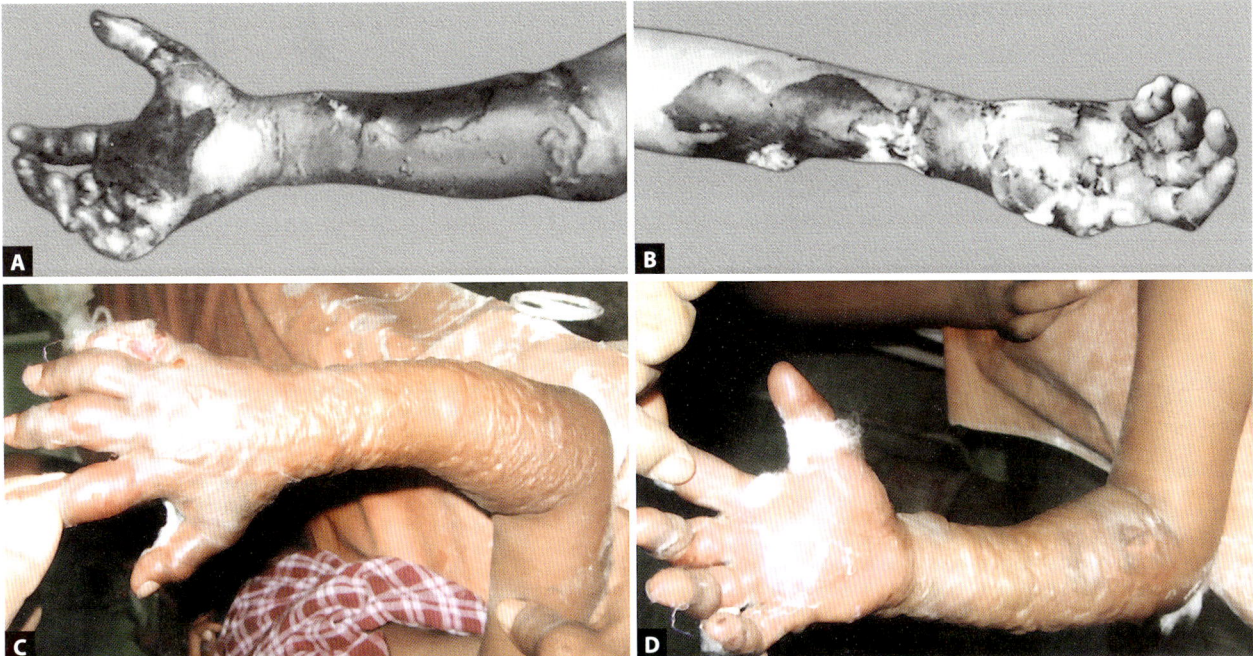

Figs. 5.22A to D: Volkmann's ischaemia
Note the swelling, blebs, necrosis and threatened gangrenous changes in forearm and hand following Volkmann's ischaemia in two cases (A & B: 1st case and C & D: 2nd case).

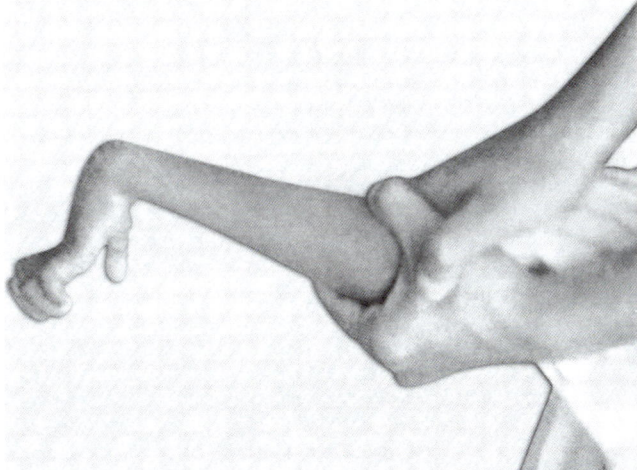

Fig. 5.23: Severe Volkmann's ischaemic contracture (VIC)
Management: From the earliest stage to advanced stage consist of proper physiotherapy; dynamic splints, occupational therapy, surgery (release, tendon transfer, joint stabilization).

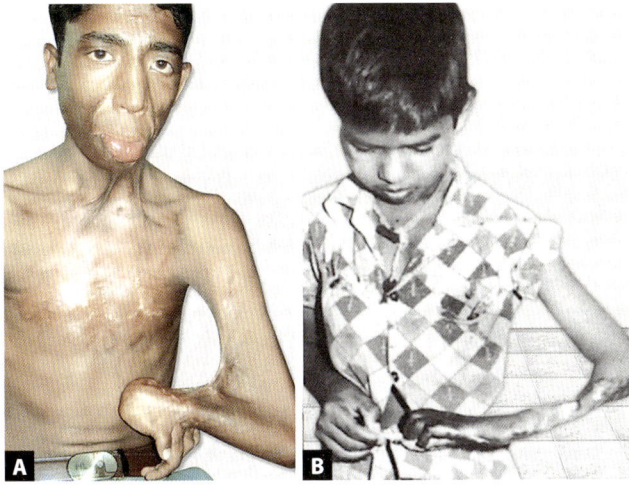

Figs. 5.24A and B: (A) Post burn contractures. Plastic surgeries in stages can improve the condition; (B) Very severe Volkmann's ischaemic contracture—After possible operative treatment—tendons released and lengthened and skin grafting—the boy is trained to button his shirt.

military recruits, elite athletes. Usually both legs are involved, in which anterior and lateral compartments are commonly affected.

Test for Lateral Epicondylitis

Lateral epicondylitis **(tennis elbow)** first described by Runge in 1873, *is an enthesopathy of the common extensor origin at the lateral epicondylar region of humerus.* It is the most common tendinitis in the elbow region and it commonly occurs around the age of 30. Its exact aetiopathogenesis is not known. However, it is being recognised as an *overuse syndrome (repetitive stress disorder)* due to repetitive tension overloading of the wrist extensor origin against resistance at the lateral epicondylar region as commonly seen in recreational tennis and racquet ball players (hence has been termed as "tennis elbow").

The pathological change is in the extensor carpi radialis brevis aponeurosis. After a tear in the tendon, this poorly vascularized area between the aponeurosis of the extensor

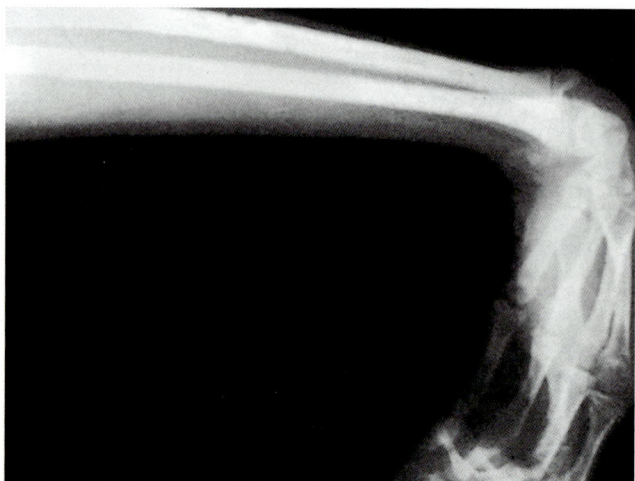

Fig. 5.25: Volkmann's ischaemic contracture—(Very severe) the X-ray picture—Management mainly by surgery (arthrodesis of wrist, capsulectomy of smaller joint, proper physiotherapy and occupational therapy).

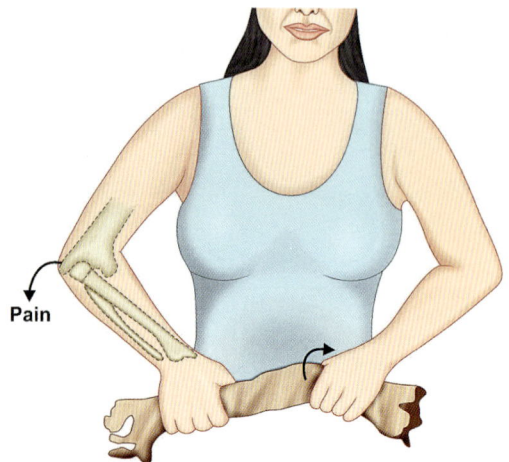

Fig. 5.26: Wringing test.

carpi radialis brevis and the cortex of humerus fills with granulation tissue rather than progressing to repair. The microscopic pathology noted in the degenerated tendon is termed angiofibroblastic hyperplasia, which denotes chronic tendinosis rather than acute inflammation.

Resisted supination and pronation increase the stresses on the lateral epicondyle, which form the basis of the tests for lateral epicondylitis.

Traction or stress injuries or vascular causes induce *osteochondritis of capitellum* (Panner's disease) which should be kept in mind while diagnosing the tennis elbow. Of course osteochondral fractures, ossification defects, avascular necrosis, accessory centre of ossification, and detachment of fragments have been suggested to be associated with osteochondritis dissecans.

Tests to Diagnose/Confirm Tennis Elbow

1. *Wringing test:* Ask the patient to wring a towel—pain will be felt at the lateral epicondylar region **(Fig. 5.26)**.
2. *Chair test:* Ask the patient to get up from a chair with both hands firmly gripping and pressing the arms of the chair. Pain is felt at the lateral epicondylar region, of the affected side.
3. *Jug test:* Ask the patient to lift a jug full of water, holding its mouth from above. Pointed pain will be felt at the lateral epicondylar region **(Fig. 5.27)**.
4. *Cozen's test:* Ask the patient to make a firm fist. While the patient maintains this position, try to passively flex the wrist. Patient will feel pain at the lateral epicondylar region **(Fig. 5.28)**.
5. *Mill's manoeuvre:* While the patient keeps her/his elbow firmly straight and wrist flexed, pronation of the forearm initiates pain at the lateral epicondylar region **(Fig. 5.29)**.
6. *Broom test:* Holding of broom firmly to sweep the floor initiates pains in the lateral epicondylar region. Ask the patient to hold a broom firmly in her hand and attempt to sweep the floor, she will complain of pain in the lateral epicondylar region.
7. *Rolling-pin test:* Rolling the dough for preparing round bread, with firmly holding the rolling-pin (*belan*), initiates pain in the lateral epicondylar region and

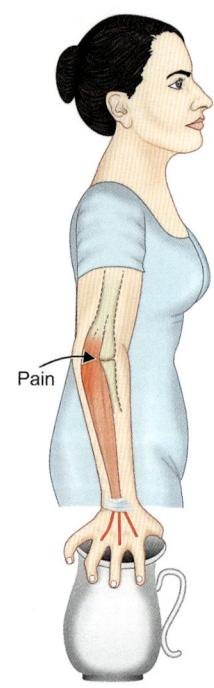

Fig. 5.27: Jug test.

NB: *Tennis leg*: It is common in middle-aged athletes in racquet sports. It occurs due to unresolved muscle strain. Classically it occurs at the musculotendinous junction of the medial head of gastrocnemius. There is focal muscle pain and tenderness at the complained-of-site and there may be palpable lump or thickening. Management consists of deep tissue massage (myofascial release) to break down the scar tissue. A medial heel wedge may be helpful.

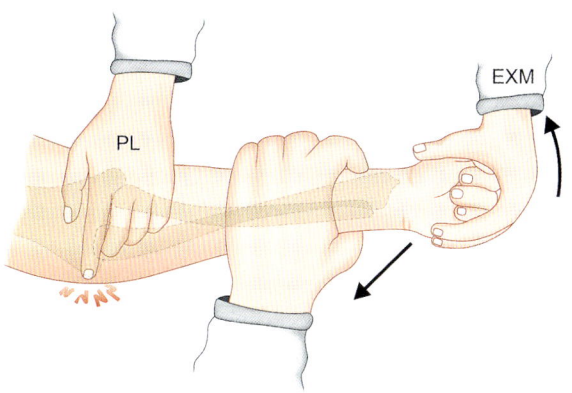

Fig. 5.28: Cozen's test.

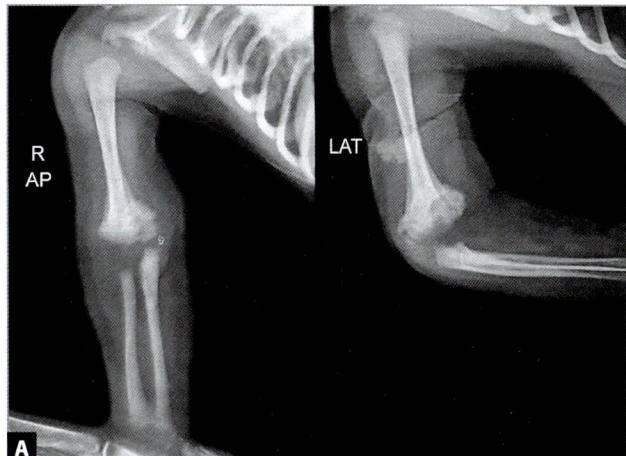

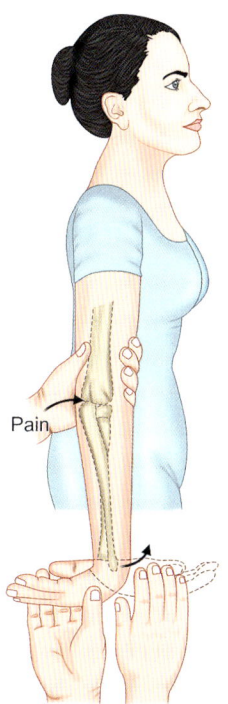

Fig. 5.29: Mill's manoeuvre.

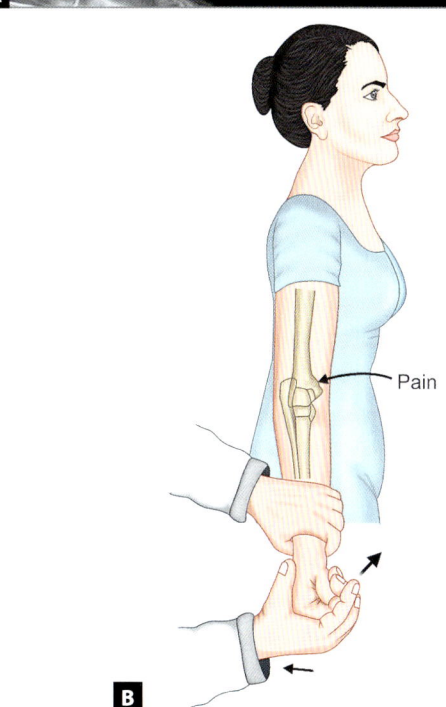

Figs. 5.30A and B: (A) Septic arthrities in neonate; (B)Test for medial epicondylitis: Anterior arrow showing active flexion at wrist by the patient and inferior arrow showing resistance offered by the examiner.

proximal portion of wrist extensors taking origin from lateral epicondyle.

8. *Stir-fry test:* While stir-frying in a pan, the patient feels pain in the lateral epicondylar region.

Test for Medial Epicondylitis (Figs. 5.30A and B)

Medial epicondylitis or golfer's elbow is an overuse syndrome caused by repetitive tension overloading of the flexor-pronator muscle at or near its origin from the medial epicondyle. Resisted pronation and flexion of the wrist increase the stresses on medial epicondyle, which form the basis of the tests for medial epicondylitis.

With the elbow extended and the forearm supinated, ask the patient to make a fist and then flex the wrist against the examiner's resistance. The patient will complain of pain at the medial epicondylar region. Medial epicondylar pain is accentuated by a valgus stress to the elbow in extension.

Test for Cubital Tunnel Syndrome

Uninterrupted prolonged flexion attitude of elbow may lead to varied compression of ulnar nerve in the tight cubital tunnel (e.g. during sleeping), symptoms of which gradually improve after extending the elbow. Keeping the elbow acutely flexed for about 5 minutes precipitates the ulnar nerve compression symptoms, if the tunnel is tight (elbow flexion test).

INVESTIGATIONS REQUIRED FOR ELBOW PATHOLOGY

- General investigations
  (As in the Chapter 1 on Introduction)
- *Radiological investigation:*
  If possible, comparative X-ray of both elbows helps in clearly delineating any pathological condition.
  - *Anteroposterior view:* Place the fully extended elbow along with the supinated forearm over the centre of the plate. The beam is to be focussed vertically, on the centre of the cubital fossa
  - *Lateral view:* Plate is placed vertically on either medial or lateral side of fully extended elbow and fully supinated forearm. The beam is to be centred on epicondylar tip from either side on the plate. It is better to take a true lateral view of X-ray in maximum possible extension and flexion of the elbow in order to record the range of movement for future reference.
- CT scan will be more helpful in delineating any bony pathology (due to trauma or disease)
- MRI will be more useful to delineate any soft tissue pathology
- *Aspiration.*
  It is easy to aspirate the joint through the anconeus triangle.

Arthrography and arthroscopy: If carefully done, it can provide useful evidences.

AFFECTIONS OF ELBOW

Congenital Conditions

- Agenesis
- Dysgenesis
- Congenital dislocation (*see* **Fig. 5.55**)/subluxation of elbow (ulnohumeral, radiohumeral, radioulnar joints)
- Congenital single bone forearm
- Congenital contractured elbow/congenital webbed elbow (*see* **Fig. 5.18A**)
- Congenital radioulnar synostosis mostly involves the proximal ends of radius and ulna, and the forearm is usually fixed in pronation. There is familial predisposition. It is more often bilateral (*see* **Fig. 5.19**).

Inflammatory

Infective
- *Acute*—Pyogenic (haematogeneous or after compound injury or iatrogenic)
- Subacute
  - Gonococcal
  - Pyogenic
  - Variolar
  - Tuberculous
- *Chronic*
  - Tuberculous
  - Pyogenic
  - Variolar
  - Syphilitic
- *Collagen-arthropathy*
  - Rheumatoid arthritis
  - Rheumatic arthritis
  - Ankylosing spondylopathy
- *Metabolic*
  - Gouty arthritis
  - Chondrocalcinosis (calcium pyrophosphate arthropathy).

Traumatic

Corresponding injuries of elbow in children and adults have been mentioned in **Table 5.2**.

TABLE 5.2: Corresponding injuries of elbow in children and adults.

Children	Adults
1. Pulled elbow (subluxation of radial head) usually occurs in childhood (younger children who are lifted by holding the forearm). Child weeps, when that elbow is touched; there is no deformity; tenderness is maximum in radial head region; flexion extension of elbow produces pain; pronation-supination causes less pain	Strained or sprained elbow

2. Supracondylar fracture
(a) Posterior
  – Posteromedial (**Figs. 5.31 and 5.32**)
  – Posterolateral
(b) Anterior
  – Anterolateral
  – Anteromedial (**Figs. 5.31 and 5.33**)
(c) 'T' Fracture very rare (0.8%)
	Comminuted supracondylar fracture (T and Y fracture)

3. Fracture-separation of lower humeral epiphysis (a very rare injury)	X

Contd...

Contd...

Children	Adults

4. Dislocation—rare in children
   (a) Posterior
   (b) Anterior
	Common in adults
	   (a) Posterior, posterolateral and posteromedial
	   (b) Anterior
	   (c) Lateral
	   (d) Medial
	   (e) Divergent
	   (f) Isolated dislocation of radial head or olecranon

5. Fracture dislocation	Fracture dislocation • Accompanying fracture may be as in baby car or sideswipe fracture dislocation (i.e. fracture dislocation of the elbow with forward displacement of both forearm bones, fracture upper ulnar shaft, fracture olecranon, fracture lower humerus) Other accompanying fractures may be: • Radial head fracture • Capitulum fracture • Olecranon fracture • Coronoid fracture • Medial epicondyle avulsion fracture (adolescent) • Supracondylar fracture • Posterior marginal fracture of condyles
6. Fracture separation of upper radial epiphysis	• Fracture head/neck of radius
7. Fracture separation or avulsions of olecranon apophysis	• Fracture olecranon
8. Monteggia fracture dislocation	• Monteggia fracture dislocation (less incidence)
9. Fracture lateral condyle (**Figs. 5.34 and 5.35**)	• Fracture capitellum
10. Avulsion fracture of the lateral epicondyle (very rare)	Hardly seen
11. Avulsion fracture of the medial epicondyle	Rare
12. Floating elbow: Ipsilateral fracture of upper or middle third forearm, along with supracondylar fracture	Floating elbow, usually in RTA

Key Diagnostic Points for Common Elbow Pathologies

Supracondylar Fracture (Figs. 5.31 to 5.33)

- Most common injury around the elbow in children (more in males, 5–8 years)
- Mostly history of fall on outstretched pronated hand
- Tenderness around supracondylar region
- If there is no swelling, irregularity of supracondylar ridges can be felt (in acute and subacute cases, this irregularity is difficult to feel because of gross swelling and organising haematoma)
- Passive movements at the elbow possible to a variable extent
- Active movements disturbed because of pain and mechanical reasons
- Arm is shortened (*not* the forearm) depending upon the amount of displacement and overriding. In late cases, cubitus varus deformity may develop if medial displacement, medial tilting and medial rotation have not been fully corrected (*See* **Figs. 5.4 and 5.5**).
  - Median, radial and ulnar nerves may be affected in that order
  - Threatened or established Volkmann's ischaemic contracture must be looked for (**Table 5.3**).
- The relationship between the three bony points on the back of the elbow is *not* disturbed.
  - Myositis ossificans is a common complication.
- In adults, supracondylar fractures are usually comminuted (communicating with the elbow joint 'T' or 'Y' fracture). Therefore, movements are grossly affected initially as well as later on.

Dislocation Elbow (Figs. 5.36 to 5.38)

Dislocations are mostly due to trauma, but may be congenital (*see* **Fig. 5.55**) or pathological (*see* **Fig. 5.54**).

- Posterior dislocation is more common
- Young adults are the usual victims
- Olecranon stands out prominently on the back of the lower arm
- The cubital fossa is occupied by a globular convex bony mass (the lower humeral articular part)
- Posterior dislocation of elbow constitutes 90 per cent of all elbow dislocations. Rarely lateral, medial, anterior, and divergent dislocations, and isolated dislocation of radial head or olecranon may occur anteriorly or posteriorly
- Triceps stands out prominently (**Fig. 5.37**)
- Movements markedly restricted initially. Later on, variable range of movements may occur
- Shortening of the forearm (not of the arm)

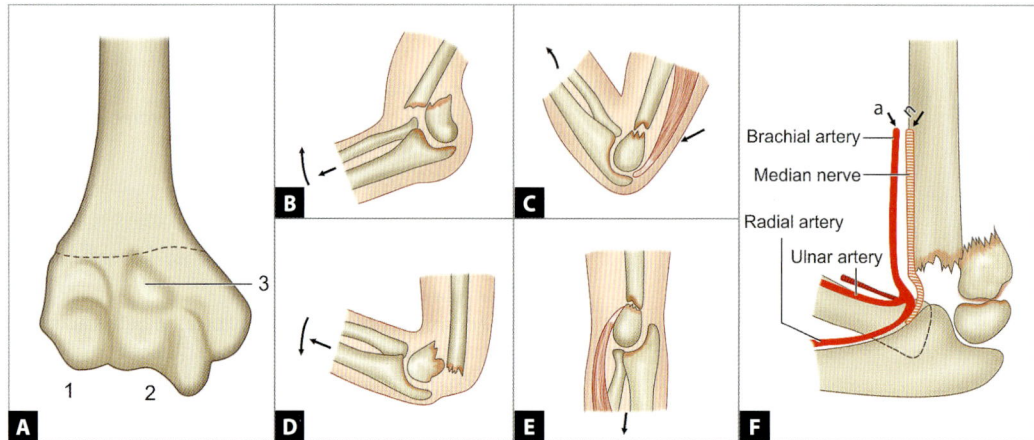

Figs. 5.31A to F: (A) the outline of normal architecture of—lower humeral end, (B and C) Pre- and post-reduction of supracondylar fracture with posterior displacement; (D and E) pre- and post-reduction of supracondylar fracture with anterior displacement, and (F) vulnerable neurovascular bundle in displaced supracondylar fracture. (A: artery; n: nerve)

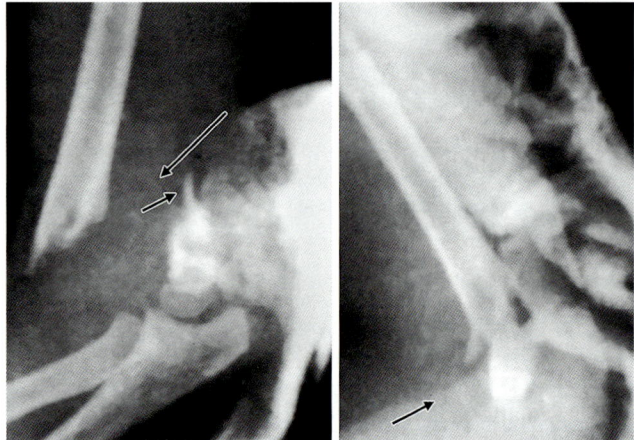

Fig. 5.32: On the left—supracondylar fracture with gross posteromedial displacement. On the right—same after closed reduction.

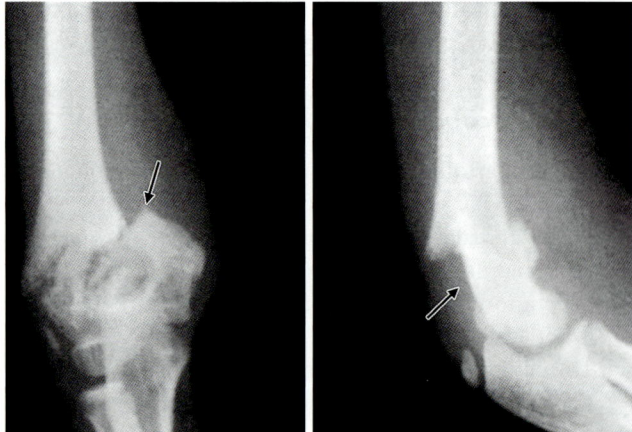

Fig. 5.33: Supracondylar fracture with anteromedial displacement.

- Relationship of the three bony points is disturbed
- Myositis ossificans is quite common complication.

An elbow dislocation is the dissociation of the joint constituted by the lower articular end of humerus proximally and the articular surface of radial head, olecranon and coronoid distally. Dislocations of elbow are of following types: Posterior (ulna and radial head displace posteriorly—posterolateral); Anterior (ulna and radius displace anteriorly with or without fracture of olecranon); Medial, lateral and divergent dislocations; Posterolateral dislocation with entrapped fracture medial epicondyle; Isolated dislocation of radial head; Fracture-dislocation or complex dislocation (dislocation associated with fracture of any articulating bone). Dislocations are mostly following trauma, however it may be congenital (*See* **Fig. 5.55**), and pathological (*See* **Fig. 5.54**).

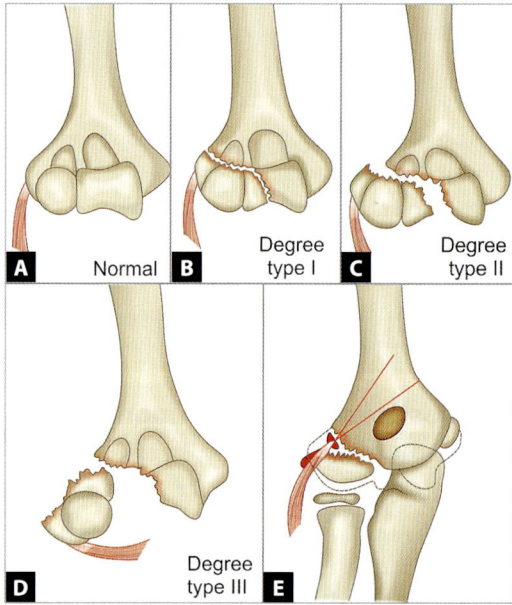

Figs. 5.34A to E: (A to D) Line sketch of different types of fracture of lateral condyle of humerus; (E), Open reduction internal fixation (ORIF) of **Figure 5.34D** (i.e. Type III).

In *fracture dislocation of elbow* (also called *complex dislocation* against simple dislocation, where there is no

TABLE 5.3: Assessment of established Volkmann's ischaemic contracture, which may be considered under four groups according to severity.

Clinical features	Mild	Moderate	Severe	Very severe
1. Deformity—				
(i) Tendency of clawing.	Negligible	Appreciable	Marked	Well marked
(ii) Flexion contracture of interphalangeal joint M.P. joint Wrist joint	+ – –	++ + –	+++ ++ + to ++	++++ +++ +++
(iii) Correctability of deformities	With slightly flexing the wrist —fully corrected	With full flexion of wrist —fully corrected	Even with full flexion of wrist —marked deformity	Wrist contracted in flexion —almost negligible effect on contracted deformities
(iv) Stretchability	Stretchable in all cases	Stretchable in majority of cases but prolonged endeavour is required, along with using the dynamic Volkmann's splint	Not stretchable	Not at all stretchable
2. Skin and subcutaneous tissue	Normal	Almost normal	Atrophic changes, may be patchy anaesthesia. Not freely pliable	Advanced atrophic changes, anaesthetic areas, adherent and parchment-like skin
3. Fingertip	Pulp normal	Stiffness of pulp	Stiff, tapering pulp	Atrophic, quite stiff pulp
4. Nailbed	Almost normal	Tapering atrophic tendency of nail	Dry look, tapering	Marked dry look, tapering, may be deformed
5. Palm	Normal	Almost normal, tendency of crowding	Crowded, atrophied thenar and hypothenar eminences	Contracted, atrophied, deep adherent creases
6. Wrist	Normal	Almost normal	Flexion contracture evident, subluxated carpals, extension not possible	Marked flexion contracture subluxated or even dislocated carpals—stiff wrist
7. Forearm	Normal	Wasted forearm specially on flexor aspect. Comparatively firm in feel in mid forearm area	Marked wasting of —forearm flexors+++ —extensors++ Firm feel of —flexor muscle+++ —extensors++ (muscles undergoing yellow degenerative and fibrotic contractures)	Negligible muscle mass in forearm (specially in lower 4/5th). Firm in feel
8. Tendon	On hyperextension of wrist contracted long flexors become obvious —Otherwise normal	Long flexors remain contracted. Contraction gradually gets exaggerated as the wrist is extended. Extensors of wrist and fingers start losing power due to less use	Both groups suffer, flexors contracted but power not completely lost. In contracted position action can be demonstrated. Extensors suffer stretch weakness, may even appear to be markedly weak	Both groups markedly suffer; are contracted and powerless. Develops adhesions at places of ulcerations
9. Radial pulse	Normal	Nearly normal	Feeble	Very feeble/absent
10. Joint	Almost normal at all levels	Palmar capsule of inter phalangeal joints and metacarpophalangeal joints contracted. Dorsal capsule has tendency of stretching	Palmar capsule of interphalangeal, metacarpophalangeal and wrist contracted. Dorsal capsule stretched. Mild tendency of subluxation at interphalangeal, metacarpophalangeal and wrist joints. Mild to moderate atrophy of synovial tissue	Palmar capsule contracted and adherent. Dorsal capsule stretched and atrophied. Marked subluxation at all levels Synovial tissue markedly atrophied

Contd...

Contd...

Clinical features	Mild	Moderate	Severe	Very severe
11. Bones	Normal	Normal; in old cases terminal phalanges rarefied	Marked rarefaction especially near the joints Thinning and tubular tendency of even the forearm bones	Marked rarefaction of bones of hand and forearm. Thinning of the forearm bones
12. Nerves (either suffer from some vascular pathology as muscles do and/or also undergo pressure changes due to entrapment and consequent pressure within the fibrotic mass)	All normal	All normal	May be features of affection of median nerve	All nerves may be affected
13. ADL— (Activities of daily living) and functions	Almost all functions possible	All ADL possible. Finer functions may be affected to variable extent	Very limited functions possible May carry on ADL anyhow	No function possible Even ADL not possible
14. Gross management	• Reassurance • Supported guarded stretching • Dynamic Volkmann's splint may be required	• Supported guarded gradual stretching • Dynamic Volkmann's splintage • Surgery for the residual deformities (soft tissue surgery— on muscles, tendons, capsule)	• Preoperative supported stretching. Surgery, first on soft tissues (muscles, tendons, capsule, neurolysis); For the residual—on joints (carpectomy, arthrodesis, arthroplasty) and/or bones (shortening of forearm bones). • Dynamic Volkmann's splint if needed	• Preoperative supported stretching • Surgery on soft tissues (muscles, tendon, neurolysis, capsule), mostly on joints (carpectomy, arthrodesis) and or bones (shortening of forearm) • Dynamic Volkmann's splint

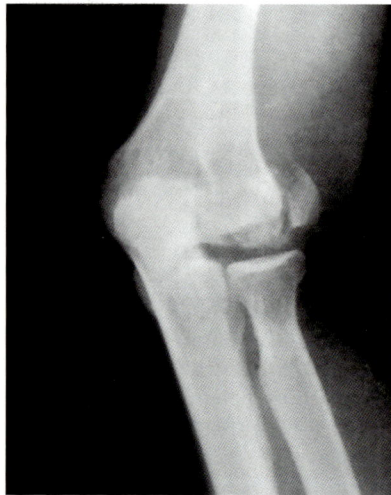

Fig. 5.35: Fracture of lateral condyle of humerus—type II. It is better to fix such fracture by screw for proper healing.

associated fracture) dislocation is associated with fracture (or fractures) of the articulating bone(s). When there is fracture of coronoid process, the threat of recurrent and chronic instability of elbow increases. Dislocation of elbow associated with fracture of radial head, and coronoid process has been named as *"terrible triad of the elbow"* by Hotchkiss and is prone to acute redislocation and chronic instability.

Myositis Ossificans (Figs. 5.39 and 5.40)

(Also refer the Chapter 2 on 'Examination of Long Bones').
- A common complication following injuries around the elbow **(Figs. 5.39 and 5.40)**, and even around hip (Refer **Fig. 12.85**). It is a benign localised non-neoplastic.

Myositis ossificans are of three types:
1. Parosteal-near shaft of long bone, most common type.
2. Periosteal-eccentric bone mass with disruption of periosteum.
3. Extraosseous – seen along tendon-rarest.
- Usually, there is a history of massage or repeated manipulations
- In the early stage, the skin is warm all round the elbow, specially anteriorly
- Firm to hard feel of the muscles in front of the elbow
- Later on, reactive warmth may not be felt but hard bony plaques may be felt
- Movements initially grossly restricted, (due to spasm and myositic activity) but gradually improves to variable extent.

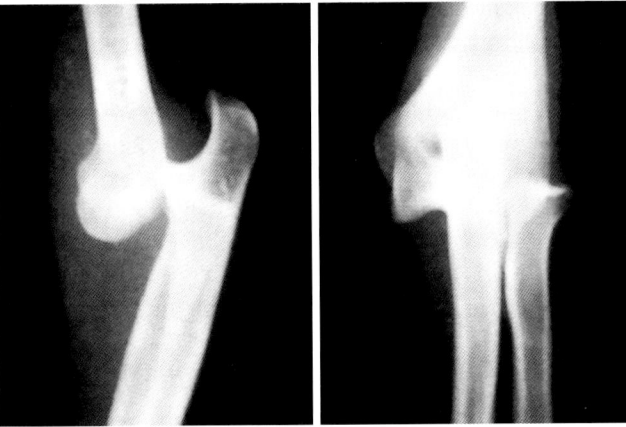

Fig. 5.36: Posterolateral dislocation of elbow joint—must be reduced, by closed method, at the earliest.

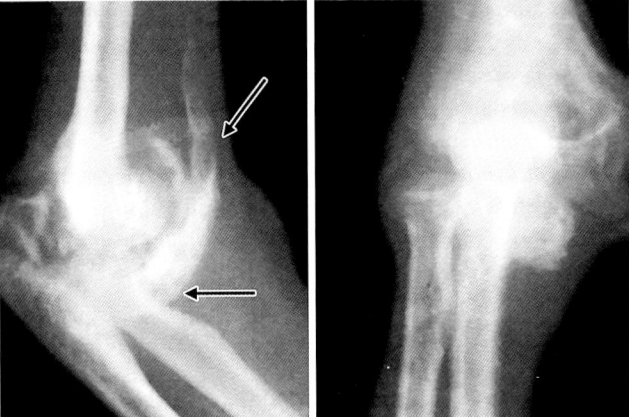

Fig. 5.39: Myositis in the cubital fossa in old dislocated elbow— It should be managed by cautions removal of myositic mass, arthrolysis, reduction of elbow joint – Prognosis remains guarded. Total free movements of elbow are difficult to achieve.

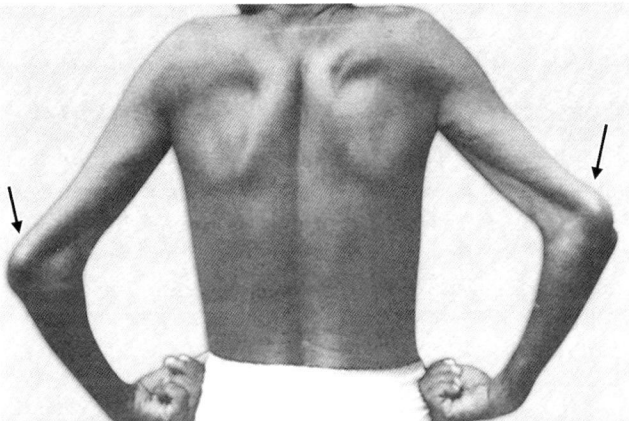

Fig. 5.37: Photograph showing bilateral unreduced posterior dislocation of elbow—note the prominent triceps on both sides.

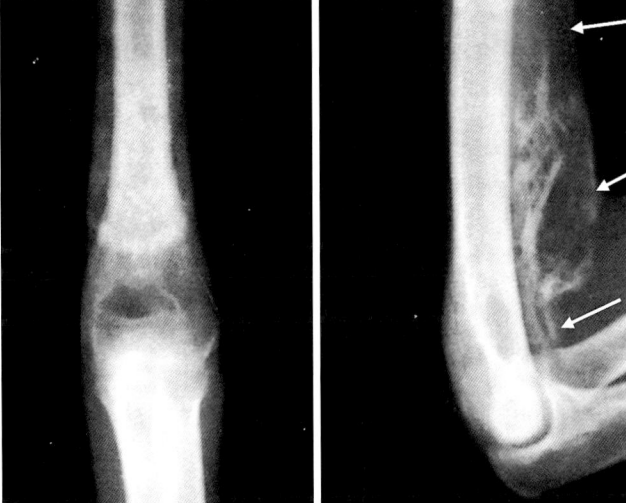

Fig. 5.40: Myositis in front of lower humerus in old injury of elbow— fibro-osseous proliferative non inflammatory lesion in the soft tissue and periosteum—Myositic mass should, be cautiously removed.

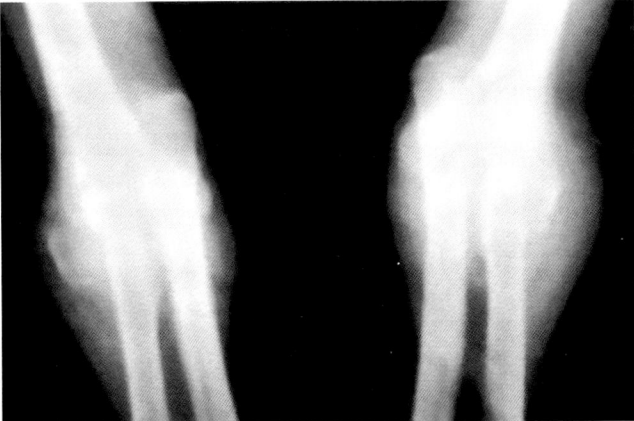

Fig. 5.38: AP view: X-ray of both sides elbow of the same patient **(Fig. 5.37).**

Heterotopic calcification/ossification:

Even there are regulatory mechanism, calcium may be abnormally deposited in extraskeletal system. Here no true bone matrix is formed. It is called heterotrophic calcification e.g. in certain hereditary and congenital conditions, calcific deposits in subacromial regions. Both extrinsic (head injuries, cerebrovascular accidents, burns, ankylosing spondylitis etc.) and intrinsic factors (injury to the abductor musculature, surgical approach, haemorrhage etc.) predispose to overall risk of heterotopic bone formation.

Heterotopic ossification may also occur around the elbow, e.g. in burn, **(Refer Fig. 12.85)** head injury patients, hypoxic brain insults.

Progressive osseous heteroplasia (POH), the term coined by Kaplan et al. (1994), is a rare distinct autosomal dominant disorder of mesenchymal differentiation characterized by dermal ossification beginning in infancy and followed by increasing and extensive bone formation in deep muscle and fascia. The causative molecular defect is the same which causes Pseudopseudo-hypoparathyroidism (PPHP). The cause of POH is an inactivating GNAS1 (guanine nucleotide-binding protein alpha-stimulating activity polypeptide 1) mutation caused only by paternal inheritance of the mutant allele.

Other causes of heterotopic ossification in childhood are fibrodysplasia ossificans progressive, pseudohypo-parathyroidism, pseudopseudohypoparathyroidism.

Fibrodysplasia ossificans progressiva (FOP) is a rare condition causing physical handicap due to intermittently progressive ectopic ossification and malformed valgoid short toes, which are often monophalangic.

Myositis ossificans progressiva (MOP) is a rare connective tissue disorder characterised by progressive ossification of the soft tissues with characteristic congenital anomalies like monophalangeal great toe, clinodactyly, short first metacarpal and reduction defects of the limb. Exact cause is not known but presumed aetiology is a causal mutation in the gene responsible for the synthesis of bone morphogenetic protein-2A (this gene is also responsible for limb patterning and ossification). Presentation by asymptomatic variant to disabling ectopic ossification causing crippling deformities, incapacitation and premature death. Out of all treatments tried, intensive physiotherapy is only variably useful. However, recently isotretinoin (13-cis-retinoic acid) in a dose of 1–2 mg/kg/day has been found to be useful.

Myositis ossificans should also be differentiated from other causes where bone formation occurs in soft tissues, such as tumoral calcinosis, dermatomyositis **(Fig. 5.41)**, polymyositis haemorrhagica, diaphyseal aclasia, Christian-Weber syndrome (relapsing nodular non-suppuratic panniculitis), etc.

Isolated excision of any ectopic bone (including heterotopic bone) should not be performed before radiographic maturation.

Medial Epicondylar Fracture (Figs. 5.42A to D)

Degrees of medial epicondylar fracture:
Degree I : Slight separation with minimal displacement.

Degree II : Avulsed fragment pulled down to joint level.
Degree III : Avulsed fragment entrapped in the elbow joint.
Degree IV : Avulsion of medial epicondyle with lateral dislocation of the elbow.

- Swelling, tenderness localised to medial epicondylar region of humerus
- Extension movements mainly limited, and in grades III and IV both movements of the elbow may be grossly limited
- In late cases, friction neuritis of the ulnar nerve may develop.

Fracture of Head and Neck of Radius

- Usually in adults
- History of fall on pronated outstretched hand
- Rotational movements of forearm markedly restricted
- Tenderness localised to just below the lateral epicondylar eminence.

Monteggia Fracture Dislocation (Figs. 5.43 and 5.44)

GB Monteggia of Milan published about the combined injury of the fracture of proximal third of ulna with anterior dislocation of radial head in 1814. Much later, JL Bado coined the term 'Monteggia lesion' to include the entire spectrum of such injuries in 1967. The classification of monteggia lesions is discussed in **Table 5**.4.

In few cases, there may be combined displacements (angulations) and dislocations (e.g. anterolateral).

- Comparatively more common in children (7–12 years) but can occur in adults also

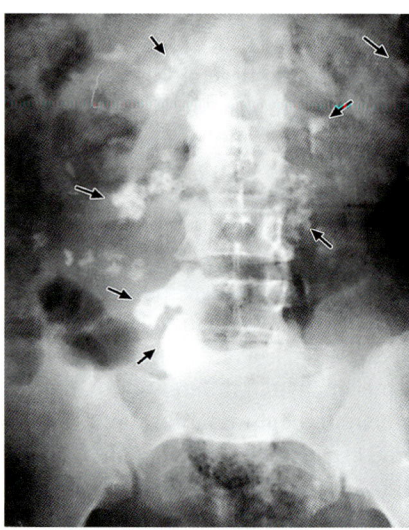

Fig. 5.41: Dermatomyositis.

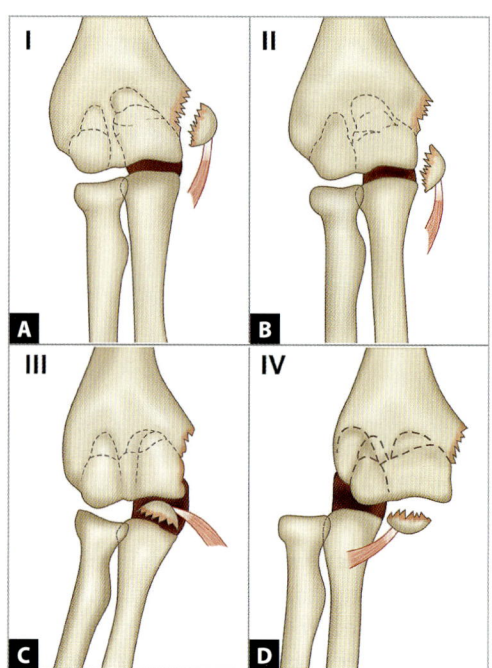

Figs. 5.42A to D: Different degrees (types) of avulsion fracture of medial epicondyle.

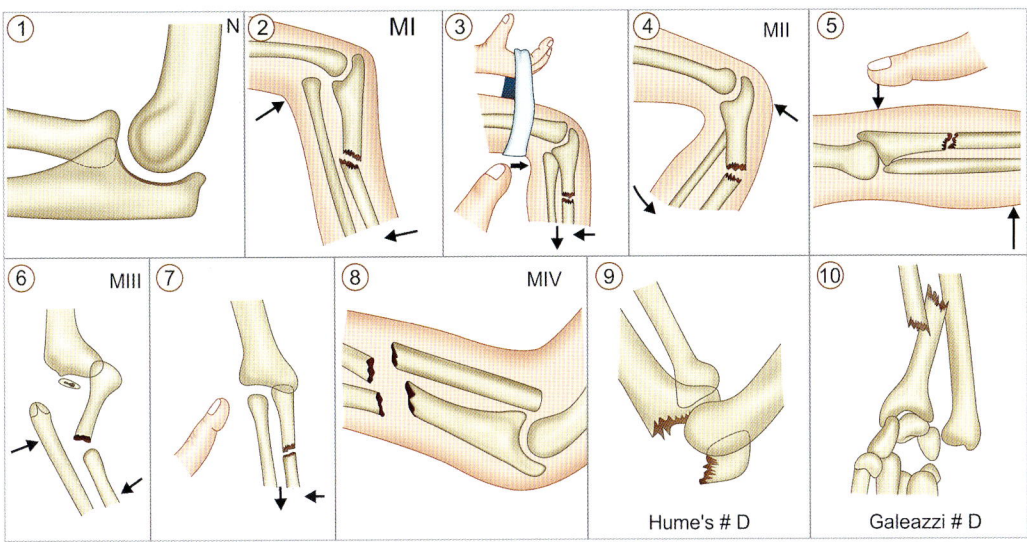

Fig. 5.43: Line sketch of four types of Monteggia fracture—dislocation with method of reduction. 1. N—normal; 2. MI—unreduced Monteggia type 1 fracture; 3. Method of reduction of –and –reduced Monteggia Type 1 fracture; 4. MII—Unreduced Monteggia Type II fracture; 5. Method of reduction– and – reduced Monteggia Type II fracture; 6. MIII—Unreduced Monteggia Type III fracture; 7. Method of reduction –and –reduced Monteggia Type III fracture; 8. MIV— Unreduced Monteggia Type IV fracture; 9. Hume's fracture; 10. Galeazzi fracture In Figures 3, 5 and 7 Figures—it has been shown where to press by thumb to reduce the fracture. (N: normal; MI: Monteggia Type I; MII: Monteggia Type II; MIII: Monteggia Type III; MIV: Monteggia Type IV)

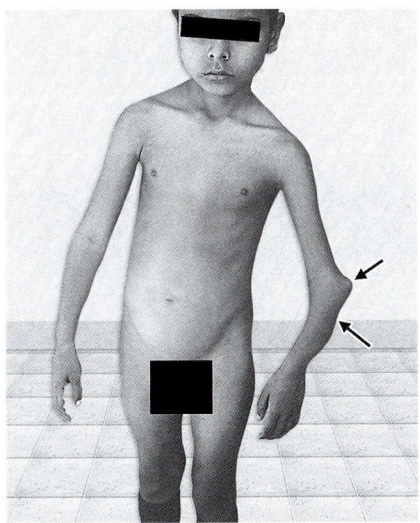

Fig. 5.44: Late presenting Monteggia fracture dislocation with unabated growth of dislocated radial head and malunited fracture of ulna. Excision of abnormally grown radial head should be done. Malunited fracture of ulna should improve by remodeling.

TABLE 5.4: Classification of Monteggia lesions (Monteggia fracture dislocations) (after Bado, Hume's 1967) (% is almost just approximate on our assessment).

Type I (Extension type) or Anterior type—60% of cases	Fracture in upper or middle third of ulna with anterior angulation	+ Anterior dislocation/ subluxation or radial head
Type II (Flexion type) or Posterior type—15% of cases	Fracture in upper or middle third of ulna with posterior angulation	+ Posterior or posterolateral dislocation/subluxation of radial head + Often a fracture of the head of radius
Type III or (Lateral type)—20% of cases	Fracture in upper or middle third of ulna (usually just distal to coronoid process	+ Lateral or anterolateral dislocation/ subluxation of radial head
Type IV —5% of cases	Fracture in upper or middle third of ulna with anterior angulation	+ Anterior dislocation of radial head + fracture in upper third of radius

- History of direct blows over ulnar aspect of the forearm or fall on pronated hand
- Rotational movements markedly restricted
- While rotating the forearm, a rounded bony mass moving under the fingers is felt either anterior, posterior or lateral to the normal radial head position, depending upon the type of Monteggia fracture dislocation
- Angulation, tenderness and swelling in the upper/middle third of the forearm mainly on ulnar side depending upon the site of fracture.

Fracture of the Lateral Condyle of Humerus
(Figs. 5.21, 5.34, 5.35 and 5.45)

Grades or degrees of lateral condylar fracture:
i. Fractured lateral condyle displaced laterally but not rotated
ii. Fractured lateral condyle displaced laterally and downward (with or without some rotation)

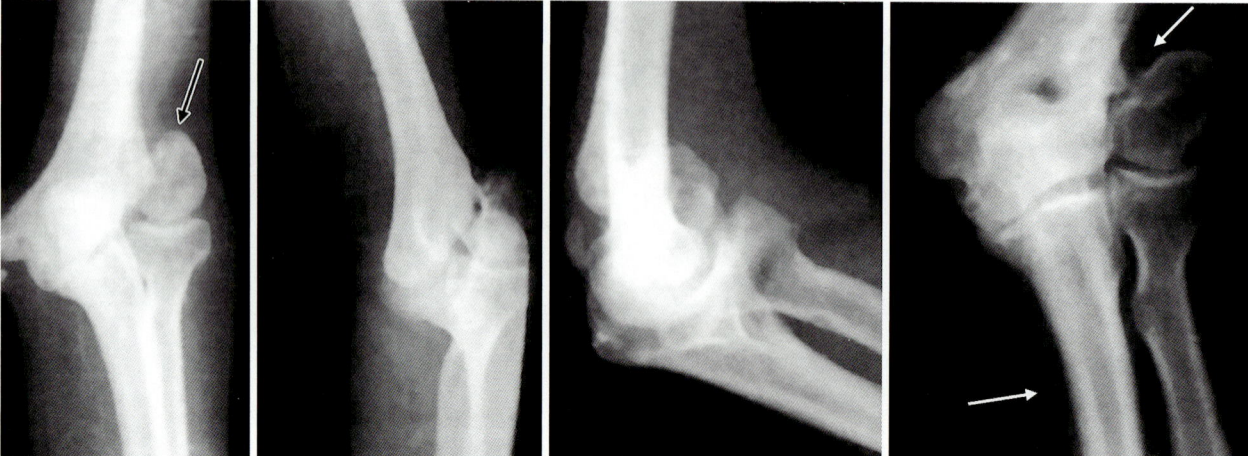

Fig. 5.45: X-ray pictures of old ununited fracture of lateral condyle of humerus with marked cubitus valgus deformity—May be treated with open reduction internal fixation and bone grafting-like bony peg. If ulnar nerve stretch is suspected/or present–anterior transposition of ulnar nerve or medical epicondylectomy will be required. Prognosis should be guarded.

iii. Fractured lateral condyle displaced and rotated around the horizontal and vertical axis. May be associated with dislocation of the elbow.
- More common between 5 and 10 years of age
- Tenderness and swelling localised to the lateral side of the lower humerus
- In Grade III—a globular, bony chunk is felt on the outer side of the elbow. In early cases, the outer rough surface can be felt, although later it gradually becomes smooth
- If neglected, it mostly goes for delayed or non-union, which leads to gradually increasing cubitus valgus (**Fig. 5.45**) with or without tardy (tardy = tarde = slow) ulnar nerve palsy. Ulnar nerve gets gradually stretched and undergoes repeated friction with extension and flexion movements of elbow leading to slow friction neuritis palsy.
- Mobility of the fragment can be demonstrated by the following method:

Method (Fig. 5.46): Hold the lower arm and elbow from the medial side in one hand while the elbow is kept flexed at 45° or at maximum possible angle (nearing 45°)in a relatively stiff elbow. With thumb and index finger of the other hand, hold the distal, displaced bony mass. In ununited fractures, this mass can be slightly moved over the parent bone.
- Medial supracondylar ridge is normal but lateral disturbed
- Movements at the elbow are fairly free, may be even complete in late cases
- Rotational motions limited to a variable extent
- In X-ray, this displaced mass appears quite small (in comparison to its clinically assessed size) because only the central ossified mass casts a shadow, the rest being cartilaginous.

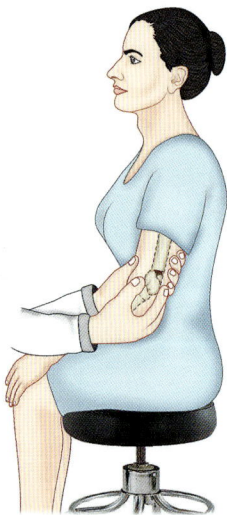

Fig. 5.46: Method of demonstrating mobility of the displaced fractured lateral condyle.

Fracture of Olecranon (Fig. 5.47)
- Common fracture in adults
- Bruises may be seen on the back of the elbow
- Irregular, tender surface of the olecranon, with or without a transverse gap. Since in most of the fractures, the olecranon process is avulsed—a transverse gap is felt at the upper end of the ulna. Patient has difficulty (even inability) in actively extending the elbow
- In late cases, triceps get contracted.

Non-traumatic

Tennis Elbow

Lateral epicondylitis (with lateral elbow pain), however, microscopic pathology noted in the degenerated tendon

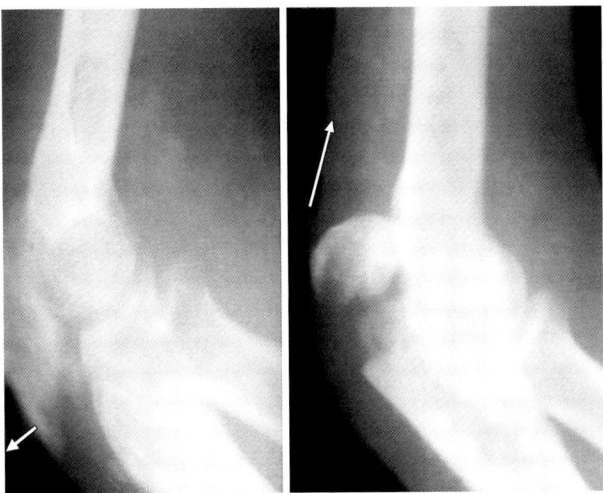

Fig. 5.47: Common varieties of fractures of olecranon (Left—oblique fracture through base; Right—transverse fracture—arrows showing direction of violence and displacement. Such fractures should be managed by open reduction and internal fixation by nail/plate.

(due to repetitive wrist extension against resistance) has been termed angiofibroblastic hyperplasia which denotes chronic tendinosis rather than acute inflammation. It is most frequently diagnosed musculoskeletal disorder in upper extremity with an incidence of 4 to 7 per 1000 per year.

- Common in ladies between 25 and 40 years of age; middle-aged athlete, e.g. game played with racket or bat
- Principal symptom is pain located at the lateral epicondyle of humerus and the common extensor origin and/or just distal to it. The pain quite often radiates distally over the extensor surface of the forearm and tends to worsen with the activities which require action of the extensor muscles
- The onset may be abrupt after an unaccustomed activity or gradual. The *course of the disease* is protracted with fluctuating symptoms
- Complains of pain in wringing movements of the forearm or lifting an object by gripping it in between the thumb and fingers or while getting up from a chair with the hands firmly pressing over the arm of the chair
- Tenderness is more or less around the lateral epicondyle
- Confirm by tests: Cozen's tests, Mill's manoeuvre, Jug test, etc.
- X-ray may demonstrate soft tissue calcifications or an exostosis from lateral epicondyle (exostosis) in about 25% of cases
- MRI may show increased signal in the musculotendinous structure at the lateral side of elbow.
- *Differential diagnosis:*
  - *Posterior interosseous nerve (PIN)* or radial tunnel syndrome (PIN syndrome caused by entrapment of PIN at the arcade of Frohse)—there is diffuse anterolateral elbow pain; maximum tenderness is at about 3–5 cm distal to the lateral epicondyle over the proximal radial forearm musculature
  - *Radio-capitellar articular disease*—patient has pain clicking with elbow movement. X-ray reveals degenerative changes at the radiocapitellar articulation.
- Treatment is mainly non-surgical that consists of NSAIDs with local analgesic application; physiotherapy (wrist extensor stretching and progressive resistance exercises); splinting; functional bracing; ultrasound; local corticosteroids PRP (with or without 2% xylocaine) infiltration into the common extensor origin and around; extracorporeal shock wave therapy (ESWT). Non-surgical treatment is successful in 85–90% of patients. If 3–6 months of non-surgical treatment fails and patient has severe pain, surgical treatment may be considered
- *Surgical treatment* consists of—Expose the origin of conjoint tendon; release its anterior and posterior edges; elevate it with underlying capsule; inspect the joint and articular cartilage; remove any loose body; debride the undersurface of tendon aponeurosis and lateral epicondyle, remove any prominent ridge of bone; irrigate the wound; reattach the tendon; close in layers; splint support for 2 weeks; passive and isometric exercises are begun at 3–4 weeks, resistive exercises by 6 weeks, full activities by 3–4 months.

Golfer's Elbow or Pitcher's Elbow or Little League Elbow Syndrome/Chronic Tension-Stress Injuries/ Medial Epicondylitis

- Common in young persons due to chronic tension stress injuries, e.g. baseball pitchers, javeline throwers, golfers, etc.
- Complains of pain in medial epicondylar region usually in valgus stress to the elbow in extension
- Significant local tenderness and mild swelling over the medial epicondylar region
- X-ray—chronic stress leads to density of the bone in the distal humerus; the physeal line (if present) is irregular and widened; the skeletal age of elbow appears greater than the patient's chronological age
- Clinical tests as given on Page 141 (*see* **Fig. 5.30**).
- Little league elbow can leave teenage pitchers with a permanent deformed arm, unless promptly and properly cared for.

Javelin Thrower's Elbow/Javelin Elbow

Miller published this entity in 1960: He observed that pain in the elbow in javelin throwers is a common complaint. "Javelin elbow" are of two types. The commonest type is caused by recurrent strain of the medial ligament usually in persons who use incorrect technique of throwing javelin. The symptoms cumulative by increase with throwing and decrease with rest. It can be treated with proper technique of throwing. However, residual symptoms are relieved by local injection of anesthetic agent with or without hydrocortisone acetate.

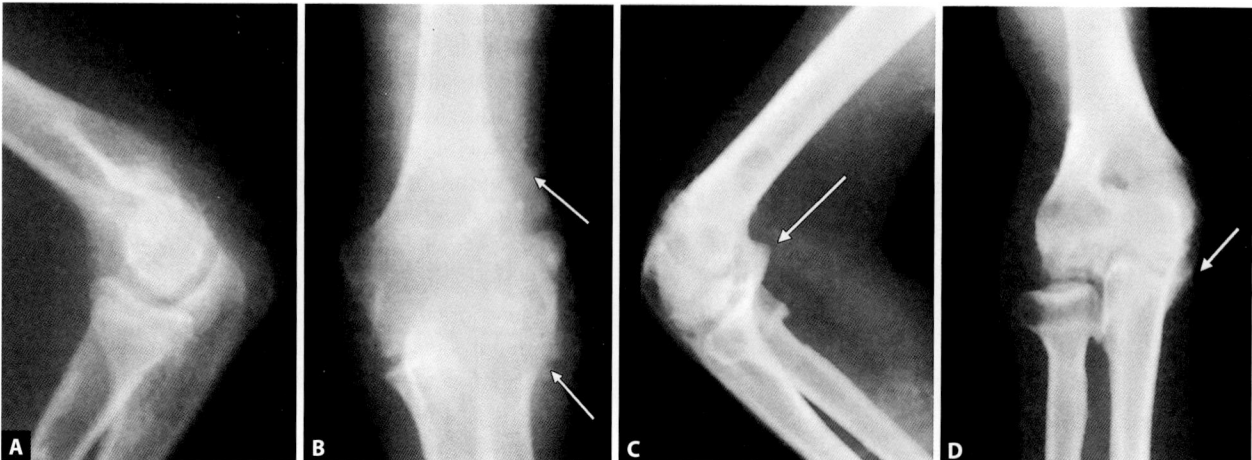

Figs. 5.48A to D: (A and B) Comparatively early tuberculous arthritis of elbow; (C and D) Advanced tuberculous arthritis of elbow Should be managed by excision of the diseased tissue, antituberculous chemotherapy, support to the joint, and guarded physiotherapy after about 6 weeks.

The second type of "Javelin elbow" occurs in expert throwers and is due to hyperextension of the elbow at the end throw, which produces an injury to the tip of olecranon. The symptoms, which may be disabling, appear even after a single throw or "malthrow", however, they resolve with rest, but may recur. The tip of olecranon may fracture, which should be removed for complete relief.

Tuberculosis of Elbow (Figs. 5.48A to D)

- Comparatively chronic history
- Forming about 2–5% of skeletal tuberculosis
- Slightly warm swelling around the elbow
- Typical tuberculous sinus
- Tenderness more at the joint line
- All movements are restricted
- Wasting of the muscles of the arm and forearm
- Flexion deformity to a varying extent
- May be fluctuant collection anywhere in relation to the elbow—usually anteriorly or a little below the elbow, even in the forearm, depending on the site of cold abscess
- Bony tenderness according to the site of primary focus i.e. usually the olecranon region, radial head, trochlear and capitular regions
- Regional lymph nodes enlarged with or without matting and tenderness
- May be evidence of active or healed tuberculosis lesion in lung.
- Management (as in any osteo-articular tuberculosis) consists of – Rest to elbow in plaster (or other) support, anti-tuberculous chemotherapy, excision of diseased tissue and gradual resumption of possible movements.

Rheumatoid Arthritis Affecting Elbow

- Rheumatoid arthritis is a chronic progressive polyarthritis affecting about 0.75% of the population.

About 70% of these patients can develop erosions in the joint and disabilities. Rheumatoid arthritis patients are on the average underweight

- Chronic history, with remissions and exacerbations
- Usually affects ladies in their 3rd and 4th decades
- Other joints, specially smaller joints of hands, wrist and foot involvement (but very rarely the distal interphalangeal joints). Joints involvement is usually bilateral
- Swelling/affection of three or more specified joints
- Flexion deformity of elbow to varying extent
- Decreased triceps skin fold thickness
- Varying restriction of movements
- Significant reduction in upper arm muscle circumference
- Mild swelling all around the elbow
- As the disease advances, ankylosis (usually fibrous—in late cases may be osseous)
- Associated with different typical rheumatoid deformities, especially in hand, wrist and foot
- Subcutaneous rheumatic nodules over the olecranon
- Repeated olecranon bursitis (*see* **Fig. 5.9**)
- Rheumatoid cachexia has been reported in patients with elevated serum levels of tumour necrosis factor-Q (TNF-Q)
- X-ray changes—periarticular osteopenia or erosion.

Septic Arthritis of the Elbow (Figs. 5.49 and 5.54)

- In young children
- Usually with other septic foci in the body
- Acute onset
- Constitutional features present
- Varying swelling depending upon collection in the joint
- Acute inflammatory features in the elbow
- Gross limitation of movements in all directions (due to pain)

Elbow Joints

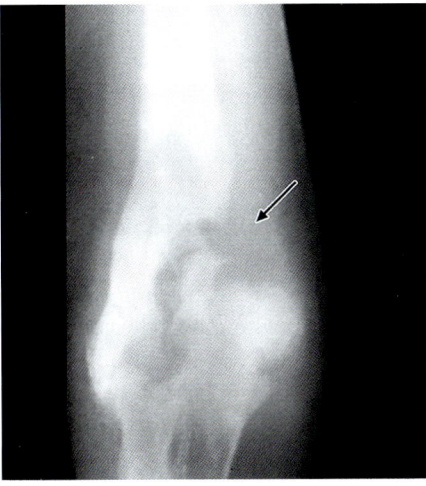

Fig. 5.49: Sequelae of chronic septic arthritis of elbow.

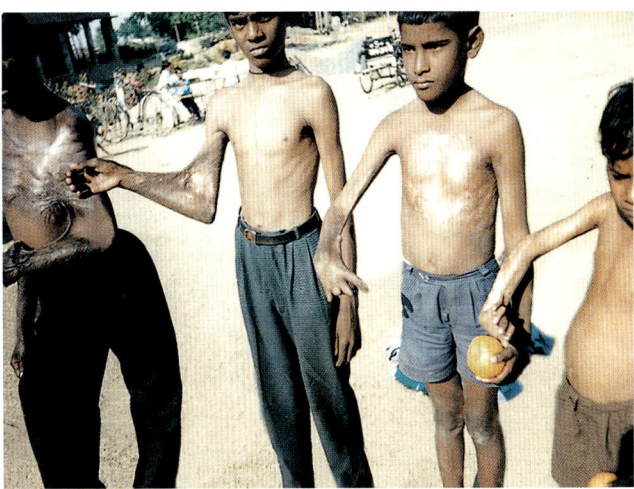

Fig. 5.52: Post-burn contracture of the elbow and allied region—elbow is the common site for such contractures after burn.

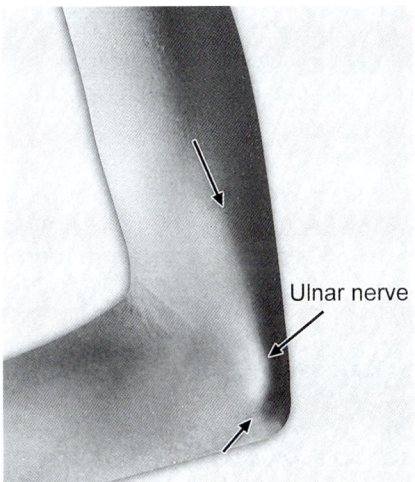

Fig. 5.50: Thickened ulnar nerve subluxating on flexing the elbow.

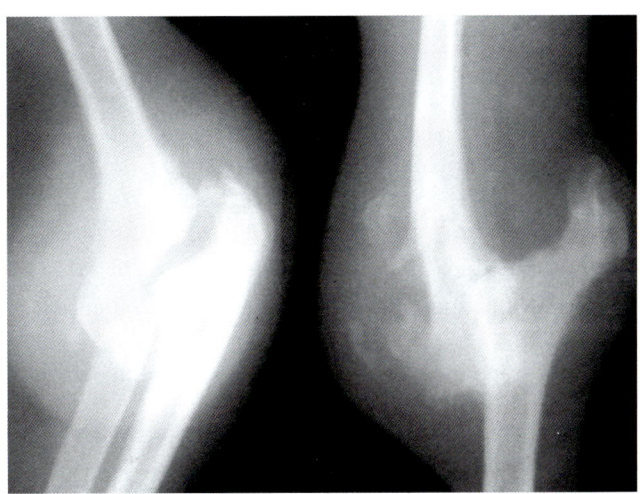

Fig. 5.53: Charcot arthropathy elbow.

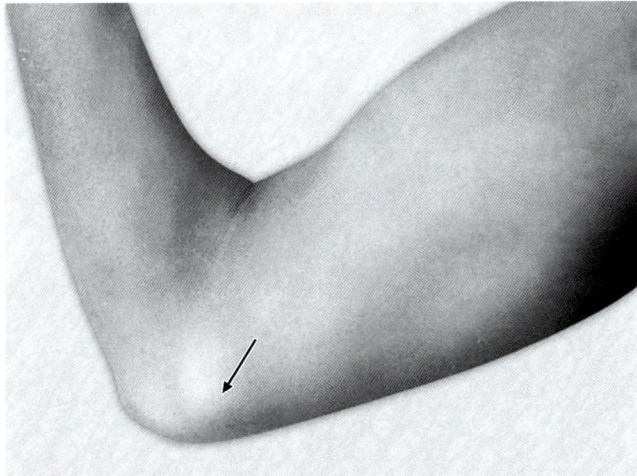

Fig. 5.51: Cold abscess in ulnar nerve in leprosy.

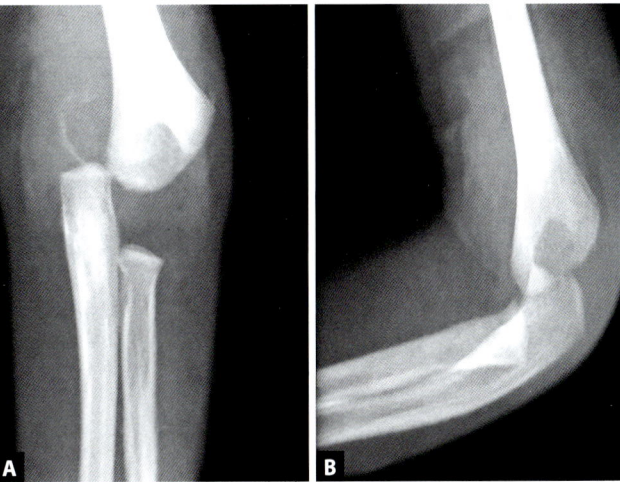

Figs. 5.54A and B: Pathological dislocation of elbow following septic arthritis of elbow along with osteomyelitis of ulna, radius and humerus in a child.

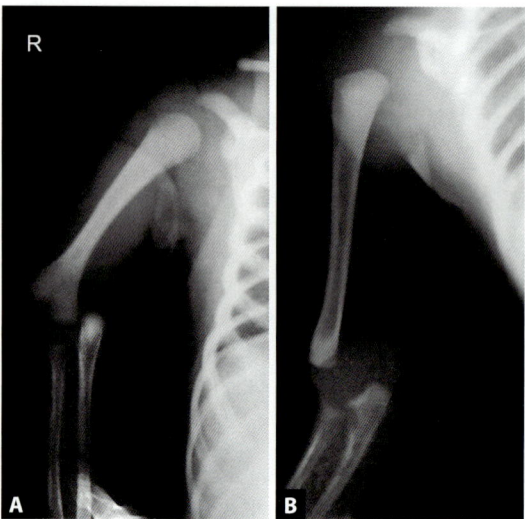

Figs. 5.55A and B: Congenital dislocation of elbow in an infant Should be managed by open reduction and intramedullary fixation for 6–8 week by k-wire to secure the reduction followed by physiotherapy.

- Aspiration of frank thick pus clinches the diagnosis. The aspirate must be sent for culture and chemosensitivity
- Regional lymph nodes enlarged, and tender.

Post-viral Arthritis (Refer Fig. 3.11) Affecting Elbow

- It was a legacy following smallpox
- Usually bilateral, more or less symmetrical affection of the elbow
- Acute stage usually corresponds to the scaling stage of smallpox
- In late stage—painless, ankylosed elbow or with gross limitation of functional movements, like old septic arthritis.

Olecranon Bursitis (see Figs. 5.5 and 5.9) (Students Elbow; Miner's Elbow)

- Olecranon bursitis is the inflammation (mostly chronic or subacute) of the bursa overlying the olecranon process and is caused by repetitive minor trauma or even acute trauma of the bursa or infection of bursa, or in gout
- It presents as a chronic soft/fluctuant swelling with variable pain and/or tenderness and limitation of movements
- True arthritis of elbow may be confused with it, however, rotation of forearm with elbow flexed at 90° will be free in olecranon bursitis whereas in true arthritis rotational movements will be painfully limited
- In olecranon bursitis, fullness will be over the tip of olecranon, whereas synovitis usually distends the normal sulcus of the ulnar groove
- Full extension is limited in arthritis, but not in olecranon bursitis
- Aspiration (usually thin/thick clear serous fluid) followed by infiltration of steroid usually clears the problem. If the aspirated fluid is cloudy, it must be sent for culture. Recurred/persistent problem needs surgical excision.

■ BIBLIOGRAPHY

1. Bado JL. The Monteggia lesion. Clin Orthopaedics. 1967; 50:71.
2. Laurence W. Supracondylar fractures of the humerus in children, a review of 100 cases. Br J of Surg. 1956;44:143.
3. Miller JE. Javelin thrower's elbow. J Bone Joint Surg. 1960; 788-92.
4. Takahara M, Shundo M, Kondo M, et al. Early detection of osteochondritis dissecans of capitellum in young baseball players. J Bone Joint Surg. 1998;80A:892-7.
5. Watson-Jones R. Primary nerve lesions in injuries of the elbow and wrist. J of Bone and Joint Surg. 1930;12:121.

CHAPTER 6

Wrist Joints

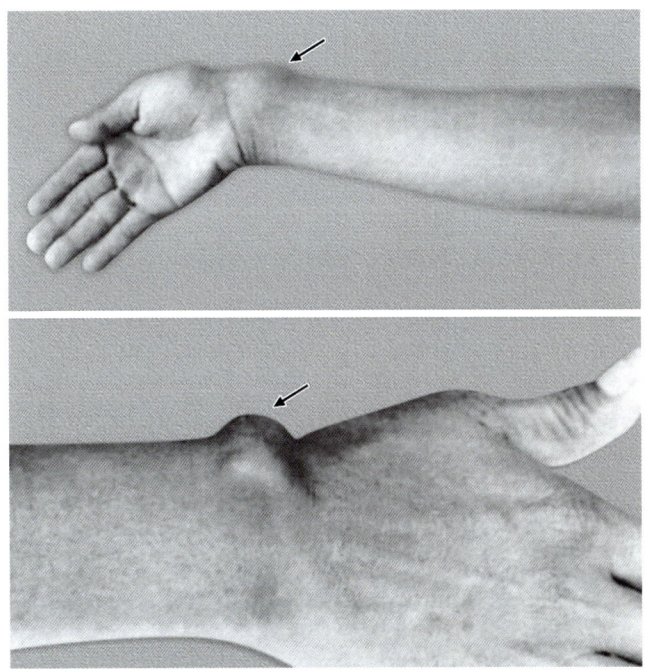

"Everyone thinks of changing the world, but no one thinks of changing himself."
—***Leo Tolstoy***
"Worry is like any other disease that attacks the weak and the confused."
—***PP Wangchuk***

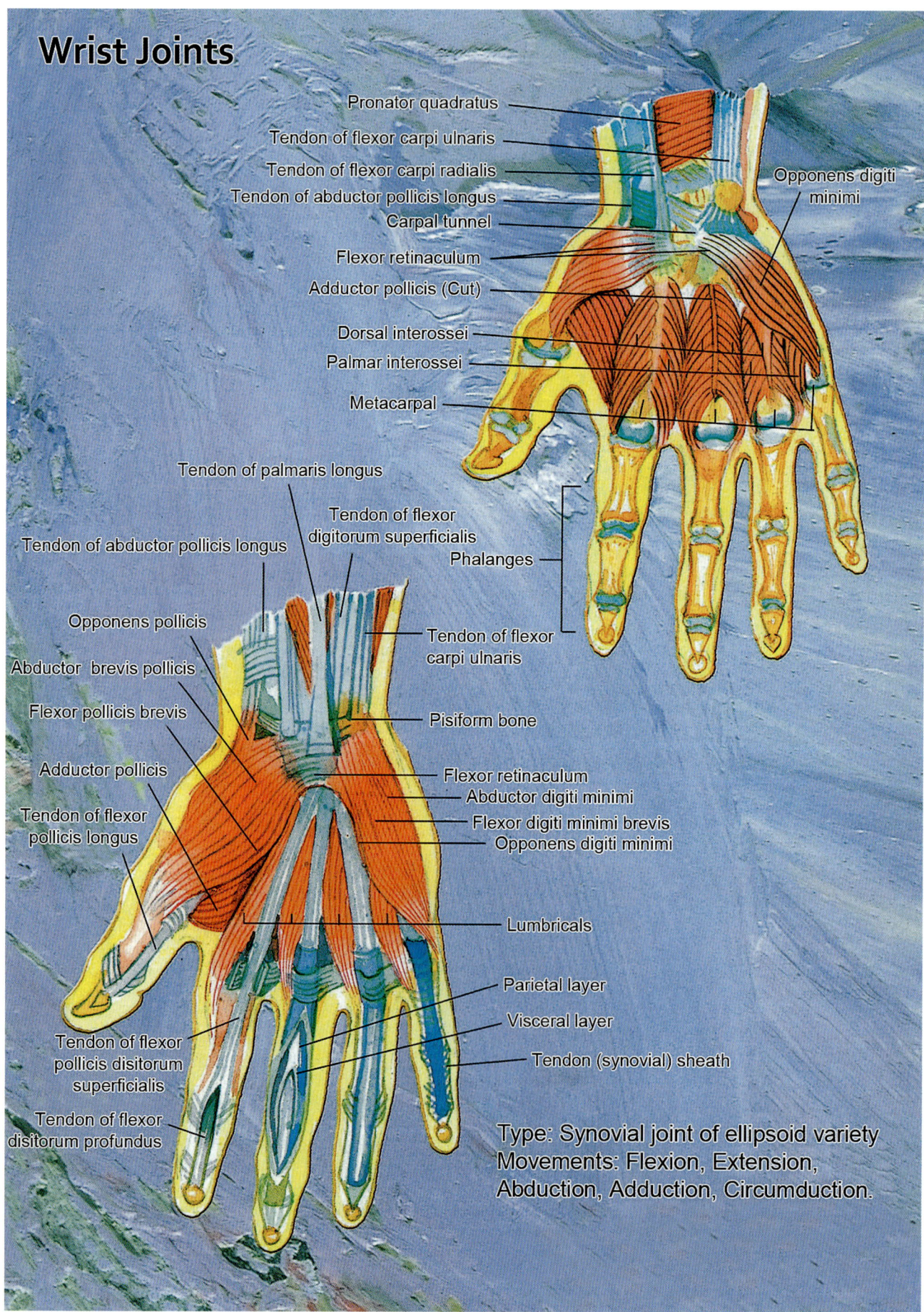

INTRODUCTION

The movements at the wrist are mainly oriented to facilitate the grip and finer movements of the hand.

For all practical purposes, in clinical assessment the local examination of the wrist, which lies in between the forearm and the hand, must include them.

ANATOMICAL CONSIDERATION

For practical considerations, the wrist should include the distal radioulnar, radiocarpal and ulnocarpal joints along with eight carpal bones and their proximal and distal articulations.

The *wrist joint proper is the articulation of the lower articular end* (concave in anteroposterior as well as lateral directions) *of the radius and the inferior surface of the triangular fibrocartilage* (extending from the medial margin of the lower end of the radius to a pit on the lateral surface of ulnar styloid process above its tip, i.e. from the rim of the sigmoid notch of radius to the ulnar styloid process) *at the proximal end.* The distal convex articulating surface consists of the curving sides of three carpal bones of the proximal row, the navicular, lunate and triquetrum (from radial to ulnar side). Since the pisiform lies on the palmar aspect of triquetrum, it is excluded from the articulation and it can be palpated as a bony prominence on the ulnar side of proximal palm, just distal to the prominent palmar crease and proximal to the base of hypothenar eminence. The intercarpal articulations *(carpals arranged in two rows in first row scaphoid, lunate, triquetrum and pisiform and in second row trapezium, trapezoid, capitate, and hamate)* participate in all movements of the wrist joint. Occasionally (about in 2%) accessory carpel bones are present – like commonly present "os centrale" amidst trapezoid, capitate and scaphoid (Gray 2008).

The synovial reflections of the wrist and the intercarpal joints are intercommunicating. As around the ankle, the wrist also has important hand-fingers-thumb controlling tendons around it, but for a difference that on the palmar aspect, just above the wrist level, the stamp-like stout pronator quadratus muscle binds the lower ends of the radius and ulna.

The lower ends of the radius and ulna articulate as a pivot joint to form the inferior radioulnar joint. Which is anatomically a diarthrodial synovial joint consisting of two parts – The bony radioulnar articulation and soft tissue stabilizers (Hagert 2010). Here, the lower end of the radius along with the triangular fibrocartilage revolves around the head of ulna. This synovial joint has its continuity with the wrist joint, therefore, this joint is likely to be affected simultaneously in all affections of the wrist proper.

The *articular surface of the distal aspect of radius* tilts 21° in the anteroposterior plane and 5–11° in the lateral plane.

The scaphoid, trapezium, first metacarpal, and thumb phalanges function conjointly as an independent unit—like 'a jointed strut'. The joints of this strut are vulnerable to degenerative arthrosis.

The dorsal cortical surface of the radius thickens to form the Lister tubercle and osseous prominences which support the extensors of the wrist in the second dorsal compartment.

On the dorsal aspect of the wrist, just beneath the extensor retinaculum (more or less blended with the dorsal capsule of the wrist joint) the following tendons are arranged in a definite order. *There are six fibro-osseous compartments lodging the following tendons* (from dorso-lateral to dorso-medial direction) **(Fig. 6.1)**.

- First compartment—Abductor pollicis longus and extensor pollicis brevis;
- Second compartment—Extensor carpi radialis longus and extensor carpi radialis brevis;
- Third compartment—Extensor pollicis longus;
- Fourth compartment—Extensor indicis and extensor digitorum;
- Fifth compartment—Extensor digiti minimi;
- Sixth compartment—Extensor carpi ulnaris.

In the fourth compartment, deep to the tendons, the posterior interosseous nerve ends as a pseudoganglion and the anterior interosseous artery ends anastomosing with the fine local articular arteries. Each compartment has a double blind ending synovial sheath around the tendon. Proximally, the sheaths extend to a variable extent and distally they end beyond the retinacular extension.

On the palmar aspect, however, none of the tendons are directly bound to the wrist surface (as on the dorsal surface) because of: (i) intervention by pronator quadratus, (ii) concave surface of the lower end of radius, and (iii) lack of separate fibro-osseous compartments which would prevent the tendons from bowstringing during flexion.

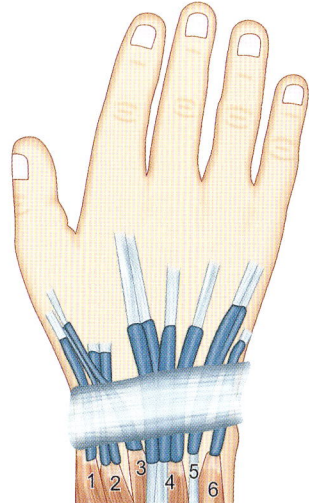

Fig. 6.1: Showing the fibro-osseous compartments on the dorsal aspect of the wrist with their contents: 1. Abductor pollicis longus and extensor pollicis brevis; 2. Extensor carpi radialis longus and brevis, 3. Extensor pollicis longus; 4. Extensor indicis, extensor digitorum, anterior interosseous artery ending and posterior interosseous nerve ending in pseudoganglion; 5. Extensor digiti minimi; 6. Extensor carpi ulnaris.

However, four tendons can be palpated and even seen, when the fingers are slightly flexed and muscles on flexor side are made tense. Three tendons (from ulnar to radial side)—flexor carpi ulnaris, palmaris longus and flexor carpi radialis—are apparently prominent in most of the person (*see* Fig. 6.42). When the fist is clenched firmly, the tendon of flexor digitorum sublimis also gets prominent between the tendons of flexor carpi ulnaris and palmaris longus.

Of the nerves, the median nerve is in closer relation to the wrist than the ulnar. The median nerve lies in between the tendons of the flexor carpi radialis and flexor digitorum sublimis and on the posterolateral aspect of the palmaris longus tendon. This nerve is likely to suffer with any encroachment of the space in between the flexor retinaculum and the wrist joint, i.e. the carpal tunnel. Normally, *carpal tunnel contains the median nerve and nine flexor tendons*— the four sublimis, four profundus and the flexor pollicis longus tendons.

The ulnar nerve becomes superficial at the wrist level. At about 5 cm above the wrist joint proper, after sending a dorsal cutaneous twig, it passes in front of the flexor retinaculum on the lateral side of the pisiform bone and posterolateral to the musculotendinous mass of the flexor carpi ulnaris where it divides into a superficial and a deep branch. The deep branch continues under cover of the hook of the hamate into the palm **(Guyon's canal)**. Guyon's canal is triangular and lies immediately ulnar to the carpal tunnel in the wrist region. Ulnar nerve and artery traverse the canal, which may be site of ulnar nerve entrapment.

The radial nerve more or less divides into 4 or 5 dorsal digital branches at about the wrist level. Clinically, it is not of much importance, as its cutaneous supply is ultimately limited to a stamp-shaped area on the back of the first web.

The creases around the wrist run almost circumferentially. The radial artery lies quite superficial on the anterolateral aspect of the lower forearm and wrist and it is not likely to be affected in common wrist affections, except for infiltrative neoplasms, glass pan cut and suicidal injuries.

The dorsal or Lister's tubercle lies on the dorsum of the lower end of the radius just lateral and proximal to the central point of the wrist. It provides a pulley-like surface on its medial aspect for the extensor pollicis longus tendon. This tendon, by passing a circuitous route around this tubercle becomes more effective in subserving its important function of extension of the thumb. On the other hand, this tendon, lying in such a close proximity to the bony tubercle, is likely to be affected in any roughness in this area (e.g. rupture of this tendon in Colles fracture).

When the thumb is actively extended firmly, a recess, bounded by the tendons of extensor pollicis longus on the ulnar side and abductor pollicis longus and extensor pollicis brevis on the radial side, becomes obvious at the dorsolateral aspect of root of thumb—it is the *anatomical snuff box.*

Fracture separation of the lower radial epiphysis (cf. Colles fracture in adult) is a very *common injury around the wrist in children.* Due to seen or unseen damage of the growth plate, it may lead to various deformities in this region **(Fig. 6.13)**.

■ METHODOLOGY

History Taking

In history taking, besides the usual points as mentioned in the Chapter 1, in case of wrist and hand (rather upper limb), the hand dominance, occupation and current work status should also be noted.

In case of trauma, ask about the mode of injury and the part of the limb which first bore the impact of violence. Usually, the wrist is involved in indirect injuries, seldom by direct violence.

General and Systemic Examinations

(*See* the Chapter 1 'Introduction')

Regional Examination

It includes overall assessment of the forelimb of the affected side with its connections to the central axis, both anatomically and neurologically. It is obligatory to examine the cervical spine, supraclavicular region, shoulder girdle, supracondylar region, elbow, forearm and up to the tip of the fingers while assessing the wrist joint.

Local Examination

Prerequisites

Both wrists must be fully exposed and examined simultaneously keeping them in identical position as far as possible, while the patient sits comfortably on a stool.

Attitude

Note any fixed attitude of the wrist and hand **(Figs. 6.2 to 6.14)**. Certain typical attitudes are significant, e.g. dinner fork deformity (or silver fork deformity) of Colles fracture; congenital manus valgus of Madelung's deformity (forward and ulnar curving of lower end of radius due to growth disturbance at the ulnar-palmar aspect of distal radial physis)—**(Otto Madelung, 1878—Figs. 6.7 and 6.8)**, arrow head deformity in diaphyseal aclasis (usually seen in X-ray **(Fig. 6.6)**, flexion and ulnar/radial deviation of the wrist and ulnar deviation of the fingers in rheumatoid arthritis; hourglass swelling on the palmar aspect both above and below the flexor retinaculum in compound palmar ganglion **(Figs. 6.15 and 6.16)**; wrist drop **(Figs. 16.19 and 16.20)** in radial nerve palsy. In established severe Volkmann's ischaemic contracture (*see* Fig. 5.23), there is a striking flexion contracture of the wrist and fingers due to the shortening of the fibrotic forearm flexor muscles. The post-burn contractures **(Fig. 6.2)** vary according to contracted structure.

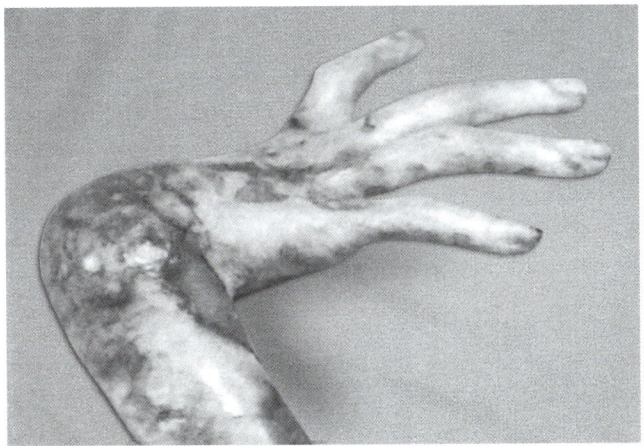

Fig. 6.2: Post-burn contracture of wrist.

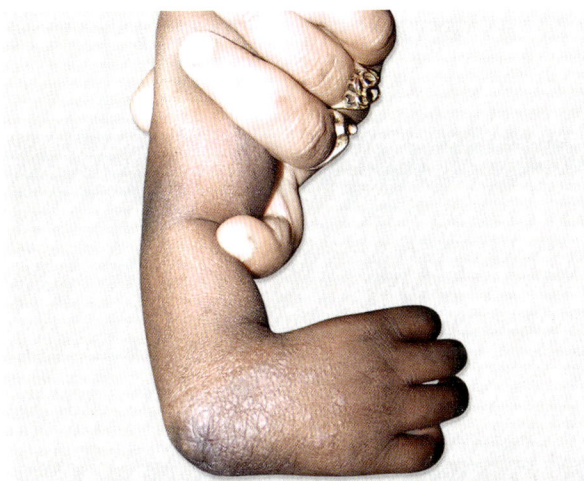

Fig. 6.3: Congenital disorganised wrist and hand.

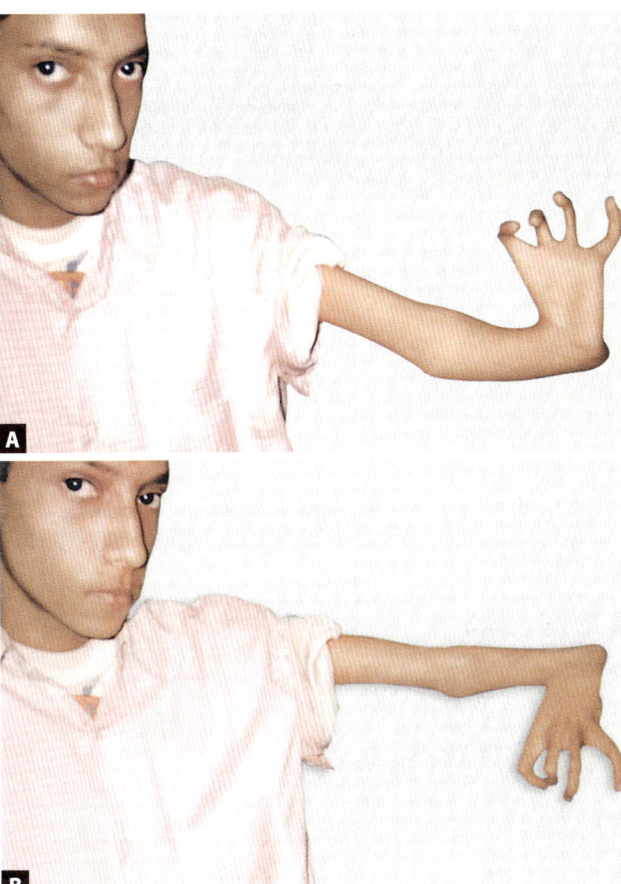

Figs. 6.5A and B: Congenital club hand with absence of radial ray. Such cases (including congenital absence of radius) can be managed by radialization of ulna, shortening of ulna (which corrects the deformity) and centralization of carpus over the digital end of ulna. These all can be done in one stage and usually provide well acceptable satisfactory result–both functional and cosmetic.

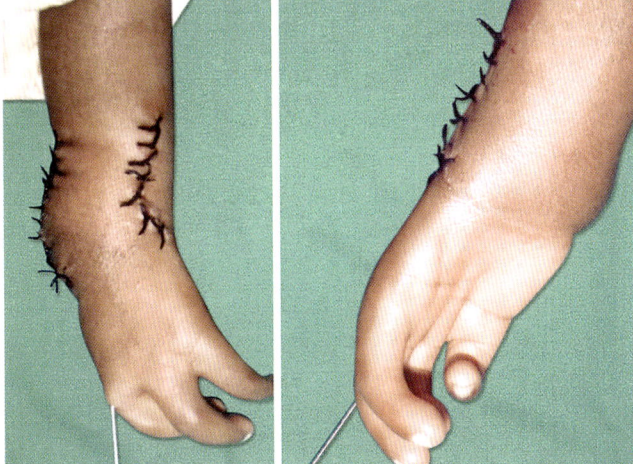

Fig. 6.4: Early post-corrective picture of the same patient (**Fig. 6.3**).

Inspection

Inspect both wrists (for comparison) in symmetrical position from the sides, dorsal and palmar aspects for asymmetry, swelling, tenderness, deformities.

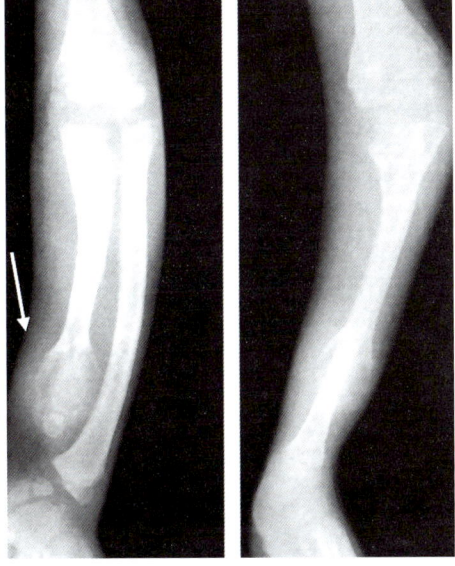

Fig. 6.6: Arrow head deformity of ulna in diaphyseal aclasis.

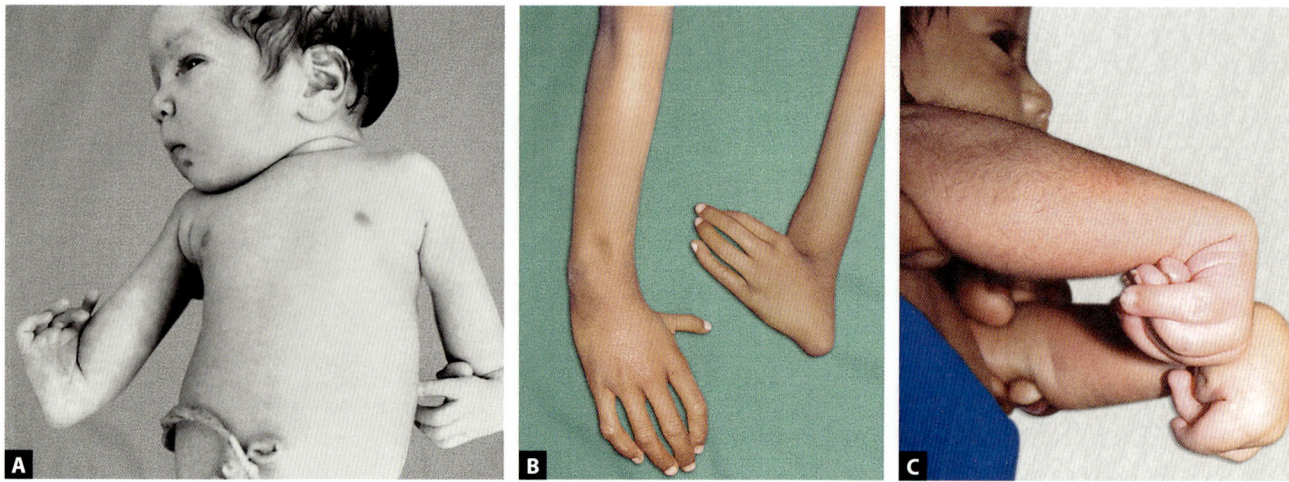

Figs. 6.7A to C: (A) Bilateral congenital Madelung's deformity (congenital subluxation of wrist); (B) Congenital solid left upper limb with Madelung's wrist on the left and mild manus valgus on the right; (C) Bilateral congenital flexion contracture of wrist, fingers and thumbs in palm deformity.

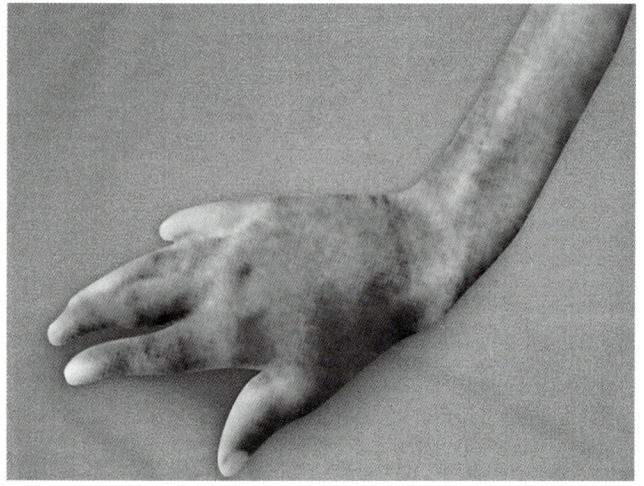

Fig. 6.8: Photograph of deformity due to osteochondroma of lower end of radius.

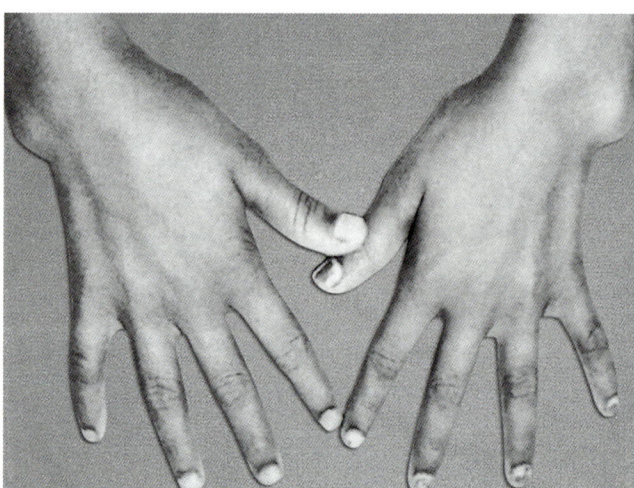

Fig. 6.10: Madelung's deformity.

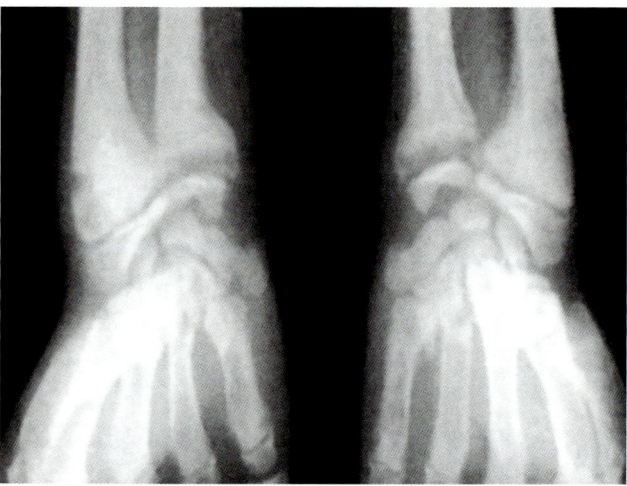

Fig. 6.9: Osteonecrosis in both wrist and hand regions.

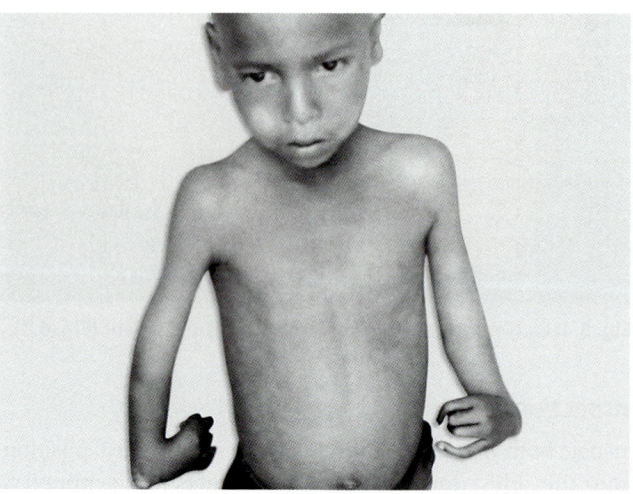

Fig. 6.11: Bilateral club hand.

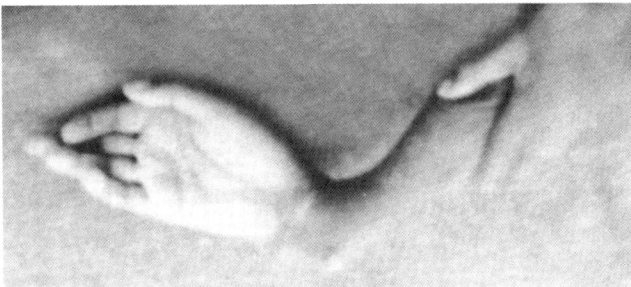

Fig. 6.12: Old epiphyseal injury of lower end of radius leading to premature closure of growth epiphysis and overgrowth of ulna.

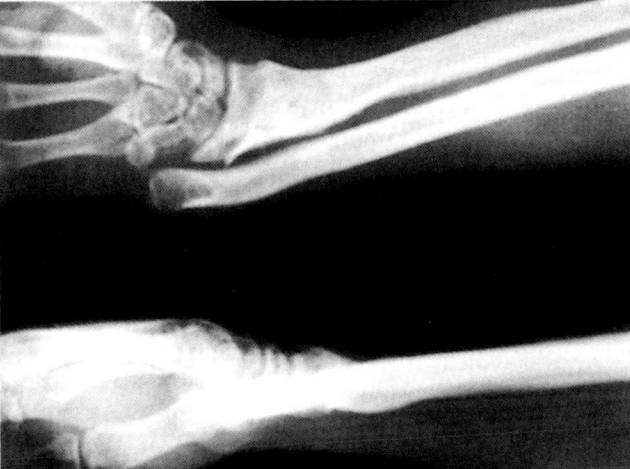

Fig. 6.13: Old epiphyseal injury of lower end of radius—premature closure of growth epiphysis and overgrowth of ulna.

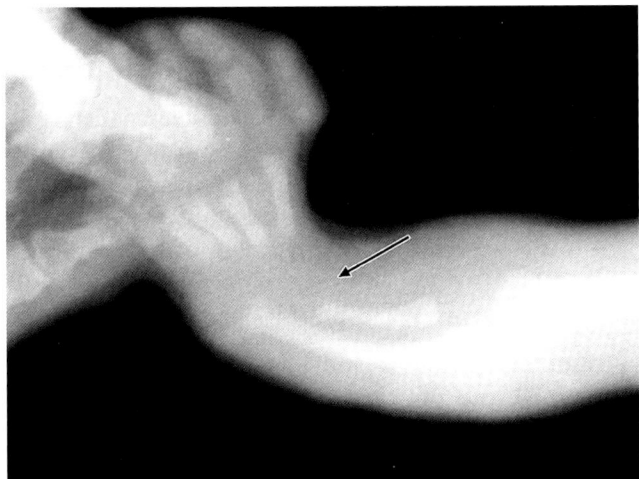

Fig. 6.14: Congenitally deficient distal radius with overgrowth of ulna and supernumerary finger.

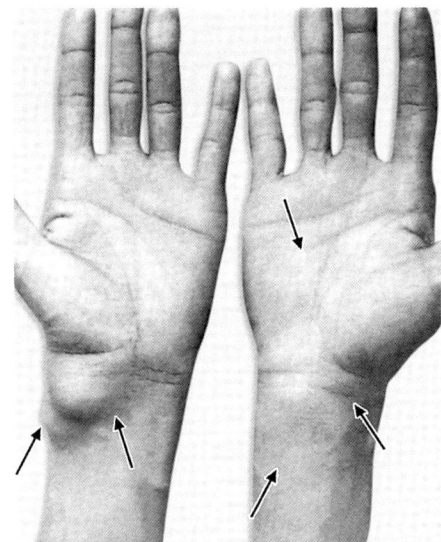

Fig. 6.15: Compound palmar ganglion on the right side and (simple) ganglion on the left side.

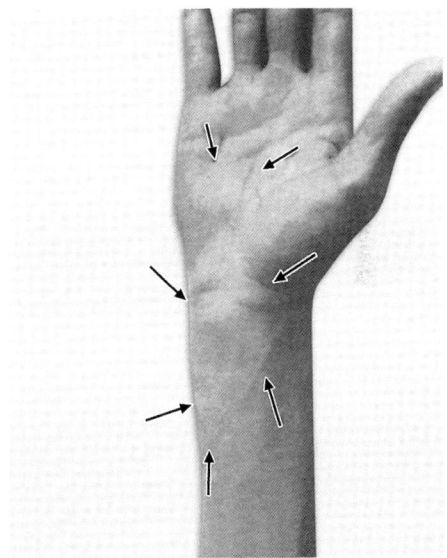

Fig. 6.16: Compound palmar ganglion more marked in oblique position of the wrist.

On the dorsal aspect: Note the normal bony and soft tissue points in systematic order, while the fingers are opened up and the patient attempts to make a fist. Look at the contour of the region, any swelling, skin condition, venous prominence, ulnar styloid prominence, creases around the joint, any swelling in relation to any tendon or the wrist joint [e.g. ganglion **(Figs. 6.15, 6.26A and B)**] and back of the forearm, any sinus, and skin contractures.

On the radial side: Ask the patient to extend the thumb and inspect the *snuffbox* (bounded by abductor pollicis longus and extensor pollicis brevis on the radial side, and extensor pollicis longus on the ulnar side) for any fullness. Note any abnormal prominence on this side of the lower radius—a typical site for de Quervain's disease **(Fig. 6.19)** and giant cell tumour **(Fig. 6.20)**.

On the palmar aspect: Look for the skin creases in relation to thenar and hypothenar eminences and at the wrist level, and note any abnormal finding—e.g. swelling, sinus, atrophy,

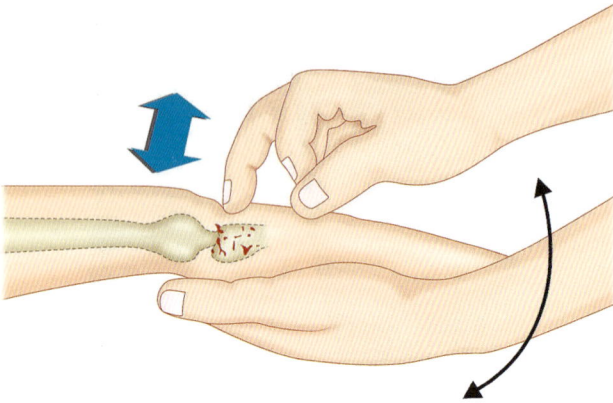

Fig. 6.17: Localisation of wrist joint line.

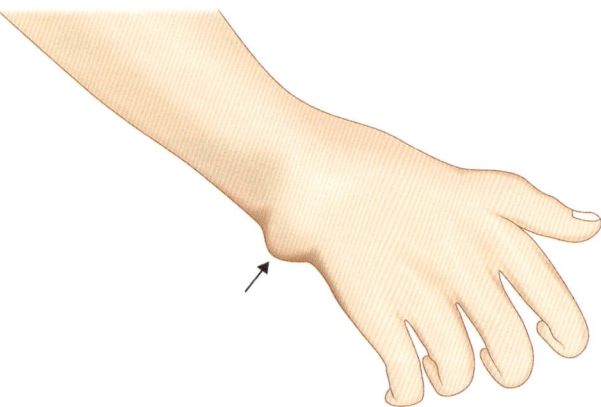

Fig. 6.18: Septic arthritis wrist with collection of pus projecting below the ulnar styloid process.

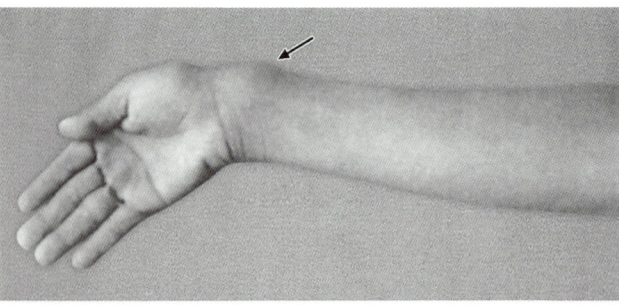

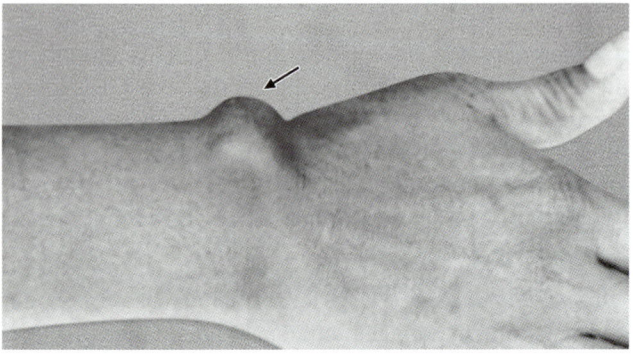

Fig. 6.19: Photographs of de Quervain's disease.

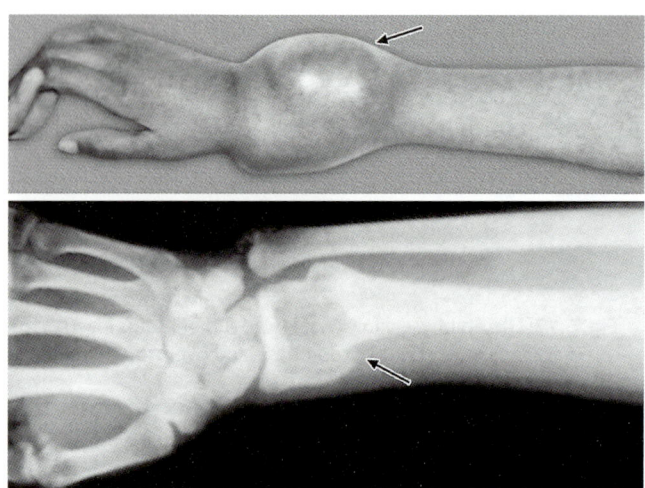

Fig. 6.20: Giant cell tumour from lower end of radius with pathological fracture.

hypertrophy, discolouration (in cervical rib syndrome), fullness in the lower forearm [compound palmar ganglion **(Figs. 6.15 and 6.16)** or Parona's space affections].

On the ulnar side: Look for the hypothenar eminence and muscular bulge of the lower forearm above the wrist. Most of the affections of the wrist, specially injuries, are associated with swelling of the hand components.

Palpation

Superficial palpation: Note the temperature, condition of the skin, any hyper- or hypoanaesthesia, any bony projection, or any other abnormal feature. Note the radial pulse with any variation, if present.

Deep palpation: Certain normal relations must be confirmed before searching for any abnormal findings. Localise the tips of the ulnar and radial styloid processes. Note their levels and compare with the other side. Normally, the tip of radial styloid process lies about 1 cm distal to that of ulnar styloid process.

Method of palpating the styloid processes **(Fig. 6.21)** with the patient's forearm pronated and the wrist in as much neutral a position as possible, support the palm in one hand. Put the thumb and index fingertips of the opposite hand on the two sides of the wrist from the dorsal aspect. In case of the right hand of the patient your right index fingertip should be in the snuffbox and the thumb tip should be distal to the head of the ulna. Gently squeeze within and at the same time shift your fingertips proximally. The pointed bony projections will be felt (the tips of the radial and ulnar styloid processes). Reverse the position of your thumb and index finger for the patient's left hand.

Method to localise the joint line on the dorsum of the wrist **(Fig. 6.17)** Support the patient's wrist on your one hand and put the tip of the index or middle finger of the opposite hand

Non-traumatic

- Diffuse swelling (soft to cystic):
  - Tuberculosis **(Figs. 6.22 and 6.23)**
  - Rheumatoid arthritis (Refer **Figs. 7.36 to 7.38**)
  - Septic arthritis (*see* **Fig. 6.18**).
- Localised swellings (either communicating with wrist joint or in relation to any tendon sheath).
  - Ganglion—round, tense, tender cystic swelling containing clear gelatinous fluid usually on dorsal, radial-palmar and ulnar-palmar aspects of the wrist **(Figs. 6.26A to C)**
  - de Quervain's disease—a firm tender swelling about 1.5 cm proximal to the radial styloid process **(Fig. 6.19)**
  - Giant cell tumour—expanded soft to bony hard swelling from lower outer aspect of the radius **(Fig. 6.20)**
  - Compound palmar ganglion—diffuse bulge above and below the flexor retinaculum (*see* **Figs. 6.15 and 6.16**).

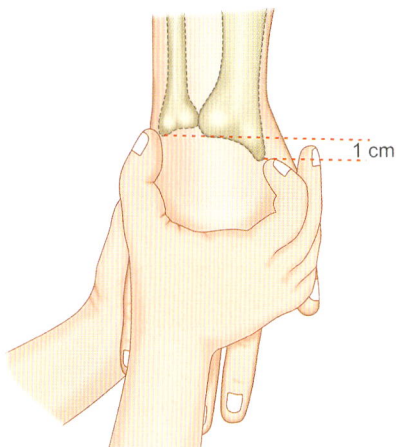

Fig. 6.21: Palpating the tips of radial and ulnar styloid processes.

Egg-Shell Crackling

The lower end of the radius is a common site for giant cell tumour. One of its cardinal clinical sign is egg-shell crackling, which is tested by the method of palpation. However, palpation to demonstrate egg-shell crackling should be avoided, since it may break the thinned out cortex through which the tumour tissue can leak out in the surroundings.

Step Sign

In case of injury, note for the step sign **(Figs. 6.27A to C)**. Pass down your index finger on the outer aspect of the forearm over the rounded radial shaft. In case of outer shift of the lower fractured fragment, your finger will suddenly step over the hard underlying structure. This 'stepping' can be felt in similar circumstances on the dorsal aspect too. This 'step sign' is of special importance in ascertaining the shift in *Colles* (posterior stepping up) and *Smith's* or *reverse Colles fractures* (posterior stepping down).

Palpation of the Snuffbox

Snuffbox lies just distal to the radial styloid process. Its radial border is formed by the abductor pollicis longus and extensor pollicis brevis tendons and ulnar border by the extensor pollicis longus tendon. The floor of snuffbox is the scaphoid bone.

Palpate carefully the snuffbox, specially in case of fall on outstretched hand. Ask the patient to extend and abduct the thumb as far as possible (thumb up position). Supporting the wrist from the ulnar side in one hand, press deeply at the floor of the snuffbox, in between the prominent tendons, and note for tenderness which usually occurs in scaphoid

in about the centre of the inter-styloid line. You will feel a gap. Confirm by gently dorsiflexing and palmar-flexing the wrist as far as practicable, the gap will slightly close and open up accordingly. Extend the fingertips along the inter-styloid line while gently moving the wrist joint, and you will assess the wrist joint line. Now, palpate for the presence of any abnormal finding, specially those which you have seen on inspection.

Bony components: Note for any bony irregularities at the lower end and posterolateral surface of the radius and the lower end of the ulna. Any abnormal swelling or bony prominence in front of the wrist should be palpated for its temperature, tenderness, size, shape, texture, consistency, relation to deeper structures and mobility.

Assessment of Instability of Distal Radioulnar Joint

Several patients present with the symptoms of instability of distal radioulnar joint even symptoms after distal radial fractures have healed. They complain of pain and abnormal motion on the ulnar side of the wrist and sometimes feeling of wrist "out of joint" in certain position, which may need manual reduction. Crepitus or clicking may be felt on rotating the forearm. *Ballottement of distal radioulnar* joint should be performed as follows:

Support the front of wrist region on one hand, and with your another thumb press over the ulnar head pushing it anteriorly and release the pressure—the ulnar head will recoil back. Note the anteroposterior excursion range of ulnar head and compare it with the normal side. The range will be more of the affected side and patient may complain of pain.

COMMON SWELLINGS AROUND THE WRIST JOINT

Traumatic

Initially diffuse, soft to hard swelling, later localise as a bony swelling.

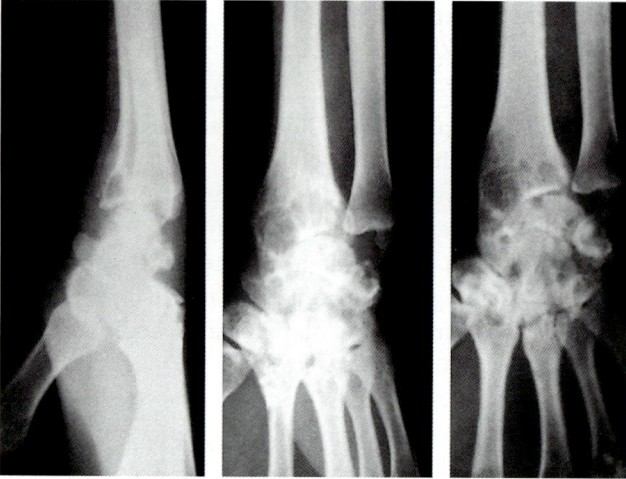

Fig. 6.22: Tuberculosis of the wrist joint with main osseous foci in lower end of radius, styloid process and scaphoid.

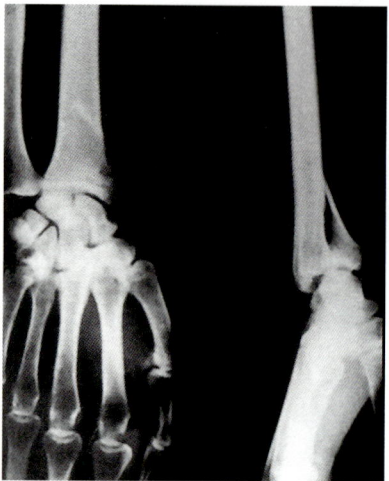

Fig. 6.24: Barton's fracture.

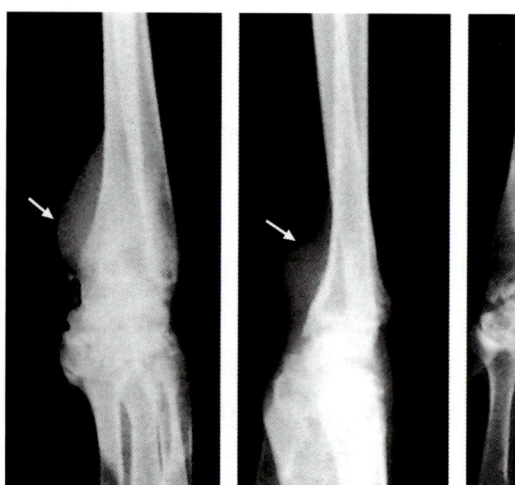

Fig. 6.23: Tuberculosis of the wrist joint with cold abscess presenting anteriorly.

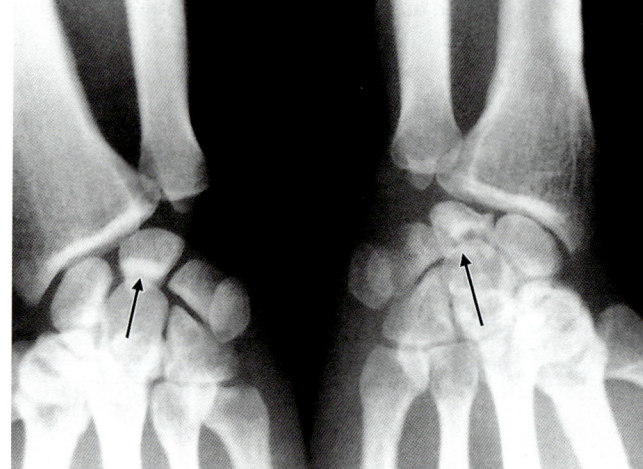

Fig. 6.25: Kienbock's disease.

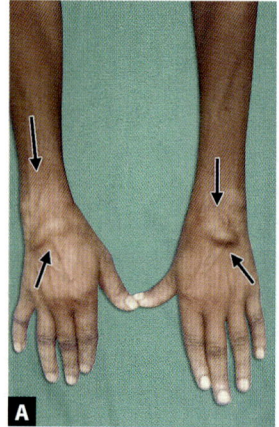
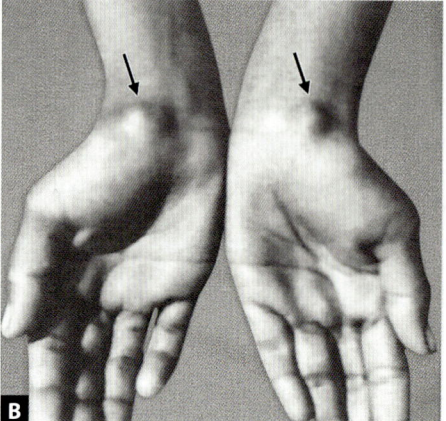
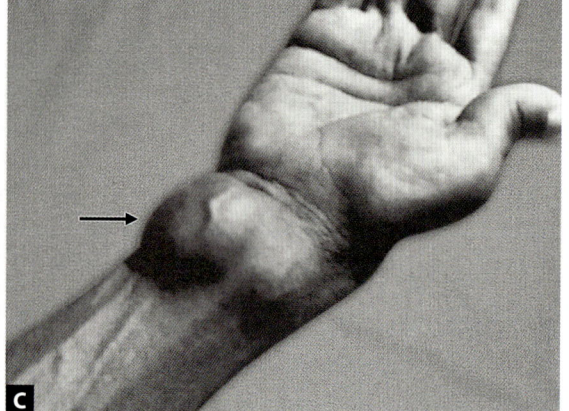

Figs. 6.26A to C: (A and B) Ganglion on dorsal and ventral aspects of both wrists; (C) Ganglion on ventral aspect of lower forearm.

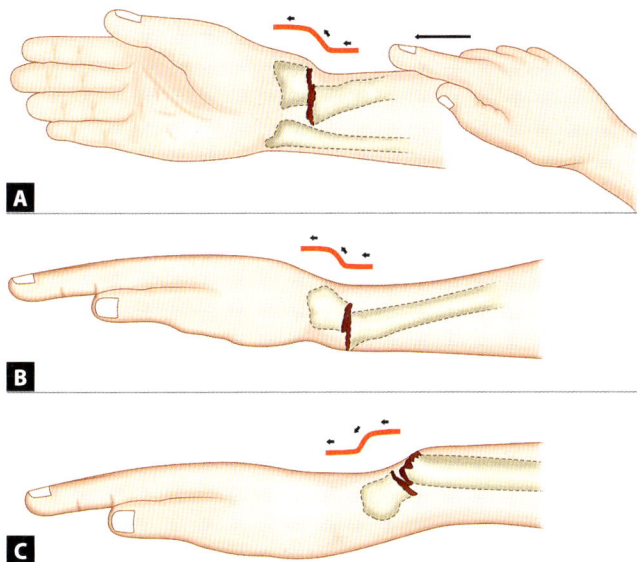

Figs. 6.27A to C: (A) Lateral step up; (B) Posterior step up—Colles fracture; (C) Posterior step down—Smith's fracture.

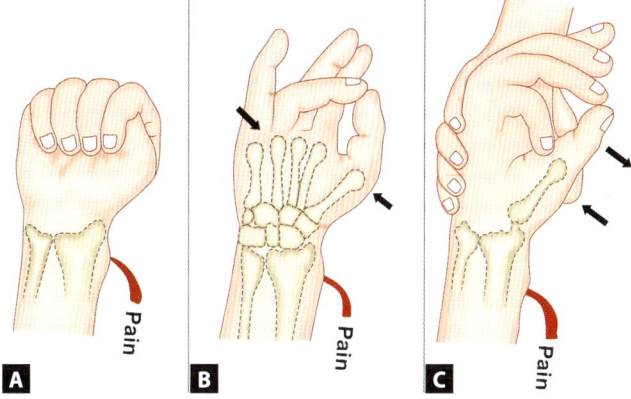

Figs. 6.28A to C: Tests for de Quervain's disease. (A) Closing firm fist triggers pain; (B) Springing over 1st and 4th metacarpal head triggers pain; (C) Active abduction and extension of thumb against resistance triggers the pain.

fracture (in case of trauma) or osteoarthritis of the wrist or intercarpal joints.

Crepitus

In a suspected case of fracture of the lower end of radius or ulna, note, if per chance crepitus is felt. Do not try to demonstrate it, even though it is diagnostic of fracture, since the manoeuvre for demonstrating crepitus is likely to break the fringes of fractured ends and thus can delay the healing of fracture.

Scaphoid shift test (Watson et al. 1988) is useful in evaluating the stability of scaphoid in an injured wrist. It involves radial deviation of the wrist with examiner's thumb opposing the normal palmar rotation of the distal scaphoid leading to the dorsal shift of scaphoid. The test is graded according to the degree of subluxation of the scaphoid and the pain felt on the dorsum of the wrist during the test.

Test for de Quervain's Disease (Chronic Stenosing Tenosynovitis)

Any suspicious swelling existing at the lower outer end of forearm, may be due to de Quervain's disease. Chronic inflammation involves all layers of tendon sheaths of abductor pollicis longus and extensor pollicis brevis. Palpate for the local tenderness. Ascertain the relation of pain with strained movements of the thumb. Test as in **Figures 6.28A to C.**

- Ask the patient to make a firm fist, keeping the thumb in palm. The patient will complain of pain just above the radial styloid process **(Fig. 6.28A)**
- In demonstrating Finkelstein's test, the patient makes a fist keeping thumb in palm. While stabilising the patient's forearm, the hand is pressed into ulnar deviation. There should be pain or extreme discomfort over the radial styloid process or anatomical snuff box or even towards the thumb and/or elbow, if the test is positive, i.e. there is *tenosynovitis of abductor pollicis longus and extensor pollicis brevis tendons.* However, even without de Quervain's disease, variable pain can be felt in that region in this manoeuvre
- While the patient keeps his thumb in opposed position towards the ring fingertip, press over the heads of 1st and 4th metacarpal with a springing action—the patient complains of pain on the outer surface of the radial styloid **(Fig. 6.28B)**.
- In the same position, ask the patient to extend and abduct the thumb against resistance. The patient will feel pain at the same site **(Fig. 6.28C).**

■ MOVEMENTS (TABLE 6.1)

Movements of the Forearm

The movements of the forearm joints result in pronation and supination of the hand. In pronation, the radius, carrying the hand with it crosses obliquely the front of ulna, so that radial upper end remains lateral, and medial end goes medial to ulna. In supination, the movement is reversed so that radius lies lateral to and parallel with the ulna. These movements occur at the **radioulnar joints:** (1) *Proximal synovial uniaxial pivot radioulnar joint* where the radial head rotates in fibro-osseous ring formed by radial notch of ulna and the annular ligament, (2) *Middle radioulnar union,* in which shafts of radius and ulna are connected by oblique cord and the interosseous membrane of the forearm; (3) *Distal synovial uniaxial pivot radioulnar joint* where there is articulation between the convex ulnar head and the concave ulnar notch on the lower medial aspect of radius.

TABLE 6.1: Normal movements at wrist.

Movement	Range of movement	Prime movers	Nerve supply	Assisted by	Limiting factors
Palmar flexion	0° to 70°–90°	• Flexor carpi radialis • Palmaris longus • Flexor carpi ulnaris	• Median nerve C6 • Ulnar nerve C8 T1	Flexor digitorum profundus, flexor digitorum superficialis	Tension of dorsal radiocarpal ligaments
Dorsiflexion	0° to 70°–90°	• Extensor carpi radialis longus • Extensor carpi radialis brevis • Extensor carpi ulnaris	Radial nerve C-6 C7	Extensor digitorum, extensor indicis, extensor pollicis longus, extensor digiti minimi, extensor pollicis brevis	• Tension of volar radiocarpal ligaments • Contact of dorsal surface of distal row of carpals to the posteriorly projected lower end of radius
Ulnar deviation	0° to 25°–35°	• Flexor carpi ulnaris • Extensor carpi ulnaris	• Ulnar nerve C8 T1 • Radial nerve C6 C7		• Tension of lateral collateral ligament of wrist joint • Contact of ulnar styloid process to the hamate
Radial deviation	0° to 15°–25°	• Flexor carpi radialis • Extensor carpi radialis longus • Extensor carpi radialis brevis	Median nerve C6 Radial nerve C6 C7	Abductor pollicis longus, extensor pollicis brevis	• Tension of ulnar collateral ligament of wrist • Contact of tip of radial styloid process to the scaphoid

For pronation—Pronator quadratus (supplied by anterior interosseous branch of median nerve, C8, TI) aided by pronator teres (supplied by median nerves, C6–C7) is responsible for rapid movement and movements against resistance.

Supination—In extended elbow for slow and unresisted supination movement, supinator may be sufficient but in flexed elbow, fast movements and movement against resistance biceps brachii (supplied by musculocutaneous nerve, C5–C6) assists the supinator (supplied by posterior interosseous nerve, C5–C6).

In *relaxed posture (anatomical rest) of the hand*, usually, the wrist is slightly extended and fingers and thumb variably flexed—the index finger is less flexed than others. In inflammation or injury of the hand, almost similar posture of hand is assumed to avoid painful tension on the involved structures, however, there may be some variation according to the tissue affected.

Palmar Flexion and Dorsiflexion (Fig. 6.29)

Method of Demonstration

The patient sits with both mid-pronated forearms supported on the table on their ulnar sides and kept parallel about 10–12" apart. The thumb and fingers are fully extended, while the forearms are firmly fixed on the table. The patient is then asked to bring his fully extended fingers towards each other in the midline as far as practicable. The outer angle subtended between the axis of the forearm and that of the hand is the angle of maximum palmar flexion. Bringing back to the zero position, the patient is asked to move the hand with fully extended fingers away from each other as far as practicable. The inner angle between the axis of the forearm and that of the hand is the angle of maximum dorsiflexion.

A quick method of comparison of dorsiflexion and palmar flexion is as follows:

Oppose the fully stretched up hands (finger-to-finger contact) and lift the elbows as far as possible. The angle sustained between the axis of the forearm and that of hand is the angle of maximum dorsiflexion. Next, the backs of the stretched hands are opposed while the elbows are depressed as far as possible, together. The angle subtended between the axis of the forearm and that of the hand will be the angle of maximum palmar flexion. However, in these manoeuvres, movement is not only at the radiocarpal joint but also includes the intercarpal and carpometacarpal joints.

Radial and Ulnar Deviation (Fig. 6.30)

The patient sits with both forearms and hands kept parallel and fully pronated about 30 cm apart on the table, the fingers and thumbs being kept fully extended. From this zero position, ask the patient to approximate the tips of extended middle fingers towards the midline as far as practicable. The outer angle between the axis of the forearm and that of the extended hand will be the angle of maximum radial deviation.

Ask the patient to move the extended fingers away from the midline as far as practicable. The inner angle between the axis of the forearm and that of the extended hand will be the angle of maximum ulnar deviation.

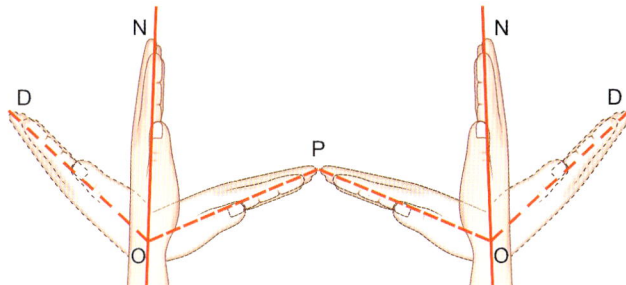

Fig. 6.29: Movements of wrist joint—palmar-flexion (<NOP), dorsiflexion (<NOD).

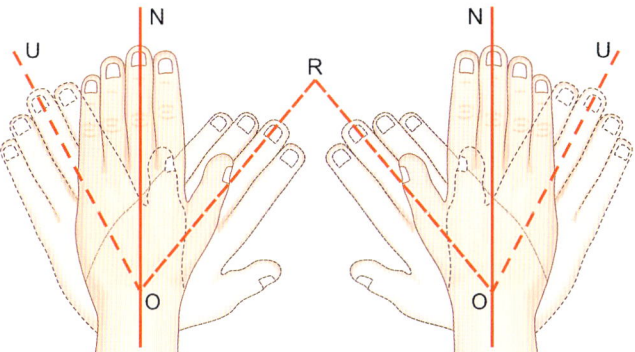

Fig. 6.30: Movements of wrist joint—Radial deviation (<NOR), Ulnar deviation (<NOU).

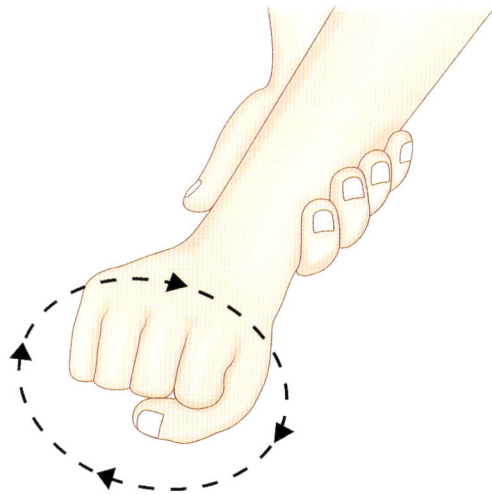

Fig. 6.31: Circumduction at the wrist joint.

Circumduction

Support the patient's pronated lower forearm from the flexor surface. Ask him to make a fist and circumduct (make a circle) in the air. This will be circumduction **(Fig. 6.31)**.

Test for Function of Important Tendons

You can perform group testing as well as individual testing.

On cursory examination, **if the patient can make a firm fist and perform circumduction, probably all tendons and**

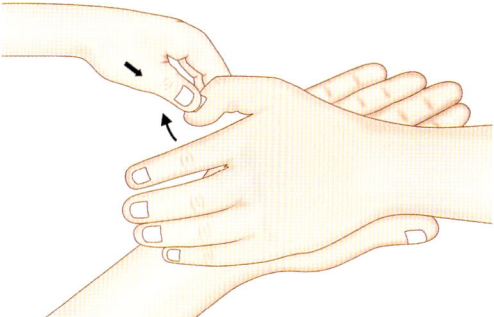

Fig. 6.32: Test for extensor pollicis longus.

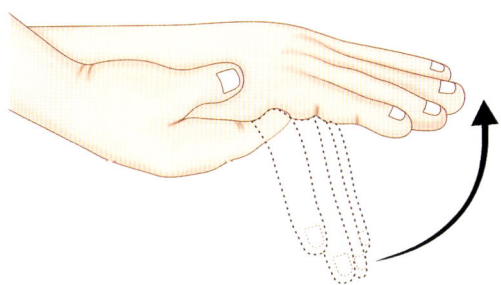

Fig. 6.33: Test for extensor digitorum.

nerves associated with the wrist and hand are normal. However, individual testing of certain tendons is important.

The flexors, extensors, radial deviators and ulnar deviators will be tested in groups when testing for these movements at the wrist joints. Important tendons to be tested are:

Extensor Pollicis Longus (Fig. 6.32)

While supporting from the flexor surface, the lower end of the forearm, wrist and proximal palm, kept in fully pronated position, ask the patient to extend the interphalangeal joint of thumb from fully flexed position as far as possible. This will be mainly by extensor pollicis longus tendon, which will stand out on the ulnar side of the snuffbox.

Ask the patient to extend the thumb both backwards and outwards. This will be by extensor pollicis brevis, abductor pollicis longus and extensor pollicis longus as a conjoint effort.

Extensor Digitorum (Fig. 6.33)

Supporting the wrist and hand as above, the patient is asked to extend the fingers, especially the middle and ring fingers, from a flexed position at the metacarpophalangeal level. In this movement, the index and little fingers are also assisted by extensor indicis and extensor digiti minimi, respectively.

Palmaris Longus (Fig. 6.34)

The fully supinated forearm and hand are placed firmly on the table. Put resistance by your hand over the palm and ask

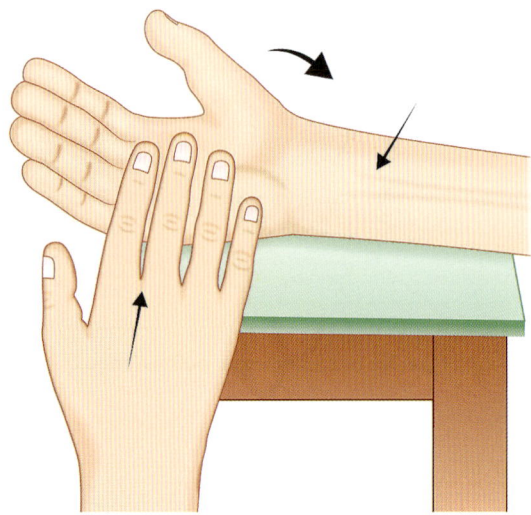

Fig. 6.34: Test for palmaris longus.

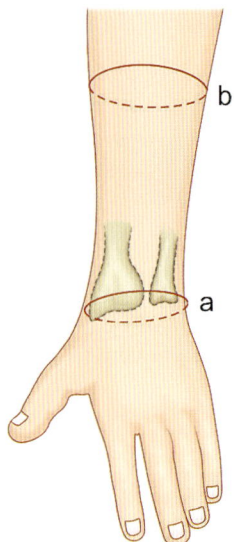

Fig. 6.35: Circumferential measurement, a = at wrist, b = at mid-forearm.

the patient to firmly flex at the wrist. Palmaris longus will become prominent near the midline of the lower forearm. About 1–1.5 cm radialwards, the tendon of flexor carpi radialis will also stand out. Keeping the wrist in zero position and interphalangeal joints of thumb and fingers fully extended with flexion at metacarpophalangeal joints, ask the patient to firmly flex the wrist against the self-imposed resistance—the three prominent flexors of the wrist will stand out, i.e. palmaris longus in the centre, flexor carpi radialis laterally and flexor carpi ulnaris medially **(Fig. 6.34)**.

Flexor Carpi Ulnaris

With the position of the forearm of the patient as described above and your hand giving resistance over the palm, ask the patient to flex with ulnar deviation tendency at the wrist level. Feel for a prominent longitudinal tight tendon—the tendon of the flexor carpi ulnaris.

■ MEASUREMENTS

Linear Measurement

The linear measurement of the wrist region is more or less the same as for that of the upper limb (both total and segmental measurements, i.e. for the arm and forearm). The measuring points are:

For total limb length—Acromion angle to tip of radial styloid process.

For the arm—From acromion angle to tip of lateral epicondyle of humerus.

For the forearm—From lateral epicondyle of the humerus to the tip of the radial styloid process.

The measurement must be comparative and both limbs must be in symmetrically aligned position (guideline will be the affected limb).

Circumferential Measurement (Fig. 6.35)

Circumferential measurement should be done at the joint level, i.e. the tape passing around both the styloid tips. The other circumferential measurement will be for increase/decrease of girth of muscle—to be measured at mid-forearm level.

Distally, the measurement of girth and size of palm will be considered in the examination of the hand.

Tests for integrity of peripheral nerves in relation to the wrist joint (median, ulnar, and radial nerves) (*See* Chapter 16 on Peripheral Nerves).

Look for the possible complications following trauma or disease in and around the wrist.

In any traumatic or non-traumatic pathology in and around wrist following clinical tests should be done besides the routine examination and tests:
1. Abduction of thumb;
2. Radial deviation of wrist;
3. Axial loading of thumb;
4. Flexion of wrist (volar flexion);
5. Extension of wrist (dorsal flexion);
6. Power grip of hand;
7. Ulnar deviation of wrist;
8. Pronation of forearm;
9. Supination of forearm;
10. Thumb-index finger pinch (Gokcen HB et al. 2018)

■ INVESTIGATIONS REQUIRED FOR WRIST PATHOLOGY

For lesions or injuries about the wrist, routine investigations more or less suffice. However, of the injuries about the wrist, a carpal fracture or dislocation or subluxation may sometimes be missed in routine posteroanterior and lateral

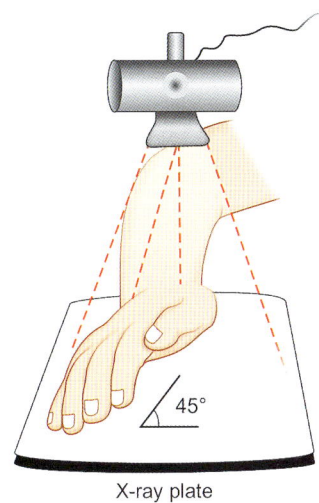

Fig. 6.36: Positioning the part for obliqueview X-ray of the wrist joint.

radiograph. An oblique and 45° semipronated oblique views are essential for such lesions, specially for the scaphoid (the most common of the carpal bones to be involved in fractures). Hence, to diagnose even a hairline fracture of the scaphoid (which unless diagnosed and treated properly has a notorious reputation of going for non-union), it is mandatory to have 45° semipronated oblique views of the wrist region with contrast exposure and development.

The differently-shaped carpal bones, arranged in rows create complex relationship with one another and with the distal forearm bones and metacarpals, which make their thorough evaluation difficult in only two views. Hence, minimum views of exposure should include posteroanterior, lateral, posteroanterior in ulnar deviation and 45° semi-pronated obliques.

MRI is helpful in evaluating the status of triangular fibrocartilage, the distal radioulnar joint, vascularity of carpals, joint surfaces and allied soft tissues, albeit with more possibilities of false-positive findings.

Arthroscopy has proved to be a more therapeutic tool than the diagnostic one.

Positioning of the Part for Oblique Projection (Fig. 6.36)

While the forearm and hand rest on its ulnar border on the X-ray plate, at an inclination of about 45° (with palm looking down) the beam is centred to the ulnar styloid process OR from the lateral position, rotate the hand backwards by 45° and centre the beam to the ulnar styloid process.

KEY DIAGNOSTIC POINTS OF COMMON WRIST PATHOLOGY

Traumatic

Fracture of the Distal end Radius-mainly consisting of Colles Fracture, Smith's Fractures, chauffeur's fracture, Barton's fracture. Fractures of the distal end of radius were historically (Hippocrates' era) considered as a part of dislocation of the wrist.

Colles Fracture (Abraham Colles, 1814) (Fig. 6.38)

- (In children before skeletal maturity, akin injury may produce 'fracture separation of lower radial epiphysis' with almost all clinical features of a Colles fracture)
- Most common injury around the wrist
- Usually elderly ladies with history of fall in courtyard or bathroom on an outstretched hand. The female:male ratio is 4:1
- Immediate pain and swelling in the wrist region
- In typical Colles fracture typical 'dinner fork' deformity (silver fork deformity) develops **(Fig. 6.27)**
- Radial styloid process recedes upwards, posteriorly and laterally
- Step sign (step up) positive
- Besides the radial fracture line, tenderness is also marked in the ulnar styloid region
- In X-ray **(Fig. 6.38)**, three typical displacements (distal fragment displaced backwards, upwards and outwards), and two typical tilts (distal fragment tilted backwards, outwards and impacted upwards into the proximal fragment). The lower fragment also supinates. The lower radial articular surface looks backwards and downwards [normally looks slightly forwards (7°) and downwards]
- If patient is taken into full confidence, variable wrist movements can be demonstrated
- Shortening of forearm
- Late cases may also be associated with Sudeck's osteodystrophy (Sudeck's atrophy, reflex sympathetic dystrophy, algodystrophy) changes in the hand and fingers (probably due to sympathetic or parasympathetic disbalance or unknown aetiology—burning pain, hyperaesthesia of skin, heaviness, and puffiness in the hand; thin shiny skin, spindle-shaped tender swelling and stiffness of the fingers' joints with varying atrophic changes in fingertips and nails, excessive hair growth)
- In late neglected cases, shoulder and/or hand becomes stiff—**shoulder hand syndrome.**

Smith's Fracture [Robert William Smith, 1847 (Figs. 6.27 and 6.39A and B)]

- Usually, due to fall on the dorsum of a flexed wrist
- Comparatively younger age group
- The distal fragment displaces outwards, upwards and forwards
- The distal fragment tilts outwards and forwards, therefore, lower radial articular surface looks more anteriorly and downwards than the normal one

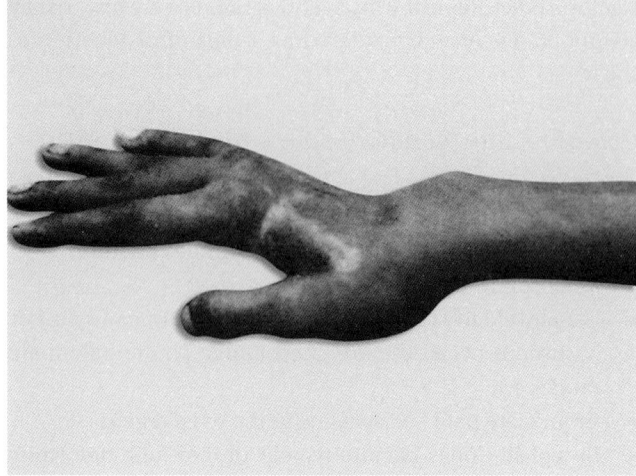

Fig. 6.37: Typical garden spade deformity of wrist and hand in reverse Colles fracture (Smith's fracture).

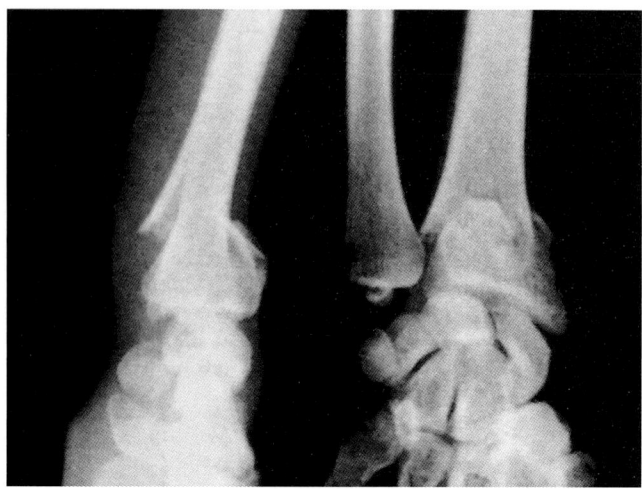

Fig. 6.38: Colles fracture.

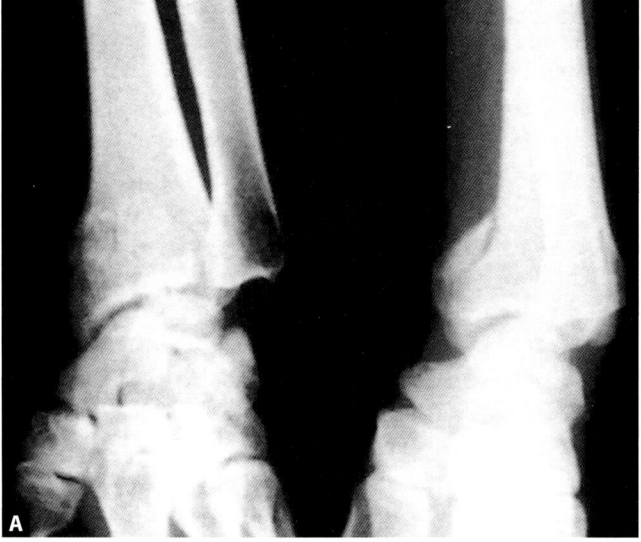

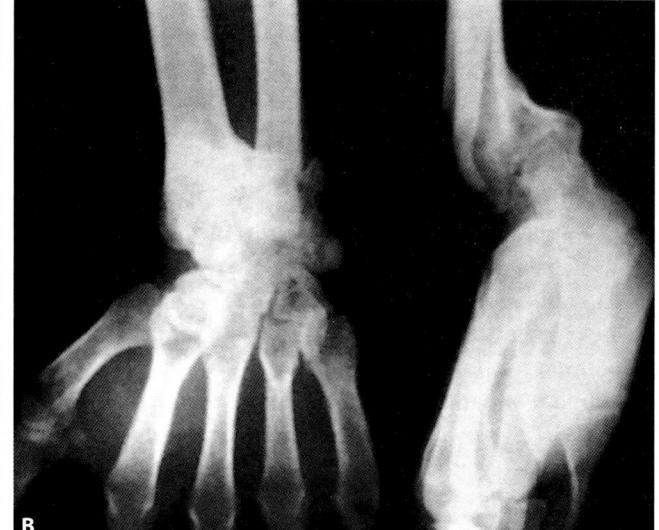

Figs. 6.39A and B: (A) Fresh Smith's fracture; (B) Grossly displaced malunited Smith's fracture.

- Clinically, many a time it is difficult to distinguish it from Colles fracture, specially when gross swelling is present. However, in fresh cases, the look of the hand (absence of dinner-fork deformity and presence of garden spade deformity **(Fig. 6.37)**, and presence of reverse posterior stepping, i.e. finger, passing from above downwards, steps down at fractured site (cf. steps up in Colles fracture) are suggestive
- With patient taken in full confidence, wrist movements can be demonstrated to a variable extent
- Shortening of forearm
- Lateral view X-ray of wrist is confirmatory.

Chauffeur's Fracture or Fracture of Radial Styloid Process (Fig. 6.40)

- History of injury, e.g. being backfire hit by recoiling car or generator handle directly over radial styloid process

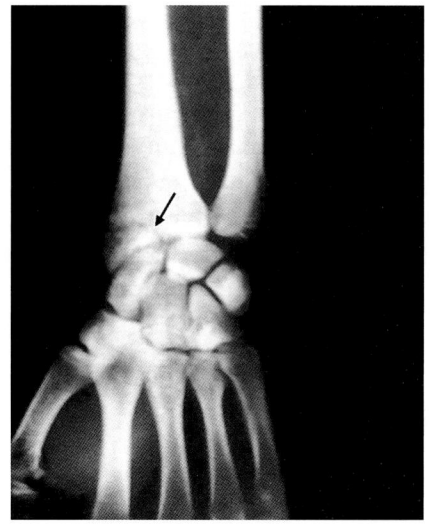

Fig. 6.40: Chauffeur's fracture (fracture of radial styloid process).

or fall on the ball of the thumb or similar injuries—commonly in young adults
- Broadening of the lower end of the forearm at the radial styloid level
- Feeling of irregularity or thickening at the junction of the radial styloid and lower radial shaft
- Maximum tenderness in this region
- Radial styloid process may recede up
- X-ray is confirmatory—fracture line enters the wrist joint between the scaphoid and the lunate bones.

Barton's Fracture (JR Barton 1838) (Fig. 6.24)
- Clinicoradiologically, more or less exaggerated picture of either Colles or Smith's fracture—thus of **two types: posterior and anterior** (very common)
- There is anterior marginal fracture of the radius
- Subluxation, both of the wrist and inferior radioulnar joints
- The fracture extends into the wrist joint, and the carpus along with the hand displaces forwards with the anterior fragment in anterior or volar Barton's fracture
- Wrist joint movements markedly painful, may be even difficult to initiate
- X-ray is confirmatory.

Fracture Scaphoid
- The scaphoid (navicular) is most commonly fractured among the carpals, because the lower articular end of radius has wider contact with it than with the lunate and the forces coming from ulnar side to the triquetrum are cushioned by the articular disc
- May be missed initially unless and until carefully examined and X-rayed in four views (anteroposterior/lateral/oblique and scaphoid). Delay in diagnosis and treatment of scaphoid fracture can lead to nonunion or malunion and may eventually lead to symptomatic osteonecrosis, carpal instability or secondary osteoarthritis
- History of injury, usually indirect (fall on outstretched hand or direct hit over the scaphoid region, specially when the hand is fisted)
- Maximum tenderness in the floor of the snuff-box, which may show comparative fullness. Snuffbox lies just distal to the radial styloid process. Its radial border is formed by the abductor pollicis longus and extensor pollicis brevis tendons and the ulnar border by extensor pollicis longus tendon
- Patient (usually young males) feels pain in actively extending the thumb fully
- Even with the slightest suspicion, oblique view X-ray of wrist region must be ordered for. In fact, in any injury of the wrist joint, it will always be rewarding to order for posteroanterior, lateral, and pronation and supination oblique views of wrist
- Crack fracture is mostly missed in recent X-rays, hence these must be repeated after 3 weeks. However, CT scan will show the fracture in the beginning itself
- Bone scan can indicate the fracture line quite early (even one hour after injecting diphosphonate).

Lunate Dislocation (Most Common Among Carpal Dislocations)
- Indirect injury—the wrist assumes a variably dorsiflexed position
- A bony mass is felt in front of the wrist
- Median nerve may be involved
- Lateral view X-ray of wrist confirmatory
- Osteochondritis of lunate due to avascular necrosis (Kienbock's disease) is a prominent cause of pain in this region.

Kienbock disease (lunate malacia) (*see* **Fig. 6.25**) is probably (as exact cause is not clearly known) caused by aseptic necrosis of the lunate. In the advanced stages of the disease, carpal collapses, joint incongruity and osteoarthritis develop. The main symptoms of Kienbock disease are pain, gradual decrease in grip strength and reduction of range of motion with the progress of the disease. Of the various treatments suggested [(e.g. excision of lunate, radial osteotomy (shortening and wedge resection), limited intercarpal arthrodesis, revascularisation, vascular bundle implantation, arthrodesis between radius and lunate, etc.], lunate excision with or without replacement, lunate excision followed by capitate osteotomy and intercarpal arthrodesis appear reliable treatment, however this disease is still poorly understood.

Osteonecrosis of scaphoid (Preiser's disease) also manifests like that of lunate, but for the more radial side and thumb oriented pain.

Robert Kienbock a noted radiologist of Vienna first described the *lunatomalacic* in 1910, and he suspected the cause of this collapse as the repetitive injury to lunate from the work activities. This cause was also supported by Muller (1920) who coined the term *occupational lunatomalacic*.

Post-traumatic Inferior Radioulnar Arthritis
- It is a common accompaniment of late Colles fracture or other injuries around the wrist
- Patient complains of pain in using the wrist as well as during rotatory movements of the forearm
- Area of maximum tenderness lies just behind and below the ulnar styloid process
- This tenderness further increases if attempt is made to displace the ulnar head forwards and backwards.
- The injury (mostly neglected ones) of triangular fibrocartilage complex is one of the most common causes

of pain in the ulnar side of wrist and distal radioulnar joint. Arthroscopically assisted repair of triangular fibrocartilage complex injury can relieve pain, improve function and stability of distal radioulnar joint.

In an old wrist injury, the unstable scaphoid can be the cause of chronic pain.

The *"scaphoid shift" test* is useful for the evaluation of the stability of the scaphoid in the injured wrist. This test (described by Watson, et al. 1988) consists of radial deviation of wrist with the examiner's thumb opposing the normal volar rotation of the distal scaphoid leading to dorsal shift of scaphoid. However, this test is difficult to perform and enough experience is needed to correctly interpret the findings. Scaphoid shift test should be considered to be positive only when the subluxation of scaphoid is accompanied with pain which is referred to the dorsum of wrist. But if the scaphoid shift test is positive in an asymptomatic wrist, then it is due to ligamentous laxity and not due to occult carpal injury.

Calcific tendinitis of flexor carpi ulnaris may present with acute symptoms (pain, swelling and redness) around the wrist joint with mildly elevated inflammatory blood examination markers—mild rise in cell count, raised ESR and CRP, X-ray shows calcific deposit on the palmar aspect of the wrist near the pisiform bone. Though it is more or less self-limiting condition, it should be treated by non-steroidal anti-inflammatory drug (NSAID), splinting of wrist—failing which local anaesthetic and corticoid injection should help.

Post-traumatic Chronic Wrist Pain

Two major causes are:
1. *Carpal instability*, which can be of two types:
   (i) Static instabilities can be identified on plain radiograph
   (ii) Dynamic instabilities need fluoroscopic examination for confirmation alongwith that of asymptomatic wrist for comparison.
   Arthrography may be useful in demonstrating defects in the interosseous ligaments, joint capsule and triangular fibrocartilage.
   Dissociated instabilities can be delineated by disruption of smooth carpal arcs.
2. *Osteonecrosis*: It affects the proximal part of scaphoid bone. Osteonecrosis is one of the most common complication of scaphoid fracture, the incidence being 10–15%. Approximately, all fractures involving the proximal fifth of the scaphoid, develop osteonecrosis of proximal pole. Although osteonecrosis of the whole scaphoid may be seen even without any trauma (*Preiser's disease*), osteonecrosis of the distal pole in the absence of trauma is extremely rare. Lunate is less commonly affected (*Kienbock's disease*, see **Fig. 6.25**) either due to trauma or abnormal repeated stresses.
   Early osteonecrosis is not delineable on plain X-ray. It can be seen as a focal area of absent uptake on isotope bone scan. During healing, it shows increased uptake. Established osteonecrosis is seen on plain X-ray as increased bone density, flattening and fragmentation. MRI is very sensitive in demonstrating osteonecrosis which is seen as diffuse areas of decreased marrow signal intensity on both T1 and T2.

Non-traumatic

Tuberculosis of Wrist (see Figs. 6.22 and 6.23)

- More common in adults
- Incidence not so uncommon
- Slow onset
- Pain in and around the wrist
- Local temperature raised
- Fullness around the wrist
- Tenderness around the joint line
- Gradual painful limitation of all wrist movements
- Wasting of the forearm muscles, and to some extent, the hand muscles too
- Supratrochlear and/or axillary glands may be enlarged and matted
- In later stage, cold abscesses or sinuses may be present (**Fig. 6.43**)
- X-ray—as in typical tuberculous lesions of any joint
- Clinicoradiological confusion with villonodular synovitis.

Rheumatoid Arthritis (Refer Figs. 7.36 to 7.39)

- Wrist is a common site, specially in ladies in their thirties
- Wrist is swollen
- Movements, specially extension, is painful. Gradually, flexion and ulnar/radial deviation deformities of the wrist develop
- Smaller joints, i.e. metacarpophalangeal and proximal interphalangeal joints of thumb and fingers may be affected (not distal interphalangeal joints of fingers as in osteoarthrosis)
- May be typical deformity in thumb and fingers (e.g. swan-neck deformity, buttonhole or boutonniere deformity).

de Quervain's Disease (At Wrist Stenosing Tenosynovitis or tendinopathy) (see Fig. 6.19)

de Quervain's disease was described by the Swiss physician de Quervain Fritz in 1895.

- Basic pathology is idiopathic stenosing tendovaginitis, in which the sheath of a tendon thickens. Common sheath of the abductor pollicis longus and extensor pollicis brevis tendons, in the first extensor compartment of the wrist, are most commonly affected. Stenosis is preceded by tenosynovitis which may also result from subclinical collagen disease or recurrent mild trauma. The stenosis develops at a point where the direction of the tendon changes. At this point the fibrous sheath, even though

gets lubricated by tenosynovium, acts like a pulley against which the repetitive movements lead to mounting of friction to the maximum
- Usually observed in ladies (6–10 times more than men) in their thirties
- In Gray's anatomy (13th edition) it was referred as *"Washer woman's sprain"* due to repeated wringing clothes
- This compartment – a fibro-osseous tunnel – is located on the posterolateral aspect of radial styloid
- Complains of painful swelling over the outer aspect of the lower end of forearm and with subjective weakness in thumb-pinch and grip
- *Eichhoff test:* The patient himself clinches his thumb in his own ipsilateral palm and then deviates the wrist ulnarwards–the patients feels pain in the first dorsal compartment.
- Pain more in squeezing type of movements by the thumb
- Firm, tender swelling about 1.5 cm proximal to the radial styloid process
- Stress tests for abductor pollicis longus and extensor pollicis brevis (as mentioned earlier) positive (Finkelstein's test). On grasping the patient's thumb and quickly abducting the hand ulnarward, the pain over the radial styloid tip is excruciating
- Hitchhiker's sign Extension and abduction of thumb causes pain in the region of first dorsal compartment
- Crepitus may be felt or heard with stethoscope.

Initially nonoperative treatment (NSAID local analgesia application, corticoid injection, splinting, (thumb spica splint) must be tried; which if fails, surgical decompression—complete release of abductor pollicis longus and extensor pollicis brevis tendon must be done. To avoid failure of surgical treatment, variations within the first dorsal compartment over the wrist should be taken care of such as for—multiple slips of abductor pollicis longus; variable insertions of abductor pollicis longus; separate compartment for the abductor pollicis longus and extensor pollicis brevis. Surgery includes the release of constricting fibrous pully with or without reconstruction surgical intervention provides significant improvement in de Quevain's tenosynovitis. However, there may be painful palmar subluxation of the tendons following release of constricting fibrous pulley only, while chances of subluxation is less in whom pulley reconstruction was done.

Giant Cell Tumour
(Fig. 6.20, also Refer Fig. 17.26)

- Most common growth at lower end of radius
- Gradual onset
- Slowly expanding the lower radial end
- Local temperature may be variably raised
- Slight tenderness present

- Yielding tendency of the expanded cortex
- Movements of the wrist remain free till very late stage
- Egg shell crackling—not to be demonstrated. However, in regular process of palpation, if one feels the crackling—it should be noted.

Ganglion Around the Wrist (see Fig. 6.26)

- Ganglions are common around the wrist, more in females between 20 and 40 years of age, and mostly appear insidiously
- Patient presents with round sessile tense translucent swelling and painful terminal movements of the wrist (when it is from the wrist joint)—a protrusion cyst of the joint capsule usually seen on the dorsum of the naviculo-lunate joint specially extension, however, the condition may be painless too
- Local tense, tender swelling in the joint line, or along the tendon
- Though cystic, but very difficult to demonstrate fluctuation
- Usually present on the dorsum of the wrist, disappears or reduces in size on extension of wrist and becomes more prominent on flexion of wrist
- May also be related to the tendons of the wrist, more between the long extensor of thumb and extensor indicis—in that case they will not disappear on movement of the wrist, rather they may slightly move up and down with movements of the particular tendon. Ganglions may also be ralated to the tendons on the dorsum of foot **(Figs. 6.43A to C)**
- If the ganglion lies deeper to the tendon, its size reduces with contraction of the particular tendon, and *vice-versa*
- When it lies superficial to the tendon, the position is reversed, i.e. becomes prominent with contraction of tendon and decreases in size with relaxation of the tendon **(Figs. 6.43A to C)**.

Carpal Tunnel Syndrome (Tardy Median Nerve Palsy) (Fig. 6.41); (Table 6.2)

- Carpel tunnel syndrome was first described as the compression/irritation syndrome of the median nerve

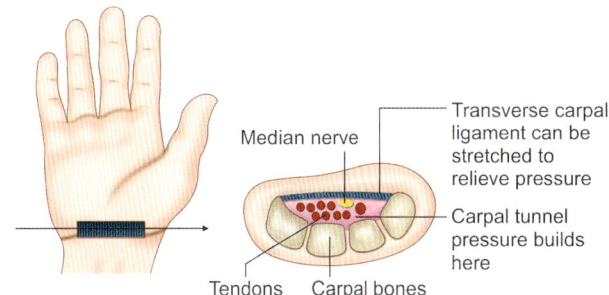

Fig. 6.41: Carpal tunnel (simplified cross-section drawing).

TABLE 6.2: Stages of carpal tunnel syndrome.

Stage	Duration of symptoms	Physical findings	Findings on electrical studies	Management
1. Early stage	• Symptoms less than 1 year	• No definite physical finding	• Electrical study negative or show some delay in sensory conduction	• Conservative; if night time paraesthesia—wrist splint for symptomatic relief • If pain, discomfort interferes with patient's work or leisure time activities—surgical decompression
2. Intermediate stage	• Symptoms more than one year • Sensory complaints are usually not disturbing • Night paraesthesia usually eliminated with the use of wrist splints	• Weakness in thenar muscles • Mild atrophy of thenar muscles	• Electrical studies show delay in sensory conduction	• Surgical decompression is indicated in this stage to avoid irreversible nerve changes
3. Advanced stage	• Symptoms for longer period (much longer beyond one year) • Sensory complaints—particularly night time paraesthesia is disabling • Persistent numbness	• Marked thenar muscles weakness • Marked atrophy of thenar muscles	• Usually irreversible nerve changes develop	• Surgical decompression does improve the condition, specially in elderly patients • Usually sensory complaints, particularly night time paraesthesia, improves, however numbness often persists

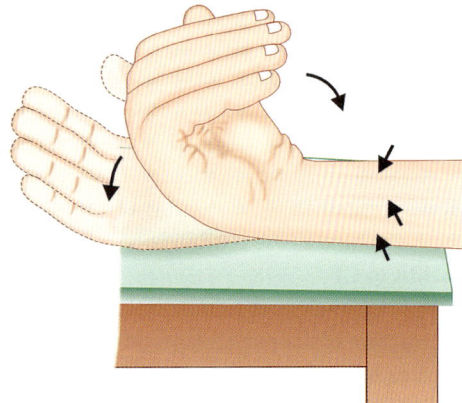

Fig. 6.42: Three prominent flexors of the wrist—palmaris longus, flexor carpi radialis and flexor carpi ulnaris.

as it transverses the carpel tunnel-by James Paget in 1865.

- Most common compressive neuropathy of the upper extremity is the carpal tunnel syndrome in which the **median nerve is compressed at the wrist in the carpal tunnel**—a fibro-osseous canal rigidly bound by the concave arch of carpal bones as floor and roofed by the transverse carpal ligament. It is a well-defined anatomic channel that *topographically extends from the wrist flexion crease to the mid-palm for a distance of about 4 cm.* This tunnel contains the median nerve and nine flexor tendons of fingers and thumb. Has depth of 10 – 13 mm, normal pressure in carpal tunnel is 2.5 mm. when pressure reaches 20 – 30 mm Hg, a decrease in epineural

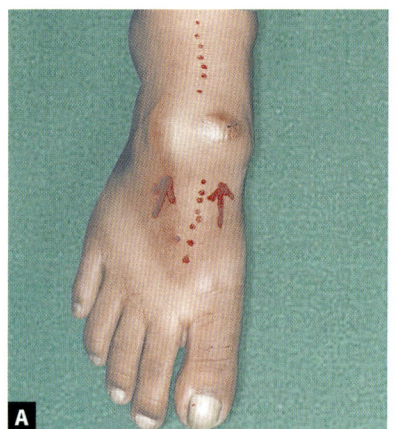 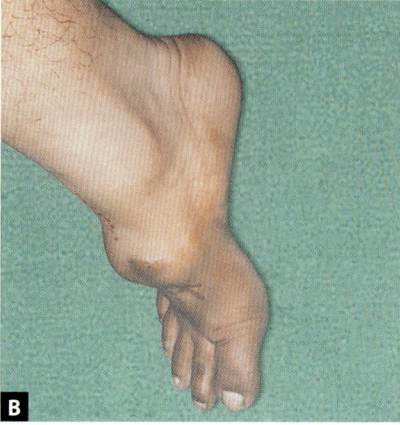 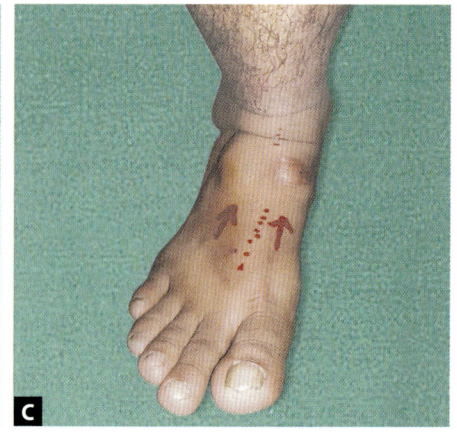

Figs. 6.43A to C: Ganglion on the dorsum of foot in relation to extensor digitorum longus tendon: (A) Note that when the person plantar flexes the foot the ganglion goes down and becomes more prominent (B), and when he dorsiflexes the foot ganglion slips upwards and becomes less prominent (C).

blood flow and oedematous changes occur. When pressure reaches 50 mm or more Hg. nerve
- Carpal tunnel syndrome is not a disease entity but rather a constellation of symptoms, which usually worsens with time. Though Sir James Paget described this condition in 1854, the term 'carpal tunnel syndrome' was coined by Moersch in 1938, and has been popularised by Phalen (1950 onwards)
- It typically affects those between 40 to 60 years of age, and about three times more in women
- Pathogenesis: The elevated pressure in the carpal tunnel produces ischaemia of the median nerve, resulting in impaired nerve conduction and associated paraesthesia and pain. In the early period, there is no morphological changes in the median nerve and the neurological findings (changes) are reversible and symptoms are intermittent. However, with prolongation or frequent episodes of raised pressure in the carpal tunnel, segmental demyelination in the nerve and more constant and severe symptoms, occasionally with weakness, occur. With prolonged ischaemia, axonal injury ensues and then nerve dysfunction usually becomes irreversible
- Based on clinical symptoms and physical findings, the carpal tunnel syndrome can be considered into 3 stages (*see* **Table 6.2**).

Causes of carpal tunnel syndrome:
- Nonspecific tenosynovial proliferation, rheumatoid arthritis; degenerative arthritis; old trauma in that region; metabolic (hypothyroidism, gout, diabetes mellitus); alcoholism; acromegaly; pregnancy; tumours; connective tissue disorders (amyloidosis; haemochromatosis); repetitive stress disorder; use of corticosteroids and estrogens; idiopathic Paget's disease
- Females in their 40-50 (middle age) are the usual victims, complaining usually in the night or early morning of feeling of heaviness, vague pain, tingling, paraesthesia, numbness in first three digits and weakness in the hand in the distribution of median nerve, specially after doing fine work
- Even without any history of earlier injury, patient complains of pain and/or tingling sensation or numbness in hand and fingers, specially in the index and middle ones
- Clumsiness or lack of dexterity is a common complaint
- Symptoms usually get relieved after rubbing the hand or hanging it over the side of the bed. However, if the hand remains in dependant position, there may be venous engorgement, which can exacerbate the symptoms

Tinel sign:
- *Percussion test* or *Tinel Sign:* The median nerve tapped from proximal to distal direction will produce tingling or electric sensation, which indicates positive test.
- Semmes-Weinstein monofilaments: Filaments with increasing diameter are touched on the palmar side of radial digits till patient can perceive its touch. This tests the slowly adapting fibers and is positive when the value is more than 2.83. (After PP kotwal and S Mittal 2016).
- *Durkan compression test*
- The symptoms get exaggerated or reappear when direct pressure is applied over the centre of the wrist from the front (this presses directly over the carpal tunnel region for 30 seconds i.e. by compressing or percussing over the carpal ligament.

Test for carpal tunnel syndrome
Phalen's test: Patient is asked to keep both wrists in flexed position, keeping the forearm vertical. Usually, pain is felt on the affected side within a minute which dramatically disappears when the wrist is extended. However, this test is positive in about 75% of cases only. There may be bulge of the flexor mass in the lower aspect of the wrist, which is characteristic of chronic tenosynovitis.

A *provocative test*, in which the *wrist flexion is combined with the median nerve compression,* appears to be clinically more useful. Here the elbow is extended, the forearm is supinated and wrist is flexed to 60°. The median nerve in the carpal tunnel is compressed evenly and constantly till numbness, pain or paraesthesia appears in the distribution of median nerve. If these symptoms occur within 30 seconds, the test is positive.

Tourniquet test: When sphygmomanometer cuff is inflated above the systolic level, patient complains of pain and paraesthesia, more on the affected side usually within a minute (as against in 2-3 minutes in normal limb). If the pressure is continued further, the sensory loss appears in 5-8 minutes in the distribution of median nerve, as against 10 minutes in the normal limb.

Local anaesthetic infiltration around the median nerve, in the carpal tunnel, relieves the symptoms if it is due to compression of the nerve here, but not if it is referred pain from anywhere else.

Demonstration of diminished median nerve conduction velocity across the wrist is almost diagnostic, of which the sensory nerve fibre conduction velocity (between finger and wrist) *test is more sensitive than motor fibre conduction.*

Local *corticoid infiltration* may provide variable relief.

Complete surgical decompression of the median nerve provides ultimate good results in majority of cases.

Complete surgical decompression of the median nerve by release of transverse carpal ligament (flexor retinaculum) through a longitudinal incision directly over it (transverse carpal ligament) provides ultimate good results. *Release may be open or single portal endoscopic carpal tunnel release.* Both have almost similar incidence of complications and similar return of hand function, however, endoscopic release is a slower technique, has a steep learning curve, has more possibilities of neurovascular and tendon injuries and incomplete release and it also involves extra costs in equipment, though more rapid recovery can be expected by this procedure. Standard open carpal tunnel release may be associated with pain in the scar and thenar and hypothenar regions, pain and weakness of pinch and grip which are difficult to treat. In an attempt to minimise the complications of open carpal tunnel release, Lee and Strickland (1998) developed a 'limited open release technique' using a small palmar incision of 1.5 cm and a set of specially designed instruments known as 'Indianatome'. This limited open carpal tunnel release (LOCTR) combines the simplicity and safety of open release with reduced tissue trauma and the potential serious complications of endoscopic release.

Flexor tenosynovectomy does not improve the results of carpal tunnel surgery in patients without inflammatory arthritis. Further the *'hourglass deformity of nerve'* a sign of chronic compression also does not correlate with the outcome.

Madelung's Deformity
[Otto Madelung 1878 (see Fig. 6.10)]

Congenital deformity manifesting during puberty, mostly bilateral and more in females, (at times a similar deformity develops following damage of inner third of lower radial growth plate due to trauma, infection or rickets). The components of this deformity (with variations) are:
- Backward and outward bowing of lower part of radius
- Backward subluxation of lower end of ulna
- Shortening of radius
- Forward and ulnar deviation of the hand
- Limitation of dorsiflexion, abduction and supination with increased flexion of wrist
- Dorsal bayonet-like deformity of radius
- In pronated position of hand a profile is produced in which the wrist is deformed by a sharp upward (dorsal) protrusion of lower end of ulna due to its subluxation.

In severe cases, pain, muscle cramps and weakness may be complained of.

Compound Palmar Ganglion
(see Figs. 6.15 and 6.16)

- Tuberculous tenosynovitis is rare and develops slowly
- In tuberculous diathesis or established tuberculous pathology or rheumatoid arthropathy
- Painless mild swelling is main complaint, very rarely also manifests as carpal tunnel syndrome
- The most common site of involvement is the flexor tendons of hand with progressive swelling and inflammation of the tendon sheath with limitation in tendon movements – e.g. compound palmar ganglion like lesion results.
- There is chronic inflammatory collection in ulnar bursa, presenting as a dumbbell appearance above and below the flexor retinaculum. There may be cross-fluctuation across the flexor retinaculum, and crepitus (probably due to melon seed bodies present in the fluid) is felt. Swellings are usually not tender nor appreciably warm.

There may be chronic pain in the wrist region (with even exacerbations) due to repetitive stress disorders (e.g. in typists) including carpal tunnel syndrome. However, now with technological advancements in typing machines, e.g. 'orbi touch keyless keyboard' such typing induced pain may be eliminated. This new typing system actually eliminates finger movement entirely and reduces wrist movement up to 80%. Such keyless board will be very much useful for patients of arthritis, partial paralysis or missing fingers.

Dejerine-Sottas Disease

Usually presenting as a painful tender mass in the wrist region, this disease is a localised enlargement of a peripheral nerve caused by interstitial neuropathy. Median nerve is usually involved. Dividing the transverse carpal ligament should help in relieving the pain and even reducing the swelling of nerve.

■ BIBLIOGRAPHY

1. Gray H, Standrings. Gray`s anatomy: the anatomical basis of clinical practice. Edinburgh: Churchill Livirostone Elsevier: 2008.
2. Gokcen HB, Akcal MA, Unay K et al. A scoring system to demonstrate the risk for bone injury in patients with clinically suspected or occult scaphoid fracture. Indian J Orthop. 2018; 52(2):184-9.
3. Hagert E, Hagert CG. Understanding stability of the distal radioulnar joint through an understanding of its anatomy. Hand Clin. 2010;26:459-66.
4. Kienböck's R. Concerning traumatic malacia of the lunate and its consequences: joint degeneration and compression. Fortsch Geb Roentgen. 1910;16:77-103.
5. Kotwal PP, Mittal S. Carpal Tunnel Syndrome. Textbook of Orthopaedies & Trauma 3rd Ed. Jaypee Ed. Kulkarni GS, Babulkar S. 2016; p. 1981.
6. Lee WP, Strickland JW. Safe carpal tunnel release via a limited Palmar incision. Plast Reconstr Surg. 1998;101:418-24.
7. Muller W. Uber die Erweichung and verdichtung des OS Lunatum, eine Typische Erkrankung des Handgelenks. Beitrage Zur Klinischen Chirurgie 1920;119-664.
8. Park MJ. Radiographic observation of the scaphoid shift test. J Bone Joint Surg (Br). 2003;85-B:358-62.
9. Phalen GS. The carpal tunnel syndrome. J Bone Joint Surg. 1966;48A:211.
10. Takase K, Imakiire A. Lunate excision, capitate osteotomy and intercarpal arthrodesis for advanced Kienböck disease. J Bone Joint Surg (Am). 2001;83A:177-83.
11. Tetro AM, Evanoff BA, Hollstien, Gelberman RH. A new provocative test for carpal tunnel syndrome. J Bone Joint Surg. 1998;80B:493–8.

CHAPTER 7

Hand

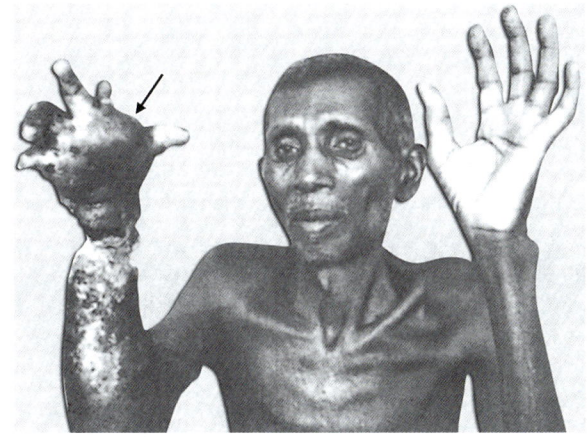
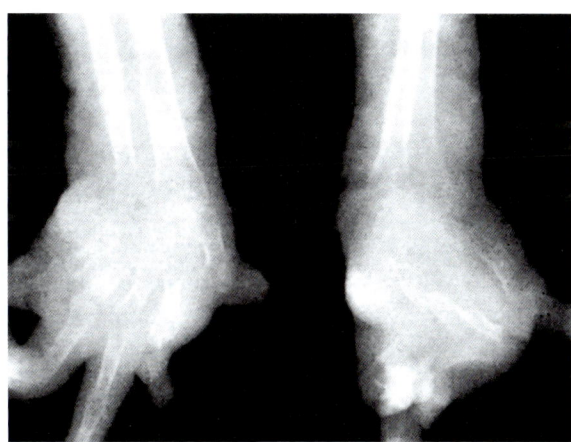

"Beauty is that which attracts your soul, and that which loves to give and not to receive."
—*Kahlil Gibran*
"A life lived for others is a life worth lived."
—*Albert Einstein*

Hand

"The hand is an organ of grasp as well as an organ of sensation and expression."
— **Sterling Bunnell**

■ INTRODUCTION

The supremacy of mankind over the animal kingdom is decided not only by the use of the lower limbs, rather more by its superiority due to its psyche and hands.

The *hand is the most developed part of the locomotor system in bipeds.* It is not only meant for performing tough jobs, e.g. holding an object firmly, added to these are very fine and delicate manoeuvres, like painting, writing and fine adjustments. Along with these, it also has an important role in sensory perception. On the whole, the hand is most complex and versatile structure of body controlled by a large area of brain space dedicated to it. Hand has been designed to serve for grasping, precise movements and as a tactile organ. On the whole it is an organ of prehension (grasp) and sensibility.

■ ANATOMICAL CONSIDERATIONS

In the process of morphological evolution, the main development in the hand has been the rotational adjustment of the thumb on the axis of the palm. This has helped in subserving the oppositional function with maximum accuracy. In human beings, the thumb does not lie in the same plane as that of the other fingers (cf, ape or chimpanzee), rather, it has rotated inwards, so that in the extended position it is placed at an angle of about 70°.

The hand, anatomically, is made up of carpals [8 carpals are arranged in proximal row (comprising of lunate, triquetrum and pisiform) and distal row (comprising of trapezium, trapezoid, capitate and hamate) and scaphoid bone links the two rows. Scaphoid (derived from the Greek word 'scaphe' which means boat) is the commonest carpal to fracture – 50 to 80%], metacarpals, and phalangeal bones **(Fig. 7.1)** (on the whole 27 bones) and their joints along with soft tissue coverings in different layers with vascular and neurological supports, more than 30 muscles and a vast web of ligaments and tendons. These all help the hand in acquiring the myriad postures to carry out the countless tasks in daily life.

The skin creases on palm and figures can serve as the rough landmarks for underlying joints and certain notable structures. The transverse carpal ligament lies at the base of the hand with its proximal boundary at the distal wrist crease. The distal palmar crease lies over the metacarpophalangeal joints of middle, ring and little fingers, and proximal palmar crease over the metacarpophalangeal joints of the index finger. The crease over the proximal interphalangeal joint more or less indicates the position of the underlying PIP joint, and that overlying the distal interphalangeal indicates the position of underlying DIP joint.

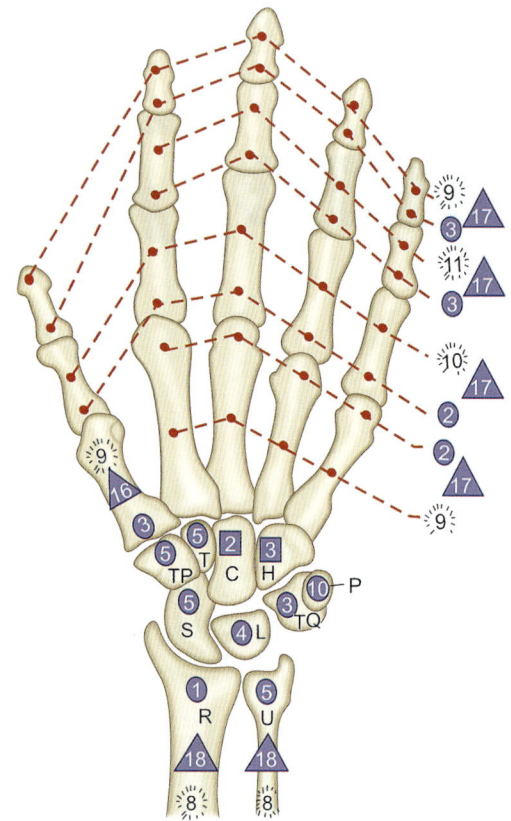

Fig. 7.1: Ossification of bones of wrist and hand; dotted circle denotes primary centre in week (IUL), complete circle denotes secondary centre in years; triangle denotes fusion of epiphysis in years.

Crude movements of the hand are controlled by the long extrinsic tendons coming from the forearm. *The basic controlling nerves for the crude functions are the radial nerve* (posterior interosseous nerve), *and the median nerve. The fine movements of the hand* are basically *controlled by the intrinsic muscles of the hand.* The concerned nerve for this is primarily the *ulnar nerve, in collaboration with the median nerve.* The extrinsic long muscles, acting synergistically, extend at the metacarpophalangeal joints and flex at the interphalangeal joints. The attachment of the intrinsic muscles, specially the lumbricals and interossei, are such as to enable them to act in balanced antagonism to the main actions of the long tendons, i.e. flexing the metacarpophalangeal and extending the interphalangeal joints.

To subserve the important functions of the hand, like holding an object and/or doing fine work, the hand must be in a position of mechanical advantage. The moment the wrist is extended, grasp position of the hand starts appearing by automatic gradually increasing flexion from the little, to index finger. In this very position of the wrist, the thumb, along with the middle and index fingers, forms an important combination for fine/precision work and sensory perception. However, combined movements at the shoulder, elbow, and wrist are essential to place the hand in an optimal position for proper functioning.

In the hand, *almost no motion occurs at the third carpometacarpal joint. It forms the central stable post for the hand and its axis is used as a reference for adduction and abduction of the digits.*

The fifth carpometacarpal joint (a saddle joint) is the most mobile of the all carpometacarpal joints.

Following any immobilisation, there is a chance of progressive fibrous contraction of the ligaments, leading to stiffness. Therefore, *in immobilising the hand, the position should be such as to keep the collateral ligaments of the metacarpophalangeal and interphalangeal joints taut.* This is achieved *by flexing the metacarpo-phalangeal joint to 90° while the interphalangeal joint is kept fully extended.*

Palmar Fascia and Fibrous Sheath

The deep fascia of the palm (palmar fascia) is divisible into three portions—the parts on both sides covering the thenar and hypothenar muscles, while the tough, triangular part covers the intermediate, central one. The central portion is attached proximally to the palmaris longus tendon, and transverse carpal ligament. At the level of the metacarpal heads it divides into four slips, one for each finger. The digital nerves, vessels and the lumbrical muscles pass distally in between these slips *(lumbrical canal)*. Each slip divides into two processes, between which pass the flexor tendons. These processes diverge and proceed deeper and distally to be attached to:

- The transverse ligament connecting the metacarpal heads
- The tough fibrous flexor sheath extending from just proximal to the metacarpal heads to the distal interphalangeal joint. This sheath firmly encases the flexor tendons in the fibro-osseous tunnel in front of the phalanges. Any pathology in this tunnel affects the working of the tendon
- The two borders of the proximal phalanx and the proximal half borders of the middle phalanx.

In Dupuytren's contracture, contraction of the palmar fascia produces acute flexion at the metacarpophalangeal and interphalangeal joints, but not at the distal interphalangeal joint (as this fascia does not extend up to it).

"NO MAN'S LAND" of the hand, first described by Bunnell, is the area where both the flexor tendons of the fingers pass through a tight fibrous tunnel. It extends *between the distal palmar crease and the insertion of the flexor digitorum sublimis at the mid portion of the middle phalanx.* Repair of the tendon injuries in this zone requires meticulous technique and care.

Spaces of the Hand

From the edges of the central portion of the palmar fascia, two septae dip down to the fascia over the interossei. Hence, three spaces are created:

- Thenar space—encasing the thenar muscles
- Hypothenar space—encasing the hypothenar muscles
- Intermediate space (mid palmar space) containing the superficial palmar arch, long flexor tendons (sublimis and profundus), lumbrical muscles and the median nerve with its branches.

On the palmar aspect, the skin is tough, tight and inelastic but at the same time very sensitive, whereas that on the dorsum is delicate, loose and elastic, accommodating even the inflammatory exudates and collections due to palmar pathology (since the dorsal subcutaneous space receives most of the lymphatics from the palm).

Space of Parona

When the radial or ulnar bursa gets distended with pus, it bursts, and pus travels up the forearm between the flexor profundus anteriorly and the pronator quadratus and interosseous membrane posteriorly—*the space of Parona.* In this space, a quantity of pus can remain collected with much swelling.

Ossification of Bones of the Hand (*See* Fig. 7.1)

Carpal Bones

Each bone usually ossifies from one centre in order of appearance:

Capitate—2nd month	Trapezium—4-5 years
Hamate—3rd month	Trapezoid—4-5 years
Triquetral—3rd year	Scaphoid—4-5 years
Lunate—4th year	Pisiform—9-12 years

Metacarpal Bones

Each bone ossifies from 2 centres, one primary for the shaft, and other secondary centre for the base of the 1st and for the head of rest of the metacarpals (2nd to 5th).

Phalanges

Each phalanx ossifies from two centres, one primary for the shaft, one secondary for the proximal end.

Synovial Sheaths of Flexor Tendons (Fig. 7.2)

Synovial sheaths of the long tendons on the palmar aspect start 2.5 cm proximal to the flexor retinaculum. One, ensheathing the flexor digitorum sublimis and profundus, proceeds as common sheath up to half way along the metacarpal bones (ulnar bursa). Except for the little finger, in which it is continuous with digital synovial sheath, the rest of the sheaths end in blind diverticulae around the tendons of the ring, middle and index fingers at mid-palm level. Another sheath for the flexor pollicis longus continues along the thumb.

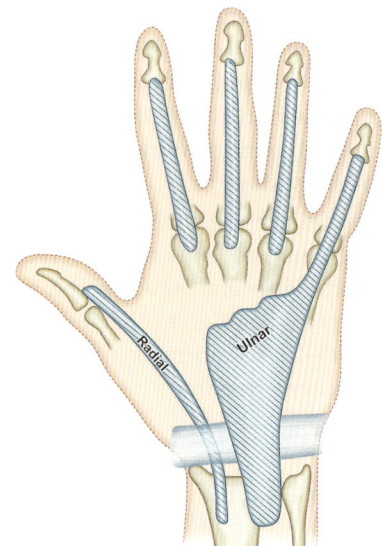

Fig. 7.2: The extent of the synovial sheaths of flexor tendons.

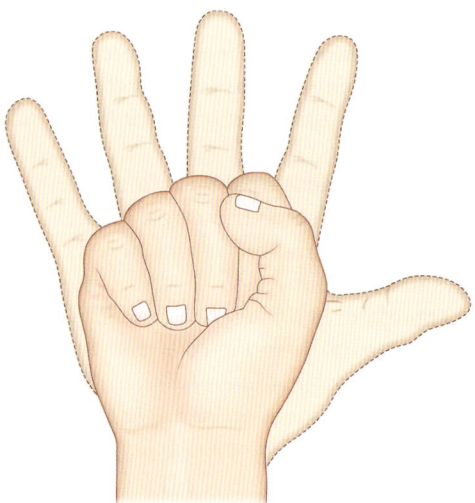

Fig. 7.3: Making a firm fist and opening of the hand with thumb and fingers extended, indicate almost normal hand.

The hand is supplied by the radial and ulnar arteries, dominantly by the latter.

■ METHODOLOGY

History Taking

(As in Chapter 1 Introduction)
The common complaints concerning the hand are pain, swelling, stiffness, deformity, weakness, and abnormal sensation. The pain may be local or referred anywhere from neck to the wrist.

Gross Assessment of Hand Functions (Figs. 7.3 and 7.4)

General and Systemic Examinations

General and systemic examinations—As described in the Chapter 1 Introduction.

Regional Examination

The cervical region, supraclavicular region, shoulder girdle, arm, elbow, forearm and wrist must be examined in any examination of the hand.

Local Examination

At the outset, the integrity of the hand should be grossly tested for. *If the patient is able to make a firm fist and open up the hand fully, and the fingers and thumb can be fully extended, it is probably a normal hand* **(Fig. 7.3)**.

Ask the patient to make a gentle fist. Observe from the back. The metacarpal heads make the proximal knuckles in the form of more or less smooth arc between index and little fingers. Depression of a knuckle indicates shortening of that metacarpal.

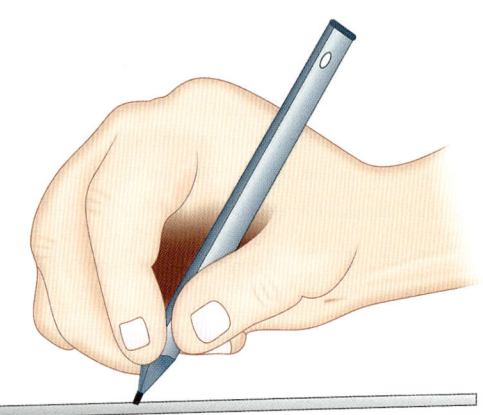

Fig. 7.4: Normal holding of a pen in writing position indicates normal intrinsics and good function of thumb and fingers.

In fully extended position of fingers, the fingertips form a regular arc with its apex at the middle finger. When the fingers flex fully, the finger-tips align at the base of the thenar eminence with the nails in the same plane.

Normally, with intact bulk of intrinsic muscles of the hand, the dorsum of hand and the web space between the thumb and index finger appear full and prominent. With the paralysis and wasting of the intrinsic muscles (e.g. after ulnar nerve lesion) the tendons and bones look more prominent on the dorsum of hand.

Jebsen-Taylor Hand Function Test: Out lines the broad assessment of the functions of hand, such as writing, card/page turning, picking up small objects, simulated feeding, stacking checkers, picking up light and heavy objects.

Prerequisites: Both the upper limbs must be comparatively assessed, in identical position, from the neck to the tips of the fingers.

Attitude and common deformities:
- Certain congenitally absent conditions (**Fig. 7.5**) or deformities of hand and finger are quite obvious, like *polydactylism*. *Polydactylism* (duplication of fingers) is a common anomaly and has been recorded even in biblical literature (3000 years ago) Many Queens of Scots also had polydactyl and it was considered as a sign of royalty (Flatt 1994). It is seen in three main types: 1. Preaxial (duplication of thumb—bifid thumb)—commoner type, 2. Central (duplication of index, middle or ring fingers), 3. Postaxial (duplication of little finger)—it is 10 times more common in Negros than Caucasians. Management mainly consists of excision of comparatively functionless digit with needed reconstruction. *Syndactylism* [(webbed or jointed fingers—It is most common congenital anomaly of hand with an incidence of one in 2,000 births, and may be hereditary. It may be complete (fingers joint from web to tip) or incomplete (fingers joined from web to any point short of tip); and simple (joined by only skin or other soft tissue) or complex (bones are also joined) (**Figs. 7.6 and 7.7**). Syndactyly mostly occurs between middle and ring fingers (*see* **Fig. 7.83**)(more than 50% of cases). In acrosyndactyly, the fingers are joined at their distal ends only. Treatment is by planned surgical separation and reconstruction at about school age. *Arachnodactyly* (= 'in the form of spider'—the fingers and toes are very long and thin, e.g. in Marfan's syndrome) or dolichostenomelia; *brachydactylism* (shortened finger); *symphalangism* (fusion of interphalangeal joint, **Fig. 7.70C**); *congenital annular grooves;* cleft hand or *lobster-claw hand* first named by J Cruveilhier (1842) and it occurs due to central deficiencies of the hand resulting from the longitudinal failure of formation of second, third or fourth ray (**Figs. 7.8 to 7.11**); *megalodactylism* (congenital hypertrophy) (**Fig. 7.12**), macrodactylism (**Figs. 7.13 and 7.14**) enlarged digits—though exact cause is not known, it may be due to abnormal blood supply or abnormal nerve supply or abnormal humoral situation) (**Fig. 7.15**); *camptodactylism* (fixed flexion deformity of the proximal interphalangeal joint, usually of little finger and mostly bilateral); *clinodactyly* [fixed contracture (usually of little finger) with angulation in radioulnar plane (*see* **Fig. 7.69**)]; *Kirner's deformity* (there is radial and palmar curving of the distal phalanx).

Brachymetacarpia (congenital shortening of the metacarpal caused by premature closure of the epiphysis.

Cleft hand is usually bilateral (**Fig. 7.11**), and is frequently associated with cleft foot, cleft lip, cleft palate and even non-cleft anomalies in cardiac and GIT systems.

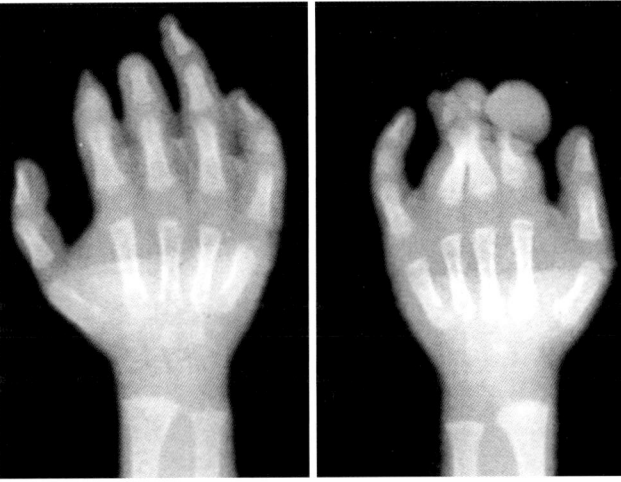

Fig. 7.6: Congenital rudimentary terminal phalanges of index and middle fingers of left hand, and distorted fusion of 3rd and 4th digits and malformations of the 2nd 3rd and 4th digits with congenital ring syndrome in right hand.

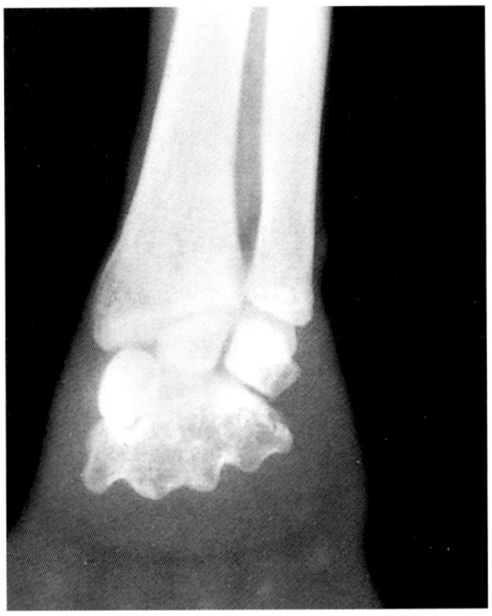

Fig. 7.5: Congenital absence of hand or digitless hand or transverse deficient hand due to severe suppression of the digital rays.

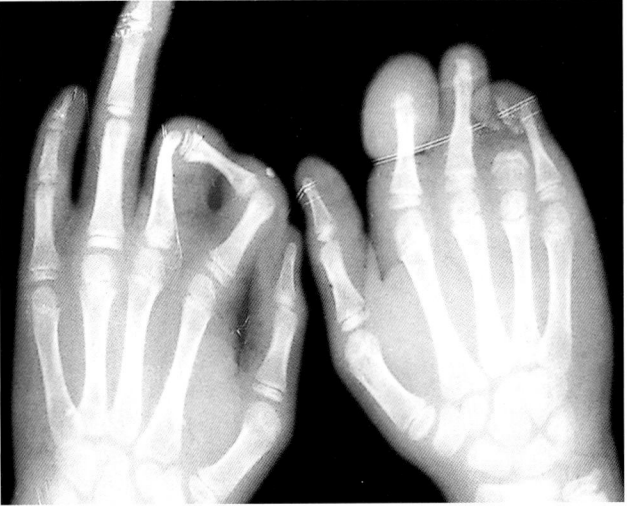

Fig. 7.7: Congenital absence of phalanges at various levels in right hand and bone-bridging between index and middle fingers of left hand.

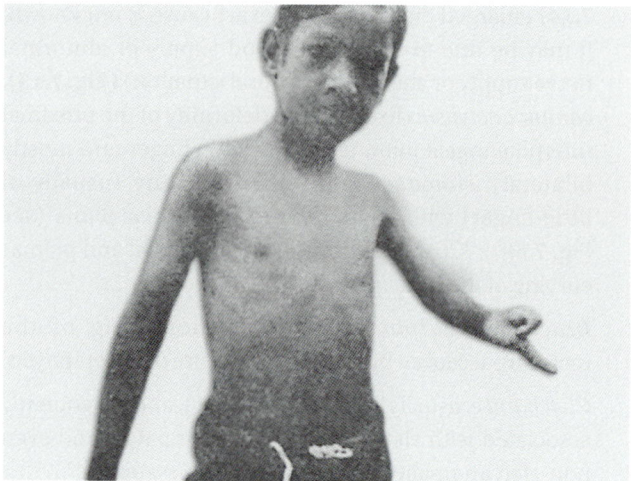

Fig. 7.8: Typical cleft hand or lobster-claw hand.

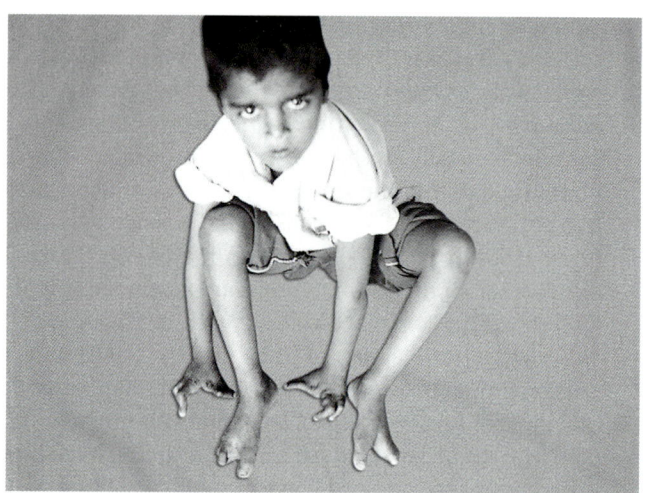

Fig. 7.11: Bilateral cleft hand (Lobster claw hand) and cleft feet.

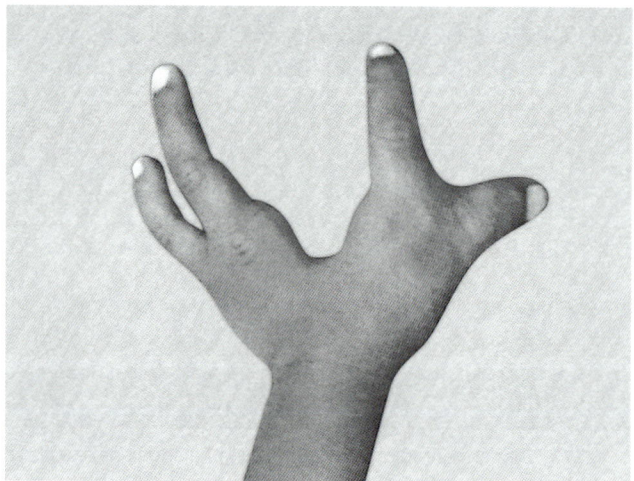

Fig. 7.9: The typical V-shaped cleft and absence of 3rd ray in lobster claw hand.

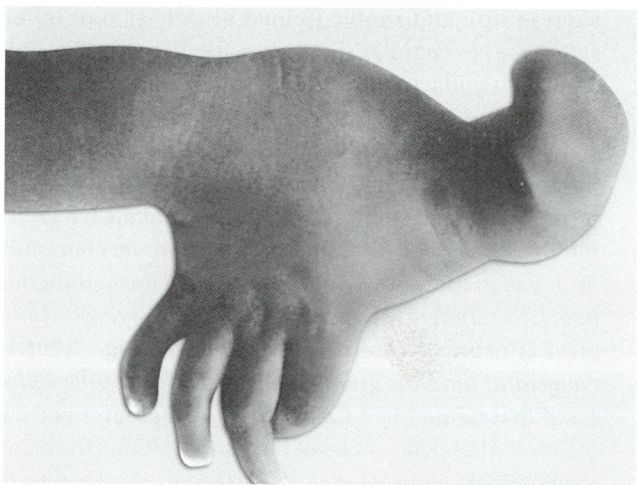

Fig. 7.12: Megalodactylism (Marked hyperplasia) of thumb and mild hyperplasia of index finger.

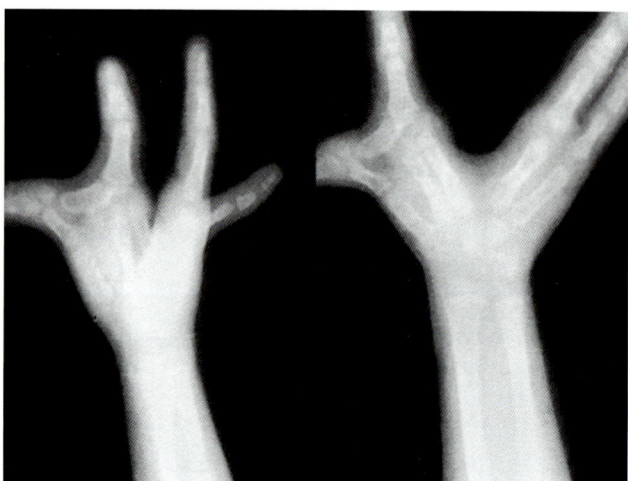

Fig. 7.10: X-ray picture of cleft hand.

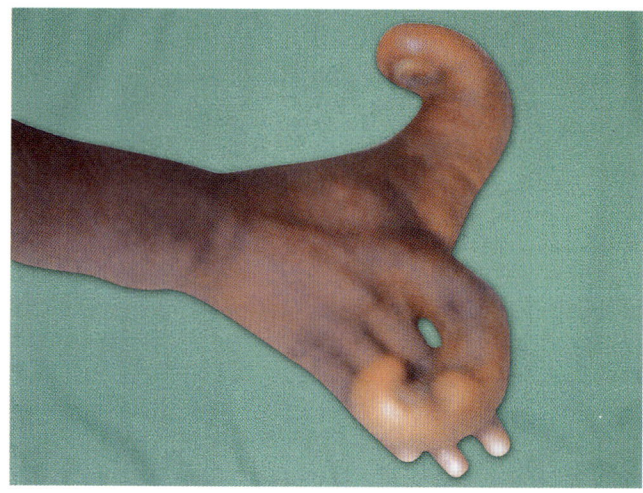

Fig. 7.13: Macrodactylism (Marked hyperplasia) of thumb and index finger.

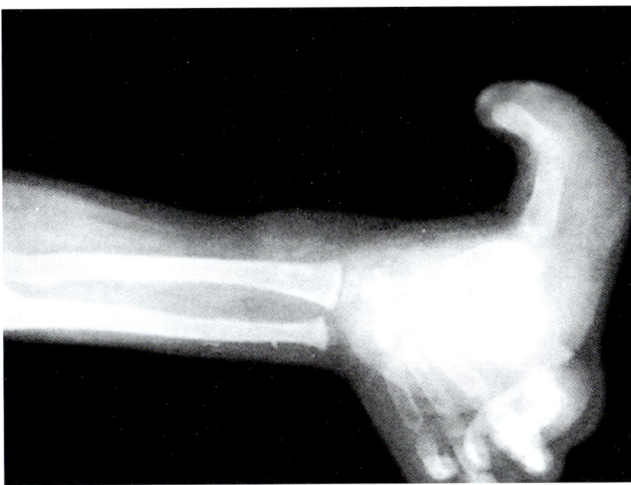

Fig. 7.14: Radiograph of same patient **(Fig. 7.13)** with macrodactylism of thumb and index finger.

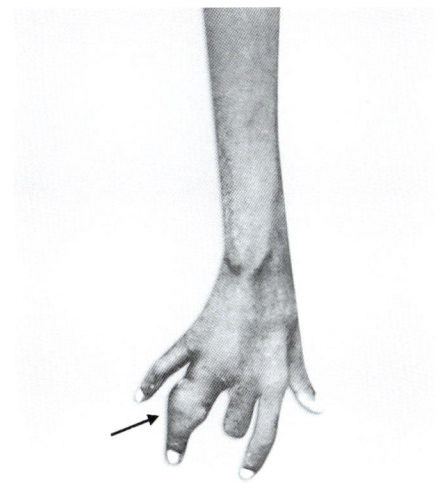

Fig. 7.17: Tuberculous dactylitis of ring finger (spina ventosa).

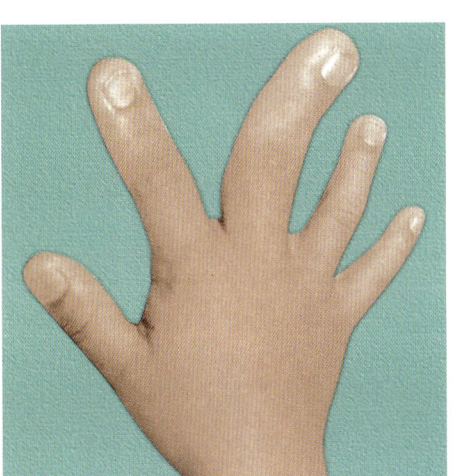

Fig. 7.15: Macrodactylism (mild to moderate) of index and middle fingers.

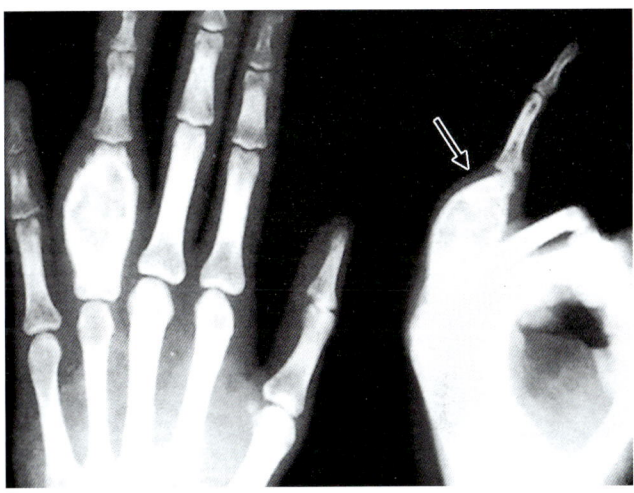

Fig. 7.18: X-ray picture—tuberculous dactylitis of ring finger (proximal phalanx).

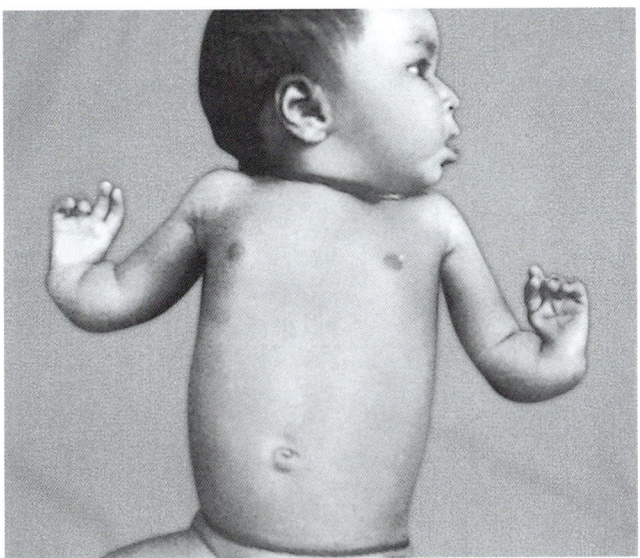

Fig. 7.16: Bilateral radial club hand.

Radial club hand (Preaxial radial hemimelia Congenital Radial deficiency – Deficiency is along the preaxial or radial side of the extremity*)* **(Fig. 7.16)** Radial club hand was first described by Petit in 1733 as bilateral club hand and absence of radii in an autopsy of a neonate (as quoted by Meht R, Thatte (2016) (absence of thumb, short index finger, entire hand deviating towards radial side, distal end of ulna quite prominent, may be associated with any deformity in the entire extremity. It may also be associated with defects in cardiovascular system, gastrointestinal tract, or genitourinary tract, aplastic anaemia and platelet defects (may be managed by centralisation of forearm and wrist and pollicisation); *ulnar club hand* (absence of small finger, ulnar deviation of the hand and wrist, short and ulnar-bowed forearm)

- Management consists of nonoperative (gradual stretching) and operative usually at about 6 month of age with an aim to centralize the wrist on the ulna.

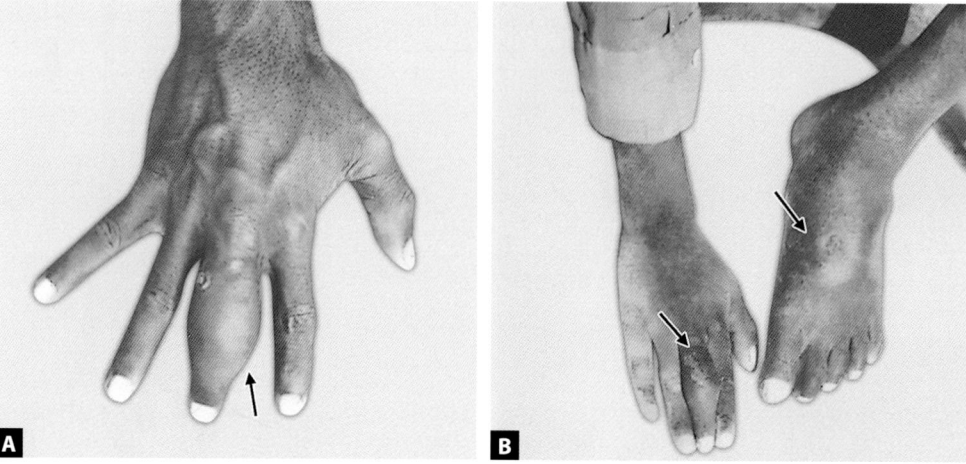

Figs. 7.19A and B: (A) Tuberculous dactylitis of right middle finger; (B) Tuberculous dactylitis of right middle finger as a part of multifocal tuberculosis, he is also having tuberculosis of left mid tarsal joints. Tuberculous infection of bone(s) of hand is not uncommon in multifocal tuberculosis—*also see* **Figs. 7.69, 7.80 and 7.81.**

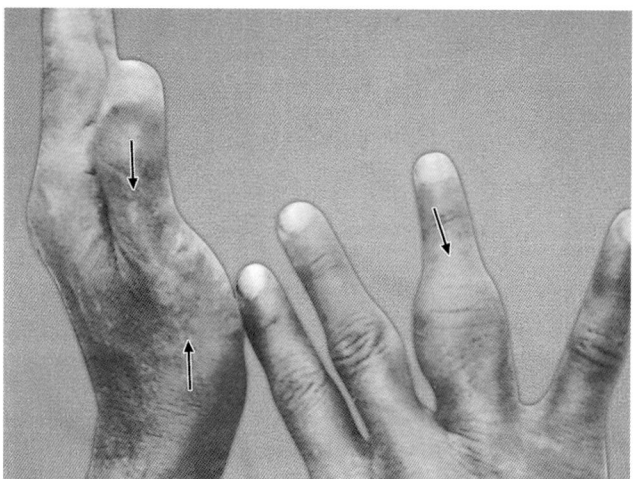

Fig. 7.20: Tuberculous dactylitis of ring finger of right hand; 3 years back he was operated for tuberculosis of metacarpo-phalangeal joint of his left hand.

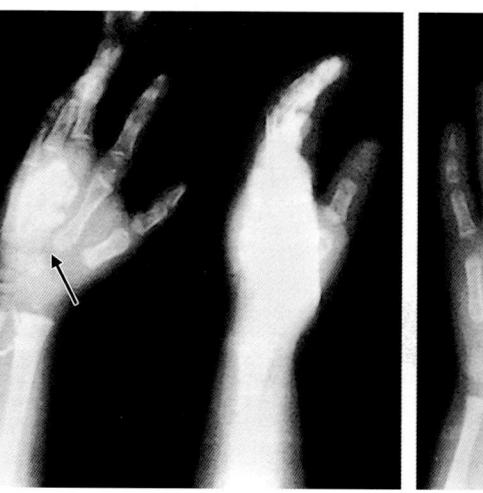

Fig. 7.22: Pyogenic dactylitis (osteomyelitis) of 3rd metacarpal.

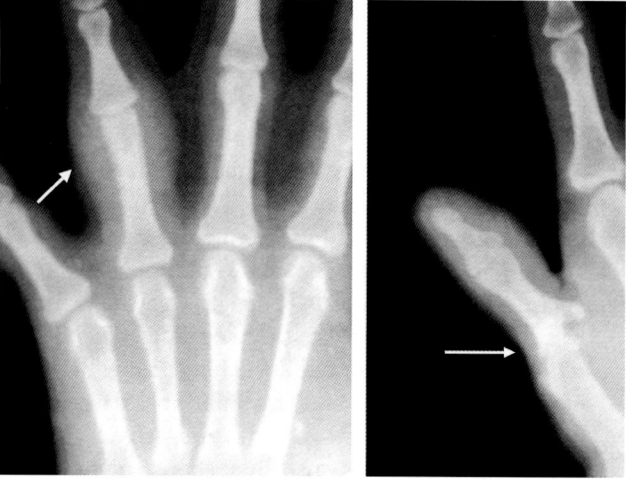

Fig. 7.21: X-ray picture of the hands shown in **Figure 7.20.**

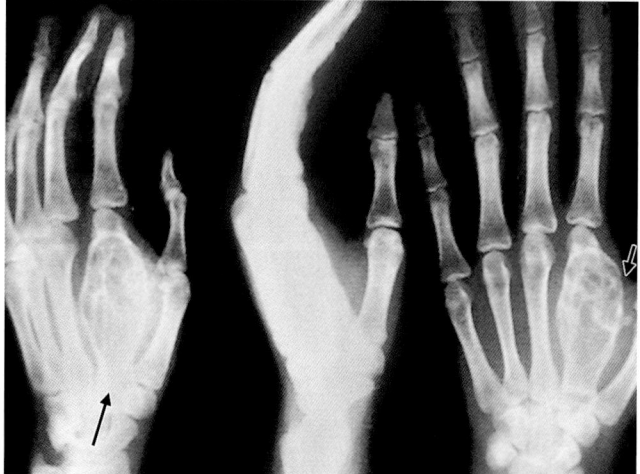

Fig. 7.23: Enchondroma of second metacarpal.

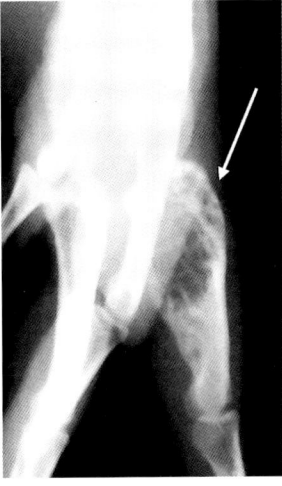 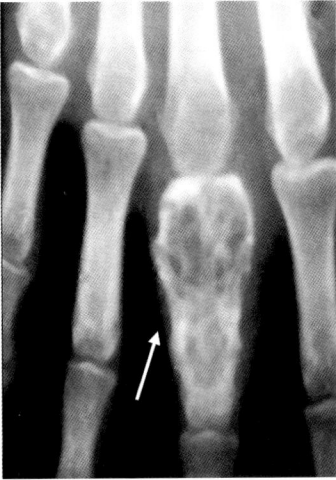

Fig. 7.24: Enchondroma of proximal phalanx of middle finger.

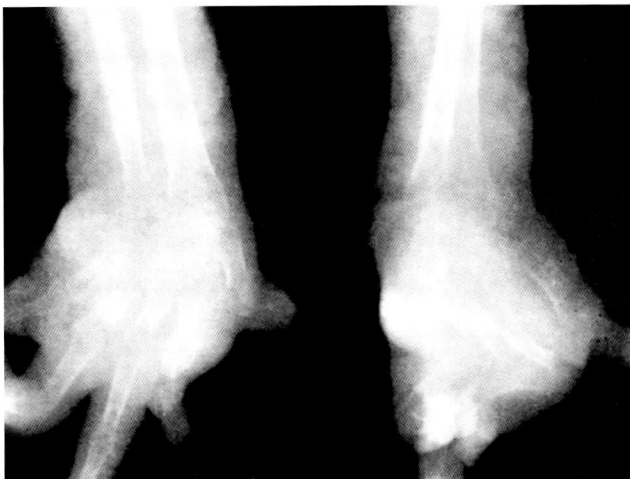

Fig. 7.26: X-ray of the same hand (mycetoma-Madura hand) shown in **Figure 7.25**. Fungal infections in the extremities may manifest as: Cutaneous infections or subcutaneous infections or deep or systemic infection. Deep infections are caused by sporotrichosis, maduromycosis coccidioidomycosis, histoplasmosis or blastomycosis. Proper medical treatment with or without surgery is necessary to manage this obstinate infection.

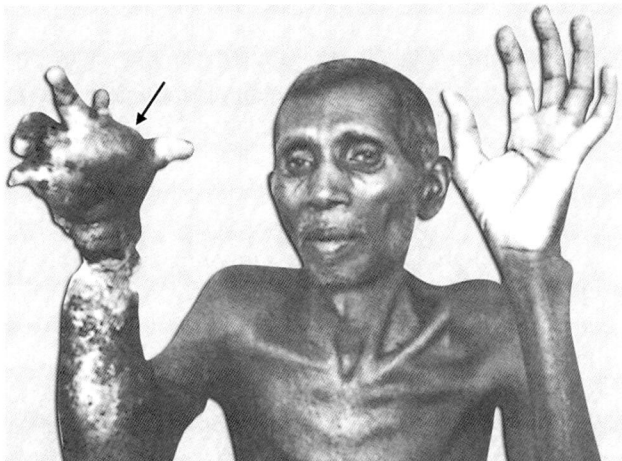

Fig. 7.25: Mycetoma of right hand—Madura hand *See also* **Figs. 15.110A, 15.111, 15.112** and the comments written below the figures.

- There may be spindle-shaped swelling at the proximal inter-phalangeal joint (rheumatoid arthritis, rupture of collateral ligaments of the joint, gout)
- Spindle-shaped swelling may occur along the phalanx, which is called *dactylitis,* e.g. in tuberculosis (spina ventosa) **(Figs. 7.17 to 7.21, 7.69 and 7.81)**, pyogenic infection **(Figs. 7.22 and 7.80)** enchondroma **(Figs. 7.23 and 7.24)**, syphilis, Madura hand **(Figs. 7.25 and 7.26)**, etc. Unless histopathologically proved, there may be confusion in proper management of dactylitis.
- Moberg (quoted by Helen et al. 2007) emphasised the importance of tactile gnosis (mystical knowledge) as the highest quality of sensibility. The fingertips are the eyes of the hand.
- Inspect and examine the profile of the terminal digit including the nail. Normally, the nail is set at an angle of about 20° with the projected line of digit the unguophalangeal angle (Lovibond angle). *Clubbing* is usually bilateral and painless. In clubbing, there

are usually three important findings—1. Floating of nail (springing back of root of nail when pressed and released), 2. Less or loss or reversal of unguophalangeal angle, 3. Increased longitudinal convexity of nail plate. Clubbing may be congenital (e.g. in cyanotic congenital heart disease, cystic fibrosis, familial); Endocrinal (e.g. in hypothyroidism); Inflammatory/Immune diseases (e.g. biliary cirrhosis, alcoholic cirrhosis, inflammatory bowel disease), Infective (e.g. in infective endocarditis, lung abscess, pulmonary tuberculosis); Vascular (e.g. in pulmonary arteriovenous malformations); Neoplastic (e.g. in lung cancer including metastatic lung cancer); Idiopathic (e.g. bronchiectasis, COPD). With proper treatment of causative disease the clubbing disappears. The tips of the fingers may present a bulbous appearance (whitlow, osteomyelitis of the terminal phalanx, hyperparathyroidism **(Figs. 7.30)**. Sometimes painless nodules develop on the interphalangeal joint, such as Heberden nodes **(Fig. 7.27)** on the distal interphalangeal joints and Bouchard nodes on the proximal interphalangeal joints. These nodules develop as a result of marginal osteophytes on the DIP and PIP joints more on the dominant hand and usually in peri- or postmenopausal women due to osteoarthritis. They are painless and very slowly progressive, without affecting the function of fingers (and hand) except sometimes slightly limiting the movements of the joint. They are hard nodules, 2–3 mm in diameter placed one on either side of midline on dorsal aspect. They may be confused with psoriasis, xanthomatosis **(Figs. 7.28 and 7.29)**, hypertrophic

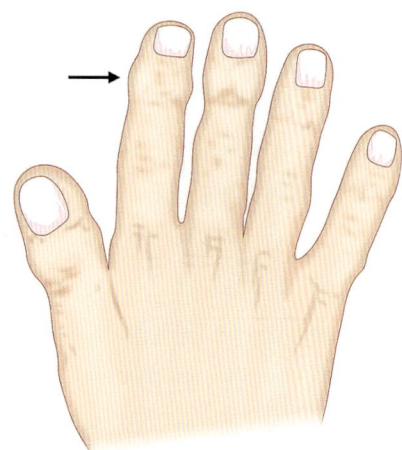

Fig. 7.27: The typical site and presentation of Heberden's node.

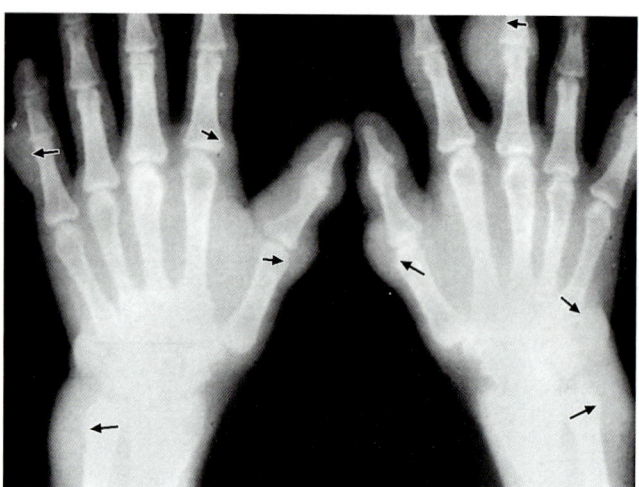

Fig. 7.29: Radiograph of synovial xanthomatosis from various joints of hand and wrist.

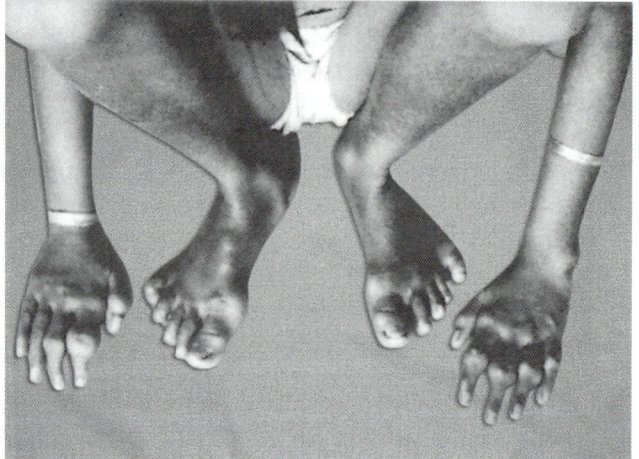

Fig. 7.28: Multiple xanthomatosis of both hands and feet. Giant cell tumour of tendon (Xanthoma) was first described by Beekman in 1915. These solid globular cellular tumour occur more frequently in hand in 1st to 7th decade of age. Multiple xanthomas may be associated with hypercholesterolemia. They are slow growing, rarely painful and benign. Histologically they contain spindle cells, fibrous tissue, cholesterol-laden histiocytes, multinucleated giant cells and hemosiderin. If needed tumour should be cleanly excised out, however, recurrence is not uncommon.

osteoarthropathy, reactive and psoriatic arthritis, hand-foot syndrome of sickle cell or sickle-thalassemia, Ollier's disease (Enchondromatosis—a developmental defect with multiple cartilaginous tumours—**Figs. 7.23 and 7.24**). The fingers may be little stiff. The spindle-shaped enlargements of the middle interphalangeal joints occur in rheumatoid arthritis

- In tendon sheath infection, the finger assumes a semiflexed position and the patient will be hesitant to extend it due to pain
- *Relation of the fingers with the thumb,* and amongst themselves and the position of the metacarpophalangeal and interphalangeal joints must be noted clearly. To evaluate the rotational alignment of the fingers, ask the patient to flex the metacarpophalangeal and the proximal interphalangeal joints and look at the alignment of the fingers. Normally, they should point towards the scaphoid bone. Subtle differences can be seen by looking at the semiflexed fingers' ends and comparing the planes of the finger-nails to those of the normal side. Even little rotational discrepancies at the base of the finger gets magnified at the finger tips leading to overlap or divergence of the digits with increasing flexion.

Look for wasting in the hands both on palmar and dorsal aspect. On the palmar aspect, look for wasting in thenar region or hypothenar region or both.

Thenar eminence is formed by opponens pollicis, abductor pollicis brevis and flexor pollicis brevis muscles—all innervated by the median nerve. Wasting in thenar eminence suggest lesion of median nerve, from higher up in its course or in carpal tunnel syndrome. There may be disuse atrophy of thenar muscle in severe osteoarthritis of first carpometacarpal joint.

Hypothenar eminence is formed by the palmaris previs, abductor digiti minimi and opponens digiti quinti—all innervated by the ulnar nerve. Wasting of this zone suggest damage of ulnar nerve. If there is wasting of both thenar and hypothenar eminences, it suggests damage of both median and ulnar nerve, or cervical myelopathy.

There are certain well-described deformities of the fingers and thumb. *Claw hand is the attitude of the hand in which the fingers become flexed at the interphalangeal joints and extended or hyperextended at metacarpophalangeal joints.*

a. *Typical claw hand develops due to paralysis of the intrinsics (ulnar,* **Figs. 7.31 and 7.32**) *or ulnar-median paralysis* **(Fig. 7.33)**. *Here, overaction of the long flexors and long extensors conjointly (predominant pull of the*

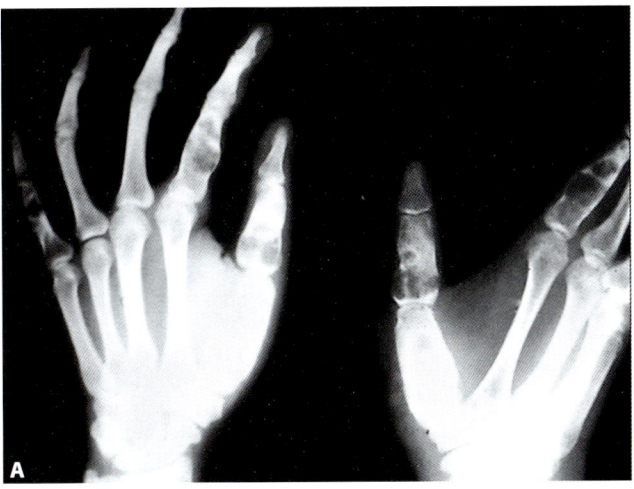
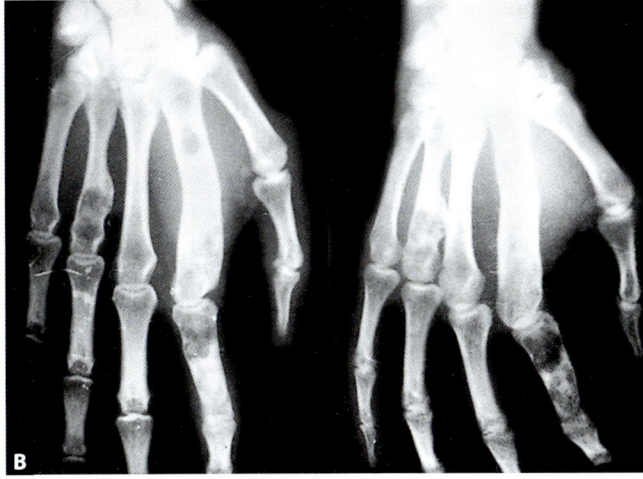

Figs. 7.30A and B: Hyperparathyroidism: In primary hyperparathyroidism (osteitis fibrosa cystica) increased production of parathyroid hormone causes bone resorption which exceeds new bone formation. It leads to hypercalcemia, hypercalciuria, hyperphosphaturia and hypophosphataemia. Usually it remains asymptomatic, except diffuse aching in muscles and bones, fatigue and weakness. Subperiosteal cysts appear in skull and long bone, which may present as tender palpable swelling *Also see* **Figure 7.72** and under-mentioned notes.

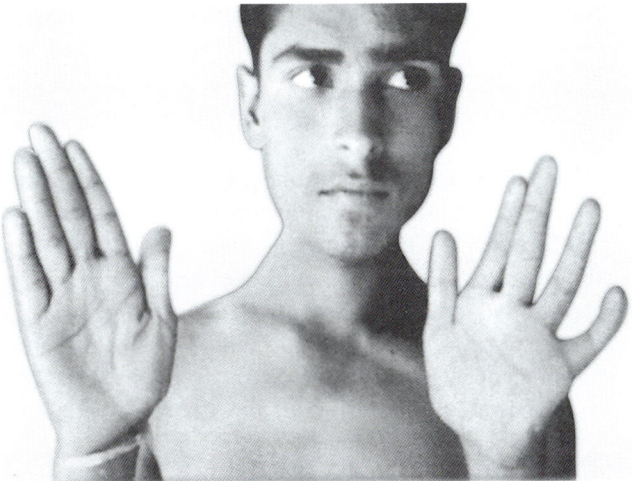

Fig. 7.31: Clawing tendency of little and ring fingers (due to ulnar nerve paralysis) patient is unable to adduct little and ring fingers.

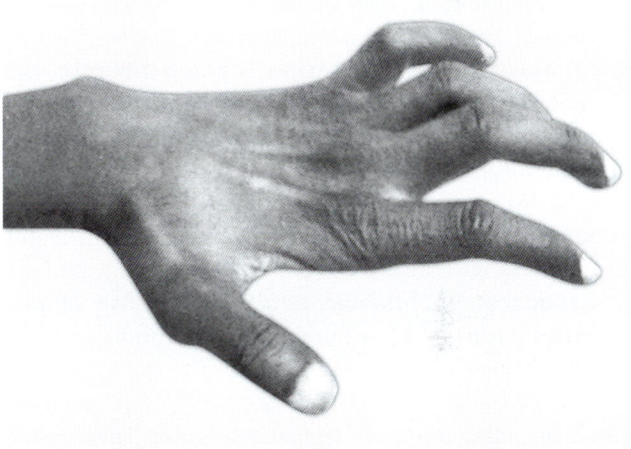

Fig. 7.33: Intrinsic minus type of claw hand due to ulnar-median nerves paralysis.

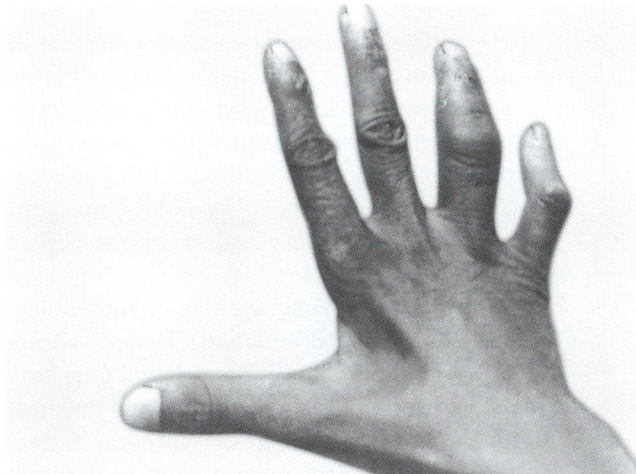

Fig. 7.32: Ulnar claw with gross wasting of first dorsal web.

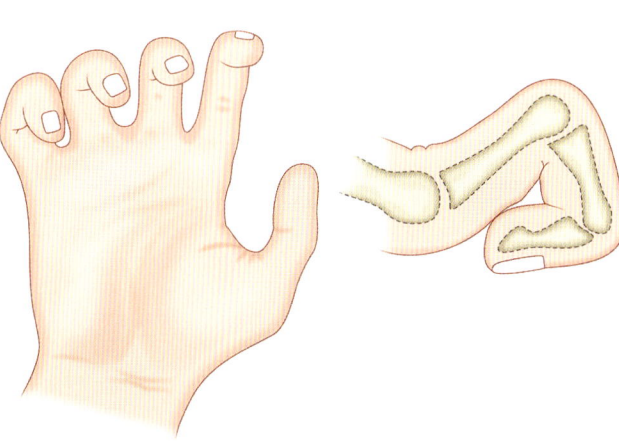

Fig. 7.34: Intrinsic minus hand.

extensor digitorum and flexor digitorum against weak or paralysed interosseus and lumbrical muscles) produce the claw hand which is of *'intrinsic minus'* type **(Figs. 7.31 to 7.34)**, e.g. in rheumatoid **(Figs. 7.74)** and leprosy **(7.75 and 7.76)**. Klumpke's paralysis, peripheral nerve injuries, syringomyelia, muscular atrophies, etc.

b. If the intrinsics are overactive, (in spasm or contracted), then the fingers present a picture which is due to overaction of the intrinsics (similar picture can be seen in less or loss of function of long tendons; skin or subcutaneous tissue contractures). The developing deformities produce an *'intrinsic plus'* hand **(Fig. 7.35)**. Basically, it is caused by intrinsic muscle tightness and contracture. Here, there will be flexion at the metacarpophalangeal joints, extension, at the interphalangeal joints and adduction of the thumb with phalangeal extension e.g. in rheumatoid hand, Volkmann's ischaemic contracture, post burn contracture, cerebral palsy (due to spasticity), trauma, fibrotic contracture following infection, Dupuytren's contracture.

The tightness of intrinsic muscles can be assessed by *Bunnell test*. In this test, the degree of passive proximal interphalangeal joint flexion is compared with the metacarpophalangeal joint in full extension (when intrinsic muscles remain stretched) and full flexion (when intrinsic muscles remain relaxed). The degree of passive proximal interphalangeal joint loss with metacarpophalangeal joint in extension indicates tightness of intrinsic muscles.

c. A concept of *'intrinsic zero'* has been developed (Srinivasan 1979), where both the lumbrical and interosseous muscles are paralysed. The extensor of the finger acts alone to produce both excessive extension of the metacarpophalangeal joint, and incomplete extension of the interphalangeal joint, thus resulting in a claw deformity.

Srinivasan (1979), has kept fingers, with paralysis of the interosseous muscle, but with functioning lumbrical, in the 'intrinsic minus' group.

Test for intrinsic plus hand: The initial or mild 'intrinsic plus' hand, which may not be producing an obvious deformity can be tested by the following method.

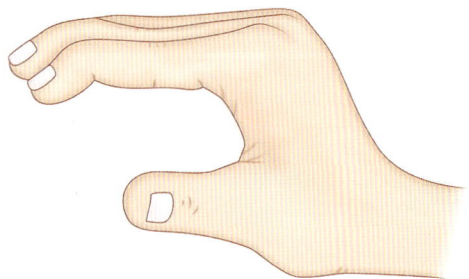

Fig. 7.35: Intrinsic plus hand.

Push the metacarpophalangeal joint into hyperextension to stretch the intrinsics. Now passively try to flex the distal interphalangeal joint. This will be very difficult, or even impossible.

Reverse intrinsic plus test: In tightness of the extensor tendon or instability of the proximal interphalangeal joint, the central slip of the extensor attachment can be relaxed by hyperextending the metacarpophalangeal joint. This allows the lateral slips to descend, resulting in flexion of the proximal interphalangeal joint.

Typical, or similar to, claw hand deformity can occur in several conditions due to lesions in:
- Cerebral cortex—cerebral palsy, tumours, hemiplegia
- Spinal cord—poliomyelitis, syringomyelia, progressive muscular atrophy, motor neuron disease
- Spinal roots (C_8 T_1) and brachial plexus—Klumpke's paralysis
- Peripheral nerves—ulnar and median nerve paralysis
- Muscular affections—myopathy
- Vascular affections—Volkmann's ischaemic contracture
- Arteriosclerotic diseases—as in Raynaud's disease and in professionals using vibrating tools
- Subcutaneous tissue and skin—congenital or burn contracture
- Miscellaneous—disuse atrophy, rheumatoid arthritis, Sudeck's osteodystrophy, post-infective contractures, post-traumatic contractures

- **Deformities of hand in rheumatoid arthritis:** Common deformities of hand in rheumatoid arthritis are:
  - Fusiform swelling (spindle-shaped) of proximal interphalangeal joints
  - Ulnar deviation of fingers with subluxation of metacarpophalangeal joint
  - Ulnar/radial deviation of wrist and ulnar deviation of fingers
  - (Severe) *Swan neck deformity* **(Figs. 7.36 and 7.37A)**: This deformity is common in rheumatoid arthritis in ladies and systemic lupus erythematosus (SLE). In SLE, swan neck deformity is usually reducible—a Jaccound deformity. In this condition, there is flexion at the distal interphalangeal joint and hyperextension at the proximal interphalangeal joint, producing a deformity resembling a swan's neck. It is caused by muscle imbalance and may be passively correctable depending upon the fixity of primary and secondary deformities.
  - *Boutonniere deformity:* Button hole or boutonniere deformity **(Figs. 7.37B and 7.38)**: Due to rupture of the central slip of dorsal expansion of finger the lateral bands drop volar to the axis of the proximal interphalangeal joint. Then they become flexors of the proximal interphalangeal joint as the joint buttonholes through the rupture. Here there is flexion

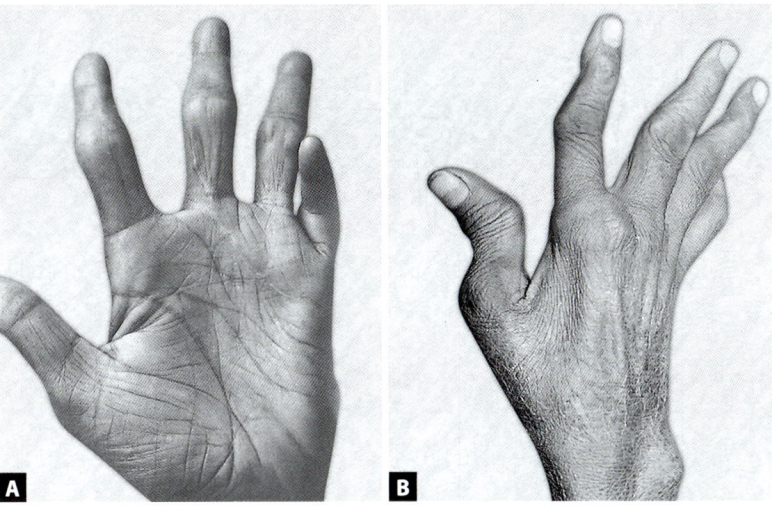

Figs. 7.36A and B: (A) Rheumatoid arthritis, (B) Bizarre combination of deformities in fingers, thumb and wrist.

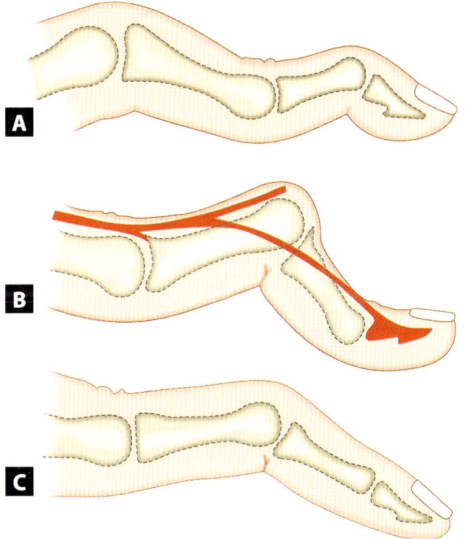

Figs. 7.37A to C: Deformities of finger: (A) Swan neck deformity; (B) Boutonniere deformity; (C) Hooding deformity.

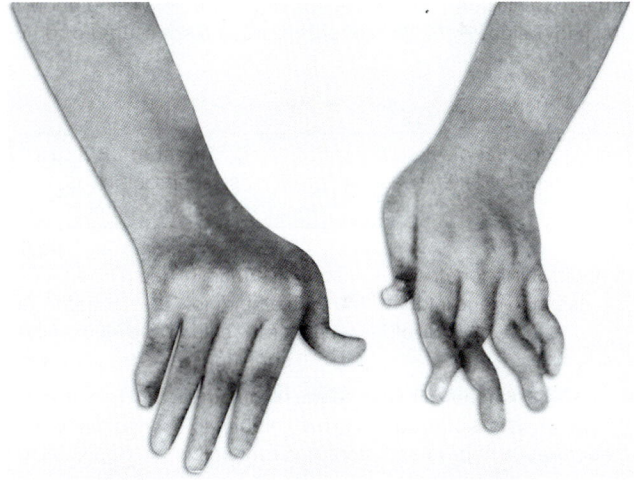

Fig. 7.38: Typical rheumatoid hand. Note ulnar deviation at wrist, swan neck deformity of fingers, boutonniere deformity of right little finger, ulnar deviation of fingers.

deformity at the proximal interphalangeal joint and hyperextension at the distal interphalangeal joint voluntary extension cannot be done (e.g. rheumatoid arthritis). Extension followed by flexion of proximal interphalangeal joint may produce a palpable and/or audible click, as the lateral bands of the distal extensor tendon diverge and slip laterally over the head of proximal phalanx.
- Piano-key ulnar head following destruction of ulnar collateral ligament.
- Sometimes bizarre deformities develop in hands and feet (*see* **Figs. 7.73 and 7.74**)
- Peculiar swellings in rheumatoid hand (**Figs. 7.39A to C**)
- Finger drop (**Fig. 7.40**) due to spontaneous rupture of the extensor tendon, usually at the wrist (e.g. rheumatoid arthritis)

- Hooding deformity (in leprosy, **Fig. 7.37C**): It consists of flexion at the proximal interphalangeal joint and either straight or hyperextended position of the distal interphalangeal joint
  Test for the presence of hooding deformity—Passively extend the fingers at the proximal interphalangeal joints and then attempt flexion of the distal interphalangeal joints. In the extended position, the distal joint presents marked resistance to flexion, whereas in flexed position of the proximal interphalangeal joint, it flexes easily
- Diabetic hand (diabetic cheiropathy): In chronic longstanding diabetes, the soft tissues of hands become thick and contracted and the fingers get slightly flexed- Ask the patient to place both palms together—a space will remain between the palms and fingers—a 'prayer position sign'

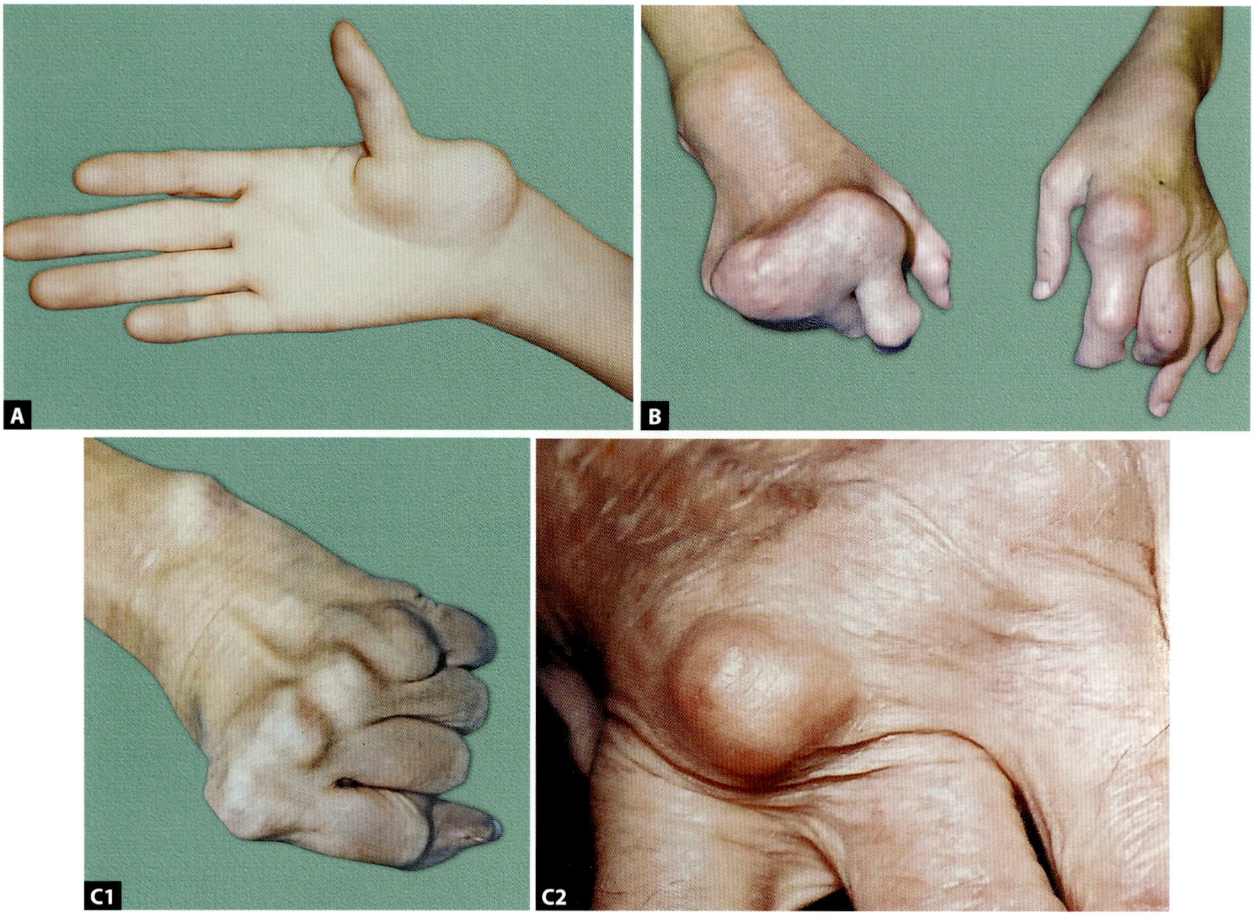

190 Hand

Figs. 7.39A to C: Peculiar swelling and deformities of MP joints in rheumatoid hands.
(By courtesy pictures provided by Sabana – GNHHC Charles A Goldfarb. My Washington University BIO)

- **Attitudes and deformities due to peripheral nerve paralysis:**
  - *Wrist drop:* In complete radial nerve paralysis, there is obvious wrist drop. Here the patient cannot dorsiflex the wrist; he cannot abduct the thumb, nor can he extend the thumb and the fingers at the metacarpophalangeal joint. The attitude of the hand remains in palmar-flexion.
  - *Benediction attitude (Preacher's hand):* In median nerve paralysis, the attitude of the hand may be typical. In long standing cases, there may be ape thumb besides wasting of the thenar eminence (Simian thumb). In this condition, the thumb lies in the same plane as that of the fingers and palm, like that of an ape. If the patient is asked to make a fist, the index finger remains prominently extended (Benediction attitude/pointing index).
  - *Claw hand:* In *ulnar nerve paralysis*, besides wasting of hypothenar eminence, the webs, as well as the intermetacarpal spaces (which are prominent from the dorsal aspect of the hand) the typical attitude of 'claw hand' develops, affecting the little and ring fingers. *When the affection of ulnar and median*

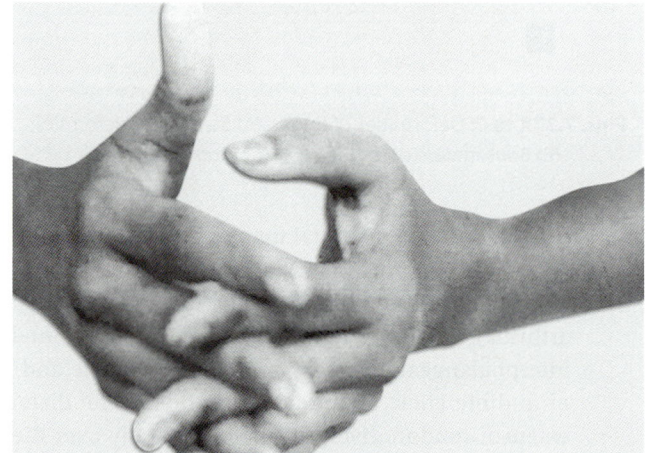

Fig. 7.40: Drop thumb deformity (left) due to rupture of extensor pollicis longus tendon in old rheumatoid arthritis (also called *Drummer's palsy* when it occurs in malunited Colles fracture due to friction attrition on the tendon). It is also called *saluting hand*—based on position of hand in American military salute—in which the thumb is simply-flexed in palm and cannot be voluntarily extended (based on description in De Gowin's Diagnostic Examinations, 2011). It is also called Mallet thumb deformity, Goose neck deformity or Flexon deformity of thumb.

nerves are combined (e.g. in leprosy), *clawing of all the four fingers* develops **(Figs. 7.41 and 7.42)**.

Dupuytren's Contracture (Figs. 7.43 to 7.47)

- *Dupuytren's disease is a benign fibroproliferative disease of unknown aetiology.* The proliferative fibroplasia of subcutaneous palmar tissue occurs in the form of nodules and cords leading to secondary progressive irreversible flexion contracture of finger joints. Gradually, there is thinning of the subcutaneous fat. The skin gets adhered followed by its pitting or dimpling. The superficial transverse palmar ligaments are not affected, only the longitudinal pretendinous bands of the palmar fascia are involved.

The Dupuytren's disease progresses through several stages—mainly being three—proliferative, involutional, and residual. It is often familial. Though not authentically proved, TGF-β1 has been implicated in Dupuytren's disease, suggesting that it may represent a candidate susceptibility gene for this condition, however, the responsible gene could not be identified as yet. Various risk factors, such as age (40-60 years), gender (male 10 times more), smoking, over alcohol intake, diabetes, cirrhosis of liver, lipid disorder (hyperlipidaemia), manual labour (working on vibratory tool), etc. have been implicated in the aetiopathology.

This disease commonly affects Northern European Caucasian men—the natives or the descendants. Dupuytren's contracture occurs in adults (40-60 years) and mostly in men (10 times more than females)

The earliest record of the disease was noted in the Icelandic sagas, in which during 12th and 13th centuries four miracle cures of putative Dupuytren's disease were effected by priests in Orkney and Iceland. *The first written description* was by Platter of Basel Switzerland in 1614, where he noted how in the hands of a master mason the tendons of ring and little fingers ceased to function. In 1777, Henry Cline proposed "palmar fasciotomy" as a cure for Dupuytren's contracture and his suggestion stands more or less true even today.

Dupuytren's contracture is the progressive contracture of the fingers due to contraction of the palmar fascia: Guillaume Dupuytren published his findings in 1831 in lancet and since then his name has been associated with this condition. Baron Dupuytren (1833) was the first to identify the cause and perform successful surgical release. Nontender, nodular thickening in the palmar fascia precedes actual contracture of fascia.

It may be associated with *Peyronie's disease* (fibrous contracture in plantar fascia leading to deformities—plantar fibromatosis)—a form of autosomal dominant disease with a high incidence of (about 80%) Dupuytren's disease, knuckle pads, *Ledderhose's disease* (fibrous contracture of penis, plastic induration of penis).

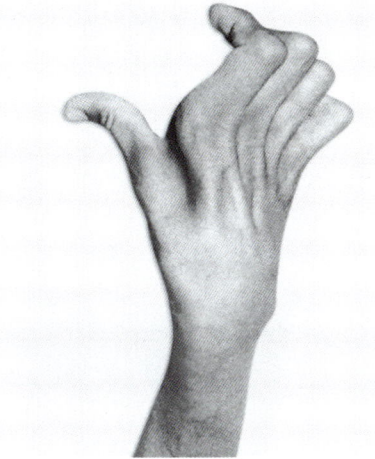

Fig. 7.41: Complete claw—combined ulnar and median nerve affections. Note the wasting of the webs.

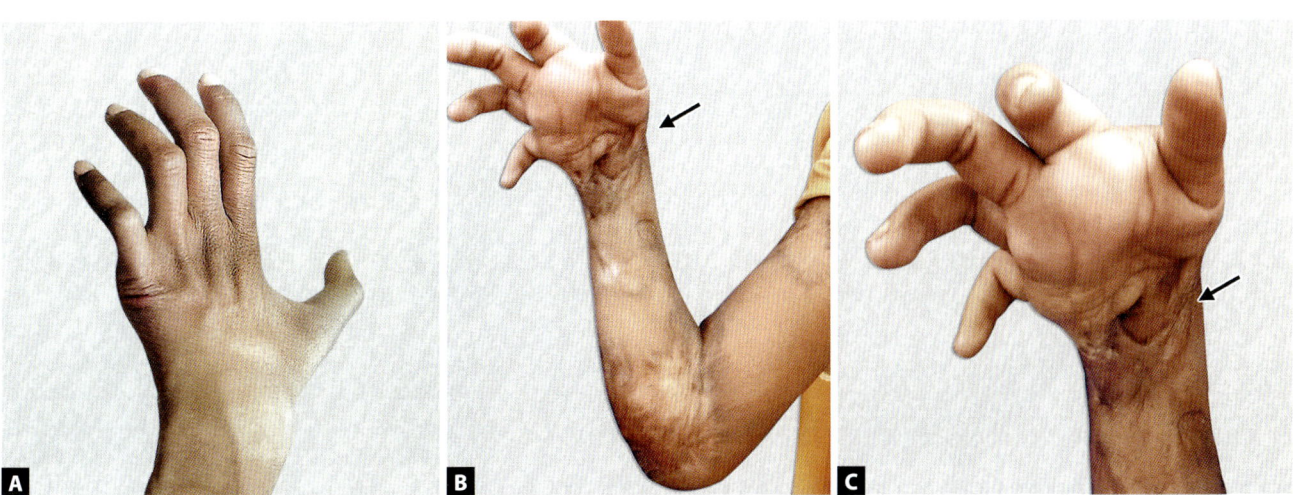

Figs. 7.42A to C: (A) Complete claw—thumb is also affected. Note the wasting of the webs; (B and C) Claw hand type deformity produced due to burn in lower region of forearm.

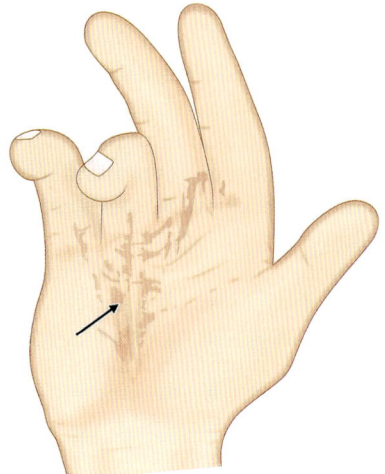

Fig. 7.43: Dupuytren's contracture.

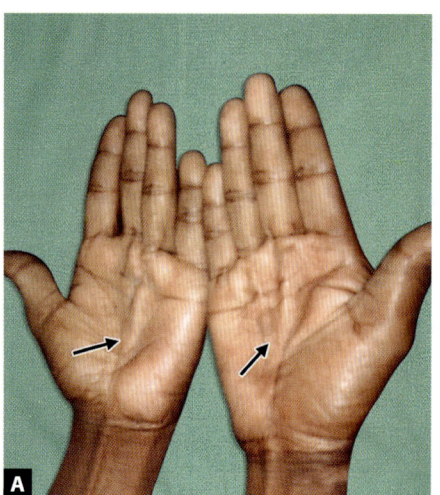

Figs. 7.44A and B: (A) Early Dupuytren's contracture in both palms; (B) Dupuytren's contractures with nodulation.

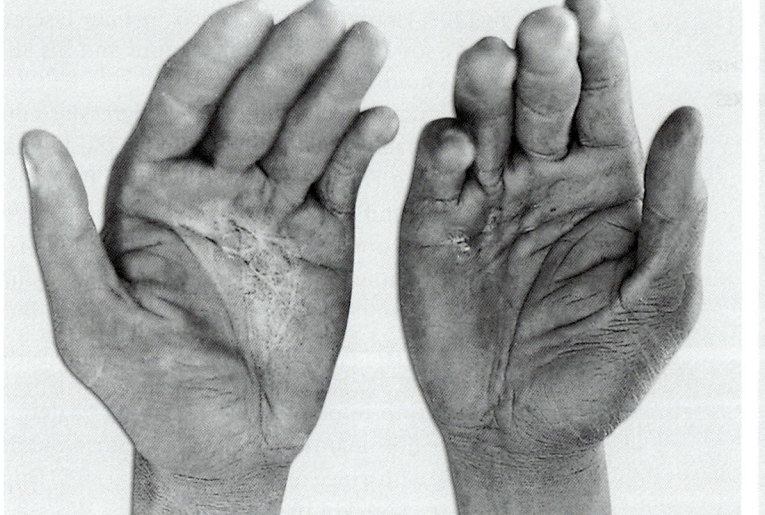
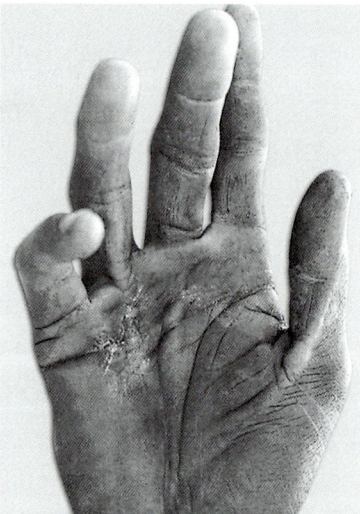

Fig. 7.45: Dupuytren's contracture in both hands. The thumb of right hand is also affected.

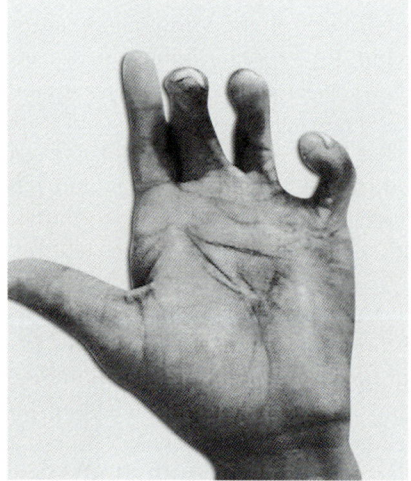

Fig. 7.46: Dupuytren's contracture of left hand with middle, ring and little fingers markedly affected but affection of index finger is in early stage.

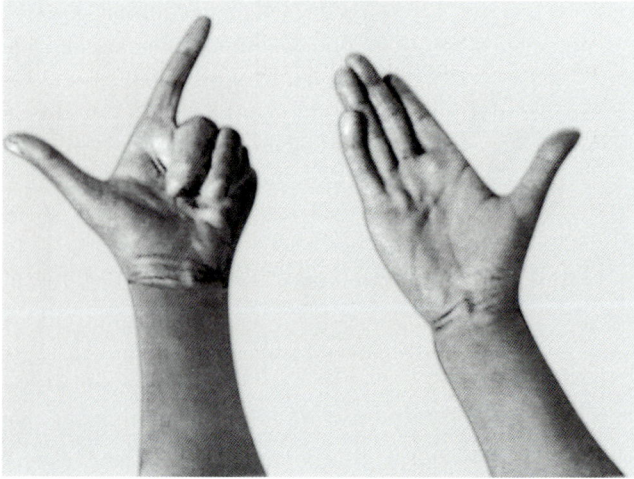

Fig. 7.47: Dupuytren's contracture in both hands—left is markedly affected with three fingers acutely flexed. On the right hand there is initial stage of affection of little, ring and middle fingers.

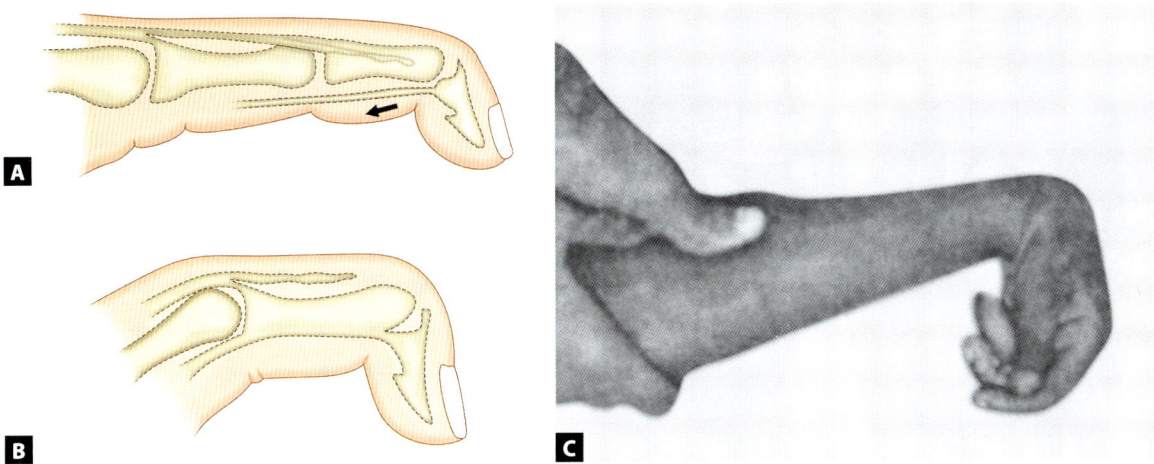

Figs. 7.48A to C: (A) Mallet finger; (B) Mallet thumb; (C) Thumb-in-palm deformity due to cerebral palsy.

The initial stage can be apparent in *'table top sign'*, i.e. ask the patient to keep the palm flat on the table, the affected finger will not touch the table all through and stands buckled back. There may be clawing tendency of the fingers but here the flexion element mainly prevails at the metacarpophalangeal joint and the proximal interphalangeal joint and rarely, the distal interphalangeal joint. This usually affects the ring finger but the little, middle, index or even thumb may also be affected in that order

Early cases may be treated by local corticoid injections and stretch-physiotherapy; more advance cases by needle aponeurotomy (percutaneous by sectioning fascial contracture with sharp edged bevel of wide bore needle followed by stretching of finger; and severe cases by planned surgical excision.

- There is a typical attitude of the *hand in brachial palsy*. In the distal type (i.e. Klumpke's type (C_8, T_1) the hand is in intrinsic minus claw hand position. In the proximal type (i.e. Erb's palsy), the hand remains in policeman's tip position, i.e. shoulder adducted and internally rotated, elbow extended, forearm pronated, wrist partially flexed, thumb in palm and fingers semiflexed
- *Mallet finger* **(Fig. 7.48A)**: It results from avulsion or rupture of the extensor digitorum tendon at the base of the terminal phalanx. Due to unopposed action of the flexor digitorum profundus, the finger gets flexed at the distal interphalangeal joint, and cannot be voluntarily extended
- *Mallet thumb* (Goose neck deformity) **(Fig. 7.48B)**: Mallet thumb results from rupture of the extensor pollicis longus tendon (usually a late complication of Colles' fracture, rheumatoid arthritis)

Trigger finger (locking finger or snapping finger): Trigger finger was first described by Notta in 1850, who coined the term 'Notta's nodule as the palpable thickening in the flexor tendon overlying the metacarpophalangeal joint. The annual incidence is reported to be about 28 cases/100 000 population (Storm 1977).

The *trigger finger* may be even congenital in neonate or acquired in infant (in first weeks to months) or in toddlers or adults (usually a female in her forties). It is generally caused by non-bacterial inflammation or repetitive trauma and swelling of the flexor tendon sheath. It causes compression of the tendon in the osteofibrotic tunnel at the level of the A_1 or A_2 pulley. Initially, the flexor muscles are strong enough to force the flexor tendon through the diminished lumen of the tunnel. Gradually, the tendon develops a constriction under the tendon sheath and due to repeated milking effect a bulging nodule develops proximal to it. Subsequently the sheath is thickened and nodule gets fixed due to fibrous changes. The patient may feel a firm nodular (knot) swelling in palm which may be the thickened zone in the first annular part of the flexor sheath or a nodule in the tendon just distal to it. The examiner can feel the nodule and its movement with the tendon.

The *trigger may be of 'primary type'* which is most common and may occur in otherwise healthy persons as well. *'Secondary trigger finger'* develops in conditions such as rheumatoid arthritis, diabetes, Dupuytren's disease, partial tendon lacerations, inflammatory arthropathies and metabolic disorders.

Due to fibrotic thickening and constriction of the fibrous flexor sheath of the long tendons, the patient (usually a female in her forties or more), complains of pain at the root of thumb or a finger with or without locking or clicking of the finger/or thumb in flexion. Any digit may be affected but thumb is commonly affected (30 to 60%) followed by the index, ring, middle and little in that order. Bilateral trigger thumbs occurs in about 25% of the time. If hand is opened up from a clenched position, then the

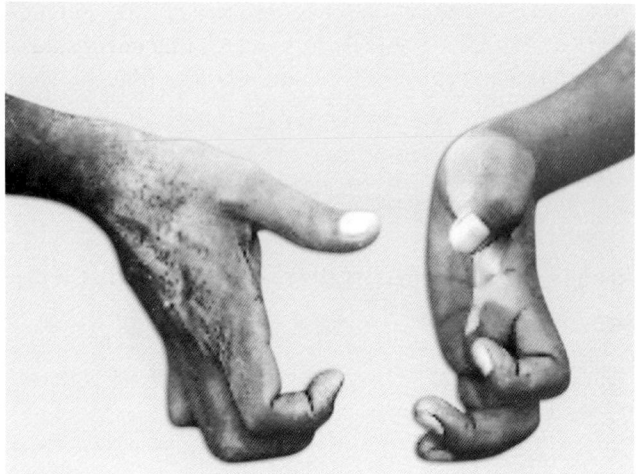

Fig. 7.49: Jersey thumb.

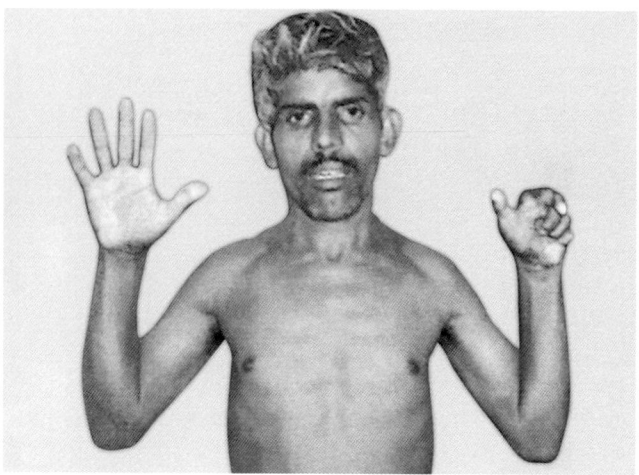

Fig. 7.50: Neglected spastic flexion deformities of fingers are is of left hand in residual hemiplegia.

affected finger remains flexed. With more forceful effort or while passively opening by other hand, it may be extended with a jerky release and often with a palpable and/or audible click. A firm tender nodule is felt in front of the metacarpophalangeal joint. It may be bilateral. Trigger thumb has been seen to produce locked flexion effect in babies (misdiagnosed as dislocation).

Management of trigger finger may be *non-invasive* (conservative), e.g. by immobilising splints, ultrasounds or pulsed electromagnetic energy; *semi-invasive,* such as local corticoids infiltration, percutaneous tenolysis; or *invasive* (surgical decompression of the constricted tendon sheath)

- *Jersey finger:* It results from avulsion of the flexor digitorum profundus (usually of ring finger, but any digit may be involved) from its insertion on the distal phalanx. It usually occurs in young males playing football and rugby. In an attempt of grasping the jersey of any opponent player, the distal interphalangeal joint is forcibly extended **(Fig. 7.49)**
- *Thumb-in-palm deformity* (**Fig. 7.48C**): It is usually seen in patients of cerebral palsy and cerebrovascular accident (stroke). The thumb is adducted and flexed into the palm, and this tendency is exaggerated by any activity.

There is flexion spasticity and contracture of the flexor pollicis longus and at times also the flexor pollicis brevis and the abductor pollicis brevis.

Sakellarides and Mitall (1984) have classified this deformity into four types. Thus, it can be due to:
- Weak or paralysed extensor pollicis longus
- Spasticity or contracture of the adductor pollicis.
- Weakness or paralysis of the abductor pollicis longus
- Spasticity or contracture of the flexor pollicis longus.

In neglected hemiplegia, there may be spastic flexion deformities of fingers **(Fig. 7.50)**.

The main aim of managing this deformity (usually by surgery) is to improve the grasp and restore the lateral or key pinch.

Bowler's Thumb (After Calandruccio JH 2013): In a regular bowler, there is possibility of repeated compression of the ulnar-side digital nerve of thumb while grasping the ball for bowling. Due to repeated compression trauma perineural fibrosis develops in the nerve which may be palpable as the markedly tender swelling. The patient complains of tingling and hyperaesthesia in the pulp of thumb, with atrophy in distal part. In the early stage, avoiding of bowling and use of protective shield or splint would help. In persistent problem, neurolysis and dorsal transfer of nerve may be needed.

Inspection

The domain of the hand starts from the distal transverse crease in front of the wrist to the finger tips. Inspect both the hands in symmetrical position. Note the *number of fingers* (if more than five—supernumerary finger); *relative length of fingers and hand* [(Marfan's syndrome—described by French paediatrician Marfan in 1896 who named it dolichostenomelia (= long, thin limb)—and is characterised by long thin limbs, generalised joint laxity, dislocation of lenses, dissecting aortic aneurysm, prolapsed cardiac valves, increased prevalence of hernia,—spider fingers and toes— the fingers and toes are very long and thin—arachnodactyly (= in the form of a spider)]; The Thumb sign (Steinberg sign), as described by Falk (1995) may be positive in Marfan's syndrome—here when the fingers are clenched over the thumb, the end of thumb protrudes beyond the ulnar margin of the hand; achondroplasia—trident hand—fingers are short, stubby and equal in length); and size of the fingers (in gigantism, the hand and fingers are enlarged and elongated). *Note the shape; size; normal anatomical bulges and creases,* e.g. hypothenar eminence, thenar eminence, hollow of the palm, creases across the palm (in Down's syndrome there is only one palmar crease), creases on the finger and finger pulps; the *web condition* (e.g. for syndactylism, club hand) and presence of any *nodule*. Skin should be inspected for its colour, texture and for presence of callosities. Inspect the *tips of the fingers and thumb,* regarding shape, presence of any deformity, atrophy, broadening, and also the *nailbeds* (shape, colour, brittleness, atrophy or degeneration of nails).

All dimensions of the hands are increased in Acromegaly and Gigantism. The overgrowth of soft tissue increases the girth of fingers and thickens the palm resulting in a paw or spade hand. In a congenital deformity called hemihypertrophy, an entire side of the body is enlarged. Due to congenital arteriovenous fistula of the upper limb local gigantism may occur. In both these conditions (*hemihypertrophy* and *local gigantism*) the hand is normally proportioned.

On the *dorsum of the hand* look for any swelling, condition of venous arches, knuckle (alignment and prominence when patient makes a fist), interosseous spaces and the webs.

The phalanges and joints of the fingers, and hand should be inspected from all aspects.

Inspect the hand with fully extended and fully flexed fingers. The *fully flexed fingers normally point towards the scaphoid, and their nails lie in one plane.* Note any abnormality.

Palpation

Superficial Palpation

Feel for the *texture* and, *sensation of the skin* (hypoaesthesia, hyperaesthesia, paraesthesia or anaesthesia).

Palpate the *finger pulps* for texture and/or tenderness and *nailbeds* for refilling of capillaries and for any tenderness.

Palpate the *webs* individually (specially the first web) and note its bulk, looseness and stretchability.

Deep Palpation

Feel for any abnormality, specially for thickening and deep tenderness in the palm, the webs, the metacarpals (from dorsal and palmar aspects), the metacarpophalangeal joints, the interphalangeal joints, the phalanges and the fingers and thumb tips.

In **glomus tumour,** (first described by Wood in 1812) pain, cold sensitivity and point tenderness are characteristic features. Masson (1924) almost defined a "glomus tumor" as that arises from a normally occurring neuromyoarterial apparatus which regulates temperature. They occur more often in hand, usually beneath the finger nail. [Glomus tumour is a well-circumscribed vascular tumour composed of a few blood vessels lined with normal endothelial cells and surrounded by a solid proliferation of round cells with uniformly sized round nuclei and scanty eosinophilic cytoplasm. The characteristic epithelioid cell of glomus tumor is derived from the pericyte of Zimmermann. There is excruciating pain if pointed pressure by a small firm object is applied on the overlying nail *(Love test)*. Meticulous complete excision of this encapsulated lesion, usually, cures it. Abnormal findings (like swellings, ulcers) must be examined thoroughly.

Feel for presence of any nodule in the line of tendons, mainly at the base of the thumb and finger, specially ring and middle—trigger thumb or finger. To confirm regarding its fixity to the tendon, ask the patient to contract the concerned tendon and ascertain the fixity of the nodule to it. On deep pressure, the nodule is tender.

Infections of the hand may remain masked for varying periods. The clinical course of hand infections is usually guided by anatomical, local and systemic factors, besides the type and virulence of bacteria. Since the fascial spaces are quite closed and tight and the skin of the palm is quite thick and tough, pus usually takes a long time to come on the surface. The manifestations are usually:

- Constitutional features
- Swelling on the dorsum of hand
- Throbbing pain in the hand

Depending upon the place for pus collection, the site of maximum tenderness can be localised **(Fig. 7.51)**. In whitlow **(Figs. 7.51 and 7.79)**, which usually develops after a puncture wound beneath the nail, there is usually not much swelling but distal nail bed becomes red and extremely painful. Maximum tenderness is at the area proximal to the free edge of nail plate at the pulp of the terminal phalanx; In *Felon* **(Fig. 7.52)** (an abscess of the finger tip pulp) the infection of the finger pad is confined within small fascial compartments attached to periosteum. The finger tip is swollen with dull pain, which becomes intense and throbbing with exquisite tenderness. With development of pus, the pulp becomes indurated. Osteomyelitis of terminal phalanx may develop **(Figs. 7.77 and 7.78)**. The flexor tendon sheath may be

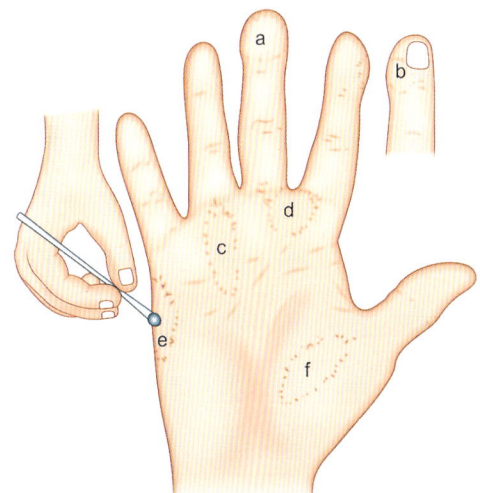

Fig. 7.51: Eliciting tenderness for infections of the hand. a = whitlow, b = paronychia, c = flexor sheath of finger, d = web infection, e = ulnar bursal infection, f = radial bursal infection.

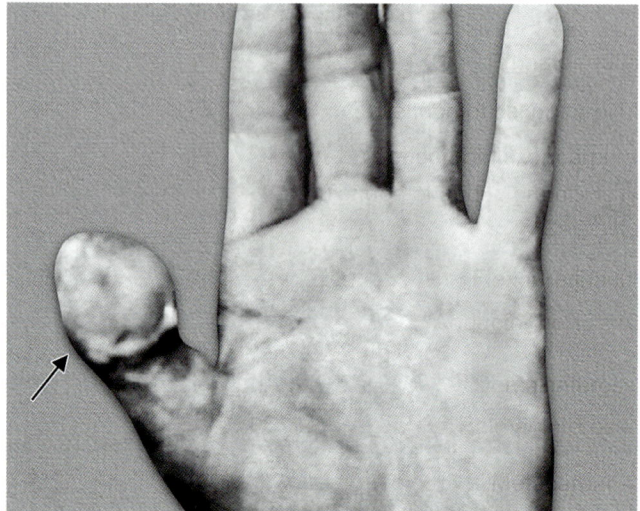

Fig. 7.52: Felon of thumb.

infected due to spread of infection from the adjacent pulp infection or through any puncture wound in the flexor creases. Besides flexor tendon sheath, the radial and ulnar bursae may also be infected at finger tip **(Fig. 7.51)**; In *paronychia* [infection of the eponychial fold—a superficial infection of epithelium (mostly caused by *Staphylococcus*) lateral to the nail plate]—on dorsolateral aspects and proximal to the nail root. The area over the matrix of nail and the lateral nail folds is swollen, inflamed, painful and tender. If there is pain on pressure over the nail plate, it indicates subungual abscess, which develops between the nail plate and periosteum. In *infection of the flexor sheaths of the fingers*—direct pressure on the centre of the finger from the palmar aspect causes pain. *In web infection*—tender point is about 1 cm proximal to the web margin on the palmar aspect. In finger webs short hair shafts may penetrate the soft skin leading to inflammation and producing *"Barber's Pilonidal Sinus".* Tender nodule(s) are felt in the web(s), looking like black dots, and it (they) may drain into sinus.

Look for nodules on the finger pads or palm. *Osler's nodes:* In patients of infective endocarditis, sometimes septic emboli lodge on the cutaneous vessels producing septic microabscesses. They present as bluish or pinkish nodules on the finger pads and/or in palms and or even in soles of feet. *Janeway Spots:* In patients of bacterial endocarditis or mycotic aneurysm small erythematous or haemorrhagic macular or nodular small spots may appear in few hours as crops in palms, soles or finger pads. The causative organism may be isolated from the lesion. They are painless and not tender, however, they may ulcerate and causative organism may be isolated from the lesion; In *ulnar bursa infection* tenderness is marked near about the centre of the ulnar margin of the palm; which in case of the *radial bursa*—at about the most prominent point of centre of thenar eminence, i.e. there is tenderness and swelling over the sheath of the flexor pollicis longus. The interphalangeal joint of the thumb is flexed and then its extension produces pain. The sheath of extensor tendons of thumb and fingers may also be infected **(*see* Fig. 7.80)**.

Tenderness in the palm should be localised either by a match stick or by a blunt pencil point **(Fig. 7.51)**.

It is not easy to demonstrate fluctuation in infections on the palmar aspect. However, in case of any suspicious swelling on the dorsum of the hand, fluctuation and induration must be demonstrated before labelling it as a pus collection. As such, any infection or trauma of the hand does manifest as swelling on dorsum of the hand. This is because the subcutaneous tissue on the dorsum is quite loose and the lymphatics of the palm drain into the dorsum.

■ MOVEMENTS

For all practical purposes, movements of the hand mean movements of the thumb and fingers **(Tables 7.1 and 7.2)**. The movements at the smaller intercarpal, carpometacarpal and intermetacarpal joints are negligible from the clinical point of view.

■ GROSS ASSESSMENT OF MOVEMENTS OF THE HAND

Ask the patient to put both hands in the shape of a cup (cupping). They should be bilaterally symmetrical. Any lag in cupping may be due to:
- Wasting of the smaller muscles of the hand, especially at thenar and hypothenar regions
- Lack of movements at the intercarpal, carpometacarpal, intermetacarpal and metacarpophalangeal joints
- Mechanical obstruction due to lesions in the palm, either following trauma, infection or neoplasm.

Gross movements of the hand can be further tested by asking the patient to make a firm fist **(Fig. 7.3)** and then open the hand fully with thumb and fingers fully extended. Making a firm fist and opening the hand fully indicates almost normal movements of the hand.

Ask the patient to hold a pen **(Fig. 7.4)** in writing position. A normal hold indicates normal functioning of the intrinsics as well as a fairly good range of motion of the thumb, index, middle, ring and little fingers in that order.

Movements of the Thumb (Table 7.1)

Clinicoanatomically, normal movements of the thumb may be grouped as:
- Abduction
- Flexion
- Extension
- Adduction
- Opposition
- Circumduction.

TABLE 7.1: Normal movements of the thumb.

Movements	Normal range	Muscle concerned	Root control	Factor limiting movement	Joint of action	How to test
Abduction	0°–60°	Abductor pollicis longus, abductor pollicis brevis	$C_{6,7}$	Tension of skin between thumb and index finger and tension of first dorsal interosseous muscle	Primarily at carpometacarpal joint, also at metacarpophalangeal joint	From thumb lying close to radial border of palm, ask the patient to open the web without producing any stretch or squeeze of the palmar skin **(Fig. 7.53)**
Adduction	60°–0°	Adductor pollicis (oblique and transverse heads)	$C_8.T_1$	The contact of ulnar border of thumb with radial border of palm	-do-	From fully abducted position, as in above, ask the patient to close the web without producing any tension or squeezing of the dorsal skin **(Fig. 7.53)**
Flexion: Metacarpophalangeal joint	0°–60°	Flexor pollicis brevis	$C_{6,7,8}$	Tension of extensor tendons of thumb	Metacarpophalangeal joint	With patient's hand resting on a table gently press over the thenar eminence. Ask the patient to bring the first phalanx of thumb towards palm, from position of easy stretch **(Fig. 7.54)**
Flexion: Carpometacarpal joint Interphalangeal joint	0°–80°–90° 0°–15°	Flexor pollicis longus	$C_8 T_1$	—	Interphalangeal joint	Hold the first phalanx from the sides. Ask the patient to bring pulp of thumb towards the palm **(Fig. 7.55)**
Extension: Metacarpophalangeal joint	60°–0°	Extensor pollicis brevis	C_7	Tension of palmar and collateral ligaments of thumb	Metacarpophalangeal joint	From fully flexed position as in above, patient is asked to bring back the first phalanx towards stretched position **(Fig. 7.54)**
Extension: Interphalangeal joint	90°–0°	Extensor pollicis longus	C_7	—	Interphalangeal joint	From fully flexed position, ask the patient to bring back the distal phalanx to extended position **(Fig. 7.55)**
Opposition: Palmar aspect of pulp of thumb rests on palmar aspect of pulp of little finger		Opponens pollicis, Opponens digiti minimi	$C_{6,7,8}$	Tension of transverse metacarpal ligament, tension of extensor tendons of thumb and little finger	Metacarpophalangeal, Carpometacarpal and intercarpal joints	The stretched thumb and little finger are brought across the palm to touch palmar aspects of terminal phalanx **(Fig. 7.56)**
Circumduction: When all movements are free, then only possible						Ask the patient to rotate the thumb so as to make a circle in the air by its tip **(Fig. 7.57)**

NB: **Osteoarthritis of the first carpometacarpal joint** is most common cause of (chronic) painful limitation of the thumb movements. Simple excision of trapezium followed by splintage for minimum period and thence early supervised mobilisation of thumb is an effective treatment. It also maintains adequate web space and thumb abduction.

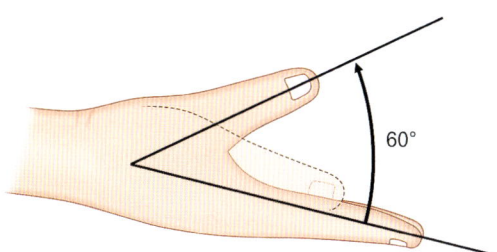

Fig. 7.53: Abduction and adduction of thumb.

Some Important Points about Thumb

- In most of the movements of the hand, the thumb acts as an active partner (functionally thumb is 40% of the hand), while the other fingers along with the palm remain comparatively passive
- Thumb has only one interphalangeal joint. Hence, most of its movements are subserved at its metacarpophalangeal and carpometacarpal joint. No wonder, these sites are predisposed to primary osteoarthritis

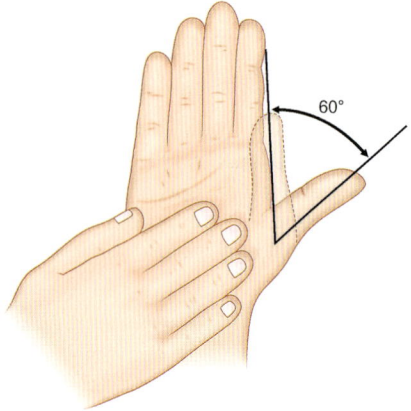

Fig. 7.54: Flexion and extension at MP joint.

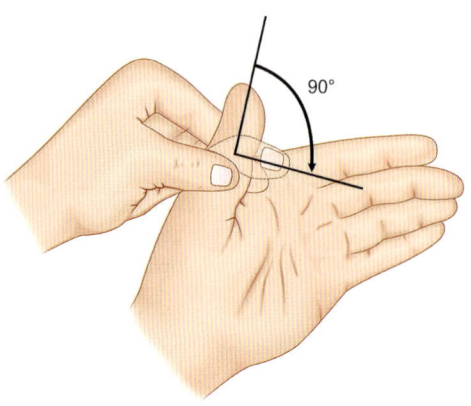

Fig. 7.55: Flexion and extension at IP joint.

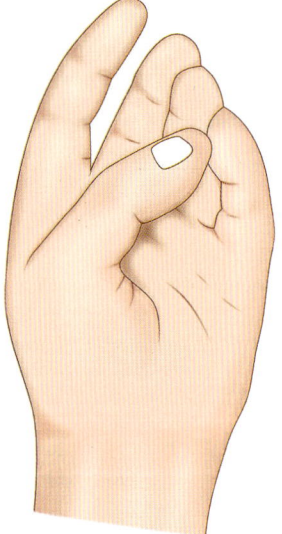

Fig. 7.56: Opposition.

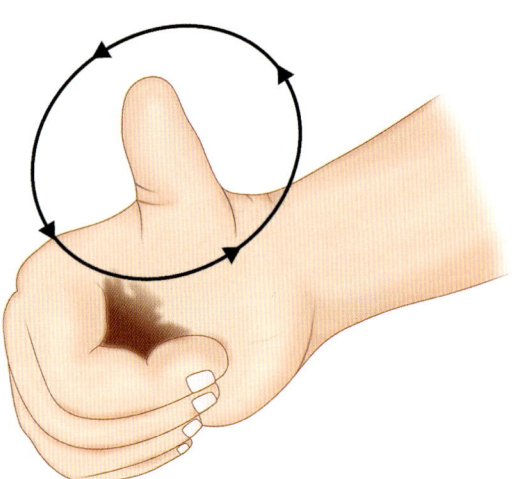

Fig. 7.57: Circumduction.

TABLE 7.2: Normal movements of fingers.						
Movements	**Normal range**	**Muscle concerned**	**Root control**	**Factors limiting movement**	**Joint of action**	**How to test**
Flexion: Metacarpophalangeal joint	0°–90°	Lumbricals, dorsal and palmar interossei. Long flexor of fingers can also influence metacarpophalangeal joint to produce flexion.	$C_{6,7,8}$ T_1	Tension of extensor expansion of the fingers	Metacarpophalangeal joint	Patient rests the dorsal aspect of the hand on table. Fix the metacarpals by your fingers at about proximal transverse palmar crease. Ask the patient to flex the extended finger to the maximum (**Fig. 7.58**)
Flexion: Proximal interphalangeal joint	0°–120°	Flexor digitorum sublimis and profundus	$C_{7,8}$ T_1	Tension of expansion of extensor digitorum tendons	Proximal interphalangeal joint	Fix the proximal phalanx between your thumb and index finger. Ask the patient to bend finger just beyond your thumb (**Fig. 7.59**)

Contd...

Contd...

Movements	Normal range	Muscle concerned	Root control	Factors limiting movement	Joint of action	How to test
Flexion: Distal inter-phalangeal joint	0°–80°	Flexor digitorum profundus	C_8 T_1	Dorsal ligaments of distal inter-phalangeal joint	Distal inter-phalangeal joint	Hold the middle phalanx between thumb and finger. Ask the patient to bend the finger just beyond your thumb (Figs. 7.60 and 7.61)
Extension: Extension at metacarpophalangeal joint not possible beyond zero position. Hence range will be flexion to zero position. In certain individuals, probably, due to laxity of the ligaments, varying degree of hyperextension may be possible at MPJ and/or PPJ (Fig. 7.62) Hyperextension—at distal interphalangeal joint	0°–30° (hyperextension). 0°–10°	Extensor digitorum, extensor indicis for index finger and extensor digiti minimi for little finger.	C_7	Palmar and collateral ligaments Flexor muscles of fingers	Metacarpophalangeal joint	Place the hand, resting on its ulnar border, on the table. Fingers being stretched more or less in the line of posterior surface of forearm. Fix the metacarpals (in between your thumb and fingers). Ask the patient to take extended finger (at interphalangeal joint) as far back as possible (Fig. 7.63)
Abduction	0°–25°	Dorsal interossei, abductor digiti minimi for little finger	$C_8 T_1$	Tension on skin and fascia in between the fingers	Metacarpophalangeal joint, carpo-metacarpal	Hold the tip of extended middle finger, with mild traction. Ask the patient to take finger (to be tested) away from middle finger in transverse direction (side ways) (Fig. 7.64). (Central axis of extended joint middle finger will be the zero position)
Adduction	25°–0°	Palmar interossei	$C_8 T_1$	Contact of fingers	Metacarpophalangeal joint, carpometacarpal joint.	After testing for abduction, ask the patient to approximate the fingers along the transverse axis (Fig. 7.64)

Testing for the flexor digitorum sublimis—Full flexion at the PIP, while other fingers are held in extension (which inactivates the flexor digitorum profundus) indicates intact flexor digitorum sublimis.

The flexion digitorum profundus muscles separate for each finger more distally than the sublimis, whose individual finger bellies separate higher. Hence profundus has mass action bellies.

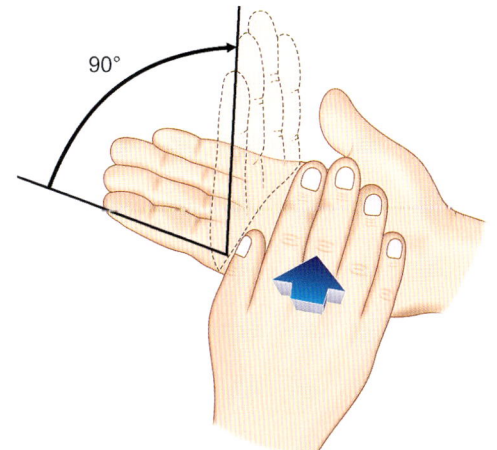

Fig. 7.58: Testing for flexion and extension at MP joint.

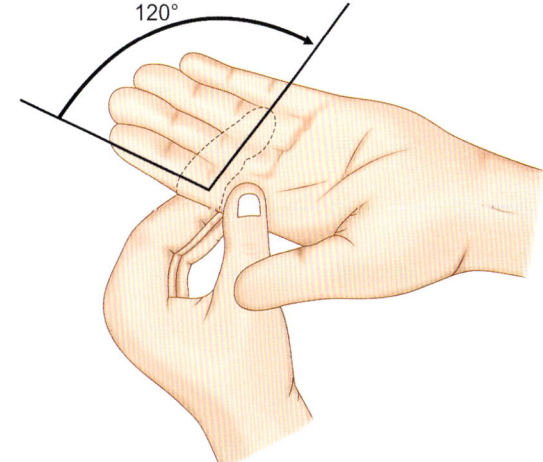

Fig. 7.59: Testing for flexion/extension at PIP joint.

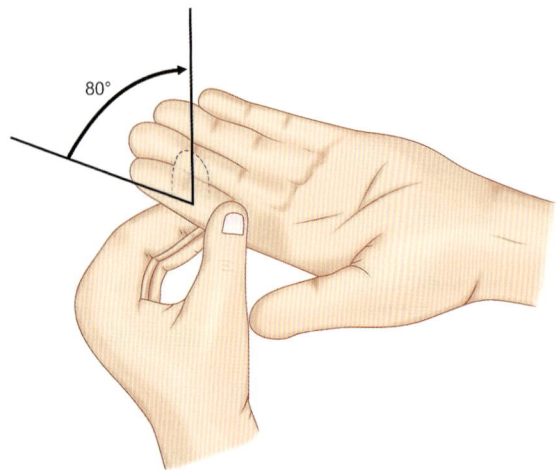

Fig. 7.60: Testing for flexion/extension at DIP joint.

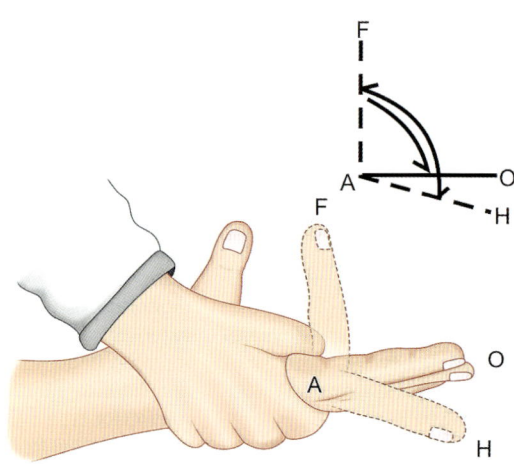

Fig. 7.63: Testing for hyperextension at MP joint.

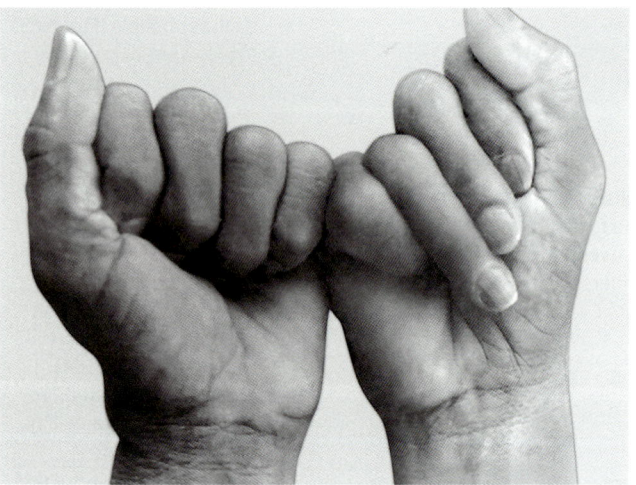

Fig. 7.61: After flexor digitorum profundus cut of right index, middle and ring fingers. Also to note that in attempt of making fist with extended fingers at distal interphalangeal joints, their tips point to scaphoid.

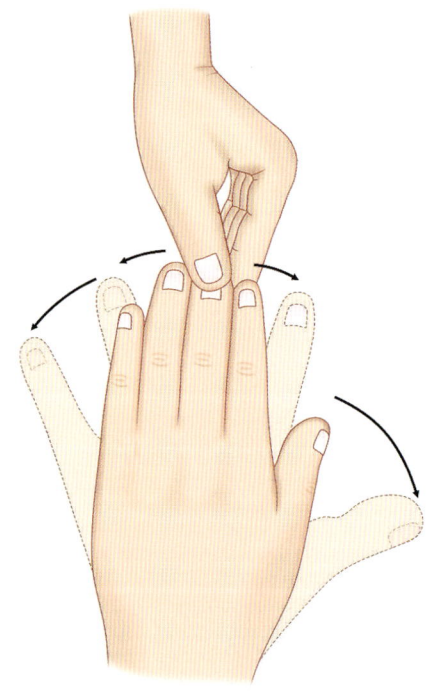

Fig. 7.64: Testing for abduction and adduction of fingers.

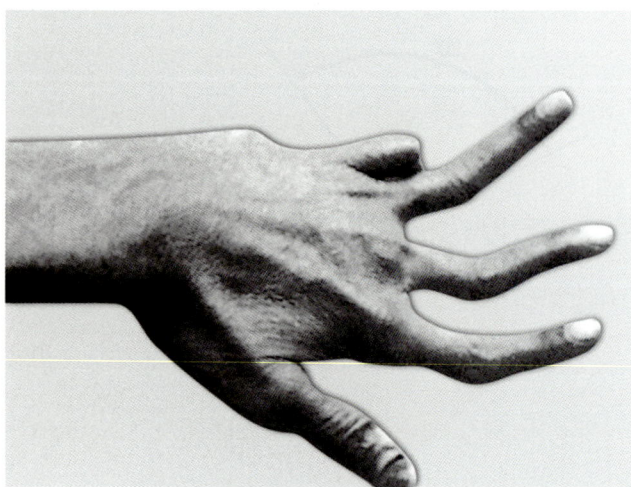

Fig. 7.62: Hyperextension at PIP joint.

- In an outstretched hand, the thumb is placed at about 80°–90° of abduction and some extension to initiate and facilitate grasp, catch, pinch and opposition movements
- Zero position of the thumb will vary according to the axis of the movement concerned
- The movements of the thumb and fingers should also be noted, as in the chapter of Introduction as far as practicable.

No examination of the hand is complete without repeated assessments for neurovascular integrity. Of course, sensibility to touch in the fingers is a most useful index of the adequacy of circulation.

Special Tests

- Test for intrinsic plus hand—*See* Page 188 (**Fig. 7.35**)
- Test for hooding deformity—*See* Page 189 (**Fig. 7.37C**)
- *Test for intrinsic minus hand*—as follows:
  - Deficient intrinsic action is mainly due to weakness of the interossei.

  Test: The patient will not be able to abduct or adduct the fingers (the middle finger being the axis).

  Further, conjoint action of the lumbricals and interossei, i.e. flexion at metacarpophalangeal joint and extension at the interphalangeal joints will also be affected to a varying extent.

  The patient is asked to stretch both his hands, keeping the fingers extended and closed to each other, if possible (with deficiency of interossei there will be lag in adduction of the fingers). Further, he is asked to flex and extend the fingers at the metacarpophalangeal joints in quick succession. Any weakness of the intrinsics will manifest by lag in flexing the extended finger.
- *Test for isolated division of flexor digitorum sublimis tendon:* Hold the adjacent fingers in full extension and ask the patient to flex the concerned proximal interphalangeal joint. This will not be possible, if the flexor digitorum sublimis is divided. The flexor digitorum profundus will not help in this action, since it gets anchored in extension with other fingers.

■ INVESTIGATION

- General investigations
- Radiological investigations

  Anteroposterior lateral and oblique views of hands and fingers, in maximum opened up position, are essential. For taking a lateral view of the individual finger, the other fingers should be flexed into the palm as far as practicable, while the finger in question should be extended as much as possible to bring it to zero-position.
- *Hand print*, as a whole and prints of the thumb and finger pulps:

  These are not only important from genetic and medicolegal point of view, but also for medical records. They also demonstrate the shape and size of hand and fingers, along with any deformities.

Traumatic conditions of the hand need careful clinical evaluation and proper investigations (both for soft tissues and bony injuries) (**Fig. 7.65**). Several of them (e.g. dislocations of small joints, fractures of the phalanges, and metacarpals tender injuries, etc.) are likely to be missed initially due to post-traumatic gross swelling of the hand. If missed, they can produce various deformities which hamper the hand functions (**Figs. 7.66 to 7.68**).

The fracture of scaphoid, if missed initially, is notorious to undergo avascular and non-union (**Figs. 7.68B and C**)

Intraosseous Keratinous Cyst

These are the rare benign lesions which commonly occur in the phalanges of hands and skull. They are very slow growing benign osseous lesion. They present with very slow growing swelling and later on with pain. Radiographs show solitary lytic lesion usually with destruction of entire dorsal cortex. Aspiration biopsy or FNAC are usually nonconclusive for diagnosis. Excision biopsy with the definite management in the form of curettage of cystic lesion and autologous iliac crest graft, confirms the diagnosis. Histopathology of the excised material shows cyst wall lined by stratified squamous epithelium with intact granular layer enclosing lamellar keratin, which confirms keratinous cyst.

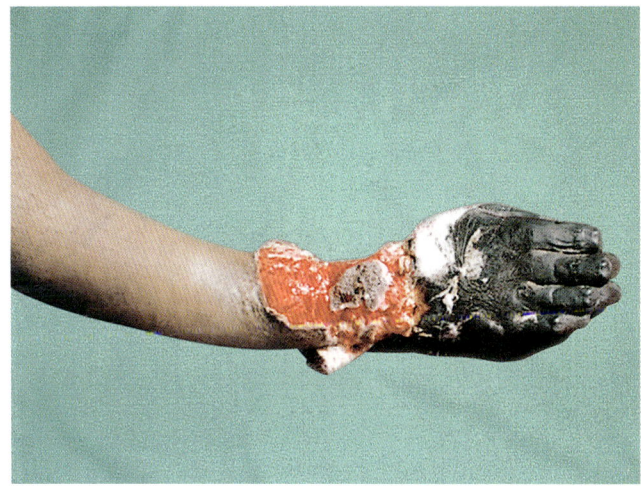

Fig. 7.65: Gangrene of the hand due to tight plaster for fracture forearm.

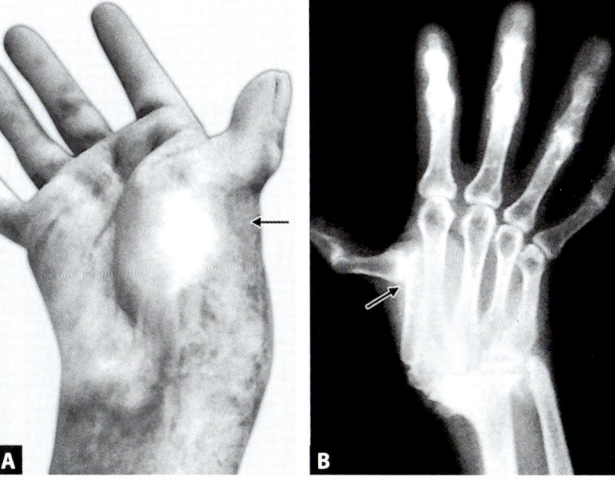

Figs. 7.66A and B: Seven years old unreduced neglected dislocation of thumb: (A) Clinical photo; (B) X-ray picture of same hand.

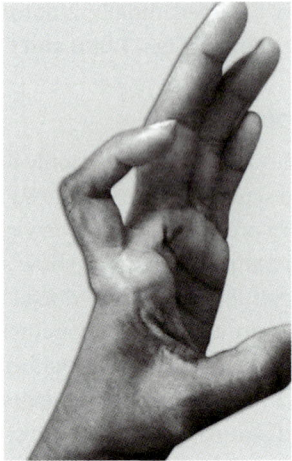

Fig. 7.67: One year old unreduced dislocation of little finger.

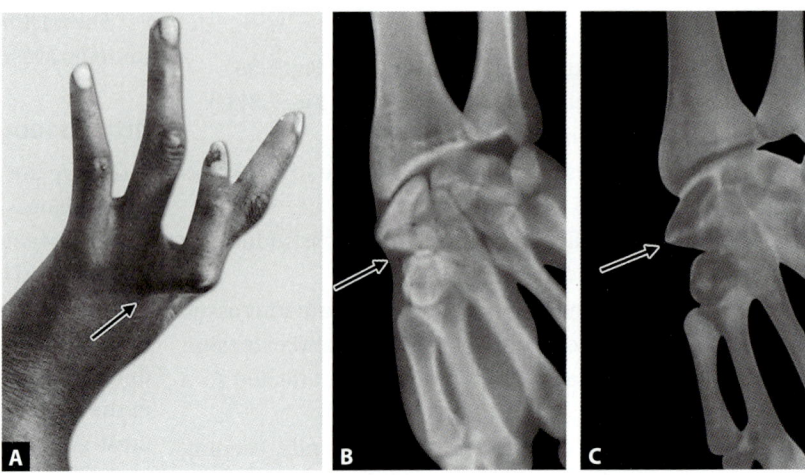

Figs. 7.68A to C: Three-year-old unreduced dislocation of middle finger; (B and C) Ununited neglected fracture scaphoid—5-month-old.

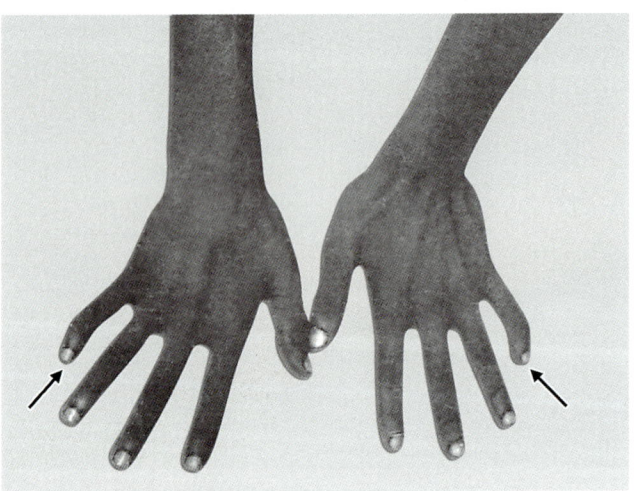

Fig. 7.69: Clinodactyly.

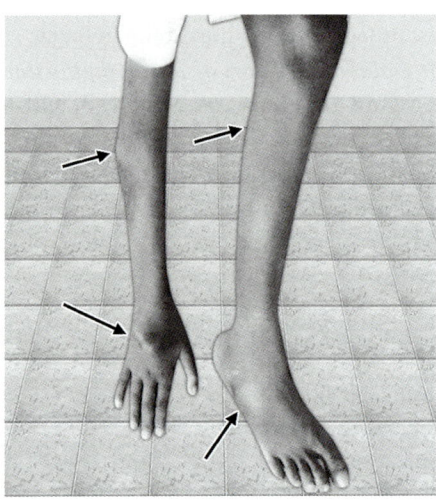

Fig. 7.70: Tuberculosis of right second metacarpal, right elbow, right cuboid and right upper tibiofibular joint—multifocal osteoarticular tuberculosis.

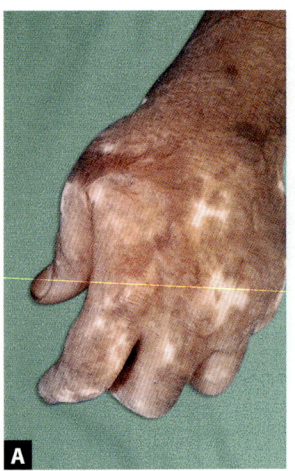
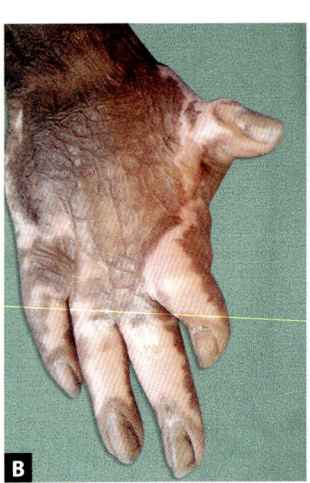
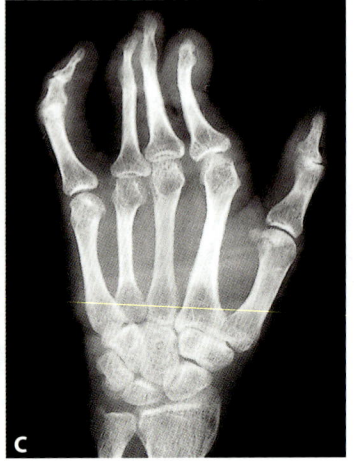

Figs. 7.71A to C: (A and B), Post-burn contracture of both hands. Such hands require expert plastic reconstruction procedures. However, this patient has been rehabilitated to use his hands for ADL and moderate earning; (C) Congenitally fused interphalangeal joints of index, middle and ring fingers—symphalangism—such problems require expert plastic surgery.

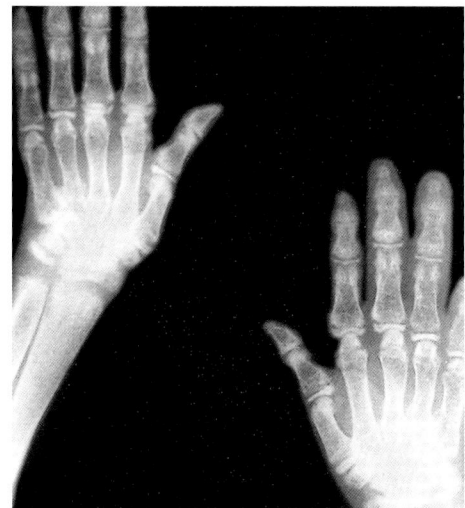

Hand bones in hyperparathyroidism

Fig. 7.72: Parathyroid glands, situated on the lateral aspect of thyroid lobes measures 6 x 4 x 2 mm weighs about 30–50 gm, have their chief parenchymal cells secreting parathyroid harmone (PTH-α polypeptide harmone 84 AA, 9500 D molecular weight). Hyperparathyroidism may be: Primary (osteitis Fibrose cystica, von Rocklinghausen's Disease), Secondary, Tertiary. Main skeletal changes are i. Bone resorption with large number of osteoclasts seen in Howship`s lacunae. Haversian canals are enlarged and cortices become like papery-thin cancellous bone. ii. Brown Tumors, which are localized accumulations of haemorrhages and osteoclasts. iii. Pathological fractures – long bones frequently bend and break under stress of weight. In primary hyperparathyroidism (osteitis fibrosa cystica Von Reckling Hausen's Disease) increased production of parathyroid hormone causes bone resorption which exceeds new bone formation. It leads to hypercalcaemia, hypercalciuria, hyperphosphatemia and hypophosphatemia, usually it remains asymptomatic, except diffuse aching in muscles and bones fatigue and weakness. Superiosteal cysts appear in skull and long bones, which may present as tender palpable swelling. Most frequently an adenoma, composed of pale clear cells is found in parathyroid gland.

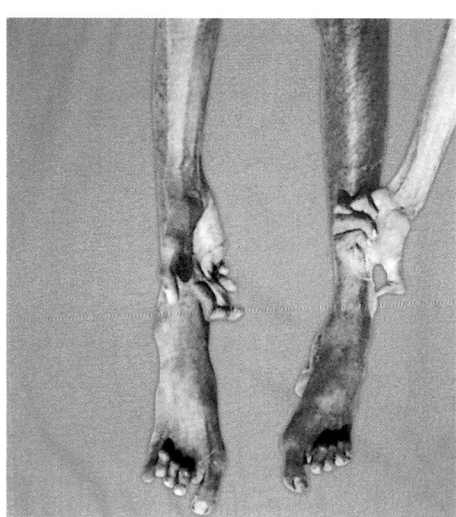

Fig. 7.73: Sometimes bizarre deformities develop in hands and feet (confusion in myopathy and rheumatoid or any condition else).

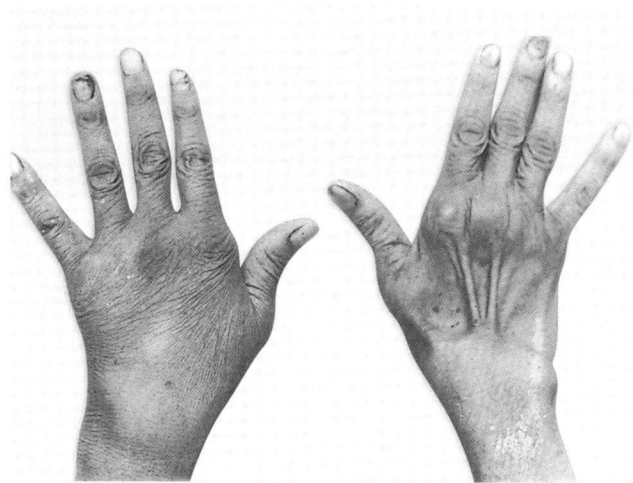

Fig. 7.74: Gross wasting of dorsal interossei muscles in rheumatoid hand. Both wrists are affected.

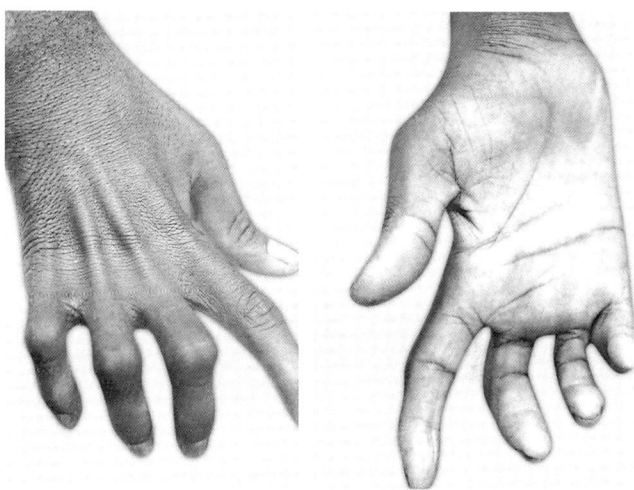

Fig. 7.75: Hansen's claw hand deformity.

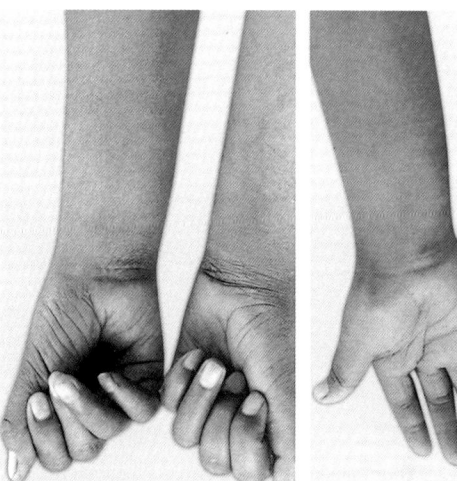
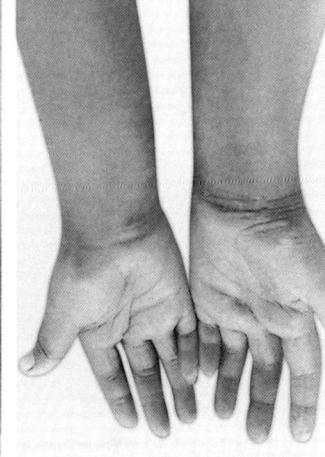

Fig. 7.76: Same figure **(Fig. 7.75)** 1 year after reconstructive surgery.

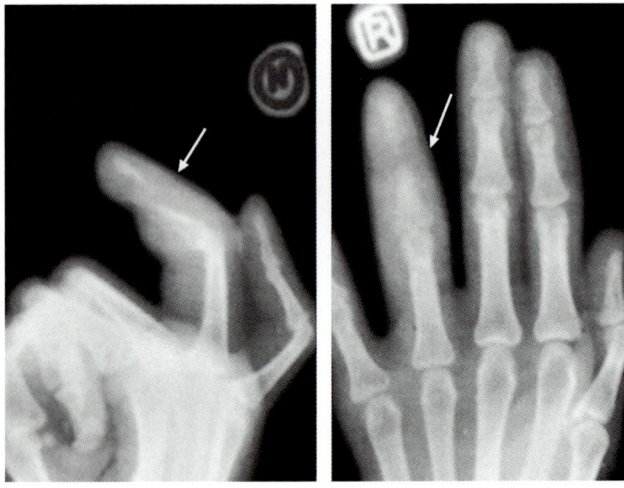

Fig. 7.77: Pyogenic abscess of finger tip which led to pyogenic arthritis of DIP joint and osteomyelitis of middle and terminal phalanges.

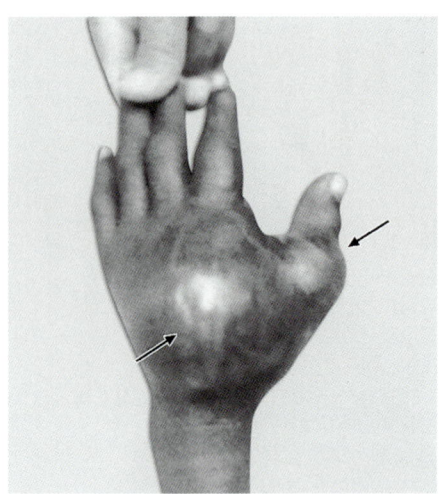

Fig. 7.80: Pyogenic abscess along the sheath of extensor tendons of thumb and index finger.

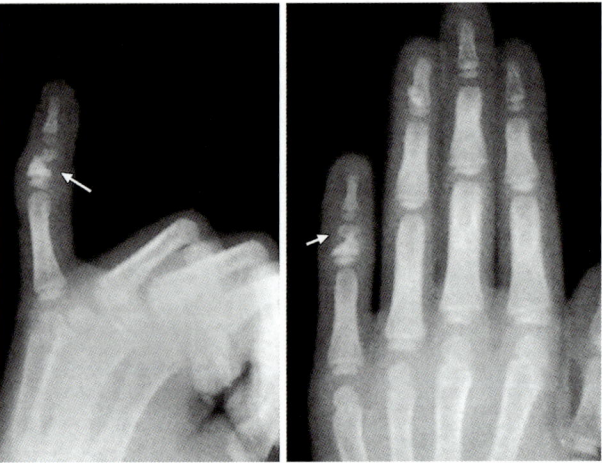

Fig. 7.78: Destruction of middle phalanx of little finger due to pyogenic osteomyelitis in infant.

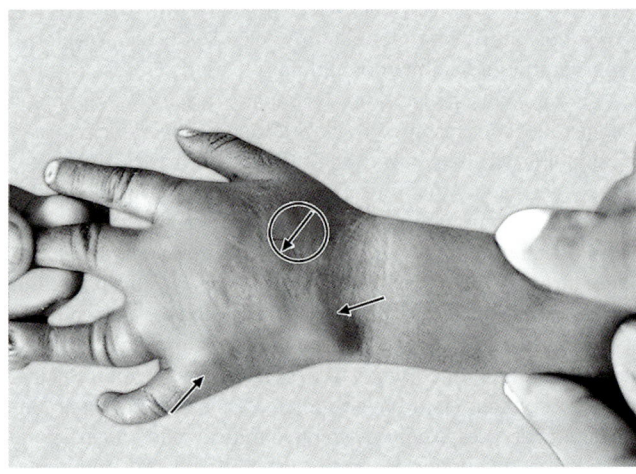

Fig. 7.81: Tuberculosis of carpometacarpal joints of 4th and 5th rays, 5th metacarpophalangeal joint with cold abscess.

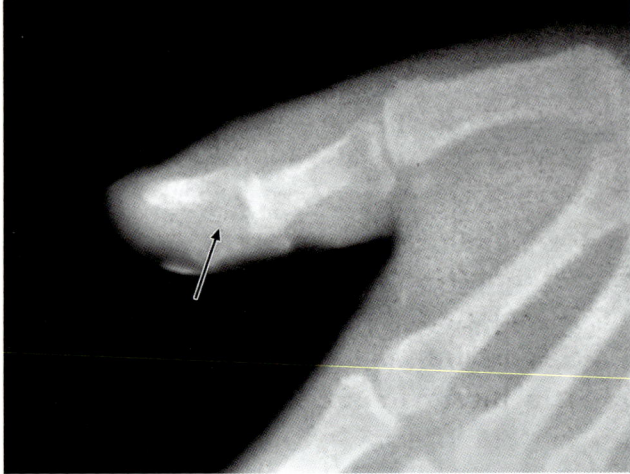

Fig. 7.79: Whitlow of thumb leading to pyogenic osteomyelitis of terminal phalanx and pyogenic arthritis of interphalangeal joint.

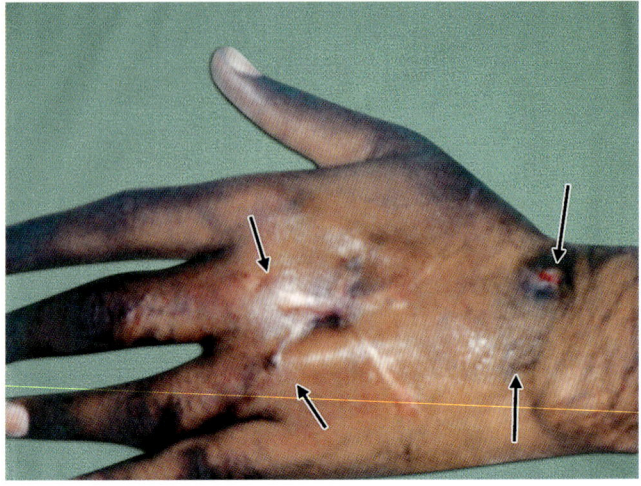

Fig. 7.82: Tuberculosis of hand affecting distal row midcarpals and 3rd and 4th metacarpals with sinuses (healed and healing). Mark the wasting of muscles.

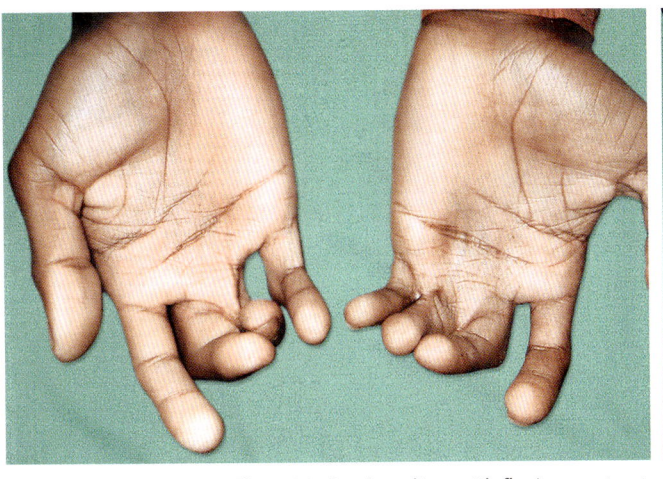 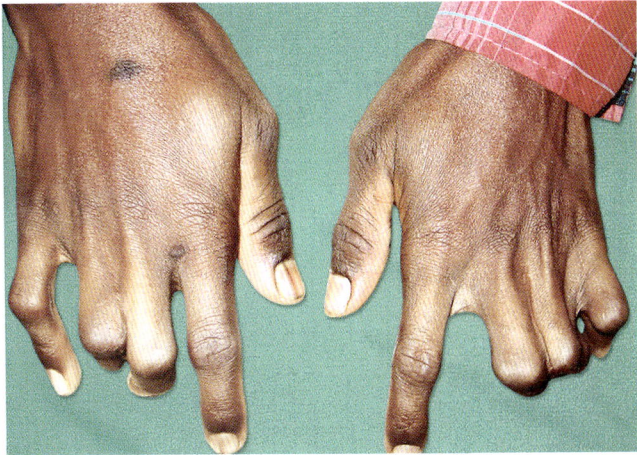

Fig. 7.83: Syndactylism with flexion contracture of fingers (mainly middle and ring fingers).

BIBLIOGRAPHY

1. Bunnel S. Surgery of the Hand (5th ed) JB Lippincott: Philadelphia, 1970.
2. Burge P. Genetics of Dupuytren's disease. Hand Clin. 1999; 15:63-72.
3. Calandruccio JH. Bowler's Thumb. In campbell's Operative Orthopaedics, 12th ed. Elsevier-Mosby, Philadelphia, 2013. p.3657.
4. Falk RH. The "thumb sign in Marfan's syndrome. N Eng J Med. 1995;333:430.
5. Froimson AI. Tenosynovitis and tennis elbow. In Green DP ed. Operative Hand Surgery, 3rd Ed. New York. Churchill Livingston. 1993;1989-2006.
6. James, JIP: Assessment and management of the injured hands. The Hand. 1970;2:97.
7. Jebsen-Taylor Hand Function Test: Quoted by Horstmann and Bleck in Orthopaedic Management in Cerebral Palsy. Mac keith Press, 2nd edition, 2007:216.
8. Lampe EW. Surgical anatomy. Ciba Clinical Symposia. 1957; 9(1):3.
9. Moberg Eric quoted by Helen M. Horstmann and Black Eugene E Orthopaedic Management in Cerebral Palsy, 2nd ed. Mac Keith Press. 2007:215.
10. Strom L. Trigger finger in diabetes. J Med Soc N J 1977; 74(11): 951-4.
11. Thurston AJ. Dupuytren's disease (review article) J Bone Joint Surg (Br). 2003;85-B:469-77.

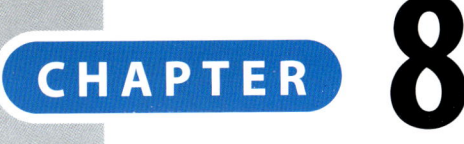

CHAPTER 8

Spine

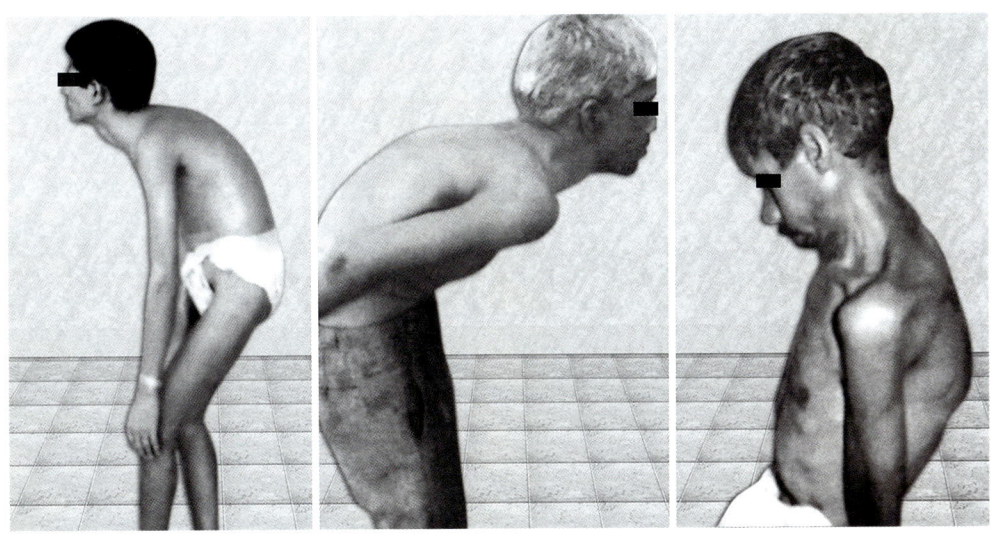

"I now recognize that the development of the nervous system is not only more complicated than we had imagined, but it may be more complicated than we can imagine."
—*Pasko Rakic*

"If you remain afraid of committing mistakes you will never be able to learn anything new."
—*SP*

"Astronauts get taller when they are in space because absence of gravity acting on their spine allows the ligaments between vertebrae to expand."

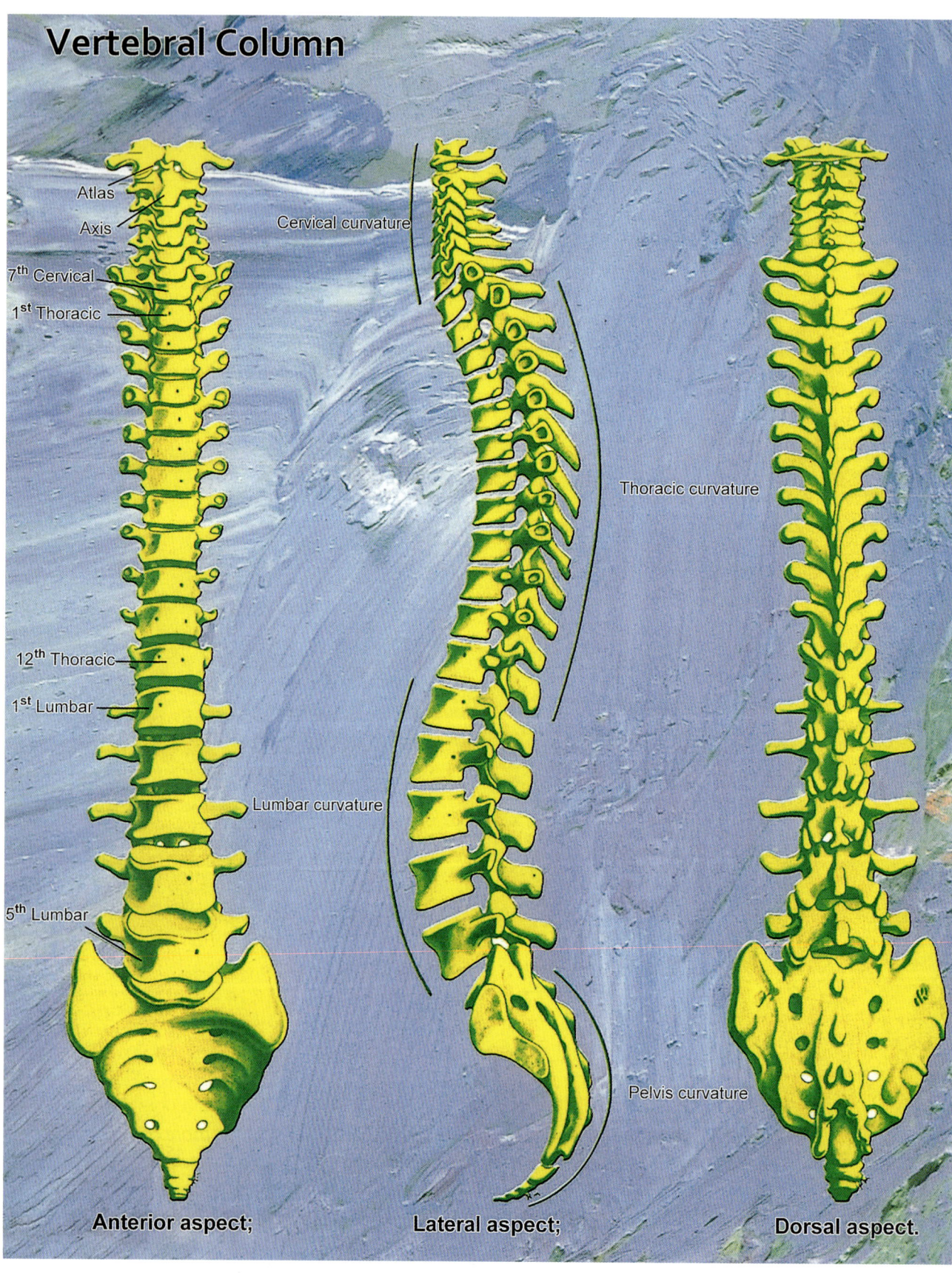

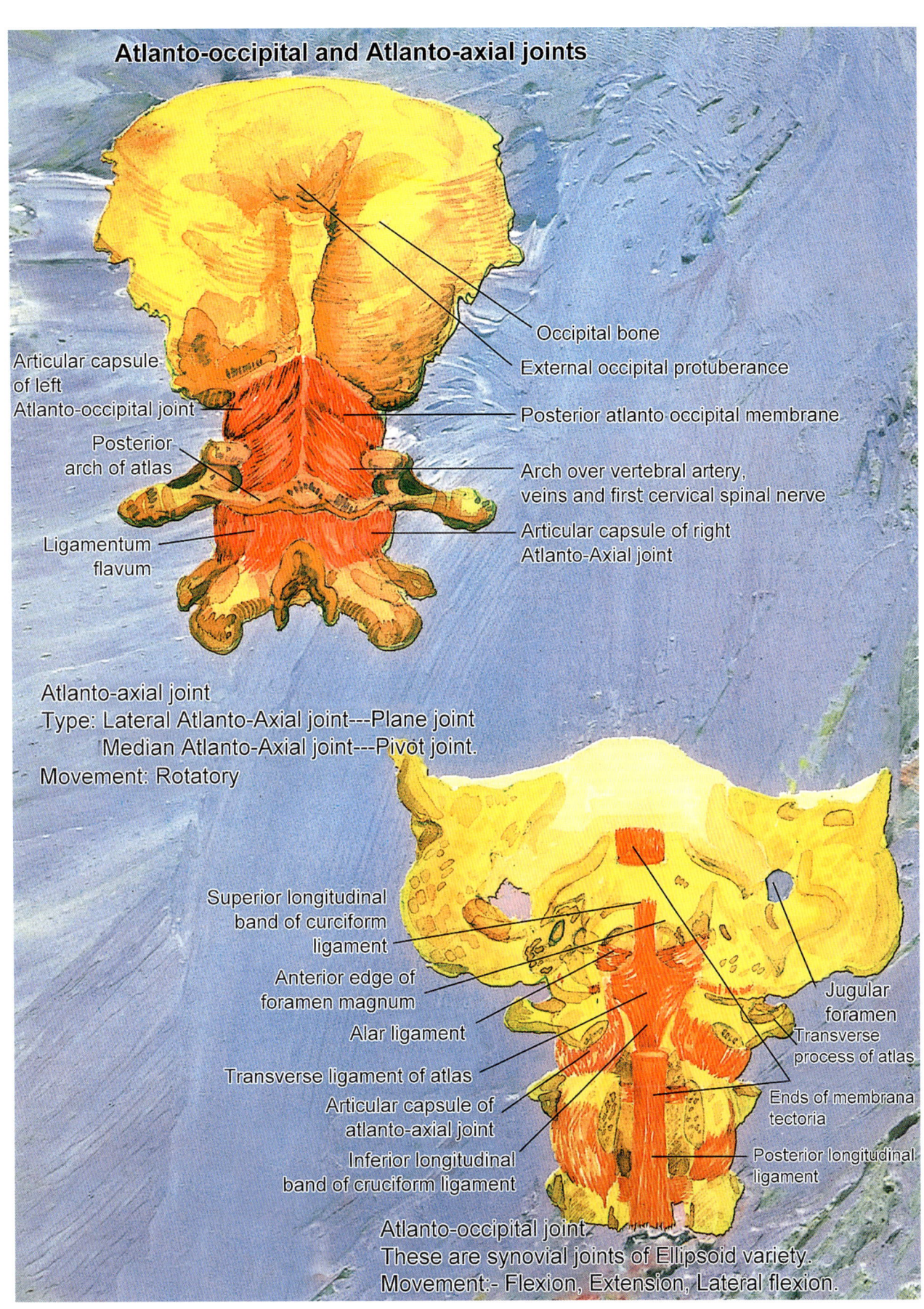

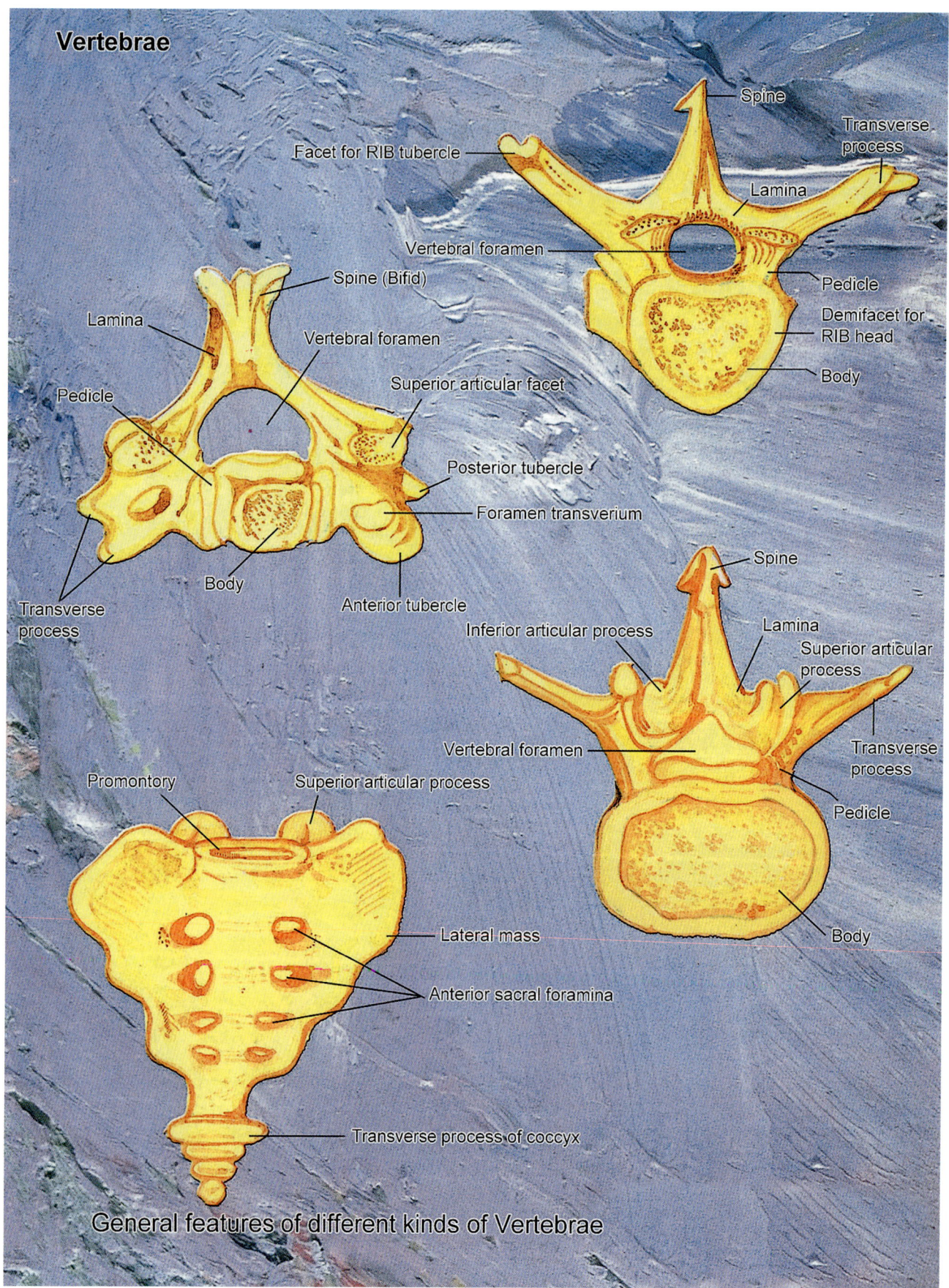

"Which of your hips has the most profound sciatica?"
—*William Shakespeare (1564-1616)*

"When a gibbosity seizes a person, it occasions a crisis of the already existing disease"
—*Hippocrates*

"The human foetus the no bigger than a Green Pea, yet is furnished with all its parts"
—*Antoni van Leeuwenhoek 1683*

"Measure twice cut once"
—*SP*

INTRODUCTION

Spine is the backbone of healthy body controlled by a healthy brain **(Fig. 8.0)**. It is indispensable and multifunctional pillar of stability. The spine is said to be in balance when the head is resting in a position directly centered over the distal sacrum and pelvis. Less muscular energy is spent in maintaining this stance; hence it is described as the cone of economy (Dubousset J 1994).

Skeletal system basically comprises of:
1. Axial skeleton—consisting of axial structures, i.e. the cranium, vertebral column and allied bones (i.e. ribs and sternum).
2. Appendicular skeleton—consisting of bones of appendages in fins, limbs or wings.

The axial endoskeleton (earlier as notochord and then as vertebral column) is the basic distinguishing feature of the phylum chordata and its subphylum the vertebrata (e.g. mankind).

In bipeds, the spinal (vertebral) column assumes following important functions:
- Encasement of the spinal cord
- Transmission of the weight of head, neck and trunk to the lower limbs through the pelvis
- Maintenance of posture
- Forming a stout back support for the vital organs of the chest and abdomen
- Providing attachment to certain important groups of muscles responsible for the maintenance of posture.

According to the functional needs, the different parts of the spine have become modified in the process of evolution in bipeds, e.g. to effect the movements of the head, the cervical spine has the maximum mobility. On the other hand, at the caudal end, the coccyx represents more or less a vestigial remnant.

Examination of the spinal column, automatically implies the examination of:
- The vertebrae
- The spinal cord (with its meninges),
- The spinal roots.

ANATOMICAL CONSIDERATIONS

Development of the Spine

The spine develops in concurrently running stages which overlap each other.

First stage—Notochord—15 days of IUL (Intrauterine life).
Second stage—Membrane stage—21 days of IUL.
Third stage—Cartilage stage—5–6 weeks and continues throughout the foetal stage.
Fourth stage—Bony stage—2nd month of IUL.

The neural tube develops from the ectoderm in the 2nd to 3rd weeks of intrauterine life.

Notochord develops from endoderm. Around the notochord, which forms the primitive axial support, formation of thirty or more somites occur. The dorsomedial part of the somite forms the skeletal muscle and is known as myotomes. The ventrolateral portion forms the vertebral body and is known as sclerotome.

The development of brain and spinal cord is complex mechanism, however, in scheduled orderly fashion right from the conception to birth **(Fig. 8.1)**.

Congenital anomalies can occur in any stage but usually occur due to defects in the membrane stage, when mesenchyme first starts forming around the notochord.

Curvatures of the Spine (Fig. 8.2)

The vertebral column comprises 33 vertebrae (cervical-7, thoracic-12, lumbar-5, sacral-5, and coccygeal-4).

The vertebral column has four curves of varying magnitude which can be assessed clearly when viewed laterally the anatomical posture of life.

The cervical curve is the least and is concave backwards extending from C2 to T2. The thoracic curve extends from T2 to T12, and is convex backward. The lumbar curve extends from T12 to lumbosacral junction and is concave backwards (also called *lumbar lordosis*) and is more prominent in females. The sacral and coccygeal regions extend from lumbosacral junction to the tip of coccyx, and along with pelvis their curve is convex backwards and downwards. On the whole the cervical and lumbar segments develop lordosis which helps in acquiring erect posture. The thoracic and sacral segments have kyphotic postures acquired from the position in utero. The thoracic segment provides attachment points for the ribcage, while the sacral segment for the pelvic girdle. The mobile vertebral body increases in size from cranial to lumbar

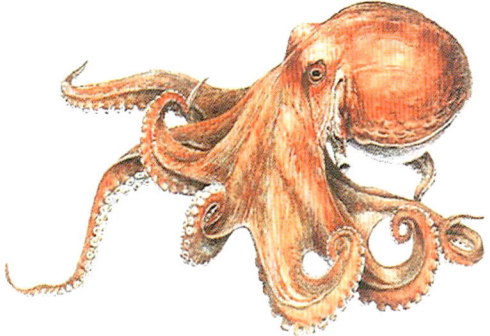

Fig. 8.1: An octopus (a sea animal with a soft body and eight long tentacles) has a "mini brain" for each arm in addition to it's main brain.

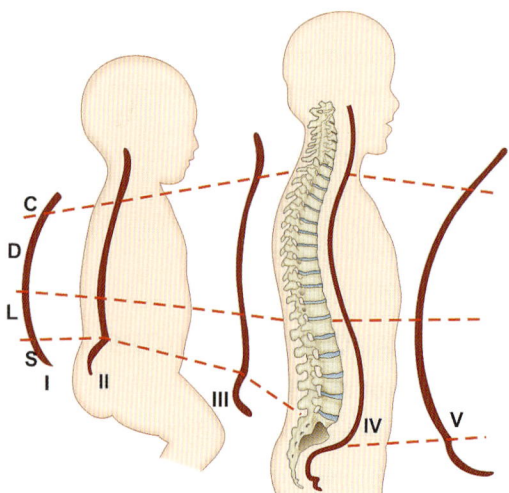

Fig. 8.2: Curvatures of spine at different ages: I—curvature in utero and early infancy; II—curvature at early childhood; III—curvature at late childhood; IV—curvature at adulthood; V—curvature of senile spine; C = cervical spine; D = dorsal spine; L = lumbar spine and S = sacral spine.

region. Astronauts got taller when they are in space, because intervertebral ligaments expand in lack of gravily.

A typical vertebra has a body anteriorly and an arch posteriorly which enclose the vertebral canal. The neural arch is composed of two pedicles laterally and two laminae posteriorly which unite to form the spinous process. On either side of the arch of vertebral body is a transverse process and superior and inferior articular processes.

A graph for recording the curves of the spinal column should be plotted—RACHIGRAPH.

Meninges of the Spinal Cord

The spinal cord is covered by three layers of meninges—*Dura mater* (only membranous layer), *Arachnoid mater* and *Pia mater*. The dura mater is a dense, strong fibrous membrane extending upward up to foramen magnum to be continuous with the membranous layer of dura mater covering the brain, and downwards it ends on the *filum terminale* at the lower border of second sacral vertebra. The dural sheath lies loosely in the vertebral canal. The *extradural space* (between dura and the wall of vertebral canal) contains loose areolar tissue and internal vertebral plexus. The inner surface of dura remain in contact with the arachnoid mater.

The *arachnoid mater*, a delicate impermeable membrane, lies between dura and pia mater and is separated from the pia mater by a wide space—*subarachnoid space* filled with cerebrospinal fluid. The arachnoid mater becomes continuous upwards with the arachnoid mater covering the brain and downwards it ends on the filum terminale.

The *pia mater*, a vascular membrane, closely covers the spinal cord and is thickened on either side between the nerve roots to form the *ligamentum denticulatum* by which the spinal cord remains suspended in the middle of the dural sheath.

Blood Vessels of the Spinal Cord and Around

Arteries of Spinal Cord

- *Main arteries (branches of vertebral artery):*
  - *Anterior spinal artery*: Runs in the anteromedial fissure (supplies anterior two-thirds of the spinal cord)
  - *Two posterior spinal arteries:* Run downwards on the dorsolateral surface, posterior to the spinal roots (supply the posterior parts of the posterior horn and column).
- *Reinforcements:* Spinal branches of vertebral, inferior thyroid, intercostal, iliolumbar, sacral or radicular arteries (at different levels from above downwards), enter through the intervertebral foramina. Largest of the radicular arteries is the arteria radicularis magna or *great spinal artery of Adamkiewcz,* which originates from the left intercostal or lumbar artery between the 4th thoracic and 4th lumbar vertebrae, with special predilection for T9 to T11. These together contribute to the formation of anastomosing channels along the cord.

Arterial Supply of Vertebrae

The vertebral bodies receive the arterial supply in corresponding embryological pattern. The branches emerge from ascending cervical, intercostal and lumbar segmental arteries. Consequently on each side upper half of vertebrae below and lower half of vertebrae above (with its intervening intervertebral disc) receive arterial supply from the same segmental supply.

Veins

Veins are principally organised in the external and internal venous plexuses (*Batson's plexus*-1940).

External vertebral venous plexus (most marked in the cervical region) consists of:
- The *anterior plexus* lies anterior to vertebral body and communicates with the basivertebral and internal vertebral venous plexus
- *Posterior plexus* lies around the posterior surface of the laminae, spinous and transverse processes, anastomosing freely with each other and with vertebral, posterior intercostal and lumbar veins.

Internal vertebral venous plexus: This lies between the dura mater and vertebrae, receiving tributaries from bone and cord and running in a vertical direction forming two anterior and two posterior veins.

The anterior internal venous plexus lies behind the posterior surface of the vertebral bodies and discs, on each side of the posterior longitudinal ligament, and are connected by transverse branches into which the basivertebral veins open. The posterior internal venous plexus lies on each side of the median plane, in front of the ligamentum flava, and anastomoses with the posterior external plexus.

Veins of the Spinal Cord

These are situated in the pia mater and form a plexus consisting of:
- Two medial longitudinal veins
- Two anterolateral longitudinal veins
- Two posterolateral longitudinal veins.

These communicate with the internal vertebral venous plexus and intervertebral vein.

Spinal Column

Spinal column remains the backbone of a healthy human body. It is indispensable and multifunctional pillar for stability.

The spinal column is composed of vertebral segments (7 cervical, 12 dorsal, 5 lumbar, 5 fused sacral and 3-4 fused/unfused coccygeal). Five fused sacral vertebrae mass articulate with the pelvic bones on either side at the sacroiliac joints. Each vertebral segment consists of an anterior solid vertebral body which has the responsibility of carrying the body load. The posterior appendages form a ring with the body of the vertebrae for encasing the spinal cord. The pedicles lie at the junction of the anterior and posterior segments. *Pars interarticularis* is the developmental region of fusion of the pedicles from front, the superior articular facets from above, laminae from behind, inferior articular facets from below and transverse processes from the sides.

In the spinal column, each vertebra has a pair of synovial joints on either side, i.e. the arthrodial joints formed by the superior articular facet of the vertebra below and the inferior articular facet of the vertebra above. These bilateral joints actually form the fulcrum of movements in between two vertebrae. However, a little movement does occur, also in between two adjacent vertebrae at the intervertebral disc level. Posteriorly, the corresponding processes of adjacent vertebrae are held together by stout ligaments.

The distance from the 7th cervical vertebra to the sacral hiatus in adults vary between 50 and 75 cm.

Important Ligaments of the Vertebral Column

- Anterior to the bodies—*The anterior longitudinal ligament* extending from basi occiput to sacrum
- Posterior to the bodies—The *posterior longitudinal ligament* extends from basi occiput to sacrum, upper end is known as *tectorial membrane* (extending from axis to occiput)
- In between adjacent laminae—The *ligamentum flava*
- In between adjacent spinous processes—The *interspinous ligament*
- Bridging the tips of the spinous processes—The *supraspinous ligament* (from vertebra prominens to occiput, is known as *ligamentum nuchae*)
- The spinal cord is more or less suspended in the vertebral canal by the *denticulate ligaments* of both sides.

The *vertebral column is controlled by a complex group of muscles*, which extend from the pelvis to the skull—the sacrospinalis—supplied by the dorsal rami of the segmental spinal nerves.

The *articular facets* and spinal appendages (transverse processes and spinous processes) of different regions may have different shape, size and directions according to their functions and required mobility (right from the atlanto-occipital zone to the lumbosacral zone).

Spinal stability is defined as the ability of the spine to maintain, under physiologic loads, the normal relationships between vertebrae in such a way that there is neither damage nor subsequent irritation to the spinal cord or nerve roots.

The *stability of spine depends upon three-column support* (Denis 1983):
- *Anterior column* consists of anterior longitudinal ligament, anterior portion of annulus, and anterior half of the vertebral body.
- *Middle column* consists of posterior longitudinal ligament, posterior portion of annulus and posterior half of vertebral body.
- *Posterior column* consists of posterior bony arch (comprising of the pedicles, facets and laminae) and the posterior ligamentous complex consisting of supraspinatus ligament, interspinus ligament, ligamentum flava, and facet joint capsules.

Spinal Cord

The spinal cord, starting as a *direct continuation of the medulla oblongata at the lower border of the foramen magnum continues as far as the lower border of L1* vertebra (in children up to L3), where it forms the *conus medullaris*. Beyond this, the bunches of the emerging roots form the cauda equina (like the hairs arranged in a horse's tail). From the tip of the conus medullaris, a delicate band continues in the centre of the cauda equina to end at S2 vertebra forming the filum terminale interna. The meninges of the cord (dura and arachnoid) blend around the filum terminale interna at the S2 level forming the filum terminale externa which runs up to the coccyx **(Fig. 8.3)**. The spinal cord has two enlargements to accommodate the roots supplying the limbs (cervicodorsal—C3 to T2, for upper limb and lumbar and sacral—T9-T12 and S1-2).

Intervertebral Disc

Normally, 23 discs exist starting from 2/3rd cervical intervertebral space to lumbosacral intervertebral space. The disc is thinner in the thoracic region and thicker in the lumbar region.

Functionally, this may be taken as a shock absorber in between two adjacent vertebral bodies. It *develops from mesoderm* (annulus fibrosis and cartilaginous plate) *and endoderm*, i.e. notochord (nucleus pulposus) and is adherent to the hyaline cartilage layer covering the adjacent surfaces of the vertebral bodies. Taken together, the discs occupy 1/5th of the total length of the spinal column

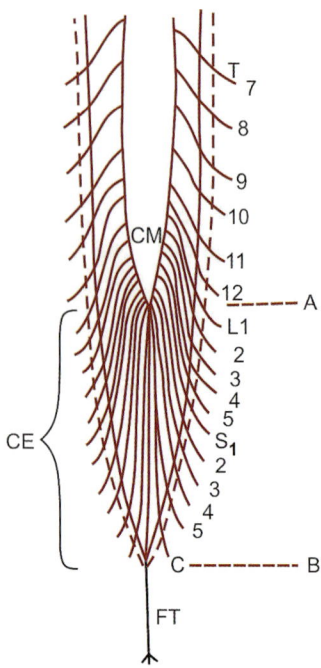

Fig. 8.3: Lower end of the spinal cord and cauda equina.
Abbreviations: CM: conus medullaris; CE: cauda equina; FT: filum terminale; A: lower border of L1 vertebra; B: lower border of S2 vertebra.

with diurnal variation in thickness of 1 cm (in women) to 1.5 cm (in men). Astronauts get taller when they are in space because absence of gravity acting on the spine allows the ligaments and intervertebral discs to expand. The discs are practically avascular by the age of about 18 years and derive their nutrition by diffusion from adjacent cancellous bones.

Structure of the Intervertebral Disc

Each disc consists of an outer laminated part called the *annulus fibrosus* (consisting of 12 concentric lamellae) and an inner part called the *nucleus pulposus*. The narrower outer zone of the annulus consists of collagenous fibres and the wider inner zone of the nucleus pulposus is fibrocartilaginous. The nucleus pulposus is well developed in the cervical and lumbar regions. At birth, it is soft, gelatinous and comparatively large, containing about 88% water, mucoid material and a few multinucleated notochordal cells. By the first decade, the notochordal cells disappear and the mucoid material is gradually replaced by a fibrocartilaginous structure. With these changes, the nucleus pulposus becomes amorphous, its water binding capacity diminished to 70% and its elasticity reduces, due to the alteration in its mucopolysaccharide and protein components. Nerve bundles have been demonstrated outside the anterior and posterior longitudinal ligaments, but not in the disc. After the second decade, degenerative changes are likely to occur, in the disc. Initially, the nucleus pulposus is a semifluid mass of mucoid material containing 70–90% water, with proteoglycan constituting 65% and collagen 15–20% of the dry weight. Gradually the water content of the nucleus pulposus decreases, converting it into a granular and friable mass. Similarly, there is a softening and weakening of the annulus fibrosus. Intervertebral disk degeneration is accompanied by the loss of extracellular matrix content due to imbalance in anabolic and catabolic pathways.

The consistency of the human foetal nucleus pulposus greatly differs from that of a healthy adult. The study of the pathway analysis, the core matrisome of the human foetal disk appears to have great potential for developing regenerative therapies in the future.

Following degeneration, even with minor strain, either the nucleus pulposus may be displaced eccentrically within the disc itself or it may bulge or burst through the annulus fibrosus, usually in a posterolateral direction. The former is responsible for unequal tension in the disc, leading to lumbago (severe acute pain and spasm) and the latter may lead to pressure upon the spinal roots.

The pathological conditions concerning intervertebral disc are expressed as follows (as suggested by Jensen et al. quoted by Witte DH in Campbells' Operative Orthopaedics, 12th ed. Elsevier: Mosby; 2013;p142):

- *Bulge of intervertebral disc:* A circumferential symmetrical extension of disc beyond the interspace around the end plates.
- *Protrusion of intervertebral disc:* A focal or asymmetrical extension of disc beyond the interspace around the end plates.
- *Extrusion of intervertebral disc:* A more extreme extension of disc beyond the interspace, with the base against the disc of origin narrower than the diameter of the extruding material itself or with no connection between the material and the disc of origin.
- *Sequestration of intervertebral disc:* A disc fragment which has completely separated from the disc of origin.

Weight Transmission along the Vertebral Column

Weight transmission along the vertebral column changes according to the posture or type/phase of mobility. In a normal stance phase, the weight is transmitted mainly along the anterior half of the spinal segments. The posterior half plays more or less a passive role and transmits very little weight (except C1 and C2). Anteriorly too, the main weight is transferred along the body surfaces. Partial weight transmission is along the diarthrodial joints. Very little weight transmission occurs along the posterior elements and processes.

APPLIED ANATOMY OF MOTOR AND SENSORY SYSTEMS

Motor System

The motor system is briefly shown in **Figure 8.4** and thoroughly discussed in **Table 8.1**.

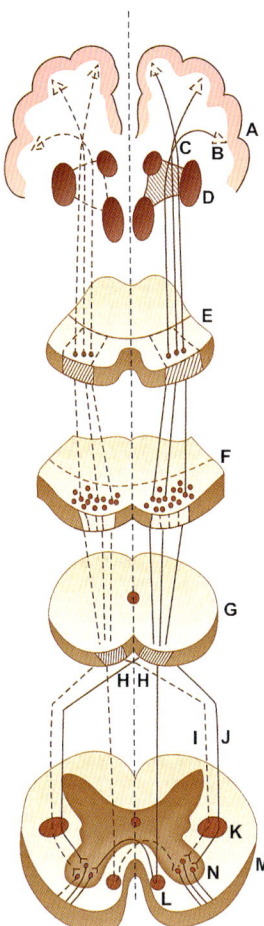

Fig. 8.4: Course of pyramidal fibres. A = motor cortex; B = pyramidal cells; C = corona radiata; D = internal capsule; E = mid brain; F = pons; G = medulla; H = medullary decussation; I = crossed fibres; J = uncrossed fibres; K = lateral white column; L = anterior white commissure; M = spinal cord; N = anterior horn cells; O = spinal nerves containing mostly crossed fibres.

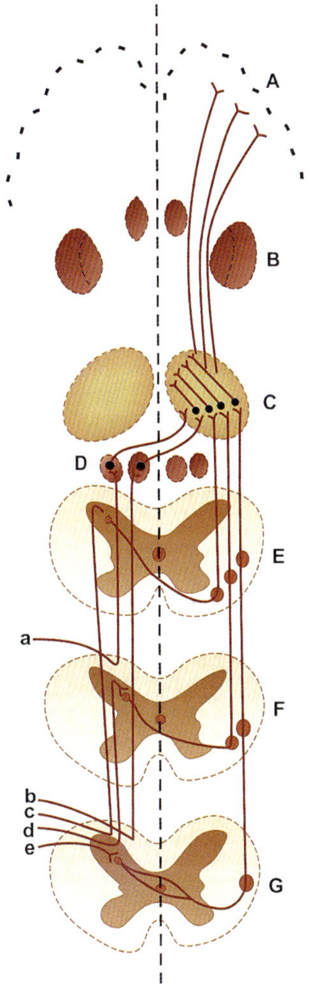

Fig. 8.5: Sensory pathways: A = posterior central gyrus; B = internal capsule; C = thalamus; D = nuclei gracilis and cuneatus; E, F and G = section of spinal cord at different levels; a = tract of Burdach; b = tract of Gall; c = touch fibres; d = thermal fibres; e = pain fibres.

Sensory System (Figs. 8.5 and 8.5A)

The first order sensory fibres for the appreciation of pain, touch and temperature terminate at the tip of the grey matter of the posterior horn. From there, second order neurons start. These fibres cross immediately, or a little above, to the opposite side in front and behind the central canal as the lateral spinothalamic tract to carry mainly pain and temperature extremes and the anterior spinothalamic tract for carrying crude touch. Both these groups of fibres terminate in the thalamus, from where the third order neurons carry impulses to the post-central gyrus.

The first order sensory fibres for the appreciation of sense of position, sense of movement, moderate temperature variation, vibration, size, shape, two point discrimination and light discriminative touch ascend directly in the posterior column and end in the nuclei gracilis and cuneatus situated in the medulla oblongata. From there, second order neurons start and terminate in the thalamus of the opposite side. The fasciculus gracilis carries fibres from the lower half of the body, whereas the fasciculus cuneatus (laterally situated) carries fibres from the upper half of the body. The third order neurons carry impulses to post-central gyrus through the internal capsule. Therefore, at any spinal cord level two major groups of sensory fibres exist.

- Those carrying pain, temperature and crude touch sensations from the opposite side of the body
- Those carrying appreciation of posture, weight, size, shape, vibration, moderate temperature variation and fine touch from the same side of the body.

Hemisection of the spinal cord results in loss of pain, thermal sensation and crude touch below the level of the lesion on the opposite side, while on the ipsilateral side there is loss of sense of position, vibration, recognition of weight, size, shape, and fine touch, besides spastic paralysis. This is called **Brown-Séquard syndrome.**

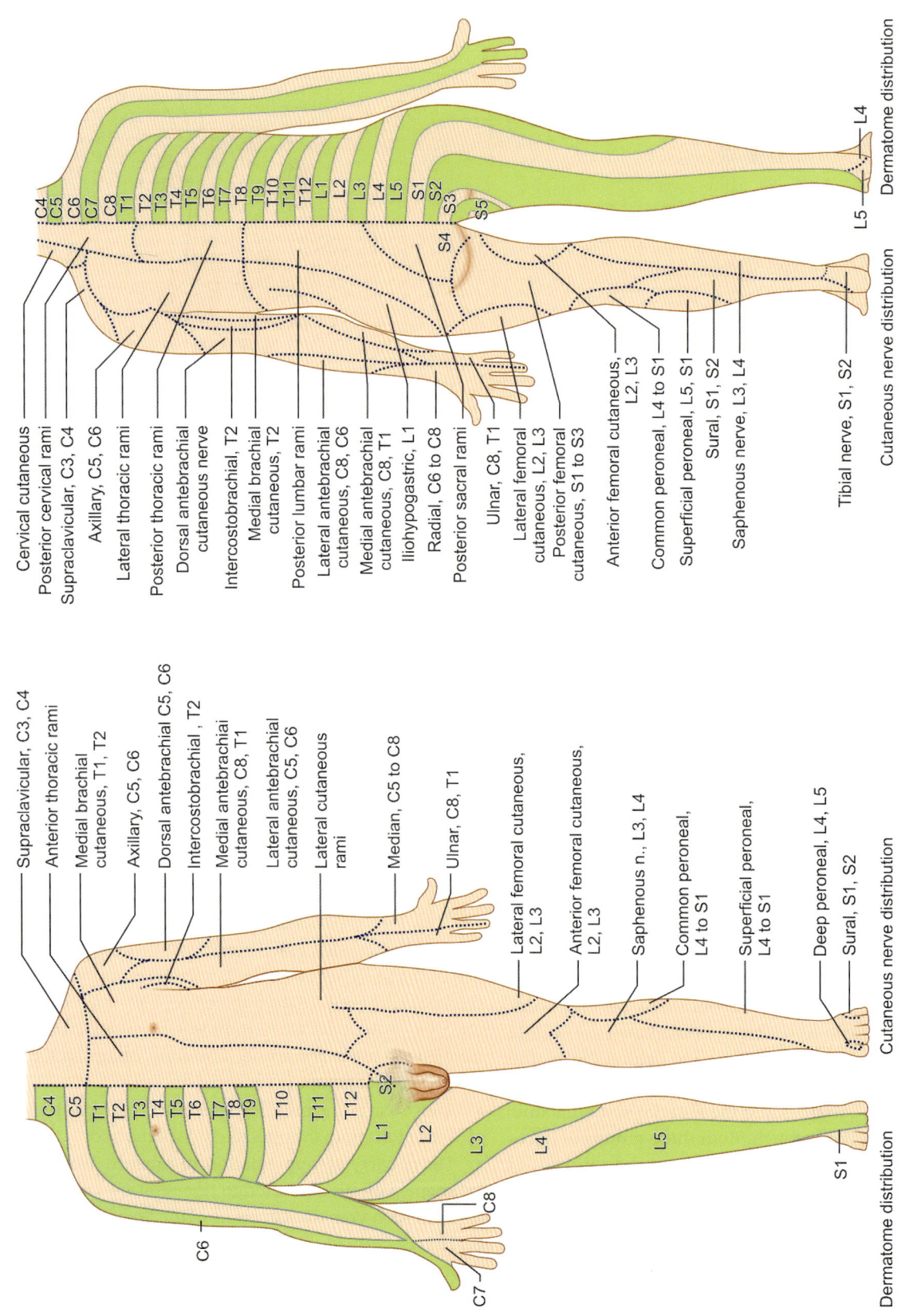

Fig. 8.5A: Cutaneous sensation mapping on the anterior and posterior aspects of body.

NB: After book by—Le Blond RF, De Gown RL, Brown DD: De Gowines Diagnostic Examination, 9th edition: http://www.access medicine.com (Pages 700 and 701)

TABLE 8.1: Applied anatomy of motor system.		
Corticospinal system	*Extrapyramidal system*	*Cerebellum*
Execution of movements of the limbs depends upon: (A) Intact higher centres (upper motor neuron)—for initiation of the impulses for voluntary movements, for maintenance of the posture		
Responsible for initiating voluntary and skilled motor activities. The following sequence illustrates this pathway. Pyramidal cells of 5th layer of motor cortex, corticospinal tract, anterior 2/3rds of posterior limb of internal capsule, middle 3/5th of the peduncles of mid brain, pons, medulla (lower part). Majority of fibres decussate with those of opposite side in the lateral column of the spinal cord as crossed corticospinal tract, few fibres which do not decussate descend downward in the anterior column as the direct corticospinal tracts and they decussate at segmental levels. A few uncrossed fibres continue as uncrossed, corticospinal tract of same side and end in the anterior horn cells of same side. The corticospinal fibres terminate at different levels in the grey matter of brain stem and the anterior horn cells of the spinal cord. *Affection of the corticospinal system is an upper motor neuron lesion* (signs—weakness, spasticity, increased tendon reflexes, extensor plantar response— except in the stage of neuronal shock; superficial reflexes are absent). (B) Lower motor neuron: Signs: Loss or less of muscle power—weakness, flaccidity, decreased/absent tendon reflexes, absent/plantar flexion-response. Lower motor neuron consists of anterior horn cells, homologous cells in brain stem and their efferent nerve fibres, which pass through anterior spinal nerve roots and peripheral nerves up to the muscles	Responsible for control of posture and initiation of movements. Specially responsible for postural mechanisms, e.g. turning to the sides, sitting, standing, walking, running, etc. It consists of—basal ganglia, subthalamic nuclei, substantia nigra, red nuclei and other structures in the brainstem These centres are connected to the lower motor neurons in spinal cord by indirect tracts—dentorubrospinal, reticulospinal, vestibulospinal, and olivospinal Affections of this system lead to: • Difficulty in initiation of voluntary movements, impairment of orientation and balancing reflexes • Alterations in muscle tone • Appearance of involuntary movements • Muscle weakness (rarely)	Receives afferents from the spinal cord, vestibular system, basal ganglia and cerebral cortex. It controls the lower motor neuron through its connections via thalamus with the basal ganglia and cerebral cortex. Lesions—cause muscular hypotonia, incoordination (ataxia)

The anatomic unit of function for the motor portion of the peripheral nervous system, i.e. a "motor unit" includes motor neuron situated in the anterior horn of the spinal cord, its axon, the neuromuscular junction, and the muscle fibres supplied by the peripheral nerve.

Bundle Arrangements and Tracts of the Spinal Cord (Fig. 8.6)

Innervation of the Urinary Bladder and its Clinical Importance (Fig. 8.7)

Sympathetics relax the detrusor and contract the internal sphincter. Urine collecting in bladder stretches the detrusor muscle. The sensation of filling passes through the sympathetic via the posterior column in the spinal cord—to higher centre. According to space and surrounding, there is either inhibition through sympathetic action, or release through parasympathetic action. When micturition is desired, parasympathetic contracts detrusor and relaxes the internal sphincter. Urine reaches the external sphincter, thereafter pudendal nerve relaxes the external sphincter.

Section of the cord above S2 leads to "**cord bladder**" or "**automatic bladder**" or "**upper motor neuron type bladder**", that is, bladder emptying is controlled by spinal centres through a spinal reflex arc. In such bladder, there is frequency and incontinence. The bladder is small and usually sensitive to small changes in intravesical pressure-volume changes.

Nerve supply of bladder consists of three main groups		
Nerve fibre groups	**Root value**	**Action**
Parasympathetic	S2–4	• Contracts detrusor muscle • Relaxes internal sphincter • Action on genitalia – Penile erection – Engorgement of clitoris
Sympathetic	L1–L2	• Relaxes detrusor • Contracts internal sphincter • Action on genitalia – Ejaculation – Orgasm
Somatic	Pudendal nerve	Relaxes the external sphincter

Section at and below S2 leads to an **autonomous or lower motor neuron type or isolated or atonic bladder** controlled by local myoneural reflexes in the bladder wall.

In such bladder, the urinary symptoms are produced usually by bilateral lesions. The bladder is flaccid, atonic and overflows without warning.

Failure of erection of penis (or engorgement of clitoris) and ejaculation (or orgasm) is caused by bilateral upper or lower

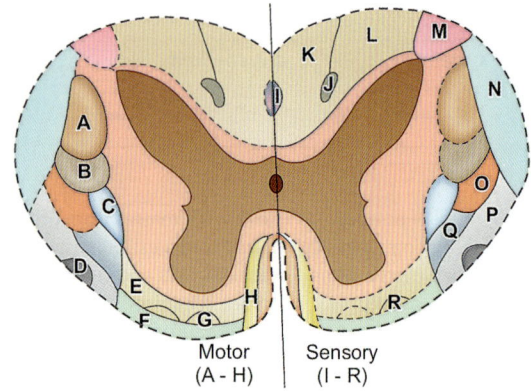

Fig. 8.6: Transverse section of spinal cord in (typical) dorsal region showing the motor (A to H) and sensory tracts (I to R) A = crossed pyramidal tract; B = rubro spinal tract; C = lateral vestibulospinal tract; D = oligospinal tract; E = reticulospinal tract; F = vestibulospinal tract; G = tectospinal tract; H = direct pyramidal tract; I = oval bundle; J = comma tract; K = tract of Gall; L = tract of Burdach; M = Lissauer's tract; N = dorsal spinocerebral tract; O = lateral spinothalamic tract; P = ventral spinocerebellar tract; Q = spinotectal tract; R = ventral spinothalamic tract.

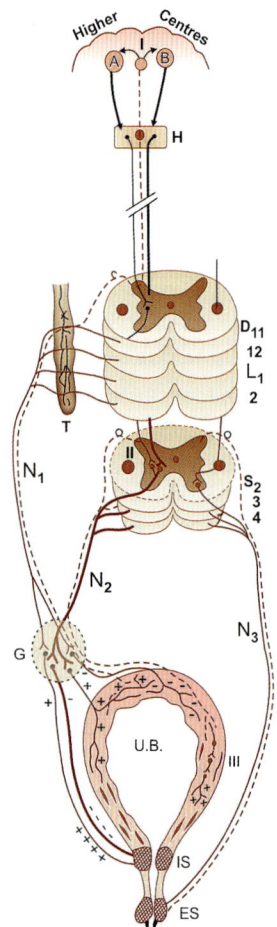

Fig. 8.7: Innervation of urinary bladder: A and B = Higher centres; H = Hypothalamus; T = Sympathetic trunk; G = Hypogastric ganglion; N_1 = Presacral nerve (sympathetic); N_2 = Nervi erigentes (parasympathetic); N_3 = Pudendal nerve (somatic); UB = Urinary bladder; IS = Internal sphincter; ES = External sphincter; '+' shows the contraction; '–' shows relaxation; Sensory pathways have been shown by interrupted line.

motor neuron lesion, besides due to mental depression which may be commonly present in such a situation.

■ METHODOLOGY

History Taking

Careful detail, history must be taken in chronological order with patience. Clinical history is not only the record of past and present suffering, but also constitutes the basis of future treatment, prognosis and possible prevention of diagnosed disease.

Besides the general mode of history taking in detail, certain important points should be given special consideration with special reference to specific pathology, e.g. (i) The patient may not have any symptoms in the spine, though the actual disease may be in it, (ii) When pain is complained of, with possible origin somewhere in the spinal column, the possibilities and course of root reference should be taken into consideration.

Spinal pain is termed as *"acute spinal pain"* when duration is less than 28 days; *"subacute spinal pain"* when duration is less than 12 weeks; *"chronic spinal pain"* when duration is more than 12 weeks.

Night pain in spine should be considered as being of probable serious pathological change.

It is being seen that if the clinician is not able to locate the cause of the spinal or any other pain, one hurries through to draw a conclusion that the patient is psychoneurotic. However, such hasty conclusion is a reflection on the examiner's diagnostic ability than on the patient, unless proven otherwise.

Patient may complain with a suggestion that he is suffering from 'sciatica' (pain along the course of sciatic nerve and its branches). Even the transfemoral amputated patient can complain pain in the sciatic distribution—**phantom sciatica** (Brown et al. 1997).

Before examining for lumbar movements, the patient should be asked for the presence of any pain and its site. If he/she indicates the lower thoracic or upper lumber area, one should be on alert. There may be serious disorders (discogenic problems are rare in this region). Therefore, this area is called *"forbidden area".*

General and Systemic Examination

Gait—If the patient can walk, the gait should be properly assessed (*see* Pages 240–246).

Regional Examination

This includes the whole spine and limbs.

Local Examination

Prerequisites: Ideally, the whole of the neck, back, chest and abdomen must be exposed. The patient should be examined in standing position (if possible), sitting on a stool (if possible) and lying on a flat bed. Most of the examination is from the back. However, most of paraplegics and quadriplegics should be examined in supine and guarded rolling lateral position in traction (except in late cases) to avoid any further damage.

Examination of the spine includes examination from the atlanto-occipital region to the coccyx. However, for all practical purposes, the sacroiliac joints examination must be taken as a part of the spinal examination.

Attitude and posture:

> *"Posture accompanies movement like a shadow; movement begins in posture and ends in posture."*
> —*Sherrington, quoted by Horstmann and Bleck 2007*

While standing, note the attitude of the patient. The posture of the patient while walking or standing can provide an important clue for reaching a diagnosis. A fixed statue-like stooping posture is characteristic of ankylosing spondylitis; standing with the legs crossed scissor like position and a tendency of equinus position may be seen in cerebral diplegia; and swaying of the body, especially while standing with feet close together is typical of cerebellar lesions.

A child with active caries spine, when asked to stand, leans forward with stiff back and supporting his body weight on his lower thighs or on something with the help of his hands **(Figs. 8.8 and 8.9)**.

Inspection

Ask the patient to stand as erect as possible. Note from behind the position of head, the hairline of scalp, length of neck and the levels of shoulders, scapulae, and iliac crests.

From posterior aspect, the shoulders and pelvis should be in level and equal and soft tissue structures on both sides should be symmetrical. The thoracic and lumber vertebrae should be vertically aligned. The inferior angle of scapulae should be in level with the seventh thoracic spinous process.

The iliac crests should be in the line with the fourth lumbar vertebrae.

Inspecting from the side and behind—note the spinal curvatures. In the midline of the back there is a longitudinal depression—the central furrow, which contains the tips of the spinous processes presenting as knob like projections. At the root of the neck, the seventh spinous process stands out quite prominently—the *vertebra prominence*. On both sides of the central furrow are the paraspinal bulges which are produced by the paraspinalis muscles. These muscles stand prominent when in *spasm* **(Figs. 8.10 and 8.90)**, (nature's attempt to prevent movements which produce pain). If they look very prominent, increasing the median furrow at about the level of the 10th thoracic vertebra, it probably indicates early caries spine in that area (Jardine). However, in advanced cases since the muscles get atrophied, there will be no spasm **(Fig. 8.9)**. On the outer side of sacrospinalis, the posterior surface of the chest wall and loin region continues. Note the levels of the

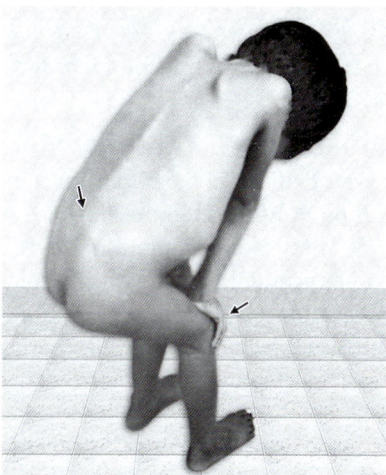

Fig. 8.9: Active caries spine L 4-5 to S1 region—when asked to stand, the child leans forward supporting his body weight on his lower thighs.

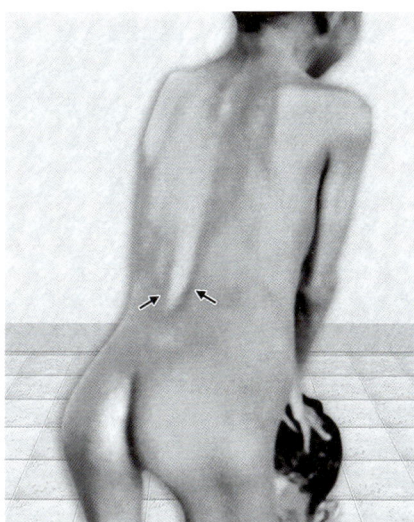

Fig. 8.8: Paraspinalis muscles go in spasm when the patient tries to flex the spine (A case of dorsolumbar caries spine). The boy stands supporting his body (hips upwards) on the head of his father.

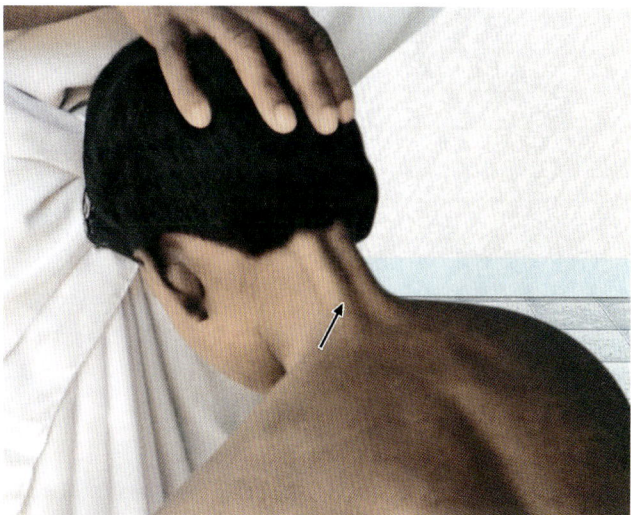

Fig. 8.10: In cervical caries with even little attempt of flexing the neck, the paraspinal muscles go in spasm.

medial and inferior scapular angles and the normal depression at the junction of the lower border of the 12th rib and the sacrospinalis muscle—the *renal angle*. The posterosuperior curvatures of the iliac crests stand prominent on both sides. The iliac crest ends posteriorly as the posterosuperior iliac spine, represented on the surface by the *dimple of Venus*, whence a vague linear depression runs downward with little outer inclination, which lies over the sacroiliac joint.

Note any deviation in the normal spinal curvature, the central furrow, the paraspinal bulge, slopes on the back of the chest, any bulge in the loin region, fullness over or below the iliac crest and any fullness or abnormality of the dimple of Venus. The pelvis should be in the neutral position, i.e., the anterior superior iliac spines should be in same vertical plane as the symphysis pubis; Hip, knee and ankle joints should be neither flexed nor hyperextended.

Look for any **dysspondylism** (an abnormality of development of the spine or vertebral column).

Abnormalities in the Curvature of the Spine

The curvatures of spine should be recorded in a graph (*Rachigraph*).

Torticollis (wry neck)(Figs. 8.11A and B): In this condition, there is side-ways bending of the neck with some rotational element resulting in head tilted to same side and chin to the opposite. It may be congenital due to—a *sternomastoid tumour* (a congenital firm mass—fibromatosis in the sternocleidomastoid—a firm mass is palpable at birth or during the first 2 weeks); fibromyositis, spasm and contracture of one sternomastoid; trauma; bony anomalies (e.g. unilateral defect in the vertebral body); Klippel-Feil syndrome; squint; or an overlying soft tissue contracture (e.g. following burn).

Acquired torticollis is mostly painful and is associated with atalantoaxial rotatory displacement usually due to frequent upper respiratory infections, inflamed adenoid and similar pathology.

Ocular torticollis is type of acquired torticollis, albeit the lesion which cause is probably congenital.

Congenital muscular torticollis, with complaints of pain and cosmetic problems is common in developing and under developed countries. Surgical bipolar release is usually beneficial in relieving pain, and cosmetic problems to variable extent.

Scoliosis (Figs. 8.12 to 8.14)

The term scoliosis was coined by Galen (131-201 AD) and was derived from Greek word meaning thereby 'crooked'.

Scoliosis is the deviation of spine in the frontal plane. In scoliosis, the spine bends sideways producing a lateral curvature but is usually accompanied by a rotational deformity (as spinal column starts to buckle it collapses — which is called scoliosis). In fact biomechanically, scoliosis can be understood as the rotated lordosis. On the whole,

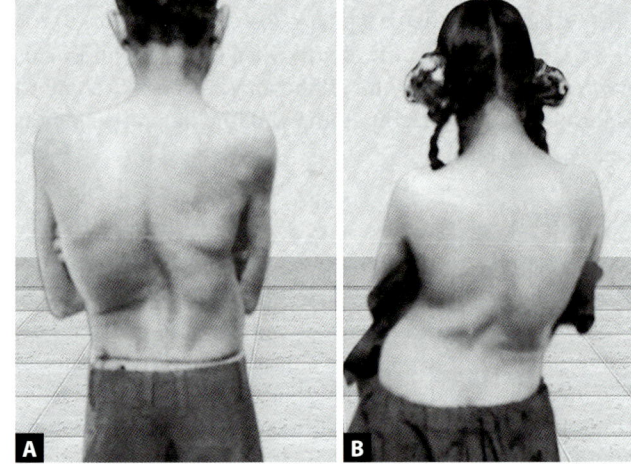

Figs. 8.12A and B: Structural dorsolumbar scoliosis in brother and sister.

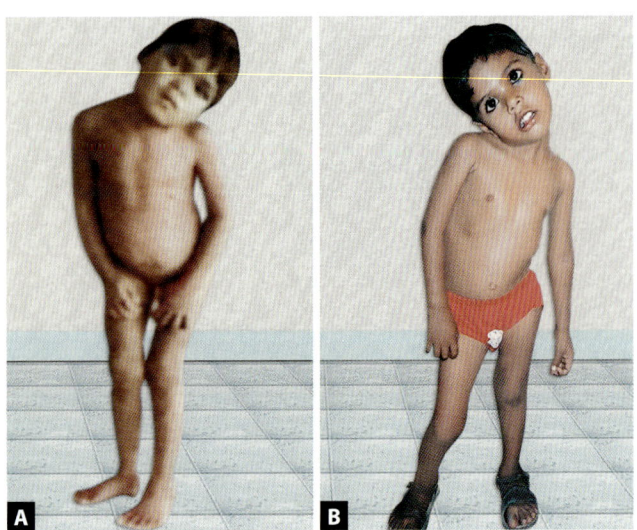

Figs. 8.11A and B: (A) Congenital torticollis on the left side, (B) Congenital torticollis on the right side, which is more common than on left.

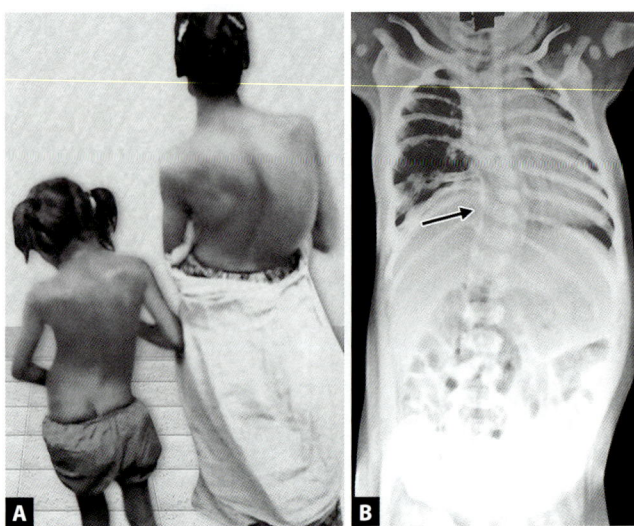

Figs. 8.13A and B: (A) Structural dorsolumbar scoliosis in mother and daughter; (B) Congenital scoliosis with skeletal deformities in ribs, vertebrae, pelvis, etc.—Infantile presentation.

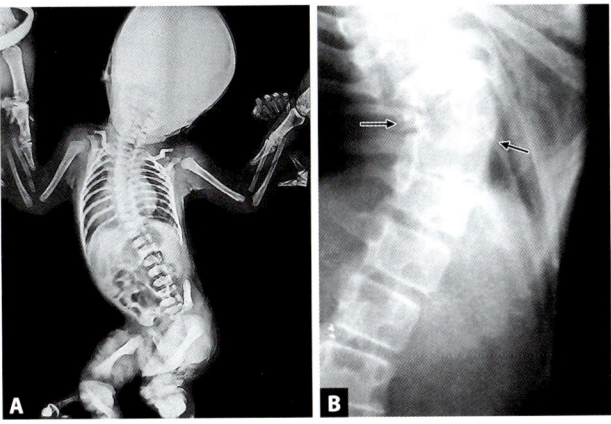

Figs. 8.14A and B: (A) Neonate with congenital scoliosis; (B) Congenital scoliosis due to hemivertebra.

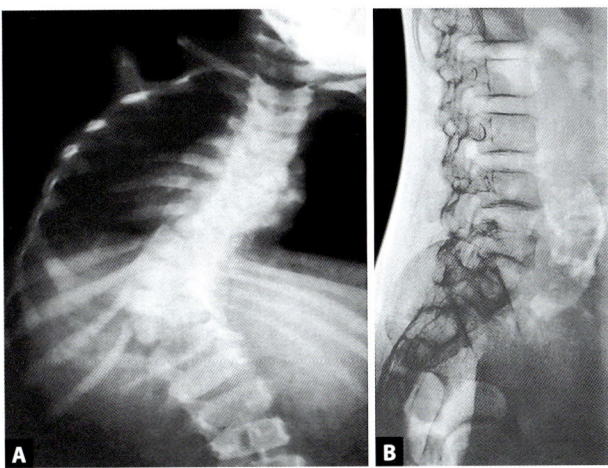

Figs. 8.15A and B: (A) Kyphoscoliosis following caries spine, (B) Calcification in aortic wall. A chance finding in chronic back pain.

scoliosis may be considered as a three-dimensional deformity with lateral deviation and torsion of the vertebrae.

On the whole females are more at risk to suffer with scoliosis with the female to male ratio of 3.5:1. This prevalence ratio increases with the increase in the magnitude of the curve and becomes more or less 7.2 to 1 for the curves more than 30°.

Scoliosis is 20 times more common in the first degree relatives of patients suffering from scoliosis.

If there is any scoliosis, note the following points: (i) the site; (ii) the persistence or disappearance of scoliosis in forward bending [functional scoliosis (sciatica, compensatory in leg length inequality, postural) disappears on forward bending and reappears when the patient becomes erect sciatic scoliosis]; (iii) the number of basic curvatures. The lateral shift caused by mechanical dysfunction and muscle spasm in the lower lumbar spine is called *semiotic scoliosis*. It usually results from painful impingement of dura mater or nerve root. *Curves are primary (major) or secondary (compensatory)* to the primary curve in an attempt to maintain spinal balance. Ponseti and Friedman classified *six main patterns of scoliosis curve:* 1. Single major lumbar curve, 2. Single major thoracolumbar curve, 3. Combined thoracic and lumbar curves (double major curves), 4. Single major thoracic curve, 5. Single major high thoracic curve, 6. Double major thoracic curve (described by Moe); (iv) appreciate upper and lower limits of the curvatures and the most prominent level of the convexity; (v) the side of the convexity; (vi) association with other deformities like kyphosis (e.g. kyphoscoliosis, **Figs. 8.15 and 8.16**); (vii) the effect on the chest. The chest bulges out posterolaterally on the convex side of the scoliosis, since in the thoracic region the ribs are attached to the vertebrae and the rotation of the vertebrae (spinal column) throws the attached ribs into prominence producing **rib hump (razor back)**, which can be better assessed in forward bending position of the patient. On the concave side of the scoliosis, there is crowding of the ribs with the appearance of a transverse furrow in the flanks **(Fig. 8.16B)**. Note the level of both iliac crests and the approximation of the last rib to the iliac crest; (viii) any change in the height of the patient due to abnormalities in the spinal curvatures, this can be assessed by

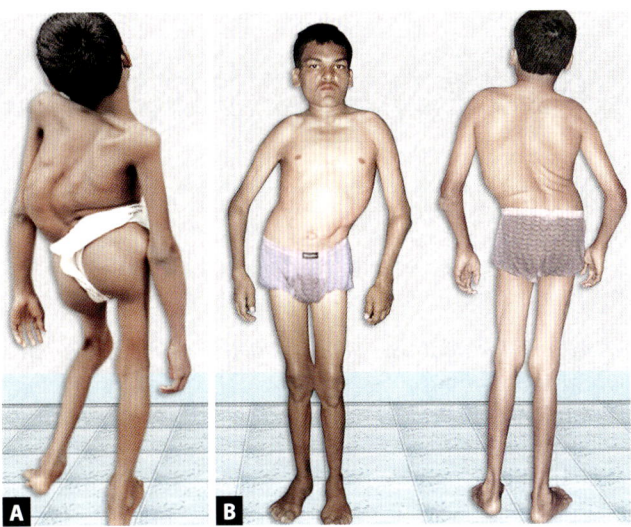

Figs. 8.16A and B: (A) Paralytic kyphoscoliosis, (B) Neglected structural scoliosis with rib hump.

the trunk/limb ratio; (ix) any facial asymmetry, deviation and prominence of the chin, squint, or difference in the level of the hair line, asymmetry in shoulder level as they may occur in certain cases of congenital or paralytic scoliosis.

Scoliosis has been described since ancient times and is defined as a lateral deviation of at least 10° from the normal coronal alignment of the spine. There is a complex three-dimensional torsion of the spinal column.

The *scoliosis is termed 'mobile'*, when normal spinal flexibility is preserved, and *'structural or fixed,'* when there is loss of normal mobility in the segment involved due to change in the shape of the vertebrae and adaptive changes in the allied soft tissue. Structural scoliosis occurs in congenital vertebral malformations **(Figs. 8.14A and B)** and paralysis of back and abdominal muscles.

The *etiology of scoliosis* as a whole is varied and that of the most common variety of scoliosis, i.e. idiopathic type is unclear. However, etiologically scoliosis may be classified as given in the **Table 8.2**.

TABLE 8.2: Etiological classification of scoliosis.

Structural		Non-structural

1. *Idiopathic:*
   – According to age:
   – Infantile (< 3 yrs)
   – Juvenile (3-10 yrs)
   – Adolescent (> 10–18 yrs)
   – Adult (> maturity)
2. *Neuromuscular:*
Neuropathic:
   – Upper motor neuron lesion, e.g. cerebral palsy, syringomyelia; spinal cord tumour
   – Lower motor neuron lesion, e.g. poliomyelitis; arthrogryposis (neurogenic); spinomuscular atrophy
   – Myopathic
Muscular dystrophy; arthrogryposis (myopathic)
3. *Congenital:*
   – Failure of formation—hemivertebrae, wedged vertebrae
   – Failure of segmentation—unilateral segmented bar
   – Associated with neural tube defect—myelomeningocoele, spinal dysraphism
4. Neurofibromatosis
5. Mesenchymal disorders, e.g. Marfan's syndrome
6. Extraspinal soft tissue contracture, e.g. post-empyema, post-burns
7. Traumatic
8. Bone dysplasia
9. Metabolic disorders, e.g. rickets, osteogenesis imperfecta
10. Neoplastic, e.g. in osteoid osteoma
11. Thoracogenic, e.g. post-thoracotomy, post-thoracoplasty; after open heart surgery in paediatric patients with congenital heart disease
	Exact cause not known, hence various theories
	• Altered melatonin production
	• Connective tissue disorder
	• Skeletal muscle abnormality
	• Thrombocytic abnormalities
	• Neural mechanism defect
	• Oculovestibular abnormality
	• Vertebral growth and developmental biomechanical factors
	• Homobex/Hox genes, etc.
		1. Functional, e.g.
		   – Postural
		   – Lower limb length inequality
		   – Pelvic obliquity
		2. Nerve root irritation, e.g. in intervertebral disc prolapse
		3. Hysterical

NB: Based on CME lecture by Johari A. IOACON 2005

Idiopathic scoliosis is the most common type (almost 80%) and according to the age of onset (first diagnosis) it may be (i) *infantile* (0–3 years), (ii) *juvenile* (4 to 9 years), and (iii) *adolescent idiopathic scoliosis* (>10–18 years). The curve of an idiopathic scoliosis, when present from childhood, differs from a lateral shift associated with recent disk problems in that it is accompanied by the lower thoracic or lumbar rotation deformity. It becomes obvious in flexion attitude.

Congenital scoliosis is supposed to be due to failure of vertebral body formation and/or segmentation during embryonic development. Formation defects include hemivertebrae and wedge vertebrae (Winter RB et al 1968).

Idiopathic scoliosis is a structural curvature of spine, the cause of which is not known. It is the most common type of structural scoliosis, accounting for almost 80% of incidence. Idiopathic scoliosis has been classified according to the age at its first diagnosis: (i) Infantile idiopathic scoliosis when children' age is less than 3 year, (ii) *Juvenile idiopathic scoliosis* – in age group of 4 to 9 year, (i) & (ii) are grouped under early-onset scoliosis. (iii) *Adolescent idiopathic scoliosis* is diagnosed in patients of 10 to 18 years of age.

Infantile idiopathic scoliosis is a lateral curvature of the spine with apical rotation and wedging, which usually presents before the age of 3 years. Some curves are progressive even leading to cardiopulmonary compromise, while remaining ones usually resolve or disappear spontaneously within initial years of life *(resolving type of infantile scoliosis*—James JIP 1951). Exact cause of infantile idiopathic scoliosis is not known, hence various theories (*see* **Table 8.2**).

Intrauterine moulding and postnatal external pressure on the spine are the simply thought causes. The cause of resolving infantile idiopathic scoliosis remains unknown.

Scoliosis is the most common and serious structural change in the spinal column of cerebral palsy patients, especially in non-walkers with total body involvement.

When the scoliosis is associated with kyphosis (kyphoscoliosis), it reduces the size of thoracic cavity leading to compromise of cardiopulmonary function **(Figs. 8.15 and 8.16)**.

Adolescent idiopathic scoliosis — These patients are more prone to chronic back pain, however, the natural history of adolescent idiopathic scoliosis does not necessarily have functional disability. The classic patient is a tall adolescent girl with the apex of the curve pointing to the right. Most of the curves are minor. Progression is usually gradual and nearly always stops with the fusion of the growth plate.

The presence of the major curves in young children is a matter of concern, since the curve may worsen in the years of growth ahead in the children. Persisting moderate to severe pain in scoliosis should be thoroughly investigated to exclude any organic pathology, e.g. neuromuscular problems.

Degenerative scoliosis: Base et al (2016) have described the secondary scoliosis developing in adult (usually after

40 years of age) as 'degenerative scoliosis. These patients do not complain of deformity, rather almost all present with pain and disability. Degenerative disk diseases, spinal canal stenosis, compression fractures can all present with scoliosis (many times named as *pseudo scoliosis*).

Hysterical scoliosis: Hysterical scoliosis should be the diagnosis of exclusion after thorough physical and neurological evaluation to rule out even the rare cause like spinal cord tumour. Here the patient presents with usually a long C-shaped curve, imbalance of trunk and a variable severity of scoliosis almost daily. Further, the curve disappears when the person lies supine. In X-ray, there is no evidence of vertebral rotation. After confirmation psychiatric consultation and therapy should be done.

Thoracic inlet narrowing with a thoracic inlet index > 5.6 compared to age matched controls (evaluated on MRI) is strongly associated with pulmonary impairment in proximal thoracic hypokyphotic curves >80°. Hence assessment in detail of pulmonary function is mandatory.

Management of scoliosis is a vast consideration, however, the practical approach should be to follow the *3-Os principles: Observe*–wait and watch for curves less than 20°; *Orthoses* for the curves 20–40°; *Operation* for the curves more than 40°.

Kyphosis

> "When a gibbosity seizes a person, it occasions a crisis of the already existing disease."
> —**Hippocrates**

There can be an abnormality in the anteroposterior curvature of the spine. Kyphosis is deviation of spine in the lateral plane. Some amount of kyphotic posture is normally present in the thoracic region and its accentuation produces hunchback, which leads to kyphotic deformity. Kyphotic posture in lumbar region is typically present in acute lumbago. If it becomes abnormally prominent (more than 45°) posteriorly, it is excessive kyphosis. These can be of two types as follows:

- *Labile kyphosis*—For example postural; due to muscle weakness (early stage of polio and myopathy), compensatory (in CDH)
- *Fixed kyphosis*—They are of two types.
  - *Angular kyphosis* (knuckle or gibbus) **(Figs. 8.17 and 8.18)**. This is due to collapse of one or two vertebrae, e.g. in tuberculosis, spinal fractures, congenital collapse, etc. Knuckle is sometimes referred as the prominence of a single spinous process indicating collapse of a single vertebra, e.g. in spinal injury, tuberculosis
  - *Gradual kyphosis* (rounded kyphosis): This is due to partial or complete collapse of more than two vertebrae, e.g. in continuous faulty posture (curve of faulty posture disappears with extension of spine), in senile kyphosis, osteomalacia, adolescent kyphosis (Scheuermann's disease) ankylosing spondylitis **(Figs. 8.19A to C)**, Paget disease, osteoporosis (Dowager's hump), acromegaly, etc. Sometimes tuberculosis of spine also produces acutely rounded kyphosis **(Figs. 8.20 and 8.21)**.

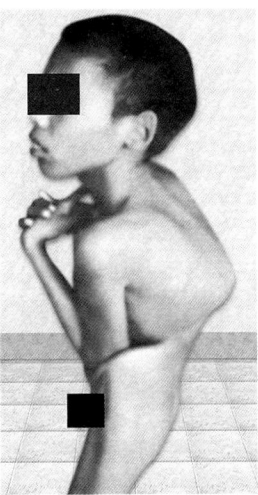

Fig. 8.17: Angular kyphosis.

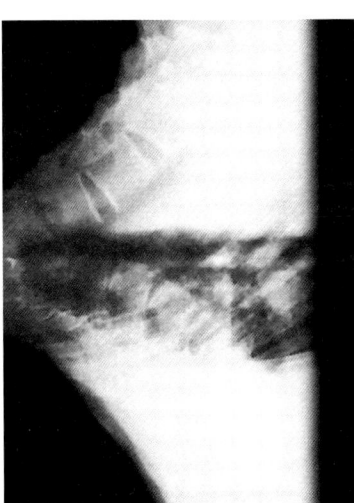

Fig. 8.18: Acute gibbus of dorsolumbar region following old caries.

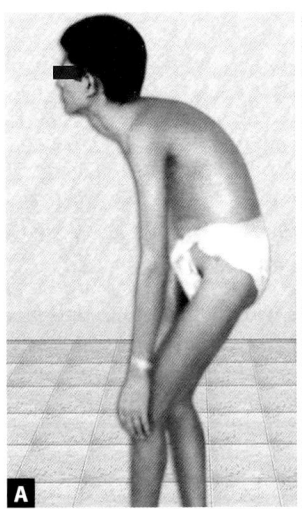

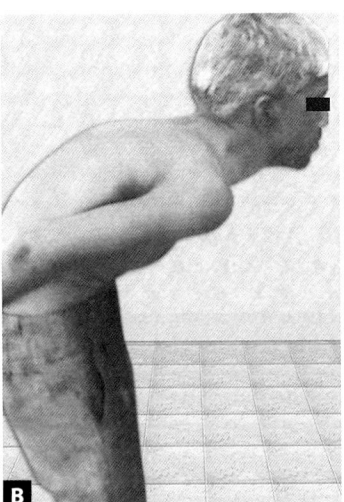

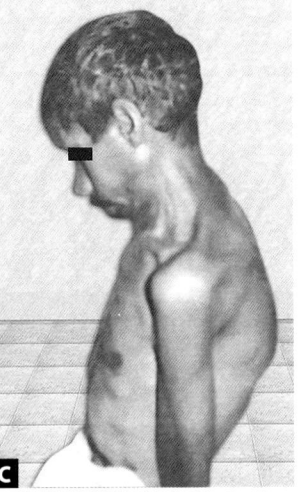

Figs. 8.19A to C: Rounded kyphosis following ankylosing spondylitis. Note also the fixed flexed back—(Pocker back in A and B) and neck in C showing *Chin-on-Chest deformity*—a highly characteristic deformity of ankylosing spondylitis.

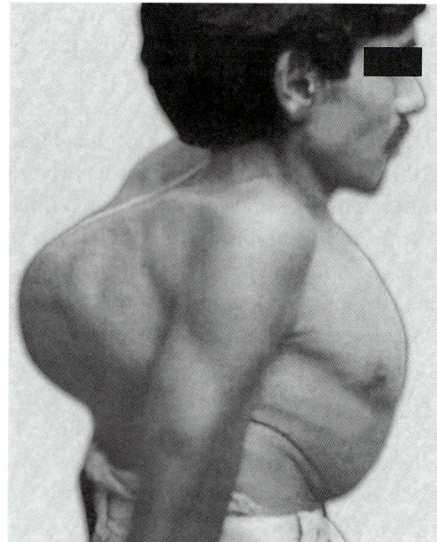

Fig. 8.20: Acutely rounded kyphosis.

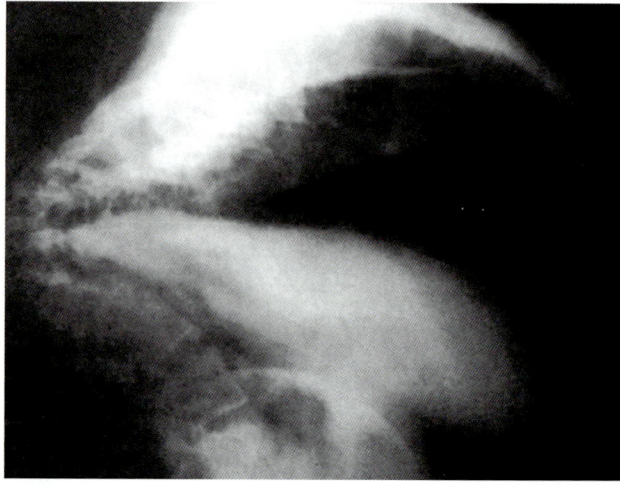

Fig. 8.21: X-ray showing acutely rounded kyphosis.

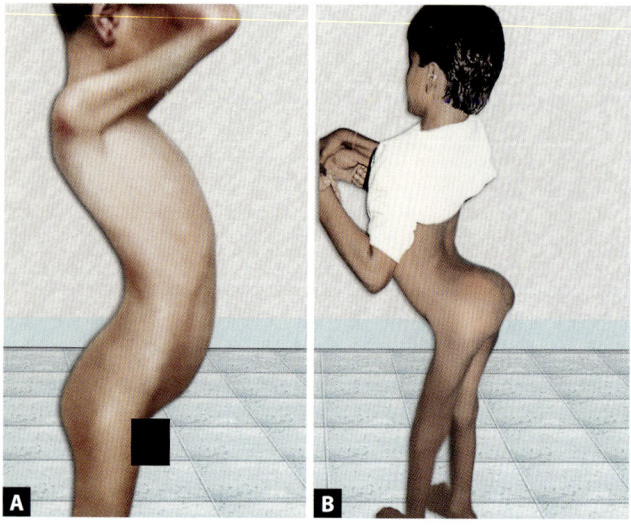

Figs. 8.22A and B: Marked lumbar lordosis.

In both these types, the flexion of spine may force the thorax to assume inspiratory position permanently with increased anteroposterior diameter and horizontal ribs. The distorted look of thorax mimics the barrel chest of pulmonary emphysema.

Congenital kyphosis is a serious condition in which progressive deformity may result in paraplegia. Congenital kyphosis can be of three types: Type I (due to failure of formation of vertebral body) has the worst prognosis with greatest risk of neurological involvement; Type II (due to failure of segmentation of vertebral body); Type III (due to failure of formation and failure of segmentation of vertebral body).

Early detection and fusion of spine are the main management for avoiding the complications. Posterior fusion is adequate for children of less than 5 years with a kyphosis less than 50°, otherwise combined anterior and posterior fusion is recommended.

In children, kyphosis is mainly due to tuberculosis and is rarely congenital. In adolescence, *adolescent kyphosis* (Scheuermann's disease) is the most common cause, followed by tuberculosis and polioparalysis. As paralytic legacy, the deformity is mostly the kyphoscoliosis.

In 1921, Scheuermann described a so-called spinal deviation—Scheuermann disease (kyphosis) distinguishable from passively correctable postural hunch back. It is characterized by fixed dorsal kyphosis with radiological changes (irregular vertebral end plates, apparently diminished disc space, wedging of the three adjacent vertebrae angled by at least 5°). Patients complain of backache (sometimes more intense), have limited/weaker extension of spine and tend to avoid energy demanding activities. Patients having kyphosis more than 100° and the apex of the curve between 1st and 8th thoracic segments may have restrictive lung disease.

Patients with less than 60° of curve may be managed by early bracing, whereas those with more than 65° of curve may require surgical correction. With increasing early care in children with curves greater than 10° only 10% require operative management while the rest can be managed non-operatively.

In adults, trauma, osteomalacia, caries spine and 'Kummell's disease account for most cases of kyphosis. In the elderly, senile kyphosis, senile osteoporosis, neoplastic collapse and Paget's disease are mainly responsible for kyphosis.

Kyphosis without scoliosis is also seen in the spine of patients of cerebral palsy. In early stage, it is flexible and looks as postural defect, but if it persists throughout the growth period, it becomes fixed structural deformity.

Flattened back: *Flattened back* is usually present in patients with lumbar spinal canal stenosis or lateral recess stenosis

Lordosis: *Kyrtorrhachic* [Gr. kyrtos = curved + rhachis = spine) means spinal curvature with concavity backwards.

When the spinal convexity becomes abnormally prominent anteriorly, this is known as lordosis (**Figs. 8.22A and B**).

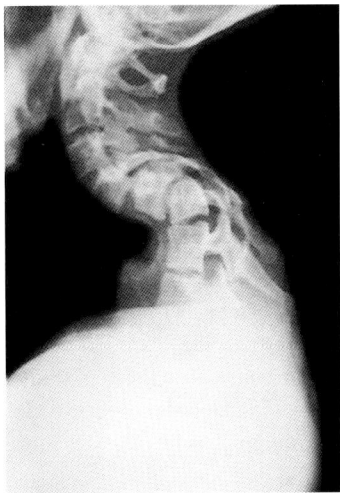

Fig. 8.23: Congenital lordosis of cervical spine.

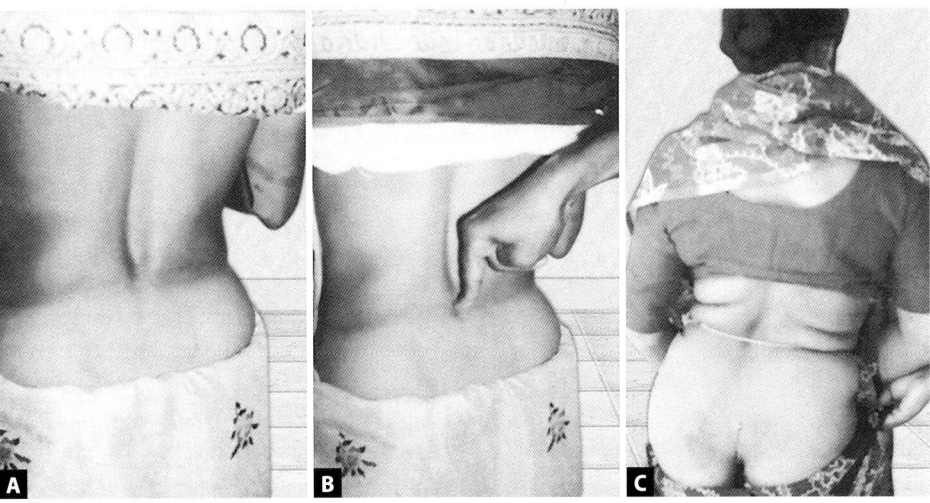

Figs. 8.24A to C: Spondylolisthesis—Note the marked deepened median furrow ending on a step (A and B). On the both flanks deep furrow are obvious (C).

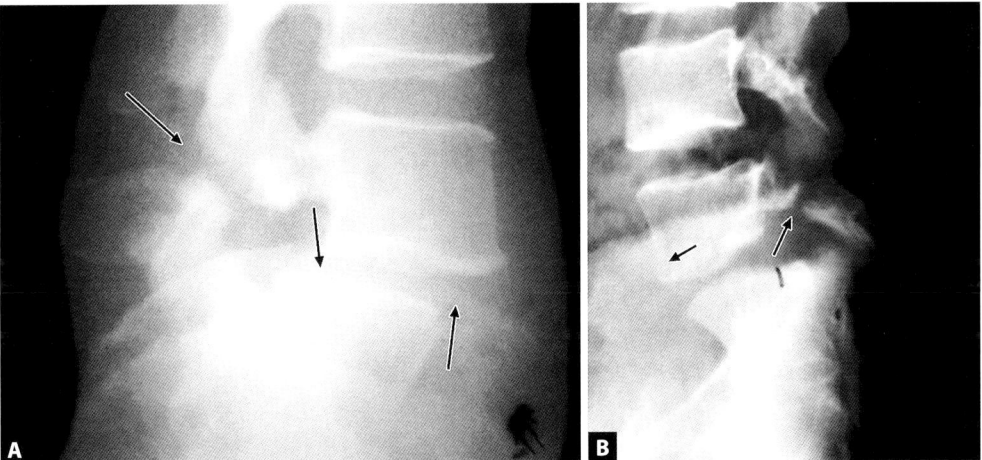

Figs. 8.25A and B: Spondylolisthesis at between L4 over L5 (B).

Weakness of anterior abdominal muscles usually produces lordosis. Lordosis also develops to counterbalance a protuberant abdomen in pregnancy, obesity and myopathy associated with swayback. Lordosis also develops as a compensatory deformity in spondylolisthesis, congenital dislocation of hip, flexion contracture of hip joint and contracted Achilles tendon. A slight amount of lordosis is normally present in the lumbar and cervical regions (In tetanus, the whole back curves posteriorly—*opisthotonus*). Rarely congenital cervical lordosis may be much marked **(Fig. 8.23)**.

In pathological lumbar lordosis, the abdomen becomes correspondingly prominent. The extent of lordosis can be assessed by visualising the central furrow. If it is deeper than normal—the *lordosis is exaggerated*. If it is about normal, the *curvature is normal*, if it is comparatively shallow—*the lordosis is obliterating*. If there is no central furrow, this is *complete obliteration of the lordosis* and *flattening of the back*; if the curvature reverses with the convexity backwards, this is *kyphosis of the lumbar spine*.

The relation between the measurements of lumbar lordosis and sacral inclination may influence the extension of hip—**"hip-spine syndrome"** (Offierski and Macnab 1983). If a patient develops a fixed flexion deformity of the hip there may be associated loss of lumbar lordosis.

In cerebral palsy patients, the flexion contracture of hips leads to increased pelvic inclination, which in turn results in lordosis.

Change in the lumbar lordosis may lead to disc degeneration and radicular pain.

In advanced degenerative arthrosis of knee, there is loss of extension of knee, which may affect lumbar lordosis and overall posture—this may be called **"knee-spine syndrome"** (Murata 2003).

The abnormal findings, such as a swelling, sinus, depression, scar, naevus, tuft of hair, specially in mid spinal line/groove/furrow etc. should be noted.

In the lumbosacral region, or adjoining one or two spaces above, note for any sudden depression in the central furrow where it tends to end. This will give an impression of

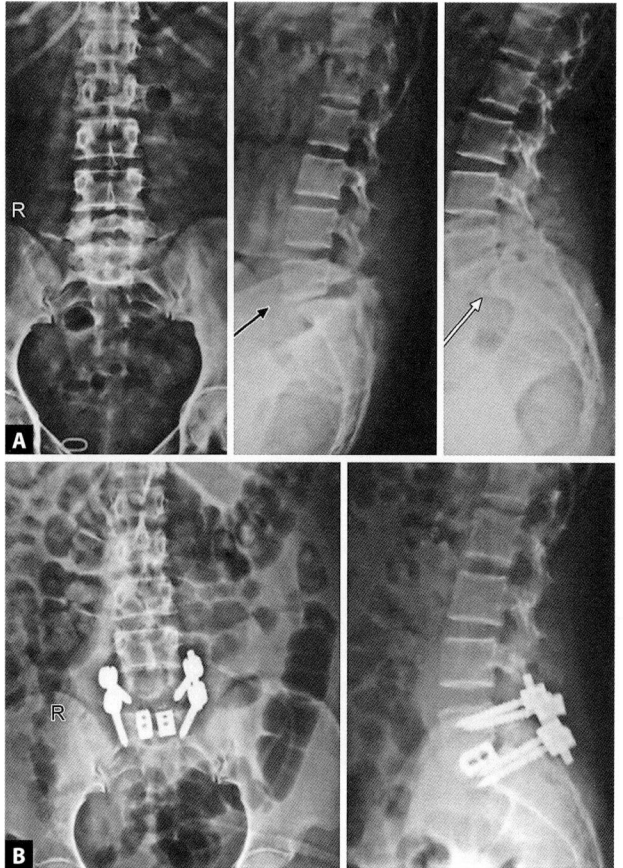

Figs. 8.26A and B: Spondylolisthesis (Gr II) of L4-L5 region. Note the complete dissolution of posterior spinal (skeletal) column (A); (B) Same patient (as in **Figure. 8.26A**) X-ray after fixation.

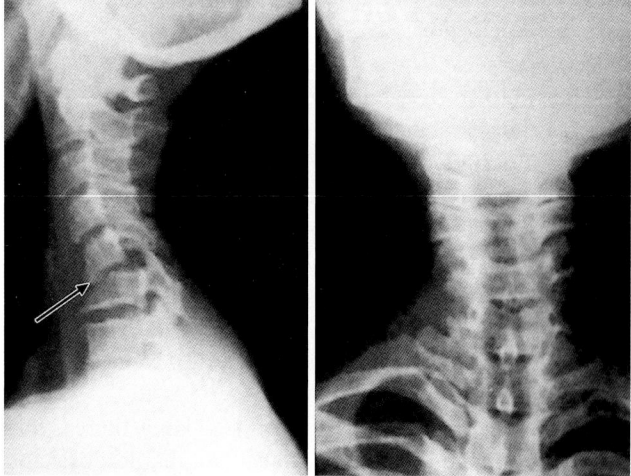

Fig. 8.27: Spondylolisthesis of cervical 5th over 6th vertebra.

a "step". This step is due to forward slipping of one vertebra with the whole column above over the vertebra below, i.e. spondylolisthesis **(Figs. 8.24 to 8.26)**. *Spondylolisthesis* also occurs in cervical region **(Fig. 8.27)**.

In certain conditions, there is a flattened appearance of the back especially the lower region. Ask the patient to bend forward. The lower half of the back, or even the upper portion, may appear uniformly flat—board like. This is described as *"boarding"* and is produced by spasm of the sacrospinalis muscle (e.g. in intervertebral disc prolapse, early ankylosing spondylitis, acute back strain).

The spinal muscles may undergo segmental spasm as a protective mechanism to avoid pain. In cases of acute trauma, the posteriorly protruded vertebral column may give a kyphotic appearance, but the spasm of sacrospinalis will be much more apparent. Above and below this particular site, sacrospinalis is mechanically stretched due to the posterior protrusion of the underlying bony projection. Hence, there cannot be local boarding.

Note any globular swelling, with or without a skin cover, especially in the lower lumbar region (*spina bifida manifesta*) **(Figs. 8.83 to 8.85)**. Search the lumbosacral region for any bulge (usually fibrofatty mass), tuft of hair **(Figs. 8.81 and 8.82)**, hyperpigmentation of skin, depression or other signs of *spina bifida occulta*.

After inspecting the back, an examination must be done from the sides and front of the trunk. The shape of the chest, any abnormality of the abdomen and any bulge or swelling should be clearly noted along with its characteristics. In case of any apparent pathology, assess the possible level and possible cause.

Palpation

Superficial Palpation

Examine for hyperaesthesia, any abnormal prominence or depression, any pulsation, or any increase in temperature.

General palpation of the whole of the back should be done by passing the palm from above downwards, right from the external occipital protuberance to the tip of the coccyx. Then start palpating the central furrow, paraspinal bulge, sides of the cervical spines, sides of the chest, the loins, iliac crests, sacroiliac region and buttocks while the patient has his arms across his chest keeping the back in as neutral a position as possible. This makes the mid-spinal line, right from the nuchal furrow to the internatal cleft, comparatively prominent. Even a minor prominence of the spinous processes can be easily palpated if the hand is passed cautiously.

Central furrow—Here palpation is mainly for the spinous processes and interspinous gaps. In a patient having wasting of the paraspinal muscles, these processes stand more prominent. On the other hand, in presence of spasm of the muscles, these processes are less prominent. Any abnormality in the pattern of spinous processes (in terms of their feel, alignment and spacing) should be noted. To avoid missing even mild sideway deviation of spinous processes, it is better to mark each spinous process with a skin pencil. If any spinous

process appears to be prominent, confirm its level, shape, size and tenderness. *Tenderness of spine can be elicited by three methods* **(Fig. 8.28)**.
- Direct pressure tenderness
- Twist tenderness
- Deep thrust tenderness.

Direct pressure tenderness (Fig. 8.28A): This is positive in any pathology in the spinous process or marked advanced pathology of the vertebral body. To elicit this tenderness, apply direct firm pressure with the thumb over the spinous processes, one by one, from cervical region to sacral region.

Twist tenderness (Fig. 8.28B): This is positive even in early pathology of the vertebral body, besides affections of the posterior vertebral elements. To elicit this tenderness apply twisting pressure/force by the thumb of the hand on the side of the spinous process (as if trying to rotate the vertebrae) and proceed from above downwards.

Deep thrust tenderness (Fig. 8.28C): This should be elicited only when the above methods have not indicated any tenderness and, therefore, the disease may be of chronic and/or less aggressive nature. It is done by applying a guarded thrust with the proximal part of the ulnar side of the fist over the spinous processes.

In younger children it is very difficult to elicit tenderness because of their general response of weeping to any stimuli. In such circumstances, demonstration of indirect tenderness has been advocated in the form of the '*anvil test*'. This is not advisable as it may produce collapse of a pathologically osteoporosed vertebral body, e.g. in caries spine. In children, elicit tenderness as far as practicable after gaining their confidence.

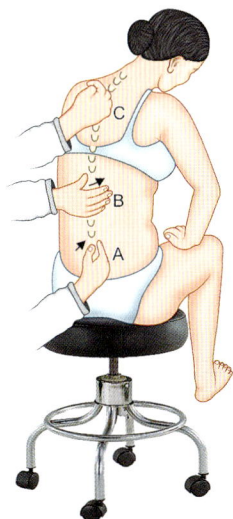

Fig. 8.28: Method of eliciting spinal tenderness: (A), direct pressure tenderness (thumb directly over spinous process); (B) twist tenderness (thumb twisting the spinous process from the side); (C) deep thrust tenderness.

In cases of spina-bifida manifesta, note the site, size, shape, content, and any impulse on coughing and perform the transillumination test.

Palpate on both sides of central furrow to note the *tone of paraspinal muscles*. If they are tight, it means they are in spasm. On deep pressure, the spasmodic muscle may even be tender. If the muscles are wasted, the bulge will be flattened and the feel will be soft. In marked wasting, it may be difficult to palpate the muscles as they are largely thinned out and the posterior portion of the ribs may be felt. In the cervical region, the sides of the neck should also be palpated. In the lumbar region, the *renal angle* should also be palpated. Pass your hands on both sides of chest and the abdomen to locate any abnormal swellings like cold abscesses. For *possible sites of cold abscesses* see **Table 8.3**.

Palpate the posterior slopes of the iliac crests on both sides. It will end in the dimples of Venus. Pass the fingers more or less vertically down for about 5 centimetres. The edges of the sacroiliac joints can be felt posteriorly. Note for any tenderness in this zone. Fibro-fatty nodules are usually felt in this region. Pressure over these nodules may elicit pain in distribution of sciatic nerve. This is called *pseudosciatica*. Deeper pressure is required to elicit the tenderness of sacroiliac joints.

If there is any sinus, its edges, tract and deeper fixations should be palpated.

Percussion

Percussion Tenderness

With rubber hammer, apply brisk tap over the spinous processes and note the points of tenderness, if any. This should be done when the above methods have not elicited tenderness. Any tenderness denotes comparatively less acute pathology.

■ MOVEMENTS (TABLE 8.4)

Movements Vary in Each Spinal Region

- *At the atlanto-occipital joint,* normal movement is nodding. Movements occur at the condyloid joint formed by the condylar processes on the both sides on the base of skull articulating with the concave articular facets on the upper surface of atlas.
- *At the atlanto-axial joint* side-to-side rotational movements occur at the pivot joint comprising of the odontoid process of the axis and fibro-osseous articular ring behind the anterior arch of the atlas.

However, initiating these movements at aforesaid joints, in extremes of these motions, all cervical joints do take part. The stress effects of rotational movements are more or less at the cervicodorsal region, it being the junction of comparatively mobile and fixed parts of spine.

TABLE 8.3: Possible sites of cold abscesses in caries spine.

Region	Pathology	Site	Remarks
1. Cervical	(i) Bursting through anterior cortex of bone as prevertebral abscess, beneath the prevertebral fascia	Retropharyngeal (central in position) may bulge in oropharynx	c.f. Acute retropharyngeal abscess which lies on one side and in front of prevertebral fascia—may burst in mouth
	(ii) Abscess tracking laterally behind the prevertebral fascia	In mediastinum	• May mimic thyroid nodule • May produce mediastinal syndrome
	(iii) Along the posterior division of spinal nerves (iv) From behind the prevertebral fascia	At back of neck on one side of the midline In posterior triangle of neck; infraclavicular region **(Fig. 8.29)** in axilla; or even down to lower part of arm along the axillary/brachial artery **(Fig. 8.30)** posterior mediastinum	• May produce mediastinal syndrome
2. Thorax	(i) Remains as prevertebral abscess (ii) May percolate on both sides of vertebral body in paravertebral gutters (iii) May perforate through parietal pleura (iv) From lower end of mediastinum, abscess may track: (a) Behind the lateral lumbocostal arch in between anterior layer of lumbodorsal fascia and quadratus lumborum. From here it may follow either of the three nerves lying behind the kidney, i.e. 12th thoracic or ilioinguinal or iliohypogastric.	• Radiologically—paravertebral abscess **(Figs. 8.31 to 8.34)** • Pyothorax • Post-renal abscess • Lower anterior abdominal parietal abscess or as rectus sheath abscess	
	Along the course of any thoracic nerve up to anterior end of intercostal space **(Figs. 8.35 to 8.39)**		
	(b) Through upper opening of psoas sheath, i.e. medial lumbocostal arch passing along the psoas muscle in the psoas sheath (c) Passing behind the median arcuate ligament along the aorta or any of its branches—branches of external iliac or branches of internal iliac	In pelvis—as psoas or iliopsoas abscess or even around lesser trochanter (i) Intraabdominal—in course of aorta (ii) Intrapelvic—may remain localised or present in gluteal region or in ischiorectal fossa	
	Along the course of one of the thoracic nerves (intercostal nerve). Along posterior division of a thoracic nerve and its branches: medial branch—2.5 cm and lateral branch—7.5 cm from spinous process	• In thorax up to anterior end of intercostal space **(Fig. 8.38)** • In abdomen—as rectus sheath abscess • Mid axillary line	
3. Lumbar	Along aorta or its branches Into the psoas sheath Into quadratus lumborum sheath Following the course of a lumbar nerve: • along femoral nerve • along obturator nerve • along sciatic nerve Extending between the posterior part of abdominal wall muscle	• As in thoracic region, i.e. iv (a) and iv (c). In front of groin or thigh (anywhere along the course) **(Figs. 8.40 and 8.38B)** Back of the thigh (anywhere along the course) Petit's triangle **(Figs. 8.41 and 8.42)**	• Abscess from thoracic disease cannot come in the Petit's triangle

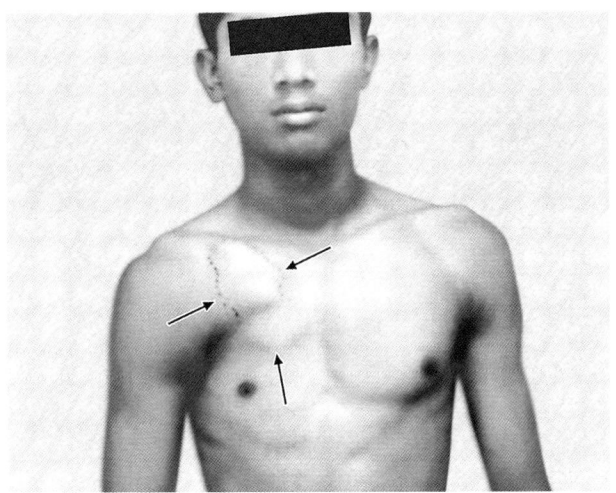

Fig. 8.29: Cold abscess tracking from cervical 5th caries vertebra along the infraclavicular nerve.

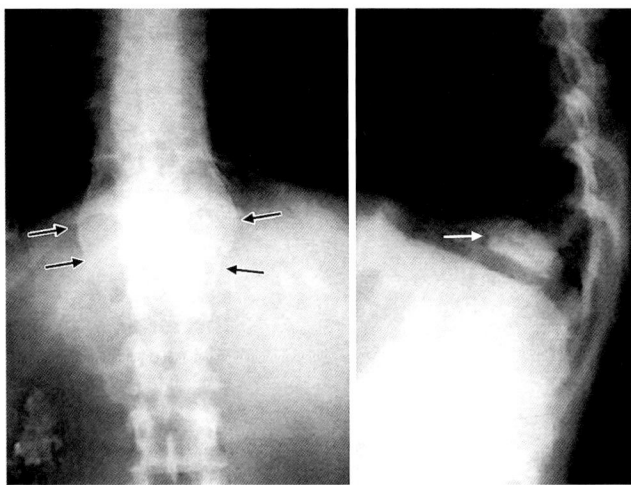

Fig. 8.32: Caries spine dorsal 11–12 vertebrae with bilateral paravertebral abscess.

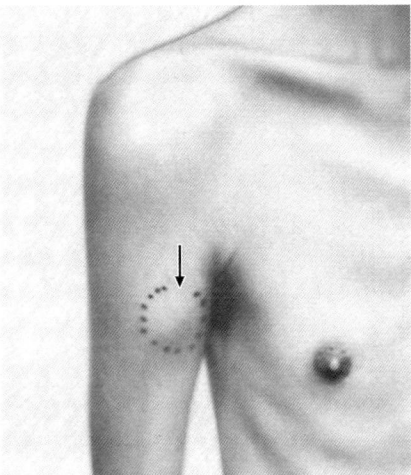

Fig. 8.30: Tracking of cold abscess along the brachial sheath from cervical caries (C4–5).

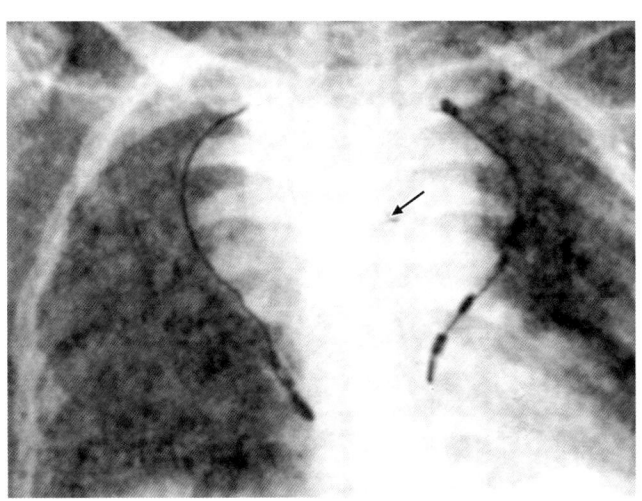

Fig. 8.33: Caries spine of dorsal 5–6 vertebrae with bilateral bird's nest type cold abscess.

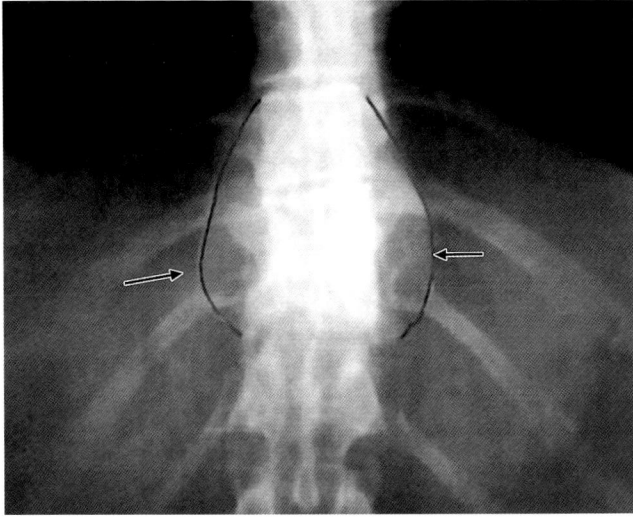

Fig. 8.31: Caries spine of dorsal 10th–11th (D10–11) vertebra, with bilateral paravertebral abscess.

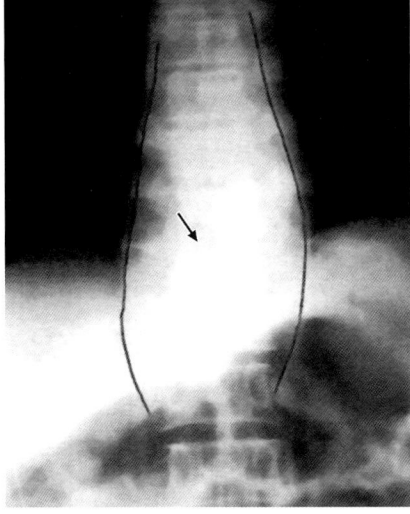

Fig. 8.34: Caries spine of dorsal 9–10 region with spindle shaped cold abscess.

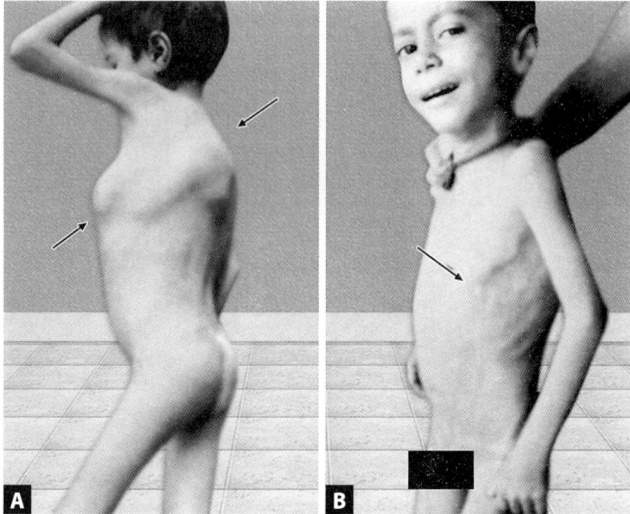

Figs. 8.35A and B: Patient of caries spine with cold abscess tracking from dorsal 6 vertebra along the rib to front of the chest (A); Same cold abscess bursted out spontaneously (B).

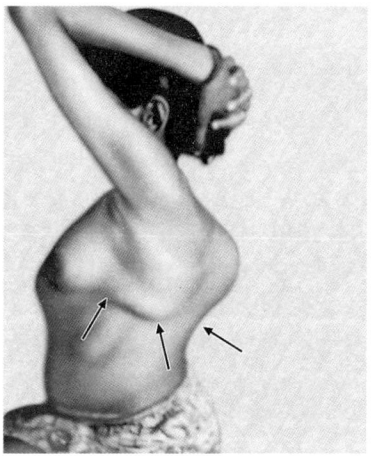

Fig. 8.36: Tracking of cold abscess from D5-6-7 caries spine along the rib.

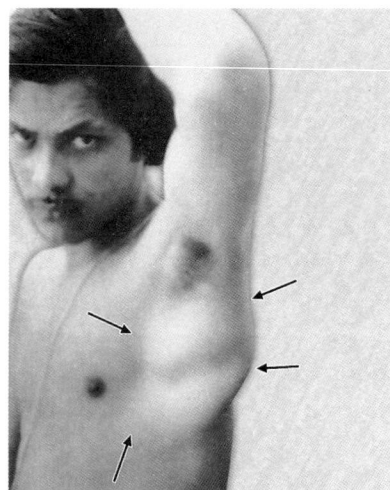

Fig. 8.37: Patient presented with the tracking of cold abscess from D4–5–6 caries spine along the rib without any complain regarding spinal problem.

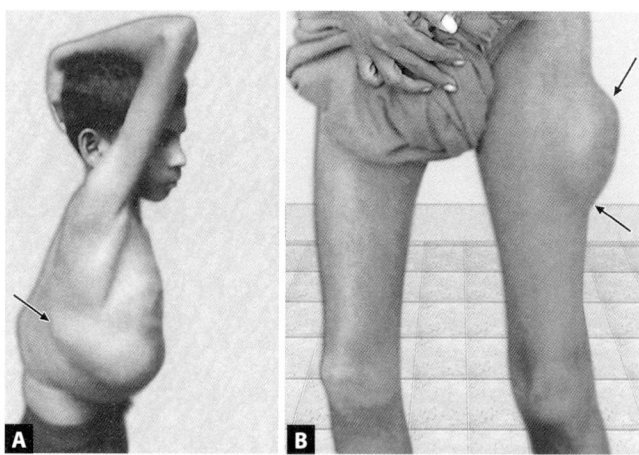

Figs. 8.38A and B: (A) Tracking of cold abscess from caries spine (at two levels—D5–6 and D11–12), (B) Cold abscess collected in upper outer thigh from L3–4–5 caries spine.

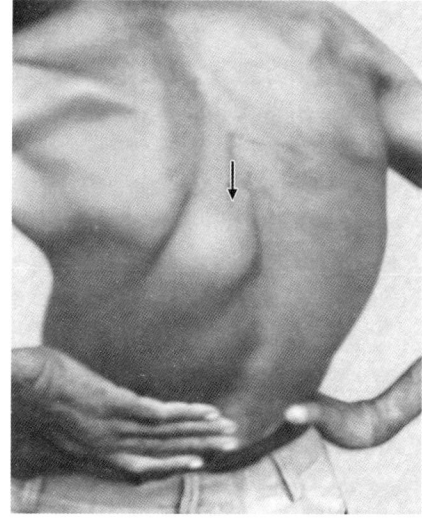

Fig. 8.39: Cold abscess tracking from dorsal 5–6 caries spine along the posterior division of spinal nerve.

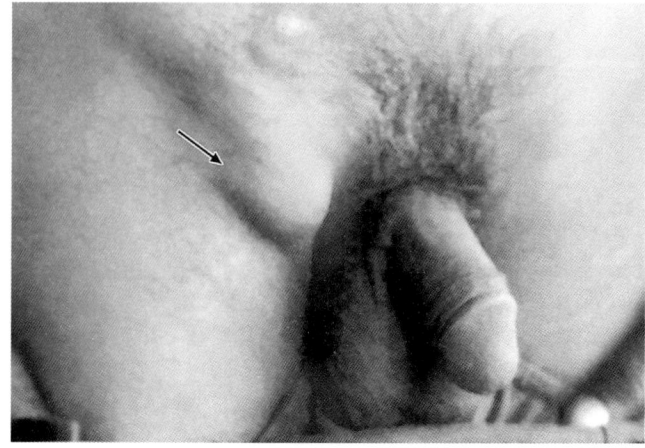

Fig. 8.40: Tracking of cold abscess in the femoral triangle along inguinal sheath from L2–3–4 caries spine.

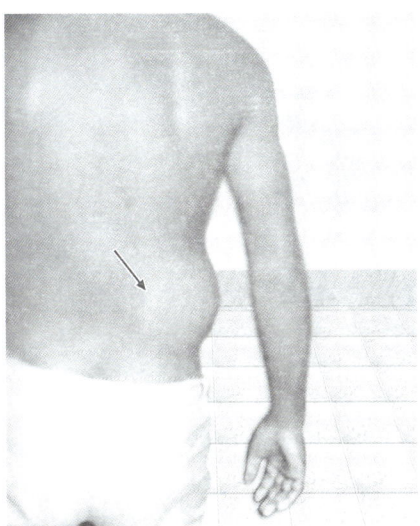

Fig. 8.41: Tracking of cold abscess in the right Petit triangle from L2–3 caries spine.

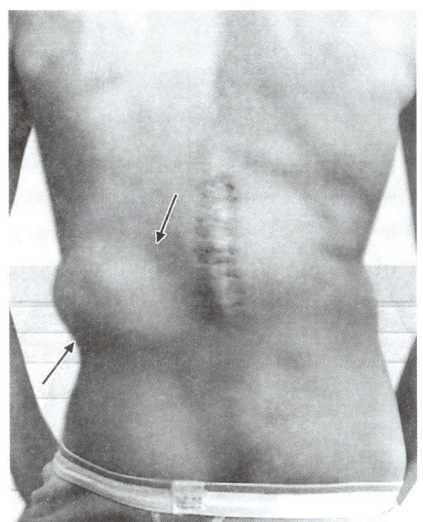

Fig. 8.42: Operated L2–3 caries spine with relapse and cold abscess in left suprailiac region—left Petit triangle.

TABLE 8.4: Normal movements at spine.

Movements	Range of movement	Prime mover	Nerve supply	Assisted by	Limiting factors
At cervical spine					
1. Flexion	With mouth closed, chin just touching manubrium sterni	Sternocleidomastoid muscles	Spinal accessory C2–3	• Scalenus anterior • Scalenus medius • Scalenus posterior • Longus capitis • Longus colli	• Tension of posterior longitudinal ligament • Tension of supraspinous and interspinous ligaments • Tension of posterior cervical muscles
2. Extension	Till head comes in contact with posterior part of upper trunk	• Trapezius • Semispinalis capitis • Splenius capitis • Splenius cervicis	Spinal accessory and C3–4 Posterior rami of spinal nerve		
3. Side bending	0°–45° on each side	Sternomastoid muscle	Spinal accessory C2,3	• Trapezius • Rhomboidus major • Rectus capitis lateralis	
At trunk					
1. Flexion	0°–90°	Rectus abdominis	Lower intercostal nerve	• Internal oblique • External oblique	
2. Extension	0°–30°	• Sacrospinalis • Quadratus lumborum	Adjacent spinal nerve D12, L1, 2	• Semispinalis • Multifidus • Rotators of spine	
3. Trunk rotators	0°–30°	• External oblique • Internal oblique	Lower intercostal nerve 1. Lower intercostal 2. Iliohypogastric 3. Ilioinguinal		
4. Side bending	0°–30°		Quadratus lumborum	T12, L1, 2	

NB: Measurement of spinal flexion as a whole—While the patient stands as much erect as possible, measure from the tip of first thoracic vertebral spine to the most prominent spine of the sacrum. Then the patient flexes the trunk by 90° at the hips, and the same span is again measured. Normally, the difference between standing and flexed position distances is 10–13 cm. A difference in measurement of 7 cm or less indicates limited flexion of the spine.

Test for Active Movement at Cervical Spine

Method (Fig. 8.43): Cervical movements should be tested, while the patient sits erect on a stool. From behind, fix both shoulders in a horizontal plane. Then ask the patient to touch the front of chest with the chin while the mouth remains closed and to take back the extended head as far as practicable **(Fig. 8.43)**; to touch ear on the shoulder top on each side (side bending **Fig. 8.44**); to look towards the right shoulder and then towards the left shoulder (rotations) **(Fig. 8.45)**.

Generally speaking real movements of the spine are flexion and extension occurring at the facet joints. Other movements, like side bending are in the true sense—stretching of the opposite ligaments.

Perhaps, it is practically impossible to elicit movements of spine at single level. Whatever we see and assess is the sum total of smaller movements at each joint level. Therefore, it is worthwhile considering the movements zone-wise.

Even in zone-wise assessment of the movements, true assessment can only be done when other more mobile segments of spine are passively fixed (rather, it is difficult to actively fix the other part).

Passive testing of cervical movements (Figs. 8.46 and 8.47): The patient should sit in maximum possible erect position on the stool. Stand behind the patient. The shoulder blades are stabilised in a horizontal plane by the left hand. Hold the chin in a neutral position, then test for backward bending and rotational movements. Now, support the chest from the front with one hand and press with the opposite hand over the occipital region to bend the cervical spine forward.

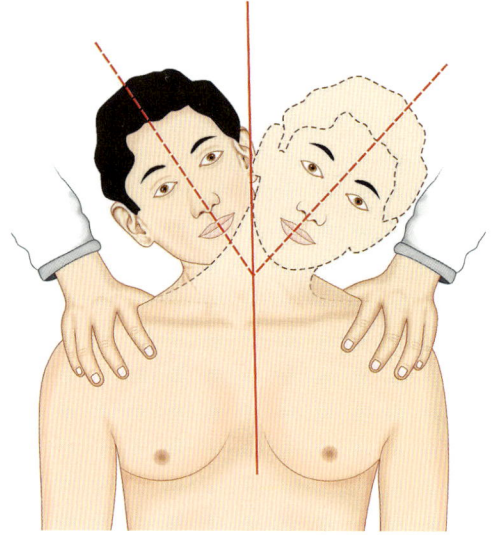

Fig. 8.44: Showing active side bending at cervical spine.

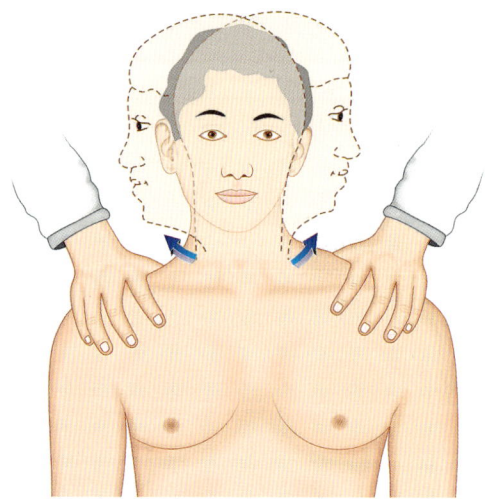

Fig. 8.45: Showing active rotations at the cervical spine.

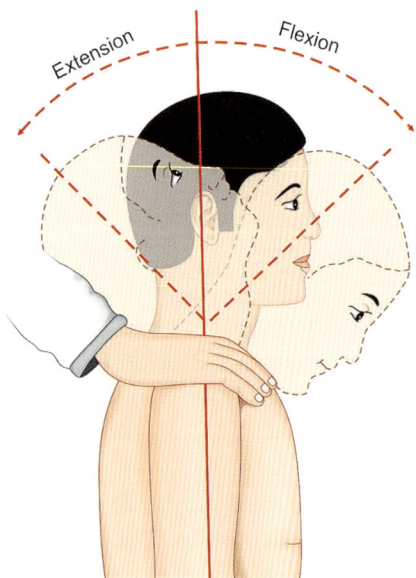

Fig. 8.43: Showing active flexion and extension at cervical spine.

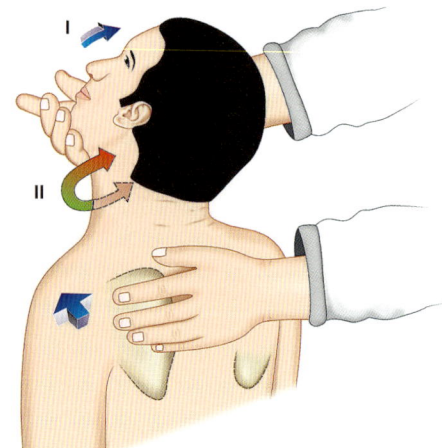

Fig. 8.46: Method of passive testing of backward bending and rotations: I = arrow showing backward bending; II = arrow showing rotations.

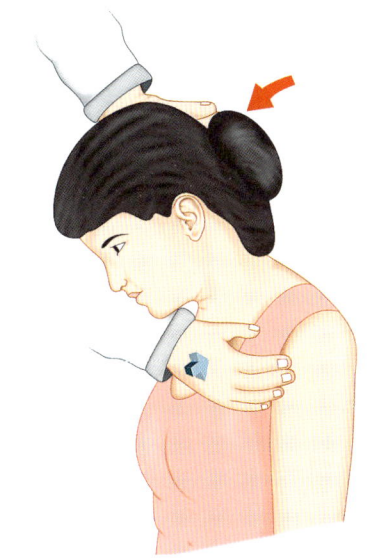

Fig. 8.47: Method of passive testing of forward bending of cervical spine.

Occiput-to-Wall Test

Loss of range of motion should be noted in each direction. Assessment of loss of extension is more important in ankylosing spondylitis which can be assessed by occiput-to-wall test or tragus-to-wall test. Normally when a person stands erect against the wall his heels and scapulae touch the wall. Any distance from the occiput to wall denotes a forward stoop of the neck, and this distance will increase according to increase in the fixed stooping (e.g. in ankylosing spondylitis).

Movements of the Trunk

Dorsal Spine

This portion of the spine is comparatively rigid, specially from cervicodorsal junction to D9. As such, all movements like flexion, extension, side bending, and rotational are possible but are much less as compared to other mobile portions of the spinal column. However, the augmented effect at each level along with the movements at the dorsolumbar spine provide an effective flexion and extension of dorsal and lumbar spines.

The dorsolumbar area (anatomically D12–L1 but clinically for all practical purposes may be taken D10–L2) is the transitional zone from a comparatively fixed to a mobile part of the spine. Hence, this area is subjected to more stress and strain by spinal movements. Effect of spinal movements at lumbar vertebrae get augmented at this level.

Lumbar Spine

Next to cervical, the lumbar region is the site where spinal movements are maximum possible. At the lowest part of the lumbar spine, i.e. lumbosacral region, again there is a transitional zone between the comparatively mobile lumbar vertebrae and the fixed sacrum. The movements in the lumbar region may not be to that extent as to which they appear. The comparatively fixed dorsal spines act like a lever-arm which gives an exaggerated effect to forward bending or backward bending. Skeletally, non-supported space below the lower costal margin provides an exaggerated effect of side bending. Here also, the dorsal spinal segment along with the chest cage provides a good leverage effect. Besides the above factors, one has to take consideration of movements at the hip in assessing movements of spines, specially lumbosacral and lumbar. Keeping the hip totally static, (e.g. bony ankylosed hips of ankylosing spondylitis) the effective forward, backward or side bending of the lower spinal column will be markedly limited. Very little gliding movements of sacroiliac joints also play a small role in augmenting the spinal movements. Therefore, while assessing purely the movements of spine, one must obliterate the movements at hips and sacroiliacs.

Method (**Fig. 8.48**): For assessing the movements of spine in general—(these movements are the movements of utility in practical life) the patient is asked to stand erect with feet approximated together. He/she then has to bend forward, keeping the knees straight and touch the ground with the tips of both middle fingers. This will be full *forward bending*. Any limitation in this movement should be noted as *distance lag from the ground to the tip of the longest finger* (**Fig. 8.48A**).

For *testing backward bending,* standing in erect posture with feet approximated, the patient has to bend backwards and go as far as practicable towards heel. Normally, the fingers should go up to about popliteal fossae level (**Fig. 8.48B**).

Side bending: The patient first stands in the same posture, i.e. erect with feet approximated and knee straight, he/she is then asked to bend towards lateral malleolus, while the other arm is diagonally opposite or closeted to the side of body. Normally, the extended middle finger can reach up to about knee level. Change the arm for opposite *side bending test* (**Fig. 8.48C**).

Fallacies

Spinal movements vary to a great extent, depending upon the obesity, the elasticity of body and gymnastic activities.

How to test for pure movements at the lumbar lumbosacral spine (**Fig. 8.48D**)?

The patient will sit on the stool, keeping her/his both thighs approximated and fully opened first web of hand adapted on both iliac crests (**Fig. 8.48D**). The patient should then be asked to bend forwards with a tendency of taking his nose in between her/his two thighs without bending at hip. The movement occurs at the lumbar and lumbosacral

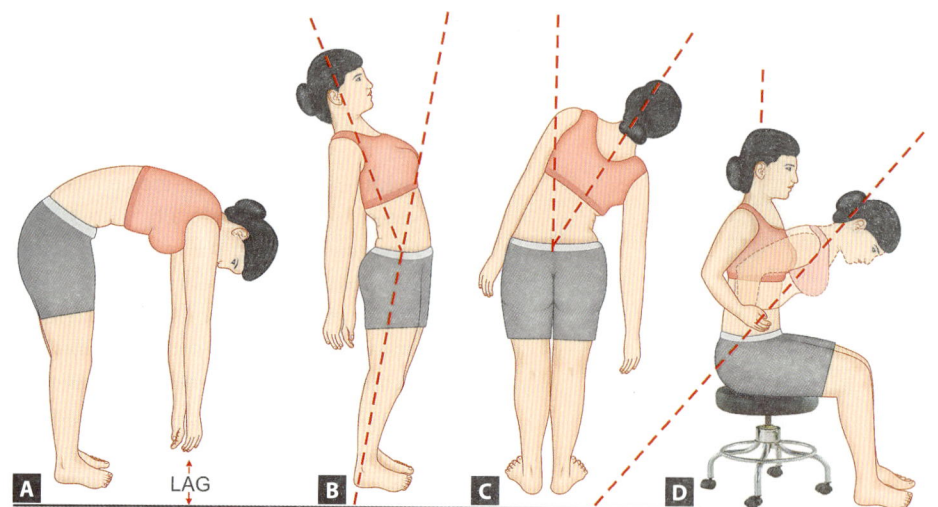

Figs. 8.48A to D: Active movements of the trunk: (A), Forward bending; (B) Backward bending; (C) Side bending; (D) Forward bending in sitting position.

region. From the erect sitting posture, she/he is then asked to bend backwards and sidewards alternately to assess these movements. While in this posture itself, the rotational movements of the spine can be tested very well. In the erect sitting posture on stool, ask her/him to look to her/his extreme right and that will be right rotation. Ask her/him to look extreme left which will be left rotation.

Schober Test

Limitation of forward flexion of the lumbar spine (as occurs in ankylosing spondylitis) can be assessed by Schober test. The person stands erect. Draw a line joining the two posterior superior iliac spines. From the midpoint of this line, mark a point 10 cm straight up in the midline. Ask the person to bend maximum forward with straight knees. In a normal person, the measured distance should increase from 10 cm to at least 15 cm.

Sacroiliac Joint

To complete the examination of spine, the sacroiliac joints must be examined. As such the movements of sacroiliac joints may be taken as invisible ones. In this joint, the bondage is mainly by tough interosseous ligaments. These ligaments are very short and allow very little of rotational movement in between the sides of the sacrum and the ear-shaped articular facets of the iliac plates. In the physiomechanics of sacroiliacs, these motions are more or less involuntary [e.g. in defecation, raising the intra-abdominal pressure, during pregnancy, straining during labour (child birth) and in locomotion].

Testing for these movements is done by indirect methods. The normal movements cannot be seen and evaluated. But if any pathology exists in this joint, especially of inflammatory nature, pain in the joint is complained of on stress tests. They are of four types:

1. Straight leg raising test (**Fig. 12.28,** Page 343)
2. Compression stress test (**Fig. 9.5**)
3. Distraction stress test (**Fig. 9.6**)
4. Pump handle test and axial rotational stress test (**Figs. 9.7**)

Also See the Chapter 9: Pelvis Pages 276, 277

■ MEASUREMENTS

Measurements of spine are not of that significance as they are for the limbs. However, in spinal deformities, specially kyphosis and scoliosis, special measurements are done to assess the degree of spinal curvatures.

Linear Measurement (Fig. 8.49)

Distance from external occipital protuberance to the tip of coccyx will be the total length of spinal column. This should be measured if possible, in erect posture of the patient. This is of value for recording in the case sheet rather than comparing. The segmental measurement of the cervical and lumbar spines are sometimes of more value. In the cervical spine—in disease like Klippel-Feil-Syndrome, the distance between external occipital protuberance to vertebra prominence is markedly reduced (the lower hair line lies almost on cervicodorsal junction). In the lumbar region, the distance from dorsolumbar spine to first sacral spine is reduced in spondylolisthesis. Another linear measurement of significance is from tip of the last rib to the highest point of iliac crest (*ilio-costal distance*). In scoliosis or even in kyphosis, these distances are accordingly reduced, while in lordosis these measurements are comparatively increased. These should be measured separately as record for the spinal deformities, localised in the upper region of lumbar spine.

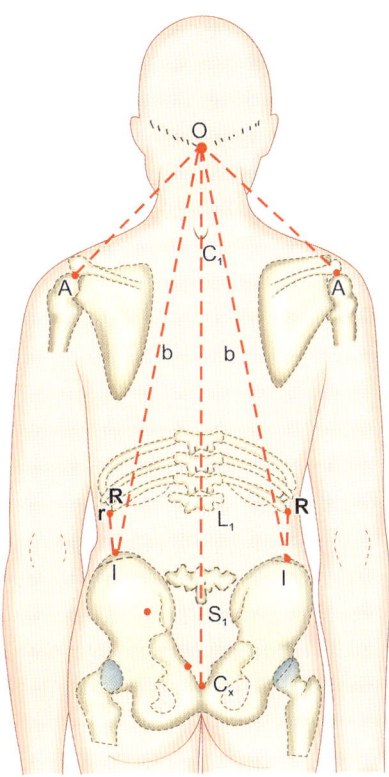

Fig. 8.49: Linear measurement of spine. O = occipital protuberance; A = acromian angle; I = iliac crest; R = tip of the last rib.

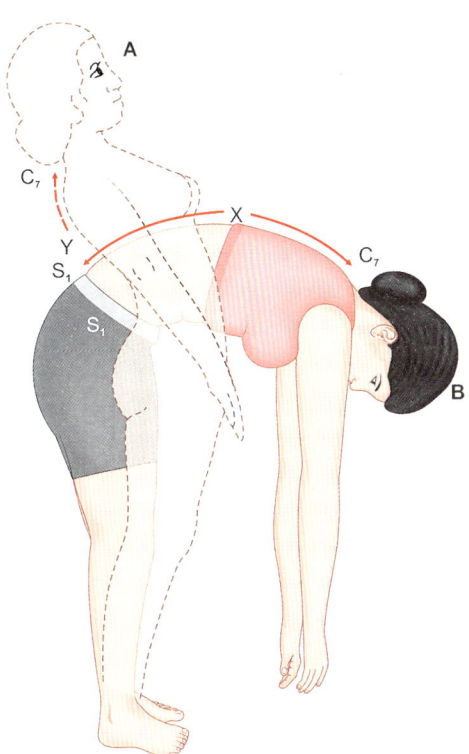

Fig. 8.50: Method of measuring the anteroposterior spinal excursion (Ex): A = full extension; B = full flexion; X = distance between C7 to S1 spinous process; Y = distance between C7 and S1 spinous process in full extension, hence anteroposterior excursion, i.e. EX = (X-Y).

The distance between external occipital protuberance to the highest point of iliac crests should be measured (*iliooccipital distance*). They are equal on both sides. Any disparity will indicate the side bending of spine. In mild scoliotic tendency, these measurements may be of value.

Method: Ask the patient to stand or sit erect or lie prone in as much neutral position as possible. Feel the external occipital protuberance at the highest point of central furrow. Pass your hands forwards over iliac crests from the dimple of Venus. Stop at a point where the slope takes a downwards turn. Measure the distances between these points and compare with other side **(Fig. 8.49)**.

To assess the anatomical integrity in neutral position of cervical spine, oblique measurements are helpful, measured from the external occipital protuberance to acromian angle **(Fig. 8.49)**. Normally they should be equal in length and inclination.

Linear measurements from vertebra prominence to S1 point in full backward bending to full forward bending indicates the range of the spinal movements in anteroposterior directions **(Fig. 8.50)**. The measurement between these two points from the position of neutral erect posture to full forward bending allow an excursion of about 10 cm.

Measurement of Chest Expansion

In ankylosing spondylitis, this measurement is of paramount importance. In a normal individual, the expansion at the level of just below the nipple is allowed by about 5–8 cm. *Limitation of this expansion to 2.5 cm in 4th intercostal space is highly suggestive of ankylosing spondylitis.*

Auscultation

Auscultation in the spinal examination may appear to be of academic importance but at times, it is of immense value. There is no harm in putting the stetho bell on both sides of spinous processes as routine examination. In conditions like aortic aneurysm or highly vascular neoplasm, patient may complain of pain in the back as presenting symptom. In such conditions, clinically palpating and/or auscultatory bruit localised in that region of spinal column may be of immense value for further probe.

■ SPECIAL TESTS

Stress Test of Spine

In case of backache, especially in youngmen, this test is of significance in diagnosing ankylosing spondylitis. Ask the patient to fully bend the spine forwards, sideways and backwards, in sequence, for 15–20 times. Then ask him to move about. He will feel relief in case of ankylosing spondylitis. However, in pathologies like, caries spine, disc prolapse, osteomyelitis and other infections of spine and spinal tumours, the patient feels his symptoms variably aggravated after the test.

Cervical Roots Stretch Test

Before performing these tests, one should rule out any instability in cervical region.

Lateral Stretch Test

In cervical spondylosis or cervical disc prolapse, lateral stretching of the cervical spine in opposite direction may lead to pain along the affected nerve root.

Cervical Compression Test

Even the initial stage of irritation of the roots can be tested by cervical compression test.

Method: Ask the patient to sit erect on the stool, keeping the head in as much neutral position as possible. Stand behind the patient with both hands placed over the vault of head, give a sudden brisk jerk in the line of spinal column **(Fig. 8.51A)**. Note the reaction of the patient specially regarding pain in cervical region and referred area. Rotate the cervical spine to about 45° to each side and ask him/her to look to the ceiling. In each rotational position, repeat the brisk compression manoeuvre and note the patient's reaction **(Fig. 8.51B)**. In positive cases, the patient will complain of augmentation of his typical symptoms in the area of root distribution which used to be felt on and off.

Avoid this test, if there is suspicion of tuberculous infection or pyogenic infection or any malignancy in the cervical region.

Distraction Test

Passively distracting (stretch-elevating) the head in neutral position, by holding it at occiput and chin, relieves the symptoms of root irritation.

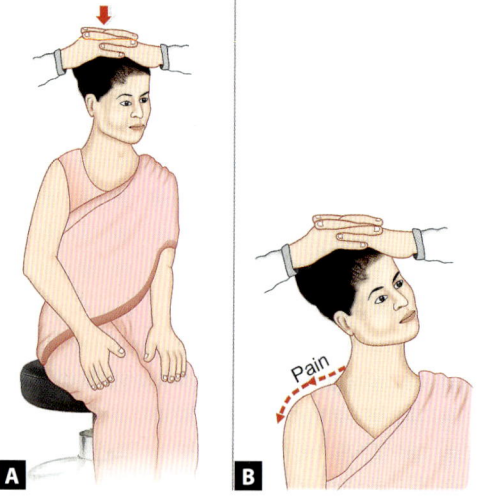

Figs. 8.51A and B: Method of eliciting cervical compression test: (A) In erect sitting position; (B) Tilted and rotated position.

Hand on Head Sign (HOH)

Patients of cervicobrachial neuralgia (brachalgia) do complain of pain with or without tingling in shoulder region, arm, forearm and even up to fingers. The symptoms of pain and tingling exaggerate when the patient stands or walks with that upper limb hanging by the side of chest (due to stretching of the nerve roots). However, when he takes the affected side hand, by holding with other hand, over the head, the symptoms decrease significantly. In acute presentation, even the patient comes with holding the affected side hand over the head (HOH). In taking the hand over the head, pain and tingling get relieved due to relaxation in the course of the nerve roots.

Hand Supporting Head Sign (HSH Sign; Rust Sign)

In tuberculous spondylitis (caries spine, Pott's disease) of cervical spine, patient may or may not complain of pain in neck, but he/she keeps neck stiff and avoids any attempt of moving (especially rotating) the neck. When seated, he/she usually supports the head with the hands (HSH sign; Rust sign) to avoid any spontaneous movement of head/neck, which produces pain.

Test for Thoracic Inlet Syndromes

The vice like compression of the neurovascular bundle has bizarre manifestations like feeling of heat, burning sensation, tingling, numbness, heaviness, congestion, bluish discolouration and even weakness in affected side upper limb, especially in the thumb and tips of the fingers. The vice compression can be clinically augmented by narrowing the angulation between the scaleni and first rib.

Method: Ask the patient to sit on the stool; stand on the side and behind the patient on which side the test has to be performed. Hold the wrist and palpate the radial pulse. Ask the patient to flex the neck on the affected side, while he elevates the chin and takes deep inspiration or with palm of the opposite hand, press the lateral side of neck towards the opposite shoulder as much as possible. At the same time, palpate the radial pulse of the extended limb. The latter is pulled downwards as far as possible **(Fig. 8.52)** while patient takes deep inspiration.

There can be three manifestations:
- No change in pulse and no complain, except some feeling of stretch over root of neck—This is *normal*
- Radial pulse may be weaker or even may get obliterated—This indicates that the *subclavian artery is getting stretched and compressed*
- The patient may complain of re-appearance or augmentation of tingling and/or numbness in the affected area—This indicates that the *brachial roots are stretched or compressed.*

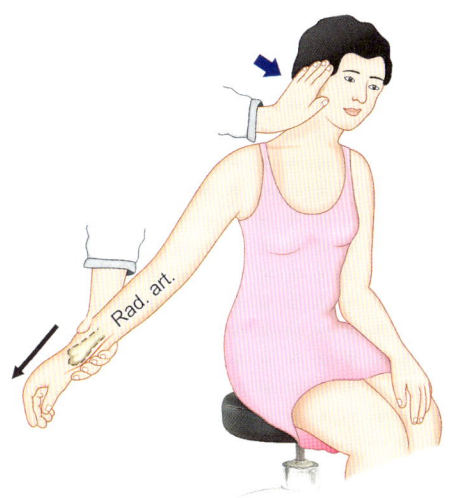

Fig. 8.52: Method of testing for thoracic inlet syndrome.

Second and third inferences should be taken as significant and corroborated with other clinical findings and investigation.

In **thoracic outlet syndrome, Adson's test** is performed to evaluate vascular compromise.

Method: The patient sits on the stool. The affected side arm is abducted, extended and externally rotated and the examiner simultaneously palpates the radial pulse. The patient is asked to look towards the side to be tested and inhale deeply. Diminution or loss of the radial pulse with development of a supraclavicular bruit suggest significant compression of subclavian artery.

Tension Tests in Lumbar Disc Prolapse

The lumber intervertebral discs are the largest in size lying almost parallel over the lumbar vertebral bodies. The L4–5, L5–S1, and L3–4 intervertebral discs are the common in that order– to undergo degeneration and their prolapse.

Tension tests are based upon the manoeuvre which tightens the sciatic nerve and thus compress the inflamed nerve root against a herniated disc. The tests are:
- Straight leg raising (SLR)
- Well leg raising test (crossed leg raising)
- Lasegue's (sign) test
- Fajersztajn test
- Lateral flexion test of spine
- Sciatic stretch test ⎫ —including sudden
- Figure of '4' test   ⎭ sciatic stretch test
- Bowstring test
- Sitting root test
- Femoral nerve stretch test is the tension test of the femoral nerve, mainly the L4 root.

Straight Leg Raising Test (SLR) (Refer Fig. 12.28)

The active straight leg raising in supine posture with extended knee, is normally possible approaching up to 90° (except in women, of Indian subcontinent, who remain very conscious in raising beyond 60° due to their clothing problems, as most of them do not use panty) without any pain. If patient cannot lie supine (as in poker back, severe kyphosis), this test should be done in lateral position alternatively. In case of sciatic radiculitis, this manoeuvre elongates the course of the sciatic nerve, putting stretch on the sciatic root. Therefore, the patient complains of pain along the course of the sciatic nerve and its branches, if there is impingement on its root, (e.g. in intervertebral disc prolapse). By and large it has been seen that *if the patient experiences pain in the course of the sciatic nerve by raising the leg up to 30°, it is diagnostic of intervertebral disc prolapse; if the pain is produced between 30 and 70°, it is suggestive of disc prolapse and pain beyond 70° is equivocal.*

This test is also of significance in assessing the stability of the hip joint, pathology of sacroiliac joint, integrity of hip flexors and quadriceps mechanism of the knee, lesions of hamstring muscle belly. However, acute/active pathology of lower lumbars and/or ipsilateral pelvis can also affect the straight leg raising. However, a completely painless SLR does not exclude the lesions of disk. The circumstances where SLR test produces negative inferences in discoarticular problem may be as follows:
- If the nerve root emerges a little higher up in the foramen and thus does not come into contact with the disk protrusion.
- Disk protrusions in between second or third lumber vertebrae and the third or fourth sacral nerve roots are not influenced in SLR test.
- Small disk protrusions are not influenced in SLR test.

Well Leg Raising Test (Crossed-Straight-Leg-Raising Test)

In supine position, if raising of the unaffected extended leg produces pain (which was not there) or exacerbates the existing pain along the sciatic distribution on the affected side, it is highly suggestive of disc prolapse, pressing on the root mostly from the medial side (well leg raising test).

Reverse Straight-Leg-Raising Test

The patient lies prone and the suspected side knee is fully flexed over the thigh. In normal situation, the person complains of quadriceps tightness in anterior region of thigh, but in intervertebral disc pathology, the patient will complain of pain in back of thigh or along sciatic distribution, because the spinal root gets tightened over the prolapsed disc and subarachnoid pressure rises due to abdominal compression in the posture adopted for the test.

Lasegue's Test

A similar test is done by elevating the straight leg by the examiner (Lasegue's test). *If it is negative, one should be sceptical in diagnosing disc prolapse.*

Method: While the patient is lying supine, the affected straight leg is elevated holding it with one hand above the ankle and pressing it by the other hand on the front of the thigh **(Fig. 8.54)**. Normal leg can be elevated up to 90° without any pain. In case of sciatic root irritation, the patient will feel pain along the course of the sciatic nerve and the lower back much earlier. Measure the angle (between back of the thigh and the bed), at which pain just starts appearing.

Fajersztajn Test

The findings of Lasegue's test can be further confirmed by passively dorsiflexing the foot while the straight leg is kept at the same angle where pain has first appeared. This manoeuvre will accentuate the pain (Fajersztajn test) **(Fig. 8.54)**.

Kernig's sign: The patient lies supine on the bed/couch. While the hip is fully flexed, the patient's knee is passively extended on either side. In patients with meningeal irritation in the lower part of spinal subarachnoid space, there will pain and spasm of the hamstrings, as the knee is extended.

Lateral Flexion Test of Spine

Ask the patient (who is standing or lying supine) with suspected disc prolapse to acutely flex the spine laterally on the affected side. Due to approximation of root to the protruded disc (from lateral side), the patient will feel a catching pain. If the symptoms are aggravated by flexing the spine on the opposite side, it indicates pressure over the root from the medial side.

Sciatic Stretch Test

Basis of the test—As suggested by Forst (1981), the basis of this test is to produce tension in the hamstring muscles, which in turn compresses the sciatic nerve. Therefore, the patient experiences acute pain at the level of sciatic notch, and along the course of sciatic nerve.

Method: (a) Ask the patient to lie supine, and support the foot of a fully extended leg in one hand and press over the ipsilateral knee by the other hand. Gradually, flex the lower limb at the hip while lifting the limb above the bed, the patient will feel pain at the level of sciatic notch in cases of sciatic radiculitis. On flexing the knee, the pain instantaneously disappears. In flexed position, the hamstrings become lax, so that the sciatic nerve is not compressed **(Fig. 8.55)**.

Sudden sciatic stretch test: Patient sits erect on the table with the legs hanging at the edge from the knees. Then ask the patient to lean back supporting herself/himself with both hands on the table. In the meantime, hold the great toe of the suspected side and suddenly lift the bent knee to straight position. In the sciatic root impingement, patient will feel bursting pain at the low back **(Fig. 8.56)**. This test can

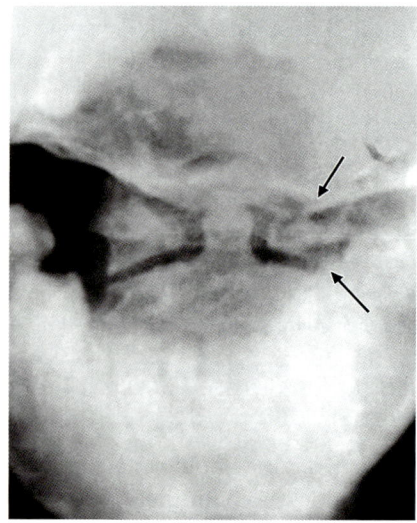

Fig. 8.53: Open mouth view X-ray of occipitoatlantoaxial region with tuberculous infection.

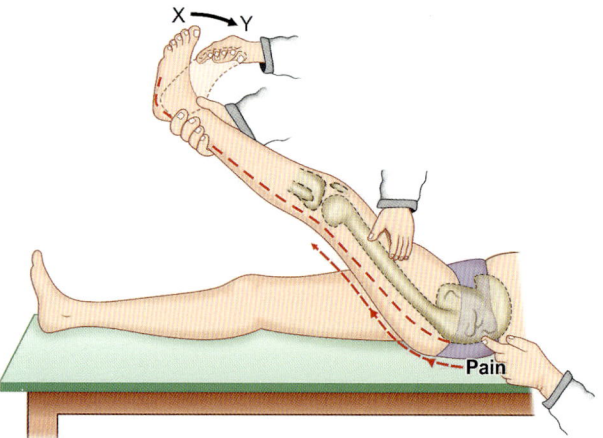

Fig. 8.54: Method of demonstration of Lasegue's test and Fajersztajn test.

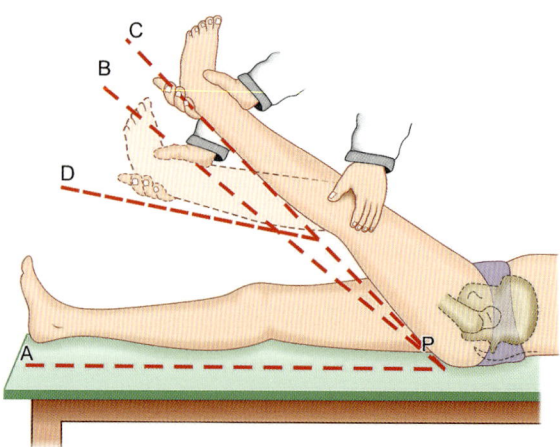

Fig. 8.55: Method of demonstration of sciatic stretch test. When limb was in position of 'A' there was no pain; in position of 'B' pain started appearing; in position of 'C' marked pain; in position of 'D' pain instantaneously disappears. 'P' indicates the site of pain at greater sciatic notch.

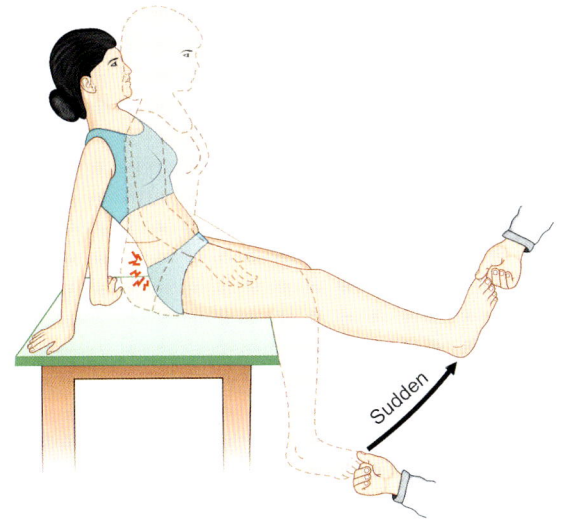

Fig. 8.56: Test to differentiate between a malingerer and a genuine patient of sciatic radiculitis—sudden sciatic stretch test.

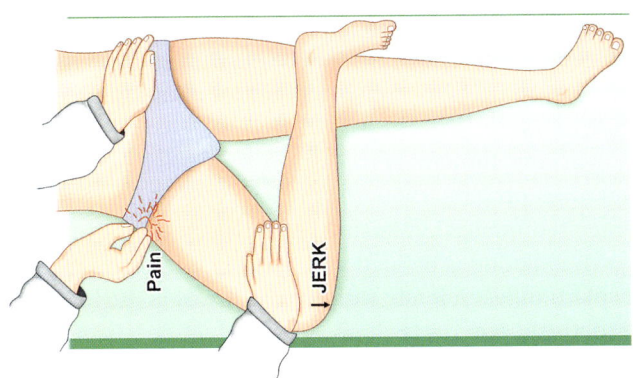

Fig. 8.57: Alternative method of sciatic stretch test (Figure of '4' test); Patrick's test or FABER manoeuvre.

differentiate between a malingerer and a genuine patient of sciatic radiculitis. A malingerer will not feel bursting pain at the low back. (Also perform Magnuson Pointing Test as described later)

Figure of '4' Test

Also called patrick Test; or **FABER Manoeuvre**-which is known by its acronym FABER (Flexion, abduction, external rotation.

Ask the patient to lie supine. Flex, abduct and externally rotate the lower limb of the suspected side at the hip and flex the knee to the extent which allows the lower part of the leg to rest on the opposite lower thigh. Now give a jerky pressure over the medial aspect of the knee. In the sciatic root impingement or affections of sciatic nerve, the patient will complain of pain pointing to greater sciatic notch and along the sciatic course **(Fig. 8.57)**. Full external rotation of limb and painless jerky pressure over knee indicates negative Patrick test and also excludes symptomatic disease of hip joint and sacroiliac joints.

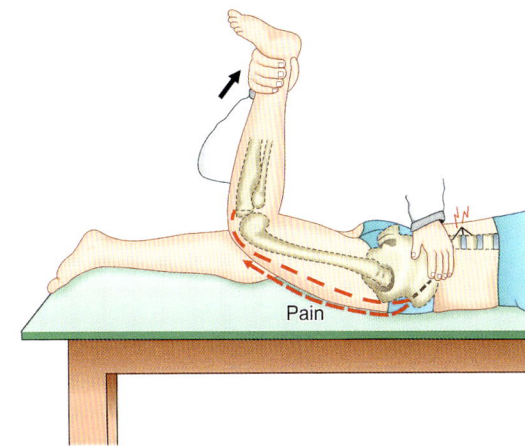

Fig. 8.58: Method of demonstrating the femoral nerve stretch test.

Bowstring Test

Patient is asked to lift the straight leg till the pain starts being felt. At this point the knee is flexed, which instantaneously reduces the pain. Pressing the terminal region of the sciatic nerve restarts the painful radicular symptoms.

Sitting Root Test

Patient sits at the edge of the table with neck bent forward. While the hip remains flexed at 90°, the knee is extended. Patient feels pain in the leg which he would like to avoid by attempting to extend the hip.

Femoral Nerve Stretch Test

Femoral nerve stretch test may be positive if the L2,3,4 roots are affected.

Method **(Fig. 8.58):** Ask the patient to lie prone. While the other leg is kept extended at the hip and knee, bend the affected side limb to 90° at knee. Hold the leg with one hand just above the ankle. The other forearm and hand should rest on the buttock at hip level, fixing the pelvis on the couch. Lift the bent leg upwards, more by stretching backwards at the hip (as passively testing for extension at hip). The femoral nerve is stretched along with the extension of hip. If the roots are pressed or over stretched, the patient may complain of pain on the front and outerside of thigh even up to knee. This is *positive femoral nerve stretch test.*

Lower lumbar sciatic compressive radiculopathy can be confused with *sciatic neuropathy* when multiple segments are involved (very rare in disc herniation). Further in straight leg raising just short of discomfort, pain caused by a sciatic neuropathy is increased by internal rotation and relieved by external rotation of the hips, which are not seen in lumbar (sciatic) radiculopathy.

Pendulum Test

It is performed to assess the spasticity in quadriceps and hamstring muscles, e.g. in cerebral palsy patients.

The patient sits on the table with the legs extended unsupported at back of the knee over the edge of the table. One by one the leg is allowed to fall from the extended position with the force of gravity. Oscillating of leg like a pendulum demonstrates the quadriceps and hamstring spasticity.

Magnuson Pointing Test for Identifying Malingerer

In a patient complaining of low back pain identify the site of pain, by asking the patient to point it and confirm by palpating the tender site. Mark the site by skin pencil. After completing other examinations, again try to locate the site by same procedures (i.e. asking the patient to point the site and palpate for tender spot). In genuine patient the spot will be more or less same but in malingerer the spot will vary each time.

Piriformis Syndrome

This syndrome is the result of *entrapment of sciatic nerve* (first described in 1928 by Yoeman; and Robinson first used the term 'Piriformis syndrome' in 1947) *by the piriformis muscle as it passes through the sciatic notch.*

Causes can be hypertrophy of piriformis muscle, trauma, excessive exercises, pseudoaneurysm of inferior gluteal artery, spasm and inflammation of piriformis muscle, anomalies of muscle, dystonia musculorum deformans, traumatic myositis ossificans.

Clinical findings: There may be history of injury to sacroiliac and/or gluteal region; pain in sacroiliac joint region, greater sciatic notch, and piriformis muscle extending down the lower limb causing difficulty in walking; acute exacerbation of the symptoms by lifting the leg or stooping; isolated atrophy of gluteus maximus; dysthesia of posterior aspect of thigh; tenderness over sciatic notch; a palpable sausage-shaped mass over the piriformis muscle, which is markedly tender during an exacerbation of symptoms. Tender mass can also be felt laterally during a rectal examination. This feature is pathognomic of the syndrome; a positive straight leg raising test, and Lasegue sign; Freiberg sign (Pain with forced internal rotation of extended thigh); and positive *sign of Pace and Nagle* (Pain with resistance to abduction and external rotation of the thigh).

The tibial nerve division of sciatic nerve is involved less often than peroneal division, since former is located more medially in the sciatic notch.

Diagnosis can be confirmed by nerve conduction studies demonstrating delayed F waves and H reflexes. CT and MRI show hypertrophy of piriformis muscle. This syndrome is managed by physiotherapy, NSAID, stretching, ultrasound, local corticoid and anaesthetic infiltration. If there is no relief, operative release of piriformis muscle is recommended.

■ NEUROLOGICAL EXAMINATION

No spinal examination is complete without thorough examination of nervous system. It should be categorically examined under the following headings:
- A quick assessment of mental state, intelligence, speech, general appearance
- Cranial nerves
- Gait
- Posture
- Motor functions
- Sensory assessments
- Vasomotor functions
- Reflexes
  - Superficial reflexes
  - Deep reflexes (tendon jerks, clonus)
- Visceral functions—assessment, specially of the bladder and bowel.

Gait (Walking) (Fig. 8.59)

"Walking—it is distinctly human; it permits us to view the world in an upright manner, though not always acting in an upright way."

Vermon Imman—Professor of Orthopaedic Surgery, Lectures on gait, 1960-70 University of California, San Francisco-quoted by Horstmann and Bleck-2007.

Ambulation is defined as the ability to walk from place to place independently with or without an assistive device (Moorhead et al 2004).

After acquiring upright posture, the normal bipedal gait was achieved at the cost of stability and speed to free the upper limbs for prehensile functions.

Walking 3,000 steps a day can lower your risk of obesity and diabetes. Increasing the daily steps over a five-year period to 10,000 can boost the benefit. Walking is a superfood—For an average person, walking 3000 to 4000 steps daily helps, however, increasing the daily steps can boost the benefit.

One of the first attempts of objective gait analysis began with the horse of the farm of Senator Lelant Stanford of California. Muybridge (1901) using time-phase photography proved that the Senator's racehorse had all four feet off the ground at times while running. The analysis and measurement of human walking began in the later part of the 19th century when Marey (1873) made records of running and walking.

Gait (Fig. 8.59)

Few Interesting Facts about Gait

- Walking is as fundamental to life as the act of breathing.
- Walking should be considered as a superfood.
- Land, air or sea birds are the masters of locomotion. The 'Ostrich' carrying its about 300 pounds body on its two legs can run at the rate of about 30 miles an hour.

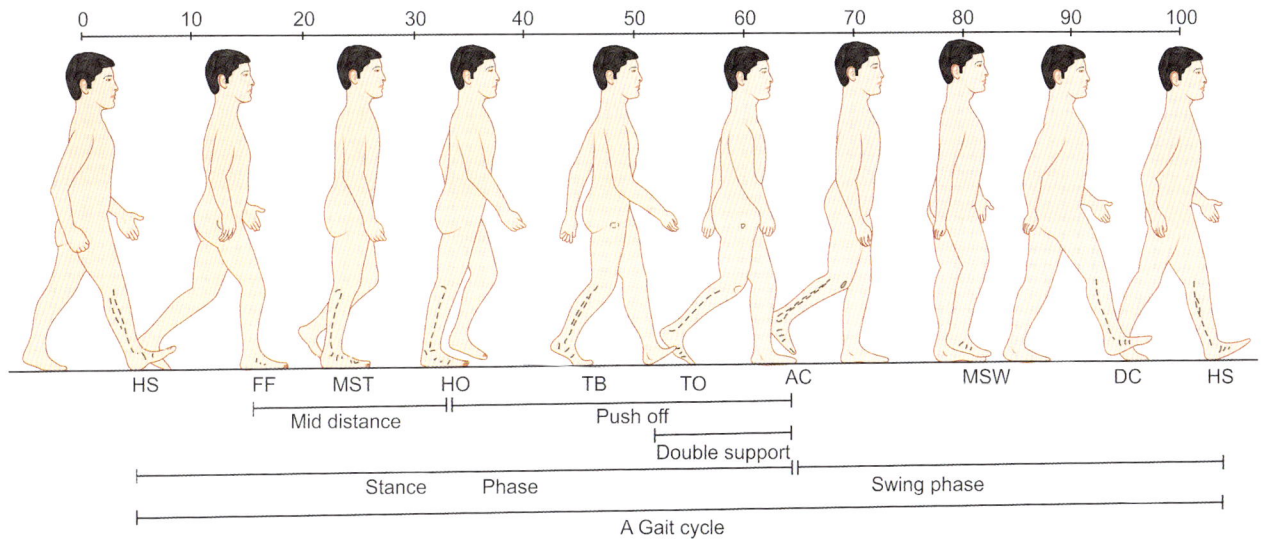

Fig. 8.59: Basics of a complete gait cycle. Stance phase 60%; Double support-11% of the gait cycle. HS = heel strike; FF = foot flat; MST = mid stance; HO = heel off; TB = toe break; TO = toe off; AC = acceleration; MSW = mid swing; DC = deceleration.

- The Kangaroo with its long muscular hind legs and weighing about 200 pounds can thrust its heavy weight into the air and clear a fence nine feet high. While airborne, this leaping marsupial uses its thick tail to counter balance and also as a rudder.
- The human being is unique in having a bipedal gait, which causes the vertical loading of the spine.
- The average fit person takes 8,000 to 10,000 steps in a day, which if added makes about 7,47,000 kilometres in a life time of an average person (on global basis)—enough to take around the planet more than four times.

All elephants walk on tip-toe because the back portion of their foot is made of no bone just only fat **(Fig. 8.60)**.

The 'gait' may be defined as the forward propulsion of body by the lower limbs in a systematic, coordinated semi-rotatory movements of the trunk, arm and head—in short gait is bipedal plantigrade progression. Human nervous system has its "unit burst generator" to control rhythmic movements, such as 'gait-cycle' in walking. The unit-burst-generators, probably, reside in spinal cord-nerve segment. When a neuron fires, it sets off a chain reaction that gives rise to rhythmic movement. Once those circuits are turned on, the body essentially goes on autopilot (Jr Neuro Sciences). The style of walking varies to an acceptable certain extent with almost each individual depending upon age, sex, body built, weight, mood, psychic status, etc. A*b*normal gaits are observed in diseased states—congenital to neoplasm, of which congenital malformations (mainly of lower limbs); neurological abnormalities; improper muscular strength; diseases and stiffness of spine, pelvis, lower limb joints; limb length disparity; and painful focus in the lower limb mainly affect the normal gait pattern.

In the normal walking, one does not place his/her one foot in front of another, rather there should be some gap between the two feet. Linear distance between the mid points of the feet varies from 5 to 10 cm and is known as *"width of base support",* i.e. the 'base of gait' as measured from heel-to-heel is 5–10 cm in a normal person.

In normal walking, the foot is placed on the ground in an angle taken from the centre of heel to second toe—*'toe-out'* or *'foot angle'* and it is on an average 70°.

Normally one flexes 35° at pre-swing stage and it must flex 70° for the foot to clear the ground.

The distance between the heel strike of one lower limb to the heel strike of the other lower limb is denoted as *"step length".* The distance between the heel strike of one lower limb to the next heel strike of the same lower limb is denoted as *"stride length".* The time taken for completion of heel strike of one lower limb to the next heel strike of same lower limb (i.e. completion of one gait cycle) is denoted as *"stride duration".* *"Cadence"* is the number of steps taken per minute which varies on several factors mainly the step length, speed of walking, sex, body built, obesity, surface on which walking is done, etc.

The velocity is meters travelled per minute. Stance phase begins with heel contact and ends with toe-off.

In the physiomechanics of gait, understanding about the centre of gravity is essential. The centre of gravity is a fixed point in a body through which the force of gravitational attraction acts.

In the human body, the centre of gravity is located just anterior to the first and second sacral segment, where all planes (coronal, sagittal and transverse) converge (Braune and Fischer 1898, cited by Brunnstrom 1962). If the lower limbs are not considered, the centre of gravity of the trunk only is located just anterior to the 11th thoracic vertebra (Hellebrant 1938, cited by Brunnstrom 1962).

The loading behaviour of the human foot during walking may vary in different regions of foot. In normal bipedal standing the heel is approximately 2.6 times more loaded than the forefoot. In pregnant women the load shift is comparatively to the heel from the forefoot.

In walking on moon, there is low oscillations of displacement of the body's walking centre of gravity. The time of swing phase increases 2½ times, thus the walking speed for a given step length remains only 40% of that of earth. Due to this, the astronauts of Apollo preferred to move on the surface of moon by taking a series of jumps to gain the speed of walking. The maximum one can jump on the moon surface is about 4 metres (MacMohan 1984).

Proper analysis of the gait pattern is mandatory for understanding it clearly. Besides careful clinical observation, modern systems of video tracking and Gait Laboratories for gait analysis are useful. However, they need to be simplified and easily understandable, so that the gait interpretations may be moved from the purview of the Gait-Lab to the physician's clinic.

Usually, gait and posture of the patient, indicates the possible diagnosis of the spinal lesion. Hence, if the patient can walk, notice carefully the type of gait and posture maintained during walking and/or standing. While assessing the gait, the legs should be adequately exposed and feet should be bare. *A normal gait must be rhythmic and soundless, having springiness in the feet which work alternatively in a definite cyclic order.* This is broadly achieved by alternate effective shortening and lengthening of lower limbs. The gait cycle begins when one foot comes into contact with the ground (initial contact) and ends when the same foot makes contact with the ground again (subsequent initial contact). The basic unit of measurement in gait analysis is the gait cycle. **A normal gait cycle is divisible into two phases for each extremity: (i) The stance phase, and (ii) The swing phase.**

As suggested at Rancho Los Angious (RLA) Medical Centre California, and also in traditional pattern—*Stance phase is further sub-divisible into: heel strike—foot flat—mid stance—heel off—toe break and—push off (toe off). Swing phase is sub-divisible into acceleration, mid-swing and deceleration phases.* In a rhythmic gait, while one foot is in the stance phase, the other passes through the swing phase. The stance phase starts with the heel of the leading extremity touching the floor (initial contact) followed by the sole of that foot. When the whole foot is in contact with the ground, this foot is supporting the whole body weight and this is the mid-stance phase. Next follows the push off phase. After momentarily stabilising the weight on the whole foot, the heel of the supporting extremity rises from the floor. In succession, the balls of toes prepare to lift-off from the ground. In the meantime, the strong action of gastrocsoleus propels the body forward. With the toes off, the entire foot leaves the ground and enters the swing phase. Once the swing phase begins, forward movement occurs entirely by the action of gravity (McMahon 1984). The leg gets accelerated forward to get in front of the body to be prepared for the next heel strike. This is the acceleration sub-phase of the swing phase. While passing in this direction, at one point the leg has to pass just beneath the body. This is the mid-swing phase. In this phase, the leg is shortened by flexing the hip and knees so that the foot completely clears the ground. Immediately after the leg goes in front of the body, the movement is restrained (deceleration). Now the foot is prepared to go for heel strike.

In the gait cycle, the role of tibialis anterior muscle has its own importance. For producing extension of ankle extensor digitorum longus, extensor hallucis longus and tibialis anterior muscles work together, of course the tibialis anterior muscle contributes most of the power. In the swing pase of gait cycle, the concentric contraction prevents stumbling. During initial contact and load bearing, the muscle provides a cushioning effect at heel strike and balances the plantigrade flexion of foot by eccentric contraction. The subsequent concentric contraction contributes mainly to the forward movement of the body by forward translation of the tibia.

During normal gait, for a moment, the two lower extremities are in simultaneous contact with the ground. This happens between push-off and toe-off on one side and between heel strike and foot flat on the contralateral side. During this period, both legs support the body weight, and this is known as *"double support".* The period of this "double support" is inversely proportional to the cadence (number of steps taken per minute) of the gait, i.e. if cadence of gait decreases, the period of double support increases and *vice versa*.

Walking can be distinguished from running by minimisation of the period of double support in running. Practically in walking, there are two periods of double support—initial heel contact in walking with the advancing limb and toe-off with the opposite limb. The two events of double support are replaced by a 'double float' when neither foot is on the ground. In running, stance is always less than swing to accommodate this period of double float (Gage 1991). In running, the duration of the stance phase is less than 50% of gait cycle. *Roughly calculated, the relative period of different phases of gait are as follows—stance phase 60%, swing phase 40% and double support 11% of the cycle.* With increase in the cadence, gradually the period spent in swing phase increases, and *vice versa*.

In physiomechanics of walking, the vertical displacement of the centre of gravity is at the core. In the human gait, the vertical displacement of the centre of gravity attempts to approximate the action of wheel which is the most efficient mechanism of motion because its centre of gravity remains perfectly in level, horizontal to the ground and without oscillation in its path of motion.

Five main determinants of the gait in the ballistic model of walking are responsible to maintain the lowest possible sinusoidal path of the centre of gravity. They are: 1. Pelvic rotation, 2. Pelvic tilt, 3. Knee flexion, 4. Plantar flexion of the stance ankle, 5. Lateral displacement of the pelvis (McMahon 1984).

In **'moon-walk',** the low oscillations of displacement of body's centre of gravity is demonstrated.

There can be several variations in a normal gait depending upon the age, sex, profession, footwear, foot shape, ground over which individual walks, clothing, posture, obesity, pathological conditions, etc. **(Table 8.5)**. Everyone (including a patient) adopts the least energy consuming style of walking. In a normal human gait, there is smooth energy efficient transfer of body through the space.

The lay description of abnormal gait can be divided into two patterns—*limping and lurching*. In 'limping' (antalgic gait) the patient avoids weight bearing on the affected side as far as possible (diminished stance phase). *Limping denotes a painful condition* on the affected side. However, in a painful hip as well, the patient may walk with an abductor lurch (lurching towards the affected side in stance phase to reduce the joint reactive forces on the hip). In lurch, the patient prolongs the stance phase to improve the stability. *Lurching denotes variable failure of abduction mechanism.* However, there are **recognised patterns of gait** which occur in particular clinical conditions:

- *Scissors gait:* Here one leg crosses directly over the other with each step, like crossing of the blades of a scissor (e.g. cerebral diplegia) due to adductor tightness. The knee

TABLE 8.5: Causes of variations and impairment in locomotion (Gait).			
1. Age:			
	6 months–1 year	Crawling stage	• More base support in quadruped position
	1–2 years	Toddler's walking • Walks on wider base to avoid falling • Reduced period of single limb support • Shorter step length • Increased cadence • More pelvic tilt	• Wide base support
	2–5 years	Gradually gait tends to become stable and advances towards normal gait pattern	Gradually base support decreases
	5–14 years	Increased stability Increased velocity Increased cadence Reduced step-length Less pelvic tilt More arm swing	Tends to acquire almost normal base support
	14 years onwards	Normal gait pattern due to developed musculoskeletal system, and strength, and proprioceptive (sensation) response	Normal base support
	Elderly person (> 60 years) or fragile person	Reduced cadence Reduced speed Decreased step length Decreased confidence in walking due to weak musculature, senility, secondary deformities in knee and feet, osteoporosis induced pain, senile nervous break down	Tends to again adopt wide base to balance the gravity and acquire confidence

2. Sex—in female		• Cadence is more in female than in male
		• Arm swinging is different and more in female due to wider pelvis
		• Pelvic rotation is visible/observed in female
		• Shorter step length leads to:
		  – Increase in number of steps in cadence
		  – Decreased stride length	

3. Profession and Habits		Prolonged adaptation of a particular posture (in any profession, job, athletic activities) may change the gait pattern	
4. Footwear		There is noticeable difference to a variable extent in bare-footed and booted walkers (especially in those who have used footwear right from childhood) In footwear also, the height of the heel, the base of the heel, height of counter, the capacity of toe box (roomy or congested or narrow) influence the pattern of gait	
5. Ground over which the individual walks			
6. Clothing used (tight fit; loose fit; too short or too long) especially in ladies affects the gait pattern			
7. Obesity		Slim persons usually walk with more velocity, increased step length, decreased steps, increased arm swings, decreased pelvic rotation Change in gait pattern is directly proportional to obesity. Obese persons usually walk with lesser velocity, decreased step length, increased steps, decreased arm swing, and increased pelvic rotation	
8. Pathological conditions		(Congenital, metabolic, developmental, traumatic, degenerative, neoplastic, psychological problems) Problems of spine, dissociated neuromuscular control, limb length discrepancies, muscular weakness, ligamentous laxity, contracture and deformities of joints, etc. can lead to abnormal gait	

may also be flexed resulting in couching, which leads to *'crouch-gait.'* During the swing phase one lower extremity crosses the other leg which is in stance phase
- *In-toeing gait (Internal rotation gait):* It is not uncommon. It may be familial. The cause of this gait is not primarily in muscle. It usually results due to metatarsus adductus, tibial bowing with tibial torsion or persistent excessive femoral anteversion. It usually resists correction by any orthotic appliances. However, if the deformity has not resolved (usually it resolves by 8 years of age) and is severe, its exact cause should be localised and treated properly
- *Out-toeing gait:* The normal range for out-toeing is from 0 to 30°; more out-toeing occurs due to relative femoral retroversion. In most infants/toddlers this out-toeing resolves spontaneously. However, when associated with lateral tibial torsion, it can become worse with growth and may need surgical correction
- *Crouch gait:* It is seen, usually in diplegics, due to cerebral palsy—its increased incidence being in adolescent years. Crouch gait is characterised by increased knee flexion in the stance phase of the gait cycle due to failure of the mechanisms responsible to maintain the body in an upright position. The body is kept in upright position by the three groups of 'antigravity muscles'—the hip extensors, the knee extensors, and the ankle plantarflexors. Failure to function adequately by any or more of these muscles results in almost collapsing of body in flexion posture leading to crouch gait. In this gait pattern, three positions are obvious—1. increased ankle dorsiflexion, 2. increased knee flexion and 3. diminished hip extension. Clinical observation and video gait analysis are sufficient to identify the established crouch gait. Patients who walk with flexed knees develop a cephalad displacement of the patella. In older patients, this can lead to disabling pain due to articular cartilage degeneration
- *High stepping (steppage) or foot-drop gait; Equinus gait:* During the heel strike attempt, the toes drop on the ground first (due to foot drop). To avoid this and to clear the ground, the patient flexes the hip and knee excessively, raises the foot and slap it on the floor forcibly. In few cases, the patient starts walking with dragging the toes on the ground without making any attempt to flex the hip and knee and raise the foot to clear the ground—*dragging gait*
- *Toe-walking:* The normal gait pattern in children is usually established by the age of 3 years. Several toddlers walk with variable equinus position (on toes) for variable period. By the age of 3 years heel strike pattern of gait must be established. If toe walking is persisting beyond 3 years, it should be taken as abnormal and pathology should be searched/investigated for. Two-thirds of toe-walker have a family history. Usual causes of persistent (beyond 3 years) toe-walking are:
  - Cerebral palsy—spastic diplegia (in 10% or persistent cases)
  - Muscular dystrophies
  - Residual polio deformities
  - Post-burn contractures
  - Post-infective (in calf muscles/regions) contractures
  - Spinal cord tumours
  - Idiopathic—it is the most common.
- *Spastic gait (Hemiplegic gait or circumduction gait):* Here, the spastic muscles do not allow the hip and knee to be flexed enough for the foot to clear the ground. Therefore, the patient partially drags his weight on the spastic leg. In this attempt, there is some circumduction effect on the lower limb (e.g. hemiplegia).

  The person rotates the hip sideways during the swing phase and places the foot in flattened manner or places the toes first before the heel strike. Gradually due to contracture of the plantar flexors, heel strike cannot be possible. On the affected side, the upper limb is usually flexed.

  Abnormality of the gait in adults who have hemiplegia is the result of equinus deformity of the ankle, decreased flexion (or hyperextension of the knee) and increased flexion of the hip. Spasm and/or contracture of gastrocnemius is the main cause of the equinus deformity (as in cerebral palsy as well). Spasticity of legs may even lead to ataxia *(paroxysmal trepidant ataxia)*
- *Helicopod gait:* A gait in which legs and feet are thrown in half circles as in hemiplegia
- *Lathyriatic gait:* In lathyriasis, there is a combination of spasticity, hyperabduction and dragging of lower limb elements in the gait
- *Waddling gait or duck gait or myopathic gait or (also referred as gluteus medius gait):* Myopathic gait is caused due to weakness of hip girdle muscles, especially the hip abductors (which are vital in stabilizing the pelvis while walking). Trendelenburg's sign is positive, i.e., there is abnormal drop of the pelvis on the side of the swing leg due to weakness of the hip abductors on the contralateral side. On the affected side the hip juts laterally as the stance leg adducts rather than maintaining its stable position. When the weakness is on both sides, there is exaggerated pelvic swing with each step as the hip droops on the side of swing leg that manifests in 'waddling' gait. When there is disturbance in the abduction mechanism of hip, there is increased lordosis. While walking the body sways from side to side on a wide base. Therefore, the patient lurches on both sides while walking like duck, e.g. in bilateral congenital dislocation of hip, osteomalacia, pregnancy, myopathy, paralysis of abductors of hips
- *Trendelenburg's gait:* It may be unilateral or bilateral. Bilateral Trendelenburg's gait is almost like the waddling gait. When unilateral, the patient lurches on the affected side and the pelvis drops on the opposite side of hip. Any condition, in which there is deficit in abduction

mechanism of the hip joint, medial deviation of the mechanical axis of the lower limb, and gross costo-pelvic impingement (e.g. CDH, fracture of femoral neck, polioparalysis), will cause this

- *Drunkers or reeling gait:* Here the patient tends to walk irregularly on a wide base, swinging sideways without stability and balance with tendency of falling with each step (seen in cerebellar incoordination, or in drunken states). In cerebellar lesion, hypotonia and ataxic gait are the main features with lack of coordination. If the patient has one side cerebellar lesion, he sways on the lesion side only with normal gait pattern on normal side.
- *Festinant gait or Festinating gait or short shuffling gait:* Due to rigidity of muscles, the patient adopts the stooping posture (flexed neck, trunk, hip and knee), in which the centre of gravity falls anteriorly. Here the patient, with stooping body, is propelled forward quickly in successions as if trying to catch up with the centre of gravity, e.g. in Parkinsonism, Wilson's disease, cerebral atherosclerosis. There will be short steps, lack of heel strike, and toe-off, loss of arm swing and lack of pelvic rotation. Since heel strike is absent, toes strike first, hence it is also called "toe-heel gait". In a few cases of parkinsonism, '**Retropulsion**' occurs, i.e. if the patient is pushed backwards, he starts walking backward involuntarily
- *Antalgic gait—Painful gait:* Due to pain anywhere from foot to hip, the patient avoids bearing weight on the affected limb (reduced stance phase, shortened step length, shortened stride length, shortened reciprocal arm swing, increased velocity of steps)
- *Stamping gait:* Occurs in sensory ataxia, e.g. tabes dorsalis, syringomyelia, diabetes mellitus, leprosy. The patient raises his feet abnormally high and jerks them forward to strike the ground slowly with a 'stamp' due to lack of kinesthetic. It looks like space-walk
- *Knock knee gait:* The gait here is also a typical one, i.e. while walking, the patient flexes the hips slightly, the knees point and appose each other, and the ankles and feet are kept apart with tendency of toe-in
- *Genu recurvatum gait:* In paralysis of the hamstring muscles (e.g. in polio), the knee goes for hyperextension (due to lack of counteraction of hamstrings) while transmitting the weight in the mid-stance phase. There is also slowing of swing during the late stage of swing phase due to paralysis of hamstrings
- *Short limb gait:* Initially, if the shortening is less than 1.5 cm, it can be compensated by pelvic tilt while walking; if shortening increases up to 5 cm it can be made up by equinus. With more shortening (usually more than 5 cm) the patient dips his body on that side due to marked pelvic tilt and equinus also increases
- *Short-leg gait (more or less as short limb gait):* Mild to moderate shortened lower limb in children is compensated by acquiring 'equinus' position (ending in equinus deformity) of the ankle and foot, when the person walks on the broadened forefoot and toes
- *Toe-tip-gait:* In persistent foot drop or contracture of the heel cord, the patient walks on the toe tips and the ball of the toes (metatarsal heads), e.g. in spastic diplegia; end stage of compensatory equinus for marked shortening of the limb
- *Quadriceps gait or hand to knee gait or five fingers quadriceps **(Refer Figs. 11.10 to 11.12)**:* Normally to transmit the weight on the lower leg during the mid-stance, the knee is locked by quadriceps contraction, but if quadriceps is much weak/paralysed, this locking is hampered. Hence, in case of very weak quadriceps, the patient stabilizes his knee for weight bearing by little leaning on the affected side and pressing over the lower thigh by his ipsilateral hand or fingers, either openly or through the pocket of the trouser
- *Quadriceps avoidance gait:* In this type of gait also the patient leans forward while walking for locking the knee which avoids the use of quadriceps on the affected side.
- *Calcaneus gait:* Patient walks on his broadened heel with a tendency of rotating the foot outwards, tendency of genu recurvatum, with no calcaneal pick up, no push off, and is due to weakness of the triceps surae or contracture of dorsiflexors of ankle and foot. There is absence of foot flat, mid-stance and toe-off stages of gait cycle
- *Gluteus medius gait:* It is more or less as Trendelenburg's gait, which is more exemplified in the paralysis of gluteus medius
- *Gluteus maximus gait:* Due to weakness in the gluteus maximus muscle, while the body propels forward during the mid-stance phase, the trunk is lurched posteriorly to effect posterior pelvic tilting and shifting the centre of gravity towards stance hip. Therefore, while walking, forward and backward movements of the trunk occur (hence it is also called *rocking horse gait*), the patient lurches backwards (mostly seen in polio paralysis)
- *Ataxic gait:* A gait in which the foot is raised higher than is necessary and brought down suddenly in a flapping manner (more or less similar to stamping gait)
- *Stiff hip gait:* Patient walks without flexing the hip (about 20° of flexing of hip is essential for normal gait). To compensate the stiffness at hip, the patient raises the pelvis and semicircumducts the limb to propel it forward. In stiff hip, the extensors of hip also becomes defunct, and to compensate it the patient does more anterior pelvic tilt with lordosis to swing the lower extremity forwards.
- *Stiff knee gait:* Normally, the knee goes in flexion during the early stage of swing phase to clear the foot from the ground. But if the knee is stiff during the swing phase, the patient has to raise the affected side pelvis to clear the foot

from the ground and swing sideways with circumduction of the limb to propel it forward to reach the heel strike
- *Circumduction gait:* If the limb is lengthened, even apparently (e.g. in fixed abduction deformity of hip) the patient has to take the affected limb in round about way to take the forward step
- *Hysterical gait:* Patient walks in bizarre fashion as if going to fall on every step, but seldom falls and that too cautiously
- *Cerebellar gait:* A staggering gait, often with a tendency to fall to one or other side, forward or backward
- *Charcot's gait:* The gait of hereditary ataxia
- *Robotic gait:* Walking like robot.
- *Gait Analysis*: In patients with wide resection (in limb salvage surgery) and endoprosthesis replacement around the knee is reported to have good functional and oncological outcomes, both objectively and subjectively, as evidenced by the symmetrical gait pattern and significant correlation with musculoskeletal tumor society score. The gait remains more or less symmetrical despite the decreased walking velocity, stride length and stance phase of the operated limb when compared to normal limbs. It indicates that the normal limb can compensate for the affected limb to achieve a symmetrical gait.
- *Varus recurvatum gait*: In this type of gait the patient hyperextends the affected knee with relative varus during the stance phase.

The typical injury-oriented gait patterns may be grouped as: Antalgic gait; Trendelenburg gait; Qudriceps avoidance gait; and *Varus recurvatum gait.*
- **Balance and posture:** Balance is a state of body in which weight is evenly distributed ensuring that a person or object does not wobble or fall over **(Fig. 8.60)**.
- **Footprints on the moon** can stay there for at least 100 million years.

Posture

"Posture accompanies movement like a shadow; movement begins in posture and ends in posture" (Sherrington, Quoted by Rusworth 1964)

Posture itself is a complex subject and requires clear understanding. For maintaining posture and balance, **(Fig. 8.60)** the proper sensory input is required from the joints, muscles, tendons and vestibular system alongwith coordinated motor outputs mediated by the cerebral cortex and basal ganglia. The particular posture adopted by the patient while walking and standing should be described clearly. There are certain postures which are very typical of particular conditions, e.g. *in parkinsonism the patient has a tendency of stooping forward with the arm adducted, elbow semiflexed, forearm semipronated and 'pill-rolling' movements in between his thumb and fingers.* Parkinson's

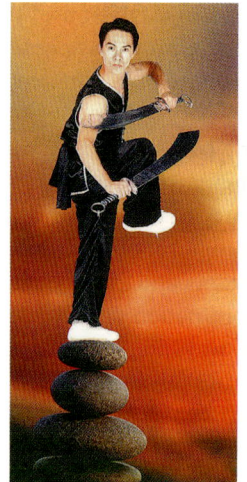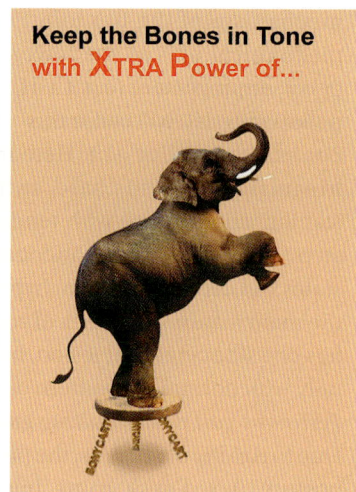

Fig. 8.60: A man balancing on stones and an elephant standing on the hind feet, in maintained posture.

disease is an extrapyramidal motor disorder presenting with abnormalities of posture and movement. It is caused by depletion of dopaminergic neurons of substantia nigra leading to decreased dopamine delivery to the striatum. In advanced ankylosing spondylitis, the patient has a typical pokerback appearance, keeping the trunk stooped forward, neck rigidly fixed and thereby has a tendency of looking towards the ground **(Refer Fig. 8.19)**.

Motor Dysfunctions

The basic functional unit of muscle, the motor unit consists of a motor neuron, the neuromuscular junction and the muscle fibres innervated by the motor neuron.

Main motor dysfunctions are:
- Loss or less of functions (Lower motor neurone type of paralysis, flaccid paralysis)
- Excess of function due to excessive unbridled neurological stimulation to muscles leads to—spasticity "There is not a clear "best test" or comprehensive quantitative measure of spasticity" (Skinner 1992)
  - Prolonged spasticity in the muscle (especially in growing age) leads to shortening of the muscle resulting in 'myostatic contracture'. Prolonged myostatic contracture leads to the contracture of the capsule and ligaments of the affected joint.
  - Spastic paraplegia
  - Upper motor neuron type of paralysis. In upper motor neuron type of paralysis, there are certain positive features, such as spasticity, hyper-reflexia and cocontraction; and negative features which include weakness, loss of selective motor control, sensory deficits and poor balance.
- **Involuntary (abnormal) movements,** e.g.
  - *Dyskinesia*—dyskinesia indicates involuntary movements of limbs, which may be of several types,

such as athetosis, ballismus, chorea, dystonia, dyskinesia, torticolis, ticks, tetany
- *Athetosis*—writhing type of motion affecting limbs, head and neck or even part of whole body
- *Ballismus* is a subtype of athetosis in which there are violent jerky movement primarily of the proximal joints
- *Chorea* (the word chorea means a dance) chorea is another subtype of athetosis characterised by random disorganised muscle contractions controlling mainly the distal joints. There are sudden abnormal discharges along the nerve cause flinging, mostly of one limb. The involuntary movements are brief, asynchronous, rapid purposeless, jerky fluid and often difficult to discern in the beginning
- *Tremor* may be considered as another subtype of athetosis in which there is almost vibratory type of involuntary movement, usually of the hands
- *Ataxia* is uncoordinated voluntary movement due to disordered cerebellar function and it results in gait disturbances and uncoordinated volitional muscle use. Simple and predominant ataxia in cerebral palsy is less common than ataxia due to predominant motor dysfunction, such as spasticity. An ataxic gait is uncoordinate and wide based. Falls are more often due to problems in standing balance
- *Dystonia*—It expresses an 'abnormally maintained posture', often associated with a plastic rigidity, e.g. flexed posture of Parkinson's disease (flexion dystonia); or the hemiplegic posture (hemiplegic dystonia)
- In *Dyskinesia*, the involuntary movements may predominantly affect the pharyngeal and facial perioral musculature (e.g. phenothiazine-induced involuntary movements)
- *Torticollis*—It is a form of dystonia in which a jerky or maintained rotational and abducted posture of neck occurs—spasmodic torticollis
- *Tics*—These are normal simple movements which become unnecessarily repeated (producing embarrassing situation). They can be easily imitated, e.g. head-nodding
- *Tetany*: Any cause of low-ionized serum calcium can lead to tetany, e.g. hypoparathyroidism, acute hyperventilation and hypomagnesemia. The threshold for muscular excitability is lowered so the involuntary sustained contractions occur, which may be painless or painful. The contracting muscles feel rigid and unyielding. Usually carpal spasm also occurs in hypocalcaemia or alkalosis in which a peculiar posture of the hand (may be also of toes) develops, in which the fingers and thumbs are held stiffly adducted and partially flexed at the metacarpophalangeal joints and interphalangeal joints are hyperextended forming the shape of a cone. All the hand muscles become rigid.

The spasm is involuntary and usually painless. It is also seen in hand dystonia associated with repetitive hand activities. In foot, the toes may be similarly effected (*carpopedal spasm*).

These effects can be reproduced or augmented by producing ischaemia of the affected limb, e.g. by inflating the sphygmomanometer cuff above the arterial pressure for three minutes—*Trousseau's sign*.

This can also be tested by eliciting *Chvostek's sign*—tap lightly with patellar hammer at the sternomastoid foramen region through which the facial nerve emerges (3-5 cm in front and below the external auditory meatus)—the facial muscles starts twitching.

Motor Function

Examine under following headings:
- Bulk of muscle
- Tone of muscle
- Power of muscle
- Rigidity
- Reflexes—A reflex is a simple motor action, stereotyped and repeatable, elicited by a sensory stimulus. The strength of the motor action is graded according to the intensity of stimulus.
    - Superficial reflexes **(Table 8.6)**
    - Deep reflexes (tendon jerks and clonus) **(Table 8.7)**
- Co-ordination of movements
- Involuntary movements
- Assessment about spasticity and its severity

"There is not a clear 'best test' or a comprehensive quantitative measure of spasticity"
—*Skinner 1992*

- Contractures.

Bulk of Muscle

- Look at and feel the bulk of the muscle and assess for any atrophy or hypertrophy. The texture, pliability and flabbiness can also be assessed simultaneously. Confirm by circumferential measurements of the bulk, comparing with the normal side. In few cases of muscular dystrophy (*Duchenne dystrophy*) due to underlying pathology, the muscle bulk increases in size and feels comparatively firm [(calf muscles **(Refer Fig. 11.9)**, glutei, infraspinate)]. Of course, they are weaker in strength.
- *Tone of muscle (state of tension found in healthy muscle and contracture)*: *Muscle tone* has two characteristics 1. slight resting tension and 2. involuntary resistance to mechanical stretch (Gamble 1988). The tension and resistance to stretch are due to viscoelastic properties and nerve impulses (McMahon 1984) Muscle tone is controlled by brain and spinal cord. Tone can be considered as the set point from which the muscle can contract to enable us to move against gravity and enable us to shift between reciprocal inhibition and cocontraction (Helsel et al. 2001).

TABLE 8.6: Main superficial reflexes.

Reflex	How to initiate	What to observe	Inference	Cord level	Fallacies
1	2	3	4	5	6
1. Trapezius reflex	• Just proximal to acromion tap the stretched trapezius	• Contraction of trapezius	Normal (Hypercontraction indicates lesion above C2 C1)	C3–C4	
2. Deltoid reflex	• Tap on upper deltoid mass just distal to acromion	• Contraction of deltoid	Normal (Hypercontraction indicates lesion above C4)	C5–C6	
3. Scapular reflex	• Scratching of skin in interscapular region	• Scapular muscle contraction	Normal	C5–T1	
4. Abdominal reflex (Fig. 8.61)	• Scratching of abdominal wall obliquely in all four quadrants, from outer aspect towards midline	• Contraction of abdominal muscles in the testing quadrant	Normal Absent in UMN lesions above their spinal level	T7–12	Obese, lax abdomen, multipara, anxious and tense patients (diminished or absent)
5. Cremasteric reflex	• With a blunt pointed needle gently scratch over the upper medial side of thigh	• Involuntary contraction of the dartos muscle of scrotum	Normal	L1	Huge filarial scrotum (diminished or absent)
6. Anal reflex	• Scratch perianal skin or insert one lubricated gloved finger in anus	• Contraction of anal sphincter • No contraction	Normal Cauda equina lesion	S3–4	Chronic perianal fistula, perianal surgery, patulous anus (diminished or absent)
7. Bulbocavernosus reflex	• Pinching dorsum of glans penis	• Contraction of bulbocavernosus muscle	Normal	S3–4	
8. Plantar reflex* (Figs. 8.62 and 8.63)	• Stroking the outer part of the sole from heel to base of outer toes (Fig. 8.62 I). • Babinski sign: Joseph Babinski, in 1896 noticed that response was best obtained when the limb was slightly flexed and the muscles were well relaxed. • Squeezing the heel cord (Gordon's sign) Fig. 8.62 III • Squeezing the calf • Pressing firmly along the medial surface of tibia (Oppenheim's sign) (Fig. 8.62 II)	1. Flexion of toes, dorsiflexion of ankle, inversion of foot (Fig. 8.63A). 2. Extension of great toe, spreading out and extension of other toes. Dorsiflexion of ankle (Fig. 8.63B) 3. Flexion of hip and knee (withdrawal reflex) (Fig. 8.63C) 4. Contraction of quadriceps (mainly anterolateral region)	Flexor plantar response (Normal) Extensor plantar responses or Babinski's sign UMN lesion UMN lesion	L5, S1	Difficult to demonstrate in anaesthetic sole, thick skin of the sole, barefoot walkers. In children below 1 year, the extension response is normal. Tense and excited individual may have extensor response
9. Throckmorton's reflex (Thomas Bentley Throckmorton, American neurologist (1885)	Percuss the dorsum of foot in metatarsophalangeal joints region	Extension of great toe and flexion of others	Normal		

NB: *In the progressive lesions, the receptive field spreads from outer part of sole over to the whole sole, the leg, knees or even the groin. Hence there also these signs can be elicited

* Chaddock's sign—A response similar to that of Babinski sign on stroking the lateral malleolus or around it and then on the lateral aspect of dorsum of foot.
* Stransky reflex—A slow but vigorous adduction of the little toe followed by its sudden release results in a dorsiflexion of the great toe.
* Schaefer's sign—Babinski like reaction on squeezing the Achilles tendon
* Infantile Reflexes and Automatisms: Infantile reflexes and automatisms may be considered as 'fixed action patterns'. They are complex motor act elicited by a sensory stimulus, e.g. Babinski sign, the Moro reflex. and tonic neck reflexes (Horstman and Black)

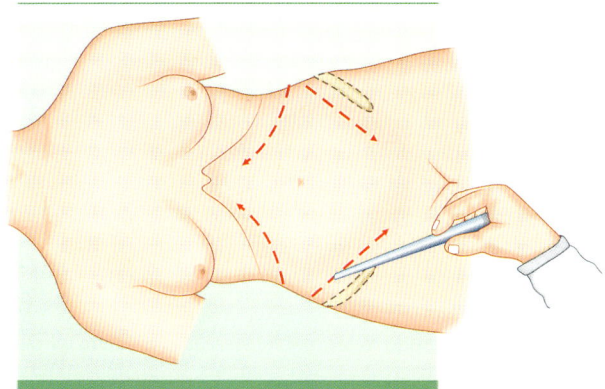

Fig. 8.61: Method of eliciting abdominal reflexes.

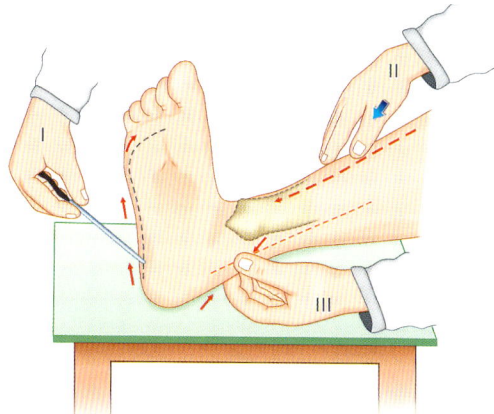

Fig. 8.62: Different methods of eliciting plantar reflex: I = by stroking the outer sole of the foot; II = by pressing firmly along the medial border of tibia (Oppenheim's sign); III = by squeezing the heel cord (Gordon's sign).

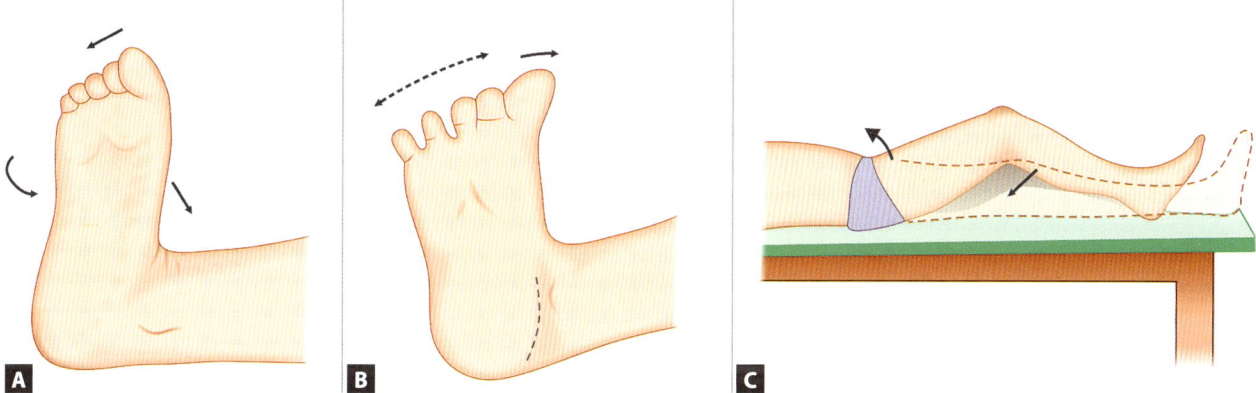

Figs. 8.63A to C: Showing different responses of plantar reflex; (A) Flexion of toes; dorsiflexion at ankle and inversion of foot; (B) Extension of big toe and fanning out of other toes; (C) Flexion of the hip and knee (In patients with amputated or fallen out toes this response should be looked for. In less severe case hamstrings can be felt and seen contracting).

Assess the tone of the muscle by palpation. Increase in tone of muscle is *hypertonia*, and decrease *hypotonia*. A hypotonic (flaccid) muscle will be soft and pliable, and provide little or no resistance to passive movements, e.g. in lower motor neuron lesions. As the tone increases in the muscle, the muscle becomes less moveable from side to side and tighter in feel. Increase and sustenance of tone leads to hypertonia.

Normally, when a particular joint is moved it can be moved freely unless the patient voluntarily resists it. But in presence of hypertonia, the patient does not have much voluntary control over the involuntary resistance offered in moving that joint.

Hypertonia can occur due to lesions of corticospinal systems or extrapyramidal pathways. Hypertonia due to pyramidal affection is called spasticity. Spasticity is a condition of increased sensitivity of the muscle to stretch resulting in contraction by recruiting all the fibres within the muscle. Spasticity is velocity dependent resistance to movement associated with exaggerated deep tendon reflexes. This spasticity produces rigidity of *clasp-knife type* (when the limb is rapidly flexed or extended, initially there is resistance, after which there is sudden yield). *Rigidity* has persistent elevated tone throughout a motion rather than extraneous movement. The persistent elevated tone can be felt while passively extending a limb with continuous resistance similar to the feeling of bending of a lead pipe.

Hypertonia, following disease of basal ganglion is termed as extrapyramidal rigidity. The rigidity is either *cogwheel type* (the resistance offered is jerky but periodic and patterned throughout as movement in a cogwheel), or *lead pipe type* (uniform rigidity throughout the movement, as in bending a lead pipe)—as found in paratonic or catatonic states, e.g. parkinsonism. It disappears during sleep. The physiological basis of this type of rigidity is not clearly known.

In hysteria also the patient offers rigidity. Here, the resistance increases proportionately to the effort applied by the examiner.

Dystonia is often confused with spasticity. Dystonic postures are usually not correctable by orthopaedic procedures.

TABLE 8.7: Deep reflexes (tendon jerks and clonus).

Reflexes	How to test	What to observe	Inference	Cord level	Fallacies
1	2	3	4	5	6
1. Knee jerk (Figs. 8.64 and 8.65)	• Patient supine, knees bent 60°, tap the patellar tendon. In the same position of the knee and heel, the forefoot is supported and tapping over the tendo-Achilles from behind elicits ankle jerk (Figs. 8.64 and 8.66) • Patient sits with leg hanging at the edge of the table, tap over patellar tendon. In the same position while one hand supports the foot at 90° to leg, tapping over the tendo-Achilles from behind elicits the ankle jerks (Fig. 8.65) • Patient sits on the stool with knee bent 90° and foot planted on the floor. Tap over the patellar tendon to elicit the knee jerk; and tap over the tendo-Achilles to elicit the ankle jerk	• Contraction of quadriceps, brief extension of knee • Diminished or absent contraction of quadriceps • May be brisk contraction of quadriceps • Exaggerated contraction of quadriceps • Leg suddenly tends to be thrown off • Sustained oscillatory contraction and relaxation of quadriceps (clonus)	Normal LMN lesion UMN lesion UMN lesion UMN lesion	L2,3,4	Anxious tense individual
2. Patellar jerk (Fig. 8.67)	• Patient supine with extended knee. Tap over your middle finger placed on upper pole of patella	Patella quickly moves upwards	UMN lesion where knee jerk is exaggerated	L2,3,4	
3. Patellar clonus (Fig. 8.68)	• Patient supine with extended knee. Hold upper pole of patella between thumb and index finger. Suddenly give a downward jerk and loosen the grip	Oscillatory up and down movements of patella	-do-	-do-	
4. Ankle jerk (Figs. 8.65, 8.66 and 8.69)	• Patient lies supine keeping the leg crossed over opposite leg; slightly dorsiflex the foot with one hand and tap over the stretched tendo-Achilles • As in knee (Fig. 8.65)	• A sharp contraction of calf muscle, foot may go in plantar flexion • The above response may be brisk/ exaggerated • Sustained oscillatory contraction and relaxation of calf muscle (clonus) • Diminished or absent contraction of calf muscles	Normal UMN lesion UMN lesion LMN lesion	S1,2	Severe spasticity, rigidity or a long-standing severe contraction of tendo-Achilles may eliminate the ankle jerk response
5. Ankle clonus (Fig. 8.70)	• Patient lies supine. Bend the knee 60°. • Hold or support the upper leg with one hand. • With another hand hold the forefoot and give sudden dorsiflexion jerk and maintain the forefoot support	Oscillatory movements of the foot due to contraction/relaxation of calf muscles	UMN lesion	S1,2	
6. Triceps jerk (Fig. 8.71)	• With one hand support patient's forearm with the elbow bent to 90° and tap over triceps tendon	• Diminished/absent • Contraction of triceps, brief extension of elbow • Brisk exaggerated contraction	LMN lesion Normal UMN lesion	C6,7	
7. Biceps jerk (Fig. 8.72)	• With one hand, support patient's semipronated forearm and elbow bent 90°. Place the supporting hand's thumb on biceps tendon. • Tap over the thumb	• Diminished/absent • Biceps contracts • Exaggerated	LMN lesion Normal. UMN lesion	C5,6	
8. Supinator jerk (Fig. 8.73)	Forearm semipronated, tap over the radial styloid process	Supinator is stretched causing supination of the forearm	Normal	C5,6	
9. Finger flexion reflex	The patient partially flexes the terminal phalanges of his fingers. The examiner then places his middle and index fingers on the palmar surfaces of the phalanges and strikes then with hammer	Flexion of the fingers will be seen and felt	Normal	C7,T1	

Contd...

Contd...

Reflexes	How to test	What to observe	Inference	Cord level	Fallacies
1	2	3	4	5	6
10. Inversion of radial jerk	Same as supinator jerk	• Brisk flexion of fingers is the only response due to hyperexcitability of anterior horn cells at C7-8 level • This is associated with absent biceps jerk	UMN lesion family; common in cervical disc lesion, trauma to cervical region, syringomyelia, cervical neoplasm	C5,6	
11. Jaw jerk (Fig. 8.74).	Patient moderately opens her mouth. Place one finger on the chin, firmly tap over it suddenly	• Muscles closing the jaw contract • Increased contraction	Normal UMN lesion	Above 5th cranial nerve	Sometimes absent in healthy person as well

N.B.
1. According to the strength of contraction, the response of deep tendon reflexes are graded as: 0 = Absent; 1 = Present but depressed; 2 = Normal; 3 = Exaggerated; 4 = Clonus
   (1) When not normally elicited, JENDRASSIK'S manoeuvre, by virtue of its increasing the excitability of anterior horn cells and stretch sensitivity of primary sensory nerve endings, helps in eliciting the deep reflexes (important for lower limbs). Here the patient does some strong voluntary effort with the upper limbs, like forcibly pulling apart the hooked fingers.
   (2) Exaggerated tendon reflexes carry pathological significance only when asymmetrical, or when supported by other UMN manifestations, since in tense and anxious persons or tetanus or thyrotoxicosis, there may be hyperreflexia
   (3) The 'ankle clonus reflex' was first described by Dimitrejevic et al as a "hyperreflexive state often associated with spasticity and upper motor neuron lesion. It is series of rhythmic contractions of muscle at a frequency of five to seven hertz in response to an abruptly and continuously applied stretch reflex". The clonus reflex requires an intact spinal stretch reflex and sustained hyperexcitability of the lower motor neurones secondary to a loss of central inhibition. In the case of this ankle clonus reflex, the first sacral nerve root mediates the spinal stretch reflex arc
2. The biceps, triceps, periosteal-radial reflexes in upper limb and the quadriceps knee jerk and ankle jerk in lower limb are hyperactive in spasticity and normal or absent in ataxia.
3. If the tapping of the patellar tendon results in adduction of opposite hip, it indicates severe spasticity, and is known as crossed adductor response.

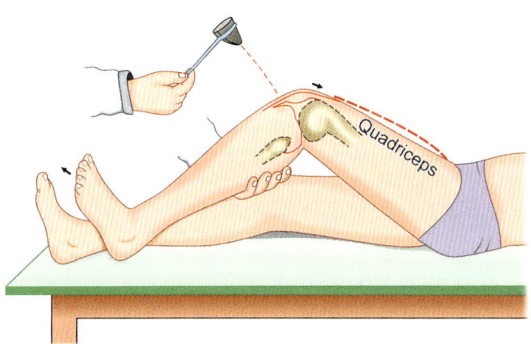

Fig. 8.64: Method of eliciting the knee jerk while patient is in supine position. Arrow is showing the movement response and the dotted line shows the contraction of quadriceps.

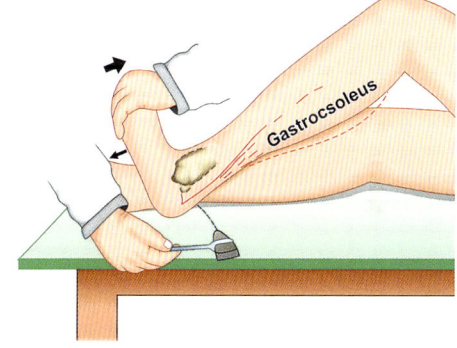

Fig. 8.66: Method of eliciting ankle jerk while the patient is lying down. Dotted line shows contraction of the gastrocsoleus as a response to ankle jerk. As a consequence a sudden plantar flexion at ankle is shown by dark arrow.

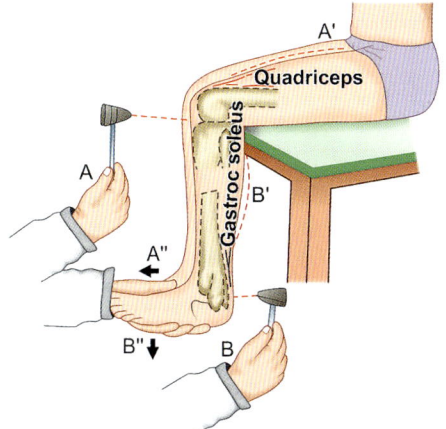

Fig. 8.65: Eliciting knee (A, A' and A") and ankle jerk (B, B' and B") while the patient is sitting at the edge of the table.

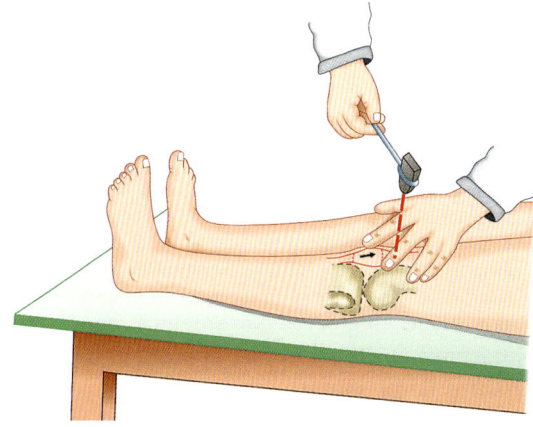

Fig. 8.67: Method of eliciting the patellar jerk. Arrow shows the sudden upward shift of patella after tapping over the upper pole.

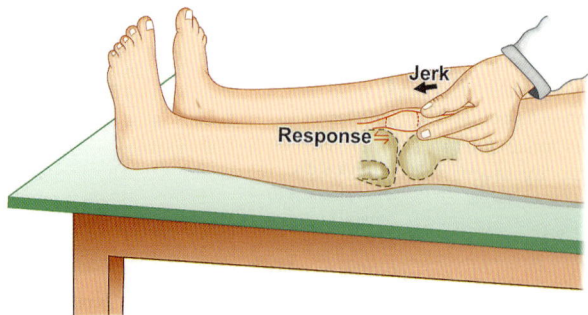

Fig. 8.68: The method of eliciting patellar clonus.

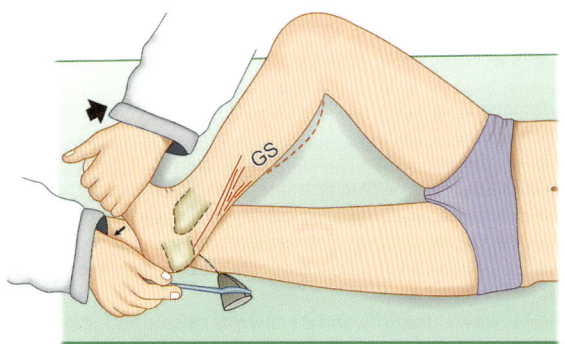

Fig. 8.69: Another method of eliciting the ankle jerk while patient is supine.
Abbreviation: GS, gastrocsoleus.

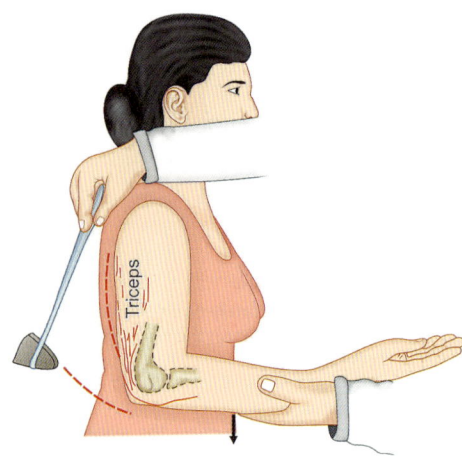

Fig. 8.71: Method of eliciting triceps jerk, dotted line represents contracted triceps after tapping over the tendon. Consequently, the elbow shows tendency of extension shown by arrow.

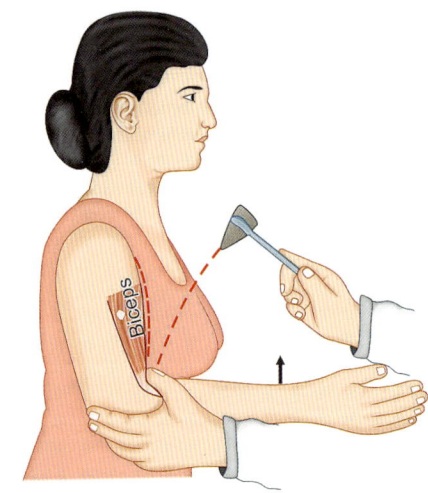

Fig. 8.72: Method of eliciting biceps jerk. Dotted line represents the contracted biceps tendon. Consequently the elbow goes in flexion as shown by arrow.

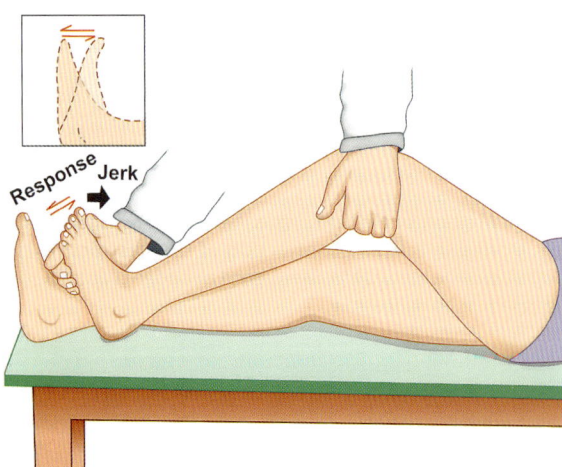

Fig. 8.70: Method of eliciting ankle clonus.

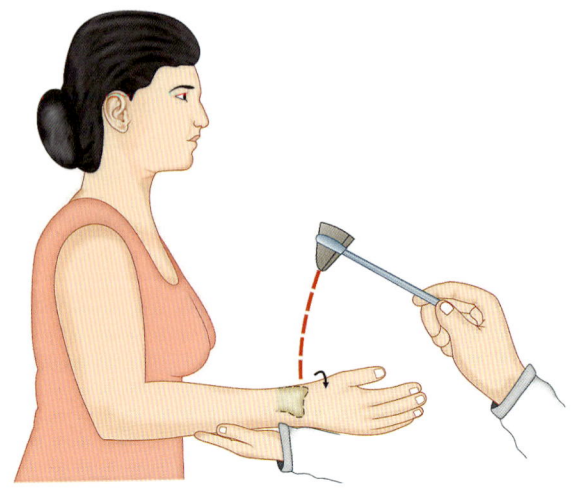

Fig. 8.73: Method of eliciting supinator jerk. Arrow showing the supination of the forearm.

Contracture—here the muscle is wasted, fibrotic and shortened. It feels firm and becomes variably unstretchable. In advanced neglected paraplegics, there may be contractures at the joints due to postural negligence or persistent flexor spasms
- *Power of muscle*: To be assessed as given in the chapter "Introduction"

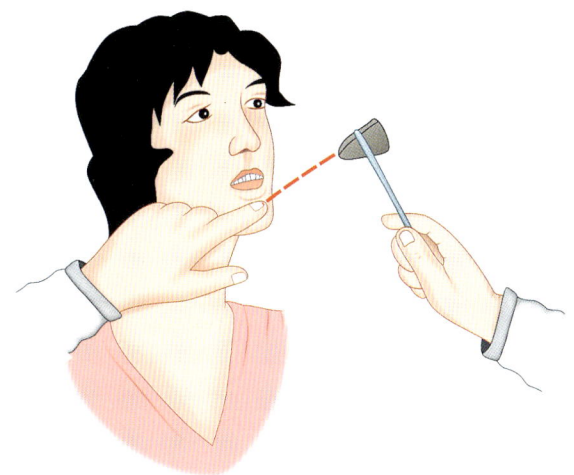

Fig. 8.74: Method of eliciting jaw jerk.

- *Reflexes:* A reflex is stereotyped and repeatable motor action, which is elicited by a sensory stimulus. The strength of the motor action is graded with the intensity of the stimulus. Actually the muscle stretch reflex is termed as tendon reflex. The muscle is stretched by a brisk tap on its taut tendon near its insertion. The muscle (tendon) stretch reflex is a reflex arc consisting of a muscle cell, a sensory and a motor neuron. The reflexes can be broadly considered into two groups:
  - Superficial reflexes **(Table 8.6)**
  - Deep reflexes (tendon jerks and clonus) **(Table 8.7)**.

  It is difficult to assess accurately the magnitude of response of eliciting the reflex, however, it may be denoted by numbers or pluses as follows:
  0—No response
  1 or + —Detectable only with reinforcement
  2 or ++—Easily detectable
  3 or +++—Brisk punctuated with occasional clonus
  4 or ++++—Sustained clonus

  Clonus is the sustained repetitive maintenance of the reflex arc with tonic stretch of the muscle.

  The diminution or loss of tendon jerks signifies the presence of a lesion affecting the afferent pathways, anterior horn cells or efferent pathways, i.e. the lower motor neuron disease. Assess clearly the diminished or lost jerk. If upper jerks are normal, then the level of cord damage will be lower to the spinal levels which control these jerks, and above the spinal level which controls the immediate lower jerk which is lost

- *Coordination of movements:* For a definite motor action, certain separate muscles or group of muscles act in synergism and cooperation to produce smooth, rhythmical, accurate activity in proper harmony and correct sequence when coordination is intact. For this, perfection in cerebellar control, neuromuscular axis, muscular tone and contractability and sense of joint position (and vision) are essential. With normal coordination, one can stop one motor action and substitute it with its opposite action. Loss of this ability (*dysdiadochokinesia*) is the feature of cerebellar disease. Proper accurate execution of skilled acts is *eupraxia* whereas the inability to translate an idea into a skilled act is *apraxia*. Lack of coordination is called 'incoordination' or 'asynergid', which can be seen in cerebellar ataxia, upper motor neuron lesions producing spasticity; lower motor neuron lesion resulting in flaccidity and loss or less of muscle power; loss of kinesthetic sensation, e.g. in neuropathic joints (e.g. Charcot's joint), tabes dorsalis, syringomyelia, leprosy, diabetes mellitus producing advanced neuropathy

Ataxia: Loss of coordination in maintaining proper posture may be defined as ataxia. Ataxia involves uncoordinated voluntary movements due to disorder in function of cerebellum and leads to gait disturbances, such as ataxic gait. The ataxic gait is uncoordinated and wide based. The person falls frequently due to difficulty in balancing himself/herself while standing or moving—it is kinetic ataxia, however, if the patient is incoordinate on lying down—it is static ataxia.

Tests

In upper limbs: Ask the patient to touch his nose tip with his index finger tip, thence with the other index finger, i.e. *finger to nose*. Similarly, ask him to touch one index finger tip to another index finger tip with arms extended. This should be repeated with his eyes closed, to assess the intactness of the sense of position of the joints of the limb.

In lower limbs: A normal gait indicates perfect coordination. However, in suspected cases, *heel to tibial shin coordination* can be tested. While lying down and with the eyes open, the patient is asked to lift one leg in the air, then to bring the heel of that leg over the upper end of the opposite tibial shin and slide it down over the shin towards the ankle.

Equilibrium reactions: If one can stand without support, this is time to test for standing-equilibrium reactions. This is of great importance in examining a developing child with suspected neuro-deficit. For quick check for balance: (i) If one can hop on one foot, the equilibrium reaction is almost perfect. (ii) Ask the child/person to stand on one foot and then on the other at least for 10 seconds, if there is inability it indicates, impaired motor function. To test for standing equilibrium reactions, while the child/person is standing erect, without support push gently from side to side and then from anteriorly and posteriorly. Normal child/person will maintain their balance with a prompt righting response to regain stability, but with deficient equilibrium reactions they will topple like a felled tree.

Romberg's sign: Truly, this sign indicates loss of position sense (sensory ataxia, e.g. tabes dorsalis). However, in advanced vertigo or cerebellar dysfunctions, this test may be positive to a varying extent. Ask the patient to stand with feet approximated and eyes closed. If the test is positive, he starts swaying and may even fall. (cf. while in cerebellar ataxia, the patient sways even with the eyes open. This can be further confirmed by observing for dysdiadochokinesia—the patient cannot perform any repeated voluntary movement rapidly)

- *Involuntary movement* (Also see *Pages 246 and 247*): Involuntary, undesired movements occur either at rest or during voluntary movements in several diseases, mostly those affecting the extrapyramidal system, e.g. basal ganglia. Few known varieties are—epilepsy, myoclonus, tremor, athetosis, chorea (meaning a 'dance'), dyskinesia—difficulty in performing voluntary movements, dystonia, tics, myokymia, hemiballismus, asterixis, tetany, etc.

Sensory Functions

Detailed sensory mapping specially for the limbs should be done for superficial touch, pain, temperature, deep touch, deep pain, and deficiencies should be noted in terms of root affections. One should note that there is a *'dynatomal' area* (a dynatome is the description of referred symptoms from root irritation), which can differ from the 'dermatomal' sensory map of that root. The strip of skin covered by the cutaneous branch of a spinal nerve is the dermatome of that spinal root.

To test the integrity of sensory component of particular spinal segment the representative area on body surface may be considered as follows:

C2 - Ear
C3 - Neck
C4 - Supraclavicular fossa
C5 - Skin over deltoid region
C6 - Thumb
C7 - Middle finger
C8 - Little finger
T1 - Inner area of arm
T2 - Infraclavicular fossa
T3 - Supramammary region
T4 - Mammary region
T5 to T9 - Respective intercostal spaces
T10 - Around the umbilicus
T11 and T12 - Infraumbilical region
L1 - Along inguinal ligament
L2 - Below inguinal ligament
L3 - Medial surface of knee
L4 - Medial malleolus area
L5 - Big toe
S1 - Lateral malleolus area
S2, S3, S4 - Gluteal region.

Superficial Touch

It should be tested with cotton wool on identical points of the two sides of body or limbs after taking the patient in full confidence. The patient's eyes should be closed or covered with a towel. In spinal lesions specially those in the lumbar region, perianal anaesthesia must be tested. In cauda equina lesion—*perianal saddle anaesthesia* is characteristic.

Test also for *two points discrimination*, which are perceived by Meissner's corpuscles and Merkel's disc and its centre is located in the sensory cortex.

Temperature

Temperature discrimination can be tested by taking two test tubes, one containing warm and the other cold water. Touch the suspected area, alternately, with the particular test tube and ask for the feeling of the patient about the temperature felt. Dissociation of different sensations should be assessed. The warmth sensation is perceived by *Raffinis end bulbi* and cold sensation is perceived by *Krause's end bulb*. However, the centre of both lies in sensory cortex.

Deep Touch

Bathyanaesthesia [Gr. bathos = deep + an = not + aisthesis = perception]—loss of deep sensations should be carefully assessed.

Note the appreciation of deep touch by sharp and blunt objects. Also test for joint sense and sense of position (by asking the patient to close the eyes and to tell about the position of the great toe, while the examiner changes its position from up → neutral → down and *vice versa*), sense of vibration (by tuning fork over bony prominence), sense of discrimination (by divider points), recognition of size, shape, form and weight of known objects *(stereognosis)*.

In *syringomyelia,* the pain and temperature sensations are lost while crude touch and postural sensibility is preserved. *Syringomyelia* is a cystic fluid-filled cavitation within the spinal cord. Scoliosis may be the first manifestation. Syringomyelia can exist with Chiari I malformations (probably due to disturbed or obstructed cerebrospinal fluid flow) or with it (described as noncommunicating syrinx). In *Brown-Sequard syndrome* (hemisection of spinal cord), there is loss of pain, temperature and deep touch sensation of opposite side while there is disturbance of sense of posture, position, movement, loss of recognition of weight, shape, size, vibration and light touch, besides spastic paralysis of same side.

Kinesthetic sensation: By kinaesthetic sensation a person becomes aware of the position and movements of different joints of the body. The impulses arising from muscles, tendons, joints and ligaments are perceived by proprioceptors, muscle spindles and Golgi bodies. The centre is located in the cerebellum. Loss of kinaesthetic sensation is called *akinesia,* loss of vibratory sensation is called *topallenesthesia,* loss of ability to recognise any known object with closed eyes due to loss of cutaneous sensations is called *astereognosis.*

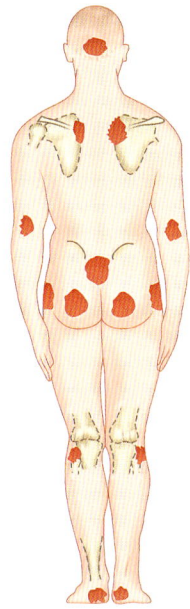

Fig. 8.75: Common sites of pressure sores shown by red-shaded area.

Paraesthesia: When the patient states that there are "*pins and needles*" sensation, it is pathognomonic of inflammation of or pressure on peripheral nervous system.

Search for Pressure Sore (Fig. 8.75)

In neurological conditions, (specially in paraplegia or quadriplegia) or following long decubitus or even short decubitus in an unconscious patient, the patient develops pressure sores. When the patient lies supine look the **common sites (Fig. 8.75) for pressure sores**—the occiput; back of shoulder blades, back of elbow joint, sacral region, buttock, and heels; over the greater trochanter when he lies on the sides, and over the anterior superior iliac spines when he lies prone.

Vasomotor Changes

Vasomotor changes should be assessed by looking for *pallor, cyanosis, redness, atrophy of skin, nailbed and subcutaneous tissues.* Presence of sweating can be assessed by observing beads of sweat through the +20 lense of ophthalmoscope as suggested by Kahn. History of *anhidrosis* (no sweating) or *oligohidrosis* (less sweating) or *hyperhidrosis* (more sweating) should be enquired for. In indeterminate or uncooperative patients, this can be found out by *certain tests*:
- *Starch iodine test:* Using iodine and starch, this can be done to map out the anaesthetic areas as dry and devoid of sweating
- *Guttman's test:* Sprinkle quinizarine powder on the skin, it will turn purple when it comes in contact with sweat. Hence, area of anhidrosis can be clearly mapped out.

Vasomotor swelling, i.e. oedema due to dependant posture, post-plaster, post-surgical, post-infective and post-traumatic conditions should be noted.

Visceral Assessment

Ask about the *bladder and bowel control*. If there is no voluntary control, enquire regarding retention of urine, retention overflow, incontinence overflow, dribbling or bed wetting. If patient has got voluntary control, ask for any scalding (burning sensation in urethra while passing urine), difficulty in initiation, frequency, precipitancy (unable to control the urge of micturition), etc.

Regarding the bowels—feeling of passage of stools, control of the sphincters, and nature of stool should be asked for.

In females urogenital assessment should be done, while in males the power of penile erection or allied complaints should be asked.

CLINICAL LOCALISATION OF THE LESION IN THE SPINAL CORD (TABLE 8.8)

Careful assessment should be done at the outset, for any other associated injury (e.g. head, chest, lung, abdomen, or extremities); extent and depth of paralysis; and for any visceral paralysis (bladder and/or bowel).

The gross idea about the involvement of the motor segment can be obtained with the help of the following anatomicophysiological facts:

- C5   controls flexion of elbow
- C6   controls extension of wrist
- C7   controls extension of elbow
- C8   controls flexion of distal interphalangeal joints of fingers (test the middle finger)
- T1   controls abduction of fingers

TABLE 8.8: Localisation of vertebrae and their relation with spinal cord segments.

Surface landmarks of certain vertebrae		Relation of spine with cord level	
Spine	Landmark	Vertebral spine	Spinal cord segment
C1	(Transverse process)—below and anterior to the mastoid process	C1–C7	Add 1
C3	At the level of the hyoid bone	T1–T6	Add 2
C4	Opposite the upper border of Thyroid cartilage	T7–T9	Add 3
C6	Opposite the cricoid cartilage	T10	L1, L2
C7	Vertebra prominence	T11	L3, L4
T2	At the level of sternal notch	T12	L5, S1
T2-3	Lies at the level of base of spinous process of scapula		
T4	Against the angle of Louis	L1	Other (if S1 is at T12) or all sacrals and coccygeal segments
T7	Inferior angle of scapula	Below L1	Cauda equina
L4	Highest point of iliac crest		
S1-2	Posterior superior iliac spine		

L2   controls flexion of hip
L3   controls extension of knee
L4   controls dorsiflexion of ankle
L5   controls extension of big toe
S1   controls plantar flexion of ankle

As the *cord proper ends at the upper border of L2 or lower border of L1 vertebra, the actual vertebral level does not correspond to the same spinal cord level. Any neurological damage below the L1 vertebra* may affect a few roots of lumbar and sacral outflow. If more roots are affected it will be a **cauda equina lesion.** The manifestation in this case will be of lower motor neuron type (i.e. weakness, flaccid paralysis, wasting of muscles, fasciculations, less/loss of tone (hypotonia/atonia), diminished or absent tendon reflexes, plantar reflex—absent or down going, perianal saddle anaesthesia, bladder and sexual dysfunction, absent ankle jerk, often accentuation of knee jerk (due to weakness of hamstrings).

Any lesion above the L1 vertebral segment will affect the cord proper. The paraplegia will be of *upper motor neuron type*, i.e. spastic type of paralysis—increased tone of muscles, spasticity, none or very little wasting of muscles, increased tendon reflexes (may be even clonus), Babinski's sign present, i.e. extensor plantar response, superficial reflexes (like abdominal) absent. *In spinal shock stage or in total damage of cord or in terminal stage, the tone may be flaccid.*

To assess the actual clinical spinal cord level, the following clinical guidelines should be observed:
- The surface mark of the vertebral bodies and their relation to that of spinal cord level are as in **Table 8.8**. Therefore, after localising the vertebral segment, additions must be made accordingly, to assess the cord level. For all practical purposes, the spinous process may be taken as the landmark for the corresponding vertebral body, except in the lower dorsals, where the tip of the spinous process is in level with the body of the vertebra below.
- If there is sensory loss, the highest level of the sensory loss should be taken as the level of cord damage
- Ascertain the hyperaesthetic skin level by passing a key end from below upward. Usually, the irritational zone of the cord affection manifests as the hyperaesthetic zone, i.e. hyperaesthetic zone area will be the lowest level of spared cord above the lesion—this is best demonstrated in viral transverse myelitis
- Rough assessment of cord level can be done by correlating with the jerks reflexes. If a particular reflex/jerk is absent, it suggests the damage of the root subserving that reflex jerk.

■ INVESTIGATIONS FOR SPINAL PATHOLOGY

Besides general investigations, there are certain special investigations which are of value in diagnosing the spinal lesions (*Also see* the "Radiological and Allied Investigations" in the Chapter 1 Introduction of this book).

Radiological Investigations

Plain X-ray must be taken in a minimum of three planes:
1. Anteroposterior view
2. Lateral view
3. Oblique view.

- *In anteroposterior view—look for:*
  - A general impression of the spinal column and of the particular vertebral segment
  - Any pedicular lesion
  - Side to side collapse
  - Lesions of transverse process
  - Paravertebral soft tissue shadows (abscess in caries spine)
  - Any deviation in the longitudinal axis of the vertebral column (e.g. scoliosis).

- *In lateral view—look for:*
  - Shape and size of the vertebral body and its relation with vertebrae above and below
  - Integrity of anterior and posterior walls
  - Wedging or compression of the body
  - Texture of the body of the vertebra
  - Any localised rarefaction or condensation of the body
  - Superior and inferior surfaces of body
  - Spinous processes (for its texture and distance from adjacent spinous processes)
  - Intervertebral space—reduction or increase in the space or any other abnormality in that region.
  - In the spinal canal—trace the posterior wall of the body of vertebra from above downwards as well as the laminar continuity at the posterior end of the spinal canal. These two lines maintain regular continuity, and in between them is the space occupied by the spinal cord and soft tissues around it. Note the dimension of the canal from above downwards and the area affected. Take note of any radiopaque space occupying shadow in the spinal canal.

OPLL is a part of family of disorders where there is calcification in ligaments. OPLL was reported by key causing spinal cord compression in 1838. It is considered to be more common in Asian countries, especially in Japanese population.

Look for any ossification of posterior longitudinal ligament (OPLL), which if present may compress the spinal cord and/or nerve roots leading to sensory and motor dysfunction, especially in cervical region and this cervical myelopathy may require surgical decompression. Japanese classified OPLL (now followed all over) on lateral plane radiography into *four types-continuous, segmental, mixed or circumscribed.*

In cervical region: Lateral view should be taken after fully flexing and fully extending the neck from the neutral position. This not only demonstrates the mobility of the spine, but also helps in delineating degenerative

changes in the diarthrodial joints, joint of Luschka, and the intervertebral foramen to a great extent.
- **Oblique views:** These views are essential to delineate the intervertebral foramina and the facet joints, specially in the cervical region. In the lumbar and lumbosacral region, this view has special importance to delineate the *integrity of pars interarticularis.* In this view, this area normally casts a shadow which mimics a *Scottish terrier's neck.* Any defect in pars interarticularis is indicated by a translucent area across the terrier's neck, as if the *terrier has been decapitated. This sign is positive in spondylolysis and spondylolisthesis.*
- For occipitoatlantoaxial region open mouth view X-ray is more informative and essential *(see* **Fig. 8.53**).

Tomography

Tomographic study (measured depth penetration X-ray) is essential to localise certain less obvious lesions in vertebra, e.g. osteoid osteoma, haemangioma.

Screening

Diagnosis and manipulation directly under screening used to be a popular method in managing fractures. But now, its value is more or less restricted to assessments in stress radiography and to observe the flow of contrast medium in myelographic or allied studies.

Cine-Radiography

To know the excursion of the spinal column and flow of contrast medium in the subarachnoid space, cineradiography is of value.

Scanogram

In the lesions which affect more or less the entire spinal column, or lesions where the relations of the different spinal zones is essential to be assessed, e.g. in scoliosis, it is useful to have a single exposure accommodating the whole of the spinal column. At least lower cervical to lumbosacral regions should be included in the exposure to know the extent of primary and/or secondary curves. This is further important to measure numerically the exact angulation of the scoliotic curves.

Methods of measuring the scoliotic curves: There are several *methods of measuring the scoliotic curves,* but the following two appear to be of practical use.
- *Cobb's method* **(Fig. 8.76)**: Locate the upper most vertebral level where the curvature ends *(superior end vertebra).* This can be delineated by the shape of disc space just above (widening on the concave side), tilt of vertebral bodies (maximum tilt towards the concavity) and the size of pedicular shadows. The pedicular shadows should be symmetrical and horizontally placed. Draw a line in continuity with the superior surface of this vertebra. Drop a perpendicular over this line outside the spinal column.

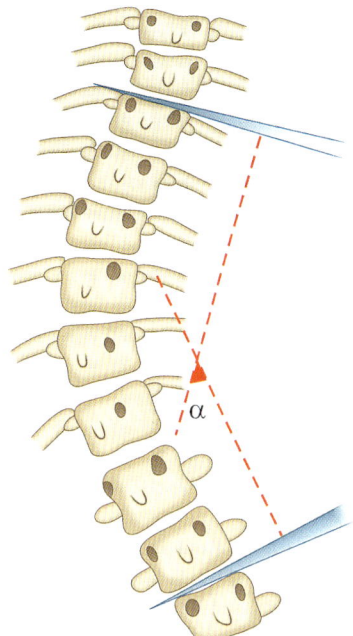

Fig. 8.76: Cobb's method of measuring the angle of scoliosis (α = angle of scoliosis).

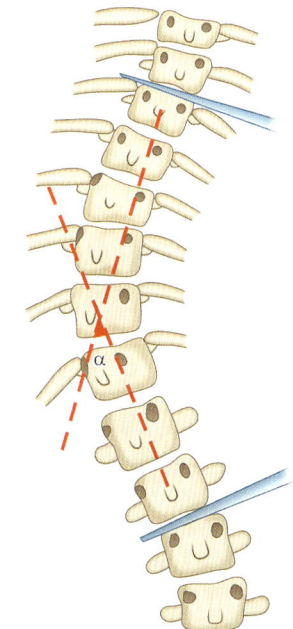

Fig. 8.77: Ferguson's method of measurement of angle of scoliosis (α = angle of scoliosis).

Elongate this perpendicular line downwards. Similarly, locate the lowest vertebra where the curve ends *(inferior end vertebra).* At the inferior surface of this vertebra, the horizontal line is prolonged to the side in which upper line was projected. Drop the perpendicular on this line outside the spinal column on the same side as above and elongate it upwards. The two perpendicular lines will cut at a point. The angle formed between these lines is Cobb's angle
- *Ferguson's method* **(Fig. 8.77):** First locate the curve end vertebrae as above. Also locate the vertebra at the apex of

the curve. Mark the centres of these vertebrae. Connect the centre of the apex vertebra to that of the centres of the superior and inferior end vertebrae and prolong them to intersect. The superior or inferior angle at the point of intersection of these lines will denote the angle of the curve
- *Computer-aided assessment of scoliosis:* Patient's spinal column is examined in three dimensions and in colour on a computer screen. To obtain these images, two X-rays of the patient (one from the back and other from the side) are placed on luminous digitising table and certain points characteristic of each vertebra are noted. Within seconds the computer shows a 3-D view of the spinal column and pelvis. Numerical and graphical data are also available. By an expert system, all possible corrective measures can be simulated, enabling the surgeon to choose the most suitable option.

Prevalence of curves measuring 10° or more is 1.9% and curves measuring 20° or more is 0.5%.

Contrast Radiography

To locate any space occupying lesion in the spinal canal, contrast radiographic studies should be done. Four methods are followed:
- Myelographic studies or contrast-dye-radiography
- Air contrast radiography
- Epidurography
- Epidural venography—to demonstrate impingement upon the epidural plexus.

Myelographic Study

Myelographic delineation is done either through lumbar route (ascending) or through cisternal puncture (descending) after injecting 5 cc of radiopaque dye into the subarachnoid space. Under fluoroscopy, the movement of the dye column is observed by tilting the X-ray table either way. Any hold up or partial/complete block is noted.

Radioactive Scanning

Radioactive phosphorus or tetracycline, or calcium or strontium are usually used for localising certain osseous growths or other space occupying lesions in the spinal canal.

Discography

Contrast studies of the disc spaces may be helpful in assessing for any prolapse of the disc material. However, the injection into the centre of the biconvex disc space should be done under image intensifier. This is not a popular method of investigation because the method is difficult and the result is not much helpful.

Needle Biopsy

The vertebral body, being deeply situated is not easily accessible for histopathological studies by open biopsy. Therefore, needle biopsy, here has more importance for:
- Biochemical studies for osteoporosis
- Cytological studies for assessing the nature of the suspected growth.

A comparatively wide bore aspiration needle is pushed from the posterolateral aspect into the suspected vertebral body, under image intensifier.

Modern Imaging Techniques

Modern imaging techniques are revolutionising the process of investigating the spinal problems. These include:
- CTS (Computerised tomography scanning)
- CTS and intrathecal low osmolality contrast media for assessment of pathology, such as tumour and dysraphic condition
- MRI (Magnetic resonance imaging) or NMR (Nuclear magnetic resonance) imaging—this technique has a great future. It is extremely sensitive and affords early detection of avascular necrosis, infection, intraspinal disorders (like disc prolapse, and can also distinguish the disc components), cord compression due to trauma and tumour. It delineates various bony and soft tissue growths without the use of contrast media, differentiation of muscular dysfunction (atrophy, paresis, and myopathy)
- Spinal cord monitoring technique to record somatosensory-evoked potentials SEP's—mainly being used during surgery on spine and spinal cord to simultaneously observe any dysfunction of spinal cord, especially while performing corrective surgery for spinal deformity.

KEY DIAGNOSTIC POINTS OF COMMON SPINAL PATHOLOGY

Cervical Spondylosis
- Middle age, males dominate
- Cervical spondylosis (cervical degenerative arthrosis; cervical osteoarthritis) results of degenerative changes in cervical discs. Osteophytes may encroach into the intervertebral neural foramina or may protrude into the spinal canal—in both sites nerve root may get irritated or even pressed
- Usual complaints—pain, tingling, numbness and even pin-prick sensations manifest along the irritated roots, more in the night. Symptoms usually start in neck or scapular region and frequently extend to shoulder, arm, forearm, wrist, and even to fingers. In upper cervical root affection, pain may extend to occiput region
- In acute root irritation, the patient usually presents with keeping his hand over the head on the affected side. Any attempt to bring the hand downwards, aggravates the symptoms *(Hand on head sign—HOH sign)*. Any attempt to cough with the head held in extension may reproduce

the pain and even other symptoms. Any attempt to rotate the extended neck initiates the pain (*Spurling's sign*). In upper root affections, the features of vertebral artery syndrome, like tinnitus, giddiness, occipital headache and transitory fainting attack may occur
- Rest in lying down position (by avoiding the weight of head) usually relieves pain to a variable extent
- Strained walking, overactivity, jerky drive, moist humid weather aggravates the symptoms
- Neck muscles are rigid on the affected side
- Movements of cervical spine variably restricted, usually at the extremes
- Cervical compression test usually positive
- Paraesthesia in periscapular region, deltoid region and in lower cervical root affections, even in the fingers
- Local tenderness in the cervical region in acute and sub-acute manifestation
- Rarely motor power weakness in the fingers and thumb and other muscles according to affection
- The biceps tendon reflex is frequently diminished or absent in C5 or C6 radiculopathy. The triceps reflex is diminished or absent in C7 root affection
- X-ray—especially the lateral and oblique views are confirmatory
- Congenital malformations may be a confusing factor **(Figs. 8.78A and B)**.
- Supraspinatus rupture, peripheral neuropathy, brachial plexus irritation should be excluded.

Klippel-Feil Syndrome (1912)

(Congenital Webbed Neck; Congenital Short Neck, Brevi Collis) **(Figs. 8.79A to D)**.
- Short or absent neck due to congenital malformation (fusion of several vertebrae) of C2 to C7 in multiple or single level of cervical vertebrae
- Hair margin quite lowered, sometimes even on shoulder level
- Marked limitation in mobility (specially lateral bending and rotation) of cervical spine
- May be associated with congenitally high-placed scapula (Sprengel's shoulder), and/or cervical spina bifida
- May be associated with mongoloid type of face
- Symptoms manifest in young adults
- Deafness may be associated in about 30% of cases
- Scoliosis (alone or with kyphosis) is commonly associated spinal deformity in about 50% of cases
- Although motion preservation is desirable in Klippel-Feil patients, mostly with stiff and fused neck, the kinematics and biomechanics of their cervical spine may hinder cervical arthroplasty. Each case should be viewed on its merit and fusion or hybrid constructs may represent more reasonable option.

Spina Bifida

Spina bifida results from failure in the fusion of the neural arch and thus neural tube defects develop.

Deficiency in the level of active folic acid (i.e. Methyl folate), and hyperhomocysteinemia (pregnant women are

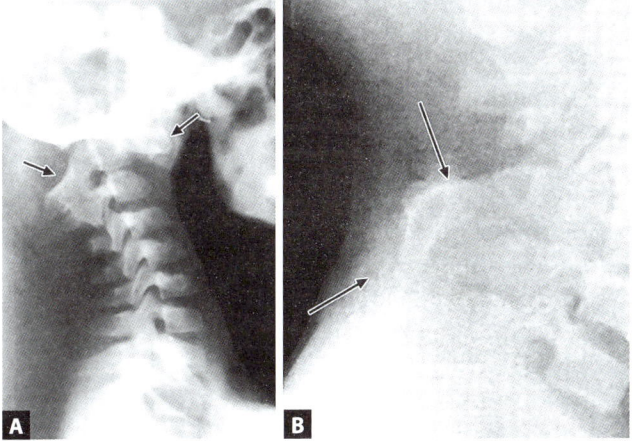

Figs. 8.78A and B: Congenital fusion of the spinal processes in cervical vertebrae.

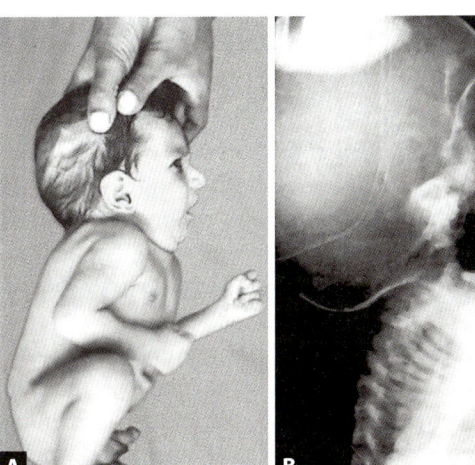 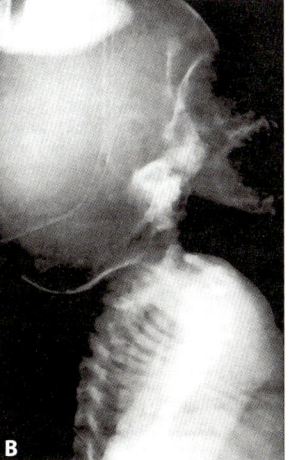 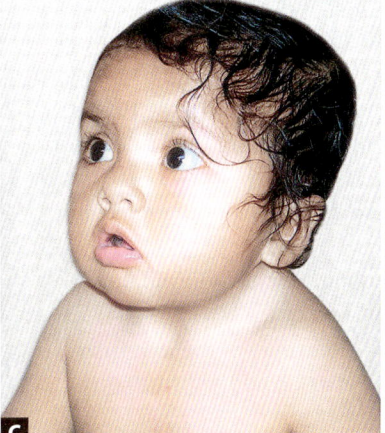 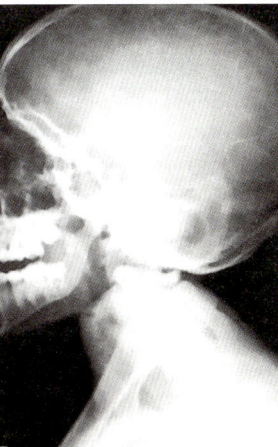

Figs. 8.79A to D: Klippel-Feil syndrome.

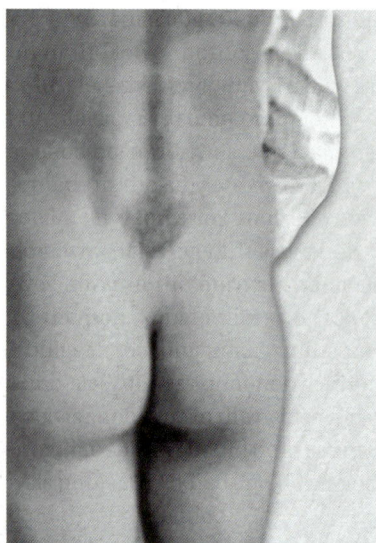

Fig. 8.80: Spina bifida occulta to be suspected by seeing the tuft of hair.

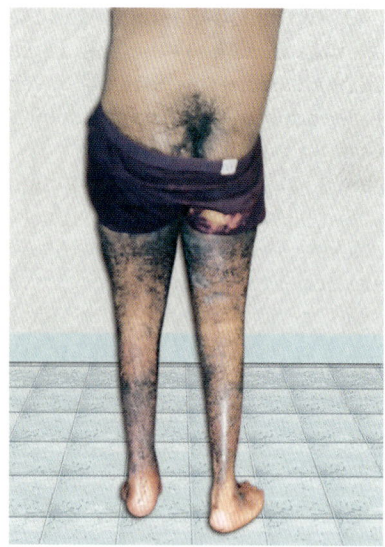

Fig. 8.81: Spina bifida occulta represented on the surface by the tuft of hair. Note the trophic ulcer (though superficial on the right buttock due to sensory impairment).

more likely to suffer due to deficiency of vitamin B9, B12 and B6) are likely to increase the risk of neural tube defects.

The incidence of *spina bifida* is about 2.5 per 10,000 live births, and there are unexplained geographical variations. *Antenatal screening is possible by using alpha fetoprotein measurements.* Spina bifida may be associated with more or less all types of foot deformities. Hence in case of congenital foot deformity, the small of the back must be examined for the signs of spina bifida (manifesta or occulta).

Any environmental or other effect may interfere with the fusion of neural tube and encasing mesenchyme, which starts from the cephalic end on the 25th intrauterine day and ends at the caudal end on the 29th intrauterine day—resulting in spina bifida.

Varieties: (a) Posterior (due to defect in the posterior bony arch: (i) occulta (ii) manifesta; (b) Anterior (due to defect in the development of bodies)—very very rare.

- **Spina Bifida Occulta (Figs. 8.80 and 8.81)**
  - Usually in lumbosacral region, it is the mildest form of spinal dysraphism.
  - Manifested by the presence of—naevus, or tuft of hair or fibro fatty mass or dimpling of skin, and the overlying skin is healthy
  - Usually symptomless, and discovered accidentally in X-ray
  - The local swelling may contain spinal fluid and then it will be fluctuant and translucent
  - May be associated with—deformity of the foot (usually bilateral equinocavovarus), bladder disturbance, sensory deficits in foot
  - Dissociated growth between cord and canal and tugging of the filum terminale with the surrounding and subcutaneous tissue lead to decreased ascent of the spinal cord; which may manifest as cord-traction or filum terminale or **Arnold-Chiari syndrome**. Clinically, symptoms like peculiar gait, features of increased intracranial pressure, spastic paralysis and cervical root pain start manifesting between 4 and 6 years of age
  - Sometimes a sinus may lead from spina bifida occulta to the skin of sacral region—a congenital sacrococcygeal sinus, which may be mistaken as pilonidal sinus.

- **Spina Bifida Manifesta (Cystica) (Figs. 8.82 to 8.85)**
  - Midline tense, cystic saccular protrusion in lumbar, dorsal, occipitocervical region, present since birth
  - Depending on level and type of lesion—variable neurological manifestations may occur
  - May be impulse on coughing
  - Transillumination may be obtained delineating the darker shadow of the cord and nerves from the bright fluid portion.

Types
- Meningocele **(Figs. 8.82 to 8.85)**—protrusion of meninges only. Here the meninges form a sac protruding through the defective neural arch mostly posteriorly. Due to breakdown of meninges secondary infection of CNS may occur; surgical repair should be done
- Myelomeningocele (most common of the three)—protrusion of a plaque of neural tissue, i.e. portion of spinal cord or cauda equina surrounded by meninges. It is more severe form of spinal dysraphisms. It includes meningocele, lipomeningocele and caudal regression syndrome. In most cases bowel, bladder, motor, and

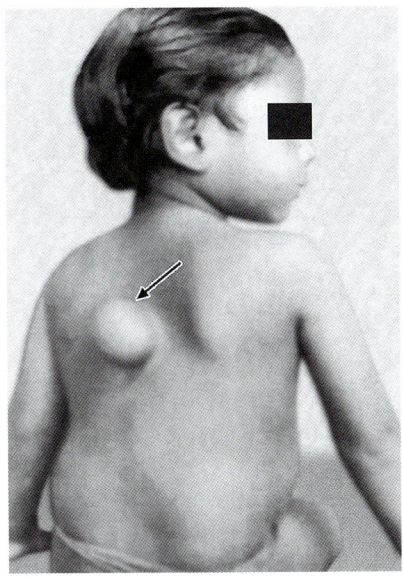 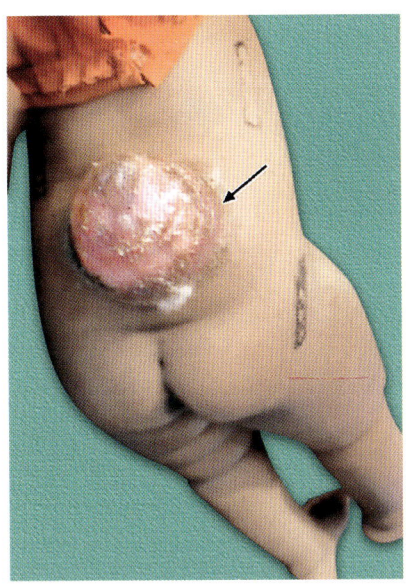 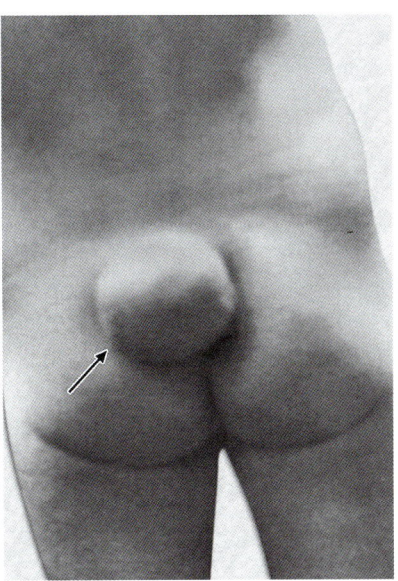

Fig. 8.82: Spina bifida manifesta (cystica).   **Fig. 8.83:** Spina bifida manifesta (cystica) covered by the thin membrane.   **Fig. 8.84:** Spina bifida manifesta (cystica).

sensory paralysis occur distal to the malformation. This developmental anomalies occur during the phase of closure of neural tube (26–28 days of gestation) or rupture of the closed neural tube. (quoted by Naik et al 2016). Early sac closure and management of hydrocephalus should be done by neurosurgeon, however, neurological involvement and its legacies variably persist throughout their life.

- Syringomyelocele—central spinal canal is dilated and the spinal cord is expanded to form the lining of sac
- Myelocele—gross spinal cord deformity, an elongated fissure surrounded by hair or telangiectasis which is in direct contact with the central canal
- Rachocele—roots spread in the walls of protrusion.

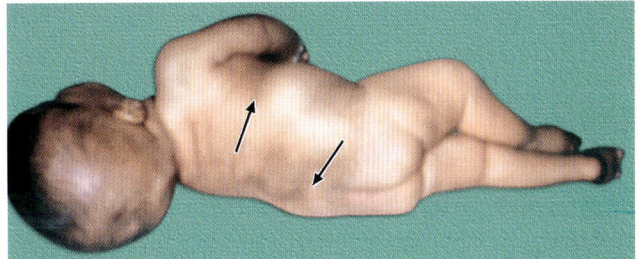

Fig. 8.85: Spina bifida with weak abdominal muscle. Note the reddish skin patches on the back and bulging of abdominal wall while the child weeps.

Caries Spine (Pott's Disease—Percival Pott 1779/Tuberculosis Spine) (*See* Figs. 8.8 to 8.10, 8.29 to 8.42, 8.91 and 8.92, Tables 8.3 and 8.9)

- Spinal tuberculosis is the most common form of skeletal tuberculosis and accounts for about 50% of all cases of tuberculosis of bones and joints, and is deep-seated paucibacillary disease.
- Today about 1/3rd of world population is affected with tuberculosis
- With increasing incidence of HIV, about 5 million new cases of tuberculosis annually in Asia
- Pain in the back or referred pain which aggravates with activities and spinal stress test
- Common sites: Lower dorsal, mid dorsal, lumbar, cervical, upper dorsal, lumbosacral
- Persistent local tenderness in the affected spine
- Spasm of muscles in early case, muscular wasting later on
- Limitation of spinal movements, especially flexion
- Presence of kyphosis, usually angular kyphosis
- Presence of cold abscess, usually distant from the primary focus
- May be associated with complications, like paraplegia (**Table 8.9**)
- Raised ESR
- Primary focus (e.g. in lungs, lymph node). In spite of advanced technology such as gas liquid chromatography and polymerase chain reaction, smear microscopy (for AFB) remains the most reliable diagnostic test (of pulmonary tuberculosis)
- Tuberculous infection of occipito-atlanto-axial region can be delineated in open mouth view X-ray of that region (*see* **Fig. 8.53**)
- In chronic, late deformed dorsal caries cases—features of cor pulmonale, due to reduced thoracic capacity
- X-ray—reduced intervertebral disc space, rarefaction/destruction (**Figs. 8.91B and 8.92**) collapse of vertebrae, paravertebral abscess shadow
- CT scan is more useful. It denotes paravertebral soft tissue swelling and abscesses more readily and can monitor changes in the size of spinal canal. Post myelogram CT

TABLE 8.9: Pott's paraplegia (caries spine) (Percival Pott 1779)—Compression paraplegia of upper motor neuron type; very rarely cauda equina lesion.

	Paraplegia of early onset	*Paraplegia of late onset*	*Paraplegia of sudden onset*
1	*2*	*3*	*4*
1. Definition	Paraplegia setting in during active stage of disease	Paraplegia setting after the disease has been cured/or remained quiescent for a pretty long time	It can come any time suddenly with or without earlier diagnosed caries spine
2. Time factor (no hard and fast rule)	Usually within 2 years of the onset of the disease	Usually after 7-10 years of the earlier diagnosed disease	-do-
3. Age	Children/adults	Adults	Any age (usually adults)
4. Common site of spinal lesion	Lower dorsal, mid-dorsal, upper dorsal, lower cervical	Mid-dorsal, lower dorsal	Dorsal lesion

5. Affections	• Motor:
	  – Staggering gait, spasticity with spastic gait
	  – Gradually increasing muscular weakness
	  – Paraplegia in extension
	  – Paraplegia in flexion
	  – Flexor spasm
	  – Mass reflexes
	• Sensory affection
	• Visceral affection
	• Contractures
	• Decubitus ulcers, chest infections
	• Urinary complication
	• Cachexia
	• Death
		• Motor and/or sensory (partly sensory)
		• Staggering gait, very slowly increasing muscular weakness
			Sudden presentation—total paralysis or variable paresis

6. Cause	Pressure over spinal cord • Tuberculous pus (paravertebral abscess® intervertebral foramen®spinal canal) • Caseous material • Tubercular sequestra • Sequestrated intervertebral disc • Pathological subluxation • Dislocation of body backward	• Recrudescence of the disease • Due to constant rubbing of spinal cord against internal gibbus	Usually vascular, i.e. tuberculous embolism or thrombotic phenomenon of segmental spinal artery
7. Depth of paraplegia	Incomplete/complete	Always incomplete	Usually complete, may be incomplete
8. Pathology in the cord	Cord is spared till very late stage	Gliosis where cord rubs against internal gibbus	Immediate no change. May suffer necrosis if collaterals do not develop quite early
9. Prognosis	Variable—usually good if treated promptly	Never good—some legacy always remains	Usually recovers
10. Treatment	Chemotherapy Conservative: rest preferably on plaster bed/ spinal frame; traction Operative— • costotransversectomy • anterolateral decompression • anterior excision with or without bone graft	Conservative Rarely operation indicated. Chemotherapy only in recurred cases	Chemotherapy Conservative

delineates compression of neural elements by abscess or bone impingement more clearly.

High quality MRI is a rapid method to identify accurately the spinal infection, albeit it does not differentiate pyogenic and nonpyogenic infection. It is of special help for posterior spinal disease, tuberculosis of craniovertebral, cervicodorsal region, sacroiliac joints, sacrum.

- Possible sites of cold abscess in caries spine (**Table 8.3**, Page 228)
- Tuli et al (2002) suggested:
  Clinical criteria to suspect **drug resistant cases of spinal tuberculosis** which include patients of spinal tuberculosis on ATT for 5 months or more showing:
  Poor clinical and radiological response OR
  Appearance of a fresh lesion of osteoarticular tuberculosis OR Deterioration of spinal deformity OR Appearance of discharging sinus OR Wound dehiscence of previously operated scar
- Discitis and vertebral osteomyelitis originate in well-perfused end plate and extend into the disc and vertebral body.
  Pyogenic osteomyelitis (mostly caused by *Staphylococcus aureus*) is more common in adult males (45–65 years). Drug abusers may have pseudomonas aeruginosa infections. Infectious spondylitis is most common in children (1–5 years)
  Pyogenic vertebral infections may occur in generalised sepsis or as a blood borne infection beginning in the capillary loop or postcapillary venous channels in the end plate.
  Bacterial infections quickly attack the intervertebral disc. In tuberculous and nonbacterial infections, the intervertebral disc is usually preserved.
  Bacterial spinal infections may also produce paralysis, which may be early (due to epidural extension of an abscess) or of late onset (caused by development of kyphosis, vertebral collapse with retropulsion of bone, and debris, or late abscess formation).

Ankylosing Spondylitis

Ankylosing spondylitis, the most common of seronegative spondylo arthropathy conditions (Marie Strumpell's or von Bachterew's disease) is a chronic systemic inflammatory disease affecting the axial skeleton (spine), the sacroiliac joints, and pelvis and frequently peripheral joints as well. Eyes (iritis, uveitis), heart and lung may be affected. The name has been derived from the Greek roots ankylos (meaning bent—cf. ankylosis means joint fusion) + spondylos (meaning spinal vertebra). If ankylosing spondylitis occurs in association with reactive arthritis, psoriasis, ulcerative colitis or Crohn's disease, it is called *"secondary ankylosing spondylitis".*

- Ankylosing spondylitis has a prevalence of 0.1 to 1.4% correlating with the frequency of HLAB27
- Age and sex predilection—males in the age group of 18–30 years are mostly affected
- Initial inflammatory process involves the enthesis (site of insertion of ligaments, tendon, and capsule into bone) followed by fibrosis/new bone formation
- Pain and stiffness, in the dorsolumbar and both sacroiliac regions, which are variably relieved by spinal stress test (cf. tuberculosis, intervertebral disc prolapse and septic arthritis where pain is increased)
- Pain and stiffness more in the morning after getting up from the bed or after getting up from prolonged rest
- Patients get comparative relief after daily routine activities, walking around or after certain exercise
- Progressive limitation of chest expansion (at 4th intercostal space if less than 2.5 cm, it is highly suggestive)
- Rest aggravates, and activity relieves the pain and stiffness
- Affection of overall range of motion and quality of life.
- Fatigue is being reported to be one of the major complaints of ankylosing spondylitis patients
- Sometimes bizarre manifestations occur, e.g. pain occurs locally or is generalised all over the body and may be over calf muscles, both heels, shoulder regions, back, and cervical spine
- Earlier, boarding of back, specially in lower region; later on pokerback in advanced cases (*see* **Figs. 8.19A and B**)
- Progressive limitation of cervical and lumbar extension movements—leading gradually to forward stooping attitude in ankylosing spondylitis. The assessment of loss of cervical range of movement should be done by occiput-to-wall test (*see* Page 233) and that of lumbar spine by Schober test (*see* Page 234). In advanced cases, Chin-on-chest deformity (*see* **Fig. 8.19C**) develops which is highly characteristic deformity of ankylosing spondylitis. The main cause is complete C1-C2 dislocation. This deformity may be post-traumatic as well. Non-traumatic progressive rigid deformity can be identified by tomography. Treatment consists of skeletal traction (halo, tongs) followed by posterior spinal fusion if and as needed
- Restricted spinal movements, especially flexion
- Formation of syndesmophytes across the disc spaces affects the mobility of the entire spine resulting in a "*bamboo spine*" (**Fig. 8.86**)
- Later on, hip, and still later, shoulder, knee, cervical region, rather all bigger joints to smaller joints, (even temporomandibular joint), become stiff (**Figs. 8.89A to C**)
- The immobility leads to secondary osteoporosis which makes the vertebral column fragile. The thoracolumbar region becomes more susceptible to fracture.
- In ankylosis spondylitis, spinal instability may develop due to spondylodiscitis (following inflammation or mechanical stress) or fractures. Spinal instability in ankylosing spondylitis is likely to develop neurological

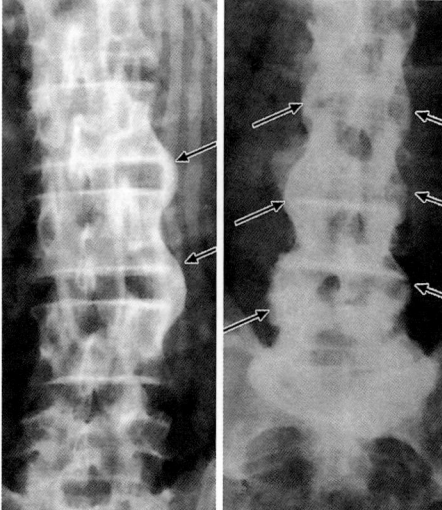 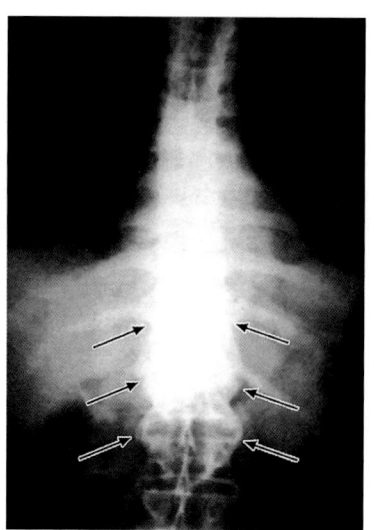 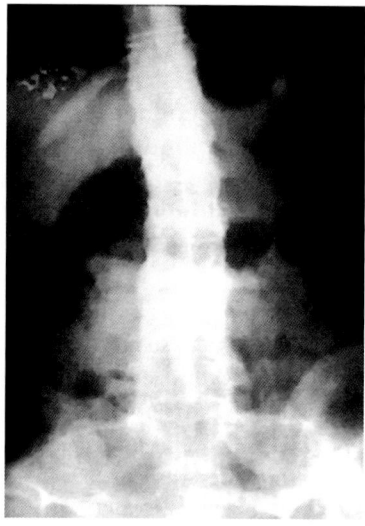

Fig. 8.86: Ankylosing spondylitis—to note the bambooing of the 1,2,3 and 4 lumbars.

Fig. 8.87: Ankylosing spondylitis—bambooing getting more marked in L_2-L_1 upwards.

Fig. 8.88: Ankylosing spondylitis—all ligaments and intervertebral spaces calcified in advanced stage of ankylosing spondylitis.

deficit, and in such cases surgery is indicated like long segment instrumentation and fusion
- May be extraskeletal manifestations
- Extraskeletal manifestations of ankylosing spondylitis may be of several organs/regions, e.g. (to remember according to):
  A = Aortic insufficiency, ascending aortitis
  N = Neurological, e.g. cauda equina syndrome, atalanto-axial subluxation with or without pressure symptoms
  K = Kidney (urinary system) urethritis, chronic prostatitis, secondary amyloidosis
  L = Large bowel—ulcerative colitis
  S = Spine—spinal stenosis, spinal osteoporosis
  P = Pulmonary—fibrotic changes in lung
  O = Ocular—uveitis, iritis
  N = Nephropathy (IgA)
  D = Discitis
- Predilection for positive HLA-B 27 individuals and their family members, especially in non-white individuals. Though strong association (92%) of HLA B27 antigen is shown in white European patients of ankylosing spondylitis, the strength of association and prevalence differ among racial groups. On the whole, HLA B27 can define the population at risk, but it is expensive and is of limited practical value for confirming the diagnosis
- X-ray: The radiological changes predominantly affect the axial skeleton (sacroiliac, apophyseal, discovertebral, costovertebral) and the sites of enthesopathy. Sacroiliitis is usually bilateral. Earliest X-ray change is erosion of iliac side of sacroiliac joint. Progressive erosion presents a picture of pseudowidening of sacroiliac joint with bony sclerosis followed by bony ankylosis.

The X-ray of ankylosing spondylitis may be confused with—osteitis condensans ilii—an asymptomatic disorder of multiparous women in which there is a triangular area of dense sclerotic bone on the iliac side and adjacent to the lower half of sacroiliac joints. *Sacroiliac joints fusion*; in AP view (mainly in the lower dorsal and lumbar region) *bamboo spine*. Prior to bamboo spine, the radiological features are initial shiny, corners —*"shiny corners"* (Romanus lesion) involvement of insertion of annulus fibrosus to the corner of vertebral bodies—*squared anterior vertebral bodies* with sclerotic anterior corners, *syndesmophytes* (ossification of the annulus fibrosus), discovertebral erosions, fusion of the apophyseal joints alongwith calcification of the spinal ligaments and *bilateral syndesmophytes* can lead to complete fusion of the vertebral column giving the appearance of the *"bamboo spine"* (**Figs. 8.86 to 8.88**). In cervical spine after fusion, it gives an appearance of *'cane-stick'* in lateral view.

Management mainly centres to regular physiotherapy; NSAID (indomethacin) sulfasalazine; surgery for fixed unacceptable joints/vertebral columns (with risks—mainly neurological damage). In advance stage of ankylosing spondylitis, patients usually present with complex primary hips for total hip arthroplasty. The commonest difficulties faced are difficulty in dislocating the hips and recreating medullary canals. Anaesthetists usually face challenge in intubating such patients. However, excisional arthroplasty of hip may provide workable hip, especially if it is unilateral problem.

Intervertebral Disc Prolapse (Fig. 8.93)

A bulging disc should be differentiated from true disc herniation/prolapse. As discs degenerate with the natural aging process, they loose water content and disc height.

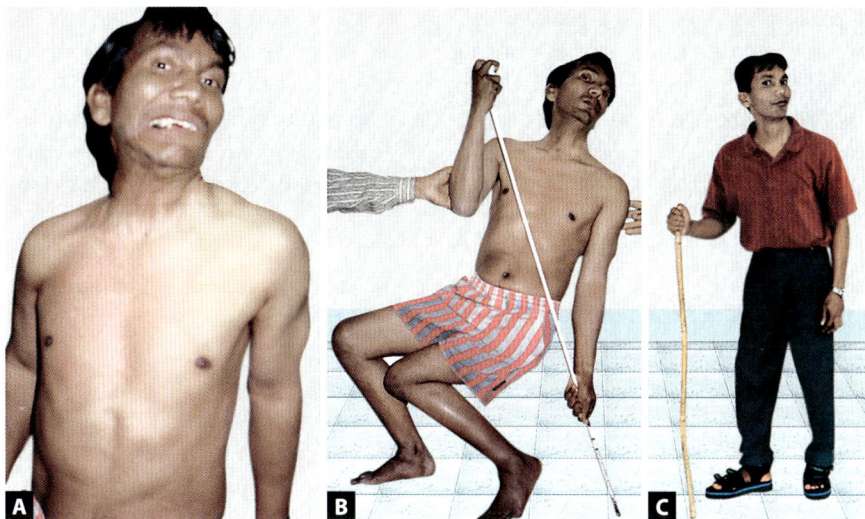

Figs. 8.89A to C: Advanced ankylosing spondylitis with fixed spine, hips, knees and temporomandibular joints—confined to bed for about 14 years. (A and B) Has also cardiac affection (not severe). After multiple operations on hips and knee now he is standing for hours, walking and running a shop of gross domestic products(C).

In this process, lateral wall of disc bulge outwards in symmetrical fashion. In a *true herniation/prolapse*, there is an *asymmetrical protrusion of disc material* outward from the normal circumference of the disc.

According to the manner in which the disc herniates, the herniated disc is commonly classified as:

- *Contained* (the nuclear material is prevented from escaping due to intact annulus or the posterior longitudinal ligament)
- *Extruded* (nucleus material escapes through deficit in annulus or posterior longitudinal ligament, but remains in contact with the nucleus pulposus)
- *Sequestrated* (nucleus material escapes and becomes separated from the remainder of the nucleus pulposus and may migrate upward or downward within the canal.

Alternatively herniated discs have been classified according to their location, which can be templated over the cross-sectional view of a disc and can be delineated in MRI as:

Central disc—	6 O'clock position
Posterolateral disc—	5.30 or 6.30 position
Intraforaminal disc—	5 to 7 O'clock position
Extraforaminal disc—	3.30 to 4.30 position
Far lateral disc—	7.30 to 8.30 position

- There is usually a history of low back pain, which may have had moderate to severe intensity, with radiation to the lower limb (usually in sciatic distribution). The onset is usually acute/subacute, following some exertive work or lifting of heavy weights. Usually symptoms are intermittent
- The symptoms increase on exertion, coughing, sneezing, changing of posture, (from standing to sitting to lying down or *vice-versa*) and on spinal stress test
- Rest relieves and activity aggravates the symptoms (cf ankylosing spondylitis)
- Neural complications may be presenting feature: variable sensory disturbances; motor weakness (extensor hallucis longus, dorsiflexors of ankle, tendo-Achilles), and even cauda equina syndrome
- Lower back muscles are usually in spasm, thus restricting the movements (mainly flexion)
- Sciatic scoliosis (antalgic or functional scoliosis) is usually present (this scoliosis gradually disappears when the patient gradually bends forward). The protruded disc usually presses the root from the lateral sides. Hence, in order to keep the root away from the disc, the spine bends to the opposite side. However, the less common pressure on the root from the medial side by disc protrusion, may produce a list on the same side. It is also to be noted that the paracaudal disc prolapse causes list to the same side, whereas the pararadicular prolapse causes tilt to opposite side.
- Grossly in lumbar disc prolapse—the following clinical criteria should be emphasised:
  - low back pain with radiation to lower limb
  - radicular pain in specific dermatome
  - nerve root tension (stretch signs)
  - presence of neurological symptoms and signs.
  - The reference of in a particular dermatome should be noted.
- Deep thrust tenderness is present usually over the L4-5 or L5-S1 region
- Straight leg raising less than normal. Lasegue's test positive
- Femoral nerve stretch test may be positive
- Ask the patient to *walk on the heels (not possible in L5 weakness) and on the toes (not possible in S1 weakness)*

alternately. In case of sciatic root stretch, the patient will complain of pain in the sciatic distribution while walking on the heel. In case of *femoral root stretch, patient may complain of pain in front of and on the medial aspect of the thigh*
- In more common S1 root compression in intervertebral disc prolapse, the ankle jerk is depressed (more easily detected and assessed when patient is in prone or sitting position) or even absent.

The relation of dermatome to the region is more or less as follows:

Dermatome	Region in which complains are done
L3	Pain and/or neurological symptoms in anterior aspect of thigh and knee
L4	Pain and/or neurological symptoms in lower knee or medial aspect of leg and ankle
L5	Pain and/or neurological symptoms in anterolateral aspect of leg and dorsum of foot
S1	Pain and/or neurological symptoms in posterior aspect of leg and/or sole of foot
Non-specific	Pain in the gluteal region or posterior aspect of thigh or in bizarre fashion

- In X-ray—*Vacuum disc sign* (indicates essentially degenerative disc disease. This sign excludes infection of disc level); osteophytes; eburnation of antero-superior edge of vertebral body are seen. Plain X-ray is also helpful in ruling out concurrent diagnosis, e.g. spondylolysis or spondylolisthesis. In few cases, flexion and extension radiographs may be required to rule out instability. In degenerative disc disease, translational motion of 3.5 mm or angular motion of 11 degrees of one vertebra over another in flexion and extension radiographs is indicative of segmental instability
- MRI is the good choice as investigation in disc herniation. Clinical findings correlate well with MRI findings. However, all MRI abnormalities need not have a clinical significance. The centrolateral disc protrusion and extrusions with gross neural foramen compromise is mostly associated with clinical signs and symptoms. Whenever there are multiple level disc lesions with neural foramen compromise, there is likelyhood to have objective neurological deficit.

  Recurrent disc herniations occur in about 3-7% of patients, usually within 6 months of surgical treatment of the primary disc herniation. Its clinical presentation may be identical to that of primary herniation. Its diagnosis is more difficult than the primary one. MRI with intravascular contrast material is usually helpful in localising the recurrent herniations. The principle of surgery for recurrent disc herniations remains almost the same as of the primary one albeit with larger surgical exposure.
- The herniated disc contains varying amounts of nucleus, annulus and hyaline cartilage. On the whole the radiological assessment can indicate the probable change in content rather than the microstructure of degenerating disc (Majeed et al 2016).
- Resistant symptomatic cervical disc compression is usually treated by traditional cervical fusion; however, cervical disc arthroplasty is being considered as a new alternative to fusion, which provides mobility similar to that of natural disk and prevents adjacent segment disease particularly in younger patients.
- Diagnosing lumber instability is difficult in clinical setting. Vertebral instability is commonly assessed on dynamic imaging finding of abnormal vertebral motion. Symptomatic lumbar disc herniation can be managed non-operatively (rest in bed, pelvic traction, analgesics, physiotherapy, belt support) or operatively (open or endoscopically). Endoscopic spine surgery (Endospine) by Destandau's Technique, introduced in 1993, is an established popular method for treatment of lumbar disc herniation. It can be performed through a small skin incision, minimal tissue dissection with excellent visualization. The technique is a safe, effective and minimal access corridor for lumbar discectomy, and it also allows early postoperative mobilization and faster return to work.

Spondylolisthesis (Figs. 8.24 to 8.27)
- Spondylolisthesis, as an entity, was first recognised and described by Belgium obstetrician Herbinaux in 1782, when he noted a bony prominence in front of sacrum, probably the body of L_5 which was lying in front of sacrum in complete type of spondylolisthesis – the 'spdyloptosis'.
- Spondylolisthesis the word coined by Killian in 1854 (GK: spondylos = spine; olisthanein = to slip or slide) is defined as slow anterior displacement (subluxation) of a vertebra at the lower lumber spine (usually L4-5 or L_5-S_1) probably due to interruption in continuity of the pars interarticularis. When the defect exists in pars interarticularis without forward slipping, it is called spondylolysis (spondylos=spine, lysis= to degenerate). Lumbar spondylolysis is virtually a non-union following a stress fracture of pars interarticularis (Wills et al. 1975)
- *Isthmic spondylolisthesis* in children principally occurs at L_5-S_1 (87%); L_4-L_5 (10%); L_3-L_4 (3%): A defect in the pars interarticularis perhaps never occur in a newborn. Spondylolysis is highly prevalent in few Native American populations. Exact etiology of spondylolysis and spondylolisthesis is not known. Probably it is multifactorial such as hereditary, traumatic, biomechanical, growth and morphologic factors. (Parent S, Labelle H 2018).
- Mostly, middle-aged (about 5.5% of males and 2.5% females) or even elderly ladies are the subjects. However, adolescents who play lot of sports, weight lifting, gymnastics or football can also have it.

- Adult Isthmic Spondylolisthesis—Spondylolisthesis is usually an acquired condition. Deformities are most progressive in childhood and are of low-grade in adults when they become almost static. In adults, two types of spondylolistheses occur—isthmic and degenerative. Isthmic type occurs more in males (with sports, gymnastics, active vocations and allied activities) than females (2:1). L5–S1 region is affected about 90% of cases. The slip is less then 50% and occurs usually due to defect in pars interarticularis
- Exact cause is unknown, but genetic and racial factor (like Inuit Eskimos), mechanical stresses (as in cricket players, weight lifters), a familial predisposition have been shown to have more incidence of pars defects.
- Bilateral stress fractures of pars interarticularis can cause spondylolisthesis
- Degenerative spondylolisthesis — as named by Newman—since it is associated with arthritic changes seen on radiographs—is mostly accompanied by spinal stenosis which further aggravates the symptoms. It is often seen in persons of more than 40 years of age. The L4–5 region is mostly affected. The posterior slip of vertebra on another is usually less than 33%.
- Complaints of persistent pain in low back with/or without radiation in lower limbs. Always suspect this condition if there is back pain in extension. No definite relation with rest or activities. In advanced cases, there may be a waddling gait
- Clinically, feeling of a step in the central furrow, in the lower lumbar region, reduction of distance between last rib and highest point of iliac crests (common sites L4–L5, L5–S1, L3–L4) **(Fig. 8.24)**
- Transverse furrows in the loin region **(Fig. 8.24)**
- Comparative limitation of movements of spine in that region, in these subjects
- Palpation through the pelvis may reveal the step because of the slipped vertebral body
- The pain along the sciatic root may be only presenting clinical symptoms, and in that case, the features of prolapse intervertebral disc will also be present
- Classical X-ray pictures—slipping of vertebra in lateral view. According to the percentage of slipping of the vertebrae HW *Myerding graded spondylolisthesis in four grades* in 1932: < 25% slip—Gr I; 26 to 50% slip—Gr II; 51 to 75% slip—Gr III; > 76% slip—Gr IV; Grade V was later added to describe ptosis i.e. *spondyloptosis* which is defined as a 100% translation of one vertebra over the next caudal vertebra. Spondyloptosis is most severe type of translational deformity and it may produce severe neurological deficits.
- Classification of spondylolisthesis: Wiltse Newman classification divides spondylolisthesis into five major types (and several subtypes) based on radiologic findings. (Wiltse LL 1976) Marchette and Bartolozzi classification is

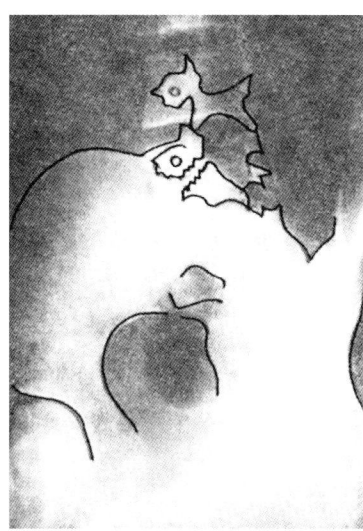

Fig. 8.90: Spondylolysis—to note the decapitated terrier sign.

an etiology-based prognosis system of spondylolisthesis, in which there are two broad categories – developmental and acquired (Marchetti & Bartolozzi 1997). Myerding grading of spondylolisthesis based on classical pictures appears to be easily understandable and non-complicated.

- Diagnosis can be further confirmed on either isotope bone scan or a single photon emission CT scan. The axial and sagittal reformatted CT images clearly delineate the pars defect. In anteroposterior view, the typical inverted Napoleon's cap sign can be visualised, which is almost diagnostic of high grade spondylolisthesis.
- Preliminary treatment is to avoid extension activities and also avoid the action and loading which precipitates the pain, and use of lumbar corset
- Decapitated Scottish terrier (dog) neck in oblique view of X-ray (in isthmic, commonest type) **(Fig. 8.90)**.

Spinal Canal Stenosis

Encroachment into the spinal canal by soft or bony tissue leads to spinal canal stenosis which produces significant effects in cervico-thoraco-lumbar or even lumbar regions Spinal Canal stenosis may be congenital or required. The effects of congenital stenosis may be aggravated by secondary acquired diseases. The stenosis may involve the central spinal canal, the lateral recesses or the neural foramen. Encroachment by soft tissue pathologies (like herniated disc, hypertrophied ligamentum flavum) or bony pathologies (like osteophyte or facetal arthropathy) can lead to symptomatic spinal canal stenosis. Measurement wise, generally, a sagittal diameter of less than 10mm significantly suggests canal stenosis. Sagittal diameter of less than 3mm of lateral recess is significant. Thickening or ossification of posterior longitudinal ligament can cause significant compromise of spinal canal mainly in cervical spinal region leading to compression myelopathy. CT demonstrates in better way the thickening and ossification of posterior

Flowchart 8.1: Spinal tumours.

```
                           Spinal tumours
                          /            \
                   Extradural        Intradural
                   /        \         /         \
            Bony (vertebral) Soft tissue  Extramedullary  Intramedullary
                              (space between  • Meningioma   • Ependymoma
                              meninges and    • Neurofibroma • Gliomas
                              the vertebrae)  • Tuberculoma  • Medullary
                              • Neurofibroma                   blastoma
                              • Meningioma
                              • Hodgkin's deposit
                              • Lymphosarcoma
                              • Leukaemic deposit
                              • Lipoma
                              • Fibroma
                              • Tuberculoma
```

Bony (vertebral):
- Benign
  - Haemangioma
  - Giant cell tumour
  - Chondroma
- Malignant
  - Primary
    - Osteosarcoma
    - Multiple myeloma
    - Ewing's tumour
    - Chordoma (sacral region, cella-tursica of base of skull)
  - Secondary
    - From breast, bronchus thyroid, prostate, stomach

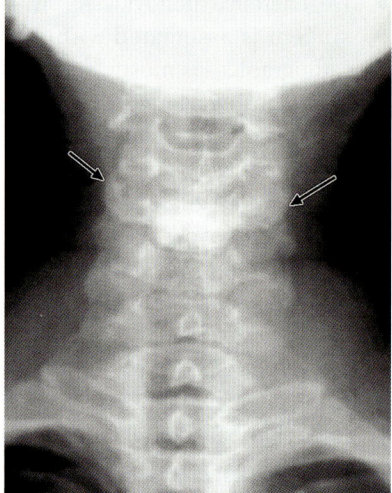

Figs. 8.91A and B: (A) Posture in caries spine of dorsolumbar region; (B) Note: the reduced intervertebral disc space between D12 and L1 and destruction of L1 vertebra—upper part.

Fig. 8.92: Caries spine of 5th cervical vertebra.

longitudinal ligament. However, conditions can be easily diagnosed on MRI.

Spinal Tumours (Flowchart 8.1)

It is very difficult to clinically diagnose authentically the benign tumours of the spine. Of the malignant conditions, secondaries are the most common, which may present with/ or without compression of the cord. Common features of secondaries:

- Elderly persons, without any history of injury, run-down conditions
- Localised or spread over tenderness, angular or no kyphosis—suspect secondaries
- Search for all possible primary sites (prostate, breast, bronchus, thyroid, gastrointestinal tract, kidney, etc.)
  - Multiple myeloma—spine is a common site of affection. Spinal presentation may be minimal or even the patient may present with compression paraplegia.
- Suspect multiple myeloma when:
  - In elderly subjects with disseminated pain in the bones, increasing weakness, anaemia, bony tenderness (specially over the flat bones)
  - Spinal tenderness at affected zone
    - Usually no deformity in spine
    - No pulmonary symptom (no pulmonary metastasis)
    - Bence Jones protein in urine (in 30% of the patients)
    - X-ray—multiple punched-out osteolytic lesions.
- Rare tumours of spine like osteosarcoma. Ewing's sarcoma, osteoclastoma and haemangioma, etc. are more or less diagnosed after histopathological investigations.

Compression Paraplegia of the Spinal Cord

Upper motor neuron (UMN) type of paraplegia resulting from compression of the dorsal segments of the spinal cord due to various causes:
- Congenital malformations (very rare)
  - e.g. Severe scoliosis.

PIVD

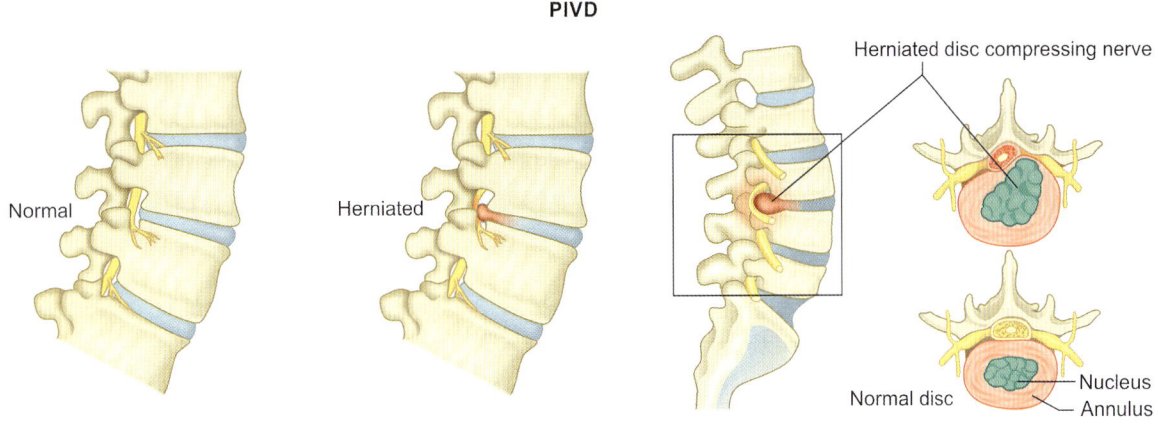

Fig. 8.93: PIVD (Herniated disc compression nerve).

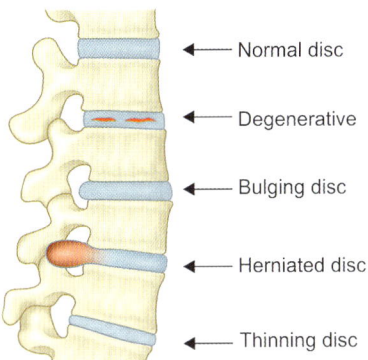

Fig. 8.94: Low back pain.

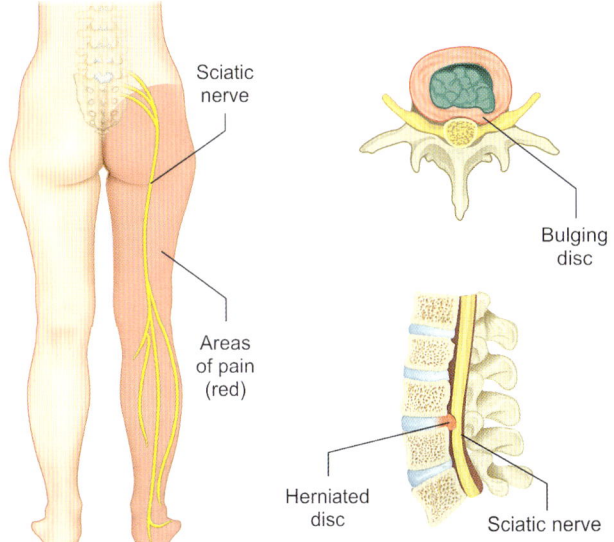

Fig. 8.95: Sciatica.

- Inflammatory (infective)—caries spine, arachnoiditis, meningitis, serosa circumscripta, epidural abscess
- Traumatic
  - Fracture, fracture-subluxation/dislocation; foreign body (bullet injury).
- Vascular
  - Vascular malformations
  - Spinal artery embolism/thrombosis
  - Aortic aneurysm.
- Miscellaneous
  - Paget's disease
  - Cysts in spinal canal, e.g. *Echinococcus granulosus*
  - Spinal cord cyst, which can be extraspinal or intraspinal, e.g. cysticercosis [infection by the larval (cysticercus) stage of the tapeworm *T. solium*].

Compression of cord in cervical region should produce compression quadriplegia/triplegia or even monoplegia of UMN type. Besides the aforesaid causes, following can also produce compression—
- Prolapsed intervertebral disc
- Cervical spondylosis
- Atlanto-axial subluxation in collagen arthropathy (e.g. rheumatoid arthritis, ankylosing spondylitis).

Cauda Equina Syndrome

It occurs due to pressure on the roots (below the level of the spinal cord termination or conus) of the cauda equina (horse's tail) due to various causes (mostly the herniated disc of central type).

Lower motor neuron (LMN) type of paraplegia produced due to compression on the cauda equina (distal to L1 vertebra) with following features:

Complains of backache, sciatica (unilateral or bilateral), sensory disturbances in feet and leg, foot drop.

Signs
- Motor—Varying (seldom complete) LMN type of weakness (usually below the knee)
- Sensory—Usually perianal saddle-shaped hyperaesthesia or hypoaesthesia or anaesthesia

- Visceral—Bladder (usually hesitancy, decreased urinary stream, urinary retention or retention overflow) and bowel involvement (sphincter laxity, absent anal wink). In males impairment of sexual functions, and impotence
- Reflexes:
  - Ankle jerk—sluggish or absent
  - Knee jerk—normal or brisk (due to weaker hamstrings)
  - Anal reflexes—sluggish or absent.

Besides varying degrees of backache, the usual diagnostic tried of cauda equina syndrome are (1) saddle anaesthesia, (2) bladder and/or bowel anaesthesia and (3) weakness in lower extremity.

Causes of Cauda Equina Syndrome

- *Acute:*
  - Trauma (fracture/fracture dislocation of lumbar vertebrae).
  - Intervertebral disc prolapse (usually central).
- *Chronic:* Spinal canal stenosis—common causes are:
  - Congenital
  - Vascular malformations
  - Degenerative
  - Iatrogenic (following fenestration or hemilaminectomy, spinal fusion)
  - Caries spine
  - Neoplastic (secondary deposits)
  - Spinal tumours (space occupying lesions in the vertebral canal—e.g. neurofibroma, meningioma, Hodgkin's deposits, lymphosarcoma, haemangioma)
  - Spondylolisthesis.

Prompt surgical decompression is rewarding in most of the cases, and any delay may result in substantial morbidity.

Is better to have overall impression of NERVE COMPRESSION DISORDERS as depicted in the following **Figures in 8.93 to 8.95**.

■ BIBLIOGRAPHY

1. Badve SA, Bhojraj SY, Nene AM et al. Spinal instability in ankylosing spondylitis. Indian J Orthop. 2010;44:270-276.
2. Basu S, Rathinvelu S, Suri T. Degenerative scoliosis. In: Kulkarni GS, Babhulkar (Eds). Textbook of Orthopaedics & Trauma, Ch. 269. Delhi: Jaypee, Delhi, 2016, p. 2458.
3. Beachesne RP, Schutzer SF. Myositis ossificans of the piriformis muscle: an unusual cause of piriformis syndrome. J Bone Joint Surg. 1997;79A:906-10.
4. Bradford FK, Sprurling RG. The Intervertebral Disc (2nd ed). Springfield II: Charles C Thomas. 1945.
5. Brown MD, Hornicek FJ, Lebwohl NH. Phantom Sciatica. J Bone Joint Surg. 1977;79A:252-53.
6. Brunnstrom S Clinical kinesiology, 1962, Philadelphia. F.A. Davies.
7. Dimitrejevic M, Sherwood A, Nathan P. Clonus, peripheral and central mechanisms. In Desmedt JF (Ed) Neurology. New York: Karger. 1978.173-82.
8. Dubousset J: Three-dimensional analysis of scoliotic deformity. In: Weinstein SL (Ed). The Paediatric Spine: Principles and Practice. New York, NY: Raven Press; 1994. pp. 479-96.
9. Horstmann HM and bleck EF. Orthopaedic management in cerebral Palsy, 2nd edn. Mackeith Press, London. 2007.p5.
10. Johari A. Paediatric spinal deformity. CME Lectures. Book IOACON. 2005;15-22.
11. Kelley BJ, Vitale MG. Early-Onset scoliosis and congenital spinal anomalies. Let`s discuss spinal deformity. American Academy of Orthopaedic Surgeons: 2018;1-21.
12. Key S A. On paraplegia depending on the ligament of spine. Guy Hosp Rep. 1838;3:17-34.
13. Majeed SA, Seshadrinath NAK, Binoy KR, Raji L. Lumbar disc herniation: Is there an association between histological and magnetic resonance imaging findings? Ind Jr Orthop. 2016;50:234-42.
14. Marchetti PG, Bartolozzi P. Classification of spondylolisthesis as a guideline for treatment. In: Bridewell KH, DeWald RL, Hammerg KW (Eds). The Textbook of Spinal Surgery, ed 2. Philadelphia PA: Lippincott - Raven, 1997, pp. 1211-54.
15. McMohan TA. Muscles, Reflexes, and locomotion. Princeton NJ: 1984 Princeton University Press—Quoted in Orthopaedic Management in cerebral Palsy 2nd edn by Horstmann HM, and Black EF, Mac Keith Press 2007.p.30.
16. Moorhead S, Johnson M, Maas M. Nursing Outcomes Classification (NOC), 3rd edition. St. Louis MO: Mosby; 2004.
17. Murata Y, Takahashi K, Yamagata M, et al. The knee-spine syndrome. J Bone Joint Surg. 2003;85-B:95-99.
18. Muybridge E (1901)- quoted Helen HM Horstmann and Eugene E Bleck. Orthopaedic Management in Cerebral Palsy, 2nd ed. London Mac Keith Press; 2007.p.56.
19. Myerding HW. Spondylolisthesis Surg Gynae and Obstet. 1932;54:371.
20. Novacheck TF. Running injuries—a biomechanical approach. J Bone Joint Surg. 1998;80A:1220-33.
21. Offierski CM, Macnab I. Hip-spine syndrome. Spine 1983;8: 316-21.
22. Parent S, Labelle H. Spondylolisthesis in children and young adults. Ronald Lehman. Jr. (Ed). Let`s Discuss Spinal Deformity. AAOS American Academy of Orthopaedic Surgeons: 2018. pp. 111-24.
23. Scheurmann H. Kyphosis dorsalis juvenilis Zeitschr. Orthop. Chir. 1921;41:305-17.
24. Schmorl G, Junghanns H. The Human Spine in Health and Disease (2nd ed). New York: Grunn Stratton. 1971.
25. Skinner SR. Direct measurement of spasticity, In Sussman, MD (ed). The diplegic child. Rosement, IL: American Academy of Orthopedic Surgeons, 1992. pp.31-34.
26. Tuli SM. Challenge of therapeutically refractory and multidrug resistant tuberculosis in orthopaedic practice. Indian J Orthop 2002:36; 211-3.
27. Wiltse LL, Widell EH Jr, Jakson DW. Fatigue fracture: The basic lesion in isthmic spondylolisthesis. J Bone Joint Surg Am. 1975;57-A:17-22.
28. Wiltse LL, Newman PH, Macnab I. Classification of spondylolysisand spondylolisthesis. Clin Orthop Relat Res. 1976;117:23-29.
29. Winter RB, Moe JH, Eilers VE: Congenital scoliosis: A study of 234 patients treated and untreated: Part 1 Natural history. J Bone Joint Surg Am. 1968;50(1):1-15.

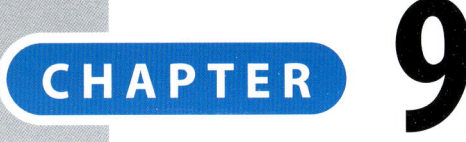

Pelvis

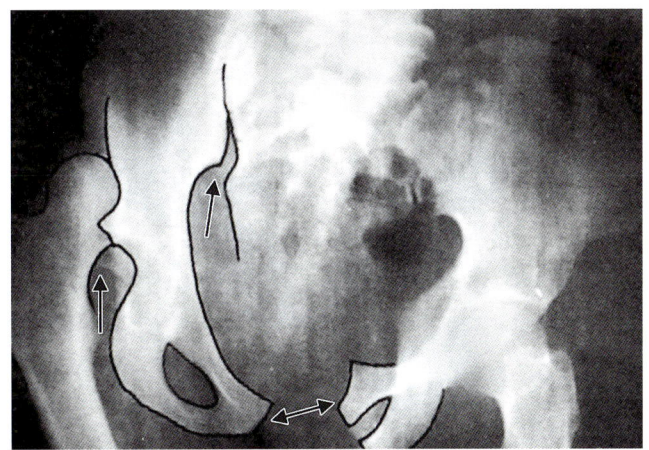

"The risk of wrong decision is preferable to the terror of indecision."
—***Maimonides***

"Nothing is more important than your smile, because when you smile, world around you starts smiling."
—***SP***

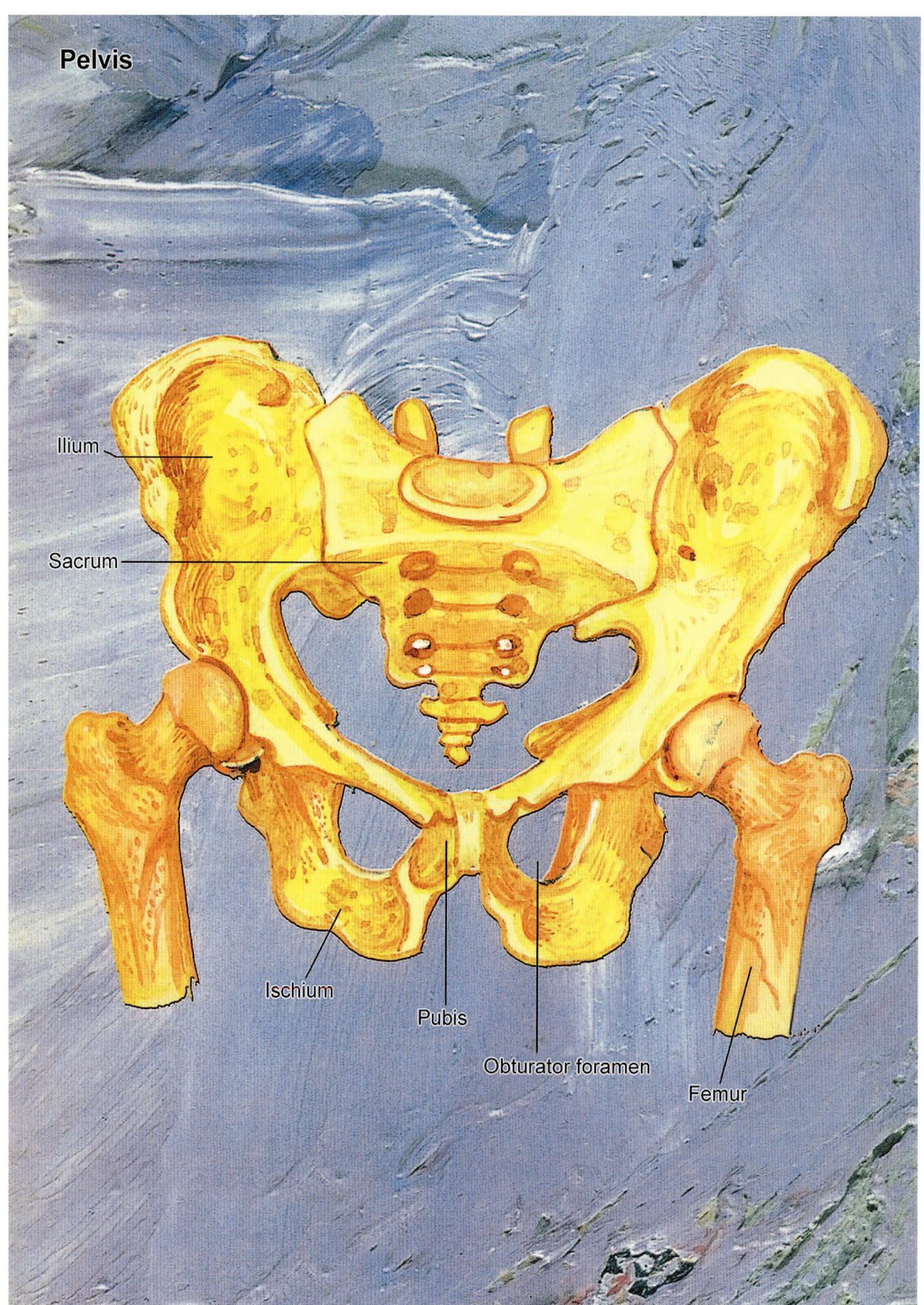

INTRODUCTION

Pelvic injuries basically comprise two sets of involvements: (i) skeletal framework of pelvis and (ii) soft tissues and visceral contents in the pelvis and around it.

Many a time, simple fractures of the pelvic bone may be insignificant from the treatment point of view. However, on the other hand, even without obvious fracture of the pelvis, visceral injuries may be so serious as to have lethal consequences, unless promptly and adequately attended to. Unfortunately, pelvic peritonitis is often severe in its manifestation.

ANATOMICAL CONSIDERATIONS

- The pelvis (means basin) is an intrinsically stable portion interposed between the movable segments of vertebral column, which it supports, and the lower limbs, upon which it rests. It is more or less in a ring form. The posterior arch of the ring, consisting of upper three sacral vertebrae and strong pillars of bone from the sacroiliac joints to acetabular fossae, is chiefly concerned in transmitting the body weight. The inlet of pelvis is broad and shallow, and the outlet is constricted and deep
- The ring comprises of two hemipelvises, with intervention of the sacrum posteriorly and a fibrocartilaginous disc anteriorly
- The adult sacroiliac joint is auricular and C-shaped with convexity anterior and somewhat inferior. The surface of sacroiliac joint at birth is about 1.5 cm^2, at puberty about 7 cm^2 and in adult about 17.5 cm^2
- The sacroiliac joint is an integral part of the *lumbo-pelvic joint complex*, where *lumbar spine, sacroiliac joint, hip joints and pubic symphysis—all work in synergism*
- The joints in between the sacrum and posterior ends of ilial plates are either amphiarthrodial (fibrocartilaginous bridging of two hyaline cartilage surfaces) or synarthrosis (articular surfaces joined by fibrous tissue) or diarthrodial (synovial joint at least in its anterior and inferior portion). Articular surfaces having irregular elevations contribute to the restricted movements and strength of the joint. The tough interosseous ligaments spread from the posterosuperior rough area of the articular surface on the ilial plates to the lateral mass of sacrum. Anteriorly, the anterior sacroiliac ligaments are thin, and thus get easily distended by any intra-articular pathology and can be felt by rectal examination. The lumbosacral nerve trunk lies anterior to it, hence any sacroiliac joint pathology can lead to inflammatory neuritis. The posterior sacroiliac ligaments are quite tough and can withstand violent trauma. These joints allow very slight anteroposterior rotational movements, occurring around a transverse axis about 7.5 cm vertically below the promontory of the sacrum. In most of the activities during locomotion, these joints have an insignificant role. Anteriorly, the two pubic bodies more or less adhere together with the intervention of a fibrocartilaginous disc, forming the pubic symphysis
- The movements of sacroiliac joint are involuntary and are caused by indirect forces like shear compression, etc. For the secondary sacroiliac joint motions, the muscles involved are erector spinae, quadratus lumborum, psoas major, psoas minor, piriformis, latissimus dorsi, obliques abdominis, gluteus maximus, gluteus medius and gluteus minimus. The weight of body and change of posture also affect the movements of sacroiliac joints. Any pathology or injury to lumbar region, specially in lower lumbar region, and also of hip region can affect the movements and functions of sacroiliac joints.

  Since, there is wide range of segmental innervation (L2 to S2) of sacroiliac joint, there are many referral zone patterns on and along the joint. The most constant referral zone has been located as 3 × 10 cm area just inferior to the same sided posterior superior iliac spine
- The normal shape of the pelvis is more or less that of a signet ring. In conditions where the bone gets softened (e.g. osteomalacia, rickets), under influence of the body weight and thrust of the two femora upwards during locomotion, the sacral promontory protrudes anteroinferiorly and the two acetabular floors project superomedially, giving a trefoil shape to the pelvis (*see* **Fig. 9.25**)
- When the hips are normal, the pelvis has almost negligible involvement, except for transmitting the weight through the acetabulofemoral head axis, but in altered situations, the pelvis accommodates disabilities, deformities, and disparities in the length of the lower limbs to a very significant extent. This postural adjustment of the pelvis leads to pelvic obliquity. Pelvic obliquity may be in anteroposterior axis (to accommodate the aforesaid effects in anteroposterior direction) or in lateral axis (to compensate the effects in the side-to-side axis)
- In pelvic injuries, following viscera and important soft tissues are affected (in order of frequency)
  - Urethra and bladder
  - Vagina and uterus
  - Sciatic nerve
  - Rectum and anal canal
  - Pelvic peritoneum
  - Iliac vessels
- If one of the bones of the hemipelvis is fractured, it is not going to affect the integrity of the pelvis in any significant way. This is because the muscles are firmly adapted to the inner and outer pelvic bone plates and act as firm splintage from both sides of the bone
- Pelvis is a common site for inflammatory pathology. Besides the complications following any abdominal and

gynaecological pathology, infections in the form of iliac abscess and psoas abscess are quite common. Being a container with a dependent position, pus and other infected materials accumulate at the bottom to present as abscesses (e.g. psoas and ilio-psoas abscess in caries spine, infected collection in pouch of Douglas)

- Even major injuries affecting the pelvis may not be of much significance in males, if the viscera and neurovascular bundles are intact. However, in females of child bearing age, any disruption of the normal anatomy or overall shape of pelvis may affect the pregnancy and delivery
- The disposition and attachment of the deeper layer of superficial fascia in the lower abdomen determines the extent of extravasation of urine due to rupture of the urethra. The deeper condensed membranous layer of the superficial fascia of abdomen (Scarpa's fascia) continues as the fascia of Colles investing the penis and the scrotum. Then it continues as the superficial fascia covering the superficial perineal muscles.
  • The attachments of Collie's fascia are as follows:
  • Above—continuous as Scarpa's fascia
  • Medially—continuous with the Collie's fascia of the opposite side
  • Laterally—attaches on the conjoint ischiopubic ramus.
  • Inferiorly—fuses with the posterior border of urogenital diaphragm.

The **spread of any extravasated urine following rupture of the urethra** in the perineum is limited below by the attachment of fascia of Colles with the urogenital diaphragm. Laterally, it can go up to the conjoint ischiopubic rami. Upwards, it may spread over the penis and scrotum. Further, it may extend over the abdominal wall passing along the spermatic cord. From the lower abdominal wall, urine may track down below the inguinal ligament up to the attachment of the Scarpa's fascia to fascia lata.

Ossification

See **Table 9.1**.

TABLE 9.1: Ossification of innominate bone or hip bone.

Primary centres	Secondary centres
Primary centres—One for ilium—8th weeks IUL One for ischium—4th month One for pubis—4–5th months At birth, acetabulum is a cartilaginous cup with a triradiate stem appearing on the pelvic surface as a 'Y'-shaped epiphyseal plate between the ilium, ischium and pubis	Secondary centres appear about puberty and join with rest of the bone between 15 and 25 years. Iliac crest—two secondary centres. Acetabular cartilage ossifies by two centres. Anterior inferior iliac spine, ischial tuberosity, pubic crest, symphyseal surfaces may have separate centres

■ METHODOLOGY

History Taking

As in Chapter 1: Introduction.

General and Systemic Examinations

As in Chapter 1: Introduction.

If there is history or suspicion of pelvic injury, the features of shock and haemorrhage must be carefully looked for. Unstable fractures of the pelvis are the third most common cause of death following road traffic accident.

Regional Examination

If the patient can walk, note the gait. Note the obvious pelvic tilt, the posture of lower back (lordosis, scoliosis, kyphosis) and any obvious deformity while standing. Perform the Trendelenburg test **(refer Fig. 12.30)**. The trauma and chronic pathology of the pelvis closely mimic the hip, sacroiliac, lumbosacral and lower lumbar involvements. Therefore, one should examine these regions separately. The corresponding lower limb should be assessed as a whole.

Most of the patients suffering from traumatic conditions are initially unable to stand due to pain. On the other hand, in most of the diseases of pelvis, except for acutely manifesting ones, the patient can stand, and walk about with a limp and deformities of varying extent.

Local Examination

Inspection: Besides looking at the surface and condition of skin, the following points must be given due attention while patient is lying supine. Note the symmetry and level of anterior superior iliac spines, iliac crests, iliac plate flares, symphysis pubis, groin folds, Scarpa's triangle, contour and bulge of abdomen, the level of umbilicus and genitalia. Usually, it is painful for the patient to turn to the lateral or to a prone position. But if possible, it should be done. While on side, note the symmetry, any bulge, prominence of iliac crest and the gluteal region, dimples of Venus, symmetrical prominences of posterior superior iliac spines, gluteal bulge, internatal cleft **(Fig. 9.1)**, gluteal folds, and back of thighs. In case of injury, look for any bruising particularly in perineum, any swelling or sinus or scar in perineum **(Figs. 9.1 to 9.4)** and any bleeding from urethra/anus/vagina.

Palpation: Palpation should be done systematically, as in inspection. Significant points to be noted in palpation:

Superficial palpation (Touch): Besides noting the findings of touch (e.g. skin sensation, temperature, tenderness, etc.) in case of any suspected pelvic injury, palpate the lower abdomen thoroughly. Note any rigidity of abdominal muscle, generalised/localised tenderness, hollowness/ fullness of iliac fossae and pelvis.

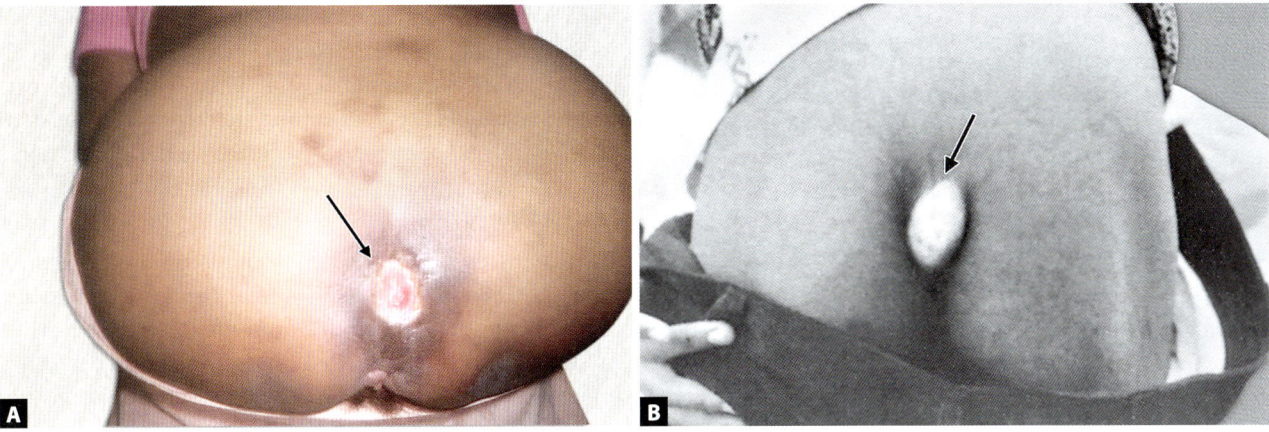

Figs. 9.1A and B: (A) Condylomatous ulcer; (B) Condylomata (syphilitic) in internatal cleft.

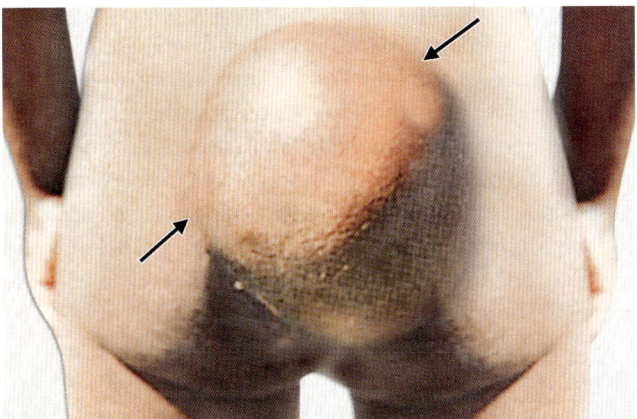

Fig. 9.2: Lipoma from sacral region.

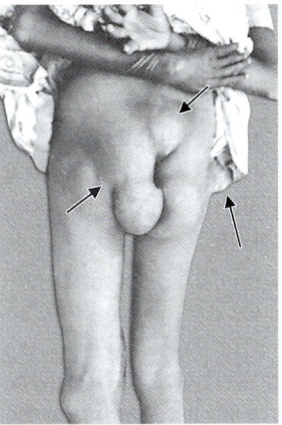

Fig. 9.3: Atypical neurofibromatous swellings in the left buttock, right back of thigh and sacral region.

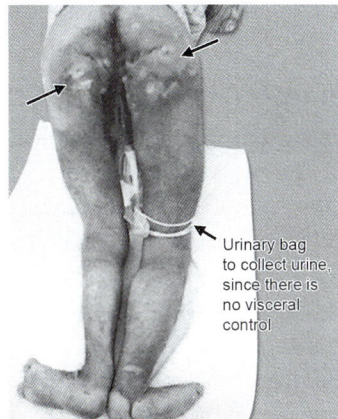

Fig. 9.4: Multiple sinuses in perineum (cf. watercan perineum) in a patient of spina bifida.

Deep palpation (Feel): Also palpate the cave of Retzius region, i.e. behind pubic symphysis. Palpate anterior superior iliac spine, the iliac crest and pubic symphysis for symmetry, regularity of surfaces or any gap in between the two halves. In disruption and any fracture dislocation of the pubic symphysis, one can insinuate a finger/fingers or even the fist if there is wide separation. In subluxation, a regular step may be felt. Palpate the inlet and outlet of pelvic margins systematically. Press each anterior superior iliac spine downwards and medially and also press over the symphysis pubis—if the patient complains of pain, it indicates the great possibility of injury or acute pathology in pelvis. The outer side and back of pelvis should be palpated on routine lines. The alignment and tenderness of sacral spines, sacroiliac joints, ischial tuberosities and coccygeal regions should be noted. Tenderness just beneath the posterior superior iliac spine and down to about 3–5 cm denotes sacroiliac joint tenderness. In very early pathology, tenderness of sacroiliac joints can be elicited by firmly tapping or guarded deep thrust applied over that region. At the bottom of the pelvis, any bulge and tenderness should be noted in the region of ischiorectal fossa.

Rectal examination: No pelvic examination is complete without per rectal and per vaginal (in adults) digital examinations. During this examination, palpate the ischiopubic rami, coccyx and inferior part of sacroiliac joints on the sides. Acetabular tenderness can also be elicited in acute pathology. In males, the condition of prostate, and, in both sexes any abnormal soft tissue bulge should be noted.

In pelvic fractures, if the patient has not passed urine smoothly, do not ask him to strain and pass urine. Check up for any extravasation of urine in the scrotum, labial region, groin and in the lower abdominal wall.

Palpation of urethra is difficult. However, gradually palpate backwards from penile urethra towards the membranous part. It is always safe to pass a sterilised rubber catheter cautiously for testing the integrity of the urethra.

Auscultation: Quadrants of abdomen must be auscultated, especially in traumatic cases. *Silent abdomen alone denotes paralytic ileus, but along with rigidity should be a definite sign of peritonitis.*

■ MOVEMENTS

In connection with pelvic examination, movements at lumbar spine, lumbosacral region, hip and sacroiliac region must be tested separately, as described in corresponding chapter. The movements of the sacroiliac joints can be tested only by indirect methods, i.e. stress tests.

Stress Tests

Stress test of four types:
1. Straight leg raising test.
2. Compression stress test.
3. Distraction stress test.
4. Axial rotation stress tests
   a. Pump handle test.
   b. Gaenslen's test.
   c. Laquer's sign.
   d. Goldthwaite's sign.

Straight Leg Raising Test (Refer Fig. 12.28)

(Also done to test sciatic radiculitis and hip-stability)

In most of the affections of the hemipelvis and corresponding sacroiliac joint, patient has difficulty or even inability in raising ipsilateral straight leg.

Method: While the patient lies supine, ask him to elevate the ipsilateral lower limb with the knee fully extended. He is asked to stop as soon as he feels pain. The angle between the back of the thigh and the bed is measured. Normally, one can lift the straight leg to about 90° without tilting the pelvis. Beyond that, it will not be possible, unless the knee is bent. Even with a normal lower limb, straight leg raising may be deficient in affections causing pain in the pelvis and sacroiliac joint.

Compression Stress Test (Fig. 9.5)

The patient lies supine on a flat bed and with the legs approximated together as far as possible. The examiner leans forwards, and compresses both anterior superior iliac spines, towards each other. Forceful compression often elicits pain in the affected sacroiliac joint, but will have no effect on lumbosacral affections. Of course, in fractures/ dislocations of pelvis, this manoeuvre will elicit pain at the affected site.

Distraction Stress Test (Fig. 9.6)

The patient lies supine with legs extended and approximated together. The examiner leans forward and presses on both anterior superior iliac spines from the inner aspect with a tendency of distracting them away from each other. The inferences will be similar, as in 'compression stress test.'

Axial Rotation Stress Test

- *Pump handle test* **(Fig. 9.7)**: The patient lies supine. Press with your left hand over patient's left shoulder. While the patient keeps the right lower limb extended, hold the left upper leg and fully flex the knee and hip (left) with a tendency to bring the left-knee towards the patients right shoulder. If right sacroiliac is diseased, the patient will feel pain on the right side in this manoeuvre (Reverse the position of the hands and test for opposite sacroiliac joint).

Pathomechanics of the test—By fully flexing the knee and hip, that side of hemipelvis is more or less locked with the sacrum. Attempts to forcibly flex the knee and hip (flexed across the abdomen) produces rotational stress at the opposite sacroiliac joint.

In this manoeuvre, even in early pathology, pain will be felt at the sacroiliac joint

- *Gaenslen's test* **(Fig. 9.8)**: The patient lies supine, with the pelvis preferably lying on the edge of examination table. On the unaffected side, hip and knee are fully flexed and pressed over the abdomen to eliminate lumbar lordosis completely. The affected side of hip is passively hyperextended. While doing so, the patient feels pain in the affected sacroiliac joint due to rotational strain

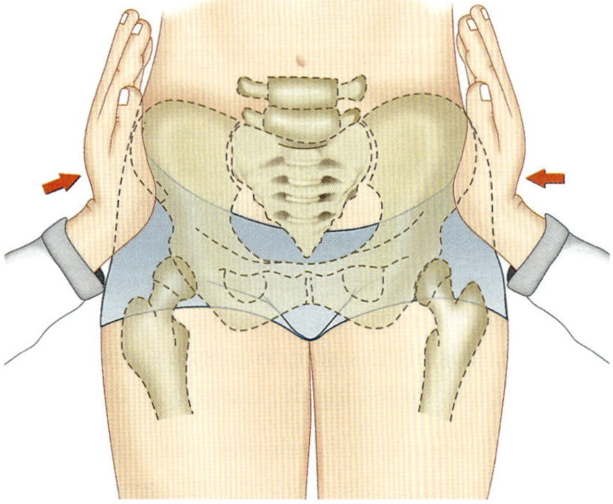

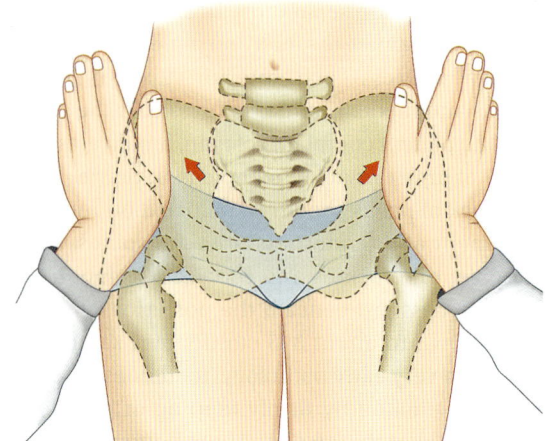

Fig. 9.5: Method of eliciting compression stress test of pelvis to elicit pain at sacroiliac joints.

Fig. 9.6: Method of eliciting distraction stress test for pelvis to elicit pain at sacroiliac joints.

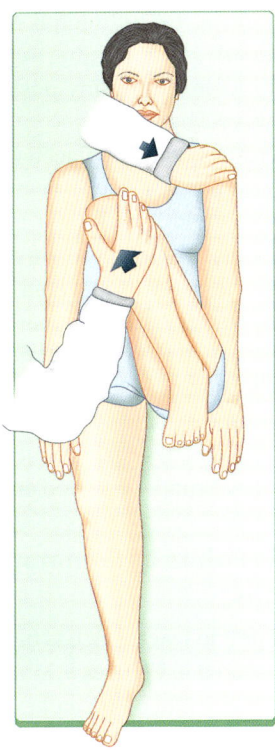

Fig. 9.7: Method of demonstration of pump handle test.

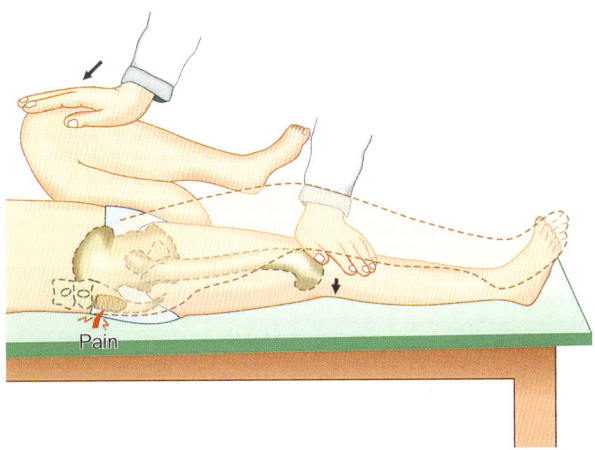

Fig. 9.8: Method of demonstration of Gaenslen's test.

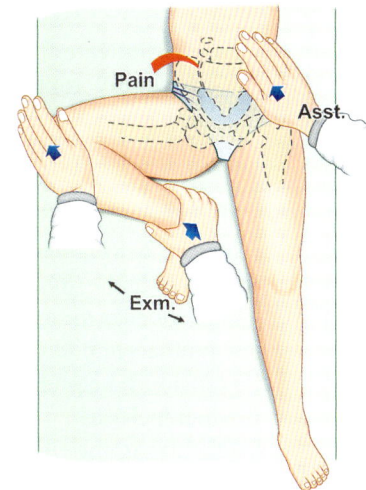

Fig. 9.9: Method of demonstration of Laquer's sign.

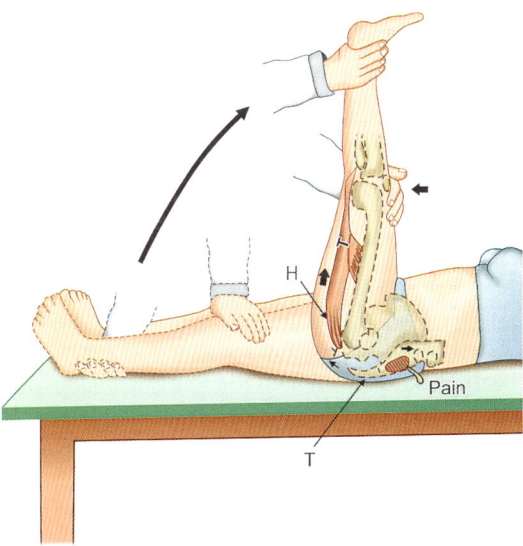

Fig. 9.10: Method of demonstration of Goldthwaite's sign. H = hamstrings; T = ischial tuberosity

- *Laquer's sign* **(Fig. 9.9)**: If the ipsilateral lower limb is forced into flexion, abduction and external rotation at the hip, the patient experiences pain in the affected sacroiliac region
- *Goldthwaite's sign* **(Fig. 9.10)**: The patient lies supine. While the knee is fully extended, the thigh is strongly flexed. The tense hamstring muscles produce rotatory strain upon the sacroiliac joint of ipsilateral side. Therefore, in sacroiliac affections, the patient feels pain on the same side on doing this manoeuvre.
- *Patrick's test* (Figure of '4' test—**refer Fig. 8.56**): With the patient's heel placed on the opposite knee, downward pressure on the flexed knee while the hip is in flexion, abduction and external rotation, leads to pain in the affected sacroiliac joint because of rotational stretch over it.

■ MEASUREMENTS

In pelvic examination, it has not much significance. The girth of the pelvis at different levels, specially at the highest points of iliac crests and supratrochanteric regions, should be noted. The linear measurements of the lower limbs should be done as described in the Chapter 12 'Hip Joint'.

Neurovascular examination of the lower limb should also be done routinely.

INVESTIGATIONS FOR PELVIC PATHOLOGY

Besides specific investigations indicated for particular pathological conditions, X-ray (in different planes) is an essential investigation for pelvic injuries and pathology.
- In taking the X-ray for pelvis, the following points must be taken into account:
- Bowel must be cleared of gases and faecal matter
- Pelvis must be centred on the X-ray table, i.e. symphysis pubis and umbilicus should be in the same vertical line
- The whole pelvis must be included in the exposure, rather, inclusion of lower three lumbars and lower down up to subtrochanteric level is very much helpful in considering the symmetry of the two hemipelvises
- In order for an X-ray of the pelvis, the clinician must be clear in his mind as to which part he wants to delineate. Anteroposterior X-rays of pelvic inlet, pelvic outlet, and sacrum—all require different positioning. One must remember that the pelvis is not placed in a plane horizontal to the long axis of the body, rather, even the fully squared up pelvis is set at an anterior inclination. Therefore, if one wants to have a true anteroposterior exposure for the pelvis, the plate should be placed in contact beneath the pelvis supported on a sandbag and the X-ray beam should be focussed at the centre of the pelvic inlet.

For Sacroiliac Joints

Place the patient on the X-ray table with a wide sandbag supporting the upper pelvis, i.e. just below the lumbo-sacral areas. The lower limbs will be in lithotomy position. The X-ray beam is to be centred on the third sacral body. In this position, the longest zone of the auricle-shaped sacroiliac joints is traversed by the X-ray beam. Confirmation of correct exposure of the sacroiliac joints can be had from the fact that the pelvic outlet will project a constricted bean-shaped impression. To expose the full length of sacrum, place a wider pillow beneath lower lumbar region transversely. Put the patient in wider lithotomy position. The beam is centred to imaginary S3 body.

Since the sacroiliac joint is placed obliquely, oblique anteroposterior and posteroanterior views are essential to visualise the joint clearly in its major extent. For oblique posteroanterior view, the patient lies prone. Then the unaffected side of the pelvis is elevated by 30°. The film is centred on the level of the anterior superior iliac spines and the beam is projected centering the midpoint of the film. For oblique anteroposterior, the patient lies supine, and the affected side is elevated by 30°.

For delineating ilial plates, ischial and pubic rami, a plain anteroposterior X-ray exposure is good enough.

Key Diagnostic Points of Common Pelvic Affections

Classification of pelvic fractures has been summarised in **Table 9.2** and presented in **Figures 9.11** and **9.12**.

An extremely rare injury—ipsilateral triple dislocation of pelvis, produces gross instability (**Fig. 9.13**).

DISEASES

Congenital Anomalies

Important congenital anomalies are:
- Undeveloped/Underdeveloped pelvis/congenital absence of any segment/zone/part of pelvis (**Figs. 9.14A and B**)
- Trefoil pelvis
- Protrusio acetabuli (**Fig. 9.15**)
- Ectopia vesicae with deficient pubic symphysis
- Morphological alterations according to associated congenital conditions, e.g. in CDH.

TABLE 9.2: Injuries of pelvis.

Skeletal (Figs. 9.11 and 9.12)

Stable (usually due to minor injury)	Unstable (due to severe injury)	Visceral (usually in severe injury)
(i) Avulsion fracture, e.g. anterior superior iliac spine (by sartorius), Anterior inferior iliac spine (by rectus femoris), ischial tuberosity (by hamstrings)	(i) Vertical—fracture of Ilium, pubis, ischium (ii) Bilateral fracture of Ilium, pubis, ischium with various combinations	• Urethra (membranous most common) Bladder • Vagina/Uterus Sciatic nerve
(ii) Fracture individual components of pelvis Fracture ilial plate Fracture pubic ramus/body Fracture sacrum Fracture coccyx	(iii) Fracture dislocation of pelvis	• Rectum and anal canal • Pelvic peritoneum with its reflections Iliac vessels
(iii) Subluxation of the joints, e.g. Pubic symphysis Sacroiliac joints Sacrococcygeal joint		

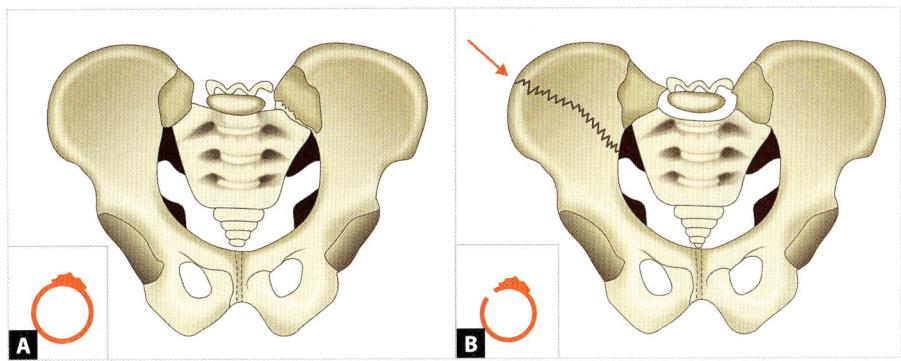

Figs. 9.11A and B: (A) Normal pelvic ring; (B) Stable fracture of pelvic ring.

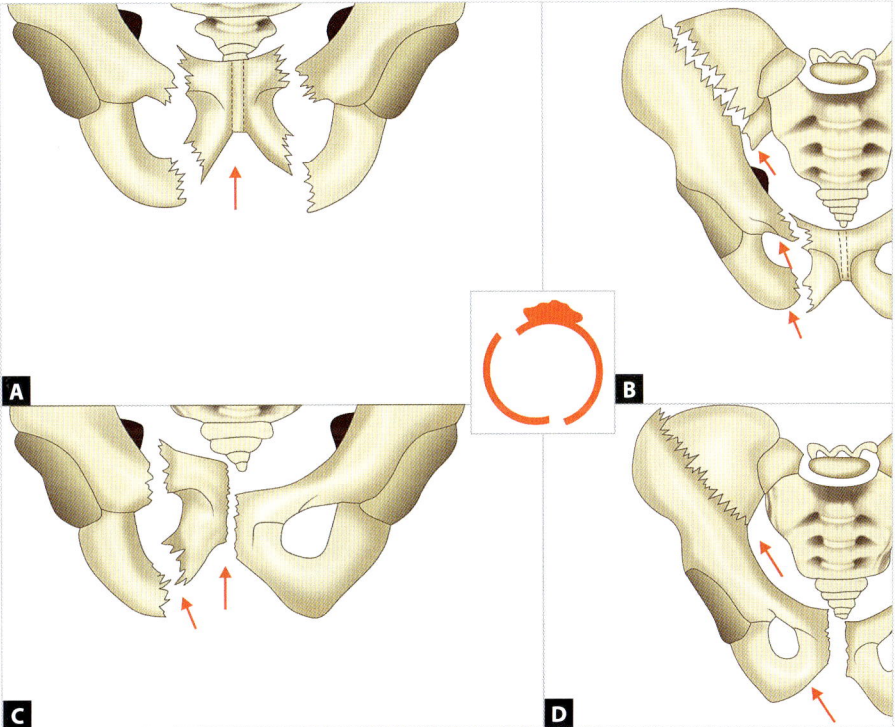

Figs. 9.12A to D: Unstable fractures of pelvic ring.

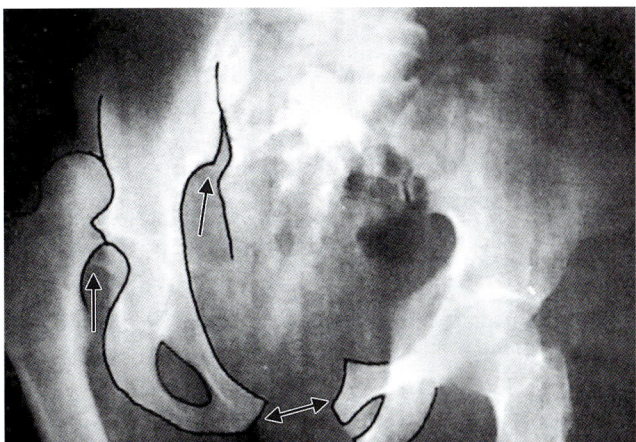

Fig. 9.13: Ipsilateral triple dislocation of pelvis: dislocations of hip, sacroiliac joint and pubic symphysis produced by run over injury by a heavy vehicle while the patient was lying down in supine posture.

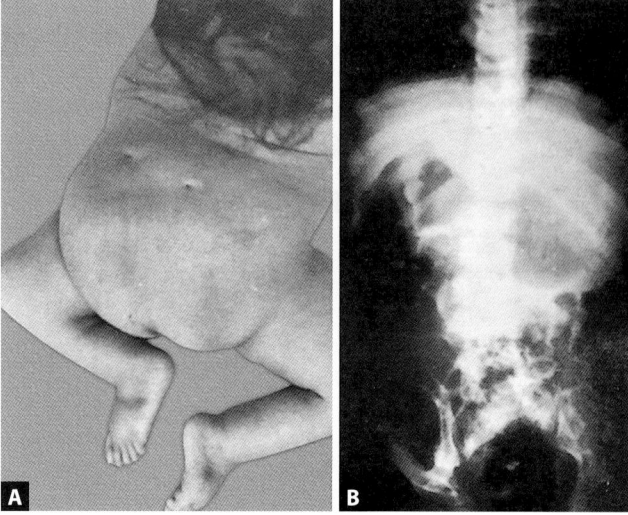

Figs. 9.14A and B: Congenital absence of sacrum.

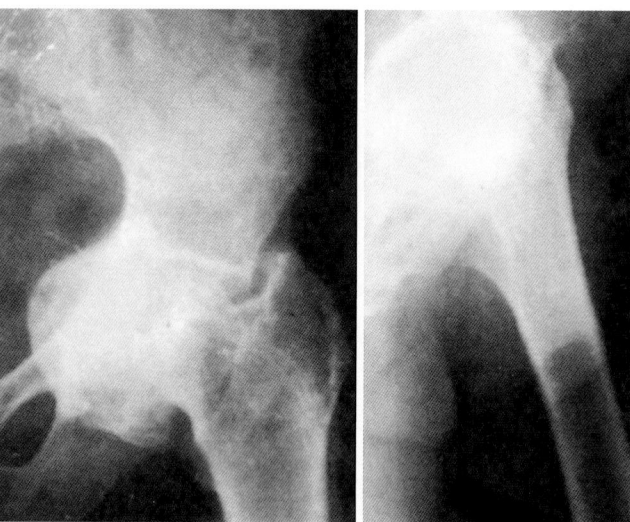

Fig. 9.16: Protrusio acetabuli.

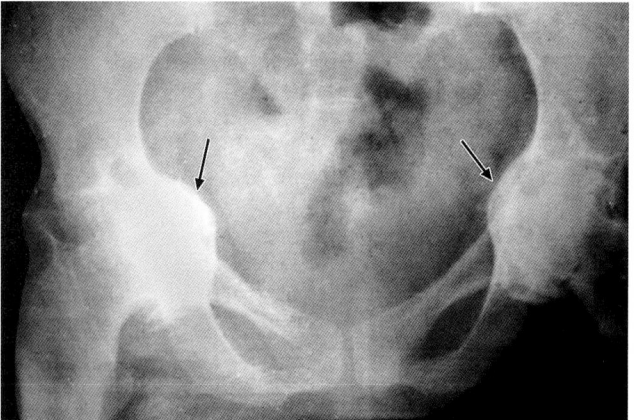

Fig. 9.15: Bilateral protrusio acetabuli due to osteomalacia.

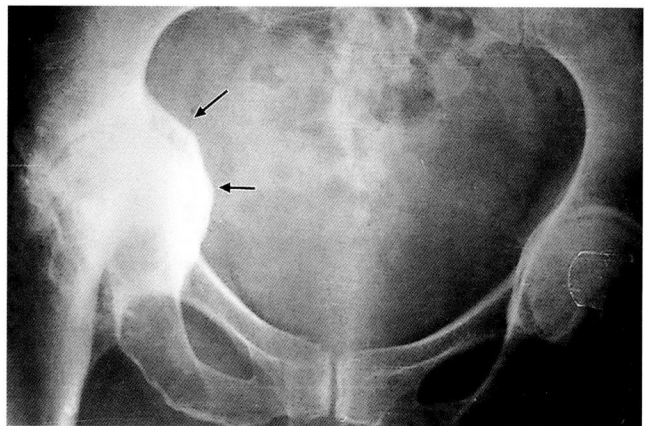

Fig. 9.17: Protrusio acetabuli following neglected central fracture dislocation of right hip (fracture acetabulum).

Inflammatory Conditions

- Tuberculous focus in acetabulum and sacroiliac joints
- Pyogenic inflammation of iliac plates, specially near about supra-acetabular zone
- Secondary involvement of pelvic bones following infective conditions of pelvic viscera, iliac abscess, compound injuries and injection abscess.

Metabolic and Deficiency States

- Rickets
- Osteomalacia **(Figs. 9.15 and 9.25)**
- Looser's zone (pseudofractures at ribs, axillary border of scapula, pubic rami, medial cortex of femur)
    - Trefoil pelvis **(Fig. 9.25)**
    - Protrusio acetabuli **(Figs. 9.15 to 9.17)**
    - Paget's disease.

Collagen Arthropathy

- Ankylosing spondylitis
- Rheumatoid arthritis.

Degenerative Conditions

Degenerative arthrosis of sacroiliac joint and acetabular margin (hip joint).

Neoplasm

- *Benign:*
    - Osteochondroma
    - Haemangioma
    - Osteoid osteoma.
- *Malignant:*
    - Chondrosarcoma
    - Multiple myelomatosis

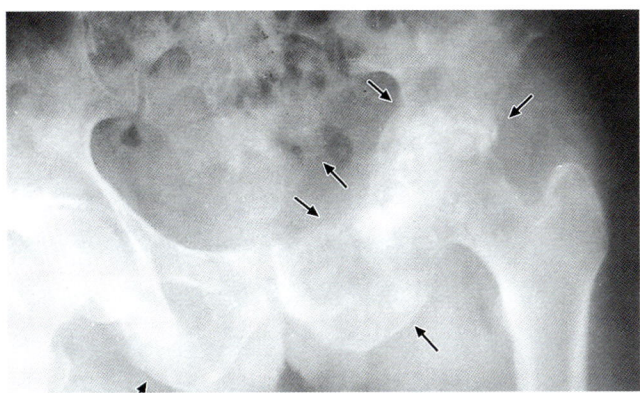

Fig. 9.18: Pelvic bone metastasis from carcinoma of prostate.

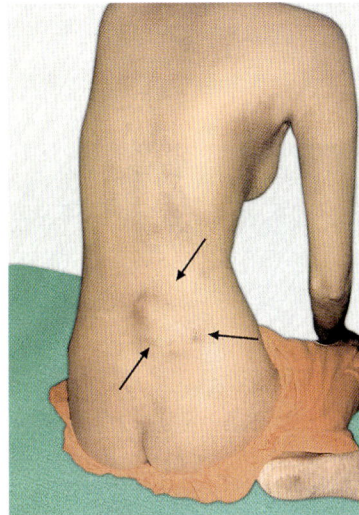

Fig. 9.19: Cold abscess from tuberculosis of right sacroiliac joint.

- Secondary carcinomatosis **(Fig. 9.18)**
- Others (rare).

Tuberculosis of Sacroiliac Joint

The patient is usually young female, with chronic history of low backache and pain in buttock region, specially on changing posture while sleeping, getting up from sitting and *vice-versa*. Sitting on the buttock of affected side is painful, whereas sitting on the opposite buttock relieves the pain. Bending forward with the knee extended is painful (tight hamstrings pulling the sacrotuberous ligament), whereas bending with the knee flexed (relaxed hamstrings) is painless.
- Little or no relief by analgesics
- Localised tenderness, fullness in sacroiliac region
- May be cold abscess—intra-pelvic/gluteal region/posterior part of iliac crest **(Fig. 9.19)**
- Stress tests positive
- Rectal examination demonstrates swelling and tenderness
- ESR usually not much raised
- X-ray—initially may be noncontributory, later on shows usual changes of tuberculosis.

Pyogenic Infection of Iliac Plate

In young children, pyogenic osteomyelitis of lower part of ilium with secondary septic arthritis of hip (and *vice versa*) is not uncommon.
- Constitutional and local inflammatory features as in any pyogenic infection
- May be local abscess
- Hip movements affected
- Pus culture and X-ray—confirmatory.

Sacroiliac Strain

Mechanical stress or traumatic strain or postpartum relaxation of the ligaments of the sacroiliac joints may lead to inflammatory changes (non-infective). The patient complains of pain in the sacroiliac region or in upper inner quadrant of buttock or the posterolateral aspect of thigh or in mixed regions to variable extent. The compression and/ or distraction stress test of pelvis produces pain in sacroiliac joint (*see* **Figs. 9.5 and 9.6)**.

Sacroiliac Arthritis

It usually occurs in spondyloarthropathies, ankylosing spondylitis (sacroiliitis). On arising from the bed, the patient complains of pain and stiffness in sacroiliac regions and low back, which improves with exercises. Pain may be referred to upper outer quadrant of buttock or posterolateral aspect of thigh. Rotational movements of spine accentuates the pain (*see also* ankylosing spondylitis).

Ankylosing Spondylitis
(Figs. 9.20 to 9.22 and 9.24)

The name 'ankylosing spondylitis' has been derived from Greek root 'ankylos' (means 'bent') (cf. ankylosis means joint fusion) and 'spondylo' (means spinal vertebra). Ankylosing spondylitis (Marie Strumpell's or von Bechterew's disease) is a chronic inflammatory disease of unknown etiology. It is a seronegative spondyloarthropathy which primarily affects the axial skeleton, the sacroiliac joints; and pelvis and not infrequently peripheral joints (*See* Chapter 8 and 10 for more informations).
- Young adults (male: female = 4:1) complaining of low backache and morning stiffness, which are relieved after exercise or activity and aggravated after prolonged rest
- Deep thrust tenderness over sacroiliac regions
- Other associated clinical findings (as in Chapter 8 Spine).
- X-ray—periarticular rarefaction, fuzziness across sacroiliac joint, sclerosis of articular margins **(Fig. 9.24)**, obliteration of joint line.

As pathology advances, trabeculations across the joint **(Refer Figs. 9.24 and 12.74A)**.

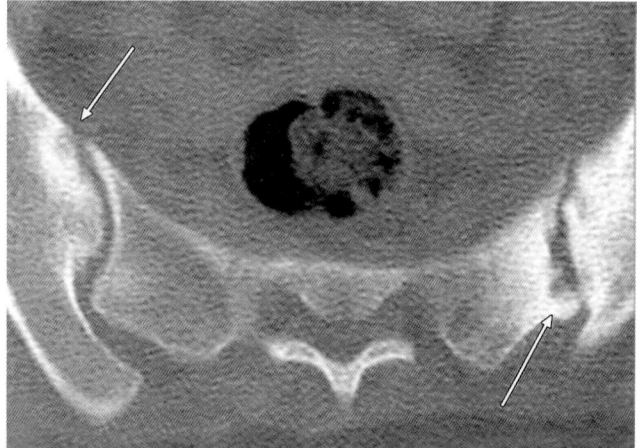

Fig. 9.20: CT scan of sacroiliac joint showing sacroiliitis with typical findings of bilateral asymmetric erosions and sclerosis.
Source: Inner Spaces Vol 1, No 1, July 2006.

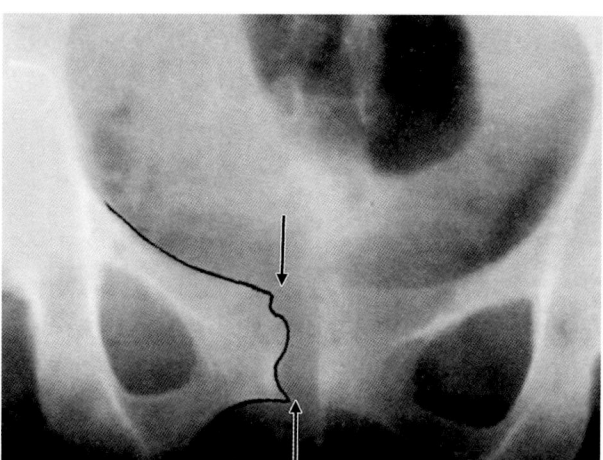

Fig. 9.23: Osteitis pubis.

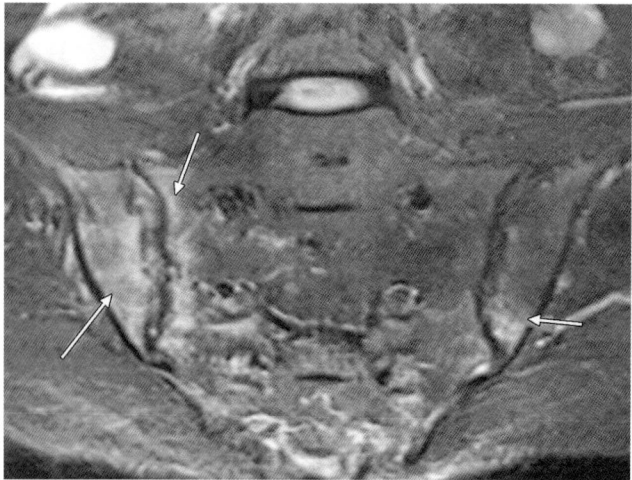

Fig. 9.21: MRI of sacroiliac joint—the special T1W fat-sat image showing bilateral asymmetric marrow oedema looking bright.
Source: Inner Spaces Vol 1, No 1, July 2006.

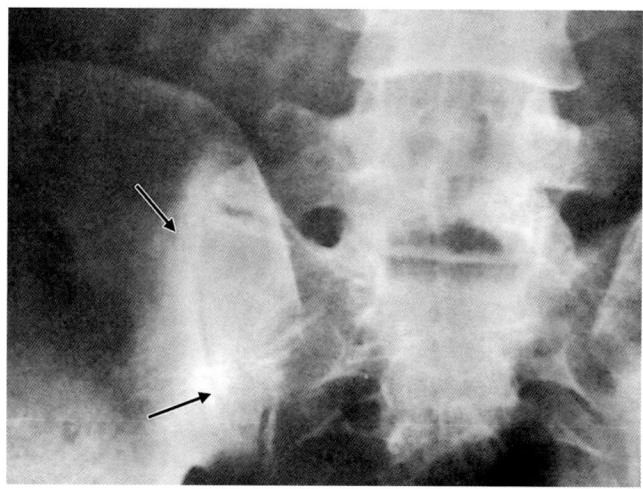

Fig. 9.24: Ankylosing spondylitis. Note the sclerosis of articular margins.

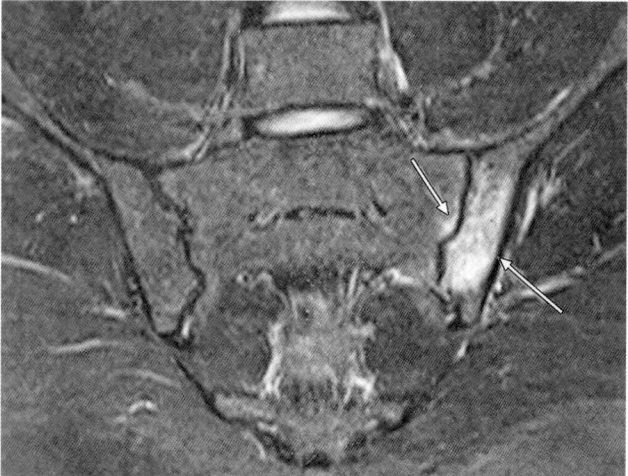

Fig.9.22: MRI of sacroiliac joint—the special T1W fat-sat image showing marrow oedema involving both surfaces of the left sacroiliac joint.
Source: Inner Spaces Vol 1, No 1, July 2006.

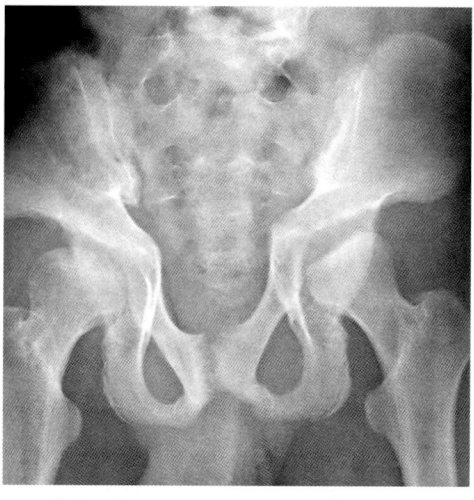

Fig. 9.25: Trefoil pelvis: Note the trefoil shape of pelvis—pelvic inlet—the acetabuli and pubic rami are pushed inwards towards the sacral promontory due to weak/soft texture of bones in osteomalacia.

Osteochondroma

- Pelvic bones are common sites
- Variable knob like irregular, hard swelling arising from bone
- Symptoms are usually due to pressure effects, cosmetic effect, or when it turns malignant, e.g. chondrosarcoma
- X-ray is highly suggestive.

Coccygodynia (Coccydynia or Coccygodynia)

- Usually, overweight ladies in their forties
- May or may not be a history of fall on buttock (on the edge of a hard object), or directly on the coccyx or subtle form of cumulative trauma which occurs due to long periods of sitting in awkward position
- Pain complained of on sitting on a hard object, or after walking a long distance, in advanced cases even when passing hard stools
- Local tenderness at sacrococcygeal junction, coccyx, coccygeal tip
- Per rectum examination elicits pain while fingertip presses posteriorly towards coccyx
- Pain in coccygeal region associated with sitting and is exacerbated while rising from a seated position
- X-rays in sitting and standing position permit measurement of the sagittal rotation of the pelvis and the coccygeal angle of incidence
- Scintigraphy (using technetium 99m) and MRI may demonstrate inflammation of sacrococcygeal area indicating coccygeal hypermobility. They also exclude serious pathology like chordoma.
- Most of the coccygeal pain respond to NSAIDs, avoiding sitting on hard object, and use of a donut cushion.

The remaining ones should respond to local (around distal third of coccyx) injection of anaesthetic and corticosteroid. In resistant cases, coccygectomy should help, especially when there is evidence of hypermobility or subluxation of coccyx in X-ray.

Osteitis Pubis

- Painful condition about the pubic symphysis with tendency to spontaneous cure
- Exact cause unknown but may follow trauma, usually surgical procedure about the pelvic region, and in women during pregnancy and vaginal delivery
- Within a period of few days, excruciating pain develops in the symphysis pubis pubic rami and adductor aspect of thighs
- Due to, probably, stress reaction to overuse or excessive mobility it develops in athletes involved in cutting sports like soccer and hockey
- Flexion movement of trunk is very painful
- Attitude becomes crouching
- Waddling gait
- Lateral compression/distraction tests are positive
- Cross leg test positive
- Direct pressure elicits tenderness over pubic symphysis and origin of adductor muscles
- Pain more on abduction of lower limb
- No local or general signs of inflammation
- X-ray—Early stage—no change. Late stage—pubic bodies look moth-eaten, rarefied and gaping widening of the symphysis (*See* **Fig. 9.23**), which gradually reossify as normal, bony architecture is restored
- In bone scan, the symphysis exhibits increased uptake
- MRI shows bone marrow oedema.

CHAPTER 10

Low Backache

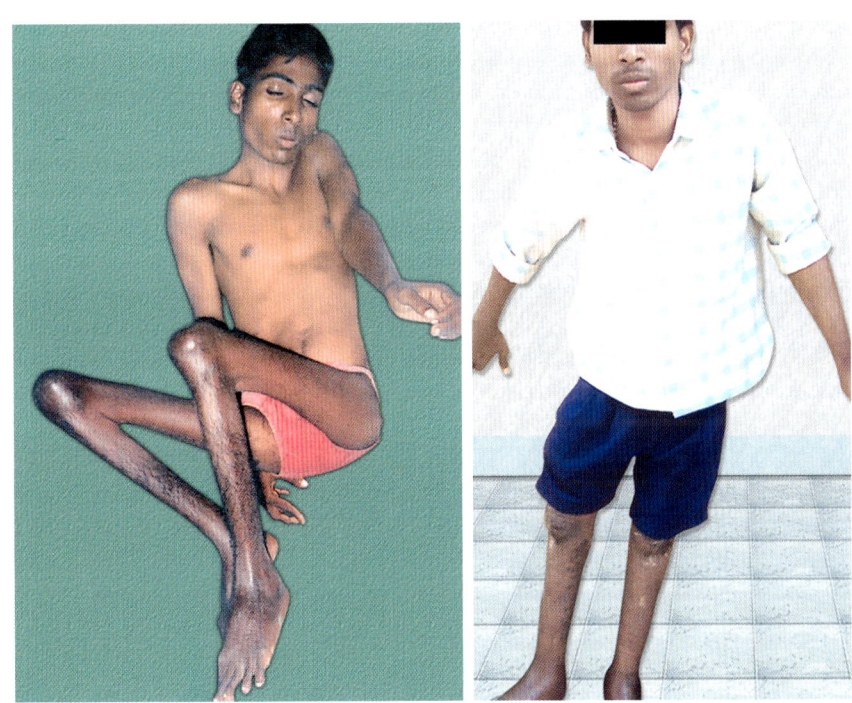

"Success is most often achieved by those who don't know that failure is inevitable."
—*Gabrielle Bonheur-Coco Chanel*

The recent discovery of a 47 million-year-old fossil (of a primate hailed by scientists as the equivalent of the Roseta stone) which resembles one of the earliest ancestors of the human race is a tremendous scientific achievement. 2,00,000 years ago the Neanderthal man did not suffer from low back pain, because he was not yet fully vertical. However, as the human being assumed upright posture, the manifestations of backache grew almost proportionately to the progress in civilization **(Fig. 10.1)**.

The human being is unique in having a bipedal gait. This causes a vertical loading of the spine and consequently varieties of low back and neck problems affect the human population. Low back pain (LBP) is experienced by 80–90% of the population, while 30–40% feel pain in the neck and arm, compared to 10–15% of the population feeling pain in the thoracic spines. LBP is second only to headache as a frequent source of pain in the body.

Lower back broadly anatomically consists of five lumbar vertebrae (stacked one upon the other connecting to the upper spine), sacrum and adjoining portion of pelvic bones; six intervertebral discs, spinal cord–cauda equina and nerves; facet joints and other small joints of spinal column; muscles, ligaments and other allied soft tissues—problems in any (or with other) of the above tissue/structure can be the cause of low backache.

Chronic low backache is proving itself as the second leading cause of disability worldwide with dramatically increasing prevalence. 60% or more people suffer from low back pain-demanding treatment in India. Low back pain patients are more prone to anxiety and depression (Wong JJ et al. 2019).

Low back pain is increasingly being recognised as one of the most common problems in orthopaedic practice today, behaving as a modern day epidemic affecting 60–75% of the working population of the world—more in developed and developing countries—probably due to altered lifestyle, increased tensions in life, lack of physical exercises/walking, prolonged sedentary lifestyle and occupations [increasing use of computers—computer backache, **(Fig. 10.1)**], increasing use of gadgetries in household works, overeating (fast food add to it), chronic alcoholism, chronic smoking, bad postures, lifting of heavy weight in bending position, heavy physical work, frequent bending, twisting, jumping, prolonged static postures, etc. Psychosocial risk factors are anxiety, depression, mental stress, distress, somatisation, work place factors.

Though low back pain is one of the most common symptom, yet it is the most elusive. *LBP may be defined as "pain, muscle tension or stiffness localised below the costal margin and above the inferior gluteal fold"* with/without leg pain [sciatica= lumbosacral radicular syndrome—(*Heijden et al. 1991*)].

Examining a patient with backache can itself cause both backache (because one must examine again and again from top to bottom performing different clinical tests) and headache to a clinician (because the cause can be numerous and intricate and malingerers are not easy to identify). The diagnostic process is mainly focussed on the triage of patients with specific or non-specific backache **(Table 10.1)**.

On no subject in orthopaedics can more controversies arise than on the problem of backache. Backache is one of the most common orthopaedic problems, and manifests as society's most expensive disease in the productive years. It is a common problem almost all over the globe. Any part of the back may ache, but the most common site is the lower back, i.e. lumbar and lumbosacral regions, followed by dorsolumbar

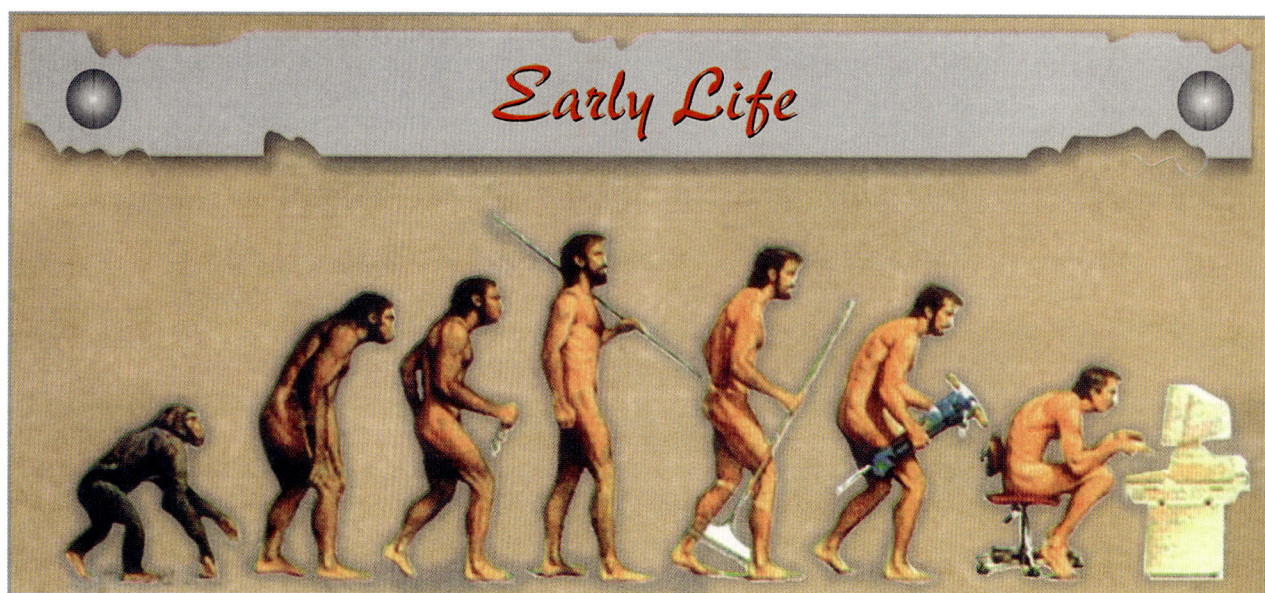

Fig. 10.1: Development of human erect posture; gradually deteriorating by modern working postures; continuous sitting over computer leads to computer backache.

TABLE 10.1: Low back pain (LBP).	
Specific LBP (10%)	**Non-specific LBP (90%)**
Symptoms caused by a specific pathophysiological mechanism, e.g. intervertebral disc prolapse, infection, osteoporosis, rheumatoid spondylitis, fracture, neoplasm, cauda-equina syndrome, etc.	Symptoms due to unrecognisable pathology and unknown cause. According to duration of LBP: LBP can be • Acute—<6 weeks • Subacute— >6 weeks, but <3 months • Chronic—>3 months

and dorsal regions. The *most common age group affected are adults and elderlies,* with the incidence *more among females.* With the march of civilisation and the consequent increasingly stressful life, the list of the causes of backache has also increased, as such that it has now assumed nearly epidemic proportions. However, increasing automation and robotisation, by helping to reduce 'backbreaking' stresses, hold promise in reducing the incidence of backache.

Five vertebral bodies and intervertebral discs withstand significant physiological loads. The vertebral bodies and discs form the *anterior column of spine,* which is concerned for resisting approximately 80% of axial compressive loads and maintaining spinal rigidity and alignment. The anterior portion of intervertebral disc is thicker than the posterior and is responsible for most of the lumbar lordosis.

The posterior column of spine, consisting of spinous process, laminae, transverse processes and facet joints, control movements and resist forces.

The main functional ligaments of lumbar spine are anterior and posterior longitudinal ligaments, interspinous ligaments and ligamentum flavum, which are oriented longitudinally along the spinal column and they resist stretch (mainly the flexion movements).

The *unit of intervertebral disc* may be considered to consist of:
- *Vertebral end plates* consisting of cortical bone in the periphery (ring apophysis of adolescents) and compressed cancellous bone in the central disc area covering about 70% of disc
- *Anulus fibrosus* consisting of multiple layers/lamellae of collagen fibres arranged circumferentially in the peripheral area of disc
- *Nucleus pulposus* is an incompressible semi-fluid jelly like material in the centre of disc space.

The cellular components of the disc are chondrocytes and fibroblastic types of cells arranged extensively in the intricate extracellular matrix of annulus fibrosus, nucleus pulposus and end plates.

Normally the water content of the disc is 70–90%.

Transitional lumbosacral anatomy (also known as *Bertolotti syndrome*) is present in 12–21% of population (Peh et al. 1999). Usually, the fifth lumbar vertebra is partially or completely sacralized or the first sacral vertebra is partially lumbarized with persistent caudal disc space.

Anatomically and functionally, the lower lumbar spine forms a more or less transitional zone from the more mobile trunk to the more static pelvic region. Thus, the lower lumbar region is the site for rotatory and shearing strains. Mechanically also, it is not suitably designed for biped weight bearing. Further this region is often a site for structural abnormalities (e.g. canal stenosis, pars inter-articularis defects). These reasons may explain the predilection of this region for disc disorders and backache.

The disabilities, length disparities and deformities of the lower limbs are accommodated to maximum possible extent by tilting of the pelvis either side ways or anteroposteriorly. This inherently puts the lower back to strain and gradually, patients start complaining of low backache.

Deformities, like scoliosis, kyphoscoliosis or even kyphosis of the spine (dorsal and/or lumbar), by changing the physiomechanics of posture and weight transmission also ultimately lead to strain at the low back.

Backache is most common in adult ladies, however, it can be the problem in any age. *Backache in young children should be a matter of concern.* In younger children, the cause is usually a serious disease (such as tuberculosis, tumour, etc.) and it should be investigated thoroughly. Children usually do not exaggerate the symptoms, nor they are malingerers. However, risk factors for LBP in children are similar to those in adults, such as heavy weight lifting, repetitive or sustained bendings, continuous sitting, obesity, cigarette smoking.

In *adolescents, Scheuermann's kyphosis* and spondylolysis should also be considered besides the common causes like tuberculosis, spondylitis, while assessing the cause of backache; pain from Scheuermann's kyphosis is localised to the midline in the scapular area, and presents with poor posture rather than pain.

■ USUAL CAUSES OF BACKACHE

Low back pain is a considerable health problem, specially in developed world. Low back pain seems to be *multifactorial in origin.* Still there are significant number of patients who do not have an identifiable cause for back pain and can be termed as non-specific back pain.

The *role of segmental instability* is now being increasingly recognised as one of the causes of low back pain.

As such, the list of causes of backache can be a very long one, but the **common causative factors** are:
- *Posture:* Certain postural defects while sitting, standing, sleeping, heavy weight lifting, prolonged standing, prolonged walking, working on heavy machines, working in stooping posture with legs close together, riding on fast

and jerky vehicles (horse riding, jeep riding, motor-bike riding) may lead to backache. Explore this possibility if no other organic cause is evident. Persons with protuberant abdomen, by virtue of constant dragging strain on the spinal ligaments, are liable to have backache, specially when they sit or stand for prolonged periods.

Individuals with tall slender physique, may develop postural defects, like gradual kyphosis in dorsolumbar region (usually in a young tall girl) or lumbar lordosis, both of which can cause dull backache.

Back pain which is exacerbated by neutral posture or lumbar extension may be originating from spondylolysis, facet degeneration or spinal stenosis

- *Congenital defects:* Defects in the vertebrae and their soft tissue allies (e.g. spina bifida, sacralisation of 5th lumbar vertebra **(Figs. 10.2A and B)** scoliosis, spondylolysis, spondylolisthesis, transitional vertebra can be potent causes of chronic backache—X-ray usually helps in the diagnosis.

Transitional vertebra (Bertolotti) Syndrome: In about 5% of general population, there may be partially sacralised or transitional vertebra at lumbosacral junction. Here the transverse process(es) get enlarged and articulates with the sacrum or pelvis as a neoarticulation

- *Injury:* Strain, sprain, ligamentous (e.g. sprung back—occurs due to tearing of all posterior supportive ligaments of lumbosacral region) and muscular injuries, fractures, dislocations, fracture-dislocation of vertebrae are common causes of backache. History of trauma and X-ray findings suggest the diagnosis.

Sometimes the history of injury is completely forgotten but the patient may suffer chronic backache due to a very old injury (Kummell's disease)

- *Intervertebral disc pathology:* In 1934, Mixter and Barr were the first to identify herniation of lumbar disc as a cause of low-back pain and sciatica.

Either due to increased turgidity or herniation (prolapse) of the nucleus pulposus, the intervertebral disc can become a potent cause for low backache. Affliction of lumbar spine can be linked to age-related changes in the intervertebral disc, zygapophyseal joints, and capsuloligamentous structures. Disc degeneration precedes all other changes, resulting in non-specific low backache, which can potentially advance into specific causes of low backache.

The pathophysiology of discogenic low back pain is not fully understood. *There are differences between degenerate discs which cause discogenic low back pain and those causing sciatica.* One must remember and analysis the statement of Cyriax – "all discs are alike, all other lesions are different".

Imaging studies have shown that radicular pain is not simply a mechanical phenomenon. It has been shown that degenerate disc tissue from patients with sciatica synthesises IL-6 and PGE. The production of the proinflammatory mediators and cytokines within the nucleus pulposus may be a major factor in the genesis of a painful lumbar disc. Sequestrated and extruded discs produce higher levels of these mediators than the intact ones.

The subject is usually a young male complaining of low backache mostly of sudden onset, with/without radiating pain in the lower limb and perhaps with some numbness and tingling.

- *SELF REDUCING' Disc lesion:* It typically occurs in young adult (20 to 40), who remain symptom free in morning to about noon even on mobility including extension of back and exertion. However, during the day backache comes on and gets worse. After going to bed pain gradually reduces and gets almost completely relieved in an hour or so.

In acute disc herniation (prolapse)—At the lower back, board like muscular rigidity and/or sciatic scoliosis are seen; coughing, sneezing, stooping, increased intra-abdominal pressure augment the symptoms (raised intra abdominal pressure during coughing and sneezing causes sudden expansion of the dura pressed against

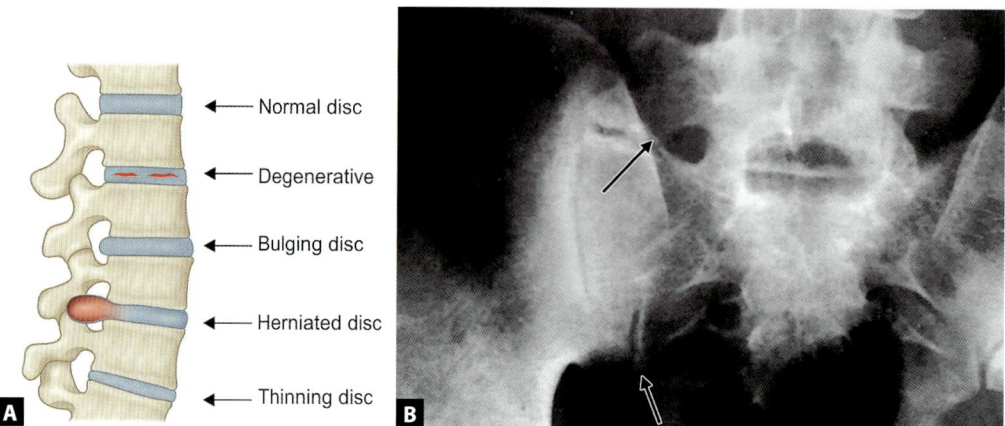

Figs. 10.2A and B: Besides intervertebral disc pathology, (Fig. 10.2A). Sacralisation of lumbar vertebrae can also cause low backache. Also note the features of sacroiliitis (Figs. 10.2A and 9.20).

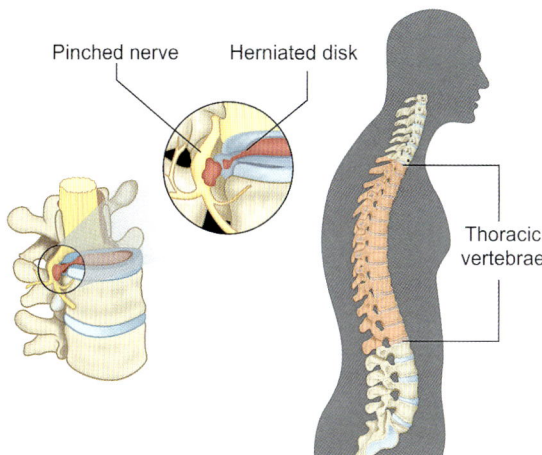

Fig. 10.3: Radiculopathy.

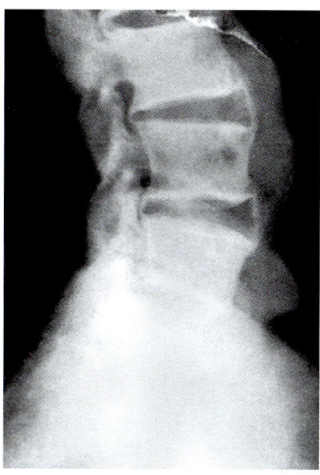

Fig. 10.4: Lumbar spondylosis.

the protrusion); straight leg raising up to or below 60°; positive sciatic stretch test and myelography confirm the pathology.

Waddell believed *"The diagnosis of disc prolapse is overused, misused and abused by both—the patients and the physicians."* The unwarranted increasing practice of ordering for MRI has undoubtedly added to this belief. Patients are also becoming overenthusiastic and ask for MRI even before get them examined for the backache.

In large posterocentral disc protrusion, the manifestations may be as acute lumbago, acute perineal pain and bilateral sciatica. In such situations, the accompaniment of *cauda equina syndrome*, should be suspected and assessed. In this syndrome the patient usually presents with typical triad of:
1. Saddle anaesthesia,
2. Bladder and/or bowel dysfunction and
3. Weakness in lower limbs. Early surgery is indicated in such cases (Gautschi et al. 1994).

Once diagnosed, discogenic low back pain, especially those associated with nerve root compression radiculitis radiculopathy **(Fig. 10.3)**, requires proper management. Most of them are amenable to non-surgical management (rest, pelvic traction, non-steroidal anti-inflammatory drugs (NSAIDs), heat therapy, lumbosacral belt, physiotherapy, epidural corticoid injection, etc.). The resistant and frequently recurred cases and those with neurodeficit, significant progressive leg pain or weakness and numbness or cauda equina syndrome require surgical management (discectomy). *Today lumbar microdiscectomy is being considered as the gold standard of discectomy techniques for the treatment of low back pain from nerve root compression* related to disc trauma or degenerative disease. However, **Ozonucleolysis** (ozone discectomy), developed in Italy, appears to be a safe and least invasive therapeutic option. It comprises of intradiscal and periradicular injections of medical ozone mixture under image guidance.

Allied conditions which may lead to backache are:
Lumbar spondylosis (degenerative changes in the lumbar region) **(Fig. 10.4)**.
Spondylolysis (weakness in pars interarticularis).
Spondylolisthesis (slipping of the vertebra along with the spinal column above, over the vertebra below)

- *Spinal stenotic syndrome:* It can be defined as the *narrowing of the osteoligamentous vertebral canal and/or the intervertebral foramina causing compression of the thecal sac and/or the caudal nerve roots;* at a single vertebral level, narrowing may affect the whole canal or part of it (Postacchini 1983).

Spinal stenosis can be categorised according to the spinal zone affected, such as cervical, thoracic or lumbar. It is most common in lumbar region followed by cervical and rare in thoracic. It may be localised or diffuse affecting multiple levels.

Radiologists have quantified stenosis to be less than 1.5 cm^2 in total area or less than 11.5 mm in AP diameter (Ulrich et al. 1980, Modie et al. 1988).

Spinal canal stenosis can be of three forms:
- *Primary stenosis*
  - Congenital
  - Developmental—postnatal defective development of vertebrae; achondroplastic and constitutional stenosis.
- *Secondary stenosis*—Compression is due to acquired causes, e.g. spondylotic changes, Fluorosis, Paget's disease, old vertebral fracture
- *Combined stenosis*—Combined causes of primary and secondary stenosis.

Causes of Stenosis

- Congenital narrowing of vertebral canal.
- Acquired causes—Traumatic, degenerative, neoplastic, iatrogenic. Degenerative spinal stenosis is a progressive disorder which involves almost entire spinal motion segment.

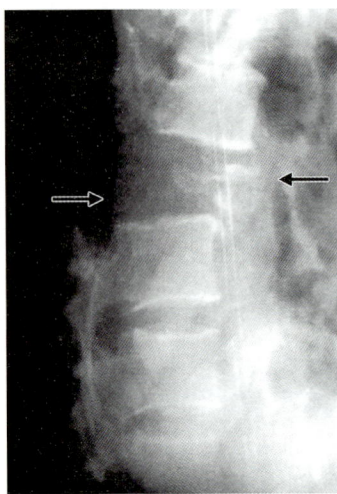

Fig. 10.5: Meningioma of L3 body presented as chronic backache. A lady of 30 years presented with chronic low back pain NOT responding to various non invasive treatment; she was also, complaining vague neurogenic pain in buttocks and lower limbs. Laminectomy approach and with cautions blunt-finger dissection revealed (tough)/soft tissue of ash-look; histopathology revealed as meningioma. By 4month she recovered and resumed the work of housewife. Gradually she lost to follow-up.

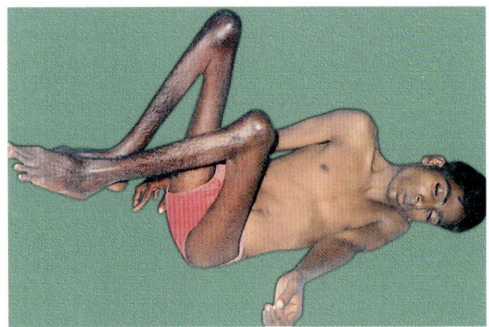

Fig. 10.6: 9 years back before presenting was treated for low backache—ultimately was bed ridden due to ankylosed spine, hips and knees for eight years.

Clinical features: Clinical features are low backache, intermittent claudications (leg cramps) and there may be deep tenderness in the affected zone.

Lumbar spinal canal stenosis remains one of the most frequently seen and clinically important degenerative spinal disorders in the aging population.

Symptoms: *Symptoms due to lumbar canal stenosis* are usually of insidious onset and progress slowly. They are as follow:

- *Vague low backache and stiffness*—worsening with activity (mechanical pain) and improving with rest
- *Pain in the leg* in the lumbar canal stenotic syndrome are of two types—(a) *Unilateral radicular type* of leg pain occurs in about 20% of patients and is more often seen with severe foraminal or lateral recess stenosis, (b) *Bilateral neurogenic claudication in leg*—symptoms of aching, cramping or burning sensation in legs starting from buttocks often progress distally to the thighs, calves and feet. These symptoms are classically exacerbated by standing and by exercising in an erect or extended posture and are relieved by sitting and forward flexion. Patients usually assume a hunched or 'semian' posture while walking. This phenomenon can be explained by the fact that *the size of spinal canal varies with different posture—single test for diagnosis of lumbar spine canal stenosis.* However, for an adequate evaluation of the cross-sectional area, CT or MRI should be performed with axial loading in patients who have symptoms of lumbar canal stenosis
- Lumbar Canal Stenosis, a common cause of low back pain, is now conventionally treated with surgical decompression with or without fusion. Transforaminal lumbar interbody fusion (TLIF) is usually performed with bilateral pedicle screw fixation and interbody cage with optimal outcome. Unilateral TLIF in selected patients provide adequate decompression and fusion.
- Ankylosing spondylitis is the most common entity of the seronegative spondyloarthropathies. Spondyloarthropathies include chronic inflammatory rheumatic diseases in which sacroiliac joints and spinal columns are mainly affected. These entities are seronegative since they are not associated with positive rheumatoid factor or other serologic auto-antibody abnormalities.
- *Ankylosing spondylitis and rheumatoid spondylitis (Sacroiliitis—see* **Figs. 9.20 and 12.74A**): Ankylosing spondylitis (derived from Greek roots ankylos — meaning bent + spondylos—meaning spinal vertebra: Marie-Strumpell's or von Bechterew's disease—both contributed to the clinical description of ankylosing spondylitis in the late 19th century) is a chronic systemic inflammatory disease affecting mainly the sacroiliac joints, spine, and sometimes also peripheral joints.

Ankylosing spondylitis most common of seronegative spondyloarthropathy conditions. **(Figs. 10.6 and 10.7)** The basic pathological lesion occurs at the entheses i.e. the sites of attachment of ligaments, tendons and joint capsule to bone. Enthesopathy (inflammation occurring at insertion sites) occurs at enthesis or subchondral bone, ultimately it results in new bone formation, calcification, and ossification.

HLA – B37 is present in 90–95% of patients of ankylosing spondylitis, however, it is neither screening test nor diagnostic test. Ankylosing spondylitis is a common condition affecting young males below 40 (male: female :: 4:1) and usually diagnosed by complaints of *morning stiffness* [more than 45 minutes (cf. in degenerative spine stiffness <30 minutes)] and even *nocturnal stiffness* which improves with exercises and movements (cf. inflammatory conditions, e.g. tuberculosis, in which pain increases with exercises and movements), pain in the

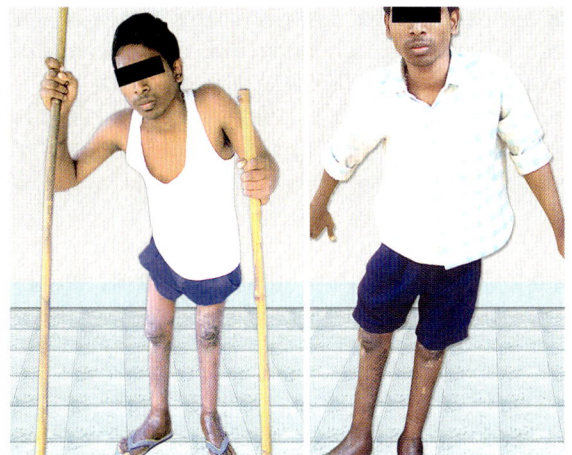

Fig. 10.7: Same patient **(Fig. 10.6)** walking with sticks in the process of physiotherapy after four stages of operations on both hips and both knees in seven months.

back (dorsolumbar or lumbar region) which gets relieved after exercises (spinal stress tests). On examination, comparatively *stiff (even flat board like) low back, sacroiliac joint tenderness (2.5 cm below posterior superior iliac spine or by direct pressure by pelvic compression test), decreased spinal mobility and limited chest expansion* (limitation below 2.5 cm expansion at the 4th intercostal space due to costovertebral joint involvement) is diagnostic. X-ray shows fuzziness, obvious erosions, mild sclerosis and later on fusion of sacroiliac joints, and bamboo spine. CT usually shows asymmetric erosions and sclerosis **(refer Fig. 9.20)** earlier and more clearly. MRI findings precede plain X-ray findings about two years. Using special MRI sequences, it is easy to look for erosions, sclerosis, fat infiltration and marrow oedema **(refer Figs. 9.21 and 9.22)**.

Iridocyclitis occurs in about 20% of cases. Aortic regurgitation may occur as a late complication in few patients.

Rheumatoid arthritis can also affect the sacroiliac joints, causing low backache

- *Infective conditions:* Acute infection presents apparently and is not a common cause. Among the chronic infections, tuberculosis of the spine is the most common cause. Other causes may be pyogenic osteomyelitis, syphilitic back, or *B. coli* infection.

  Osteoporotic compression fractures (e.g. in osteoporosis, osteolytic vertebral metastasis, myeloma, vertebral haemangioma, etc.) has emerged as a major cause of persistant backache. In patients with pain unresponsive to standard medical treatment, vertebral body cement augmentation in the form of *percutaneous vertebroplasty* has been found to be relatively safe and effective procedure by significant pain relief, increased function and quality of life. Success rate of vertebroplasty, on overall assessment, exceeds 90% with less than 1% of complication

- *Neoplastic conditions*
  In the benign group
  - Osteoid osteoma, aneurysmal bone cyst, haemangioma, neurofibroma and meningioma **(*see* Fig. 10.5)**

  In the malignant group
  - Secondary carcinomatosis, multiple myeloma, Hodgkins deposit, lymphosarcoma, giant cell tumour, osteogenic sarcoma.

  Apart from these, malformations (angiomatous) and neoplasms of the spinal cord may also be responsible for backache.

- *Degenerative arthrosis of spine:* In elderly subjects, low backache, usually variably relieved after some activities and massage, may be due to degenerative changes in the spine, with/without primary healed pathology and/or deformity

- *Senile osteoporosis:* Elderly subjects, usually ladies complain of constant mild backache. With typical rounded kyphosis X-ray is confirmatory

- *Other causes in ladies:* Leucorrhoea, pelvic inflammatory diseases, repeated pregnancy, uterine disorders (prolapse, growths), and intrauterine contraceptive devices

- *Metabolic:* Osteomalacia **(Fig. 9.25)**, alkaptonuria **(Fig. 10.8)**
  Osteomalacia (analogue of rickets occurring in the adult skeleton)—Usually child bearing-age group mother, with multiple quick succession of pregnancies, complains of constant dull boring pain. Flat bones are tender. Pelvis may be deformed (trefoil pelvis), classical Looser's zone in X-rays (especially of femur and tibia), which are transverse radiolucent lines surrounded by a small amount of sclerotic bone. In advanced cases, typical 'trifoil pelvis' develops

- *Malingerer's backache:* This is a usual problem in industrial workers, which can be suspected in lack of any organic pathology, and confirmed by their bizarre manifestations (mostly unrelated), and watching the patients activities at home and in society

- *Compensation backache:* With a view to exploit the employer and/or insurance company for undue compensation, several workers keep on complaining about backache with no definite and discernible organic pathology. Low back pain is a favourite complain of malingerers

- *Abdominal and pelvic causes:* Backache may be a manifestation of abdominal visceral or pelvic (genitourinary) pathologies. Upper abdominal conditions can cause pain in the dorsolumbar region; lower abdominal conditions in lumbar region; and pelvic pathologies in lumbosacral, sacral and sacroiliac regions. Nowhere in the spine, any accountable pathology can be delineated

- *General (miscellaneous) causes:* Exposure to cold, viral infections (e.g. influenza virus), fibrositis, myositis, chronic constipation, febrile illness, depressive psychosis

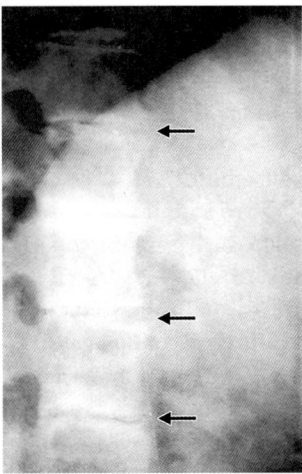

Fig. 10.8: Alkaptonuria (Ochronosis, Ochronotic arthritis). Note the degenerative calcification of the intervertebral discs. Alkaptonuria is a rare hereditary disorder of tyrosine metabolism, where there is deficiency of homogentisic acid oxidase enzyme resulting in increased excretion of homogentisic acid in urine (approximately 3–7 g per day) and accumulation of oxidised homogentisic acid and its polymers in soft tissues resulting in degenerative arthritis. The musculoskeletal manifestation of alkaptonuria is called 'ochronosis' (coined by Rudolf Virchow because of the ochra or yellow appearance of cartilage). The patients are usually asymptomatic until early adulthood. It is a congenital and inherited as Mendelian recessive trait mostly occurring in offsprings of consanguineous marriages. Homogentisic acid is deposited in tissues like sclerae, ligaments, tendons, cartilage, intervertebral disc which turn black due to the pigment. Homogentisic acid is present in urine turns black on heating or dark brown on standing or in adding an oxidation agent. Bluish green colouration of urine with the addition of a drop of dilute ferric chloride solution is diagnostic. Almost all alkaptonuries develop ochronosis by the midlife age – i.e. pigmentation – yellow appearance of cartilage and fibrous tissue of body. Alkaptonuria usually progress to ochronosis and arthropathy of hips, knees, shoulders, sternoclavicular joints with pain and limitation of movements. There may be associated CVS, genitourinary and upper respiratory tract involvement. Management is mainly symptomatic. Joint involvement if crippling, requires reconstruction.

- Working women with fast life are liable to suffer *"fanatic life syndrome"* (FLS) manifesting as exhaustion, burnout feeling, backache, etc. due to greater pressure to juggle work on demanding career and home commitments for a nuclear family
- *Ligamentous postural syndrome*: Back pain occurs and pain occurs and increases by maintaining a particular posture and relieves by altering the posture. Barber (1964) termed this ligamentous, postural syndrome as *'the theatre cocktail party syndrome'* – which is typically seen in young adults, in which due to discomfort/pain in ligaments, it becomes impossible to sit in the theatre or stand in the cocktail party.
- *Idiopathic:* While examining a patient with low backache, one should follow the method of examination of the spine. However, as seen in the above mentioned causes of low backache, one will be obliged to examine the lower limbs, abdomen and pelvic region. Diagnosis by 'exclusion' is markedly helpful in coming to a conclusion. Of course, corroboratory investigations should also be done in order to clinch the diagnosis.

If no obvious cause (e.g. caries spine, spondylolisthesis, or advanced ankylosing spondylitis) is detected on routine examinations, it is worth while to put the lower back to stress and recommended postural exercises and note the results. In backache, due to postural defects, spondylotic changes and in early ankylosing spondylitis, patient definitely feels better after doing the exercises.

Referred (pain) backache should also be kept in mind, if no obvious musculoskeletal cause is detected. Referred backache may be even from pathologies like oesophageal carcinoma, peptic ulcer, pancreatitis (acute or chronic), pancreatic carcinoma, renal pathology including carcinoma, retroperitoneal pathology (e.g. lymphoma), aortic aneurysm, spinal cord pathology including tumour.

Before starting the clinical examination of patients of backache, understanding about the followings should help:

Backache is the symptom complex which should be unleased and analysed by proper clinical examination and proper investigations. A careful history, detailed in chronological sequence must be taken – Not in a hurry History is the record and story of the past and present suffering and it constitutes the basis and proper planning of future treatment, prognosis and prevention.

Symptoms, concerning backache, can be broadly grouped under three headings:

Lumbago—is a sudden attack of severe low back pain leading to some extent of fixation and twinges on attempted movement.

Backache—is a vague word denoting any discomfort or pain (usually dull and chronic in nature) in the lower back.

Sciatica **(Fig. 8.94)** *(Pain in the distribution of sciatic nerve)*—It denotes pain which was originally described by Hippocrates in 400 BC. radiates from buttock to the posterior region of thigh and calf. It usually is limited to a specific dermatome (like L_4, L_5, S_1 or S_2). It may be accompanied by paraesthesia and sensory and/or motor deficit. In sciatica, unilateral pain in the concerned dermatome usually results by pressure on dural sleeve of one of lower lumbar nerve roots.

In patients under 60 years of age sciatica usually recovers within 12 month of the onset of radicular pain.

In sciatica, it is important to distinguish radicular pain from dural pain. The latter is extrasegmentally referred, hence is experienced over a large area than a dermatome. All the different aspects of pain should be explored like, on set, localization, progression radiation with its direction, duration, influence of posture and movements on pain, continuous or intermittent effects of stepping, walking, climbing stairs, squatting, Buddha-sitting, getting up straight from sitting, coughing, sneezing, stooping (forward bending), backward and side bendings, attempts of lifting some weight etc.- on the pain. If the patient complains of paraesthesia, especially *"pins and needles"* sensation – it is pathognomonic of pressure on or inflammation of the peripheral nervous system.

Enquire about time of starting of pain – morning, daytime, while going to bed, lying flat or an sides, turning in bed on sides.

Onset of pain—sudden, gradual, on some activity

Nature of pain, duration of pain – momentary, continuous, pain free intervals, site of pain-upper lumbar, central, unilateral, bilateral, low back, buttock(s), thigh(s), leg(s), ankle(s), foot(feet), toe(toes), sole(s).

A genuine patient usually places his/her palm at the site of maximum pain. A psychological unstable patient does not touch the painful area, but only points the site vaguely with the thumb.

Bilateral vague leg pain is usually dural pain.

Segmental pain in both legs may occur due to two protrusions.

Radicular pain in both lower limbs usually occurs in spinal stenosis, lateral recess stenosis, spondylolisthesis or even metastatic neoplasm

Iliac arteries thrombosis and even osteoarthritis of hip joint may produce intermittent claudication and pain in both legs.

The level and site of pain in the back and buttock may help in indicating the cause and guiding the treatment to variable extent.

In backache with dural reference, pain is usually located in the lumbo-sacral region and may radiate to one or even both buttocks.

Pain in the upper lumbar area may be referred from some abdominal pathologies including aortic aneurysm and even malignant conditions.

Pain and numbness in sacral, coccygeal and perineal region may be due to compression or affection of S_4 root.

Pain in *lower buttock* indicates a segmental reference from S_2.

Early morning pain – during or just after leaving the bed and which gradually eases out with activities and/or exercise is suggestive of ankylosing spondylitis. Sometimes early morning pain is caused by *discodural interaction*, in which case the increased hydration of disc, in lying down position, probably increases as existing small posterior bulge, which slowly compresses the dura mater leading to gradual increase in pain much earlier in morning with a disc prolapse, the patient complains of pain and stiffness in back in the morning.

■ INVESTIGATION

Investigation for back pain is determined by the nature of pain, age of patient, clinical history and provisional diagnosis. Relevant investigations include blood tests, nerve conduction test, imaging (X-ray, CT scanning, MRI, dual energy X-ray absorptiometry, myelography). Plain X-ray is almost always done, however, subsequent tests should be ordered according to the suspected responsible tissue (i.e. whether of neurological, or soft tissues, or bony origin). Other imaging technique like, computed tomography (CT), magnetic resonance imaging (MRI) or single-photon emission computed tomography (SPECT) should be ordered according to indication. MRI is most useful in disc-related problems. Provocative discography is useful investigation for diagnosing discogenic low back pain. It is a subjective test relying, on the radiologist's and patients perceptions to determine the result. Bone scanning is useful in assessing the age of vertebral fracture, suspected infection, metastasis, etc. Along with SPECT scan provides sensitive analysis of metastatic disease.

■ SUMMARY OF MANAGEMENT OF LBP

Management of low back pain should be started after localizing its, site and cause. *Management* of low back pain may be:

A. Nonsurgical—Medications (NSAID, muscle relaxants, oral steroids, analgesic; injections— myofascial tender trigger points injections of lidocaine, steroids, normal saline; Facet joint injections—fluoroscopically-guided local anaesthetic blocks of joints or its nerve supply; Epidural injection of steroid; short-term bed rest and to remain active; physiotherapy; electric stimulation — transcutaneous electric nerve stimulation (TENS); traction; manipulation and mobilization; exercises; acupuncture and massage.

B. Surgical—Surgical arthrodesis is gold standard for failed non-surgically treated cases.

Recent surgical trial treatments for degenerative lumbar disc are: Annuloplasty—intradiscal electrothermal therapy (use of radiofrequency to alter or shorten collagen fibres in capsulorrhaphy procedures in peripheral joints (Saal and Saal 2002); Percutaneous nucleotomy and nucleoplasty; dynamic stabilization devices—stabilizing the degenerative segment without associated arthrodesis; Artificial disc replacement [(a) Artificial nucleus replacement, (b) Total disc replacement].

Management of low back pain, specially the non-specific ones is more complex than the understanding their etiology and risk factors.

Low backache is being treated with variable effectiveness as follows:

- Drugs—Non-narcotic analgesics, aspirin, analgesics; NSAIDs; Muscle relaxants; Antidepressants; Mood elevators
- Local application—Analgesic; counter irritants; oil massage
- Heat therapy—Dry heat, moist heat, electric pad, mud pack, infrared, short wave diathermy
- Physiotherapy—Back muscle exercise, massage, manipulation, TENS, ultrasonics, magnetic therapy. Manipulation Should be avoided in any inflammatory or neoplastic lesion or compression of S_4 root.
- Back supports—Lumbosacral belt, magnetic belt

- Acupuncture, moxibustion, tattooing
- Traction—pelvic traction
- Injection therapy
  - Epidural injection
  - Facet joint injections
  - Local (at pain site injections; injection over iliac crest for iliac crest pain; injection over iliolumbar ligament for non-specific low back pain)
  - Trigger point injections for myofascial pain syndrome
- Intradiscal electrothermal therapy
- Radiofrequency denervation
- Surgical treatment
  - Fusion surgery
  - Artificial disc replacement
- Miscellaneous
  - Postural adjustment while working, sitting, standing, walking **(Fig. 10.10)**
  - Adjustments of bed, mattress, pillow
  - Adjustments, improving or change in profession, job, and work environment

- Back schools; back care education
- Ergonomics
- Behavioural therapy
- Electromyographic biofeedback
- Intensive multidisciplinary treatment programmes.

The normal cross-sectional area of lumber spine is 150–200 mm^2 and a decrease to less than 100 mm^2 may be a more reliable indicator of the lumber canal stenosis (Schonstrom et al. 1985). Disc herniation can produce central canal stenosis.

■ PREVENTION OF LOW BACKACHE

Low back pain is a dynamic entity with rates of incidence, recurrence and recovery. Conservative care of LBP is just an effort to help patients manage their predicament when they are at their worst rather than to cure them of this affliction.

Except for the low backache due to organic causes (such as neoplasm, infection, trauma, congenital defects) most of the low backache can be prevented by:

- Regular exercises to maintain spine strong and flexible **(Fig. 10.9)** (Help taken from M/s Jenburkt Leaflet).

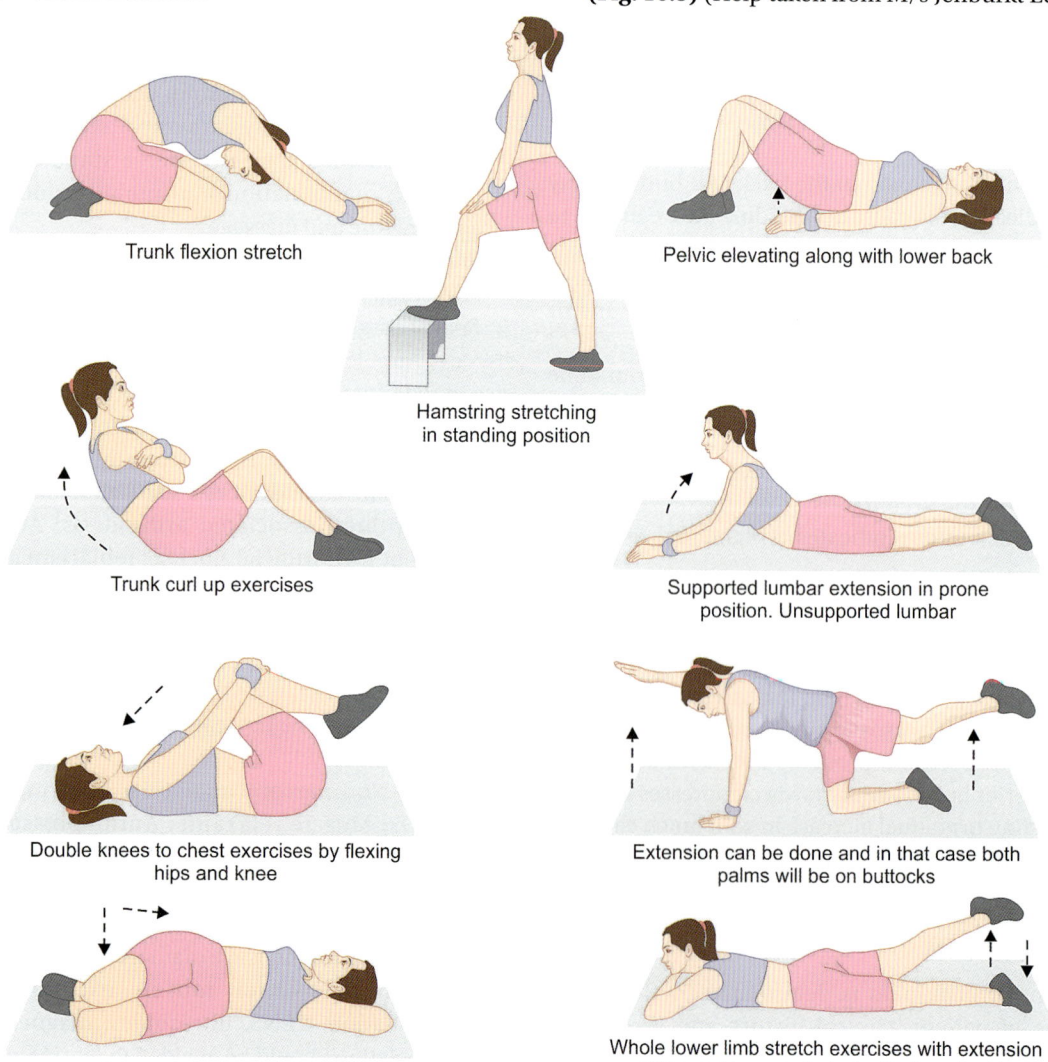

Fig. 10.9: Shows the exercises to be done regulary to keep the back (Spine) strong and flexible.

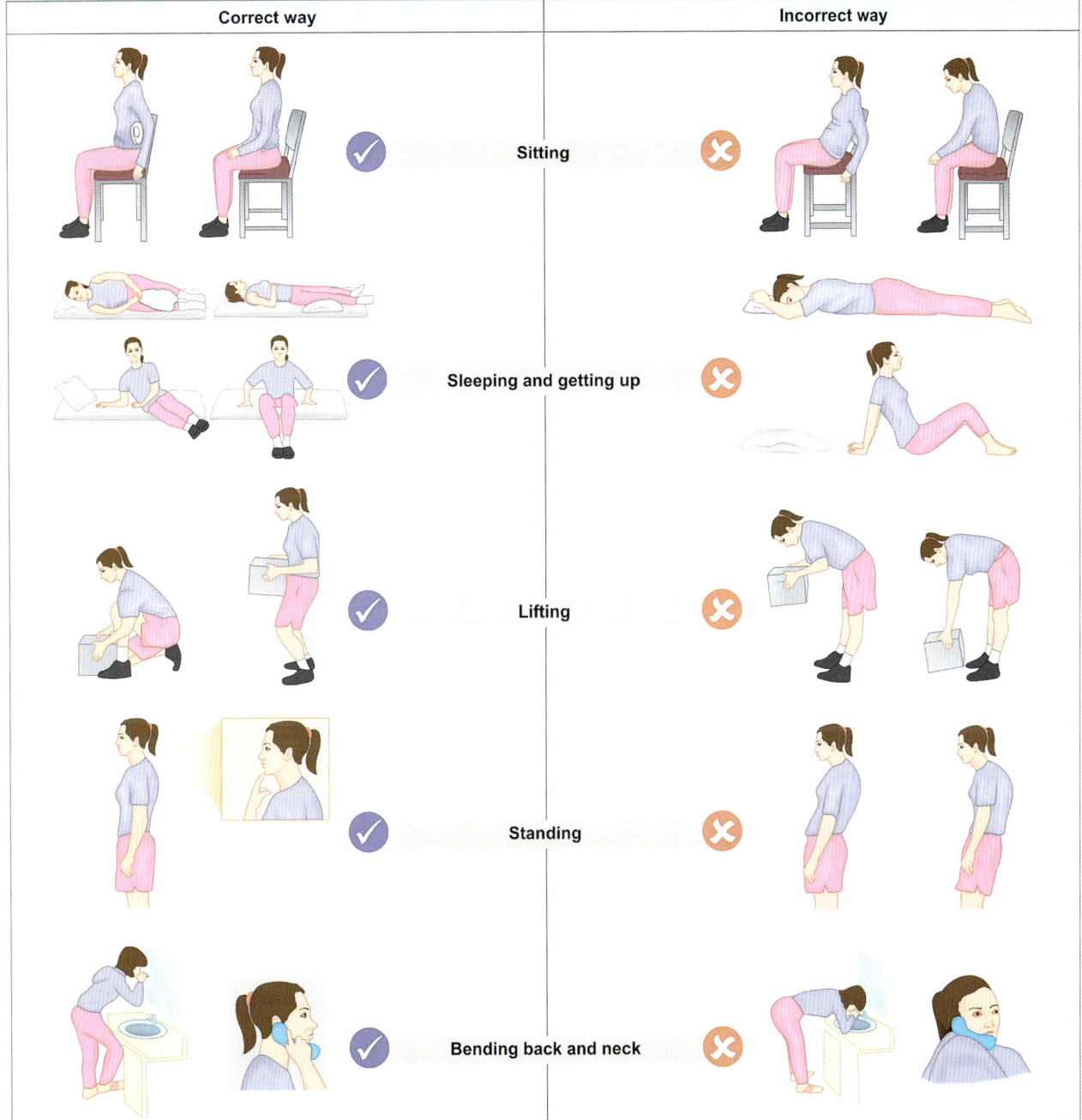

Fig. 10.10: Shows correct and incorrect ways of adopting posture of back for regular (common activities).

- Maintaining the proper posture while sitting, standing, walking, sleeping and other activities. One should not slouch

Using the correct way of sitting, standing, lifting, bending, sleeping, and moving techniques **(Fig. 10.10)**
- Maintaining proper body weight; being overweight puts a strain on the back muscles, ligaments, and spinal joints
- Proper nutrition and care to avoid developing osteoporosis
- Avoiding sagging bed and posture while sleeping
- Avoiding improper and overuse of back
- Avoiding smoking, too much alcohol and chronic constipation (specially due to nonvegetarian diet and fast foods).

Psychological and social factors, e.g. working habits, profession, domestic environment and associated compensation claims have definitely influenced the problems of low back pain and are rather better predictors of outcome of the management than the clinical and imaging findings. Patients with somatisation and doctor shopping are at a higher risk for a poor outcome of the management.

BIBLIOGRAPHY

1. Barbor R. Treatment for chronic low back pain. Proceedings of the IVth International Congress on Physical Medicine, Paris 1964.
2. Colhoun E, McCall IW, Williams L, Cassar Pullicino VN. Provocative discography as a guide to planning operations on the spine. J Bone Joint Surg (Br). 1988;70B:267-71.
3. Gautschi OP, Cadosch D, Hildebrandt G. Emergency scenario: Cauda equina syndrome- assessment and management. Praxis (Bern 1994). 2008;97:305-12.
4. Harrold AJ. Alkaptonuric arthritis. J Bone Joint Surg. 1956; 38:532.
5. Kang JD, Georgescu HI, McIntyre-Larkin L, et al. Herniated lumbar intervertebral discs spontaneously produce matrix metalloproteinases, nitric oxide interleukin-6 and prostaglandin E2 spine. 1996;21:271-7.
6. Mixter WJ, Barr JS. Rupture of the intervertebral disc with involvement of the spinal canal. New England J Med. 1934; 211:210-5.
7. O'Donnell JL, O'Donnell AL. Prostaglandin E2 content in herniated lumbar disc disease. Spine. 1996;21:1653-5.
8. Postacchine F. Lumbar stenosis and pseudostenosis: Definition and classification of pathology. Inl J Orhop Traumatol. 1983;9: 939-50.
9. Schonstrom NS, Bolender NF, Spengler DM. The pathomorphology of spinal, stenosis as seen on CT scans of the lumbar spine. Spine (Philadelphia PA 1976), 1985;10(9): 806-11.
10. Spivak JM. Degenerative lumbar spinal stenosis. J Bone Joint Surg. 1998;80A:1053-66.
11. Van der Heijden GJMG, Bouter LM, Terpstra-lindeman E. The efficacy of traction for low back pain. Results of a pilot study. (In Dutch) Ned T Fysiotherapie. 1991;101:37-43.
12. Waddell G, Mani CJ, Morris EU, et al. Normality and reliability in the clinical assessment of backache. Br Med J. 1982;284: 1519-23.
13. Wong JJ, Cote P, Tricco AC et al. Examining the effects of low back pain and mental health symptoms on healthcare utilisation and costs: a protocol for a population – based cohort study BMJ Open 2019; 9: e031749. dol: 10.1136/bmj open – 2019 – 031749.

CHAPTER 11

Examination of Paralytic Patients*

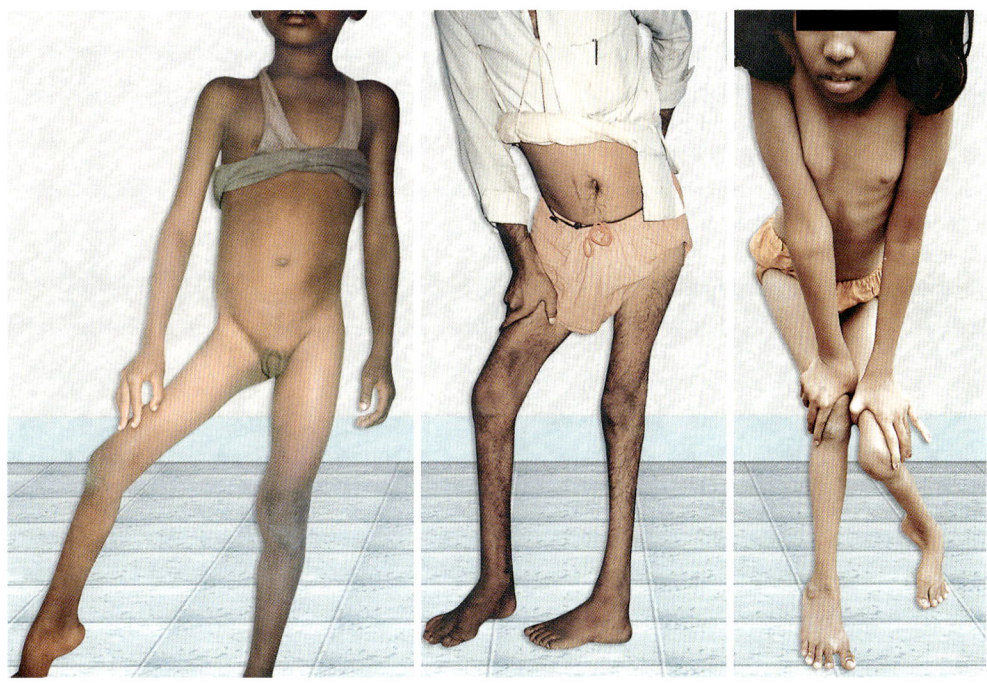

"You can't get attention of one who focussed on himself."
Everything should be made as simple as possible, but NOT simpler.
—SP

*Also see Chapters on Spine and Low Backache

"The human foetus, though no bigger than a green pea, yet is furnished with all its part."
—*(Antonj van Leeuwenhoek, 1683)*

■ INTRODUCTION

Global status report of WHO (quoted by Dash D 2017) has categorized cardiovascular diseases (including coronary artery disease, stroke, artherosclerosis and heart failure) as leading causes of death and disabilities, followed by menace of diabetes—these have more or less replaced the position of infectious diseases which led to death and persistent disabilities and dependency.

The examination and assessment of a paralytic and dependent disabled persons must be rehabilitation-oriented from the very beginning.

Most of the paralytic conditions do not recover fully. Assessment should be psychologically, socially, economically and rehabilitation oriented. The assessment must aim not only at finding out the disability of the patient, rather, the functional capabilities with which the patient has been left, and the potentiality of improvement must be fully explored. Even with residual powers, tremendous, sometimes unbelievable functional capacities (gains) can be achieved. One should remember that a tiny 'ant' bestowing tremendous strength can boost a burden 50 times its weight.

In examining such a patient hitherto, the main aim has been to find out the cause of paralysis by assessing as discussed in the chapter on spine. This chapter mainly aims at assessing the extent of residual disabilities and the potential for improvement.

The assessment of a handicapped person should aim to find out his/her disabilities and potential abilities. *The National Centre for Medical Rehabilitation and Research has developed a model to translate* medical findings into clinical benefits for individuals with disabling conditions by *describing five domains of disabilities:*
1. *Pathophysiology*
2. *Impairment*
3. *Functional limitation*
4. *Disability*
5. *Societal limitation (NCMRR 1993).*

In the International Classification of Impairment, Disabilities and Handicaps of world the World Health Organisation also widens the perspective from a narrow focus on disability to an emphasis on health and function in society (ICIDH-2 1999).

Syzygiology (the study of interrelationships or interdependencies specially of the whole, as opposed to the study of separate parts or isolated functions)—is of great importance in these paralytic patients **(Figs. 11.1 to 11.3)**.

To project the positivity of handicapped persons', in India this word has been replaced by 'DIVYANG' (which Denotes–Connected with a God a Goddess–'DIVYA'. This word was suggested by Hon'ble Prime Minister of India Shri Narendra Modi *'Man Ki Bat'* episode in 2015.

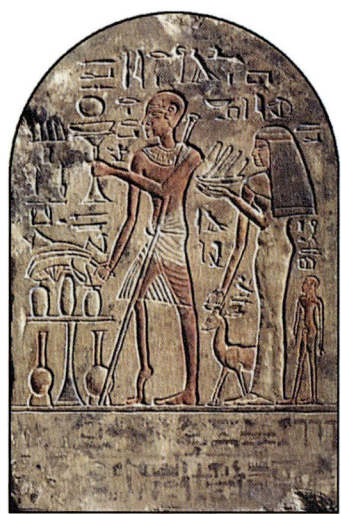

Fig. 11.1: Roma (eighteenth dynasty), door-keeper and priest of the temple of Astarte at Memphis, who suffered from poliomyelitis of the right lower limb (still kept at the Ny Carlsberg Museum, Copenhagen).

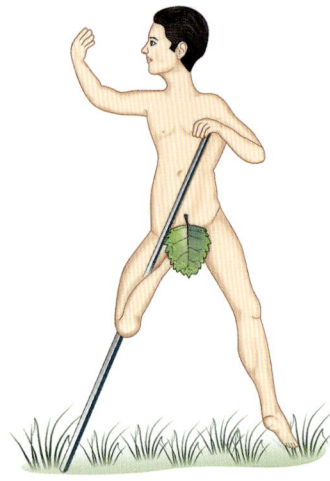

Fig. 11.2: Poliomyelitic deformities of the lower limbs drawn on an antique Italian jar dating from the fourth century BC. (Musée du Louvre, Paris).

■ ANATOMICAL CONSIDERATION

There are approximately 640 muscles constituting up to 40% of adult body mass.

Skeletal muscle consists of cells called *fibres*, which are grouped into *fascicles*. The *motor unit* consists of a *lower motor neuron* originating from an anterior horn cell in spinal cord, and all the muscle fibres it innervates. Each muscle fibre is surrounded by a plasma membrane called sarcolemma. Muscle fibres contain myofilaments called actin, troponin, tropomyosin and myosin, which are contractile proteins.

Muscular contraction, and relaxation occurs as follows: Muscle contraction occurs by shortening of myofilaments within muscle fibres. Stimulation causes an *action potential* to be transmitted along the sarcolemma then through the 'T' tubule system to the sarcoplasmic reticulum. This causes release of calcium into the sarcoplasm. As the

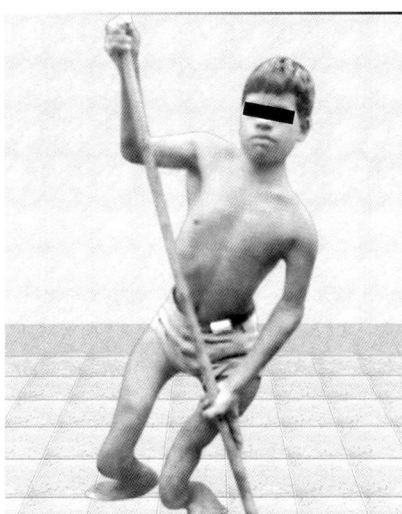

Fig. 11.3: Judge ability more than disability of a physically handicapped person (divyang). In spite of gross deformities he is in job.

calcium concentration increases, actin is released from a state of inhibition allowing actin-myosin cross-linkage and shortening of the myofilaments. The muscle fibre shortens until calcium is actively pumped back into the sarcoplasmic reticulum which breaks the cross-links, leading to relaxation of fibres.

Paralysis

Loss or less of power of muscles has been defined as follows:
- 'Paralysis' for complete loss of power
- 'Paresis' for diminution (incomplete loss) of power
- 'Palsy' is a non-specific (loosely spoken) descriptive term which indicates varying degrees of paralysis and/or paresis.

Paralysis is broadly of two types:
1. Loss or less of function of muscles with wasting of muscles occur in lower motor neuron type of paralysis and peripheral nerve lesions (muscle wasting is less)—it is called *flaccid paralysis (paraplegia)*. Here the muscle tone is reduced and response to tendon reflexes are lessened or lost. Fasciculations are seen in lower motor neuron lesions. Damage of the nerve supplying a muscle leads to spontaneous motor unit firing which is visible as a twitching of muscle fibres.
2. Excess of function, increased tone of muscle and uninhibited reflexes occur due to excessive unbridled neurological stimulation to muscles, which leads to spasticity—it is called *spastic paralysis (paraplegia)* that occurs due to upper motor neuron lesions. Fasciculations are absent in these lesions.

Muscles Commonly Affected in Polio-Paralysis

Poliomyelitis is a highly infections viral disease exclusive to humans. Causing degeneration of the anterior horn cells and ventral nerve roots and certain brainstem motor nuclei leading to the lower motor neuron type of paralysis of the affected muscles. One of the three polio viruses transmitted primarily via faecal-oral route spreads to the central nervous system through haematogenous route.

Since the extensive immunisation by Sabin oral vaccine, containing all three types of attenuated virus, the incidence of poliomyelitis has markedly decreased almost all over, (except certain African Countries, Pakistan, Bangladesh, etc.). India has been declared now as polio-free country. However, legacies of polio (weakness of muscles, deformities, limb-length disparities, etc.) will require proper management for more than further 30 to 50 years (*see* **Figs. 11.23 to 11.30**).

- *In lower limb* (in order of frequency and severity of affection) of muscles commonly affected are:
  - Tibialis anterior
  - Quadriceps femoris
  - Gluteus medius
  - Gastrosoleus
  - Gluteus maximus
  - Tibialis posterior
  - Peroneus tertius
  - Hamstrings
  - Peroneus longus and brevis.
- *In upper limb* (in order of frequency and severity of affection) muscles commonly affected are:
  - Deltoid
  - Biceps brachii
  - Short rotators of shoulder
  - Extensor carpi ulnaris
  - Extensor pollicis longus
  - Extensor digitorum
  - Supinator
  - Flexor digitorum profundus
  - Flexor digitorum sublimis.
- *In Trunk* (in order of frequency and severity of affection) muscles commonly affected are:
  - Sacrospinalis
  - Pectoralis major
  - Latissimus dorsi
  - External oblique abdominis
  - Internal oblique.

Muscles Commonly Escaping Polio-Paralysis

- Tensor fascia femoris
- Iliopsoas
- Pronator teres
- Trapezius
- Subscapularis
- Intrinsics of foot and hand.

The muscles having wider representation at the neural level usually escape unless the affection is of very severe magnitude.

■ METHODOLOGY

History Taking

Besides general considerations, the main stress should be given to:
- Complaints—Congenital (e.g. for spina bifida)/acquired (in case of trauma—mode of injury and management)
- Any familial tendency (may be positive history in myopathy)
- *Social and economic background:*
  - Geographical topography
  - Place of residence and its surroundings
  - Structural barriers around residence.
- Any constitutional features (e.g. for febrile onset in poliomyelitis)
- Immunization status
- Chronological history of milestones of development
- *Pregnancy and delivery:*
  - Antenatal period
  - Mode of delivery
  - Any problem during or after delivery
  - Drugs taken during pregnancy.

General Examination

(Besides general and systemic examination as written in Chapter 1 'Introduction'). Most of the paralytic patients are carried to the clinician by attendants. However, if they can walk, note the following:
- The effect of disability on general posture of the patient
- The apparent mode of compensation for the residual disabilities, deformities and limb length discrepancy
- Mode of stabilisation while standing **(Fig. 11.3)**
- Mode of walking
- Aids required for walking
- Mode of clearing hurdles and negotiating steps.

The examiner must look for and note the expression, mental alertness, approximate IQ, any change in facial appearance, salivation, tongue position.

Regional Examination

Usually the disabilities are initially localised to a particular region, but with the passage of time the patient develops associated deformities and disabilities of the adjoining joints or even the contralateral limb and trunk. Therefore, general assessment of the patient as a whole is necessary. Try to identify the primary site of lesion and then assess the deformities which chronologically developed as a mechanism of compensation to achieve functional gain. In long-standing paralysis, natural compensatory mechanisms may be present and give a grotesque, ugly look, but they may be of immense functional value to the patient in helping to meet his/her bare minimum needs **(Figs. 11.3 to 11.5)**. This can be very well exemplified while assessing a neglected patient.

Local Examination

This should be done at the different sites of deformities and residual disabilities.

Prerequisites

- Expose the affected regional zone and the contralateral limb completely.
  - The patient should be examined in the compensated position which he/she assumes for his/her daily activities.

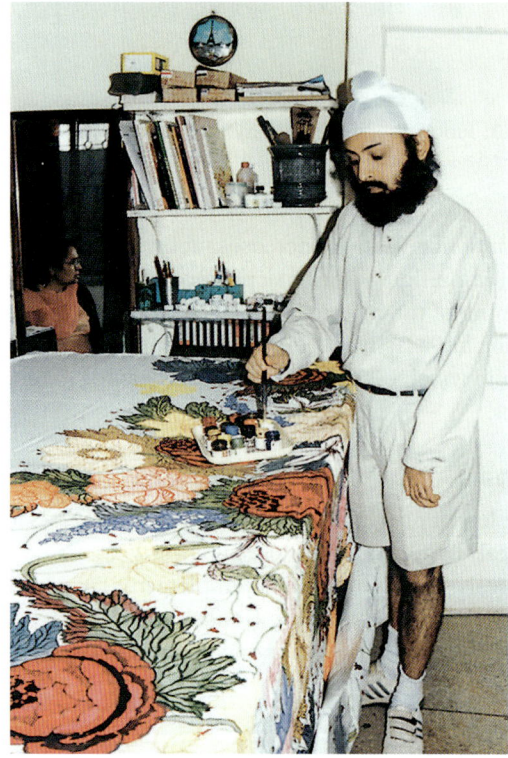

Fig. 11.4: Self-rehabilitated polio-paralytic disabled person with left upper limb flail, left lower limb and right lower limbs variously affected (operated)—doing excellent painting work. Judge his abilities.

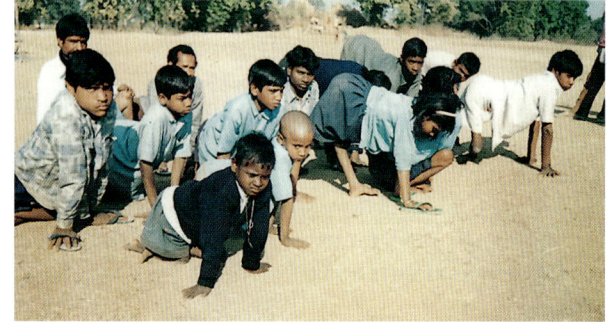

Fig. 11.5: A group of divyang children collected at a rural camp for management by surgery and rehabilitation procedures (*see* **Figs. 11.22 to 11.25**).

Attitude and Gait

In such patients, attitude depends upon:
- The type and extent of paralysis
- The period of paralysis
- Compensatory mechanisms developed by the patient to combat the disabilities, deformities and limb length disparities.

Certain common attitudes: [Specially in neglected polio and cerebral palsy (a group of disorders resulting in non-progressive brain damage) patients].

The tensor fascia femoris deformities complex (TFFCD). This is the most common deformity complex of the lower limb in neglected polio **(Figs. 11.6 and 11.7A to G)** and myopathy patients **(Fig. 11.8)**.

Testing for the Tightness of Iliotibial Tract

Before contractual stage, the tightness of the iliotibial band can be evaluated by **Ober's test.** For this test, the patient lies in lateral position, and with the hip extended and abducted and knee flexed at 90°, the proximal part of the leg is allowed to drop passively on the contralateral limb on table top. Normally, it should fall. The test is considered positive when the leg fails to drop. This indicates iliotibial band tightness which can lead to altered gait, low back pain, recurrent trochanteric bursitis and lateral knee pain due to snapping of iliotibial band over the lateral femoral condyle causing iliotibial bursitis.

Tensor fascia femoris complex deformities (TFFCD) develop due to contracture of tensor fascia femoris muscle-iliotibial tract axis. By virtue of its alignment on the anterolateral aspect of hip and posterolateral aspect of knee, it primarily produces flexion, external rotation and abduction at the hip and flexion at the knee. Further assisted by contracture of outer hamstring and gravity, posterolateral subluxation of knee develops. If further neglected, postero-lateral rotation and genu valgum of leg develop. Secondarily, equinovarus deformity develops at ankle and foot.

In severely neglected cases, pelvic obliquity, lordosis, fixed lower lumbar scoliosis and varying shortening of the affected limb develop.

According to severity tensor fascia femoris complex deformities (TFFCD) patients may be grouped under five grades **(Figs. 11.7A to G)**. Grade I and II can be well improved by graduated stretching and physiotherapy. Most of the grade III patients require soft tissue surgical release along with physiotherapy. In grade IV, about 20% require bony operation as well for correction. All grade V patients compulsorily require combined soft tissue and bony operations for possible correction.

Hand to Knee Gait [Five Fingers Quadriceps (Figs. 11.10 to 11.12)]

It is usually to be seen while the patient is walking. The affected limb is always kept forward in stepping, with the body leaning towards it anteriorly. With weak quadriceps, the patient gradually learns to stabilise his knee by directly transferring his body weight over the lower thigh, through his ipsilateral hand, usually by keeping the knee in variably flexed position. With markedly weak quadriceps, specially when it is associated with shortening of the limb, the foot is in equinus, the knee flexed and the fingers and thumb of the ipsilateral hand are firmly anchored on the front of the lower thigh. The skin of that region of thigh may become hyperkeratotic, even warty, tough and hyperpigmented **(Fig. 11.12)** while the underlying quadriceps mass is markedly atrophied. In moderately weak quadriceps, even two finger support over the region helps the patient in stabilising the knee joint. The intelligent patient adopts this function by keeping his hand in ipsilateral pant-pocket and pressing over the thigh through it.

The weak quadriceps is compensated by equinus position and/or hand to knee gait (which produces hyperkeratotic skin at the lower quadriceps region **(as in Figs. 11.10D and 11.12)**.

Gluteal Lurch

Gluteus medius or gluteus maximus or both paralysis lead to an unstable hip and unsightly and flinging lurch. In isolated paralysis of gluteus medius, the trunk sways towards the affected side and the pelvis sags on the opposite side. When gluteus maximus is paralysed alone, the body lurches backwards. Trendelenburg test will be positive in gluteal paralysis. However, when the gluteal paralysis is severe, the test cannot be performed, as it will become impossible to balance on the affected side.

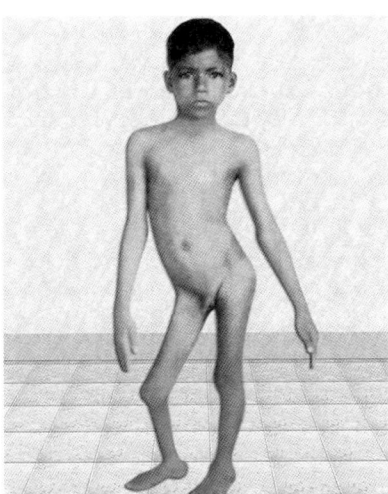

Fig. 11.6: Boy with mild tensor fascia femoris (TFF) complex deformity (Similar posture is usually adopted in iliac abscess). Note flexion, abduction and external rotation deformity at hip, mild flexion at knee, secondary equinus tendency at ankle, secondary scoliosis tendency at spine to compensate the pelvic tilt.

Examination of Paralytic Patients

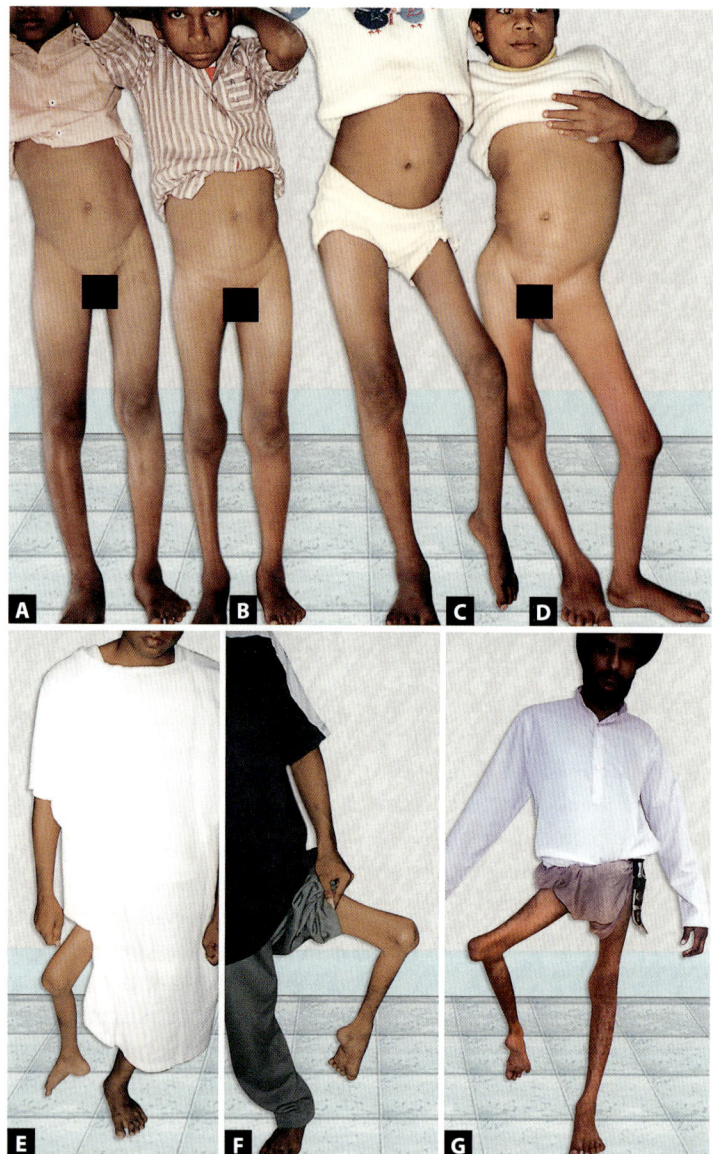

Figs. 11.7A to G: Various stages of tensor fascia femoris contracture (TFF complex deformities) due to polio-paralysis. Contracture in ascending order—very mild to very severe degree. A—GI, B—GII, C—GIII, D—GIV, E,F,G—GV— All can be corrected: A & B by physiotherapy; C & D by physiotherapy and operative release of contracted ligaments and fascia; E, F & G by—Operative release of contracted ligaments, fascia and joint capsule + Traction + Physiotherapy.

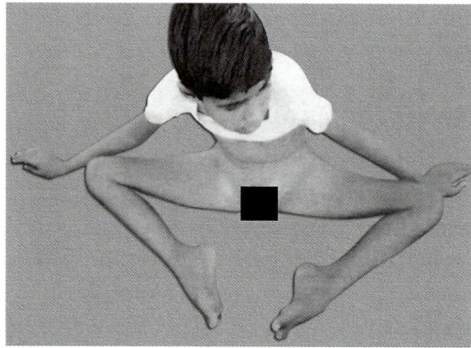

Fig. 11.8: Boy of myopathy developed bilateral tensor fascia femoris complexes deformities due to neglected posture. Upper limbs and trunks are also weak.

Totally flail lower limb can be made stable for weight bearing by pantalar arthrodesis and knee arthrodesis **(Figs. 11.13 and 11.14)**. However, the bones of lower limb should be stout enough to sustain the weight (Cf. the leg bones of bat are so thin that no bat can walk). External support is essential, if bones are too thin to avoid any fracture.

Typical Attitudes of Foot Deformities (Vide Chapter on the Foot)

With the decline in the incidence of poliomyelitis, cerebral palsy has now taken over as a major cause of disability in children.

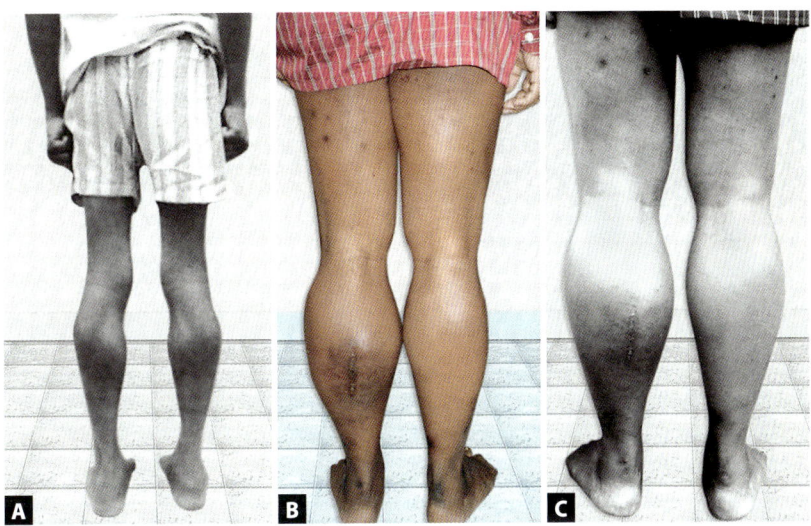

Figs. 11.9A to C: (A) Pseudomuscular hypertrophy in myopathy—Early (mild). Note the wasted thigh muscles, (B) Pseudomuscular hypertrophy—severe. Note that after surgery for biopsy, the hypertrophy has increased in both cases (left calf of B & C), (C) Myopathy with pseudomuscular hypertrophy of calf muscles. Hypertrophy of muscle may also occur with anabolic steroid use, hypothyroidism, congenital myotonia. The bulk of normal muscle may also increase after exercises against resistance.

Cerebral Palsy

"The child with cerebral palsy becomes the adult with cerebral palsy." (Terver et al. 1981).

The term cerebral palsy' was coined by Sir William Osler in 1987 in Pennsylvania. William John Little published the first clinical report of cerebral palsy in 1843. Little had an equinovarus deformity of his left foot due to polio-paralysis.

The exact incidence of cerebral palsy is not clear however the annual frequency is approximately two per 1000 live birth (Jope 2013).

Cerebral palsy (a group of permanent disorders of the development of movement and posture) is the most common childhood motor disorder. The motor disorders are usually accompanied by disturbances of sensation, perception, cognition, communication, epileptic attacks, behavioural abnormality or secondary musculoskeletal problems, visual, hearing proprioceptive and equilibrium impairments.

Cerebral palsy is not a single entity but a heterogenous collection of clinical syndromes characterised by abnormal motor patterns due to permanent disorders of the development of movements and postures. Actually it consists of a group of disorders resulting in non-progressive brain damage. Basically, it is a neuromuscular disorder of cerebral origin occurring due to injury or insult to the developing brain in prenatal, natal or neonatal (postnatal) period and is non-progressive. Exact etiology remaining uncertain, it hovered around the brain damage, birth trauma and lack of oxygen" and certain risk factor such as very preterm (before 32 weeks of gestation) and extreme preterm birth, (before 28 weeks of gestation), intrauterine growth restriction, birth asphyxia, multiple pregnancy, infections (meningitis, septicaemia), deficiencies (like iodine), toxicity, Rh factor incompatibility;

TORCH group of infections (*Toxoplasma gondii*, rubella, cytomegalovirus, herpes)—transmitted from mother to foetus—led to cause brain malformations during 1st and 2nd trimester. Ultrasonography is perhaps the most powerful predictor of cerebral palsy in low birth weight baby. *Cerebral palsy is the most common cause of the upper motor neurone syndrome in childhood.* Usually, there is hypertonicity, however, hypotonia (usually with motor weakness) may be noted transiently in cerebral palsy, which may even persist for a variable period.

Certain aspects of cerebral palsy must be basically clear. It is not a diagnosis. Its etiology and pathology are not clearly established. Its prognosis cannot be pronounced. It may be taken as an 'umbrella term' covering a group of non-progressive, but often changing, motor impairment syndromes secondary to lesions or anomalies of the brain arising in the early stage of its development (Mutch et al. 1992).

As expressed by Terver et al. (1981), the fact is that 'the child, with cerebral palsy, becomes the adult with cerebral palsy'. These children are brought to the orthopaedic surgeons for their obvious motor disabilities. However, a systemic evaluation and management based on rational guidelines involving a multidisciplinary approach is essential. *Neurologically cerebral palsy patients are mostly of six types*:

1. Spastic (about 60–70%)
2. Ataxia
3. Athetoid
4. Rigid
5. Mixed types (about 10–15%)
6. Atonic.

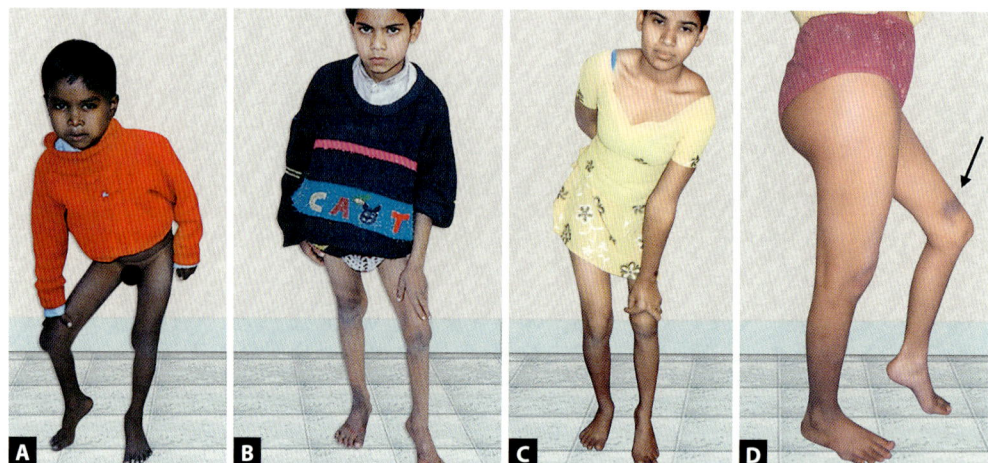

Figs. 11.10A to D: Hand to knee gait (five fingers quadriceps) in children of polio-paralysis with weak quadriceps—managing to walk. The weak quadriceps is compensated by equinus position and/or hand to knee gait (which produces hyperkeratotic skin at the lower quadriceps **(as in Figure 11.10D).**

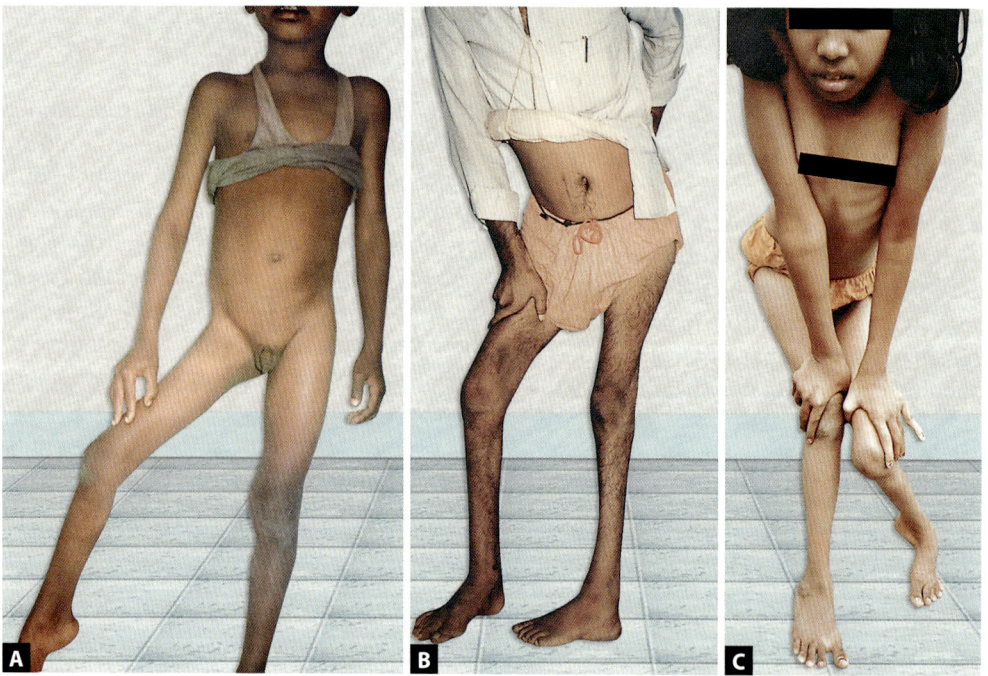

Figs. 11.11A to C: (A) Hand to knee gait—five fingers quadriceps; (B) Hand to knee gait; (C) Bilateral hand to knee gait.

The key features of the musculoskeletal pathology is a failure of longitudinal growth of skeletal muscle, and so orthopaedic synonym for cerebral palsy is aptly *"short muscle disease"*. The musculoskeletal pathology and accompanied gait disorder are progressive during childhood.

Clinically, cerebral palsy may be monoplegic (rare), *diplegic* (most common), *hemiplegic, triplegic* (more theoretically) or *quadriplegic or whole body involvement.*

- The cerebral palsy patients **(Figs. 11.15 to 11.21)** with mental retardation are usually microcephalic with/without dribbling of saliva **(Fig. 11.41)**. In a few cases, there may be squint or nystagmus. Typically, they show flexion, adduction and internal rotation at the hip, flexion at the knee, mild tendo-Achilles tightness and valgus of the foot with or without toe-in
- In the upper limb, the shoulder is adducted and internally rotated; the elbow is kept variably flexed; the forearm is in pronation; flexion and ulnar deviation develop at the wrist with fanning tendency of the fingers. In hand, the fingers also have the tendency for hyperextension at the metacarpophalangeal joints (usually affecting the index and ring fingers) and *thumb in palm deformity* **(Fig. 11.15A)**. However, presentations may be mild to severe

Examination of Paralytic Patients

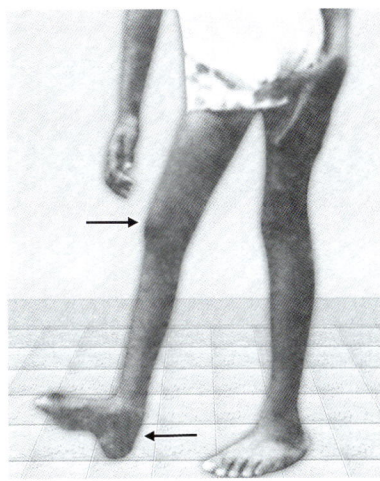

Fig. 11.12: Note the hyperkeratotic, tough and warty skin in front of lower right thigh of a polio-paralysis patient walking for years with five finger quadriceps. He has also calcaneo-cavo-valgus deformity of right foot.

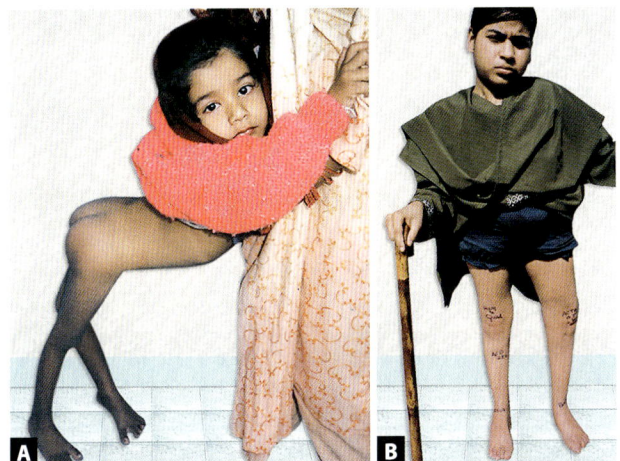

Figs. 11.13A and B: A quadruped like girl due to weakness in both lower limbs and spine can be made to biped, after multiple operations on both almost flail lower limbs. Left knee Pandey's trans epiphyseal (**Refr Fig. 11.31**) fusion; Left pantalar arthrodesis; Hamstrings to quadriceps transfer in right side; Pandey's calcaneal sling sliding osteotomy in right foot. She is using spinal support for more stability of trunk.

- In cerebral diplegia, the lower limbs assume a typical *"scissor-gait"* on attempts at stepping, mainly due to spasticity of the adductors of the thigh (**Figs. 11.15 and 11.16**)
- In hemiplegics, the foot develops equinovarus deformity and the shoulder may be adducted and internally rotated with/without other aforesaid deformities of upper limb. The patient walks with spastic gait.

Before the typical features of cerebral palsy develop, even the early cases can be clinically diagnosed by carefully assessing the response to certain primitive reflexes, as charted in **Table 11.1**.

To prognosticate about the sitting and walking abilities of a CP child, the following observations may be of help (After Paine, 1966):
- If the child starts sitting even by the age of 2 years, it should be considered a favourable sign for his walking
- If sitting of its own comes between 2 and 4 years, the chances of standing and walking independently are about 50%
- If independent sitting is not learnt before 4 years, independent standing or walking will hardly be possible
- If a cerebral palsy (CP) child, without severe contracture, cannot walk by the age of 8 years, there is hardly any chance of his ever walking in future.

Besides doing proper physical examination observa-tion should be made on child's behaviour, verbal ability, facial configuration and expression, head control, general build, nutritional status, drooling, general mood, eye contact, eyeball position, hand preference.

The parents' attitude towards the CP child should also be noted—whether they are supportive, depressed or hostile?

A cerebral palsy patient should be assessed for functional abilities, including:
- *Sitting ability:* Can sit independently/can sit only when propped/cannot sit
- *Walking ability:* (a) Community walker—can move about independently in society, (b) can walk about inside the house only independently, (c) can walk with some assistance or aids, (d) cannot walk
- *Eating ability:* (a) Can eat with his hand independently, (b) can eat only with the help of some aids and/or appliances, (c) cannot eat of his own even with aids and/or appliances and, (d) has to be fed
- *ADL* (Activities of daily living): (a) Can manage ADL independently, (b) can manage ADL with some assistance, (c) cannot carry out ADL and, (d) has to be helped by others.

The neonate with cerebral palsy usually have no deformities or musculoskeletal abnormalities at birth. Deformities like dislocation of the hip and fixed contractures, scoliosis, etc. develop during the rapid growth of childhood.

The position in infancy and childhood like asymmetrical postures and position (which must be prevented and taken care of) might be responsible for developing deformities in cerebral palsy like windblown hips, windswept lower limbs, facial asymmetry, a bat ear and plagiocephaly. The initial deformity usually develops as dislocation of hip followed by scoliosis and then pelvic obliquely.

The *gait in spastic diplegic children* may be variable, however, the most common pattern includes problems in the sagittal, coronal and transverse planes. Characteristically, there is anterior pelvic tilt with compensatory lumbar lordosis; flexed internally rotated and adducted hips; flexed stiff knees and equinus at the ankle, and in-toeing.

Examination of Paralytic Patients

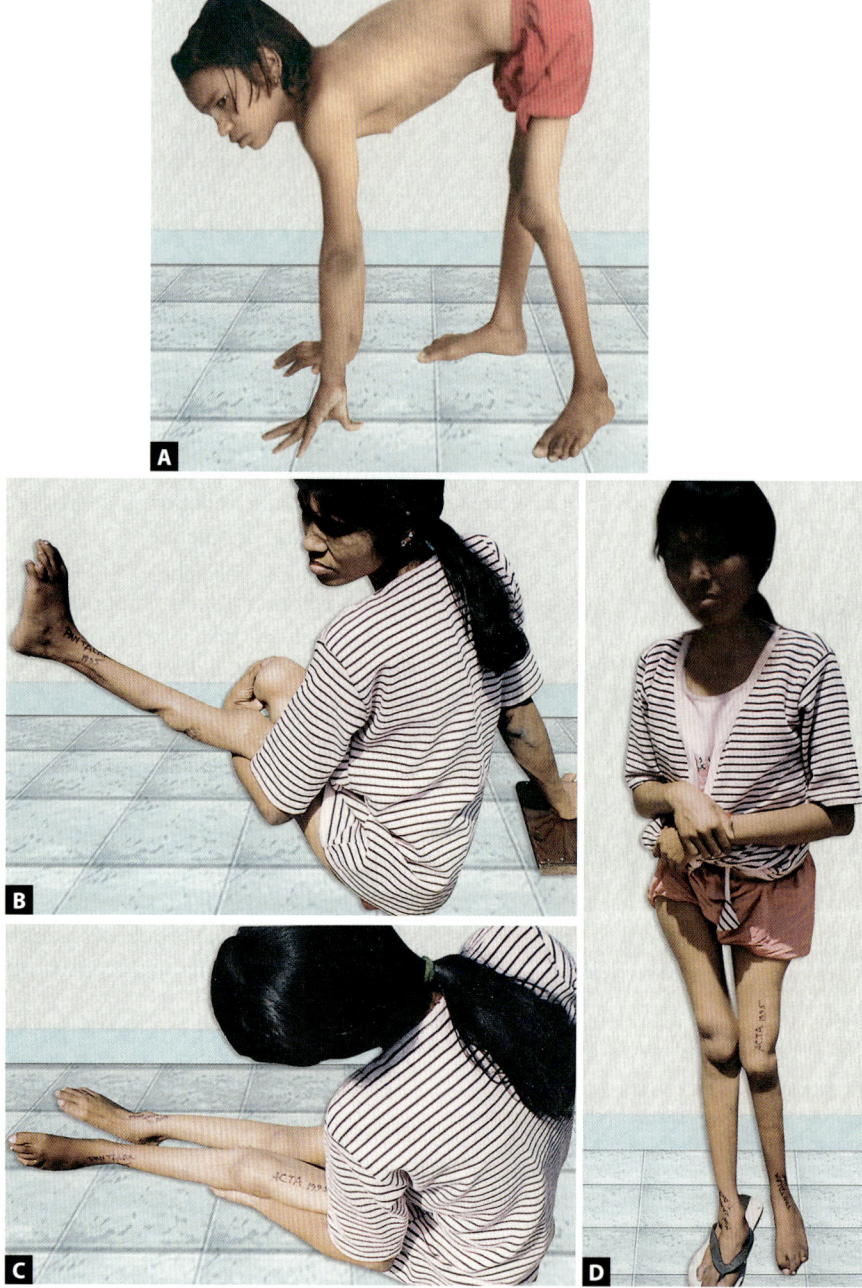

Figs. 11.14A to D: Polio-paralysis patient—came as quadruped (A) Operated in stages; (B) Knee transepiphyeal **(Fig. 11.31)** arthrodesis; (C) Modified triple arthrodesis; (D) Now she is walking with stability.

The gait in this attitude is awkward, inefficient and more energy consumable. With internal rotation and adduction of the hips there is knocking of the knees. While walking the patient oftenly falls due to frequent tripping. There is poor foot clearance and footwear wears excessively. These peculiar attitude, deformities and gait pattern (especially the in-toeing gait) are more or less due to 'lever arm disease' (i.e. dynamic and static problems due to abnormal muscle tone, musculotendinous contractures and medial femoral torsion).

All children with spastic hemiplegia walk independently without any aid. Most of the spastic diplegics do walk but assistive devices may be required by many (most common being two or one stick). However, spastic quadriplegics rarely have functional walking.

On the whole functions and quality of life can be improved in most of the cerebral palsy patients by addressing the different disabling aspects of the disease such as:

- **Tackling the spasticity**—By injecting (a) *Phenol*—a neurolytic agent used for motor nerves, e.g. the obturator

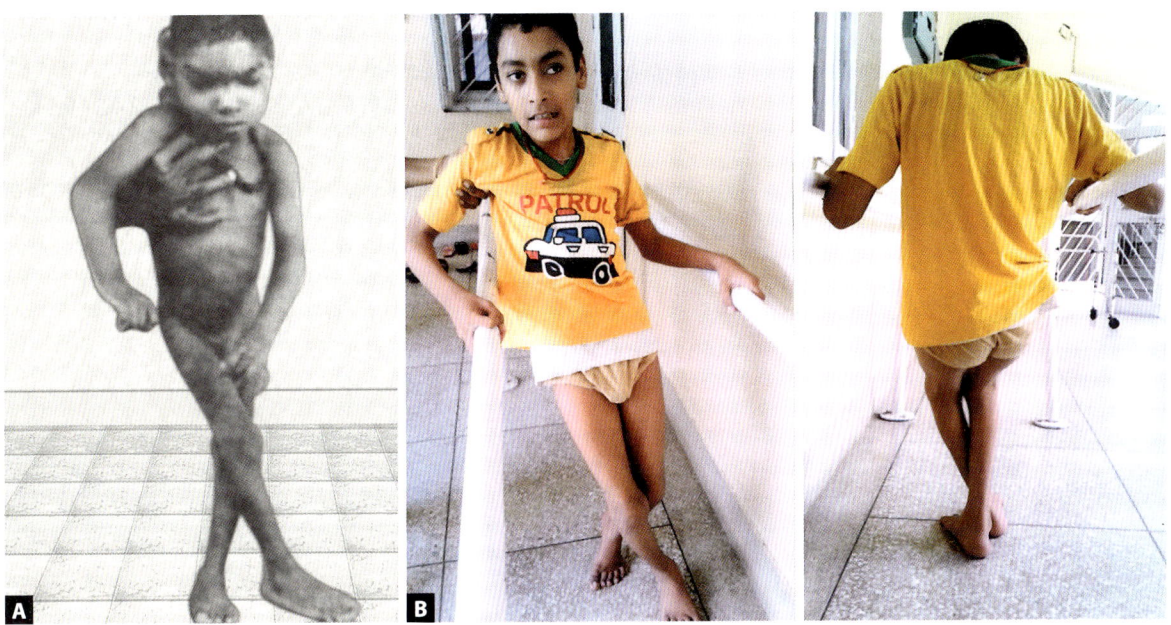

Figs. 11.15A and B: Typical cerebral palsy child, note the scissoring of the legs in attempt of standing (A)/walking (B); microcephaly; thumb in palm deformity (A).

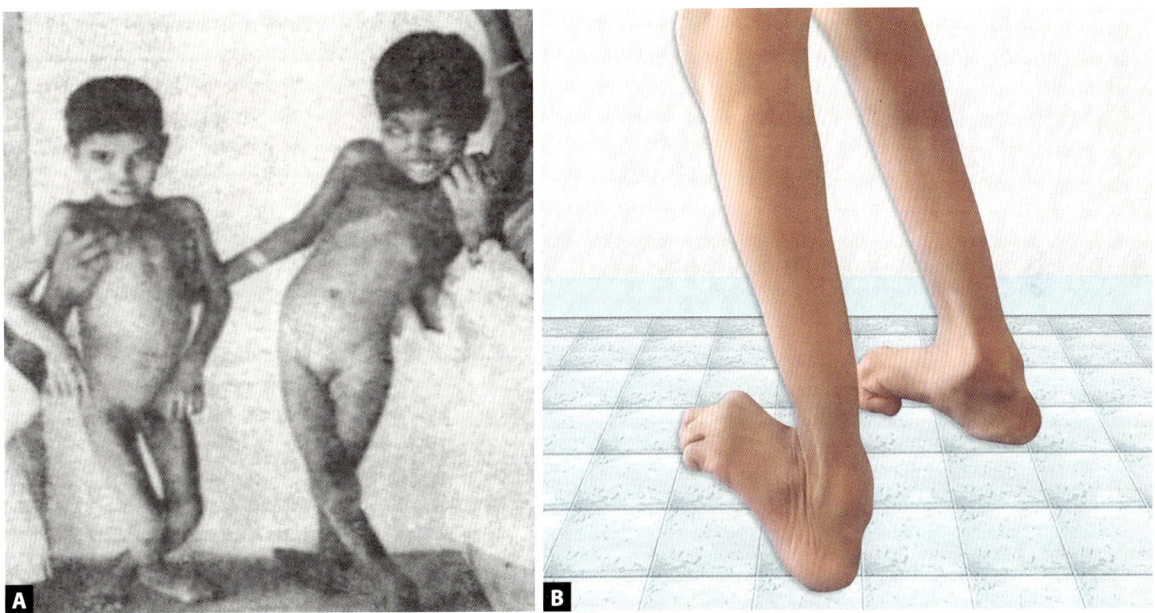

Figs. 11.16A and B: (A) Cerebral palsy in both—brother and sister; (B) In cerebral palsy acute spasmodic flexion deformity contracture of toes.

nerve for adductor spasticity and musculocutaneous nerve for spasticity of the elbow-flexors, (b) *BTX-A* (a potent neurotoxin produced by *bacterium clostridium botulinum* under anaerobic conditions) is considered to be focal or regional intervention, and its effect is pharmacologically completely reversible. It is mainly used for dynamic equinus (toe walking), adductor spasticity (scissoring), hamstring spasticity (crouching gait); (c) *Intrathecal baclofen* is powerful for managing severe generalised spasticity, of course it is expensive, invasive and has high rate of complications, even life-threatening; (d) Surgically *selective dorsal rhizotomy* can be done to manage generalised spasticity of the lower limbs. Of course with marked reduction in spasticity, weakness of the lower limbs also ensues, which requires intensive physiotherapy to regain functional strength.

- **Correction of fixed deformities**—Despite effective means of managing spasticity, most of the spastic cerebral palsy

Examination of Paralytic Patients

TABLE. 11.1: Reflexes of neonates.

Name of reflex	When to appear/disappear	How to elicit	What to observe	Inference
Tonic neck reflex	Appears at 2 months and disappears at 6 months	Neck flexion	Arms flex and legs extend	Presence of this reflex is incompatible with independent standing and walking
Asymmetric tonic neck reflex		Head is turned to one side and then to the other	Flexion of upper and lower limbs on skull side and extension on the face side	Absent reflex indicates poor prognostic signs for walking
Moro's reflex	Appears at birth, disappears at 3 months	Neck is suddenly extended	Upper limbs extend away from body and then come together in embracing pattern	Persistence indicates bad prognosis for walking
Neck righting reflex	Appears at 4–6 months, disappears at 24 months	Head is turned to one side	Shoulder, trunk, pelvis and lower limb follow the turned head	Persistence indicates bad prognosis for walking
Parachute reaction	Appears at 9 months and persists forever	Child is lifted horizontally by the waist and suddenly lowered on the table	Arms and hands fan out towards the table as though to protect from fall	Absence indicates bad prognosis for walking
Palmar grasp reflex	Appears at birth and disappears at 6 months	A pencil is passed along the medial side of palm	Tries to grasp the pencil	Persistence indicates bad prognosis for walking
Extensor thrust	—	Lift the child by axilla and suspend and then lower so that feet touch the table top	Normal infants will flex their legs	If there is definite and progressive extension of lower limbs and even trunk—it is abnormal

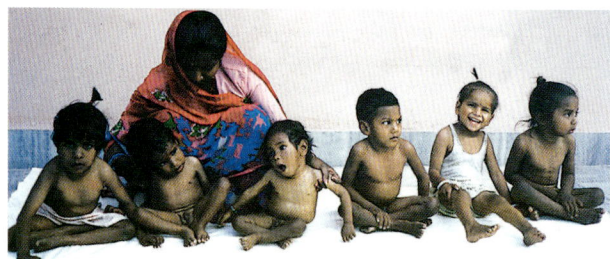

Fig. 11.17: Cerebral palsy patients in group—in various stages of exercises, rehabilitation and training.

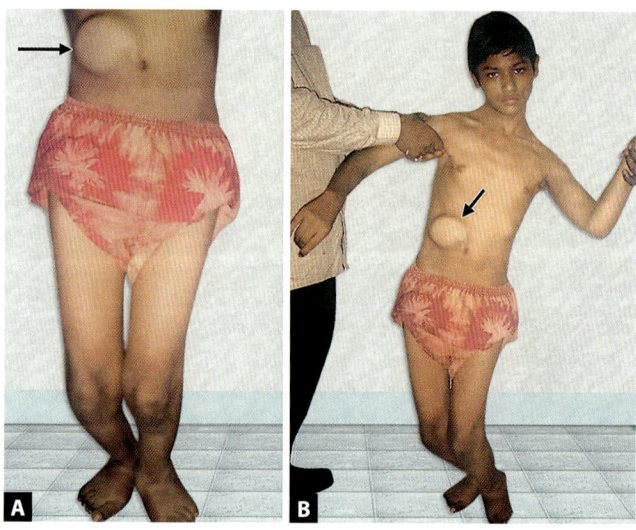

Figs. 11.19A and B: Medicines hardly work in CP patients. Botulinum-A toxin injected intramuscularly in selected muscles decreases muscle tone, chances of contractures, increases range of motion and motor function, decreases scissoring on standing. On the whole it is costly, improvement after injection starts in 1–3 weeks and lasts for about 12 weeks but on the whole effect is temporary. This patient implanted with diclofenac/baclofen pump in the abdominal wall has also hardly any lasting benefit.

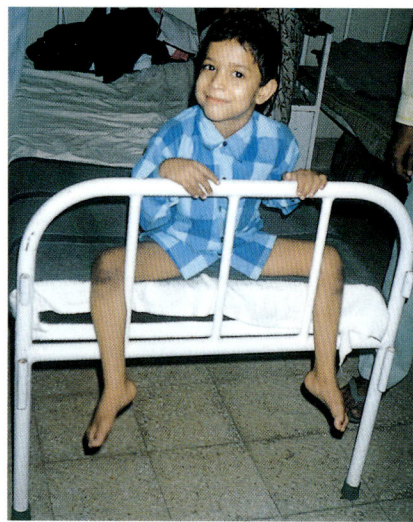

Fig. 11.18: Autocorrection of adductor tightness in cerebral palsy patients. This position also counters the internal rotational tendency of hips along with adduction (due to spasm and contracture of adductor muscles).

patients develop progressive musculoskeletal deformities with their growth, such as fixed contractures of the two joint muscles and, a range of bony deformities collectively designated as 'lever arm disease'. These contractures and deformities can be improved/corrected by proper surgery. To correct gait problems all deformities should be corrected simultaneously if possible. Derotation osteotomy of femur at (proximal) intertrochanteric or/

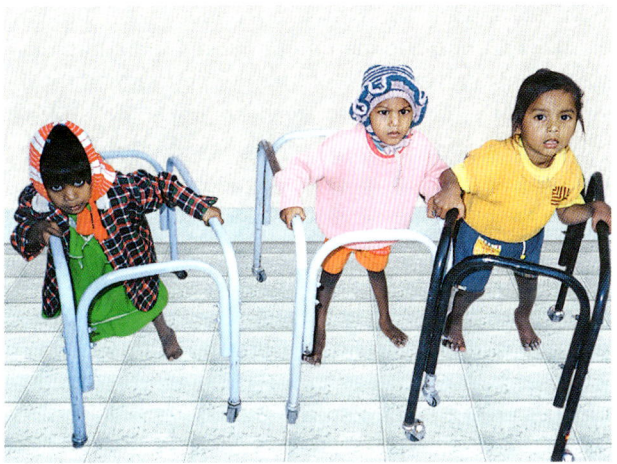

Fig. 11.20: Cerebral palsy children undergoing postoperative physiotherapy after adductor release, and high tendo-Achilles lengthening.

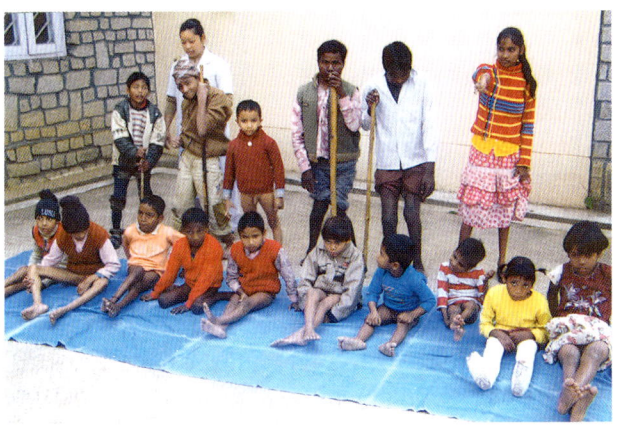

Fig. 11.21: Cerebral palsy children in group after adductor release and high tendo-Achilles lengthening—undergoing rehabilitation physiotherapy.

and (distal) supracondylar levels very well corrects the rotation of the hip and thereby foot progression angles in spastic diplegic children.
- **Improving the weakness in the cerebral palsies—**It has been believed that the assessment of muscle power and their strengthening exercises are neither possible nor desirable in spastic cerebral palsy patient, since the strengthening exercises have been apprehended to increase the spasticity/or may even actually increase the spasticity. However, if carefully done, the assessment of the muscle power is possible. Further, the management of spasticity and correction of deformity should be combined with optimum strengthening exercises and proper training to improve the functional gains.
- Proper Physiotherapy, Occupational therapy and Rehabilitation Programmes.
- Mental Development Activities.

Inspection

Besides the apparent position due to unbalanced contracture of opposite groups of muscles of the limb, a rough idea of the extent of involvement of the muscles can be obtained by inspection. In the abdominal wall, a definite ballooning of the particular sector in which the muscle is paralysed, can be noted (*see* **Figs. 11.19A, 15.63,** Page 455).

Palpation

Besides general consideration, palpation should particularly ascertain including:
- The bulk of the muscles
- The tone of muscles
- Any affection of contralateral muscles and tendons
- The extent and thickness of callosities at the joints due to abnormal weight bearing.

In acute cases (mainly in polio), muscle tenderness should be elicited, since this will give a guideline to the depth of involvement.

■ MEASUREMENTS

This must be a routine procedure even in the early follow-up of a paralytic patient, specially in polio patients in growing age. It has been found that:
- The earlier the age of affection—the more is the limb length discrepancy
- The more extensive is the affection (specially if it has been neglected) the more is the disparity—unless a balance between the paralysed and unaffected opposing group of muscles has been maintained (by physiotherapy—stretching, splintage and/or operation). The presence of severe deformities in paralytic patients, specially bilateral affections, sometimes presents a real problem in measuring the true limb length discrepancy. However, in such circumstances the nearest possible value should be worked out in as far identical position as possible.

Mode of Measurement (*see* relevant chapter)

In poliotics, with the involvement of hip region, it is difficult to do exact true measurement mainly because of ill-developed hemipelvis. Even without any fixed deformity anterior-superior iliac spines are not at the same level, and further, it is not possible to levelise them. However, the *measurement can be done in the following manner.*

The patient lies comfortably supine, stretching both his lower limbs in as much neutral a position as possible. Identify the fixed deformity on the affected side. Keep the opposite limb in identical position. In bilateral affections keep both lower limbs in as much identical position as possible. Measure the total and segmental lengths (distances) on one side (which appears to be normal or nearly normal). From the anterior-superior iliac spine of other side (which is lower), draw a horizontal line towards the opposite anterior-superior iliac spine. Draw another horizontal line from other anterior-superior iliac spine up to the midline. The difference between the two lines at the midline will indicate the structural deficiency in developing the anterior-superior iliac spine. This difference is subtracted from the measurement done on the side in which the anterior-superior iliac spine is high up. For all practical purposes, the remaining length will indicate the total length of that limb.

Circumferential Measurement

A paralysed limb is invariably wasted. Hence, circumferential measurement is mostly for compilation of records.

Linear Measurement

This measurement has its main importance for lower limb. However, measurement should be done as described in concerned chapters.

■ MOVEMENTS

(*See* Chapter 3: Joints)
Since in a limb, several joints may be affected due to paralysis of the controlling muscles, the movements at each individual joint must be charted separately.

Flail joints are hypermobile and mostly subluxated. Paralytic dislocation usually occurs in hip and shoulder.

Muscle Assessment Chart

While assessing muscle power, a rough estimation of the group action should be done (e.g. the dorsiflexion and palmar flexion at the wrist, the flexion and extension at the elbow, and so on). Thence individual muscles should be tested and its power charted in proper proforma (*see* Pages 318 to 320). For testing the power of individual muscle, one should proceed as follows:

Ask the patient to perform the normal actions which can be done by that functioning muscle against standard resistance and gravity. If this is not possible, then he should be asked to complete the functional action of that muscle against only gravity, which if not possible should be done with gravity eliminated. In all these procedures, note the extent of action (movement) achieved. If initiation of movement is not possible, look at and feel the contracting muscle as it attempts to perform its function. After testing as above power should accordingly be graded from 5 to 1. If even flickering of the muscle is not appreciated then it is graded as '0'. Power between grades 5-4, 4-3, 3-2 can be subgrouped as indicated in the Chapter 1: Introduction.

Grading of Muscle Power

As in the Chapter 1: Introduction.

Assessment of Contractures (Table 11.2)

This examination is essential to:
- Reveal the degree of contractures
- Assess whether the contracture is stretchable or not
- Know the effect of the contractures on the underlying joint
- Know the effect of the contracture on the vascularity of distal joints.

Special Test for Particular Joint (see *Chapter 3: Joints*).

Assessment of Early Polio Cases and Allied Condition

Any paralysed patient, but specially the polio cases, must be assessed thoroughly to form a base line. Of course, this will be a specialised job for the physiotherapist, but as a clinician, one should have an overall picture of the regions affected, along with the extent and complications of the affection. Problems in assessment arise in very young children, i.e. below the age of 2 years. In such cases, proceed as follows:

TABLE 11.2: Grading of contractures: Depending upon the given criteria, contractures can be graded as mild, moderate or severe.

Criteria	Mild	Moderate	Severe
Skin	Normal	Callosity on convex surface starts appearing	Callosities almost always present
Pain on stretching	None or very mild	Pain on stretching beyond 25%	Pain almost from the beginning of stretching
Stretchability	Full or almost full	25–50%	0–25%
Effect of stretching on vascularity	No blanching on full stretching	Blanching beyond 50% stretching	Blanching in range of 0–25% stretching
Effect on the underlying joint	No effect	It starts subluxating after stretching beyond 50%	Underlying joint mostly remains subluxated and/or presents tendency of subluxation on attempts of stretching

Ask the attendant of the child to hold the baby's upper chest from the sides and keep the child away from him so that the limbs hang in the air. Observe from the front and do mild continuous pinching over the lower quadrants of the abdomen and observe the movements at each joint of lower limbs and the working of the muscle groups/important individual muscles. If only one lower limb is affected, it provides a good comparison. However, even if both lower limbs are affected the overall functions of the limbs, movement at the joints, group actions of the muscles and individual action of important muscles can be assessed while the child screams. Weakness of the abdominal muscle becomes apparent by ballooning of a sector of the abdominal wall when the child cries **(Refer Fig. 15.65A)**.

Now the child is held from the front and observed from the back. Give a mild continuous pinch on both sides of the lower back and assess as above. Besides the movements and power in the lower limbs, the power of the spinal muscles can be assessed while the child is wriggling the back.

For the upper limbs—the child is held at the lower chest from the sides, while the upper limbs are hanging by the side of the chest. Pinch at the upper medial aspect of the arm and observe, as for the lower limbs.

In extensive and very early affections, the child should not be examined as above, rather, observe the movements while the patient is lying comfortably on the bed. Muscle tenderness should be elicited gently in the suspected areas. If power is markedly weak (grade 2 or less) assess while the patient is lying in such a way as to eliminate the effect of gravity.

Assessment of the Tensor Fascia Femoris (TFF) Complex Deformities (*see* Figs. 11.7A to G)

By and large, this is the most common deformity complex affecting the lower limbs in poliomyelitis and in myopathy. It also starts appearing quite early in neglected convalescent cases (even by 3-4 weeks). If detected early, guarded stretching usually corrects it.

Method of Detecting Early Deformity

Ask the attendant to hold the child at the chest from the sides with the legs hanging in the air. The deformed limb will not hang straight. If the other lower limb is normal even the earliest deformity of the affected side will be obvious. Hold the opposite buttock with one hand and with the other hand hold the suspected limb at the knee level (thumb over the knee, index and middle fingers above the popliteal fossa, and ring and little fingers below the popliteal fossa). While the knee is kept in maximum extension, the lower limb is moved medially and backwards. Resistance will be felt. Simultaneously, palpate along the iliotibial band for any tightness (compare with other side). In advanced cases, a subluxating tendency of the head of the femur can be felt during manoeuvre.

Second method—The child is laid on the bed on his side with the side to be tested kept up. The trunk is held straight with one hand fixing the buttock. With the other hand holding the knee as above, the lower limb is taken medially and backwards. Observations are made as above by comparing with the opposite side.

To confirm that abduction contracture is only due to iliotibial tightness, the following observation is useful: when the patient lies supine with extended hip and knee, the abduction contracture is present, but it disappears with flexion of hip and knee.

Iliotibial band contracture can be assessed quantitatively by the following test:

The patient lies prone. The examiner, standing on the opposite side of the limb to be tested, holds with one hand the affected limb just above the ankle with knee at 90° flexion, hip in maximum abduction and the limb in neutral rotation, while his other hand presses over the buttock to keep pelvis fixed on the table. The limb is then gradually adducted till the firm resistance is encountered. The angle subtended between the vertical axis of the body and the limb is the angle of abduction.

Testing for Tightness of Tendo-Achilles

Individually, this is the most common deformity of the lower limb, specially in polio-paralysis and cerebral palsy. Even in flail ankle and foot (with 0-2 powers of the tendo-Achilles) tightness occurs due to gravity.

Method of Testing

The child is held and the knee fixed as in testing for TFF deformity. Hold the foot in the other hand in neutral position (mid-patella, mid-ankle and second web in one line) and try to dorsiflex it at the ankle. In case of tightness, resistance will be felt. In further advanced cases, rocking of the foot at the ankle to one side can be felt while performing the above manoeuvre. Once rocking is felt, the foot should not be subjected to forceful stretching lest the developing talus will be compressed and damaged.

In neglected cases of mild tendo-Achilles tightness, the child is brought with the following complaints—inability to squat, pain in the calf, pain in the heel, thinning of the calf and small size of the heel and even foot. Observe the patient while walking—he will walk with a tendency of high stepping and later on with an equinus tendency of the foot. On asking him/her to walk on his/her heels, he/she will not be able to do so on the affected side. On asking him to squat, he will do so by keeping his affected foot in front and away from the other foot. If he/she is then asked to bring the affected foot to the level of the normal foot, he/she will either lose his/her balance and tend to fall backwards and therefore, support himself/herself with his/her hand kept on the ground behind his/her body, or he/she will balance himself/herself by raising the heel, thereby transferring the weight just on the forefoot.

The calf is comparatively thin and firm, the heel is small and comparatively clean looking than the other as it does not touch the ground.

Severe cases of tightness of tendo-Achilles result in equinus deformity of the foot.

Assessment of Instability

The main problem in a paralytic patient is instability at different joints, which should be assessed individually. The sum total of instabilities at different joints of a limb may result in the grotesque unstable disabilities for that patient. Hence, the degree of instability of that limb in carrying out the different grades of function should be assessed.

Grades of function are basically:
- *ADL (Activity of daily living)*—Mainly consist of eating, attending the natural calls and bare minimum dressing
- *Critical functions:* At every joint, certain range of movements are critically needed for basic functions, e.g. at wrist 0°–20° dorsiflexion to hold and grasp; at right elbow 30°–100° of movement for eating; at left elbow 20°–40° of movement for cleaning the private parts; at the knee 0°–30° of movement for walking, etc.
- *Job-oriented function*
- *Full function.*

NEUROLOGICAL EXAMINATION

(*As in Chapter 8: Spine*).

Investigation

The principle investigation in a paralysed patient is to keep a proper photographic record and prepare a detail neuromuscular-sensory chart on the first visit (and also on subsequent visits), which not only helps in diagnosis but also forms a baseline for comparison in future.

Radiology

This is the other important investigation. In case of lower limb, radiograph should be done of both sides in as much symmetrical a position as possible.

For practical assessment of any trunk deformity, radiograph should be taken in standing weight-bearing position—specially to assess paralytic scoliosis and pelvic obliquity. For the hips, weight-bearing position is much useful, to know its exact position under the stress of body weight and the ground reaction against it.

For the knees, lateral view is more useful, in which flexion deformity and any subluxation of upper tibia will be clear.

For the ankle and foot, it is also beneficial to expose the film while weight bearing, keeping the ankle-foot relation at right angles (or as much as possible towards right angle). Both feet should be simultaneously exposed in superoinferior projection. In lateral view, lower half of the leg, ankle and the foot should be exposed in the same film for charting the different angles and measurements, keeping the leg-foot angle at 90° or as nearly 90° as position.

To assess exact lower limb discrepancy, radiologically both the lower limbs should be exposed together in standing position right from hips to ankles, if possible, in one film or in two films, after keeping a common metallic marker to be included in both films.

Serum enzyme: Serum creatine phosphokinase estimation in early myopathy is more specific and is 200–300 times the normal value.

Blood and urine chemistry: In muscular dystrophy, serum creatinine and urinary creatinine estimation is an important aid to the diagnosis, serum creatinine is increased.

KEY DIAGNOSTIC POINTS OF CERTAIN PARALYTIC DISEASES

Poliomyelitis (Figs. 11.22 to 11.35 and 11.13 and 11.14)

- History of fever, gastrointestinal upset or respiratory tract infection
- Onset—acute and mostly in early childhood
- Lower motor neuron type of asymmetrical paralysis
- Nonprogressive muscle weakness
- Practically no sensory loss (except in very early stage for varying period)
- In neglected cases, various deformities in lower limbs, trunk and in upper limbs.

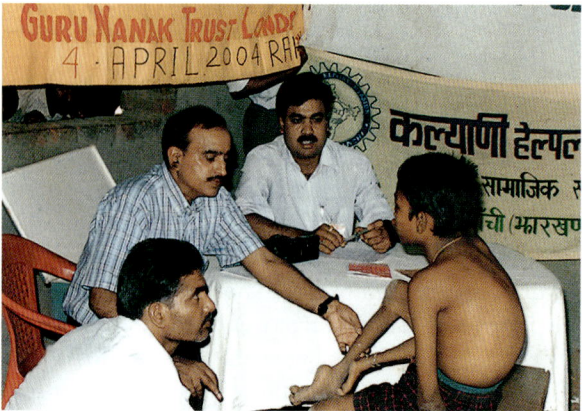

Fig. 11.22: Physically handicapped children are being screened in disability detection camp.

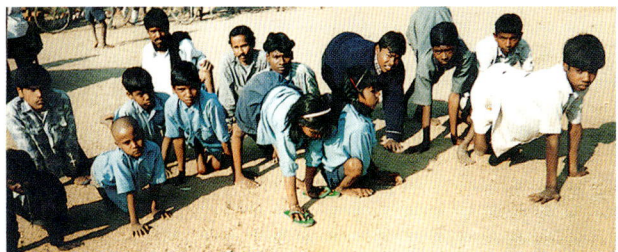

Fig. 11.23: Problems of polio-paralysis in rural India till early first decade of 21st century. However, the deformities already developed will need care, correction and rehabilitation for more than three decades to come.

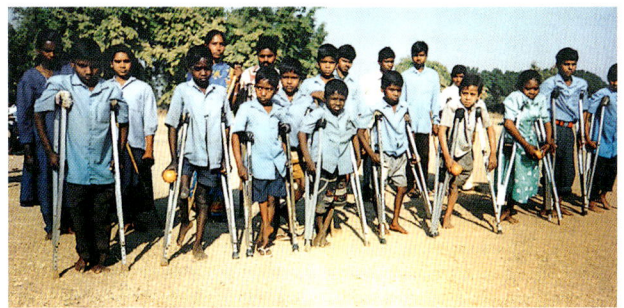

Fig. 11.24: Polio-paralysis problems which will challenge the medical profession for at least 4 decades to come.

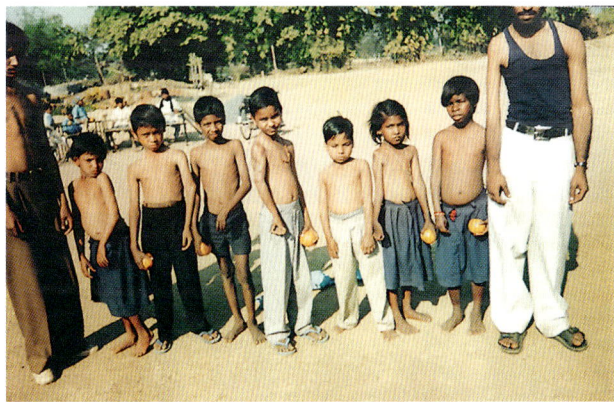

Fig. 11.25: Polio-paralysis in upper limbs—shoulder region is commonly affected.

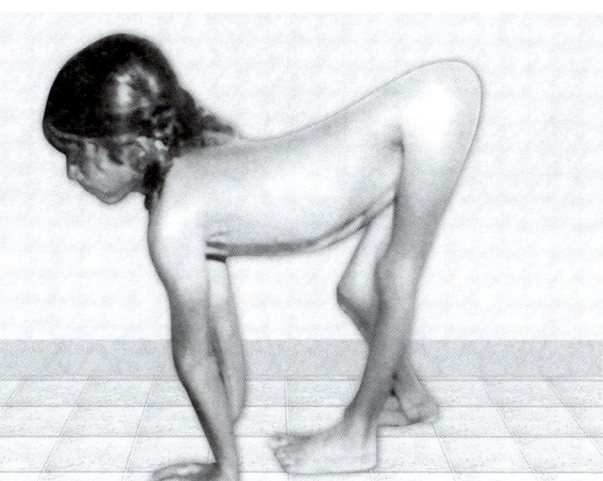

Fig. 11.26: Due to polio-paralysis with gross weakness in hip, pelvic girdle and lumbar regions, the child is walking like quadruped. She should be managed like the girt in Figures 11.13A and B.

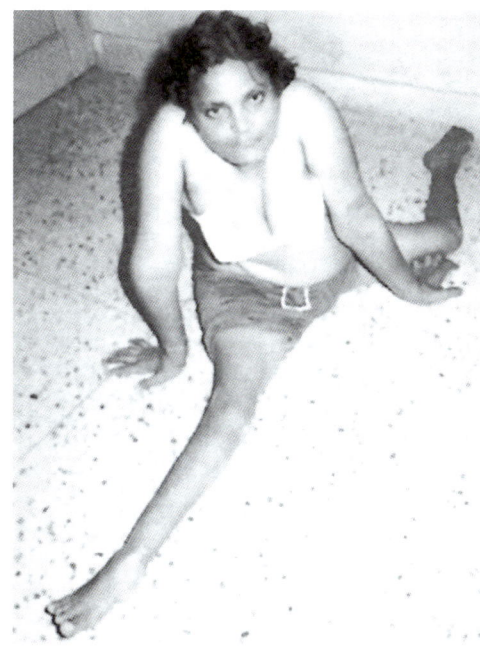

Fig. 11.27: Due to polio-paralysis with gross weakness in both lower limbs and lumbar region, the girl is managing to sit and also to glide on wider base and supporting herself on her both upper limbs (note the hypertrophy of upper limb muscles). In such patients fusion of knees with pan-talar arthrodesis should help to stablise her in erect position of course some aid must be given according to need.

Guillain-Barrè Syndrome

Guillain-Barré syndrome (described by three French neurologists—Georges Guillain, Jean Alexandre Barrie and Andre Strohl in two soldiers with acute areflexic paralysis followed by recovery).
- It is an eponym for a heterogeneous group of immune mediated (demyelinating peripheral neuropathic disorder occurring 1–3 weeks after viral infection, gastroenteritis, etc.) peripheral neuropathies
- There is usually rapidly progressive ascending symmetrical motor paralysis with/without sensory and autonomic disturbances, with pain in back and limbs, and distal numbness and tingling
- Cranial nerve may be involved affecting airway maintenance, facial muscles, swallowing, eye movements
- There is ascending flaccid paralysis with diminished deep and superficial reflexes
- With chest wall involvement, respiratory failure may occur
- Pain is common in about 50% cases and may be even severe
- Cases are mostly sporadic, but may be in cluster

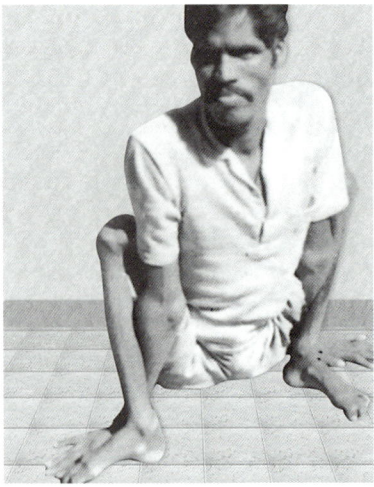

Fig. 11.28: In flail lower limb arthrodesis of knee (which preserves the growing potentiality of lower end of femur and upper end of tibia) in even children (beyond the age of 7 years) provides sound stability in limb which can prevent the disabilities like in **Fig. 11.27**—*see also* **Figs. 11.13 and 11.14.**

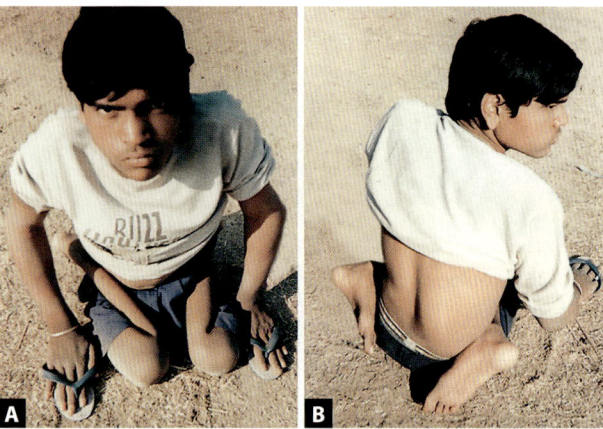

Figs. 11.30A and B: Complete polio-paralysis—Lumbar region downwards. He is mobile on his both hands (A) managing to stabilize lower back with both ankles and feet (B).

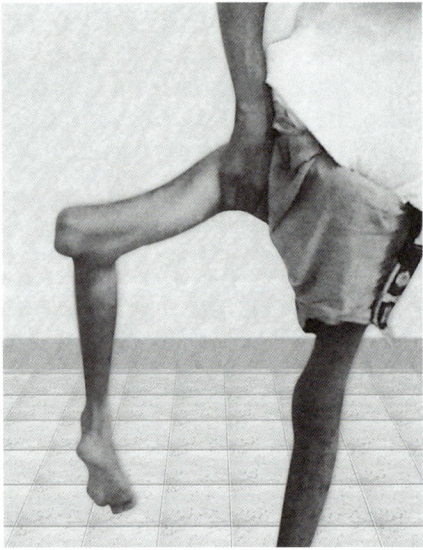

Fig. 11.29: Neglected flail right lower limb (due to polio-paralysis) with bizarre deformities. He is managing to walk with one crutch and supporting his flail lower limb with other hand. He can be improved to the extent of using his right lower limb for weight bearing and manageable walking by surgery (knee arthrodesis and pantalar arthrodesis).

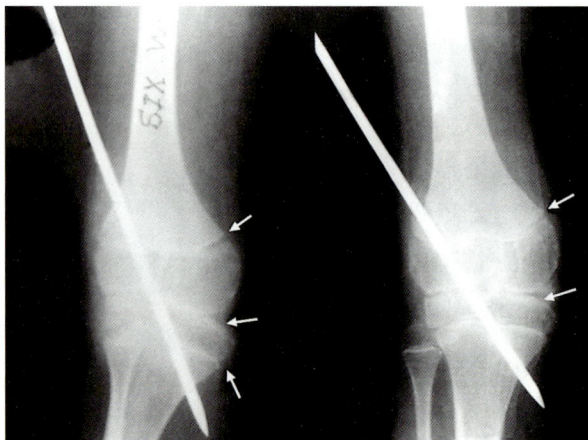
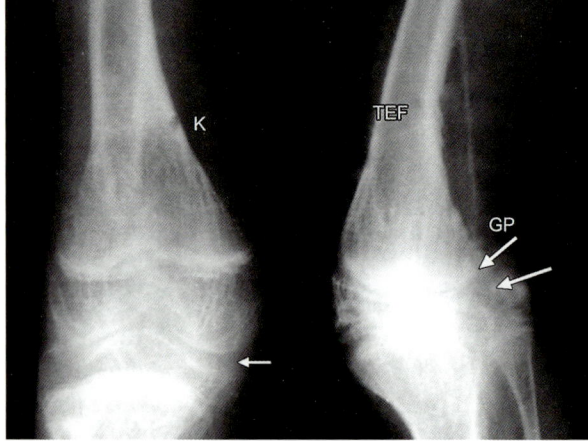

Fig. 11.31: In flail knee of child transepiphyseal arthrodesis of knee. The epiphyseal growth plates are not affected and both femur and tibia keep on growing even after arthrodesis. (K: kirschner; TFF: tensor fascia femoris; GP–growth plate)

- Supportive care is the corner-stone of management
- There is mostly variable recovery in 6–12 months.

Cerebral Palsy

Neuro developmental disorders (NDDs) include cerebral palsy, autism, attention deficit hyperactivity disorder (ADHD) and intellectual disability, epilepsy, autoimmune disorders including autoimmune encephalitis and neuromuscular disorders and muscular dystrophy. NDDs prevail alone or in combinations in 2–9 year old children in about 12% in India (Gulati 2017).

The London physician, William John Little (1810–1894) published the first clinical report of cerebral palsy in 1843.

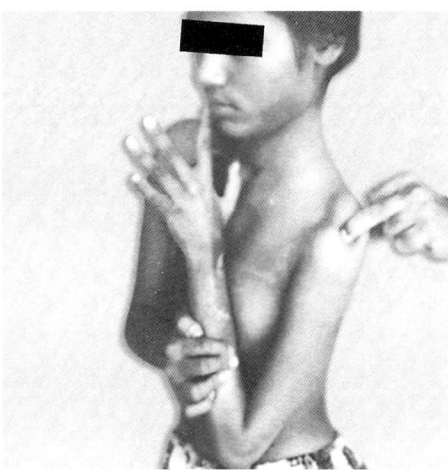

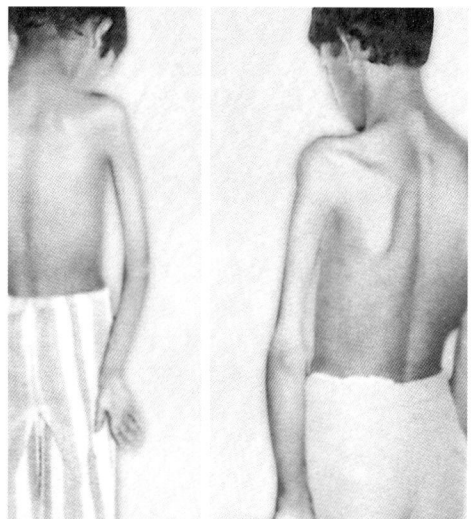

Fig. 11.32: Polio-paralysis of left upper limb. Note the wasting of paralysed deltoid and the humeral head can be subluxed out with a finger pressure. Left wrist has been arthrodesed for the gross weakness, after which the latent functions of the fingers and thumb have markedly improved. She can make fist and open fingers fully **(Fig. 11.33)**.

Fig. 11.34: In polio-paralysis of upper limb the shoulder is the commonest site of paralysis.

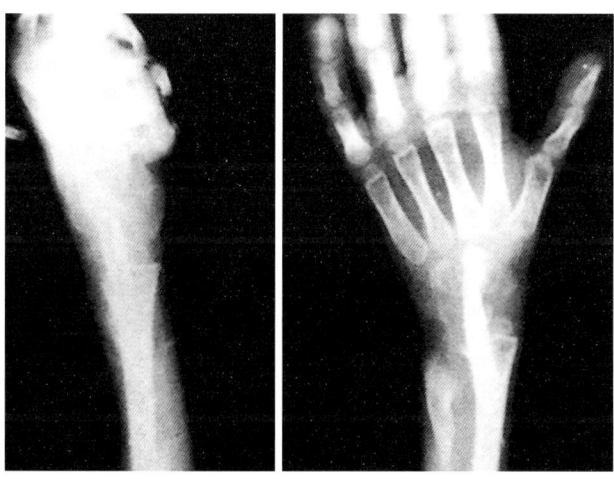

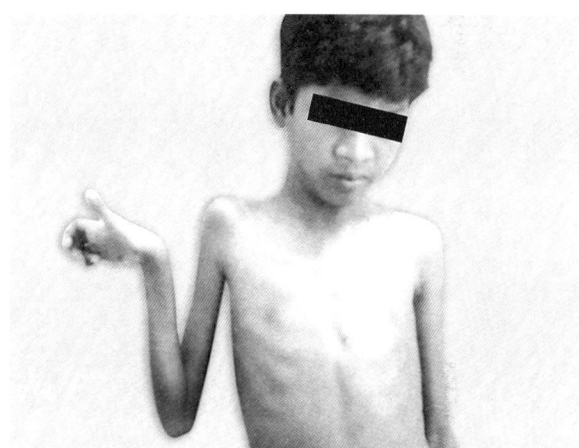

Fig. 11.33: Same child **(Fig. 11.32)**. X-ray in fisted (L) and opened fingers position (R) showing arthrodesed wrist using ipsilateral ulnar graf.

Fig. 11.35: In polio-paralysis affecting the upper limb, the common combination of affected regions (with magnitude of affection in that order) is the shoulder, wrist, hand, elbow even after arthrodesis.

After he presented in 1862, his accurate and robust paper entitled "On the influence of abnormal parturition, difficult labors, premature birth, and asphyxia neonatorum on the mental and physical condition of the child especially in relation to deformities" before the obstetrical society of London, the description of this syndrome was widely recognised as 'Little Disease' by the end of 19th century.

In simple words *Cerebral Palsy* may be considered as a group of nonprogressive neurological disorders caused by an insult/injury to the area of brain which controls movements of muscles and posture. The insult/injury of the brain may occur in prenatal, natal or postnatal (in the first two years of life) phase of foetus baby. Broadly *CLINICAL FEATURES* of cerebral palsy consist of:

- Delayed disappearance of congenital reflexes (few may even persist much longer)
- Usually spastic bilateral and almost symmetrical deformities, affecting all four or any three or any two or even one limb
- Upper motor neuron type of paralysis
- Varying mental retardation (In about 25% of cases)
- May be associated microcephaly, squint and dribbling of saliva. **(Fig. 11.41)**, strabismus, hyperopia (long sightedness)
- About 35% of all children of cerebral palsy will have seizures, which usually happen due to electrical misfiring in the brain (triggered after brain damage, head injuries, infections, dehydration, tumors, genetic factors)
- **Dysphagia** (problems in swallowing) – Cerebral palsy children remain at risk of dysphagia due to poor muscle and motor function control

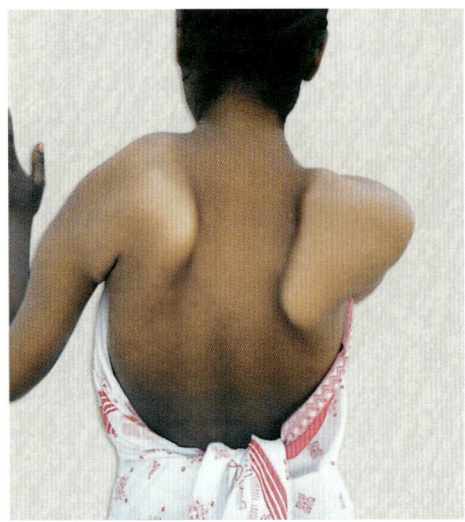

Fig. 11.36: Gross wasting of scapular muscles in myopathy with winging out of scapulae in lady aged 23 years.

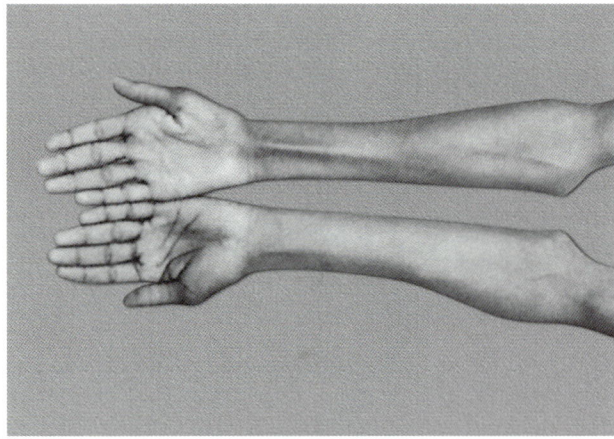

Fig. 11.38: Myopathy: note the wasting of muscles in both distal forearm and hands (right more than the left).

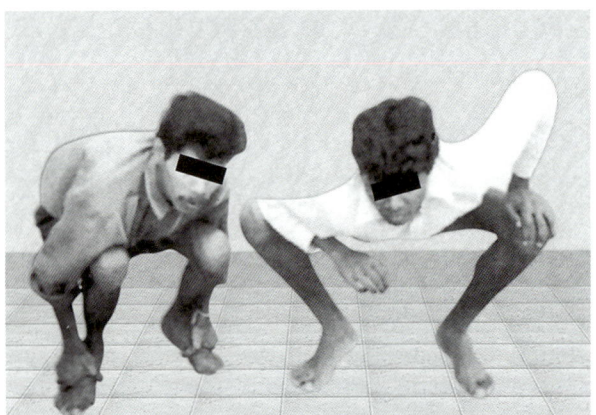

Fig. 11.37: Affected by myopathy—the boys are climbing up on their own lower limbs—knees to get up from the sitting posture (Gower's sign).

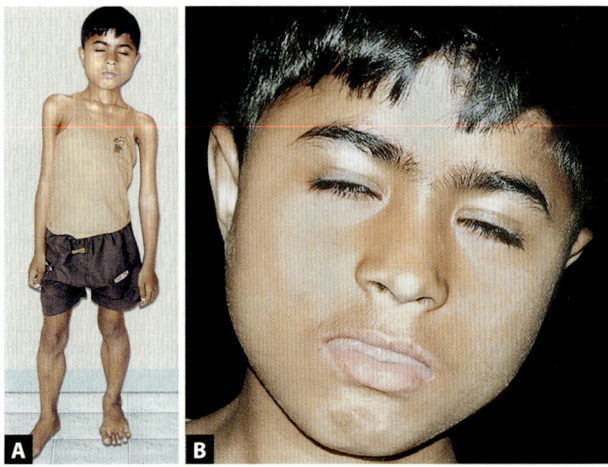

Figs. 11.39A and B: Tongue sign—In advanced case of myopathy the tongue-tip remains semiprotruded quite often.

- **Cognitive and Behavioral Issues** like, recognition issues, memory and learning issues, problems with comprehension and decision-making skills
- **Digestive problems** like constipation, incontinence, vomiting, aspiration
- Physical and Mobility problems
- **Autism** About 7% of cerebral palsy children have autism (mild to severe).
- **ADHD** (Attention Deficit Hyperactivity Disorder) Cerebral palsy children remain at risk of developing ADHD – attention deficit hyperactive disorder like hyperactive, and impulsive, as well as inattentive.

Myopathy (Figs. 11.36 to 11.39)

Myopathy is a general term referring to any disease that affects the voluntary muscles. Patients experience muscle weakness due to dysfunction of muscle fibres. Muscular dystrophy, is a heterogenous group of inherited disorders, prevalent all over, affects males, and is characterized by progressive weakness and wasting of mainly the skeletal muscles, however, diaphragm and heart muscles are often affected.

Muscular dystrophies are of three groups:
- Duchenne muscular dystrophy, characterized by progressive muscular weakness and degeneration, starts at about the age of 5 years and presents with waddling gait and difficulty in climbing the stairs. Becker muscular dystrophy has milder features of Duchene muscular dystrophy, and they start usually after 16 years of age.
- Congenital muscular dystrophy (In this group are also, limb girdle muscular dystrophy, muscle eye brain muscular dystrophy etc)
- Autosomal dominant group involving the scapuloperoneal dystrophy and facioscapulohumeral dystrophy.

Duchenne muscular dystrophy:
- May be familial history of disease
- Manifestation usually after 5 years of age

- Lower motor neuron type of mostly bilateral symmetrical lesion (in fascioscapulohumeral or Landouzy-Dejerine myopathy only one side is affected)
- No sensory loss
- Pseudomuscular hypertrophy of muscle may be present (*see* **Figs. 11.9A to C**)
- *Gower's sign:* Mild degrees of muscular weakness in lower extremity are easily missed. This can be assessed by Gower's sign: Ask the person to sit on the floor. Initially, the person (usually the children) hesitates to sit (to conceal the weakness). Then ask him/her to get up and watch the mode of getting up. The patient uses both arms or raises the buttocks first by taking purchase (by hands) on the floor towards the feet and then climbs up the legs. It is typically seen in patients with proximal lower extremity muscular weakness due to myopathy (**Fig. 11.37**)
- Increased blood creatinine level. Decreased creatinine level in urine is characteristic of the disease
- Much increase of serum creatinine phosphokinase is diagnostic of myopathy. However, serum creatinine phosphokinase may also be elevated in—muscle crush injury, intramuscular injections, recent strenuous exercises, myocardial infarction, racial variation, e.g. healthy Negroes
- *Tongue sign*—In advanced cases, the child keeps the tongue semiprotruded, with mouth partially opened (**Figs. 11.39A and B**).

There is no definitive treatment of muscular dystrophies. Physiotherapy and occupational therapy should be carried out to minimise the disabilities and maximise the possible functions.

Duchenne Muscular Dystrophy

It is an inherited X-linked recessive disease caused by a frameshift mutation in the dystrophin gene at the Xp 21.2 locus of the X chromosome. There is progressive weakness and by the age of 10–14 years, the patient becomes unable to walk and becomes confined to wheelchair. Gradually, pulmonary and cardiac complications develop by third decade which may lead to death usually scoliosis develops.

Motor Neuron Disease

- Usually, young adults presenting with gradual weakness, atrophy and fibrillation in the shoulder girdle muscles
- May be lower motor neuron type of lesion in the upper limbs and associated upper motor neuron type of lesion in lower limbs
- No sensory loss.

Polyneuritis

- Usually, adult female complaining of sensory disturbances which may be bilateral or unilateral
- Lower motor neuron type of lesion
- Variable muscular weakness and sensory disturbances affecting more than one site.

Examination of Paralytic Patients

In the patients with paresis/paralysis, the record of muscle power and allied neuro-musculo-sensory assessments must be maintained in systemic way at regular intervals, which reflects the improvement or deterioration of the patient's condition. In cerebral palsy muscle power testing will be altered, due to lack of voluntary control, or limited due to spasticity and/or contracture, however, at least some idea of the muscle function can be gained. It is also relevant, because recently muscle strengthening exercises have been shown to be important in improving the function in spastic diplegia.

■ PROFORMA TO RECORD THE MUSCLE POWER

Po/SpD—/PND—/My/MND/Others........ No

Group 0,1,2,3,4

Prophylactic vaccines: Po/Wh.cgh/Dep/Tet/Meas/any other

Name of patient_____ Age_____ Sex_____ Ward_____ Hospital No._____
Complete address_____ Tel:_____ Fax:_____ e-mail:_____

LEFT							RIGHT				
					Therapist's signature						
				Dates		Wh. cough					
				Action	Name of muscle	Nerve root supply					
					Head, Neck and Trunk						
					Facial muscles	Cr. VII					
				Flex	Sternocleidomastoid	Cr. IX					
				Ext	Neck extensors	C1-T1					
				Flex	Rectus abdominis	T7-L1					
				Ext	Dorsal spinal muscles	Segmental supply, Post- div. of spinal nerves					
					Lumbar spinal muscles						
				Rot	To the right						
					To the left						
				El Pel	Quad lumb	T12,L1,2,3					
					Scoliosis						
					Lordosis						
					General posture						
					Spine flat or flexed						
					Lower Limbs						
					Hip						
					Iliopsoas	L1,2,3,4					
				Flex	Sartorius	L2-4					
					Rectus femoris	L2,3,4					
				Ext	Gluteus maximus	L5, S1,2					
				Abd	Gluteus medius, minimus	L4,5 S1					
					Tensors fascia lata	L4,5 S1					
				Add	Adductor longus, brevis, magnus	L2,3,4					
				Rot	Ext rotators	L2-5, S1,2					
					Int rotators	L4,5, S1,2					
					Knee						
				Flex	Inn-hamstring	L4,5, S1,2					
					Out-hamstring	L5, S1,2,3					
					Gracilis	L2-4					
				Ext	Quadriceps	L2,3,4					
					Ankle						
				Plant Flex	Gastrocnemius and soleus	S1,2					
					Soleus	L5, S1,2					
				Dorsi Flex	Tibialis anterior	L4,5 S1					
					Peroneus tertius	L4,5 S1					
				Inversion in dorsiflexion	Tibialis anterior	L4,5, S1					
				Inversion in plantar flexion	Tibialis posterior	L4,5 S1,2					
				Everters	Peroneals—longus, brevis, and tertius	L4,5, S1 L5, S1					
				Eversion in dorsiflexion	Peroneus tertius	L4,5, S1					
				Eversion in plantar flexion	Peroneus longus Peroneus brevis	L4,5, S1 L5,S1,S2					

LEFT			Action	Name of the Muscle	Nerve Root Supply	RIGHT			
				Toes					
				Lumbricals	L4,5, S1				
			Flex	Fl dig Longus	S2 S3				
				Fl dig brevis	S2 S3				

Contd...

Contd...

			Ext	Ext. digit longus	L5 S1				
				Ext. digit brevis					
				Hallux					
			Flex	Fl hall brevis	S2 S3				
				Fl hall longus	S2 S3				
			Ext.	Ext hall longus	L5 S1				
				Ext hall brevis (a part of Ext digit brevis)					
				Measurements in Lower Limbs					
				Ant Sup iliac spine to med malleolus					
				Ant Sup iliac spine to knee jt line					
				Knee jt line to Med malleolus					
				Apparent shortening / lengthening					
				Mid thigh circumference					
				Mid calf circumference					
				Upper Limb					
				Scapula					
			Abd	Serrat anterior	C5-7				
			Elev	Upper trapezius	C2-4				
			Add	Mid trapezius	C2-4				
				Rhomboids	C4-5				
			Depr	Lower trapezius	C2-4				
				Shoulder					
			Flex	Coracobrachialis and ant deltoid	C5-6				
			Ext	Latissimus dorsi	C6-8				
				Teres major and post deltoid	C5-7				
			Abd	Deltoid and supraspinatus	C4-6				
			H Abd	Post deltoid	C5-6				
			H ADD	Pect major	C5-8, T1				
			Rot	Ext rotator					
				Int rotator					
				Elbow					
			Flex	Biceps brachii	C5,6				
				Brachioradialis	C5,6				
			Ext	Triceps	C6-8				
				Forearm					
			Sup	Biceps	C5,6				
				Supinator	C6				
			Pron	Pronators	C6				
				Wrist					
			Flex	Fl carp rad	C8				
				Fl carp uln	C8				
			Ext	Ext carp rad	C6,7				
				Ext carp uln	C7				
				Fingers					
				Lumbricals	C7,8 T1				
			Flex	Fle dig subl	C7,8 T1				
				Fle dig prof	C8, T1				
			Ext	Finger exten	C7				
			Abd	Dorsal int and Abd digiti minimi	C8, T1				
			Add	Palm Inteross	C8				
				Thumb					
			Flex	Fl pol brev	C6-8				
				Fl pol long	C8, T1				
			Ext	Ext pol brev	C7				
				Ext pol long	C7				
			Abd	Abductor poll	C7				
			Add	Adductor poll	C6,7				
			Oppos	Thumb to tip of little finger	C6-8, T1				
				Respiration					
				Intercostals					
				Diaphragm	C4,5,6				

Po = Poliomyelitis	I = Injury	PN = Peripheral Nerve	ND = Motor Neuron Disease
Sp = Spinal Injury	D = Diseases	My = Myopathy	Wh Cough = Whooping Cough
Dep = Diphtheria	Tet = Tetanus	Meas = Measles	Sup = Superior
Rot = Rotator	Flex = Flexor	Ext = Extensor	
El Pel = Elevator Pelvis	Abd = Abductor	Elev = Elevator	
Depr = Depressor	H Abd = High Abductor	H Add = High Adductor	
Pron = Pronator			
Add = Adductor			

Contd...

Examination of Paralytic Patients

Additional Data: Eyes _____ Hearing _____ Face _____ Tongue _____ Speech _____
Mastication _____ Swallowing _____ Diaphragm _____ Intercostals _____

Sitting Status (Figs. 40A to D)

'W' sitting position	...........(more or less Muslim prayer position; common in neglected CP patients)............	Present / Not present
Church prayer position	................(kneeling on both knees)...............	Possible / Not possible
Buddha position	.................(sitting crossed legs)................	Possible / Not possible
Bajrangbali position	...........(sitting with one knee in kneeling position, while other knee is bent at 90° with foot firmly planted on the ground)............	Possible / Not possible
Standing to squatting	....	Aided / Unaided
Squatting to standing	....	Aided / Unaided

Walking Status

Cannot stand	Date_____	Walks in parallel bar		Date_____
Stands with support	Date_____	Walks with invalid walker		Date_____
Stands without support	Date_____	Walks with crutches		Date_____
Cannot walk	Date_____	Walks with canes		Date_____
Walks with braces	Date_____	Walks unaided		Date_____
Walks with corset	Date_____	Walking on toes		Possible/Not possible
		Walking on heels		Possible/Not possible
		Climbs stairs with support		Date_____
		Climbs stairs without support		Date_____
Contractures and Deformities	Upper limb:	Rt _____		Lt _____
	Lower limb	Rt _____		Lt _____
		Gait _____ Normal/Abnormal—Type of gait		

Scoliosis and trunk deformities:

Key to grouping of the extent of paresis/paralysis

Group 0   Cases which have a general residual weakness with functional value just below normal.
Group 1   Cases with involvements of face or neck or trunk or one limb only.
Group 2   Cases where two limbs are affected either wholly or partially. The paralysed limbs may be both upper limbs or both lower limbs or one upper limb and one lower limb or one limb and the trunk.
Group 3   Cases where three limbs are affected either wholly or partially or it may be two limbs with trunk or neck or face and so on.
Group 4   Cases where all four limbs are affected wholly or partially, or it may be three limbs with trunk or face or neck and so on.

Scaling of Muscle Power

0. No contraction
1. Flicker
2. Joint motion with gravity eliminated
3. Joint movement—antigravity
4. Joint movement—antigravity with resistance
5. Normal.

Any **sensory disturbance** should be depicted in diagrammatic dermatomal distribution.
Any **vasomotor changes** should be noted clearly.

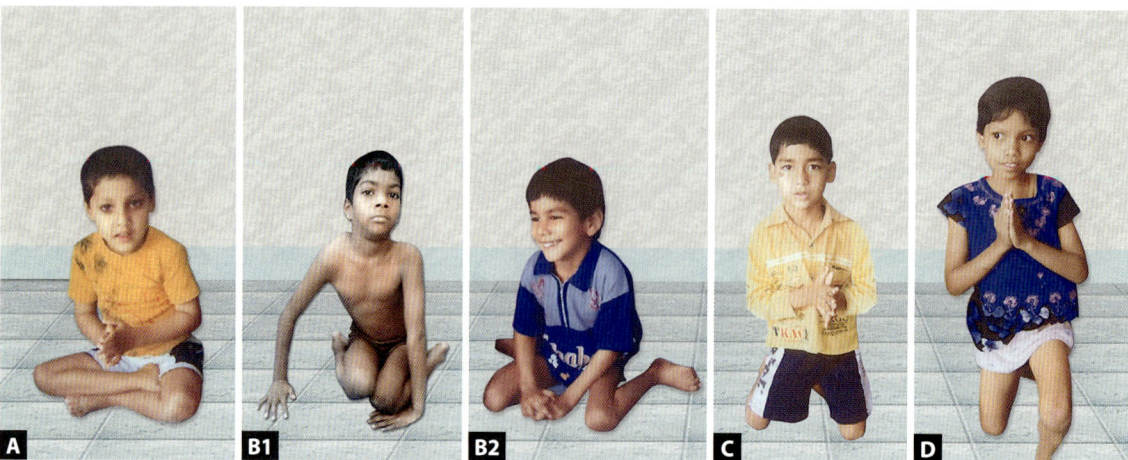

Figs. 11.40A to D: A—More or less Buddha sitting position; B1 and B2—'W' sitting position; C—Church prayer sitting position; D—Bajrangbali sitting position. If one can sit painlessly in all four positions besides squatting and he/she can walk painlessly on toes and heels for all practical purposes, his/her spine, sacroiliacs, hips, knees and ankles are almost within normal acceptable limits.

■ CEREBRAL PALSY – CASE RECORD

Patient's name. . . . . Hosp No. . . . . CP No. Age. . . . . Sex. . . . . .Weight. . . . . .Height. . . . .

Complete address. . . . .   Telephone No. . . . .

Prophylactic vaccinations with dates . . . .

Whooping cough and diphtheria. . . . . .Tetanus toxoid. . . . .

Any other sera or protective vaccines . . . .

Complain . . . .

1. Mother's health during pregnancy
    a. Any drug taken during pregnancy
    b. Any trauma or stresses during pregnancy
    c. History of TORCH infection during pregnancy
2. Length of pregnancy
3. Special features of labour and presentation
4. Delivery at hospital or home.
    a. Type of delivery (Forceps, Vacuum, Caesarean)
    b. Presentation of Child (Head/Breech/Shoulder/any other)
    c. Length (Time) of labour.
5. Age and any blood relation in between the parents at time of birth of child: Father. . . . . Mother. . . . .
6. Condition of baby at birth:
    a. Cried   b. History of asphyxia at birth   c. Blue baby   d. Suck when
    e. Temperature   f. Jaundice
    g. Transfusion given or not
    h. Twitching
    i. Convulsion
    j. Rh factor: Mother   Father   Child
    k. W.R. Kahn or allied tests
    l. Weight at birth
7. Milestones

	Normal			Normal
i. Gross:	Within	Delayed		Within
Neck holding	4 Months		Crawling	7-½ Months
Rolling over	6 Months		Standing	15 Months
Sitting	7 Months		Walking	18 Months

   ii. Details

Mental	Age	Motor	Age
Smiles		Turns on sides.	
Recognize familiar faces.		Raises head prone.	
Grasp.		Raises head supine.	
Waves bye bye		Rolls over.	
Throws		Crawls	
Monosyllables.		Sits up	
Speaks in sentences.		Stands up	
Articulation.		Walks with/without support.	
Drools.		Teething. . . . .,.	
Control over bladder and bowel		When achieved.	
Handedness (right/left)			
Hearing.		Vision.	
Behaviour.		I.Q.	

8. Primitive Reflexes
9. Habits:
    a. Sleep
    b. Appetite: Good Farr Poor   Fair   Poor
    c. Feeding habits: Breast Fed   Weaned when
                                                                                            Weaned how
    d. Diet: Liquid   Any difficulty
        Swallowing   Solid   Chewing

e. Eating: With hand   Spoon
f. Dressing
10. Previous Illness
11. Previous Treatment
12. Schooling: Ordinary school   Special school/Home education
13. Family history of congenital deformities . . . .
    a. Abortion
    b. Still birth
    c. Premature birth
    d. Brothers and sisters with ages
    e. Casualties among children and cause of death
    f. Epilepsy in family
    g. Mental disease in family
    h. C.P. in family
14. When and how did the parents aware of child's condition
15. Clinical Examination:
    a. General examination
    b. Type of CP

Modified Ashworth Scale—the most universally accepted clinical tool used to measure the increase of muscle tone		
Score	Ashworth scale (1964)	Modified Ashworth scale Bohannon and Smith (1987)
0 (0)	No increase in tone	No increase in muscle tone
1 (1)	Slight increase in tone catch when limb moved	Slight increase in muscle tone, manifested by a catch and release or by minimal resistance at the end of the range of motion when the affected part(s) is moved in flexion or extension
1 + (2)		Slight increase in muscle tone, manifested by a catch, followed by minimal resistance throughout the remainder (less than half) of the ROM (range of movement)
2 (3)	Marked increase in tone limb easily flexed	More marked increase in muscle tone through most of the ROM, but affected part(s) easily moved
3 (4)	Passive movement difficult	Considerable increase in muscle tone, passive movement difficult
4 (5)	Limb rigid	Affected part(s) rigid in flexion or extension

c. Motor system
d. Degree of muscle tone
e. Voluntary movements
f. Involuntary movements
g. Abnormal reflex postures
h. Contractures
i. Deformities
j. Co-ordination
k. Gait
l. Sensations
m. Test for cerebellar disease - (a) Diadochokinesia
n. What is interfering?
         Cognitive impairment
         Poor head control
         Asymmetry
         Floppy trunk
16. Urine test for phenyl pyruvic acid
17. Management plan:
    Therapy ....   Physical
                                                               Occupational
                                                               Speech
                                                               Vocational
                                                               Any other

    Drugs
    Aids/orthosis
    Surgery
    Follow-ups
18. Additional information (if any) ....
19. Remarks ....

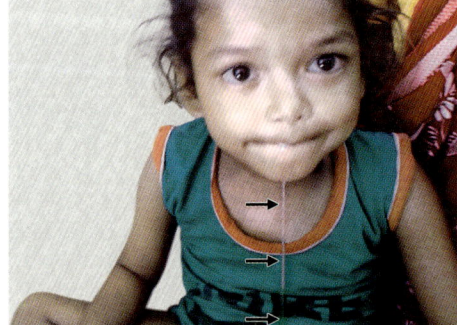

Fig. 11.41: Note the continuous drooling string of saliva in a CP child.

Therapists signature

Primitive Reflexes							
Reflex	Present	Absent	Age				
	months	months	Date				Comments
Spinal Level (Apedal stage)							
(Primitive reflexes)							
1. Flexor withdrawal	Up to 2	After 2					
2. Extensor thrust	Up to 2	After 2					
3. Crossed extension	Up to 2	After 2					
Brainstem Level (Apedal stage)							
(Primitive reflexes)							
1. ATNR	Up to 4-6	After 4–6					
2. STNR	Up to 4-6	After 4–6					
3. Tonic Labyrinthine	Up to 4	After 4					
4. Associated reaction	Absent	Absent					
5. Positive supporting reaction	Up to 4	After 4					
6. Negative supporting reaction	Up to 4	After 4					
Midbrain Level							
(Quadrupedal stage)							
(Righting reaction)							
1. Neck Righting	Up to 6	After 6					
2. Body Righting	6 onwards	From 6					
3. Labyrinthine on head prone	1–2 onwards	From 0–1–2					
4. Labyrinthine on head supine	6 onwards	From 0–6					
5. Labyrinthine on head lateral	6–8 onwards	From 0–8					
6. Optical righting	1–2 onwards	From 0–1–2					
Automatic reaction:							
1. Moro	Up to 4–6	After 4–6					
2. Landau	From 6–30	After 0–6–30					
3. Protective extensor thrust	6 onwards	From 0–6					
Cortical Level							
Equilibrium reaction							
(Bipedal stage)							
1. Supine	6 onwards	From 0–6					
2. Prone	6 onwards	From 0–6					
3. All fours	8 onwards	From 0–8					
4. Sitting	10–12 onwards	From 0–10–12					
5. Kneeling-standing	15 onwards	From 0 15					
6. Hopping	15–18 onwards	From 0–18					
7. Sea saw	15–18 onwards	From 0–18					
8. Squatting	15–18 onwards	From 0–18					
9. Walking	18 onwards	From 0–18					

BIBLIOGRAPHY

1. Gage JR, Deluca PA, Renshow TS. Gait analysis. Principles and applications: Emphasis on its use in Cerebral Palsy J Bone Joint Surg (An). 1995;77A:1607-23.
2. Gautam VK, Anand S. A new test for estimating iliotibial band contracture. J Bone Joint Surg (B). 1998;80-B:474-5.
3. Graham HK, Selber P. Musculoskeletal aspects of cerebral palsy. J Bone Joint Surg. 2003;85-B:157-66.
4. Gulati S. Neurodevelopmental disorders: The journey, the dreams, and their Realization. Ann Natl Acad Med Sci (India). 2017; 53(1): 30–35.
5. ICIDH-2 International classification of Impairments, Disabilities, and Handicaps—beta draft 2. World Health Organisation, Geneva, Switzerland; 1999.
6. Jobe MT Cerebral palsy of the hand. In campbell's operative orthopoudies twefifth Edition Volume four. Elsevier—Masby; 2013.pp.3535
7. Mutch L, Alberman E, Hagberg B, Kodama K, Perat MV. Cerebral palsy epidemiology: where are we now and where are we going? Dev Med Child Neurol. 1992;34:547-55.
8. NCMRR Research Plan for the Centre for Medical Rehabilitation. NIH Publication 1993;93:3509. US Department of Health and Human Services Public Health Service. National Institutes of Health. National Institute of Child Health and Human Development.
9. Pirpiris M, Trivett A, Baker R et al. Femoral derotation osteotomy in spastic diplegia. J Bone Joint Surg. 2003;85-B: 265-72.

CHAPTER 12

Hip

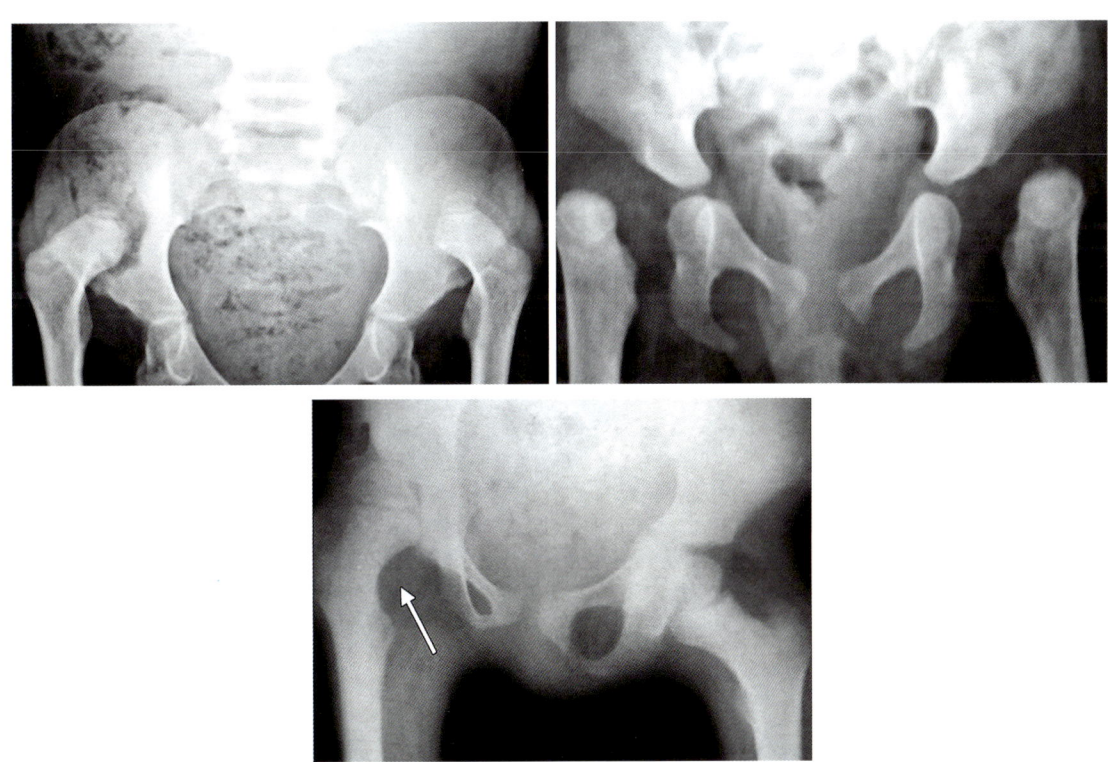

"What do we live for, if not to make life less difficult for each other."
—*George Elliot*
"We must accept finite disappointment, but never loose infinite hope."
—*Martin Luther King Jr.*

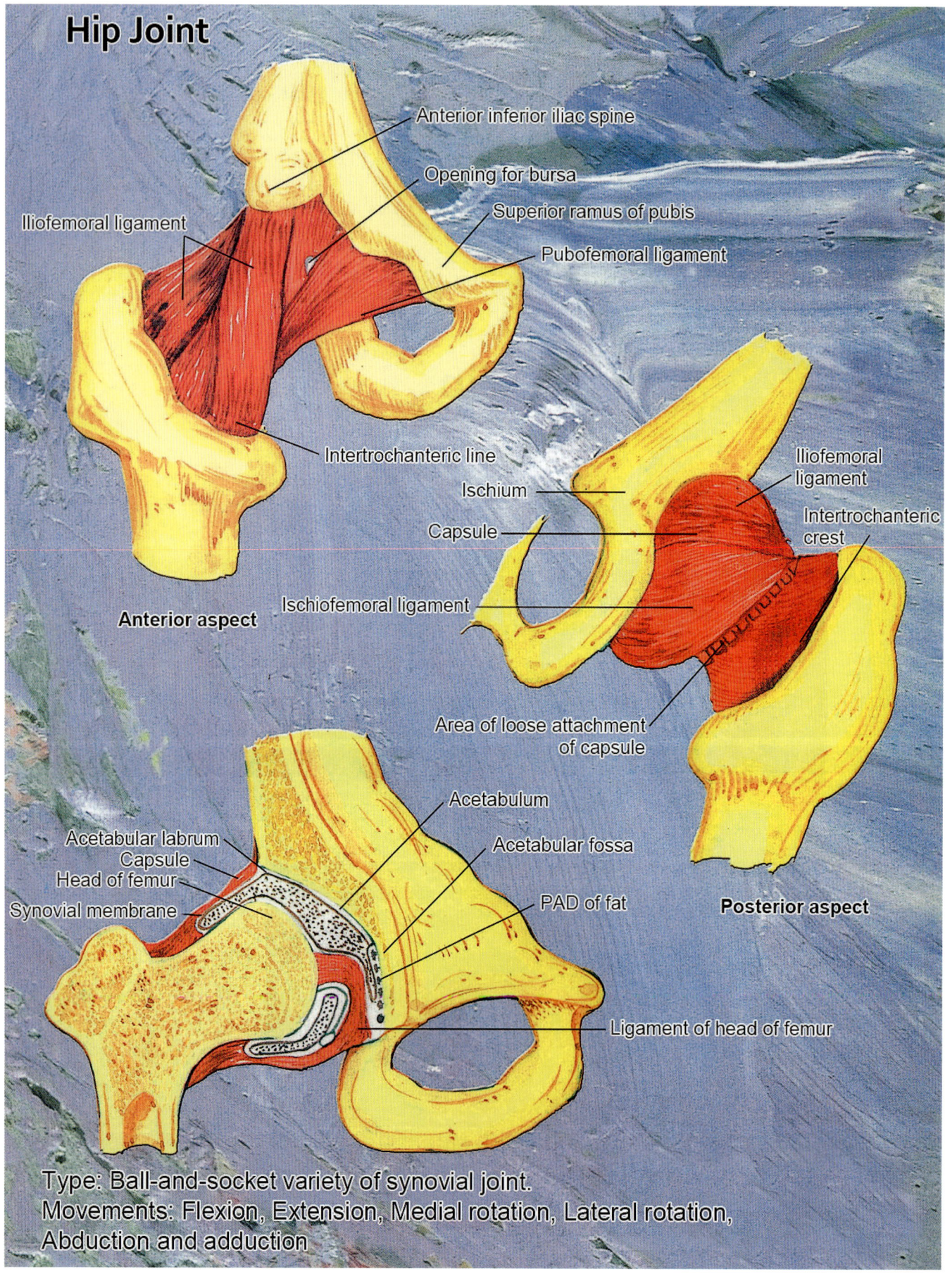

"There is only one thing that is more painful than learning from experience, and that is, not learning from experience."
—*Archibald Mcleish*

INTRODUCTION

In bipeds, the hips have the great responsibility of transmitting the ground reaction against the body weight while at the same time preserving mobility. To mechanically accommodate this postural change, the head and neck of femur undergo angulation and rotation at the base. Any affection of the hip is of much concern to the patient since it affects locomotion from the very beginning. The patient mostly tries to accommodate the disabilities following such pathology, as far as practicable, by various compensatory mechanisms.

ANATOMICAL CONSIDERATIONS

- The hip joint—formed by head of femur and acetabulum—is one of the largest and most stable synovial ball and socket (enarthrosis) variety of joint in the body with great range of motion. If it is injured or suffers any pathology, it is usually manifested by affecting the normal gait.
- Compensations for deficits at the hip are usually made by various tiltings at the (i) pelvis, (ii) lower spine, (iii) ankle and foot, and (iv) knee.
- Early pathology at the hip may manifest as pain on the anteromedial aspect of the knee (being referred along the anterior division of the obturator nerve). Hence, it is imperative to examine the hip fully for any unexplained pain in the knee.
- At birth a single proximal growth plate is present; with medial portion forming the capital epiphyseal plate and the lateral portion the greater trochanteric apophyseal plate (Morgan and Somerville 1960). The capital epiphysis ossifies at about 4–6 months and is responsible primarily for metaphyseal growth of the neck of femur and less for the appositional growth of the head of femur (Canole and King 1984). The trochanteric apophysis ossifies at about 4 years of age and is primarily responsible for the appositional growth of the greater trochanter and less for the metaphyseal growth of femur (Canoe and King 1984).
- Development of neck-shaft angle (upward inclination) and the femoral torsion: Arising between the trochanters, the femoral neck slants proximally and medially forming an angle with the femoral axis which is called the neck-shaft angle. The neck-shaft angles are more or less constant varying from 130°–140° in embryonic life settling at the age of 4–6 years to about 135°. Neck shaft angle greater than this is called 'coxa valga', and lesser than this is 'coxa vara'. The angle of femoral torsion is the angle formed by the plane of the transcondylar axis and the plane of the central axis of the femoral neck. Normally, the neck lies in anterior oblique direction, i.e. anteversion of neck (forward inclination of the neck relative to the shaft by 15°–20°). When the angle of anteversion is greatly reduced or goes to a negative value it is the retroversion of the neck. The newborns have femoral anteversion of a mean of 38° (range–60°), which decreases with normal growth and development to the adult mean of 19°. Increased femoral neck anteversion during childhood is associated with the cosmetic deformity of intoeing gait (*Also see* Page 244 and **Figs. 12.38 and 12.39**). The gain in morphological evolution, has to pay its price by making the neck very much susceptible to rotational shearing stress.
- The arterial supply (retinacular, metaphyseal and that through ligamentum teres) of the head and neck of the femur is such as to make it very vulnerable in intracapsular injuries of the hip.
- Calcar femorale (an oblique longitudinal condensation of the compact trabeculae on inferomedial aspect of the neck, trochanteric region and upper shaft) provides an internal support for the mechanically disadvantageously placed head and neck of the femur. It also determines to a great extent, the displacement of subcapital and trochanteric fractures.
  The distance between the centre of the femoral head to the tip of greater trochanter is usually two and a half times the radius of the femoral head.
- Capsular reflections of the hip encases the whole of the neck anteriorly. Posteriorly, it is deficient by about 1.5 cm from intertrochanteric crest, thereby encasing most part of the upper metaphyseal end of the femur. Hence, infective pathology (e.g. pyogenic infections) is very much likely to affect the hip joint quite early.
  The capsule is reinforced by the ligaments almost all around, strongest of which is anteriorly placed as the iliofemoral ligament *('Y' ligament of Biglow)*
- The hip is a ball and socket joint. This joint permits flexion-extension, abduction-adduction, internal rotation-external rotation and to a varying extent the circumduction. Since the femoral head has to transmit the ground reactions against the body weight, it becomes vulnerable to dislocation. However, the watershed created by the reinforced margins of deep acetabulum (except for the posteroinferior region) mostly prevents this. Further, the acetabular surface is inclined (oriented) 45° downward and 15° anteriorly
- Fortunately, the hip is surrounded by thick layers of stout muscles, which can take the greater load of hip functions even when there is deficit in the intracapsular bony lever.
- The hip is commonly vulnerable for the congenital deformities, i.e. dysplasia/subluxation/dislocations; infective pathology—pyogenic/tuberculosis; fractures —fracture neck of femur (intracapsular)/trochanteric fracture (extracapsular); dislocations and degenerative arthrosis, besides a host of other pathologies. Hence, at almost all ages, detail assessment of the hip is essential. In hip involvements, the first movement to be lost is extension, the hip gradually assuming a varying flexion

attitude with progress of the underlying pathology. With erosion of the articular cartilage, rotational movements, besides extension, are lost early.
- The hip joint space becomes most accommodative in the posture of flexion, abduction and external rotation. Hence, this is the most common postural attitude in case of pathologies where there is a collection in the joint.
- The protective natural splint for the painful conditions of hip is by spasm of the powerful flexors (iliopsoas) and adductors. Therefore, in any erosive pathology, these deformities are commonly seen. However, the effect of prolonged decubitus in a particular posture and compensatory mechanisms by the patient, do affect the ultimate posture of the limb.

Certain Important Anatomical Landmarks

- *Pubic tubercle*: In adults, pubic tubercles are about 2.5 cm on either side of pubic symphysis. A line joining them and prolonged on either side crosses the normal femoral head in the normal pelvis
- Anterior landmark of femoral head is about 1 cm below and out to the mid-inguinal point
- From a central point at the base of the greater trochanter, a line drawn to the ipsilateral mid-inguinal point (or to opposite anterior superior iliac spine) represents the femoral neck.
- A line joining the posterior superior iliac spines in normal pelvis crosses at the second sacral segment (where spinal dura ends) and if prolonged on either side, this line transects the sacroiliac joint almost in the middle.
- A line joining the most prominent point of ischial tuberosities lies almost at the level of the base of greater trochanter.
- The femoral axis slants medially from hip to knee.

■ METHODOLOGY

History Taking

Besides as given in the Chapter 1 'Introduction', certain leading questions are essential to elicit certain points, specially in early pathology and that too in children. The main complaints in a hip disease are pain, limp (may be after some activity), stiffness, deformities, limb length disparity, swelling and paralytic disabilities.

Truly, the hip pain is felt in the groin region in about 90% of cases (in adductor tendinitis also the pain is felt in the groin).

Pain in the lateral hip region or buttock is usually the referred pain from the lumbar spine or trochanteric bursa. However, hip pain may radiate from the groin to the anteromedial aspect of thigh, greater trochanter, buttock and knee (mainly on medial aspect of knee). Rotational movements (passive or active) of hip are limited in hip pathologies mainly due to pain and spasm of muscles related to hip movements.

Pain in posterosuperior iliac spine region and buttock is usually referred from the lumbar spine and sacroiliac joint. If this pain radiates down along the back of thigh and knee and goes further down mostly it is radicular pain. Pain in lateral side of hip is mostly peritrochanteric and it may radiate down along lateral part of thigh as occurs in tendinitis of iliotibial band. Pain in lateral hip region may be also from inflamed trochanteric bursa, a snapping iliotibial band, gluteus medius and minimus tendinosis, hip joint pathology.

In hip intra-articular pathology, patient tries to denote the site of pain by his/her hand placed as if surrounding the hip in the shape of 'C' with the thumb placed in the groin crease and the fingers on the buttock (Byrd 'C' sign quoted by Gutyon JL, 2013 in cambell's operative orthopaedics, 12th Edn: Elsevier Mosby: p. 335).

Pain of hip appearing after sitting for longer period and minimising on standing or walking is usually due to some impingement in hip. Femur-acetabular impingement (FAI Cam and Pincer types) is common cause of hip pain, and if left untreated end up in hip arthritis; early treatment by arthroscopic debridement, CAM excision and labrum repair saves the hip from undergoing arthritis. Pain occurring with popping or snapping sensation is usually caused by snapping psoas tendon or iliotibial band or by the labral tear. Snapping of posterior edge of iliotibial band or anterior edge of gluteus maximus over the greater trochanter during the flexion and extension of hip and repeated snapping may lead to inflammation of trochanteric bursa—"*external snapping hip*". This usually occurs in ballet dancers, runners, soccer players and allied strains.

The "*internal snapping hip*" is produced due to snapping of iliopsoas tendon over the iliopectineal eminence or the anterior hip capsule. In flexion of hip, the psoas tendon lies lateral to iliopectineal eminence, but when the hip is extended, the tendon slips across the iliopectineal eminence and anterior hip capsule, during which a snapping sensation and an audible gentle thud is produced with/without some pain in the groin.

Most of the pathologies affecting the hip (traumatic or non-traumatic) can be roughly guessed by seeing the attitude of the patient and taking his age into consideration.

Common Pathologies (According to Different Age Groups)

Traumatic
- Up to 5 years of age, fracture or dislocation involving the hip joint is very rare
- In 5–20 years of age—fracture neck of femur (intracapsular) is seen
- In sportsmen, there is a possibility of avulsion of the lesser/greater trochanter
- In young adults, the injuries around hip are dislocations; fracture of neck of femur (intracapsular); fracture pelvis; fracture of trochanteric region (extracapsular)

- In the middle age, the usual incidence is of fracture of neck of femur (intracapsular), fracture of trochanteric region (extracapsular), dislocation, fracture pelvis
- In the elderly, fracture of trochanteric region (extracapsular), fracture of neck of femur (intracapsular), pathological fractures and fracture pelvis commonly occur.

Non-traumatic
- 0–5 years of age—(Congenital) Developmental hip dysplasias/(DDH); Tom Smith arthritis (transient synovitis), pyogenic infections, tuberculous infection
- 5–10 years—Perthes' disease, tuberculous infection, pyogenic infection
- 10–15 years—Adolescent coxa vara, Perthes' disease, tuberculous infection, pyogenic infection and bone cysts
- 15–35 years—Ankylosing spondylitis, rheumatoid arthritis, tuberculous infection, idiopathic osteonecrosis, secondary osteoarthrosis and bone cysts
- Elderly—Degenerative osteoarthrosis (primary or secondary osteoarthritis), secondaries from any primary malignant tumour, tuberculous infection.

In case of trauma, hip is usually involved in indirect violence (e.g. slip in the bathroom, tripping, missing of step, etc.), which mostly results in the unsolved problems of fracture of the neck of femur. The immediate status of the patient, specially as regards standing, weight bearing and using the affected limb in locomotion, should be enquired into.

General and Systemic Examination

It is done as usual, with a special emphasis on the type of gait (refer to the Chapter 7 'Spine'), if the patient can walk; and mode of weight bearing, if the patient can stand.

An overall assessment of the patient and the hip condition should be noted while the patient is walking, standing and sitting on a stool. Any particular attitude or abnormal finding should be noted, such as scoliosis of the lower back **(Refer Figs. 8.11 to 8.13)**, elevation of the buttock region and prominence of trochanters. Five fingers quadriceps purchase **(Refer Figs. 11.10 and 11.11)** in polio patient can only be marked while the patient is standing and walking.

Regional Examination

Since various compensatory mechanisms right from the lower lumbar spine to the ankle and foot can occur to accommodate the hip pathology, these regions must be examined in any hip involvement.

Local Examination Prerequisites

Prerequisites of hip examination:
- Patient should be supine on a flat bed or couch
- Both lower limbs, hips and abdomen must be exposed (a narrow strip to be placed over private parts, specially in females). A female attendant must be by the side while examining a female patient
- To note the attitude, patient should be asked to lie comfortably in as far neutral a position as possible.

Attitude

Although attitude of the limb varies in various stages of different pathological and traumatic conditions, certain attitudes may be considered as typical.

In congenital dislocation of the hip—broadening at trochanteric level, widening of the perineum, asymmetry and/or duplication of gluteal fold **(Figs. 12.1 and 12.2)**.

The term "congenital dislocation of hip" was introduced in about 1920 by Hilgenreiner. After that various (more than 15) names have been suggested. Klisic P recommended for changing the terminology to *"developmental displacement of*

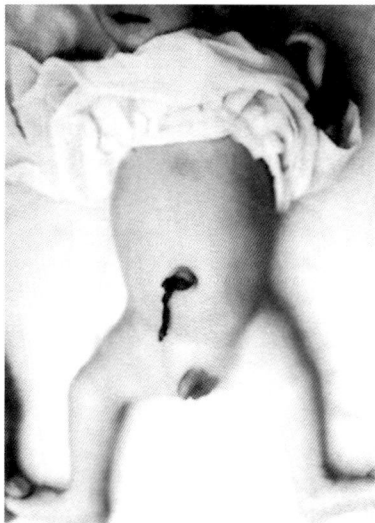

Fig. 12.1: Photograph of the child with CDH showing widening of perineum (also has duplication and asymmetry of gluteal fold and shortening).

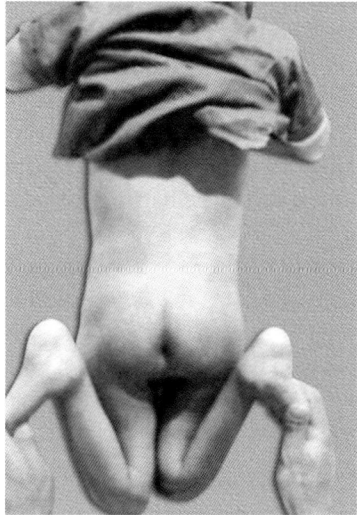

Fig. 12.2: Marked dissociation in gluteal folds in CDH.

the hip", based on the different pathological manifestations of the condition, embracing all variants of the disorder (dislocations, subluxation, dysplasia, hypoplasia and instability) whether they occur prenatally or postnatally.

Developmental dysplasia of the hip (DDH) denotes a wide spectrum of pathological conditions, ranging from subtle acetabular dysplasia to irreducible hip dislocation (Michael et al. 2001).

In synovitis of hip joint—mild flexion, abduction and external rotation, with apparent lengthening of the limb.

In true arthritis of hip joint—flexion, adduction and internal rotation with/without true shortening of the limb.

In pure posterior dislocation—flexion, marked adduction and internal rotation with apparent and true shortening.

In anterior dislocation—flexion, abduction, and external rotation, with apparent lengthening of the limb in low type, whereas in the high type there is marked external rotation in full extension and some abduction.

In trochanteric fracture, marked external rotation (outer part of foot mostly touching the bed) of the lower limb, is characteristic. *In fracture neck of femur* also, there is external rotation but not so marked (due to catch in the capsule due to irritation by the fractured end); in late cases variable flexion and adduction may be superadded except where patient has managed to walk where there may be even abduction of the limb.

Inspection (Table 12.1)

It should be done from the front, side and the back **(Figs. 12.3A to D)**.

Palpation

As in the Chapter 1 Introduction, confirm the findings of inspection from different sides. While palpating, *mark with a skin pencil the bony points* (anterior superior iliac spine, tip of greater trochanter, pubic tubercle, ischial tuberosity) required for assessing measurements and movements. It is more convenient and accurate to localise the sharp bony points by the metal end of the measuring tape.

If the presentations of the hip pathology are vague: (i) *Percussion on the heel pad* with firm fist (Heel thrust test) in the extended position of leg, and over the trochanter usually induces discomfort and/or pain in the groin region if there is any disease or injury in the hip, (ii) Keep your clenched fist between the patient's knees and ask the patient to squeeze your fist from the sides. In any painful condition (disease or injury) of pelvis or hip or even femora or knee, the patient will complain of pain pointing to the approximate site.

Superficial Palpation (Touch)

Touch and assess the temperature, skin surface (smooth/rough), any hyperaesthesia/anaesthesia, venous prominence, sharp bony points.

TABLE 12.1: Inspection of the hip joint.

	Fixed bony points	Soft tissue region	Abnormal findings
From front (Fig. 12.3A)	Anterior superior iliac spine, pubic symphysis and pubic tubercle	Iliac fossae, inguinal ligament, groin fold, femoral triangle (Scarpa's triangle), front of the thigh	Muscular wasting, any swelling, sinuses, scar marks, ulcers, obvious pulsations, abnormal skin conditions, level of anterior superior iliac spine
From the side (Fig. 12.3B)	Iliac crest and trochanteric region	Gluteal bulge, supratrochanteric depression, infratrochanteric depression, lateral thigh muscle mass	Same as above and level of tip of trochanter in relation to the anterior superior iliac spine
From the back (Fig. 12.3C)	Back of iliac crest, posterior superior iliac spine represented by dimple of Venus, ischial tuberosity region	Gluteal bulges, gluteal folds, back of the thigh	Muscular wasting, any swelling, sinuses, ulcers, obvious pulsations, abnormal skin condition, contracture **(Figs. 12.4 to 12.7)**

Deep Palpation

Besides that in Chapter 1 Introduction, note the hollowness/fullness/tenderness of the iliac fossae and site and volume of femoral pulsation at the base of the Scarpa's triangle. In conditions like posterior dislocation of hip, excised or dissolved head and neck of femur, Buerger's disease the femoral arterial pulsation is weak, or sometimes not palpable (Positive Narath's sign).

Points to be palpated (by applying deep finger pressure) to locate tenderness of the hip joint **(Figs. 12.8A to C)**:

- *Anteriorly:* Just below and lateral to the mid inguinal point at the base of the Scarpa's triangle
- *Laterally:* Just above the tip of the greater trochanter by giving direct pressure or thrust over the trochanter. The patient points towards the hip joint, if it is tender. *Intensities of trochanteric tenderness can hint towards underlying pathology,* for example:
  - *Touch tenderness*—fresh trochanteric fracture, acute inflammatory lesion in that area
  - *Deep pressure tenderness*—healing trochanteric fracture, trochanteric bursitis, trochanteric cyst, fracture neck femur
- Trochanteric bursitis is inflammation of the bursa lying between the tendon of gluteus maximus and posterolateral surface of greater trochanter. It causes pain around trochanter which may be confused with the pain of herniated disc. They can be differentiated by eliciting

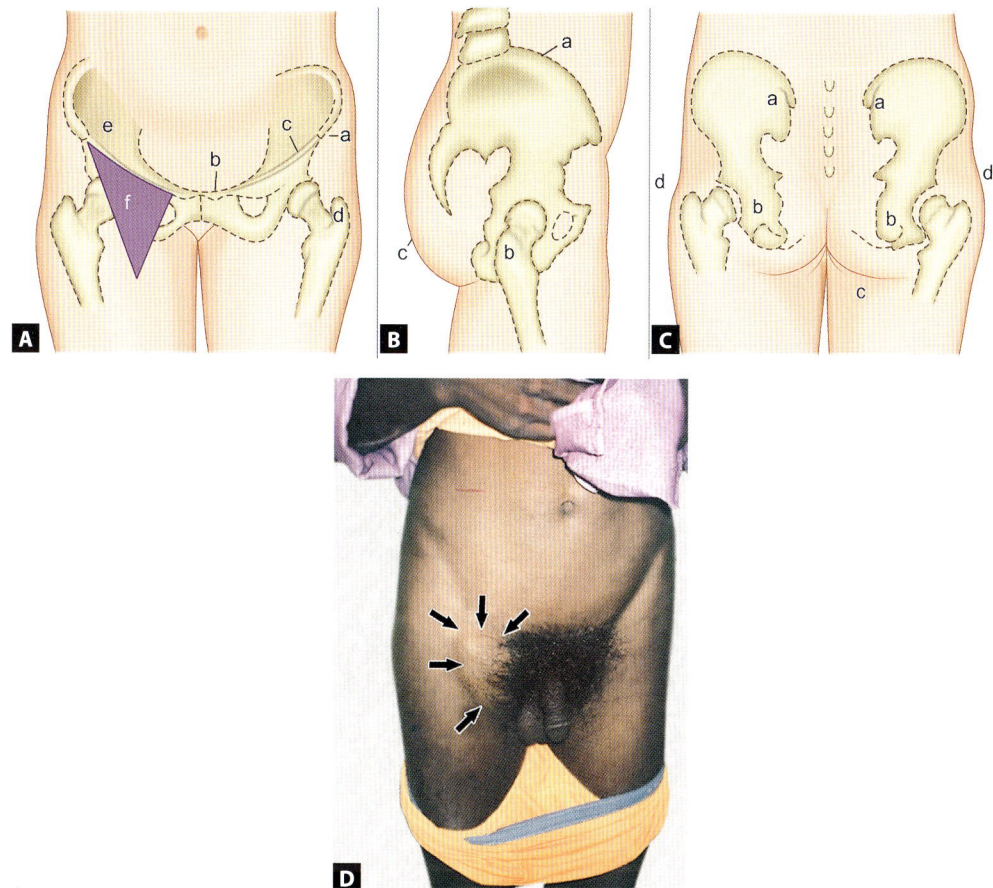

Figs. 12.3A to D: (A) Inspection from front. Note the following: a = anterior superior iliac spine; b = pubic tubercle; c = inguinal ligament; d = greater trochanter; e = iliac fossae; f = Scarpa's triangle, (B) Inspection from side: a= iliac crest; b = trochanteric region; c= gluteal bulge, (C) Inspection from back. Note the following: a = posterior superior iliac spine; b = ischial tuberosity; c = gluteal fold; d = supratrochanteric depression; (D) A rounded or oblong swelling in the base of right Scarpa's triangle may be femoral hernia (or cold abscess as in **Figure 8.39**).

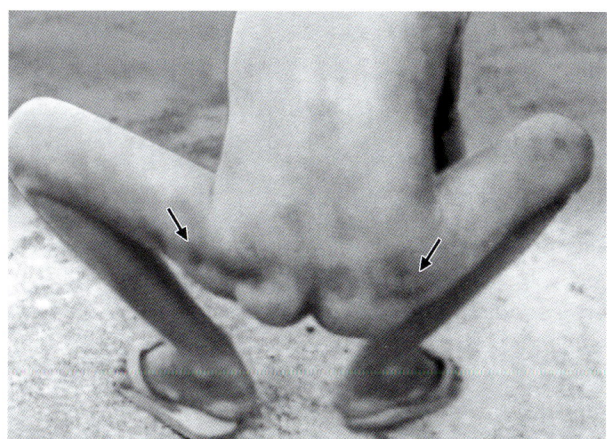

Fig. 12.4: Bilateral gluteus maximus contracture—Photograph showing puckering in the buttock and thigh due to fibrosis along the line of gluteus maximus, specially when the patient attempts to squat or stoop forewards.

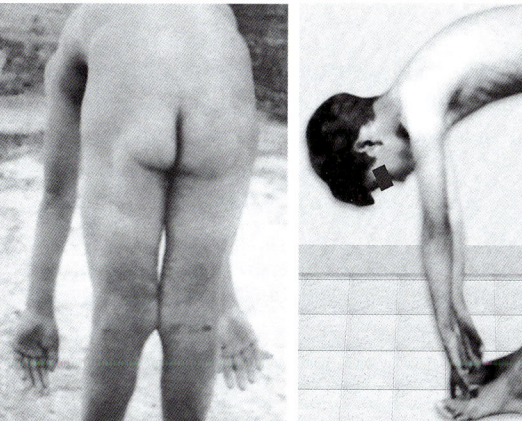

Fig. 12.5: Due to gluteus maximus contracture the patient is not able to stoop fully.

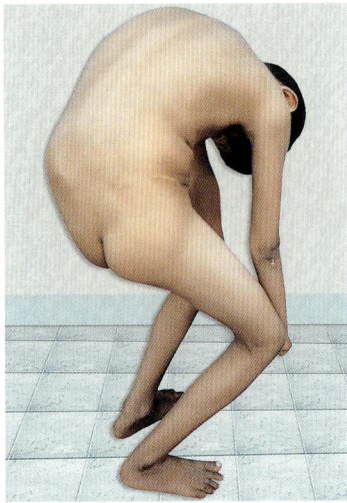

Fig. 12.6: Marked gluteus maximus contracture.

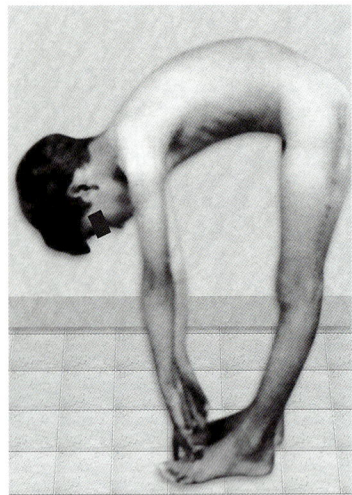

Fig. 12.7: Same **(Figs. 12.4 and 12.5)** patient, after operative release of the fibrotic contracture, he is able to stoop fully and there is no puckering.

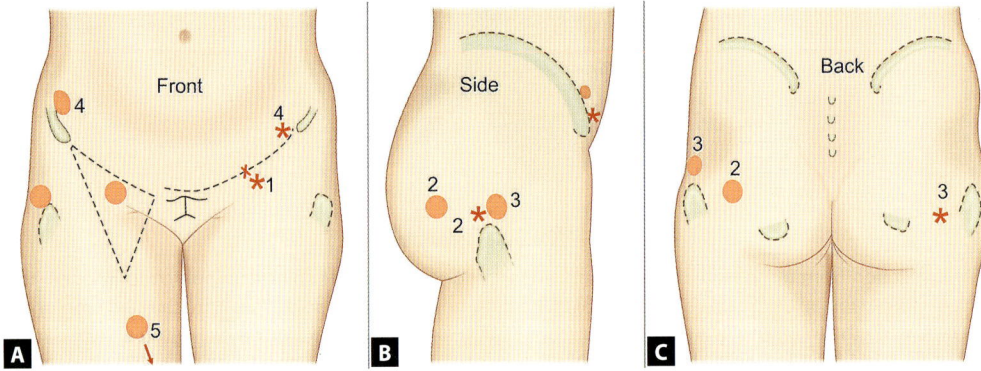

Figs. 12.8A to C: Points to be palpated to locate the tenderness (shown by stars—*) of hip joint; and sites to be suspected/palpated for cold abscess originating in hip joint (shown by circle containing dots—•).

tenderness around posterior aspect of greater trochanter in trochanteric bursitis and in sciatic notch in herniated disc.
  • *Thrust tenderness*—transmitted tenderness in fracture neck femur, fracture acetabulum, tuberculosis hip and other chronic inflammatory hip involvements.
- *Posteriorly*
  • About the centre of a line joining the trochanteric tip to the ischial tuberosity
  • About the centre of a line joining the ischial tuberosity and posterior superior iliac spine.
- *Iliac fossa:* In the base of iliac fossa more inferiorly
- *Medially:* At the junction of the groin with the medial aspect of the thigh.

Sites to be inspected and palpated for cold abscess or for any collection from the hip joint **(Figs. 12.8A to C)**
- Base of Scarpa's triangle
- Gluteal region
- Supratrochanteric region
- Iliac fossa
- Anteromedial aspect of mid-thigh even up to knee joint, in that direction.

Heel Thrust Test

When the local clinical findings are inconclusive about the involvement of hip, the heel thrust test can indirectly suggest it. Patient lies supine with suspected side lower limb fully extended. A firm thrust is applied over the heel by fist. The patient will complain of varying pain/discomfort in the hip region if it is involved in any pathology.

Allied, to hip, places should also be examined (palpated), such as, tenderness at the pubic symphysis indicates osteitis pubis. Tenderness along inguinal canal may be due to inguinal hernia; Deficiency with/without tenderness in the abdominal wall may be due to sports hernia; Tenderness over the greater trochanter and abductor tendon may be due to trochanteric bursitis and partial tear of gluteus medius.

Lymph Nodes

Inguinal and external iliac groups of lymph nodes should be examined.

■ MOVEMENTS (TABLE 12.2)

In examining the hip joint, two aspects which present maximum difficulties to young clinicians and students are:
- Eliciting the range of different movements of the hip joint
- Measurement of the limb for limb length disparity.

It is essential to know the normal range of movements in the different directions.

For measuring opposing movements (e.g. flexion-extension; abduction-adduction; internal rotation-external rotation) there must be a zero position of the joint for that group from where it will be convenient and accurate to measure the range of motion in that particular direction.

Normal Range of Movements

For flexion-extension: The back of the thigh, calf and heel points must touch the bed (zero position). The fully extended (or as far as possible extended) limb going above, or in front, will be flexion (to be measured from zero position onwards). While lying prone or on the side, the extended limb going posteriorly is extension. While lying on the sides, the long axis of the extended limb as a whole should be in line with the trunk and parallel to the bed (zero position).

TABLE 12.2: Normal movements of hip.

Movements	Axis	Range of movement	Prime mover	Nerve supply	Assisted by	Limiting factor
Flexion	—	0°–110° to 130°	Psoas major	L 2–3	Rectus femoris, Sartorius, Pectineus, Tensor fascia lata Adductor longus Adductor brevis Adductor magnus (Oblique fibres)	With extended knee—tension on hamstrings With flexed knee—contact of thigh with abdomen
Extension (Extension beyond zero position)	—	0°–20°	Gluteus maximus Semitendinosus Semimembranosus Biceps femoris	Inferior gluteal (L5, S1–2) Sciatic nerve (L4, 5, S1, 2, 3)		Tension of anterior capsule is re-enforced by iliofemoral ligament Tension of hip flexors
Abduction	Anteroposterior axis passing through head of femur	0° to 45°–55°	Gluteus medius	Superior Gluteal nerve (L4, 5, S1)	Gluteus minimus Gluteus maximus (Upper fibres) Tensor fascia lata	Tension of hip adductors, tension of medial band of iliofemoral ligament and adjoining capsule
Adduction	Do	0° to 35°–45°	Adductor longus Adductor magnus Adductor brevis Pectineus Gracilis	Obturator nerve (L3, 4) Femoral nerve (L2, 3, 4)		With extended knee—contact of upper part of thigh with the opposite one With flexed knee—tension of abductors and tension of lateral band of iliofemoral ligament
External rotation	Vertical axis, passing through centre of head of femur and mid-patellar point	0° to 40°–50° (except in persons not used to Budha sitting position) (e.g. Europeans, Americans, etc.) in whom the terminal 10°–20° are limited on either side	Obturator externus Obturator Internus Quadratus femoris Piriformis Gemelli superior Gemelli inferior	S3, 4 S1, 2, 3 L5, S1 S1, 2 S1, 2, 3 L5, S1	Sartorius, long head of biceps femoris	Tension of internal rotators of hip Tension of iliofemoral ligament

Contd...

Contd...

Movements	Axis	Range of movement	Prime mover	Nerve supply	Assisted by	Limiting factor
Internal rotation	-do-	0° to 30°–40°	Gluteus minimus Tensor fascia lata	Superior gluteal nerve (L4, 5, S1)	Gluteus medius (anterior fibres) Semimembranosus Semitendinosus	With flexed hip, tension of ischio-femoral ligament Tension of hip external rotators With extended hip, tension of iliofemoral ligament
Flexion, abduction and external rotation of hip, while knee is flexed			Sartorius (Tailor's muscle)	L2, 3, 4	Hip flexors Knee flexors Hip abductors	
Abduction of hip in flexion			Tensor fascia lata	L4, 5, S1	Hip external rotators Gluteus medius Gluteus minimus	

Circumduction:
Limitation of any of above mentioned movements will not allow free range of circumduction

For abduction-adduction: The long axis of the limb must be parallel to each other and to the axis of the trunk [the line joining the mid-inguinal point (practically anterior superior iliac spine may also be taken), mid-patellar point, midpoint on anterior aspect of ankle joint and second web of the foot, is the long axis of the limb]. From this zero position, abduction, i.e. the limb moving outwards and adduction, i.e. the limb moving towards the opposite limb or inwards without moving the pelvis, are measured.

For internal rotation-external rotation: For this, the zero position is that in which the patella is almost horizontal and the great toe is pointing vertically upwards (except in toe-out and toe-in deformities). From this zero position, the rotational movement in either direction (internal and external) are measured.

■ FIXED DEFORMITIES OF HIP

Persistent muscular spasm; persistent posture assumed to avoid pain or to conceal any obvious deformity/disparity of the limb-lengths; destructive changes in the joint; fibrotic contractures in periarticular soft tissues and surgical interventions may lead to particular fixed positions of a joint, from where limb cannot be brought back to neutral position, but further movement in the same axis may be possible—"fixed deformity."

The hip joint commonly gets fixed in flexion, adduction or abduction, internal rotation or external rotations, either singly or in various combinations. Common fixed deformities are flexion, abduction, external rotation, in that order. The *combination of fixed deformities* are flexion, adduction and internal rotation; flexion, abduction and external rotation; adduction and external rotation in that order.

For understanding the pathomechanics of these deformities, one must clearly understand the following points:

- The hip being a ball and socket joint, allows a certain range of motion in all directions. Beyond that normal range, if one tries, either actively or passively, to move the hip, it is not that the femoral head is moving in the acetabular socket, rather the head is fixed in the acetabulum and the opposite ligaments get tighter and thereby both the head and acetabulum move as one unit moving the hemipelvis. Thus, beyond the normal range, movements are achieved by moving the pelvis. In case of limitation of the terminal movements, this situation will come early, i.e. short of the normal range. In presence of any fixed deformity in that direction, if we attempt to bring the limb to zero position, the pelvis will start moving from the very point of fixity
- Beyond the position of fixed deformity, it may be possible to have some free range of the same motion
- If the joint is fixed in a particular direction, the opposite motion is automatically not possible
- In measuring this fixed range, one should measure from the zero position
- The pelvis must be fixed to the bed while testing for the range of motion. The moment the pelvis starts moving (manifested by movement of the anterior superior iliac spine), one must stop and bring the limb back to just short of this situation. Then measure the range from the zero position
- Even though a patient may have a fixed deformity, he usually adopts some compensatory measures in order to:
  • Conceal the deformities
  • Maintain the equilibrium by shifting the centre of gravity

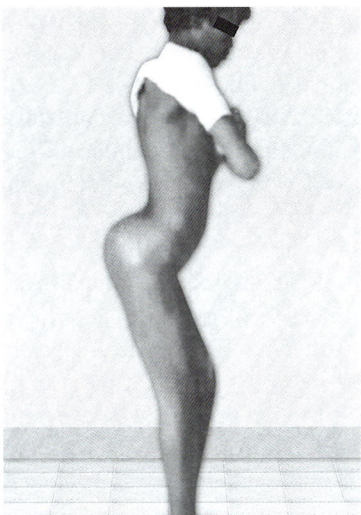

Fig. 12.9: Photograph showing lumbar lordosis due to fixed flexion deformity at hip.

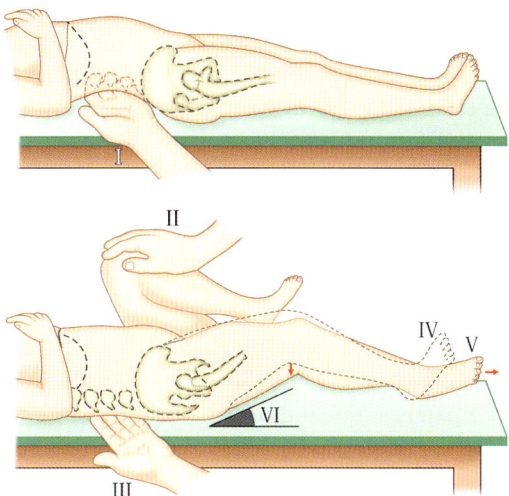

Fig. 12.10: Method of eliciting fixed flexion deformity at hip by Thomas test.

- Apparently make up the disparity of the limb length
- Stabilise the unstable hip.

Therefore, in most of the fixed deformities, there are compensatory, secondary functional (postural) deformities, e.g. in fixed flexion deformity of hip—lordosis at the lumbar spine **(Fig. 12.9)**; in fixed abduction deformity of hip—lowering of the pelvis on that side and scoliosis with convexity towards the affected side; in fixed adduction deformity of hip—raising of the pelvis on that side and scoliosis with convexity towards the unaffected side.

Fixed external/internal rotation deformities remain more or less revealed because of lack of proper compensation. Any attempt to properly compensate these deformities produces stress at the lumbar and lumbosacral region, as well as on the knee, ankle and foot.

Hence, in assessing the fixed deformities first of all it is essential to neutralise the postural compensatory deformities.

With a painful hip, flexion contracture or fixed flexion deformity, the patient stands with hyperextension of lumbar spine (as a compensatory posture). When he/she attempts to walk, the lumbar spine further goes for extension. In hip flexion contracture, the pelvis also rotates towards the affected side during the extension of hip to accommodate the inadequate extension of hip. This combination of asymmetric external rotation of pelvis during extension of hip along with flexion contracture is called a *pelvic wink*.

Fixed Flexion Deformity of Hip

In most of the pathological conditions of the hip, the first movement to be lost is extension, i.e. the backward movement from the zero position. Thereafter, the hip goes in for increasing flexion deformity with progress of the disease. If there is fixed flexion deformity at the hip, there will be compensatory lumbar lordosis to conceal it. This must be obliterated to see the actual fixed flexion deformity.

For assessing the fixed flexion deformity, the whole credit goes to Hugh Owen Thomas who described this test in the year 1876.

Methods (Fig. 12.10)

The patient lies supine on a firm flat surface. The examiner gradually flexes the normal hip, holding the bent knee till the compensatory lordosis is obliterated. This should be judged by insinuating the hand between back and the bed. When the fingers can no longer be insinuated, flexion of the normal hip is stopped. In this manoeuvre, the affected hip, if in fixed flexion deformity, will automatically be lifted anteriorly up to a certain angle. While the normal hip is kept in the flexed position, the affected hip is actively or passively extended as far as possible keeping the limb in neutral longitudinal alignment (i.e. '0' position in between abduction and adduction, and '0' position in rotation)—which cannot be extended beyond the angle of fixed flexion. Now the angle subtended between the back of the thigh and the bed, will be the angle of fixed flexion deformity.

Severity of the flexion contracture at the hip will not be appreciated if the hip is allowed to abduct while the Thomas test is performed.

Criticism of Thomas test

- The patient is hurt further in a painful hip
- In obese or heavily built individuals, it is not easy to perform this test, because of improper appreciation of obliteration of lumbar lordosis
- In bilateral fixed flexion deformity of the hip, it is difficult to perform this test. Since the unaffected side is necessarily manoeuvred to elicit this test it would never facilitate comparative evaluation in bilateral cases

- Quite often, inappropriate amount of force is applied in flexing the thigh over the abdomen, which leads to anterior tilting of the pelvis. Then the actual measurement would be of the angle made in the long axis of the distal part of the pelvis and the bed, rather than the long axis of the thigh and the bed, leading to fallacious measurement
- In presence of ankylosed knee (in extension), it is difficult to perform this test.

Prone Hip-extension Test (Staheli 1977)

The patient lies prone with the pelvis lying at the edge of the table and the lower limbs hanging free in flexion. The examiner places one hand on the posterior superior iliac spines and the other hand gradually brings the affected limb into extension. The point at which the pelvis begins to move anteriorly, stop there and measure the angle subtended between femur and the horizontal plane—this is the angle of fixed flexion deformity.

Alternative Methods (Fig. 12.11)

This method is more useful in bilateral fixed flexion deformities of hip. Put the patient prone on the couch in such a fashion that the trunk lies fully supported on the couch and the hip region is at the edge of the couch. Support both the knees with your hands to avoid hurting the patient. Then, passively, extend the hips by lifting the knees till resistance is felt. No force should be used. Keeping the thighs in this position, the angle made between the long axis of the trunk (easily manifested, by putting the forearm on the back with hand projected beyond the buttock) and the thigh would be the angle of fixed flexion deformity. In the same attempt, flexion deformities of both the hips can be evaluated.

If there is superadded cause for lordosis, like spondylolisthesis, this can be evaluated more easily in a prone position than a supine. If there is simultaneous fixed flexion deformity of the knee, that also can be measured easily in this position. While the knees are kept supported, the legs are allowed to fall towards '0' position (i.e. fully extended position) of the knee. If the *fixed flexion deformity* is more

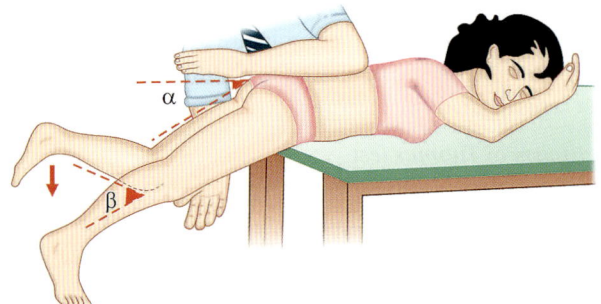

Fig. 12.11: Alternative method of assessing fixed flexion deformity of hip joint, specially useful in bilateral cases; simultaneously fixed flexion deformity at knee can also be assessed. (α = angle of fixed flexion deformity at hip; β = angle of fixed flexion deformity at knee).

than 90°, gently take the leg passively towards zero position. In presence of fixed flexion deformity, the knee cannot be extended beyond the angle of fixity.

Once the fixed flexion deformity is measured, the patient is asked to flex the hip further as much as he can—this will be the *free active flexion* range. Then holding the flexed knee, further flexion is attempted till either the front of the thigh touches the lower abdomen, or the pelvis just starts tilting forward—this will be *free passive flexion range*.

So, the ultimate picture of flexion at the hip will be the sum total of fixed flexion deformity + free active flexion + free passive flexion. Beyond the attempt of passive flexion of the hip, if the front of upper thigh does not touch front of lower abdomen, it is due to terminal limitation. The angle by which the front of the upper thigh is not touching the lower abdomen, will be the amount of terminal limitation of flexion.

All newborn infants have a flexion contracture of the hip with a mean value of 28° (Haas et al. 1973). It gradually decreases (19° at 6 weeks and 7° at 3–6 months of age).

Fixed Abduction Deformity of Hip

Consequent to this deformity, there is downward tilt of the pelvis, i.e. anterior superior iliac spine is at a lower level as compared to the other side.

To measure the amount of fixed abduction, the affected limb is passively abducted till the ipsilateral anterior superior iliac spine is in the same horizontal line to that of the opposite (i.e. normal) side. In this manoeuvre, the ipsilateral hemipelvis (represented by the anterior superior iliac spine) with hip fixed in abduction, i.e. the hemipelvis and the limb moving as one, tilts upward. When the line joining, the two anterior superior iliac spines cuts the midline at right angles (or the anterior superior iliac spines should be equidistant from the umbilicus or xiphisternum)—the *pelvis has been squared up*. While the limb is kept in this position, draw a vertical line from the anterior superior iliac spine—the angle subtended between this line (or midline of body) and the long axis of the thigh will be the *fixed abduction deformity* **(Fig. 12.12A)**.

Alternative Method (Fig. 12.12B)

While the affected limb is in position of maximum comfort, join both anterior superior iliac spines. From either side of these iliac spines, draw a perpendicular on the midline. The angle subtended between the two lines will be the angle of fixed abduction deformity (After ML Kothari).

Fixed abduction is commonly complimentary to a shortened limb. *Roughly for each centimetre of true shortening there should be 10° of fixed abduction deformity*.

To know the free range of abduction, the patient is then asked to actively abduct the limb, following which the limb is passively abducted as far as possible, (there must not be any movement of the pelvis). The ultimate range of possible

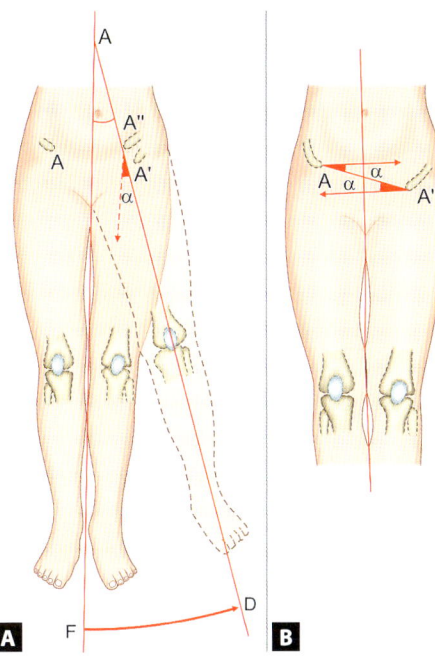

Figs. 12.12A and B: (A) Assessment of pelvic tilt—here α is the angle of fixed abduction deformity (A, A', A" = anterior superior iliac spines); (B) Pelvic tilt can also be assessed without altering the position of lower limb by measuring *"Kothari's angle"* (If affected side ASIS is lowered, α = angle of fixed abduction deformity); A and A' = anterior superior iliac spines.

abduction will be the sum total of fixed abduction + free active abduction + free passive abduction.

Fixed Adduction Deformity of Hip

This is the reverse of fixed abduction deformity. Here the anterior superior iliac spine of the affected side is elevated as compared to the opposite side.

To measure the angle of fixed adduction, the affected limb is further adducted, leading to lowering of anterior superior iliac spine, till both anterior superior iliac spines are in the same horizontal plane. *The pelvis is thus squared up.* In this very position of the limb, draw a vertical line from the anterior superior iliac spine. The angle between this line and the long axis of the thigh will be the angle of fixed adduction.

Alternative Method (Fig. 12.12B)

While the affected limb is in position of maximum comfort, join the two anterior superior iliac spines. Draw a perpendicular from any anterior superior iliac spine over the midline. The angle formed between these two lines is the angle of fixed adduction (After ML Kothari).

Fallacies

- Squaring is not possible in fixed scoliosis, due to fixed obliquity of the pelvis
- Iatrogenic, e.g. when the anterior superior iliac spine has been removed for bone grafting

- Mal/or ill development of hemipelvis (e.g. in residual polio deformities)
- Unreduced dislocation of sacroiliac joint
- Malunited/unreduced vertical fracture of ilium.

Fixed Rotational Deformities of Hip

These can be measured by noting the angle subtended between the imaginary perpendicular over the centre of anterior surface of patella and a plumb line over the same point.

These rotational deformities can also be deduced by noting the direction and amount of inclination of the normal big toe provided there are no fixed deformities at the knee and ankle.

■ NORMAL MOVEMENTS AT HIP

Methods of Eliciting Different Movements (*see* Table 12.2)

To get a gross idea of the hip movements, *ask the patient to stand erect, to sit in squatting and in cross-legged position. If he can do these fully, for all practical purposes the hips are normal.*

Extension (Figs. 12.13 and 12.14)

This can be tested with the patient lying either on his side, or in a prone position with extended lower limbs. While lying on one side, the patient is asked to take back the limb of other side. While in the prone position, the patient is asked to take back his extended lower limb, keeping his knee straight (the pelvis must not move). The range of posterior movement of the limb from the zero position, will be the angle of extension. Usually, additional degree of extension may be elicited (passive range) by passively extending his hip beyond the active range.

Flexion (Fig. 12.15)

Keeping the one lower limb extended, the patient is asked to flex his/her other lower limb at the hip with knee fully flexed till the front of the upper thigh touches the front of the abdomen, or the pelvis just starts moving. With the knee extended normally one can flex up to 90°.

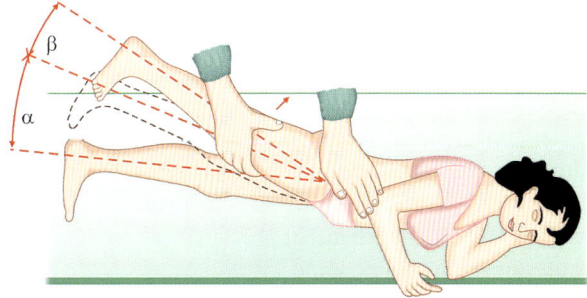

Fig. 12.13: Showing the active extension at hip while the patient is lying on side; further extension will be possible by passive backward pressure with examiner's other hand. α = range of active extension; β = possible passive extension.

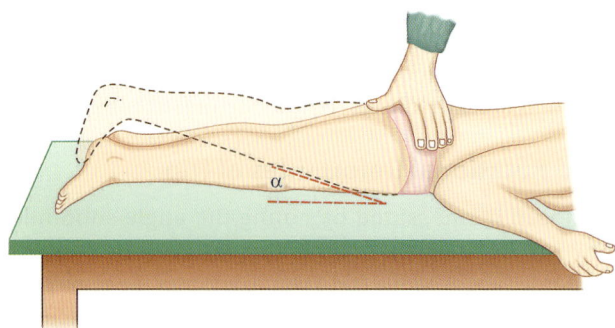

Fig. 12.14: Showing the active extension at the hip while patient is lying prone. Note the fixation of pelvis by examiner's hand during movement. α = range of active extension at hip. Further few degrees of passive extension can be achieved when the examiner assists by lifting up the extended thigh.

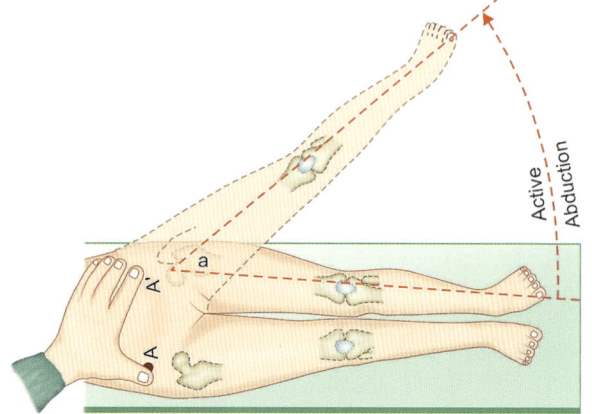

Fig. 12.16: Showing the active abduction at hip with hip and knee extended α-range of active abduction at hip. A and A'= anterior superior iliac spines.

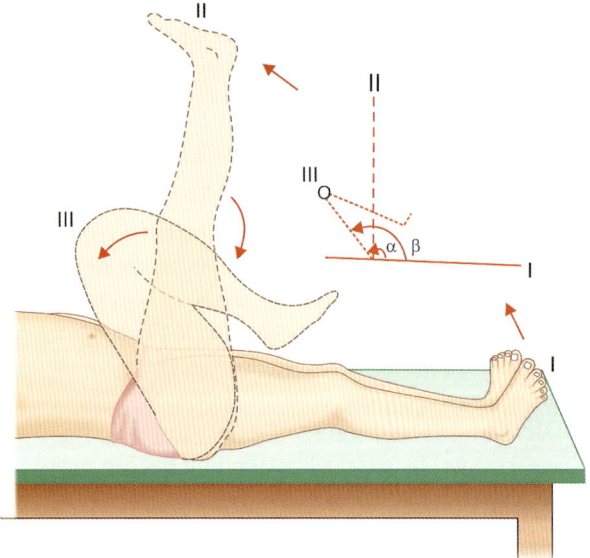

Fig. 12.15: Showing the method of active flexion at hip; α = with knee extension (II); β = with the knee flexed (III).

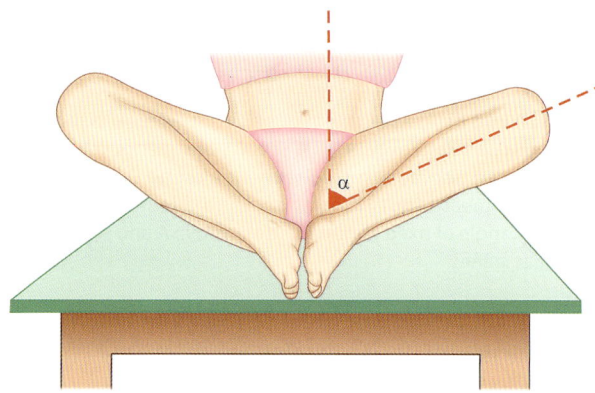

Fig. 12.17: Showing the active abduction at hip with hip and knee flexed; α = range of active abduction at hip.

Abduction (Fig. 12.16)

Hold the ipsilateral iliac crest by the spread out hand so that thumb is on anterior superior iliac spine (in children the same hand can hold both anterior superior iliac spines, i.e. the pelvis). Ask the patient to move out his extended limb in the horizontal plane till the thumb just appreciates movement of the anterior superior iliac spine (limit of normal abduction). If patient cannot reach this point (end of active movement), hold the lower part of the leg with the other hand and gradually move it out till the thumb just appreciates any movement of the anterior superior iliac spine.

Abduction in Flexion (Fig. 12.17)

Ask the patient to flex both the hips as far as possible up to 90° (optimum). In this position, with the soles of his/her feet approximated together, the patient is asked to touch the couch with the outer aspect of his knees. Note the deficit. Normal range in children is 80°–90°, which gradually decreases to 60°–70° in adults.

Restriction of this movement occurs in congenital dislocation of the hip, Perthes' disease, tuberculosis of hip.

Adduction (Fig. 12.18)

Holding the pelvis, as in testing for abduction **(Fig. 12.16)**, ask the patient to cross his opposite neutrally placed extended limb till the pelvis just starts moving (normally the middle third of the opposite thigh is crossed before the pelvis moves).

External/Internal Rotation (Figs. 12.19 and 12.20)

For clarity, rotational movements should be tested passively. To get an approximate idea, the extended limb is rolled in and out holding at the junction of the middle and lower third of the thigh by the palm **(Fig. 12.19)**. However, to measure these, hip and knee are flexed to about 90°. Fixing the knee by the left hand, and securing the heel by the right, with the

Hip

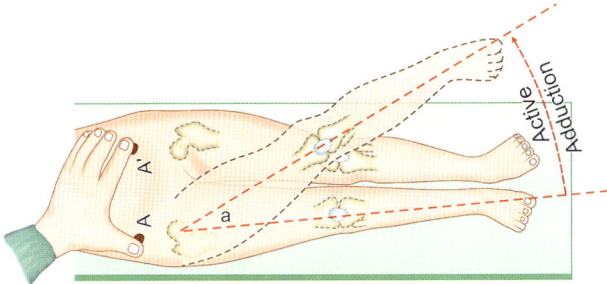

Fig. 12.18: Showing the active adduction at hip = α-range of active adduction at hip.

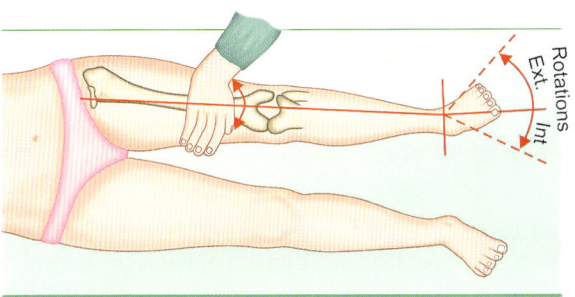

Fig. 12.19: Quick method of eliciting rotations at hip.

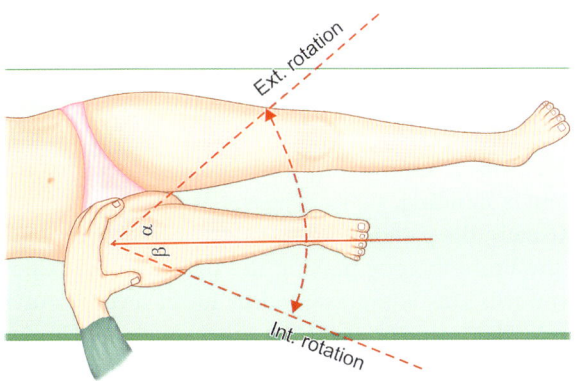

Fig. 12.20: Method of exact assessment of rotational movement at hip; α = angle of external rotation at hip; β = angle of internal rotation at hip.

hip as fulcrum, the leg is taken in and out to elicit the external and internal rotations of the hip correspondingly. The range through which the foot moves in, will be the angle of external rotation and the range through which the foot moves out, will be the range of internal rotation **(Fig. 12.20)**. After a certain range the rotational movements are limited by feeling of a terminal catch and then if force is applied in the same direction, patient lifts his buttocks simultaneously. Therefore, one should stop just short of this.

The rotational deformities can also be assessed by similar manoeuvres in prone position of the patient (position the patient as in alternative method of measuring fixed flexion deformity of hip, **Fig. 12.11**).

Circumduction

This can only be possible when all movements are free, hence, as a corollary it may be taken that a *hip having full circumduction is almost a normal hip*. For getting a rough idea about hip pathology, *if the hip can be fully flexed and extended and rotational movements are free, in most of the cases this should be taken as a normal hip.*

Snapping hip syndrome: This is mostly of extra-articular type, in which a snap is heard and felt when the knee is flexed and the hip is rotated medially.

■ MEASUREMENTS

Linear Measurements

Shortening in one lower limb is usually compensated (while walking) by:
- Tilting the pelvis down (i.e. anterior superior iliac spine dips at lower level)
- Gradual acquiring of equinus position of foot
- Flexing the opposite lower limb at hip and knee when shortening is beyond the compensatory capacity of pelvic tilt and equinus posture.

Linear measurements are of two types:
1. Apparent measurement
2. True measurement

Apparent Measurement

This measurement helps in assessing the extent of natural compensation developed for concealing the actual deformity/disability/disparity at the hip joint, and lower limb length disparity specially by tilting the pelvis sidewards (fixed abduction and fixed adduction deformity).

While standing, the patient with a hip or hips involvement unawarely tries to assume a posture, by developing natural compensations, which would broadly aim at:
- Concealment of the deformities
- Bringing the centre of gravity towards the median plane
- Postural equalisation of the limbs
- Stabilising the unstable hip.

Thus, apparent or functional limb length discrepancy is primarily measurement of *pelvic tilt* typically induced by scoliosis or hip contractures **(Fig. 12.21)**.

Method
Prerequisites
- Apparent measurement should be done while the patient is lying supine in a comfortable posture with the affected limb in the line of the trunk **(Fig. 12.22)**
- The lower limbs should be in parallel position. To achieve this, handle the unaffected limb to make the limbs parallel. In bilateral affections, apparent measurement is not of much significance.

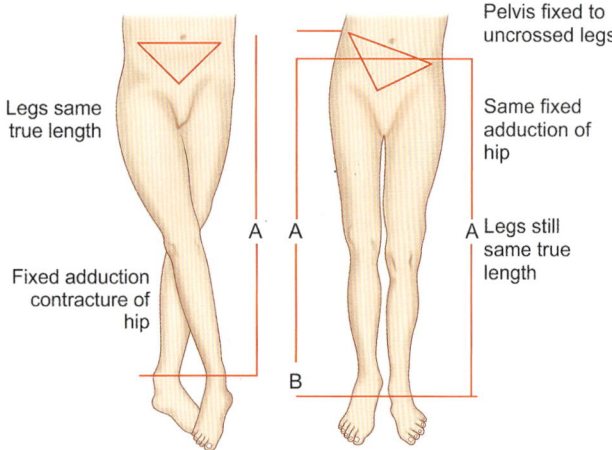

Fig. 12.21: Functional shortening.

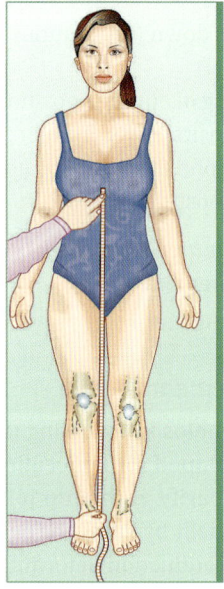

Fig. 12.22: Method of apparent measurement of lower limb. Note that the limbs are in parallel position and body is aligned to the limbs.

The measurement should be taken from any central fixed point on the trunk (e.g. central point of suprasternal notch, xiphisternum, umbilicus) distally *to the sharp bony point of the medial malleolus.*

Significance of apparent measurement
- Assessment of the compensations that the patient has developed to conceal any fixed deformity of hip and/or disparity of the limb lengths
- On many occasions, this natural compensation also improves the cosmetic aspect.

True Measurement (Fig. 12.23)
It is the measurement taken from anterior superior iliac spine to the medial malleolar tip while both lower limbs are kept in identical position and pelvis is squared. This can be done either in standing or in lying down position.

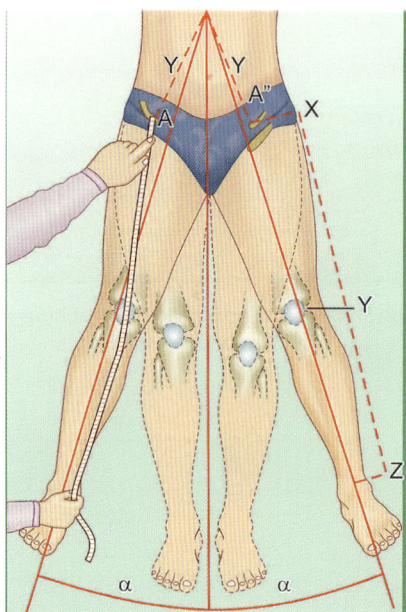

Fig. 12.23: Method of true measurement of lower limb. XZ = Total length of the lower limb; XY = length of thigh component; YZ = length of the leg component; α = angle of abduction required for squaring the pelvis, the normal limb has also to be taken out by α angle to make it identical.

In a suspected case of limb length disparity, its effective assessment should be done in ambulatory patients by block adjustment method (*see* **Fig. 2.18**) in standing weight bearing position.

Method of measuring limb length disparity while patient is standing.

Usually, the patient compensates shortening by abducting the limb, thereby making the pelvis on that side tilt downward. This is represented by lower level of anterior superior iliac spine on that side. Ask the patient to bring the abducted lower limb to as far as the zero position, while the trunk is erect. He is able to do so by gradually lifting the heel, in the process of which the anterior superior iliac spine starts moving upwards. As soon as it comes in the horizontal plane, insert the measured wooden block beneath the foot so as to keep up that level. The height of the wooden block required, is the limb length disparity.

Similarly, if there is lengthening of the limbs, anterior superior iliac spine remains higher up. Insert the measured wooden block beneath the opposite foot to the extent that it brings anterior superior iliac spines in horizontal level. The height of wooden block required will be the amount of lengthening of the opposite affected limb.

Measurement in Lying Down Position
Prerequisites
- Patient must be fully exposed.
- The bony points must be distinctly marked with a skin pencil. The bony points are the anterior superior iliac

spines, medial central or lateral central point of the knee joint line (or tibial flare), distal sharp bony point on the inferoposterior aspects of the medial malleolus, sharp point on the posterosuperior aspect of the greater trochanter, sharpest point on the ischial tuberosity, which can be marked conveniently by flexing the hip joint and knee at 90°
- The concealed fixed abduction or adduction deformity must be accurately revealed by squaring up the pelvis, i.e. where the line joining the tips of the two anterior superior iliac spines is horizontal, i.e. it should cut the central line at right angles or the anterior superior iliac spines should be equidistant from the umbilicus or any other central fixed point
- The limbs must be kept in identical position
- The affected limb should be handled to square up the pelvis (level the pelvis) by exaggerating the noted abduction/adduction deformity. The normal limb should then be handled to keep it in identical position to the affected limb
- For localising any bony point or joint line, palpation by fingertip may be misleading and may cause some false recording due to stretching of the skin. The metal end of the measuring tape is best utilised for this purpose, for example:
    - For the anterior superior iliac spine, the metal end of the measuring tape should be gently slided over the inguinal ligament towards the anterior superior iliac spine and the first bony resistance catching the metal tip should be marked without squeezing or stretching the skin
    - For the trochanteric tip, the metal end of the tape is passed down and laterally over the gluteus medius till it is obstructed by a sharp bony resistance. This point is marked
    - At the knee, the adductor tubercle may be difficult to mark, specially in a fatty or a heavily muscular limb. Hence, mark the joint line which can be very easily located by sliding the metal tip of the tape upwards over the medial surface of medial tibial condyle, till it engages into a transverse slit, i.e. the joint line. The central point of the joint line, on the medial surface of the joint, should be taken as the fixed point at the knee
    - For the medial malleolus, the metal tip should be slided up vertically towards the medial malleolus, and the first bony point catch should be taken as the point and marked.

Total Length

A quick assessment of limb length disparity can be done by eliciting Allis or Galeazzi sign. Here the hips are flexed, as much as possible, up to about 60° and the knees are bent at 90° with feet planted over the bed. Both the closeted knees should normally be in same horizontal level. Any disparity in level indicates limb length disparity.

Actual measurement should be done first on the normal side. Total length is measured from the anterior superior iliac spine to the tip of medial malleolus or lateral malleolus. If the true shortening is equal to earlier done apparent shortening, it indicates that there is no compensation. **If the true shortening is more than the apparent one, it indicates that part of the shortening has been compensated by tilting the pelvis downwards (fixed abduction deformity). If the true shortening is less than the apparent shortening, it indicates fixed adduction deformity besides shortening without any compensation.**

Any disparity in the limb lengths can be localised by taking the *segmental measurement*.
- *Leg length*: Central point on medial knee joint line to tip of medial malleolus.
- *Thigh length*: It is divisible into two segments:
    - *Infratrochanteric* (from the tip of the greater trochanter to the knee joint line).
    - *Supratrochanteric* (measurement for the length of the neck and head of femur).

Supratrochanteric Measurement

A quick approximate assessment of the supratrochanteric disparity can be done by comparing the limbs by *"digital Bryant's triangle"*. Here the tips of the thumbs are placed on anterior superior iliac spines, the tips of the middle fingers over the trochanteric tips and the tips of the index fingers over the imaginary points of intersection of the perpendiculars dropped from anterior superior iliac spines over the bed and from the trochanteric tips over the first line.

By drawing the **geometrical Bryant's triangles** on both the sides, the quantitative supratrochanteric disparity can be assessed.

Method (Fig. 12.24)

In already squared-up pelvis, a perpendicular line is drawn down from the anterior superior iliac spine, to the bed/couch (A–C line in **Figure 12.24**). From the tip of the greater trochanter, draw a perpendicular line over the first line (B–C line—base of the triangle). Join the tip of the greater trochanter to the anterior superior iliac spine (A–B line—hypotenuse). Each side of this right-angled triangle is compared with its counterpart on the other normal side.

Interpretation

Any shortening of the line drawn from the tip of the greater trochanter—i.e. base (i.e. more or less femoral axis continuation line)—(b) indicates riding up of the trochanter, which may be due to the shortening in the neck, head, joint proper or dislocation of the joint. In gross overriding

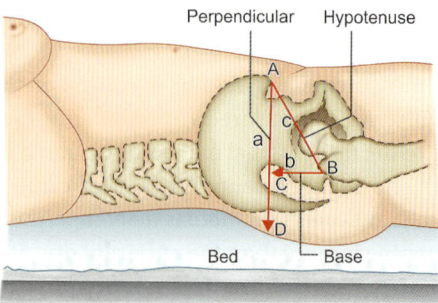

Fig. 12.24: Method of drawing the Bryant's triangle (ABC): Line 'AD' is the perpendicular drawn from anterior superior iliac spine on bed which cuts the baseline 'BC', which is the perpendicular line, drawn from the tip of greater trochanter on the first drawn line, i.e. AD: The line AB is joining the anterior superior iliac spine to the tip of the greater trochanter and it forms the hypotenuse (C).

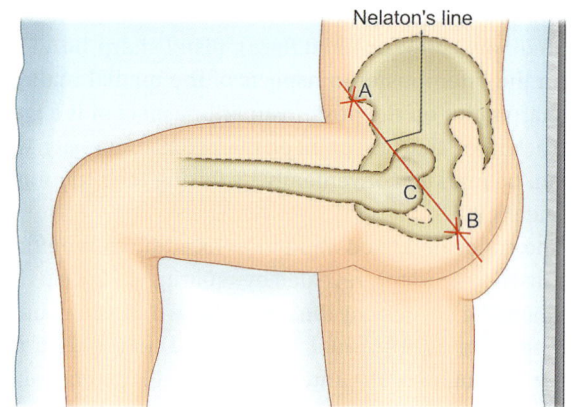

Fig. 12.25: Method of drawing the Nelaton's line; note that line joining anterior superior iliac spine (A) to ischial tuberosity (B) is just touching the tip of the greater trochanter (C).

of the trochanter, the trochanteric tip may lie above the perpendicular line drawn from the anterior superior iliac spine over the bed. Here, Bryant's triangle will be drawn above this perpendicular line—thus it is *reversed Bryant's triangle*, and the shortening will be the sum total of extent of overridden trochanteric tip above the perpendicular line dropped from anterior superior iliac spine (A–C line) and the base (BC line in **Figure 12.24**) of the Bryant's triangle of the normal side.

Any shortening of the perpendicular line (a) drawn from the anterior superior iliac spine over the bed, i.e. the base line of triangle—(b), indicates anterior sliding or tilting or internal rotation of the trochanter/or head of the femur (e.g. in posterior and central dislocation of the hip joint). In flexion contractures of the hip, following old fractures or destructive lesion of the joint, and in trochanteric fractures, the length of this line (b) will increase.

Any shortening of the hypotenuse (c) indicates approximation of the trochanter towards the central point of the body, e.g. in central fracture-dislocation of the hip, old fracture neck femur with neck absorption, absence of head due to disease or surgery, protrusio acetabuli.

Fallacies of Bryant's triangle: In bilateral affection of the hip; excision of anterior superior iliac spine, e.g. for bone graft; a limb disarticulated at the hip. Bryant's triangle has no significance nor can be drawn on the affected side.

The *quantitative measurement of the Bryant's triangle can be confirmed by the qualitative assessment done by following drawing:*
- Nelaton's line
- Schoemaker's line
- Chiene's test
- Morris's bitrochanteric test

Nelaton's line (Fig. 12.25): Turn the patient on the normal/opposite side, the limb preferably bent 90° at the hip and knee. A line is drawn from the sharpest bony point on the ischial

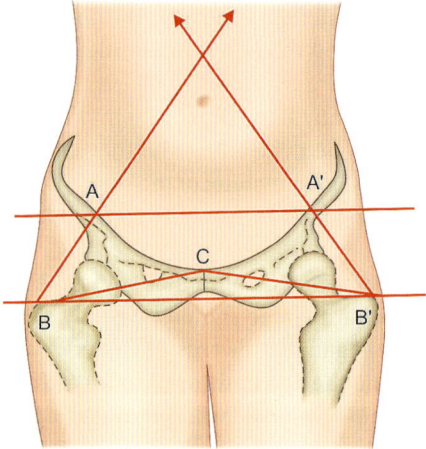

Fig. 12.26: Method of drawing Schoemaker's line (BA and B'A'); Chiene's test (AA' and BB' are parallel); Morris's bitrochanteric test (CB and CB' are equidistant).

tuberosity to the anterior superior iliac spine. Normally, this line should pass through the tip of the greater trochanter. In the case of supratrochanteric shortening, the trochanter will be above this line. This line is to be drawn on the affected side only.

Schoemaker's line (Fig. 12.26): The patient lies supine. A line joining the trochanteric tip and anterior superior iliac spine is prolonged in its direction on the abdomen on each side. Normally, these should meet in the central line at, or above the umbilicus. In case of riding up of the trochanter, the line on that side will meet its counterpart below the umbilicus and on the opposite side. *In a bilateral coxa vara or congenital dislocation of the hip, both lines will meet in the centre, but below the umbilicus.*

Chiene's test (Fig. 12.26): The lines joining the two anterior superior iliac spines and tips of greater trochanter should be parallel. If the tip of the trochanter is upridden, then the lines will converge on that side.

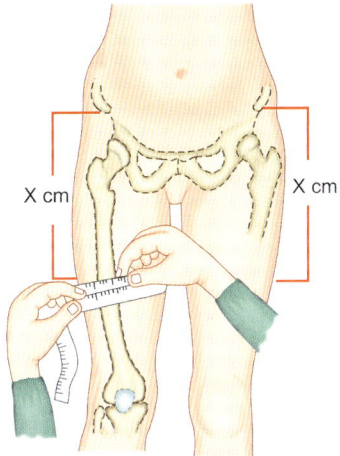

Fig. 12.27: Method of circumferential measurement of thigh.

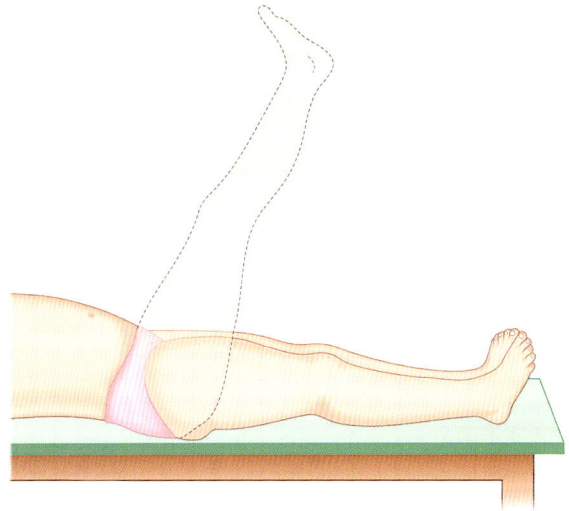

Fig. 12.28: Showing the straight leg raising test.

Morris's bitrochanteric test (Fig. 12.26): The distance from the tip of the trochanter to the pubic symphysis should be equal. If the trochanter is externally rotated or displaced back, on that side distance will be increased, and *vice versa*. These distances should be measured by using graduated callipers.

In bilateral hip affections, true measurement is inconclusive. In such cases, do segmental measurement (supra- and infratrochanteric thigh components, and leg component). Add them and compare with the other side measurement. Then corroborate with indirect evidences about the shortened side (e.g., if trochanter is ridden up—that will be the shorter side).

Circumferential Measurements (Fig. 12.27)

- At the affected sites—to indicate swelling or widening or collections or wasting
- Ideally at the mid thigh on both sides to indicate any muscular wasting or hypertrophy, however, it can also be taken at equidistant points, from a fixed point, e.g. 10 or 15 cm from the apex of patella on either side and the measurements are compared.

■ SPECIAL TESTS

Tests for Stability of Hip

Straight Leg Raising Test (Fig. 12.28)

If the acetabulum, hip joint space, head, neck of femur and rest of the lower limb are normal, the patient can easily raise his straight leg up to about 80°–90°. In any affection of the aforesaid regions or even the sacroiliac and adjoining areas or in sciatic root irritation, or acute painful lumbar pathology straight leg raising is affected. In performing active straight leg raise, the person has to use force about double of his/her body weight due to the joint reactive force generated by the hip flexors. Hence according to the severity of disease, the patient will get pain in active straight leg raise. The method will be the same as given in the Chapter 8 Spine.

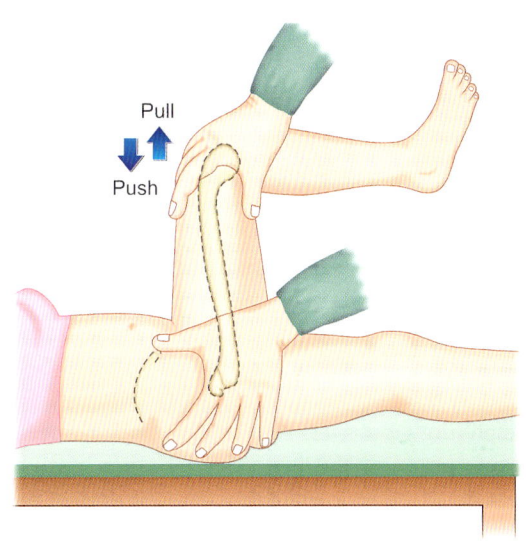

Fig. 12.29: Showing the method of demonstration of telescopic test.

Telescopic Test (Fig. 12.29)

By this method, the intactness and adaptation of the head and acetabulum are assessed.

Method: Patient lies supine. Flex the knee and hip as much towards 90° position as possible. For the patient's right hip, put your opened up left hand closely adapted to the trochanter and outer part of the buttock. The right hand, while firmly holding the lower end of femur, pulls up and pushes down the thigh away from and towards the bed. Even in normal condition, a slight amount of excursion of trochanter can be felt underneath the palpating hand. If the excursion is more, it indicates instability of the hip joint (e.g. in old unreduced posterior dislocation, paralytic hip, loss of neck and/or head).

Trendelenburg's Test

Friedrich Trendelenburg described this test in the year 1895 for assessment of congenital dislocation of hip. This test is done while the patient is standing.

Basically, a positive Trendelenburg's test indicates weakness of the gluteus medius muscle, which may also reveal hip joint pathology.

Principle of the test: *It is done to* assess the *integrity of the* **abductor mechanism of the hip**, which constitutes of the fulcrum, lever arm and power. *Intact abduction mechanism ensures stability of the hip joint.* With the fulcrum at the hip joint, normal lever arm of the intact head, neck and shaft of femur, and good power in controlling group of muscles, specially in the gluteus medius, one can have a normal rhythmic gait with alternate almost measured and controlled steps and load bearing on the hips. With affection of any of the aforesaid, the normal mechanism of weight bearing is disturbed and a gluteal or Trendelenburg lurch develops.

Method (Figs. 12.30A and B): While one stands on one leg, the opposite part of the body, pelvis [represented on the surface by anterior superior iliac spine (ASIS)] and the lower limb are lifted up to clear the ground. This is effected by the force of contraction of the ipsilateral gluteus medius, with an intact lever arm and fulcrum, working from below and pulling the upper part of the pelvis down. Therefore, the opposite pelvis is lifted up. This is indicated on the surface by elevation of the gluteal fold, the iliac crest, the level of the scapula and the shoulder top on the other side. This should be better observed by standing behind the patient. While performing Trendelenburg's test, ask the patient to stand on one leg, and keep your thumbs on the iliac crests, by which it will be easy to assess the dipping down of the pelvis. 5° drop of pelvis or gluteal fold may be taken to be within normal limits. More than 5° is definitely abnormal.

If this gluteal mechanism does not work, the opposite pelvis sags down which is indicated by lowering down of the gluteal fold (iliac crest, scapula/shoulder top), on that side. This is *Trendelenburg's positive test.* This test is positive in the conditions in which any of the above three (fulcrum, lever and power) is affected, e.g. congenital dislocation of hip, fracture neck femur, abductor paralysis due to poliomyelitis, etc.

Fallacies

- The intact quadratus lumborum muscle plays its role in effecting the normal gluteal mechanism. The ipsilateral quadratus lumborum working from below pulls down that side of the trunk, while the opposite quadratus lumborum working from above lifts up the iliac crest, i.e. pelvis. Hence, affection of the quadratus lumborum can also give a positive Trendelenburg's test.
- In certain congenital conditions, where there is dissociation of coordination of different groups of controlling muscles of joints (even other than the hip), there may be affection of these mechanism, e.g. cerebral palsy, congenital dysplasia of hip
- Affections of sacroiliac joints by virtue of producing pain may produce a *pseudo-positive Trendelenburg's test*
- The medial shift of the mechanical axis of leg below the hip (e.g. in bow knee, bow leg, malunited fracture of femur or tibia) the test may be pseudo-positive
- In obese and bulky persons, the test may be pseudo-positive.

Detecting hip instability in newborns is one of the most difficult examinations of the musculoskeletal system. Jones D (1998) has highlighted the problems of detecting neonatal clinical instability and dislocability of hip through Ortolani and Barlow tests. Though these tests have a high specificity (100%) but a low sensitivity (<60%), specially when it is performed by the less experienced ones. Their value is in hip surveillance not in screening.

Ortolani's Sign

Ortolani's sign was described by Marino Ortolani in the year 1937 to diagnose congenital dislocation of hip even in the neonates.

Principle: Ortolani's sign is almost similar in principle and manoeuvre as that of Barlow's test (1962). Here, when attempt is made to reduce the dislocated hip, the head enters the original acetabulum after jumping over the acetabular labrum, giving a sensation of snapping.

Method (Fig. 12.31): The child lies supine in as much relaxed a position as possible. Flex both hips to right angles, slightly internally rotate and hold the bent knees by both palms, with the thumb placed over the upper inner side of the knees. Both thighs are abducted and externally rotated, while the

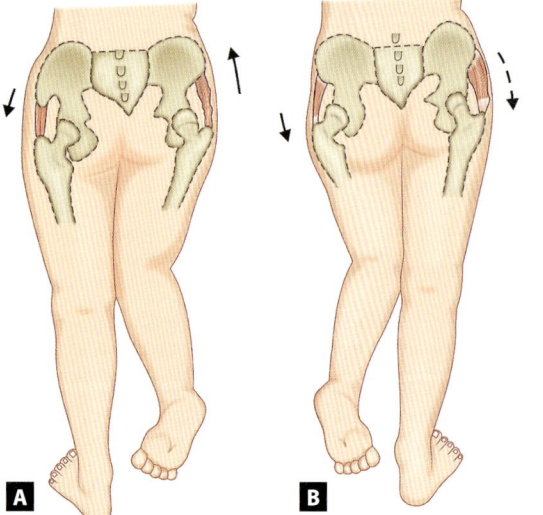

Figs. 12.30A and B: Demonstration of Trendelenburg's test: (A) patient is standing on the normal limb; (B) patient is standing on the affected limb (positive Trendelenburg's test).

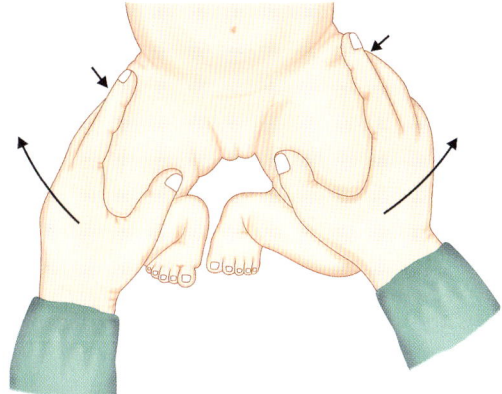

Fig. 12.31: Demonstration of Ortolani's sign.

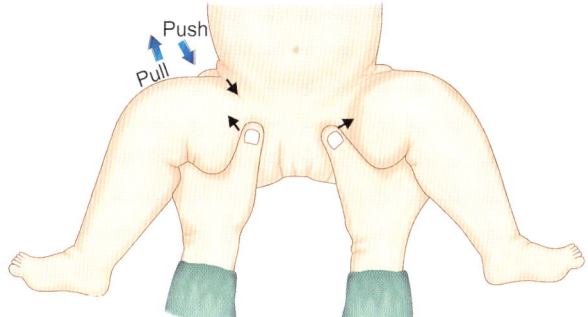

Fig. 12.32: Demonstration of Barlow's test.

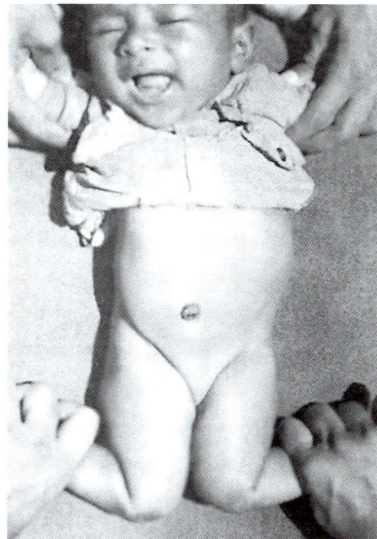

Fig. 12.33: Pandey's test in supine position.

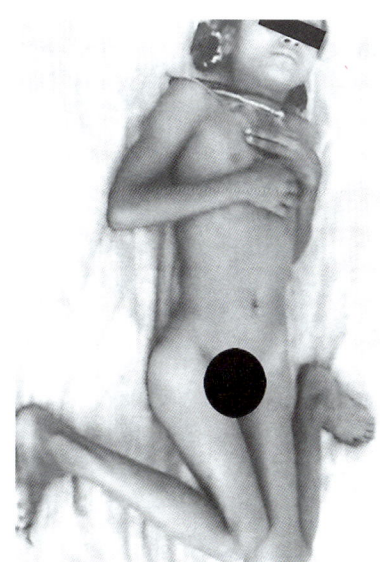

Fig. 12.34: In older children this Pandey's test can be demonstrated even without assistance.

spread up fingers press inwards and medially over the greater trochanter. As the head jumps over the labrum, snapping is felt and/or heard.

Barlow's Test (Fig. 12.32)

Patient lies supine, the flexed hips are abducted as much as possible. Hold the upper femur with the middle finger on the greater trochanter and the thumb in the groin. Using alternate pressure from both sides, the head can be levered in and out of the acetabulum.

Pandey's Test for Early Detecting Developmental Disorders of Hip (DDH—Dysplasia/Subluxation/Dislocation of Hip (Figs. 12.2, 12.33 to 12.36)

The child lies supine. Both thighs are approximated together in the midline. Holding the lower leg, flex the knees symmetrically as far as possible beyond 90°. Now internally rotate and extend the hips as much as possible. In this position, note for:

- Any resistance felt in terminal internal rotation, specially on the affected side of the hip
- Any widening of the perineum (*see* Fig. 12.1)
- Any abnormal crease in the groin (may be seen on the affected side)
- The level of the groin folds/labial folds (may be raised on the affected side)
- The trochanteric prominences (obviously prominent and up on the affected side)
- The level of the bent knees—a stiff flat sheet placed tangentially over the normal knee will not touch the affected knee and the deficient distance will give a rough measurement of the shortening of the affected thigh.

The same test can be done by putting the child in prone position **(Figs. 12.35 and 12.36)**. Put the child in prone position. Approximate the extended thigh in the midline. Holding at the lower leg, bend the knees symmetrically as far as possible beyond 90°. Now, internally rotate the hips to the maximum possible extent. In this position, note for:

- The level of the gluteal folds—on the affected side, the gluteal fold may be higher
- Widening of perineum if present

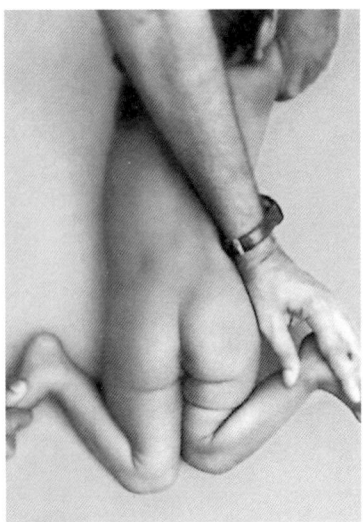

Fig. 12.35: Pandey's test in prone position of the patient.

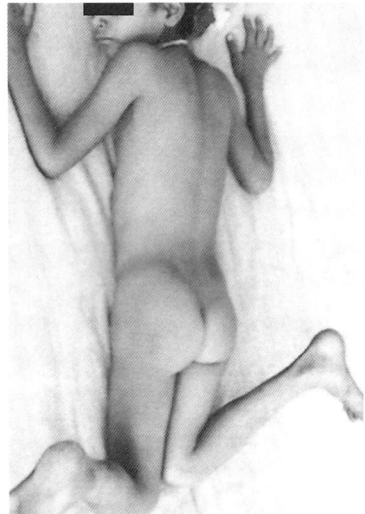

Fig. 12.36: Same Pandey's test can be demonstrated even without assistance.

- Presence of abnormal gluteal folds, which may appear on the affected side
- Level of the knees—on the affected side the knee may fall short of the tangential (horizontal) level of the normal knee. The deficient distance gives the rough estimate of the shortening of thigh component.

Impingement Tests

(After Guyton JL 2013 in Campbell's Operative Orthopaedics 12th Ed p. 335)

In performing anterior impingement test, after flexing the hip to 90° it is adducted across the midline and fully internally rotated (FADIR). In symptomatic anterior impingement, the internal rotation is limited and painful (in performing the manoeuvre).

In lateral and posterior impingement, even pure abduction of hip may produce pain, besides in performing FABER test (Flexion, Abduction, External Rotation). FABER test may produce pain in sacroiliac or lumbosacral affection).

Limitation of Hip Abduction

Limitation of hip abduction (LHA) is a common clinical sign in late dislocation of the hip. Limitation of the range of abduction more than 20° is most important clinical sign of a pathological hip (Terjesent 1996).

Limitation of hip abduction should be tested in supine position with both hips flexed to 90° and attempt to fully abduct the both hips. If there is limitation of hip abduction, the test should be recorded as positive, otherwise it is negative. Any limitation of abduction is noted and the angle of limitation is measured from the horizontal. This test of LHA is considered to be positive if the angle of limitation is more than 20° as compared with the contralateral side. Although it is not a quantifiable test, but is definitely useful in unilateral developmental dysplasias of hip (DDH) but not in bilateral cases where LHA is difficult to assess and compare.

LHA unilateral sign has specificity and reasonable sensitivity (more than Ortolani's test) specially if it is detected by the age of 3–4 months, when further investigations must be done to confirm.

Measuring Abduction of Hip in Flexion

The patient lies supine on the couch. Both hips are flexed by 45° with the knees and ankles closeted together. Then the knees are 'opened apart' aiming the outer side of the knees to touch the couch. In any limitation of abduction that side knee will remain at higher level resisting any further going down.

Other Tests

Gauvain's Sign

Sir Henry Gauvain described it in the year 1910. This is of *value in early doubtful cases of tuberculosis hip.*

Principle: In active tuberculosis of the hip, on initiating its rotatory movements, the muscles around the hip and lower abdomen go into spasm.

Method: Holding the lower end of femur, the thigh is rotated at the joint inwards and outwards. After the movement is checked, any further slight sharp rotation is followed by spasmodic contraction of the muscles of the joint as well as those of the lower abdomen. The reason of abdominal muscles going into spasm is that in this manoeuvre, the rotational movements of the femur is transmitted to the ipsilateral iliac spine.

Sciatic Stretch Test (See the Chapter 8: Spine)

Though it is important for eliciting the sciatic stretch, it will also be positive where external rotation of the hip is limited.

Narath's Sign

Normally, femoral arterial pulsation can be felt, just below the mid-inguinal ligament region, quite appreciably on both sides. But when the head is not in the acetabular socket, e.g. in posterior dislocation of the hip joint, the vessels fall back unsupported so femoral arterial pulsation, which is felt against the head of the femur, will be feeble or even may not be palpable—positive Narath's sign.

Patrick's Test (Faber Manoeuvre)

The patient lies supine, and the examiner places the patient's test leg in such a manner that the foot of the test-leg lies more or less in Figure '4' manner and the foot of the test-leg is on top of the knee of the opposite side. The examiner then slowly lowers the test side knee-thigh, kept in abduction, towards the examination table. A negative test is indicated by the test side knee-thigh falling to the table or at least remaining parallel to the opposite side. A positive test is indicated by the test side knee-thigh remaining above the opposite straight leg. If positive, the test indicates that the hip joint may be affected **(Fig. 12.37)**, with limitation of movement(s) of hip.

Craig's Test

In Craig's test, the patient lies prone with the knee flexed to 90°. The examiner palpates the posterior aspect of the greater trochanter of the femur. The hip is then passively rotated medially and laterally until the greater trochanter is parallel with the examining table or reaches its most lateral position. The degree of anteversion can then be estimated, based on the angle of the lower leg with the vertical. The test is also called the *Ryder method for measuring anteversion or retroversion* **(Figs. 12.38 and 12.39)**.

Galeazzi's Sign

The Galeazzi's sign is good only for assessing unilateral congenital dislocation of the hip and may be used in children from 3–18 months of age. The child lies supine with the knees flexed and the hips flexed to 90°. A positive test is indicated by one knee being higher than the other **(Figs. 12.40 and 12.41)**.

Rectus Femoris Contracture Test (Ely's Test)

The patient lies prone and the examiner passively flexes the patient's knee. On flexion of the knee, the patient's hip on the same side will spontaneously flex, indicating that the rectus femoris muscle is tight on that side and that the test is positive. The two sides should be tested and compared.

Noble Compression Test

This test is used to determine whether *iliotibial band friction syndrome* exists near the knee. The patient lies supine, and the knee is flexed to 90° accompanied by hip flexion.

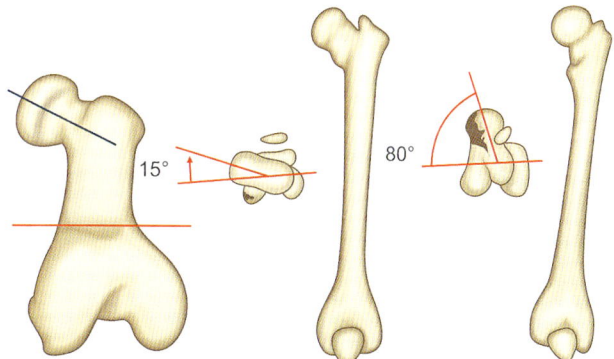

Fig. 12.38: Assessment of anteversion of femoral neck.

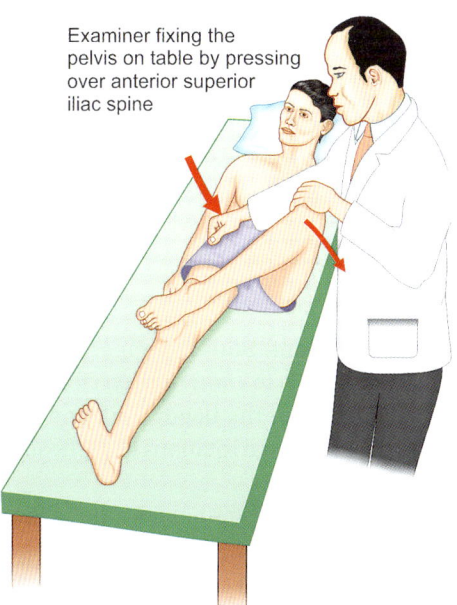

Fig. 12.37: Detection of limitation of motion in the hip.

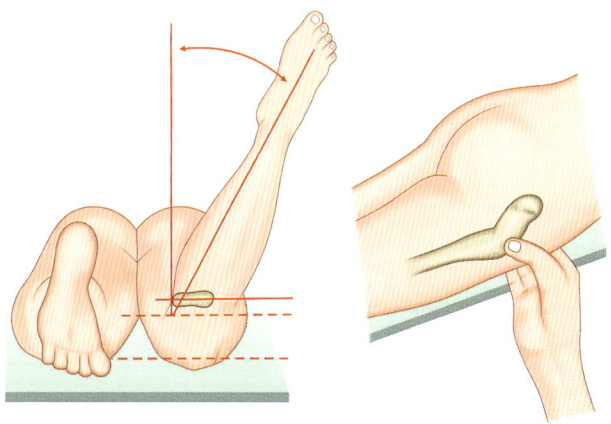

Fig. 12.39: Degree of anteversion and palpation of greater trochanter parallel to table.

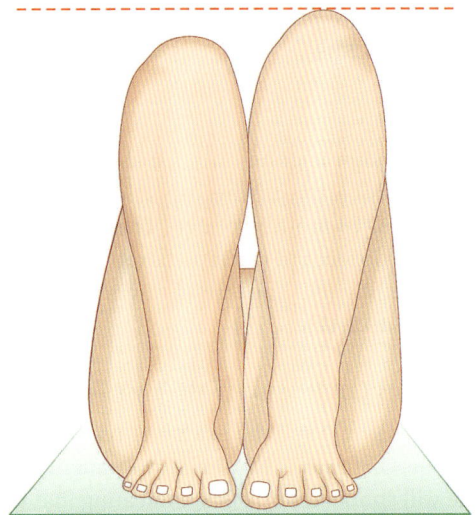

Fig. 12.40: Galeazzi's sign (Allis' test).

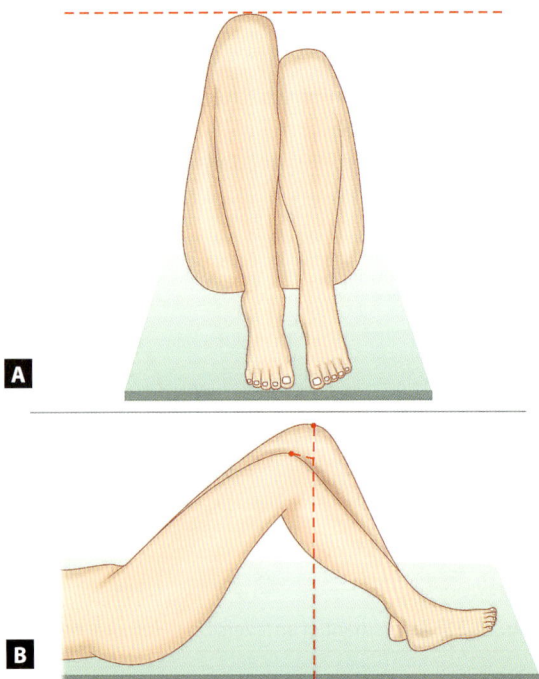

Figs. 12.41A and B: Left shortened tibia (A) and right shortened femur (B).

The examiner then applies pressure with the thumb to the lateral femoral epicondyle or 1–2 cm proximal to it. While the pressure is maintained, the patient slowly extends the knee. At approximately 30° of flexion (zero degree being a straight leg), if the patient complains of severe pain over the lateral femoral condyle, a positive test is indicated. The patient will say it is the same pain that accompanies the patient's activity (e.g. running).

Testing for Normal Flexibility in Hamstrings

The patient flexes the hip to 90° while the knee is bent. The patient then grasps behind the knee with both hands to stabilise the hips at 90° of flexion. The patient actively extends each knee in turn as much as possible. For normal flexibility in the hamstrings, knee extension should be within 20° of full extension.

Erichson's Sign

When the iliac bones are sharply pressed toward each other, pain is felt in sacroiliac disease, but not in hip disease.

Hart's Sign

Hart's sign is the limitation of abduction of the hips seen in congenital dislocation of the hip.

Per Rectal Examination

In suspected central fracture of dislocation, fracture of floor of acetabulum, pathological affection of acetabular floor, protrusio acetabuli (Otto pelvis), per rectal examination will elicit tenderness with/without abnormal bulge in that region.

Examination of Related Peripheral Nerves and Vessels

The sciatic nerve may be involved in several pathologies of the hip, e.g. dislocation of the hip, fracture of acetabular margin, or in surgery on the hip, etc. Hence, it is imperative to examine for integrity of this nerve.

Ask the patient to dorsiflex and plantarflex the ankle. If he can do so properly, the sciatic nerve, for all practical purposes is intact.

Fortunately, affections of the hip are less likely to affect the main blood vessels of the lower limb, i.e. femoral blood vessels.

However, peripheral vascular diseases sometimes present with *baffling* symptoms, even mimicking a hip pathology. Exclude them by palpating the dorsalis pedis, anterior tibial, posterior tibial and popliteal arteries.

■ INVESTIGATIONS

- General investigations—as in Chapter 1 Introduction
- Special investigations.

Special Investigations

X-Ray

X-ray is most important. Both anteroposterior, and lateral projections are essential to know the exact femoroacetabular relations; conditions of the head, neck and acetabulum; neck-shaft angulation; axial rotations of the head, and length of the neck.
- While taking anteroposterior view, the following points must be kept in mind:
  • Keeping the pelvis in as much symmetrical a position as possible, comparative view of both the hips must be taken

- Both lower limbs should be kept in zero position in as far as rotation, adduction and abduction are concerned (i.e. hips extended, legs parallel, and patellae in neutral positions)
- Contrast radiography will be helpful in delineating early infective pathology of the hip and its surrounding structures.

Special points to be noted in AP projections

- *Continuity of Shenton's arc*—The lower margins of the neck of femur and superior pubic ramus make up parts of the same arc. Any breakage of continuity suggests dislocation of hip or disruption of neck of femur
- The relation of capital epiphysis to the femoral neck
- Relations of capital epiphysis/femoral neck to the acetabular cup.

Proper lateral view of the hip is often a difficult task for projection, though it is mandatory (e.g. to diagnose and also to assess for perfect reduction after the femoral capital epiphysis slip; to assess perfect reduction, positioning and fixation of fracture neck of the femur).

Method: The extended limb is abducted to about 20°. The X-ray tube is focussed on the groin at midpoint of anteroposterior plane. The plate is placed closely adapted to the outer aspect of the hip region.

Alternative method: Patient is put in lithotomy position (hip flexed, abducted and externally rotated). X-ray tube is centred on the mid-inguinal point, while the cassette is kept behind the hip. In this very position lateral view, X-ray of both hips can be exposed if X-ray tube is focussed on the mid sacral point and the cassette is placed behind the pelvis

- *Oblique projection of the hip:* Three quarters internally and externally rotated views—essential for detail assessment of fracture and displacement in central fracture dislocation
- In comparatively *old fracture neck of femur,* X-ray should be taken in 15° abduction and 15° internal rotation of lower limb (at least thigh) to neutralise the anteversion of femoral neck (to assess the length of neck)
- In coxa plana or *Legg-Calves-Perthes disease* (LCPD), anteroposterior projection, keeping the hip maximally abducted and internally rotated gives an assessment about containment of the flattened head in the acetabulum.

Monitoring at regular intervals by plain radiography and CT (and if needed by scintigraphy) is essential to determine the natural history of Legg-Calves-Perthes disease (LCPD) and the progress in revascularisation of the necrosed femoral head, and further to know about the fate of the osteochondral fragments in LCPD, though osteochondritis dissecans after LCPD is rare (it was first described by Haas A in 1937). Early changes of LCPD are not apparent until 6 weeks or more from the onset of disease, however scintigraphy and MRI may be helpful.

Arthrography

It is of special importance in conditions like congenital dislocation of hip, Perthes' disease.

Arthroscopy

It is not of much value for hip, except in the hands of devoted arthroscopists.

Aspiration and Aspiration Biopsy (Anterior or Lateral Route)

Except where the capsule is distended due to collection of fluid, it is difficult to aspirate the contents of the hip joint.

Ultrasound

Presence of fluid inside the joint and unossified articular cartilage can be evaluated. It is important in case of hip dysplasias in neonates and septic arthritis in children.

Assessment of overall functions of the hip is essential in every case, and much more of the hip, which has been operated upon, specially after total hip replacement. For this purpose **Table 12.3** (based on Harris hip function scale) is useful.

Avascular necrosis [(AVN, osteonecrosis)] of femoral head occurs when intraosseous microcirculation is disturbed. Vascular insufficiency in the head causes prolonged ischaemia which leads to *osteonecrosis*. There is circulatory impairment of a zone in bone leading to its eventual death. The *femoral head, humeral head, scaphoid, femoral condyle, talus, lunate and proximal tibia are the sites of predilection for osteonecrosis.*

Osteonecrosis of femoral head may occur in young adults secondary to childhood disorders like slipped capital epiphysis or some trauma.

■ BROAD ASSESSMENT OF HIP FUNCTIONS

Harris hip score (HHS) was developed to assess the results of hip surgery and also to evaluate various hip disabilities and methods of treatment in adult population. The original scoring system was published in 1969. Other systems have also been developed like: Hip Disability and Osteoarthritis Outcome Score (HOOS); Oxford Hip Score (OHS); Lequesne Index of Severity for Osteoarthritis of the Hip (LISOH); and American Academy of Orthopaedic Surgeons (AAOS) Hip and Knee Questionnaire. However HHS has more acceptability.

It is a progressive pathology that usually affects persons in 3rd to 4th decade. *Osteonecrosis of femoral head* is reported in 10,000–20,000 in adults every year in USA (Deqiang Li et al 2016). Gradually, it leads to almost complete destruction of hip joint. Patients usually remain asymptomatic in early course of disease. Gradually pain develops on walking, in the groin region. As the disease progresses, limping starts

TABLE 12.3: Harris hip function scale.

Harris hip function scale
(Circle one in each group)

Pain (44 points maximum)

None, ignores	44
Slight, occasional, on compromise in activity	40
Mild, no effect on ordinary activity, pain after unusual activity, uses aspirin	30
Moderate, tolerable, makes concessions, occasional codeine	20
Marked, serious limitations	10
Totally disabled	0

Function (47 points maximum)
Gait (walking maximum distance) (33 points maximum)

1. Limp:
None	11
Slight	8
Moderate	5
Unable to walk	0

2. Support:
None	11
Cane, long walks	7
Cane, full time	5
Crutch	4
Two canes	2
Two crutches	0
Unable to walk	0

3. Distance walked:
Unlimited	11
Six blocks	8
Two to three blocks	5
Indoors only	2
Bed and chair	0

Functional Activities (14 points maximum)

1. Starts:
Normally	4
Normally with banister	2
Any method	1
Not able	0

2. Socks and tie shoes:
With ease	4
With difficulty	2
Unable	0

3. Sitting:
Any chair, 1 hour	5
High chair, 1/2 hour	3
Unable to sit 1/2 hour any chair	0

4. Enter public transport
Able to use public transportation	1
Not able to use public transportation	0

Absence of Deformity *(requires all four)* **(4 points maximum)**

1. Fixed adduction <10 — 4
2. Fixed internal rotation in extension <10 — 0
3. Leg length discrepancy less than 1 1/4 inch
4. Pelvic flexion contracture <30°

Range of Motion (5 points maximum)

Instructions

Record 10° of fixed adduction as "–10° abduction, adduction to 10°"

Similarly, 10° of fixed external rotation as "–10° internal rotation, external rotation to 10°"

Similarly, 10° of fixed external rotation with 10° further external rotation as "–10° internal rotation, external rotation to 20°"

Permanent flexion

	Range	Index Factor	Index Value*
A. Flexion to	_____°		
(0–45°)		1.0	
(45–90°)		0.6	
(90–120°)		0.3	
(120–140°)		0.0	
B. Abduction to	_____°		
(0–15°)		0.8	
(15–30°)		0.3	
(30–60°)		0.0	
C. Adduction to	_____°		
(0–15°)		0.2	
(15–60°)		0.0	
D. External rotation in extension to	_____°		
(0–30°)		0.4	
(30–60°)		0.0	
E. Internal rotation in extension to	_____°		
(0–60°)		0.0	

*Index Value = Range × Index Factor

Total index value (A + B + C + D + E) _____

Total range of motion points (multiply total index value × 0.05) _____

Pain points: _____

Function points: _____

Absence of deformity points: _____

Range of Motion points: _____

Total points (100 points maximum) _____

<70 = poor, 70–80 = fair, 80–90 = good, 90–100 = excellent

Harris WH. Traumatic arthritis of the hip after dislocation and acetabular fractures: treatment by mold arthroplasty. *J Bone Jt Surg* 1969;51A: 737–755.

Hall & Brody: Therapeutic Exercise: Moving Toward Function, 2nd Edition
©2005, Lippincott Williams and Wilkins

KEY DIAGNOSTIC POINTS OF COMMON HIP PATHOLOGY

Vide Tables 12.4 to 12.7.

TABLE 12.4: Traumatic hip—differential diagnosis.

	Capsular tear haematoma	Fracture neck femur	Fracture trochanter	Anterior dislocation	Posterior dislocation	Central fracture dislocation	Fracture pelvis
1	2	3	4	5	6	7	8
Age (more common)	Adults/elderly	Elderly ->50 years	>65 years	Young 20–40 years	30–50 years	20–45 years	20–50 years
Sex (more common)	Male	Female	Male	Male	Male	Male	Male
Violence	Indirect twist	Indirect twist	Direct/indirect	Forced external rotation and abduction in flexion produces low type; forced external rotation and abduction in extension produces high type	Internal rotation adduction strain on flexed hip	Internal rotational, abduction. Direct fall on the heels. Indirect violence along the shaft of femur with direct violence from the trochanteric region (e.g. thrown from dashboard injury) Produce type I. Main violence transmitted along the femur while hip in slight internal rotation and some abduction in extended limb (fall from height produces type II)	Fall from height or direct run over by automobile
Presentation	Pain on walking and standing	Walking/standing—not possible. Sometimes in abduction type or impacted type of fracture—patient can walk guardedly with some support for initial few days.	Bed ridden, Swelling ++ Ecchymosis + After few weeks patient may take steps or even walk slowly with support	Initially in bed; later on, even if not treated, may walk about with deformity and limp	Initially in bed. Later on, even if not treated, may walk about with deformity and limp	Not able to stand/or walk for pretty long time Swelling and bruises/abrasion over trochanteric region and knee	Varying presentation, depending upon planes and severity of fracture may not be able to walk
Pain	Pain ± (in certain movements +)	Pain ++	Pain +++	Pain +	Pain +	Pain ++	Pain ±
Attitude	Not particular	Spasmodic adduction with slight external rotation. In old neglected fracture—mild flexion, adduction and even internal rotation	Limb lies extended and externally rotated almost till the outer side of the foot touches the bed	In low type—marked abduction and external rotation with some flexion In high type—some abduction and external rotation with full extension	Hip flexion, adduction, internal rotation	Internal rotation with adduction	Nothing particular
Limb length	Not affected	Shortening (in fresh cases usually 1 cm and usually 3 cm in late presenting cases)	Shortening usually 1–2 cm; in unstable type or neglected cases, may be even up to 5 cm or more	Lengthening of limb	True shortening may be about 5 cm	True shortening 0.5–2 cm	None except in displaced vertical fracture of ipsilateral ilium, pubis and ischium

Contd...

352 Hip

Contd...

	Capsular tear haematoma	Fracture neck femur	Fracture trochanter	Anterior dislocation	Posterior dislocation	Central fracture dislocation	Fracture pelvis
1	2	3	4	5	6	7	8
Movements	Fairly free, only extreme of rotations, painful	Painful, in impacted type variable range of movements possible	All movements restricted	Variable range of movements possible	Limitation of all movements	Very short range. Except for flexion, other movements may be possible, to variable extent	Hip movements free except in terminal range, which produces stress pain in pelvic region
Tenderness	Centre of the base of femoral triangle (mid inguinal vicinity)	Mid inguinal region, Trochanteric thrust tenderness, Ipsilateral iliac fossa, Medial and posterior hip points	Trochanteric region	Anterior hip region	Posterior and postero-superior to hip	Ipsilateral iliac fossa, trochanteric thrust	In region of pelvic fractures
Bony abnormality on palpation	None	None	Trochanter broadened, thickened, irregular	Anteriorly globular head with transmitted movements	Posteriorly in gluteal region globular head with transmitted movements	In thin subjects comparative bony fullness in ipsilateral iliac fossa	Rarely iliac fracture involving crest produces an irregular feel. Symphysis disruption may be felt
X-ray	Nothing particular	Confirmatory	Confirmatory	Confirmatory	Confirmatory	Confirmatory	Confirmatory
Classification	—None	see below	As on page 353 Flowchart 12.1	As on page 340 Table 12.7	As on page 340 Table 12.7	As on page 340 Table 12.7	(See in Chapter on Pelvic Injury Pages 266, 267)
Complications	Very rarely avascular necrosis	— Nonunion — Malunion — Shortening — Stiffness of hip — Avascular necrosis — Degenerative arthrosis	— Malunion — Shortening — Residual external rotation deformity — Coxa vara — Stiffness	— Stiffness — Myositis ossificans — Avascular necrosis — Degenerative arthrosis — Vessels and nerve injuries	— Stiffness — Myositis ossificans (see Figs. 12.84 and 12.85) — Sciatic nerve damage — Avascular necrosis — Degenerative arthritis	— Haemorrhage, shock — Degenerative arthritis — Possibilities of damage of pelvic viscera	— Haemorrhage — Shock — Damage to urethra — Damage to pelvic viscera — Obstetrical problems

TABLE 12.5: Classification of fracture neck femur (Interrelation with other classifications).

	Types	Abd/Add.	Pauwel's	Garden (Figs. 12.42A and B)	Treatment	
A.	Undisplaced (which comprise impacted, valgus, Garden I and certain Garden II—form approximately 25% of intracapsular fractures)	Abduction (mostly)	I	II (Fig. 43B)	Children	— Conservative, very rarely operative
					Adult	— Operative; conservative in selected cases
B.	Displaced Impacted	— Abduction	I	akin to I (Fig. 43A)	Children	— Conservative, very rarely operative
					Adult	— Conservative or operative according to age, choice, facilities (fixation in impacted position)
	Unimpacted	— Adduction	II or III	III or IV (Figs. 43C and D)	Children	— Operative (reduction and fixation)
					Adult	— Operative (reduction and fixation; displacement osteotomy; replacement arthroplasty; removal of head)

Flowchart 12.1: Classification of fractures in trochanteric region (Based on Evan's classification).

```
                    Type I                                          Type II (Fig. 12.44)
        Fracture line running from superolateral          Fracture line running from superomedial to
              to inferomedial direction                    inferolateral direction—always unstable.
                                                         (Treatment: Possible reduction and internal fixation)

    Undisplaced (always stable-                         Displaced
    (Treatment: Conservative;                       (Figs 12.45 and 12.46)
    internal fixation may be done)

                        Reducible                                   Non-reducible
                (Stable—treatment: fixation                  (Not stable—treatment:
                preferable; properly done conservative       possible reduction and internal fixation;
                also satisfactory)                           or osteotomy + internal fixation)
```

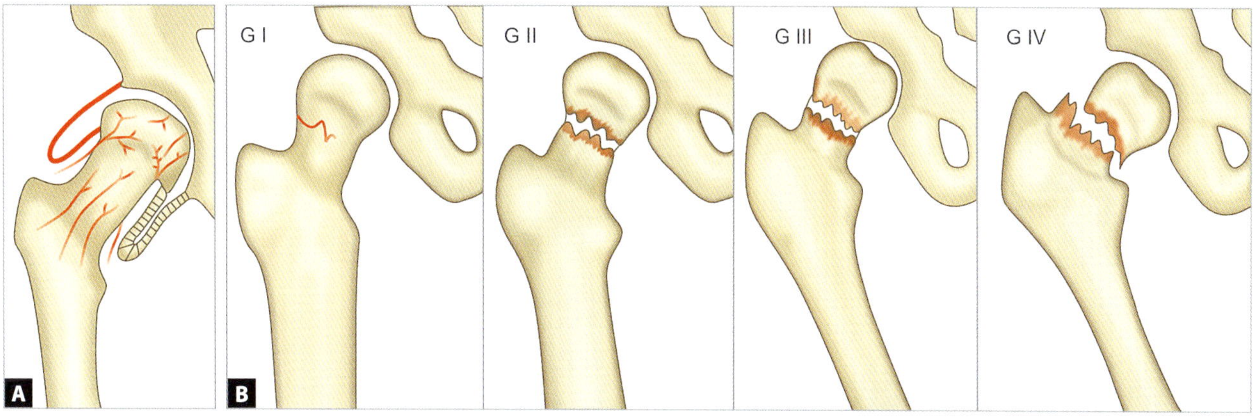

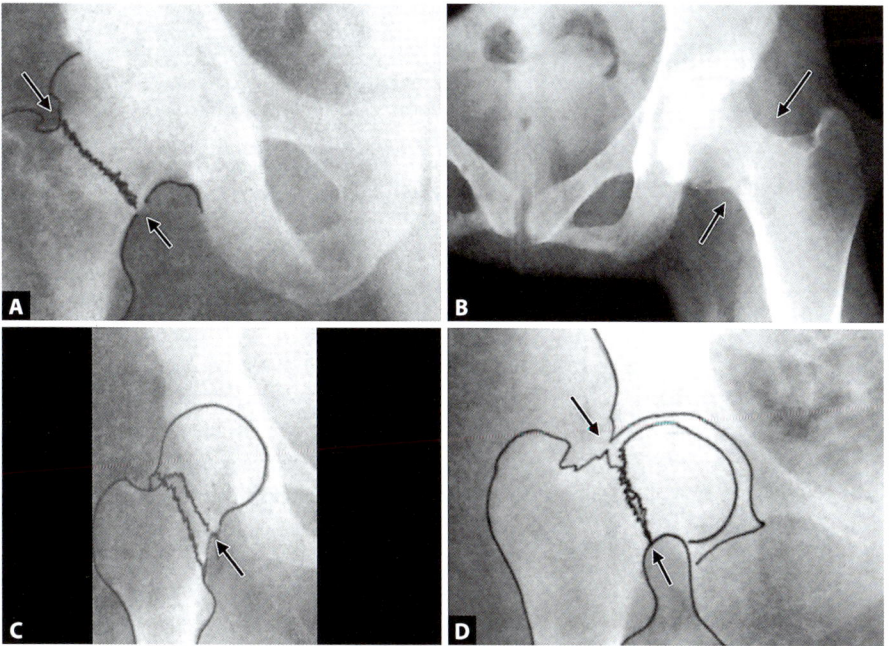

Figs. 12.42A and B: (A) Vascular supply of femoral head; (B) G I to G IV Garden's four grades (types) of fracture of neck of femur.

Figs. 12.43A to D: (A) Garden type I fracture of neck of femur; (B) Garden type II fracture of neck of femur; (C) Garden type III fracture of neck of femur; (D) Garden type IV fracture of neck of femur.

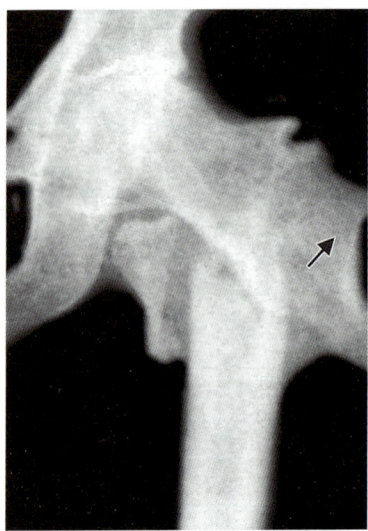

Fig. 12.44: Fracture trochanter with fracture line running from superomedial to inferolateral direction (all are unstable fractures). Such fractures should be treated by (open) reduction and internal fixation.

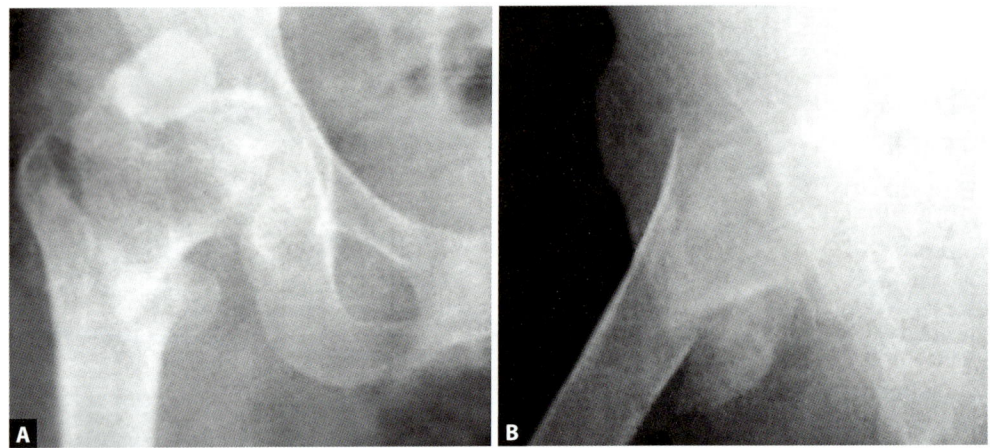

Figs. 12.45A and B: Fracture trochanter—fracture line running from upper outer to inferomedial direction. (A) All such fractures are stable, except the grossly comminuted ones; (B) like in (A).

TABLE 12.6: Classification of dislocation of hip joint.			
A	Traumatic	— Posterior	Ilial type **(Figs. 12.47 and 12.48)**
			Sciatic type **(Fig. 12.49)**
		— Anterior	Low type **(Figs. 12.51 and 12.52)** (Obturator type)
			High type **(Fig. 12.53)** (Pubic type)
		— Central	Type I— Where weight bearing articular area is intact **(Figs. 12.54A to D)**
			Type II— Where weight-bearing area is fractured, but not grossly displaced
			Type III— Where acetabulum is grossly comminuted
		— Fracture dislocation	— With fracture of posterosuperior rim of acetabulum **(Fig. 12.55)**
			— With chip fracture of head
			— With fracture neck of femur
B	Non-traumatic		— Congenital dislocation of hip **(Fig. 12.56)**
			— Paralytic (Poliomyelitis) **(Figs. 12.50, 12.57)**
			— Pathological (septic arthritis) **(Fig. 12.58)**
			— Spastic (cerebral palsy)

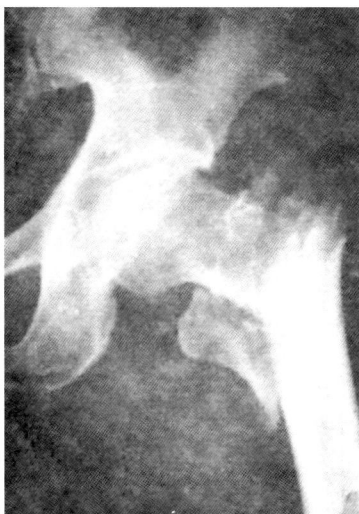

Fig. 12.46: Fracture trochanter with fracture line running from upper outer to inferomedial direction with comminution (mostly stable fracture).

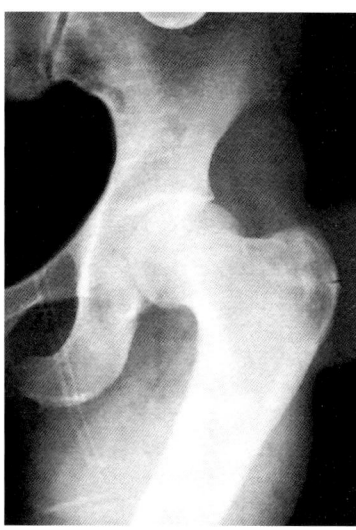

Fig. 12.49: Posterior dislocation of hip joint (low type; sciatic type).

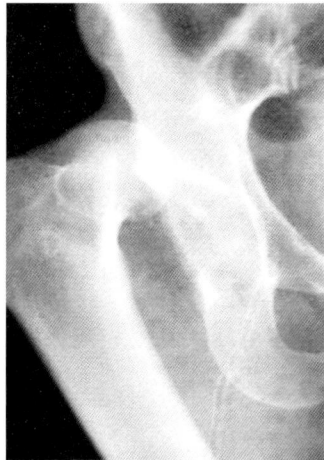

Fig. 12.47: Posterior dislocation of hip joint (typical high type; ilial type) in adult.

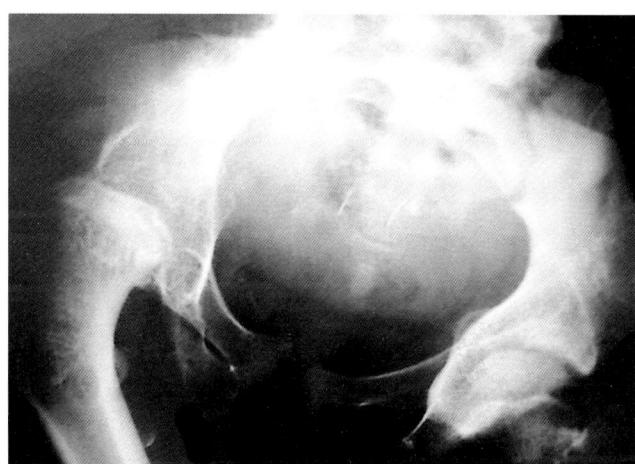

Fig. 12.50: Neglected posterior subluxation/dislocation of right hip in a polio-paralysis patient.

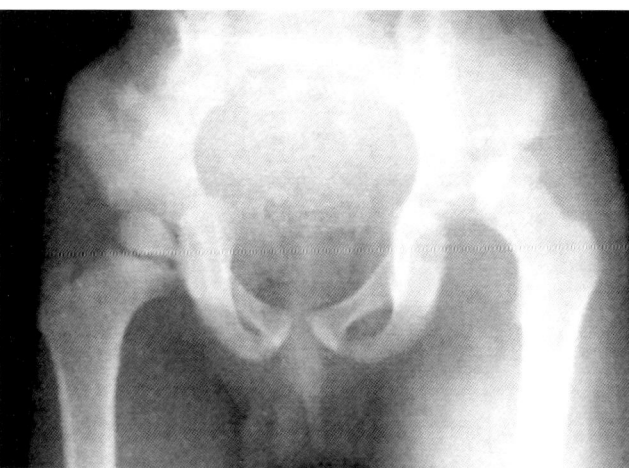

Fig. 12.48: Neglected posterior dislocation of hip (high or ilial type) in a boy aged 11 years.

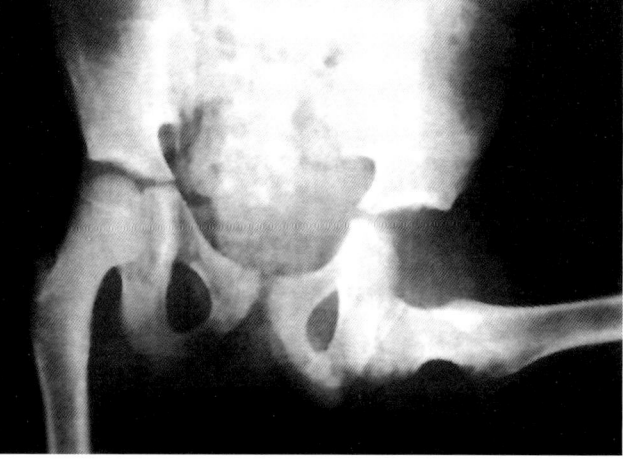

Fig. 12.51: Anterior dislocation of hip joint (obturator type).

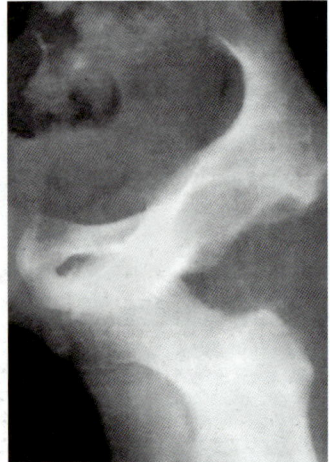

Fig. 12.52: Anterior dislocation of hip joint (obturator type).

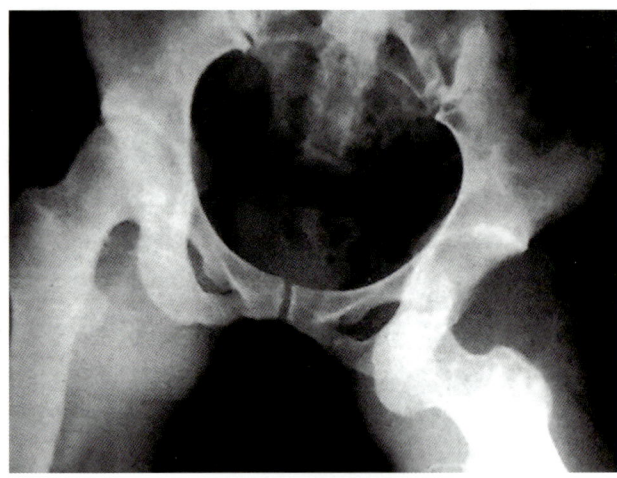

Fig. 12.53: Anterior dislocation of hip joint in adult (pubic type).

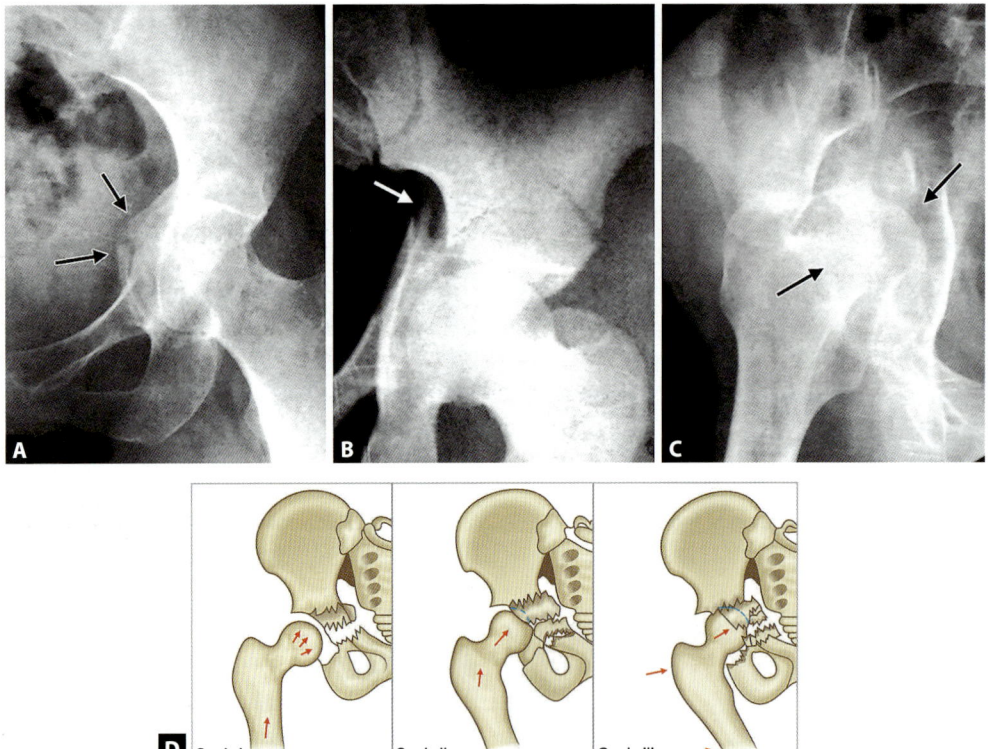

Grade I representing A (above X-ray)   Grade II representing B (above X-ray)   Grade III representing C (above X-ray).

Figs. 12.54A to D: Central-fracture dislocation of hip joint: (A) Grade I, (B) Grade II, (C) Grade III, (D) Line drawing representation of central fracture dislocation of hip joint.

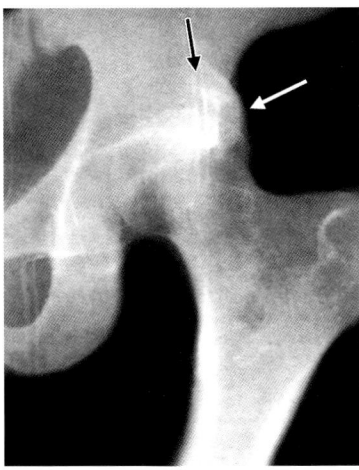

Fig. 12.55: Fracture-dislocation (fracture of posterosuperior rim of acetabulum) of hip joint.

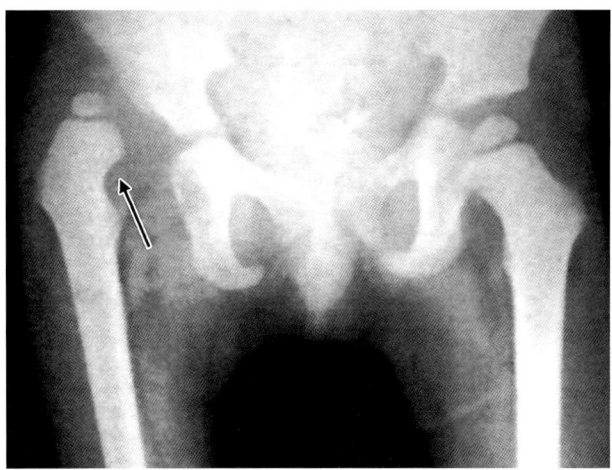

Fig. 12.56A: Neglected congenital dislocation of right hip joint.

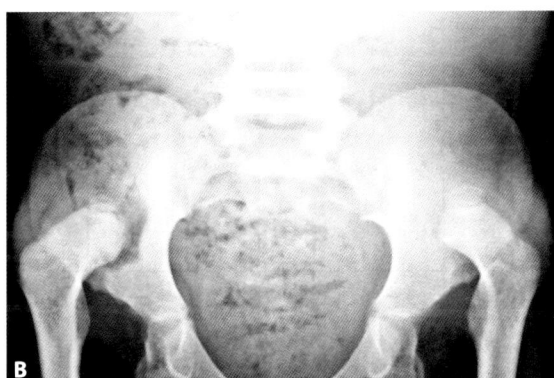

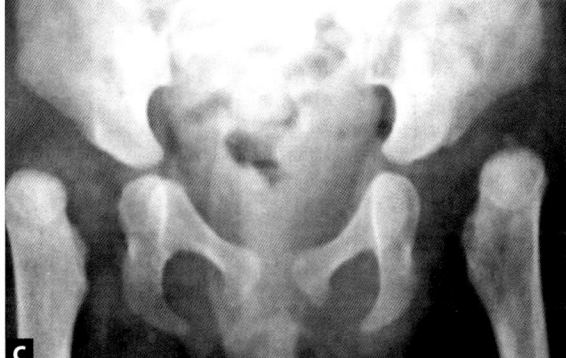

Figs. 12.56B and C: Neglected bilateral congenital dislocation of hips.

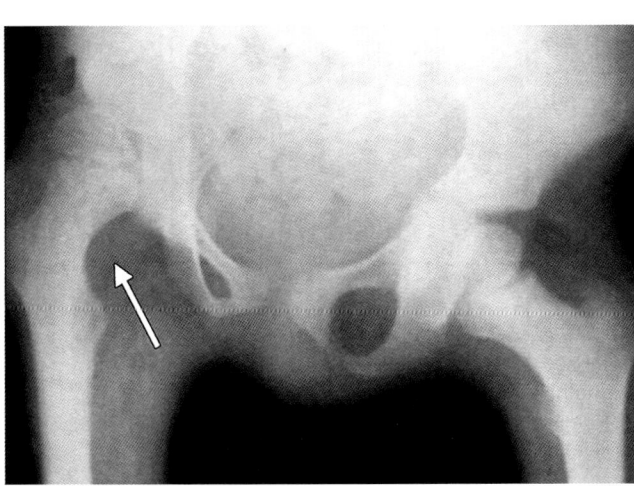

Fig. 12.57: Paralytic subluxation of right hip joint (unilateral).

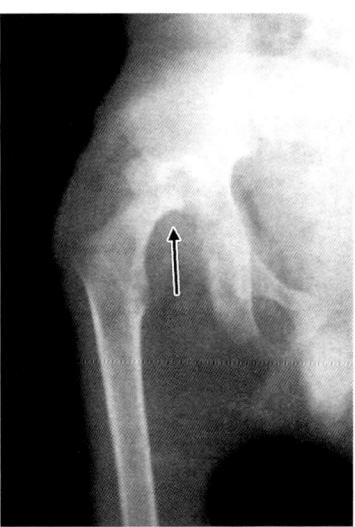

Fig. 12.58: Septic arthritis hip—sequestrating capital epiphysis dislocating out—Pathological dislocation.

TABLE 12.7: Non-traumatic hip affections—differential diagnosis.

Developmental dysplasia of hip (DDH) Congenital dislocation of hip (Fig. 12.56) Recognised by Hippocrates more than 2000 years ago. Term was coined by Hollgenreiner in about 1920	Tuberculous hip (Figs. 12.64 to 12.68)	Septic arthritis hip (Figs. 12.58 to 12.63)	Perthes hip (Legg-Calves-Perthes Disease LCPD) (Figs. 12.69 to 12.71)	Adolescent coxa vara+ Slipped capital femoral epiphysis (Fig. 12.72)°	Ankylosing spondylitis (Figs. 12.73 and 12.74A)	Rheumatoid hip	Degenerative arthrosis	Paralytic hip (Fig. 12.57)
2	3	4	5	6	7	8	9	10
Developmental dysplasia of hip denotes a wide spectrum of pathological conditions ranging from subtle acetabular dysplasia to irreducible hip dislocation	—	—	LCPD is a self-limiting disease of childhood with avascular necrosis of proximal femoral capital epiphysis. It may be a part of generalised constitutional disorder associated with a disturbance of growth of bone and cartilage in various areas of body. The main feature of Perthes hip is ischaemic necrosis of ossification centre of femoral head. The cause of ischaemia, fragmentation and protracted reformation of the femoral head observed in this disease is unknown. Several sites of osteochondritis may be observed in the same patient. Children of Perthes hip have delayed skeletal maturity and abnormalities in the proportion of growth in various regions of body. The age of onset has a bearing on the long-term outcome—the younger patients have better prognosis	Slipped capital epiphysis is a disorder in which there is gradual or acute displacement through the capital physeal plate. The physiolysis is through a widened hypertrophic zone, which is weakened as a result of altered chondrocyte maturation and enchondral ossification The child is often obese with delayed sexual and skeletal maturity. The epiphysis probably slips as a result of high shear forces in the hip at the time of the adolescent growth	Ankylosing spondylitis is a chronic systemic inflammatory disease affecting mainly the sacroiliac joint, spine and frequently peripheral joints as well	—	—	—

Note:
+ Congenital coxa vara is a developmental abnormality usually not detectable at birth and recognisable in later childhood or even in adolescent age. The abnormality is a primary cartilaginous defect in the femoral neck with abnormal decrease in femoral neck-shaft angle, shortening of femoral neck, comparative overgrowth of greater trochanter and shortening of the involved limb
° The terminology "slipped capital femoral epiphysis" appears to be technically incorrect, since the femoral epiphysis normally remains in acetabulum and it is the proximal femoral metaphysis [femoral neck and shaft] metaphysis which relatively displace in relation to femoral epiphysis and acetabulum rotates externally with anterosuperior translation:
Transient synovitis (exact cause not known), is one of the most common causes of pain and limb in one hip in toddler and teenager 3 to 10 years with acute onset without any history of injury nor any systemic illness. Symptoms gradually resolve completely. Pathologically there may be some synovial effusion, synovial hypertrophy with nonpyogenic, nonspecific inflammatory reaction. Management: rest in bed, restricted weight bearing, symptomatic drugs.

Contd...

Hip

1	2	3	4	5	6	7	8	9	10
Age	Newborn	3–10 years age	Newborn to 5 ++ 5 to 15 +	3 to 10 years	10-16 years	18-30 years	25–35 years	Primary >40 years Secondary >20 years	1–4 or more years
Sex	Female > male Affects the left side more severely	Male	Male = Female	Male > Female	Male > Female, average male 14; female 12	Male > Female	Female > Male	Male > Female	Female > Male
Geographical distribution.	More in cold countries (Caucasians)	Third world—	Third world	More in white race	—	—	More in cold climate	More in cold climate.	Third world
Presenting symptoms	Initially detected by doctor. May be other associated congenital deformities. Later on, waddling gait, still later on, pain in hip or exertion	Developing/undeveloped countries Limp, pain, deformity, abscess, sinus, constitutional features, stiffness limb length disparity (LLD) +	Constitutional features, pain, swelling, spasm, local inflammatory features, deformity, stiffness, LLD ++	Limp after exertion, vague pain, stiffness LLD ±	Pain, limp, LLD ±, 30% are bilateral. In preadolescent period-hormonal changes of puberty. Most of the patients are obese, with delayed sexual and skeletal maturity The epiphysis probably slips as a result of high shear forces in the hip at the time of adolescent growth spurt	Pain, stiffness, limp Pain may be in knee	Pain, limp	Pain after rest, stiffness, gradual limp	Weakness, deformity, LLD
Salient features	Trendelenburg's test +, gluteal fold asymmetry, Ortolani's, Barlow's and Pandey's tests +, painless movements, abduction in flexion limited to varying extent, adduction excessive, telescopic test positive, Galeazzi's test positive, Infants with clinical instability (Ortolani's, Barlow, Pandey's tests positive); considered to be at risk as a result of breech presentation; family history; postural and structural foot deformity, torticollis, and oligohydramnios should be assessed; ultrasonographically by six to nine weeks of age	Spasm +, all movements restricted. Typical attitude— *Synovitis stage— flexion, abduction, external rotation, *Arthritis stage — flexion, adduction, internal rotation. Later on flexion, adduction, internal rotation +, with true shortening pseudo-dislocation (if patient has been walking—abduction instead of adduction)	In collection stage, initially-flexion, abduction, external rotation. Later on flexion, adduction, internal rotation. All movements restricted. Thickening and tenderness in trochanteric or ileal region	85% unilateral. Abduction and internal rotation limited. Abduction in flexion limited, antalgic gait	Abduction and internal rotation limited. External rotation and adduction may be excessive Gradually, fixed adduction and external rotation deformities. Trendelenburg's test/gait	Mostly bilateral affection, marked stiffness Active hip flexion causes lateral hip rotation, and resisted internal rotation is painful, ankylosis develops in flexion, external rotation and abduction (mostly due to posture) Trendelenburg gait	Flexion, adduction and internal rotation limited	Initially limited extension, abduction and external rotation, later on, all movements may be restricted	Hypermobility, gross wasting

Contd...

	1	2	3	4	5	6	7	8	9	10
Investigations: a. X-ray: Both hips must be X-rayed in as much comparative position as possible	Up to 6 months—no diagnostic X-rays picture. Dysplastic feature, shallow acetabulum, capital epiphysis up and out, Shenton's arc broken (Fig. 12.56)	General rarefaction Localised destruction, reduction in joint space, wandering acetabulum, sequestration. (Figs. 12.64 to 12.68)	Soft tissues shadow, osteomyelitic changes in adjacent ileum or trochanter, bone formation, bone destruction, sequestrum, pathological dislocation, damage of capital epiphysis (Figs. 12.58 to 12.63)	In early stage, head-socket distance increased Flattening, fragmentation and mushrooming of femoral head. Broadening of neck Areas of avascular necrosis in denser areas. X-ray must be taken in full abduction and internal rotation to see the containment (Figs. 12.69 to 12.71) Changes in plain X-ray are not apparent till 6 weeks or more of onset of disease. Scintigraphy and MRI can establish diagnosis earlier	Posteroinferior slipping of capital epiphysis, neck shaft angle reduced. It is femoral neck which drifts anteriorly and superiorly and the femoral head remains inferiorly and posteriorly stable in the acetabulum Thus name of the disease appears misnomer Rarely the femoral neck migrates in the opposite direction so that the femoral head rests more anteriorly and superiorly Dividing the physis in thirds, the amount of slip is graded as I (starting from lateral side slip is in the third); II (2nd 1/3rd); III (Last 1/3rd complete slip). Slips may be stable (more common, patient can walk, no risk of AVN) or unstable (patient unable to bear weight, high risk of AVN	Reduced joint space, condensation at joint margin, tendency of cross trabeculation, associated sacroiliac ankylosis (Figs. 12.73 and 12.74)	Marked osteoporosis, thinning of cortex, later on—joint space reduction, subchondral cysts, tendency of ankylosis	Reduction in joint space, subchondral osteophytes, subarticular sclerosis	Osteoporotic and thin bone, dislocation/ subluxation, push-pull films can detect abnormal excursion of head
b. Blood and others	Nothing particular		ESR-raised lymphocytosis	Total WBC count increased, poly-morph count markedly raised Aspiration of pus from joint	Nothing particular	Nothing particular	ESR raised, Rose-Waaler negative HLA B 27 antigen present	Rose-Waaler positive	Nothing particular	Nothing particular
Classification	1. Dysplasia 2. Congenital subluxation 3. Congenital dislocation		Earlier classification of staging of tuberculosis hip is more academic rather than practical • Stage of synovitis • Stage of arthritis • Arthritis with gross destruction and pathological dislocation Shanmugasundaram (1983) suggested a clinicoradiological classification of tuberculosis of hip. Applicable for the lesions in children (C) and adults (A): Following radiological types: "normal appearance (C); Traveling acetabulum (C & A); Dislocated hip (C); Perthes type (C); Protrusio acetabuli (C, A); Atrophic type (A); Mortar and pestle type (C, A).	Stage of • Collection in joint (exudate + pus) • Sequestration of capital epiphysis • Pathological dislocation • Ankylosis	Catterall's radiological classification based on area of epiphyseal involvement, its collapse and metaphyseal reaction—into four grades—is most popular	—	—	—	• Primary (Idiopathic) • Secondary to – trauma – infection – Perthes' disease – coxa vara – osteonecrosis in adults – Obesity	• Subluxation • Dislocation

Contd...

1	2	3	4	5	6	7	8	9	10
Manage-ment	Conservative 1.—Splints (Pavlik harnesses, e.g. Von-Rosen's splint), 2. Reduction and plaster in 60° abduction Operation on pelvis—acetabuloplasty, pelvic osteotomy —On upper shaft-osteotomy. Total hip replacement	Conservative: General rest, local rest by POP, splint, traction. Chemotherapy. Operative: Excision[(5)], excision arthrodesis. Later on may go for total hip replacement after 5 years of complete quiescence	Conservative: Rest, antibiotics, aspiration of pus and installation of antibiotics Operative: Drainage, excision of diseased tissues sequestrum and granulation, etc.	All modes of treatment aim to prevent the femoral head from deformity by its containment before the revascularisation stage sets in (Waldenstrom H 1938) Conservative: Splint, POP cast (Broom stick type), Physiotherapy, traction, Operative: Adduction osteotomy of femur, varus derotation osteotomy involves varus angulation and correction of rotation, thus increasing the coverage of femoral head in the acetabulum and redirecting medially and anteriorly to control the lateral displacement of femoral head (Saini et al. 2009) pelvic osteotomy. Later on abduction osteotomy of femur, total hip replacement (THR)	Conservative: close reduction and POP cast. Operative: Regardless of the severity of the slip, pinning in situ provides the best long-term functional result and delay in the development of degenerative arthritis with a low risk of complications But marked slipping should be prevented by early diagnosis and prompt stabilization of epiphysis	Conservative: Physiotherapy, analgesics, corticosteroids, deep X-ray. Operative: Girdlestone arthroplasty, Total hip replacement (THR) Corrective high femoral osteotomy	Conservative: Analgesic, (NSAID), Corticosteroid, gold salts, heat therapy, physiotherapy, rest by traction Operative: Synovectomy, cup arthroplasty, THR	Conservative: Stick support, physiotherapy, analgesics, postural adjustments. Operative: Abduction displacement type osteotomy of femur, THR, Girdlestone arthroplasty	Conservative: Physiotherapy, orthotics Operative: Tendon transfer to improve stability, osteotomy, arthrodesis

Note

1. In children, the criteria for treatment should be based on measurements on both ultrasound and radiography; both should show abnormality before intervention is considered necessary.
   Total hip replacement, for the patient with a *dysplastic hip* is difficult—more difficult for dislocated (type 2 and 5) hips than subluxed ones (Type 1). Hartofilakidis et al practica classification into 3 types of *congenital hip diseases* in adults is a good guideline for replacement of hip: Type I— Dysplasia in which femoral head is still within the true acetabulum; Type 2—hips are with low dislocation in which the femoral head is in false acetabulum, the inferior lip of which is in contact with or overlaps the true acetabulum; Type 3—hips are with high dislocation in which false acetabulum has no contact with the true acetabulum. Types 2 and 3 present technical problems in performing THR.
2. *Neoplasms* and allied conditions **(Fig. 12.82)** in and around hip region manifest in bizarre fashion, depending upon the site of onset, nature of neoplasm and aggressiveness of the growth. Presenting features are mainly pain and limp. Later on, pathological fractures, swelling, deformities develop.
3. Certain rare but typical photographs: Figs 12.74 to 12.83 on Pages 365-367
4. Best prognostic indicator for hip in *Perthes disease* is the shape of femoral head at skeletal maturity. Normal or flattened spherical heads present few problems. Greater the deformity of femoral head at the end of active period, the greater is the chance of degenerative changes.
5. B Mukhopadhyay (1956) has emphasized the role of *excisional surgery in bone and joint tuberculosis*, which along with antituberculous chemotherapy can cure the disease.

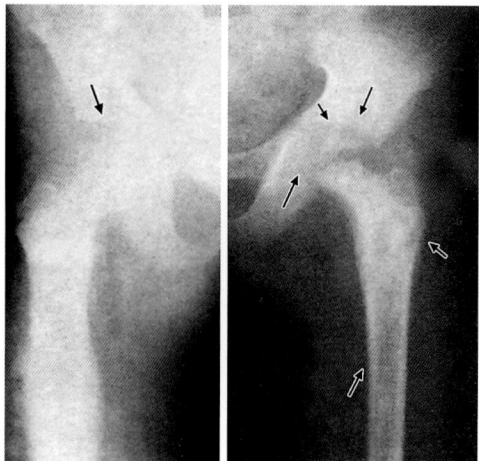

Fig. 12.59: Septic arthritis hip, sequestrating capital epiphysis.

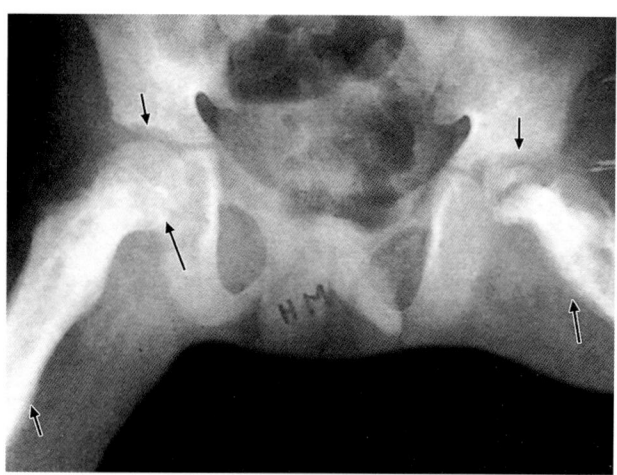

Fig. 12.62: Septic arthritis hip—bilateral septic arthritis of hip (left more affected).

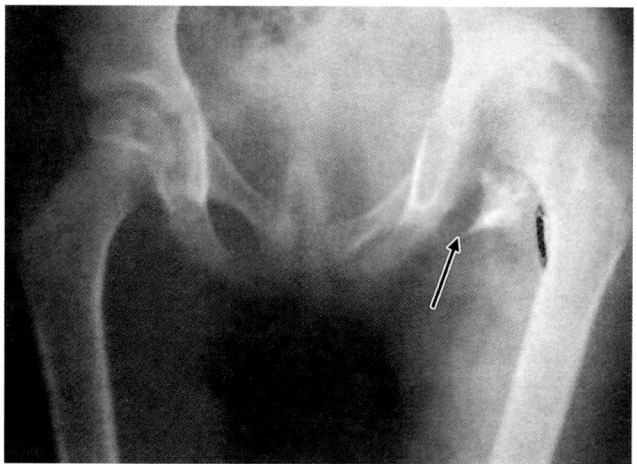

Fig. 12.60: Pathological dislocation of hip joint following old septic arthritis.

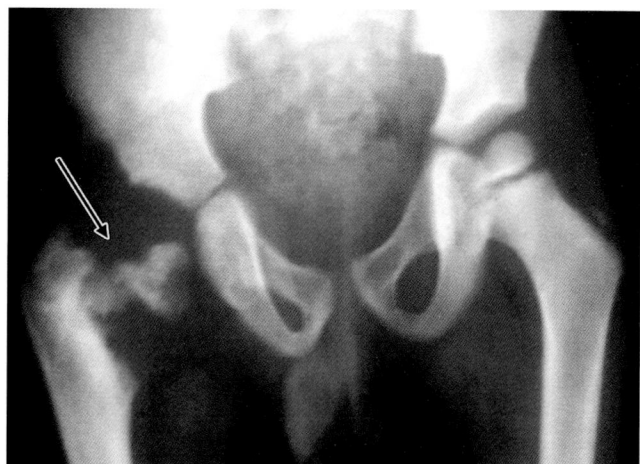

Fig. 12.63: Septic arthritis in a child with gross damage of femoral head and neck and huge pus in the right hip joint.

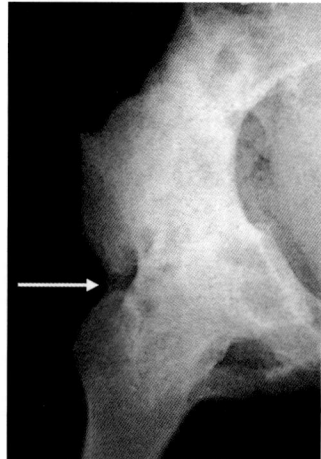

Fig. 12.61: Septic arthritis hip with bony ankylosis in deformed position of abduction.

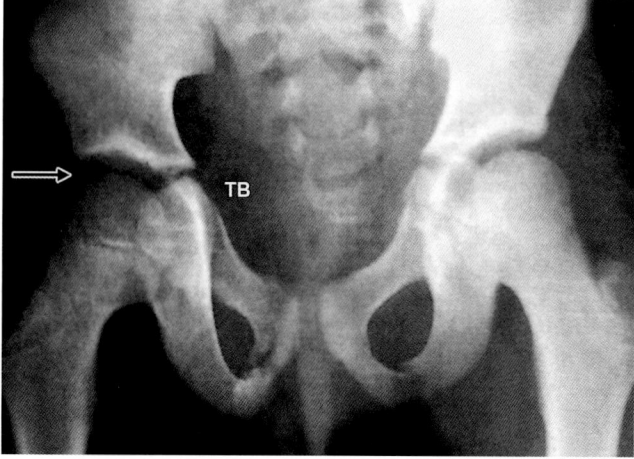

Fig. 12.64: Tuberculous synovitis of right hip. Note the increase in joint space and rarefaction of adjoining bones.

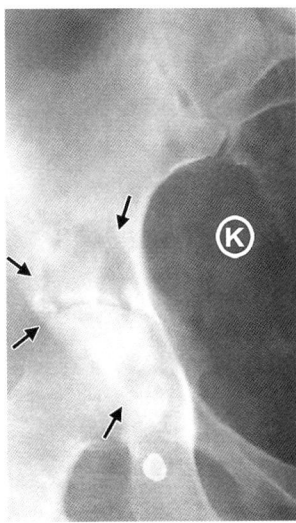

Fig. 12.65: Tuberculous arthritis hip with primary focus in upper part of acetabulum.

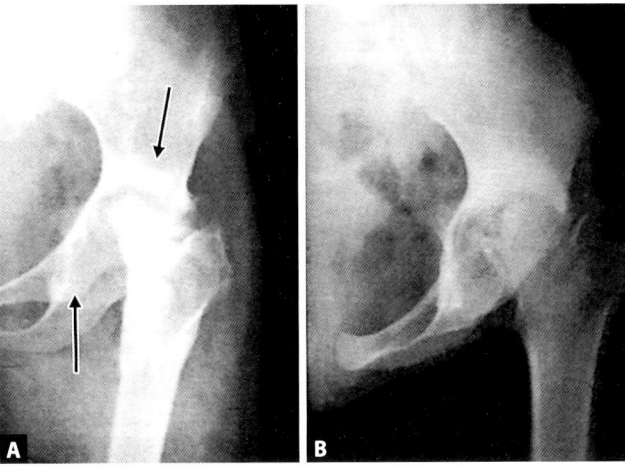

Figs. 12.67A and B: Advanced tuberculous arthritis of hip joint, with destruction of head and wandering acetabulum.

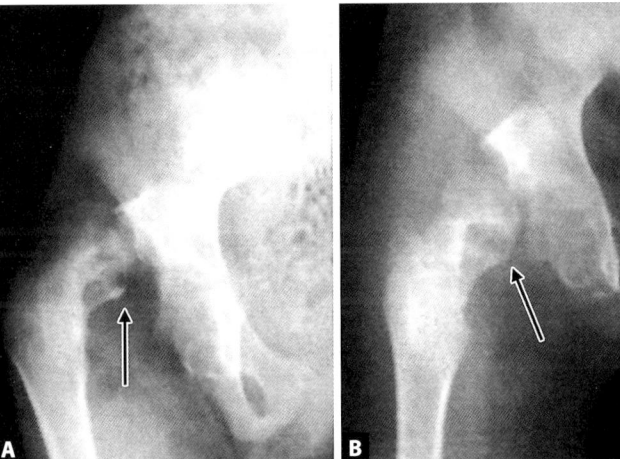

Figs. 12.66A and B: Advanced tuberculous arthritis of right hip joint with encysted lesion in cervical area and pseudodislocation.

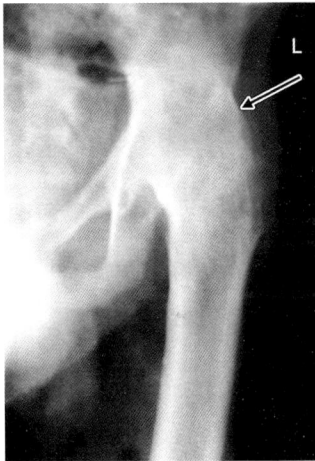

Fig. 12.68: Tuberculous arthritis of hip ankylosed in acceptable functional aligned position.

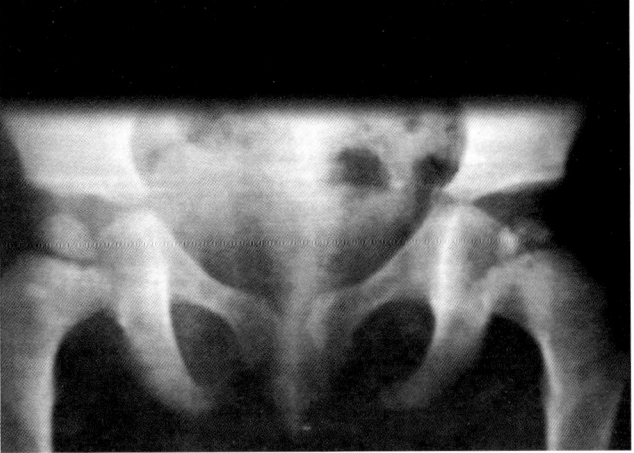

Fig. 12.69: Legg-Calve-Perthes' disease getting vascularised (left side).

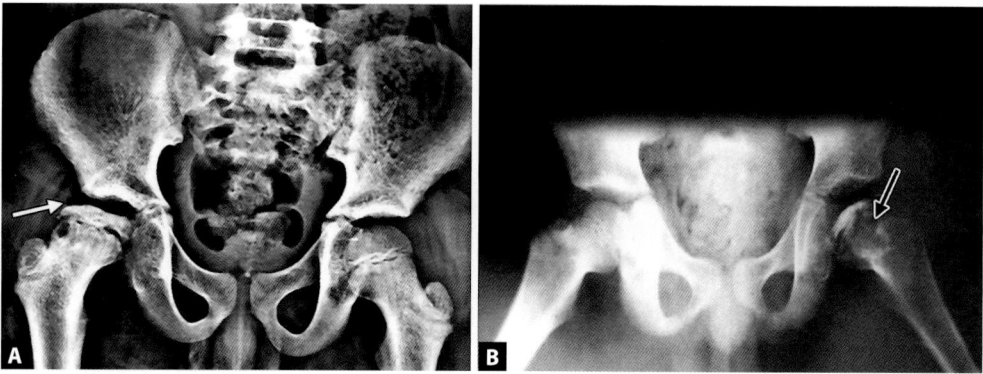

Figs. 12.70A and B: (A) Perthes' disease healed with deformed femoral head; (B) Legg-Calve-Perthes' disease with markedly collapsed capital epiphyses on left side.

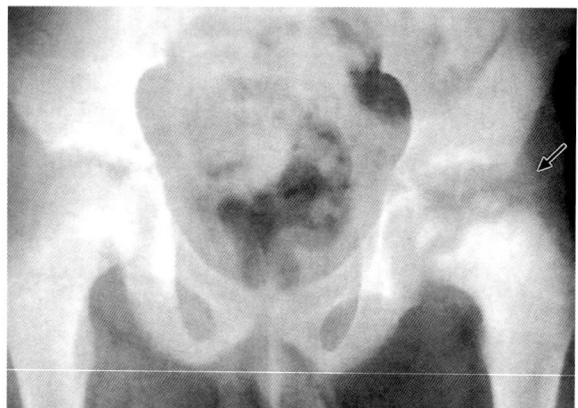

Fig. 12.71: Legg-Calve-Perthes' disease—advanced stage (left side).

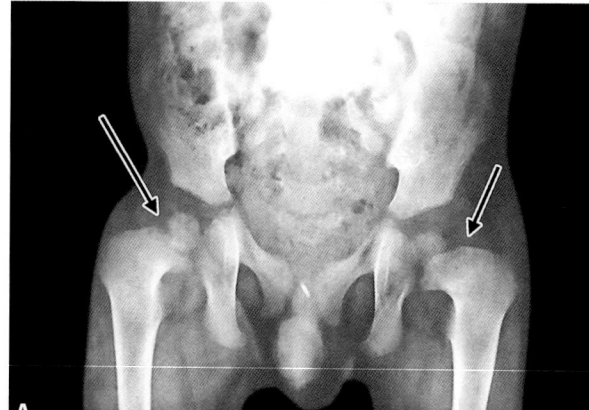

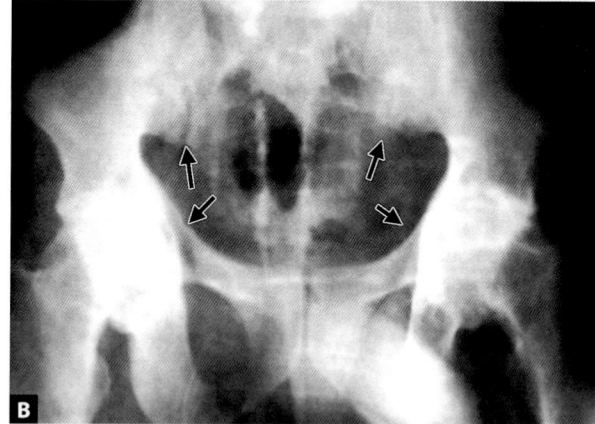

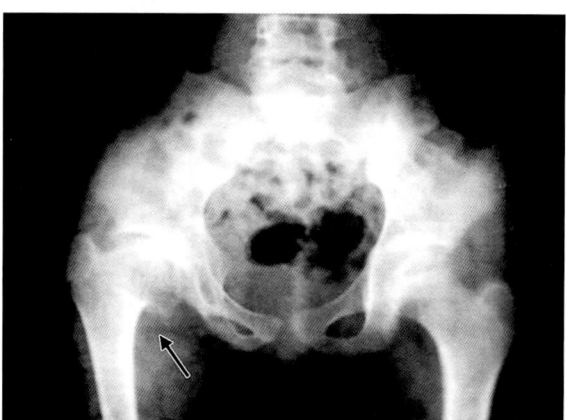

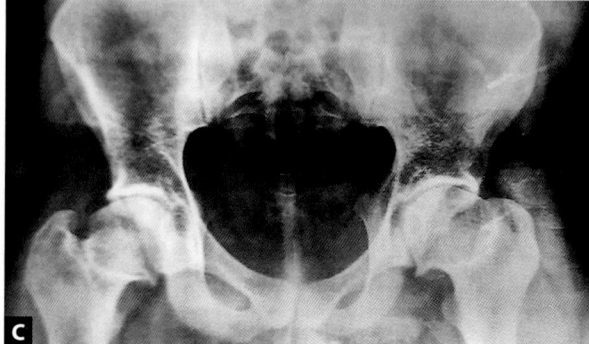

Fig. 12.72: Slipped capital epiphysis of right hip. It is a developmental disorder affecting adolescent hips. There is deformity of proximal femur at the level of growth plate which usually gets displaced posteromedially resulting in coxa vara (reduced femoral neck-shaft angle – normal being 135°). The capital femoral epiphysis lies in posteroinferior position in relation to the metaphysis. In this condition, the femoral capital epiphysis does not slip (as its name indicates), rather it is the proximal femoral metaphysis, which rotates externally with anterosuperior translation. It is most common in North America. Blacks are more affected than Caucasians. Exact cause is not known, but probably the proximal femoral growth plate fails due to excessive shearing stress. Once diagnosed and confirmed with X-ray, strict bed rest and non weight bearing should be enforced, of the various treatments pin/cannulated screw fixation in situ should be preferred.

Figs. 12.73A to C: (A) Bilateral slipped capital epiphysis; (B) Pre-bony ankylosis stage of ankylosing spondylitis; (C) Bilateral slipped capital epiphysis with avascular necrosis (more in right hip).

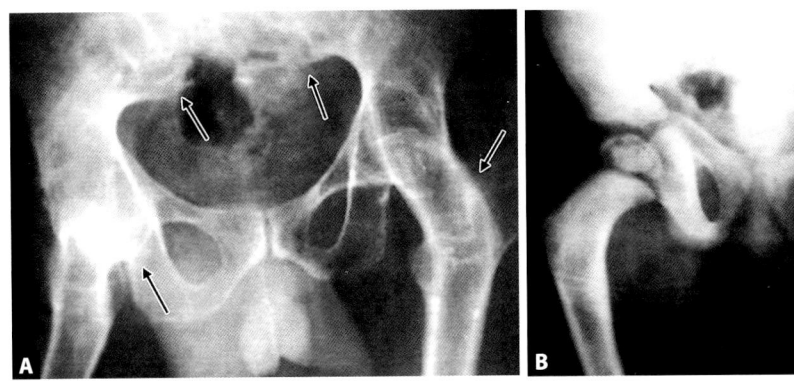

Figs. 12.74A and B: (A) Ankylosing spondylitis with markedly advanced totally fused hips and sacroiliac joints; (B) A typical affection of hip in **cretinism** (note fragmentation of capital epiphysis).

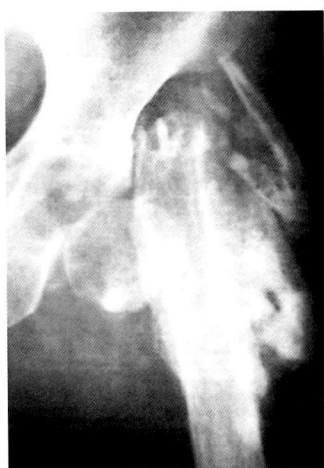

Fig. 12.75: Charcot's disease of hip. Charcot neuroarthropaths is a progressive condition. It affects bones, joints, and soft tissues of the affected joints like hip, knee, ankle, and foot. Regarding its origin, their are several theories like neuropathic, repetitive microtrauma, or increased blood flow leading to washout of bone and their breakdown mostly occurs in patients with diabetes mellitus and diabetic neuropathy. It is considered as an end-stage complication of diabetes mellitus. *Also see* **Figs. 13.48B –13.49** on Pages 391–392 X-ray picture of *Charcot' arthropathy of knee*; **Fig. 5.53**—*charcot arthropathy elbow.*

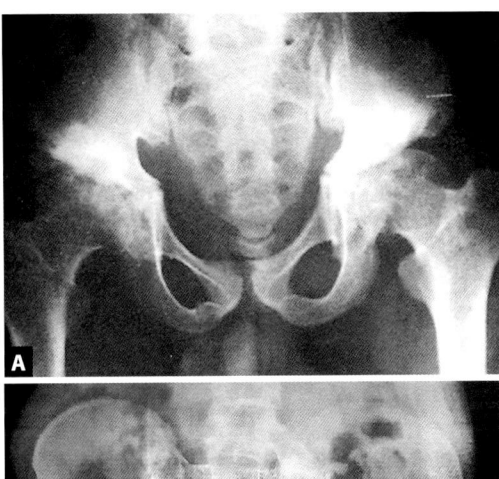

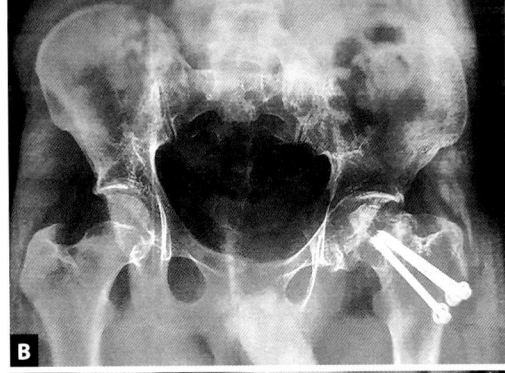

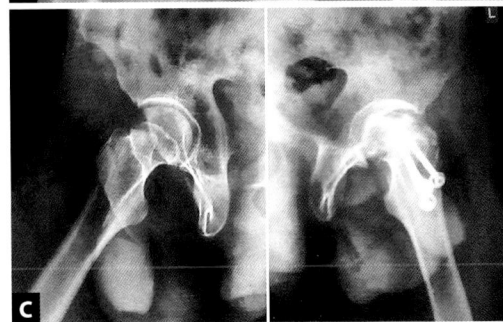

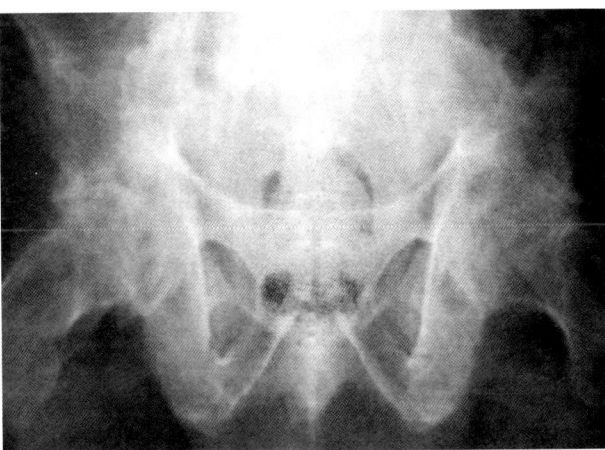

Fig. 12.76: Bilateral **idiopathic avascular necrosis of hip** joint (right more than left).

Figs. 12.77A to C: Bilateral **avascular necrosis (osteonecrosis)** of femoral head in a chronic alcoholic. ONFH is a disabling condition of hip joint that primarily affects the young individuals with male predominates. Prolonged steroid intake, idiopathic, chronic alcohol consumption and trauma are believed to be predisposing causative factors. Steroids and alcoholism usually affect both hips. It may be after fracture neck of femur and even after its fixation **(Fig. 12.77B)**; (C) Lateral view of hips.

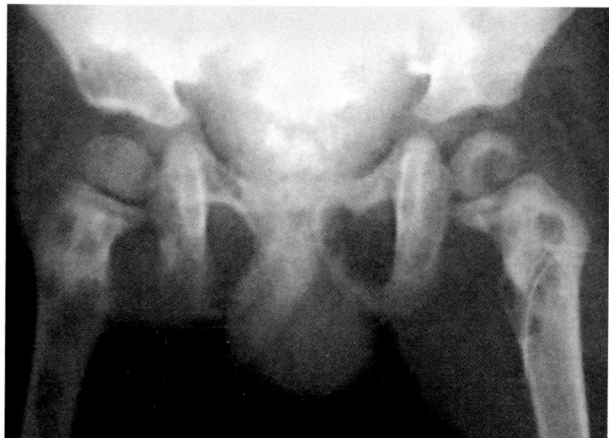

Fig. 12.78: Sickle cell (anaemia) disease—manifestations in pelvis, hips and femora. *Also see* **Figs. 12.79, 12.80, 12.81**.

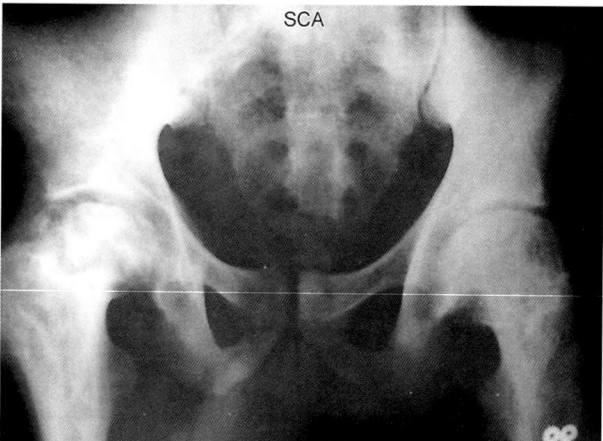

Fig. 12.79: Sickle cell (anaemia) disease—manifestations in hips and femora. Herrick, a Chicago-based cardiologist, was the first to describe sickle cell anaemia as a separate entity in 1910; however, Graham observed the skeletal changes in this disease in 1924. Sickle cell disease is an inherited blood disorder which affects the red cells which then contain sickle haemoglobin.

with variable limitation of movements specially of internal rotation and abduction.

In early stage, X-ray looks normal. As the disease advances, changes like density or lucent appears in femoral head, and further the diagnostic 'crescent sign' develops. Ultimately variable collapse of femoral head occurs. Ficat (1985) has suggested radiographic staging of osteonecrosis of femoral head, which is mostly accepted.

Etiopathogenesis is not explainable in all cases, however, intraosseous hypertension and abnormalities of blood supply are more acceptable concepts. *Possible causes* can be grouped under following headings:
- Post-traumatic, e.g. in fracture of neck of femur, scaphoid, talus, humeral head
- Extrinsic vascular pressure, e.g. marrow hypertrophy; marrow replacement; increased intraosseous pressure; dislocations; joint effusion

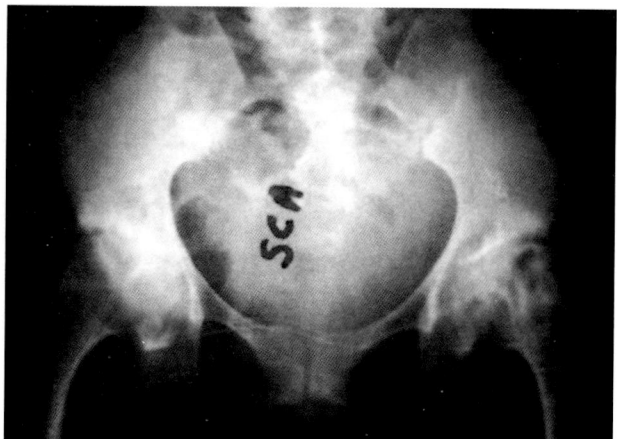

Fig. 12.80: Sickle cell (anaemia) disease—advanced changes (painful avascular necrosis of femoral head – **sickle cell** disease in hips: Sickle cell hemoglobinopathy is a common genetic disorder with a typical topographical and racial distribution. It is hereditary familial chronic disease with mild to severe symptoms (frequent painful) episodes, anaemia, weakness, bone joint pains, infection, etc), with normal life span to reduced life expectancy. Sickle cell disease includes related molecular disorders like-sickle cell anaemia, sickle cell trait, sickle cell hemoglobin C disease, sickle cell thalassemia, sickle cell haemoglobin D and D and G disorder, etc. In sickle cell disease changes on haemoglobin associates alteration on the surface of RBC – the red cell membrane takes the typical shape of a sickle in stress conditions like dehydration, acidosis and anoxia. Treatment mainly consists: of treat precipitating, infection, anaemia (even by infusion of packed red cells, genetic counselling of patient and sickle community. Patients should regularly take folic acid (5 mg daily) and consume much water. Indian Government has set a target to eradicate sickle cell by 2047.

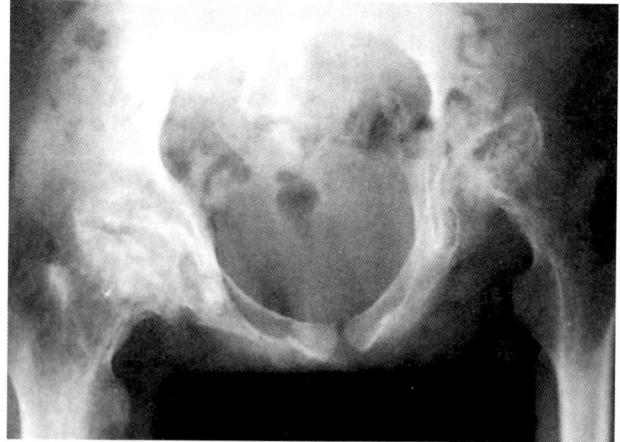

Fig. 12.81: Bilateral avascular necrosis of femoral head with collapse (left more than right) in **sickle cell (anaemia) disease.**

- Intrinsic occlusion (microembolisation), e.g. by blood clots, fat droplets, sickle cells, nitrogen bubbles
- Thrombosis, e.g. in vascular disorders (vasculitis, coagulation defects)
- Cytotoxicity, e.g. in chronic alcoholics, prolonged steroid therapy

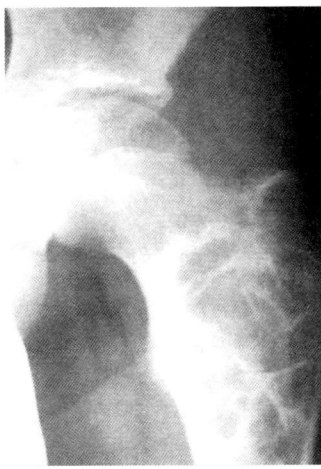

Fig. 12.82: **Fibrous dysplasia** of trochanter with threatened pathological fracture.

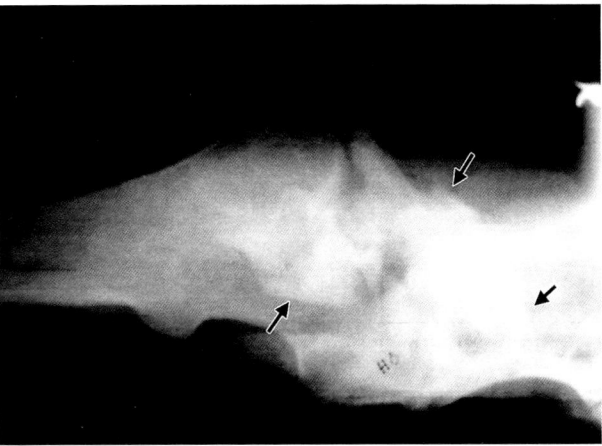

Fig. 12.85: **Myositic mass** around hip in an extensive burn case.

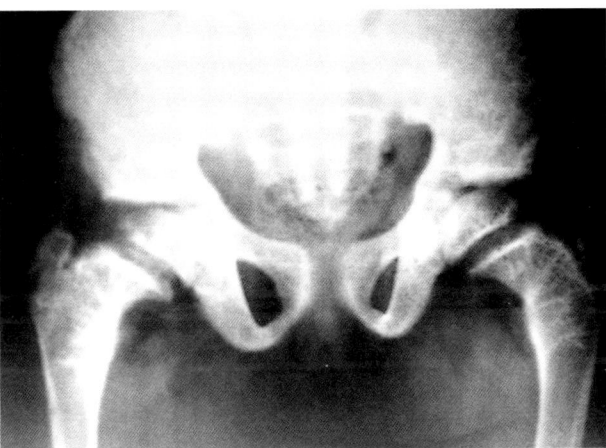

Fig. 12.83: **Renal rickets.**

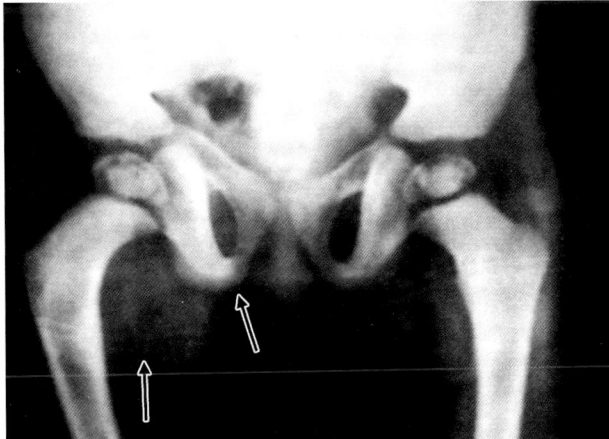

Fig. 12.84: **Myositic mass** around hip in a neglected posterior dislocation.

- Osteopaenia with microfractures
- Multifactorial
- Idiopathic.

Conditions where AVN commonly occurs: After trauma; prolonged (high doses) steroid therapy, testosterone, lipid lowering drugs, renal transplant, cirrhosis liver; Caisson's disease; sickle cell disease; pancreatitis; collagen vascular disorders and SLE; Gaucher's disease; sarcoidosis; hyperlipidaemias; radiation therapy; coagulopathy; cancer chemotherapy; patients with HIV infection; alcohol abuse.

Legg-Calve Perthes Disease was first described by Waldenstrom, mistakenly as tuberculosis in 1909. However, Legg AT, Calve J and Perthes GC described this condition independently in 1910, and since then it is known as Leg-Calve-Perthes disease. It is also called coxa plana or osteochondrosis of hip joint. It occurs due to interruption of blood supply of femoral capital epiphysis due to no known exact cause.

In Legg-Calve-Perthes Disease, rarely, osteochondritis dissecans may develop (first described by Hass in 1937). It is a self-limiting disease of hip, of unknown etiology occurring mainly in white male children of poor families in UK (rare in blacks, Indians, except in southwest coastal, Polynesians) in the age group of 3-10 years of age. It is characterised by avascular necrosis of the ossification centre of the femoral capital epiphysis which is ultimately resorbed and replaced. The natural history of disease can be considered in two phases: evolution phase (in which the affected region is painful) and healing of epiphysis phase. In the evolution phase the small femoral head epiphysis is radio dense, the epiphyseal plate is uneven and metaphysis is blurred. A crescentic fracture line may be seen in the subchondral region.

In the second phase, there is healing of the epiphysis, gradual repair of the fragmented femoral head to a homogeneous epiphysis with continuous growth and ossification of femoral head. However, even though the quality of bone becomes normal, the femoral head and neck and acetabulum may become deformed. After revascularization of bone there is no pain in the affected zone. Ultimate result in most of the cases is slight shortening, variable deformity, restricted movements of hip and premature osteoarthritis. It may remain asymptomatic for long period only to be diagnosed by plain X-ray and or CT. Osteochondritis fragment may become separated and lies as loose body in the joint. It should be managed under 'supervised neglect scheme' till it interferes with the mechanics of hip, when it should be removed.

Avascular necrosis (AVN) is preceded by bone marrow oedema, which can be seen in MRI. In the early stage (Stage I), hyperbaric oxygen improves tissue oxygenation, reduces oedema and induces angioneogenesis. By reducing the intraosseous pressure, venous drainage is restored and the microcirculation improves.

Progressive collapse is the main complication of osteonecrosis of femoral head which leads to disabilities in patients, who are young and active.

Gaucher's disease is a rare genetic disease, usually occurring in children born to the couples in a community where inbreeding (near relative or close family marriage) is common. The Jewish doctor Gaucher discovered the storage of fat disease which was prevalent among Jews who fled Hitler's oppression, and settled down as a community and inbreeding became common to keep the race afloat.

In this metabolic disease, there is abnormal metabolism and storage of fat. It results in bone fragility, neurological disturbances, anaemia, and enlargement of liver and spleen. Splenectomy may save such children.

■ BIBLIOGRAPHY

1. Chung SMK. The arterial supply of developing proximal end of the human femur. J Bone Joint Surg. 1976;58A.
2. Deqiang Li, Ming Li, Peilai Liu, et al. Core decompression or quadratus femoris muscle pedicle bone grafting for nontraumatic osteonecrosis of the femoral head: A randomized control study. Ind. Jr of Orthopaedics. 2016;50:629-35.
3. Fahey JJ, O Brien, ET. Acute slipped femoral epiphysis. J Bone Joint Surg. 1965;47A:1105.
4. Ficat RP. Idiopathic bone necrosis of the femoral head. Early diagnosis and treatment. J Bone Joint Surg Br. 1985;67:3-9.
5. Graham GS (1924) – (Quoted by Babhulkar SS) Textbook of Orthopedics and Trauma, 3rd edition. New Delhi: Jaypee Brothers; 2016. p. 484.
6. Green WB. Treatment of hip and knee problems in myelomeningocele. J Bone Joint Surg. 1998;80-A:1068-82.
7. Handerson RS. Traumatic anterior dislocation of the hip. J Bone Joint Surg. 338-602.
8. Harris WH. J Bone Joint Surg. 1969;51:737-55.
9. Hartofilakidis G. Stamos K, Karachalios T, et al. Congenital hip diseases in adult. Classification of acetabular deficiencies and operative treatment with acetabuloplasty combined with total hip arthroplasty. J Bone Joint Surg (Am). 1996;78: 683-92.
10. Harty M. Anatomy of the hip joint. In: Tronzo RG (Ed): Surgery of the Hip Joint Lea Philadelphia Febrger; 1973.
11. Herricle JB (1910) – (Quoted by Babhulkar SS) Textbook of Orthopedics and Trauma, 3rd edition. New Delhi: Jaypee Brothers; 2016. p. 484.
12. Jones D. Neonatal detection of developmental dysplasia of hip. J Bone Joint Surg (Br). 1998;80-B, 943-5.
13. Joshi N, Mohapatra SS, Goyal MP, et al. Short term outcome of varus derotation.
14. Klisic PJ. Congenital dislocation of the hips: A misleading term [brief report]. J Bone Join Surg (Br). 1989;71:136.
15. Lai CH. Avascular necrosis in rheumatic diseases, aetiology, pathogenesis and clinical features. Orthopaedic Update (India). 2000;10(3):26-8.
16. Mukhopadhyay B. Role of excisional surgery in Bone and joint tuberculosis – Hunterian Lecture. Ann R Coll Surg Eng 1956; 18:288-313.
17. Pandey S. Congenital bilateral contracture of Gluteus maximum. Int. Surg. Vol 61. No. 1 Chicago 1976.
18. Reis ND, Schwartz O, Militianu D, et al. Hyperbaric Oxygen Therapy as a treatment for stage I avascular necrosis of the femoral head. J Bone Joint Surg (Br). 2003;85-B:371-5.
19. Saini R, Goyal T, Dhillon MS, et al. Outcome of varus derotation closed wedge osteotomy in Perthes disease. Acta Orthop Belg 2009;75:34-9.
20. Shanmugasundaram TK. A clinicoradiological classification of tuberculosis of hip. Current concepts in Bone and Joint Tuberculosis 1983.
21. Terjesen T. Ultrasound as the primary imaging method in the diagnosis of hip dysplasia in children aged less than 2 years. J Pediatric Orthop. 1993;05:123-8.
22. Trendelenburg F. Dtsh Med Wochenscher. 1895;21:21.
23. Trueta J. Normal anatomy of human femoral head and its clinical importance. J Bone Joint Surg. 1965;318:82.
24. Vasudevan PN, Vaidyalingam KV, Nair B. Can Trendelenburg's sign be positive if the hip is normal? J Bone Joint Surg (Br). 1997; 79B:462-6.
25. Vitale MG, Skaggs DL. Developmental dysplasia of the hip from six months to four years of age. J Am Acad Orthop Surg. 2001;9(6):401-11.
26. Waldenstrom H. The first stages of coxaplana. J Bone Joint Surg 1938;20:559-66.

CHAPTER 13

Knee

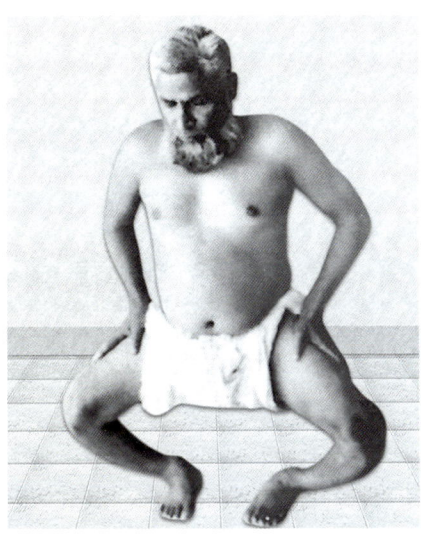
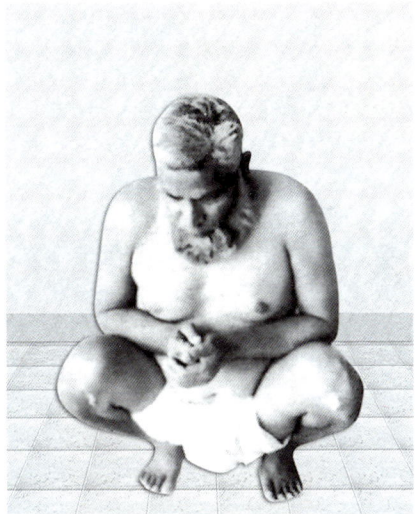

"Friendship improves happiness and abates misery, by the doubling of our joy and dividing of our grief."
—***Cicero***

"Honesty and clear communication are crucial for a healthy long-term relationship."
—***SP***

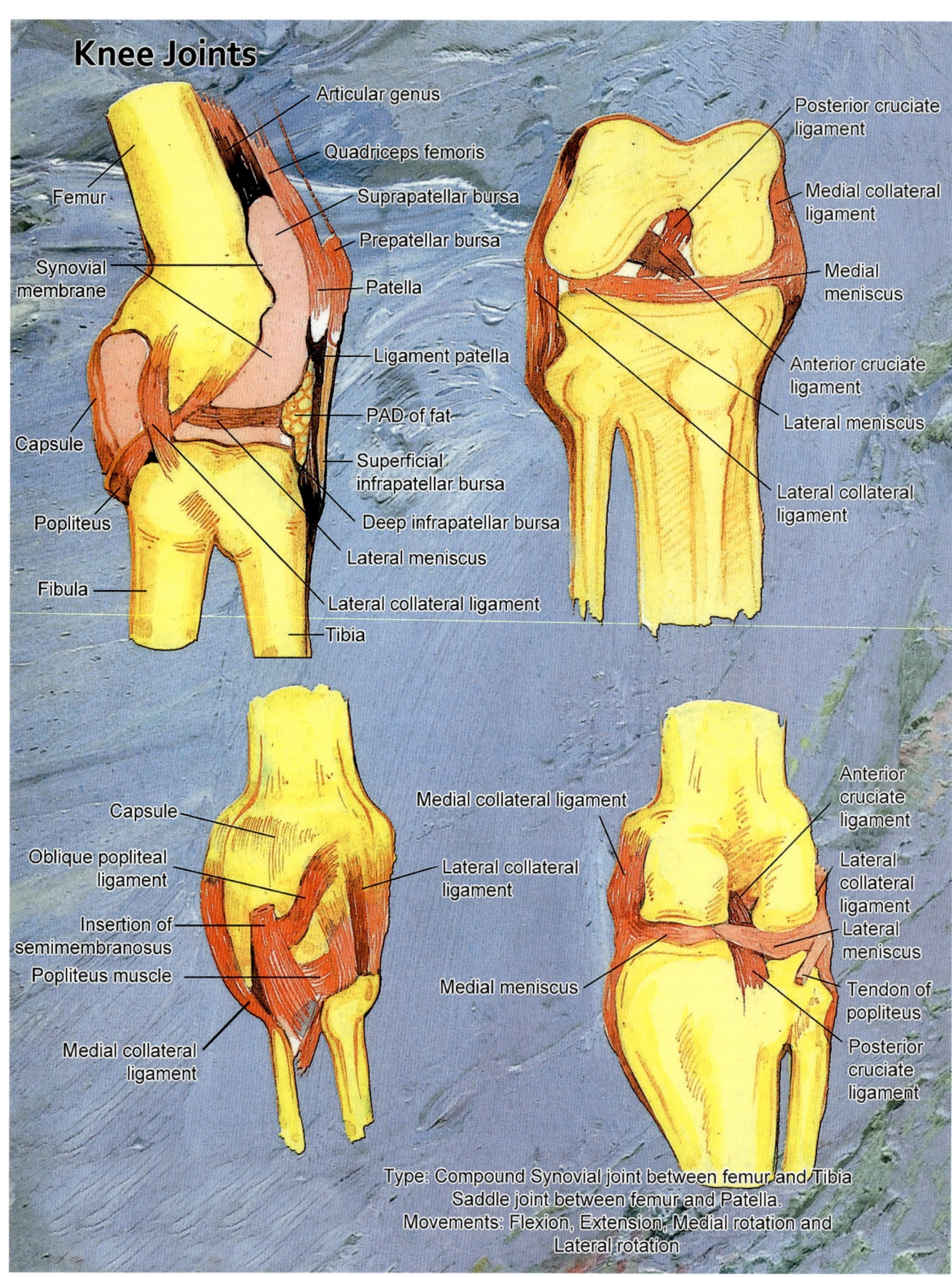

INTRODUCTION

Evolutionwise the basic characteristics of the human knee were present almost 300 million years ago. Broadly the knee is a triaxial joint having three sets of interrelated articulations, i.e. tibiofemoral, patellofemoral and upper tibiofibular.

The knee is the *largest joint in the human body* and is most frequently injured.

The knee, being one of the *most exposed joints*, is much more vulnerable to trauma and disease, specially in sports activities. With the advancements in the sports medicine, the knees are becoming more and more important. Accurate clinical diagnosis is essential to provide an adequate base for arthroscopic surgery, which plays a major role in the management of the lesions of the knee.

The function of the knee may be summarised as a biological transmission system in which it receives, redirects and dissipates a range of biomechanical loads.

ANATOMICAL CONSIDERATIONS

Anatomically the *knee joint is a compound joint* composed of three articulations: Two condyloid joints (medial and lateral articulations of the distal femur and proximal tibia) The medial femoral condyle has larger surface area but the lateral femoral condyle is longer and one sellar joint (articulation of posterior surface of patella with anterior aspect of lower end of femur). It is the largest synovial major weight bearing joint whose stability depends not only on ligaments but also on surrounding muscles. The patellar tendon inserts into tibial tuberosity. The iliotibial band attaches onto the Gerdy tubercle. The medial epicondyle provides attachment to the medial collateral ligament AND lateral epicondyle to the lateral collateral ligament.

The intercondylar area provides attachment to the cruciate ligaments – the anterior cruciate ligament laterally and posterior cruciate ligament medially. The tibial medial condyle is broad and concave, whereas lateral tibial condyle is smaller, more circular and convex. The tibia has also medial and lateral condyles to articulate with the corresponding femoral condyles.

The head of fibula articulates with lateral tibial condyle forming an arthrodial joint, which is at little lower level to the knee joint and is quite separate from it. The fibula is held to the tibia by the joint capsule and anterior and posterior ligaments.

- The knee is a *complex synovial joint*, in which fibrocartilaginous menisci are present. It is mainly comprised of: (i) femorotibial compartments (lateral and medial which are separated by vertical fibroligamentous structures attached to the intercondylar eminence of the tibia and the intercondylar notch of the femur), and (ii) patellofemoral compartment.

  The capsule of knee joint is complex fibrous sheet reinforced by bands and tendons crossing the joint
- The *synovial reflections of the joint* are quite extensive and complicated. Therefore, (i) any synovial affection (or infection) can remain synovial for a pretty long time before invading the articular components, (ii) most of the pathologies of the knee joint first manifest either as synovial swelling and/or as a swelling produced from synovial secretions, (iii) diseases which have more predilection for synovial affection are much more common in this joint

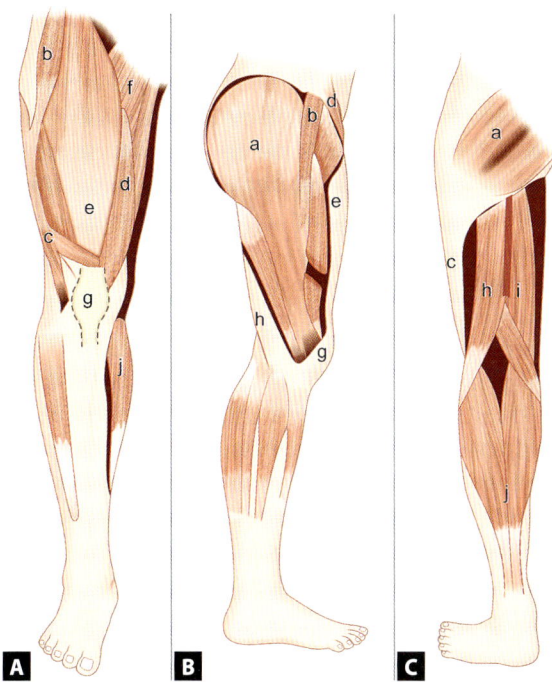

Figs. 13.1A to C: Contour of the limb around, above and below the knee—(A) from front, (B) from side, (C) from back. a = gluteus maximus, b = tensor fascia femoris, c = iliotibial tract, d = sartorius, e = quadriceps, f = adductors, g = patella, h = biceps femoris, i = medial hamstrings, j = gastrocsoleus.

- The *articular surfaces* of knee are not congruent. On medial side, the femoral condyle with its larger surface area articulates with tibia like a wheel on a flat surface, while on lateral side femoral condyle with its larger surface area articulates like a wheel on a dome. Thus, they are so oriented that their adaptations are vulnerable in any horizontal and/or rotatory stress, like abduction, adduction, anteroposterior or rotatory stresses
- Except posteriorly, the joint is quite superficial in its other aspects
- The integrity of the joint is dependent mainly on the ligaments and muscles in and around the knee joint
- Of all the muscles, the vastus medialis is the main dynamic stabiliser of the knee
- There is no other joint in the body which contains *so much of intra-articular ligaments or cartilaginous structures and bony prominences* as the knee joint. Therefore, internal derangements of the knee joint are quite common
- There is no other joint which is associated with such a *big sesamoid bone, i.e. patella, which* is more or less flat triangular in shape and is embedded in the tendon

of quadriceps femoris. Patella has thickest articular cartilage in the body. The distal extension of this tendon is the patellar ligament, which is attached to the tibial tuberosity. In flexion, the patella opposes the lateral part of the medial femoral condyle; in passive extension, the patella loosely rides in front of distal femur, while in active extension it is often pulled up against the lateral femoral condyle. The patella *subserves several important functions*—(i) It acts as a natural knee cap protecting the joint proper from direct external violence; (ii) It acts as a buffer to the violent quadriceps contractions; (iii) Acting on a pulley like mechanism, it augments the action of the quadriceps apparatus, transmitting the forceful quadriceps contractions to tibial tuberosity through the ligamentum patellae; (iv) It prevents unwanted friction of the quadriceps tendon over the femoral condyle thereby mechanically easing the quadriceps mechanism; (v) It aids in the nourishment of the articular surface of the femur; (vi) Patients after total patellectomy feel difficulty in suddenly getting up from a fully crouched position, perhaps due to comparative diminution in the power of extension (from a fully flexed position). This indicates the importance of the patella.

The blood supply of patella is from patellar plexus formed by the branches of superior, medial and inferior geniculate arteries.

- The *vestigial synovial folds* can be a cause of internal derangement of the knee joint, like impingement of the infrapatellar pad of fat even with a trivial injury
- Being superficial, even any insignificant prick can lead to severe infective arthritis of the joint
- *Movements:* From the stability point of view (for securing stability), the knee joint has been allowed only one axial movement, i.e. flexion and extension. Rather, it should be taken as only one movement, i.e. flexion from zero degree of full extension—the anatomical position (of full extension). However, the kinematics in the human knee encompass much more than flexion and extension, the important one being medial pivoting kinematics. Therefore, from trauma point of view, rotational stresses on the knee joint produce more damage. The anatomically provided checks do not allow the leg component to go beyond the zero position and are probably not strong enough to withstand moderate to severe rotational strains (e.g. in missing a step or while running or playing)
- The iliotibial band attaches in the Gerdy tubercle. Summarily, it can be deduced that articulation in knee allows flexion and extension of the joint along with rolling (screw home) motion during terminal extension.
- The main *neurovascular bundle* of the leg and foot lies in close vicinity of the posterior capsule of the knee joint. Hence, it is quite vulnerable to certain types of injuries around the knee (specially dislocations of the knee joint, displaced supracondylar fractures of femur and displaced fractures of tibial condyles). However, extensive collateral network around the knee may make it possible to obliterate the popliteal artery without jeopardising the circulation of distal portion of the extremity. Therefore, it is imperative to assess the integrity of these vital structures in affections of the knee joint, especially after trauma
- Whatever may be the pathology, traumatic or cold, the methodology of examination remains the same. However, in traumatic cases, more importance should be given to stress-integrity of the knee joint, while in cold cases, the condition of the articular components is more important
- *Bursae around the knee joint*: These are situated in between the tendons and the coverings of the joints. They are quite often affected by pathologies, varying right from non-specific to malignant neoplastic conditions. In these conditions, the patient presents with knee complaints. (*See* Pages 388–389)
- *Menisci*: Menisci, the wedge shaped fibrocartilaginous structures lie in the outer region of the tibiofemoral component of the knee joint. The *medial and lateral menisci* are flattened crescents of fibrocartilage which rim the peripheral borders of the tibial condyles. Their radial cross-sections are wedge-shaped with the base—the thickest part—lying outward. This configuration deepens the articular surfaces of the tibial condyles and fills the space between the convex femoral condyles and the flatter tibial surface. The ends of the crescents of menisci are anchored firmly to the slopes of the tibial spine, their outer margins are attached to the upper end of tibia by the coronary ligaments, and have their inner margins free. The range of excursion of medial meniscus is less than that of the lateral, hence it is more vulnerable to rotational strains. The internal structure of both menisci is primarily collagen with a small amount of proteoglycan.

The blood supply of the medial and lateral menisci is from the medial and lateral genicular arteries.

Earlier, when the functions of the menisci were not fully studied, they were considered by the anatomists as fillers of the vacant joint space, and as working for spreading of the synovial fluid in between the articular surfaces. With these considerations in mind, the treatment of meniscus tear was excision at the earliest. Therefore, even on clinical suspicion, meniscectomy was done as a routine. Now, the *functions of menisci in human being* have been very well studied. Besides the aforesaid functions, other functions are:

- By virtue of its location, it prevents synovial and capsular impingement during flexion extension movement
- Helps in stabilising the joint in all planes, especially during rotatory strains
- About 50% of the insignificant weight bearing or load transmitting forces are carried by the menisci
- Mechanically, it deepens the tibial condylar surface

- Acts as shock absorber.

  Thus, based on better understanding of functions of the menisci, and supported by the arthrographic and arthroscopic findings, now the aim is to save and repair the torn menisci than to excise it

- The *anterior cruciate ligament* (ACL) is an intra-articular and extrasynovial ligament of an average length of 31–38 mm and width of 11 mm. ACL is composed of longitudinally oriented bundles of collagen tissue arranged in fascicular subunits within larger functional bands—mainly two main bundles—an anteromedial bundle (which becomes taught in flexion and lax in extension) and a posterolateral bundle (which becomes taut in extension and lax in flexion). *ACL acts as the primary restraint to anterior translation of knee*

- The *long axis of the thigh and leg* (i.e. femorotibial angle) are not in the same line, rather, the leg axis is placed at 7° ± 3° valgus to the thigh axis. The thigh axis is placed at an angle of 81° on the outer side over the horizontal line, whereas the leg axis makes an angle of 87° over the horizontal knee axis on the inner side **(Fig. 13.2)**

- Long cassette posteroanterior weight-bearing X-ray views can be helpful to assess limb mechanical and anatomic alignment, especially in advance degenerative and destructive diseases and in patients with congenital or acquired femoral and tibial deformities.

- In a normal knee, approximately *60% of the weight bearing forces are transmitted along the medial compartment and 40% through the lateral compartment*. In a knee with unicompartmental arthritis limb alignment is altered and gradually more load is distributed to the affected compartment causing further degenerative changes and angular deformity.

Ossification around knee joint—**(Fig. 13.3) (Table 13.1)**

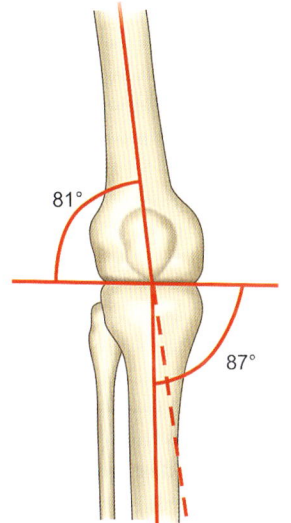
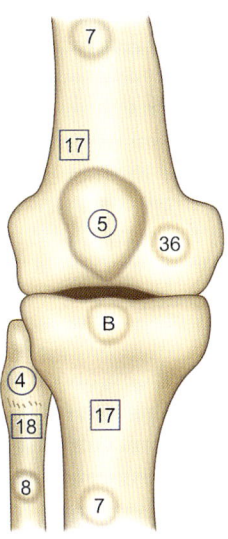
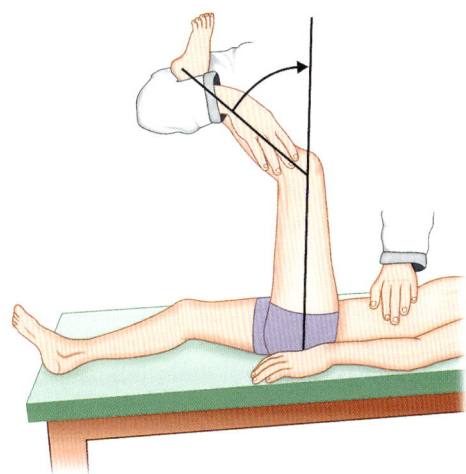

Fig. 13.2: Showing normal longitudinal axis of femur and tibia (femorotibial angle).

Fig. 13.3: Ossification around the knee. Dotted circle—primary centre in weeks IUL. Complete circle—secondary centres in year. Square—fusion in years. B—at birth.

Fig. 13.3A: Test for spasm and/or contracture of hamstrings and measurement of "popliteal angle"

NB: Figure drawn after HELEN M HORSTMANN and EUGENE E BLECK in their book. Orthopaedic Management in Cerebral Palsy, 2nd Edn. Page 38. 2007, Mackeith Press.

TABLE 13.1: Ossification of bones around the knee.

Bone	Primary for shaft	Secondary	Unites with shaft
Tibia	7th week IUL	• For the lower end, early in 1st year	15th year in female / 16th year in male
		• For upper end, usually present at birth	16–18 years
Fibula	8th week IUL	• For lower end 1st year	17th year in male / 15th year in female
		• For upper end 3-4 years	19th year in male / 17th year in female
Patella		Ossifies from several centres which appear at 3-6 years and quickly coalesce. Accessory marginal centres appear later and fuse with the central mass	
Femur	7th week IUL	Secondary centres—one each for head 3-6 months, greater trochanter—4th year, lesser trochanter—12-14th year.	14-17th year
		For the lower end at 9th months IUL	16th year in female / 18th year in male

METHODOLOGY

History Taking

Usual complaints in case of knee pathologies are pain, swelling, limitation of movements (usually painful), problems and pain in weight bearing, and deformity. Though history taking will be as usual, however, certain factors should be particularly ascertained. In recurrent swellings of the knee in a child, history of bleeding from gums and any increase in duration of bleeding due to any cut, if present, must be noted. In case of injury to the knee, the nature of violence, immediate effect of injury on the patient as a whole and the knee in particular should be noted. In older knee injuries, history of locking of joint, sense of 'giving way' at the knee on walking or running should be ascertained. Any other relevant point should be categorically noted.

An inflamed knee may be due to intra-articular or extra-articular pathology. In acute inflammatory arthritis of the knee, there is spasmodic flexion of knee and loss of extension with an associated effusion. However, if in an inflamed knee full extension can be achieved without pain and a negative bulge sign, the cause is likely to be extra-articular.

When younger patients develop severe knee pain, the causes are usually injury (e.g. fracture and/or ligamentous injury), infection/inflammation/generalised joint diseases (e.g. gout or psoariasis, etc.).

General and Systemic Examinations

These should be done as in the Chapter 1: Introduction. In case of pain or swelling of the knee joint, one must enquire about involvement of other joints, especially the smaller joints, because knee is a common site for collagen arthropathy. Besides, any obvious generalised pathology and clinical manifestation must be noted.

Regional Examination

In regional examination, at least the hip and the ankle are to be examined, since the involvement of either can have an impact on the knee, thus confusing the clinical examination. However, it will be much informative and desirable if lumbosacral to foot region is examined in the purview of regional examination.

Analysis of Knee Complaints Due to Regional Pathology

Occasionally, the patient complains of pain in the knee, specially on the anteromedial aspect, though there is no pathology in the knee joint itself. This is the referred pain from the hip joint (especially where the superomedial aspect of femoral head is affected) through the anterior division of the obturator nerve which also supplies a twig to the hip joint, e.g. in Legg-Calve-Perthes disease, slipped femoral capital epiphysis, early tuberculous infection, etc.

In the affections of sacroiliac joint, pain referred along the sciatic nerve, either due to sciatic radiculitis or fibro-fatty nodules over the sacroiliac region, may be felt mainly at the back of the knee.

In ankle pathology or painful hindfoot syndrome, sometimes the patient complains of pain in the knee, specially in the anteromedial compartment. This is because, in these conditions, the patient wants to avoid weight on hindfoot, so the ankle and foot are put in equinus position, which automatically has an external rotational tendency of the knee joint. With continued effort in this posture, the knee is strained more and more, resulting in stretch pain sensation.

In spastics, spasm of the hamstrings gets an upper hand over the quadriceps. This sustained spasm leads to pain in the back of the knee joint. In the long run, degenerative changes manifest quite early in such a knee, leading to actual pain in the knee proper.

Local Examination

Prerequisites

- Both the knees must be examined simultaneously for comparative study
- Pelvis to toes must be exposed with covered genital region
- Patient must be examined on a hard couch
- Examine the patient in walking, standing, sitting, squatting and lying down position (if possible). Observe gait from the side. Watch the attitude of the knee in full weight bearing and in the relaxed position
- While patient is sitting, attitude should be noted in as far as extended and flexed positions of the affected knee. The normal knee should be kept in identical position for comparison.

Flexion Deformity of Knee

Flexion deformity of knee occurs due to spasm and/or contracture of the hamstrings and in neglected cases, there is also contracture of posterior capsule of the knee. The deformity becomes obvious when the patient attempts to do straight leg-raising and it can be measured by 'popliteal angle' as follows:

The patient lies supine. The affected side lower limb is flexed at hip by 90° and knee is extended to point of resistance. The angle subtended between long axis of leg and distally extended long axis of thigh will be the "popliteal angle" **(Fig. 13.3A)**.

- In acute injury, the pain, muscle spasm and hemarthrosis/effusion limit flexion and full extension and in such cases complete examination is not possible. Such knees should be supported in comfortable position or put in traction for a day or two, unless vital problems like vascular or neural damage (e.g. in knee dislocation are suspected.

Attitude

While examining in lying down posture, supine position should be adopted. Back should be relaxed by resting it on the couch. Mark the attitude of the affected knee from the front and the side. Normal limb must be kept in identical position for comparison. In most of the cases with recent pathology or trauma, the joint is swollen all around, more so anteriorly, and assumes an attitude of about 30° flexion. In most of the chronic diseases, the knee goes for a peculiar deformity complex, i.e. triple deformity. Here in flexed position of the knee, the tibia subluxates posteriorly and laterally and also rotates laterally over the femoral condyle. Gradually, leg also goes in valgus. Thus, though it has been identified as *"triple subluxation deformity,"* in its full form, actually it is a *"quadruple deformity complex"*. It is common in advanced tuberculosis and rheumatoid arthritis, but even postural contractures can produce such deformity and subluxation.

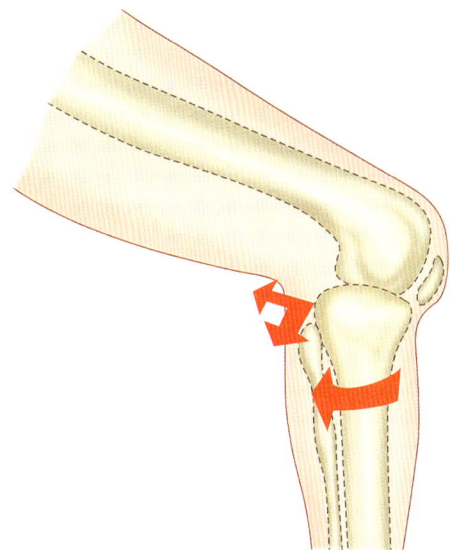

Fig. 13.4: Diagrammatic representation of the mechanism of triple deformity of the knee.

Pathodynamics of Triple Deformity of Knee (Figs. 13.4 to 13.6)

The flexed attitude of the knee joint is a protective position and position of rest. Therefore, following any painful condition there is early tendency of spasm of the hamstring group of muscles. This position allows enough of posterior space in the knee joint for collection of blood or exudates. With constant flexed attitude of varying extent, the posterior capsule starts contracting. This flexion provides further mechanical advantage to the hamstrings, specially the biceps femoris and iliotibial band which now become important flexors of the joint. While lying down, the patient tries to keep the hip in external rotation, till the outer part of the knee rests on a support or the couch. In this position, gravity-assisted contraction of the iliotibial band helps in outer subluxation of the tibiofibular component. Taking further mechanical advantage, the biceps femoris and iliotibial band further keep on contracting, the fibulotibial component, therefore, rotates laterally. These three conjoint and successive deformities are grouped together as triple deformity of the knee joint. Besides the above, deforming forces also pull the leg outwards, i.e. in valgus.

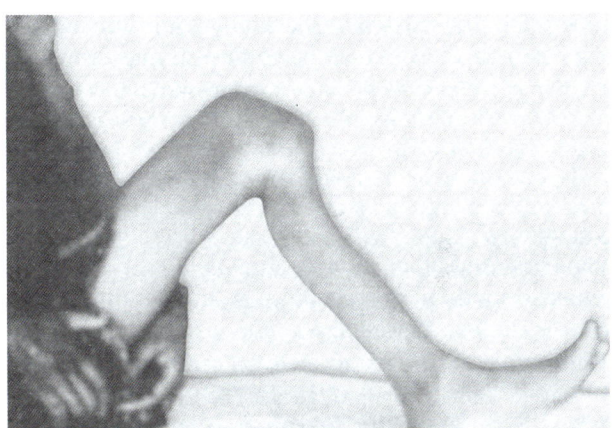

Fig. 13.5: Triple deformity of knee joint showing flexion contracture of knee, in which tibia has subluxated posteriorly and rotated laterally.

Clinical Assessment of Triple Deformity of Knee

In observing from the outer side, the flexion of knee will be obvious. Simultaneously comparing with the equally flexed normal knee, depression of the upper tibial end denotes posterior subluxation, which can be further confirmed by palpating the subluxated posterior upper end of the tibia through the popliteal fossa. In this position, the distal end of the condyles of femur are more prominent and more palpable anteriorly as compared to the other side (specially the medial one).

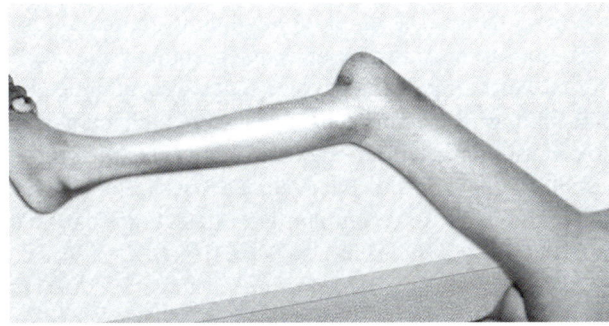

Fig. 13.6: Triple deformity of knee joint showing flexion contracture of knee, in which tibia has subluxated posteriorly and rotated laterally with genu valgum (thus quadruple deformity complex).

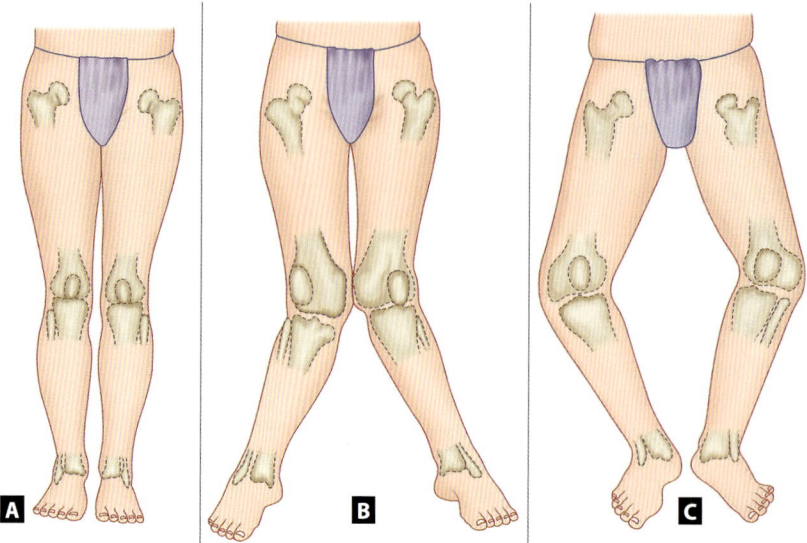

Figs. 13.7A to C: (A) Normal alignment of thigh and leg; (B) Genu valgum; (C) Genu varum.

In case of outward subluxation of the upper end of tibia, observing from the front, the tibial tubercle will be placed more outward, the tibial shin will be aligned more outwards and the fibular head will be placed more posterolaterally. Valgus of the leg can be confirmed by measuring the outward drift of the medial malleolar tip from the midline.

Genu Valgum/Varum

Observe the alignment of the leg component to the thigh component. Normally, the mid-inguinal point, centre of patella and mid-ankle joint are in one line. If this line is prolonged to the foot, it should pass through the second web **(Fig. 13.7A)**. Deviation of the leg axis (for all practical purposes from centre of the knee, i.e. centre of the patella) outwards is called valgus **(Figs. 13.7B, 13.8 to 13.17)** and inwards as varus **(Figs. 13.7C, 13.18 to 13.27)**. This must be tested in both lower limbs.

In lower extremity the angular changes of three joints (knee, ankle and subtalar) are closely related. Varus deformity of knee is variably compensated by ankle and foot. Varus deformity of knees are usually associated with valgus hindfoot alignment. On the other hand, valgus deformity of knees are associated with varus hindfoot alignment. Hence in knee joint deformity and arthritis, ankle joint is oftenly affected by arthritis. Furthermore, the subtalar joint is also influenced by ankle joint arthritis. This explains why the patients of knee joint deformity and arthritis experience and complain of more multiple pain in foot and ankle regions as well. Hence in the knee pathologies (and complaints) proper examination of hindfoot (or even whole foot) is essential.

In the first 2 years of life, some medial bowing of tibia and some genu varum should be taken as normal. It resolves by the age of 2 years. After the age of 2 years, genu valgum becomes apparent, which may even increase up to the age of 4 years.

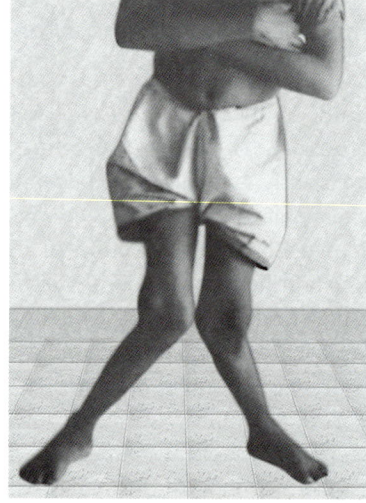

Fig. 13.8: Photograph of rachitic bilateral marked genu valgum.

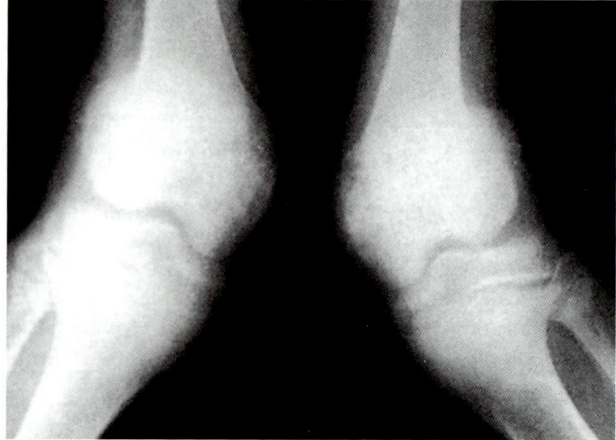

Fig. 13.9: X-ray of both knees of same patient **(Fig. 13.8)**. Such deformities can be corrected by femoral supracondylar osteotomy. Supplemental calcium and vitamin D should be given according to need.

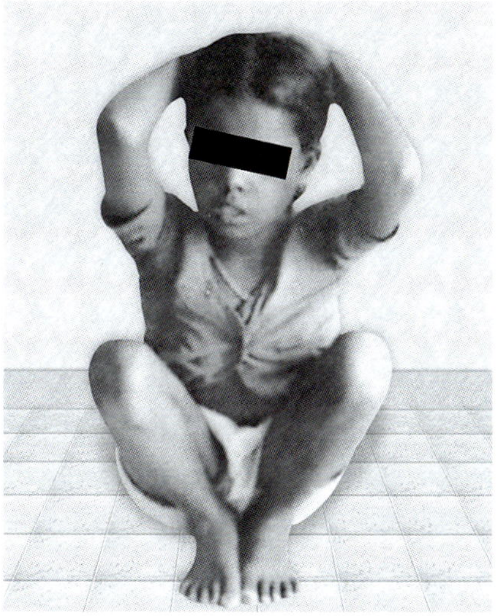

Knee

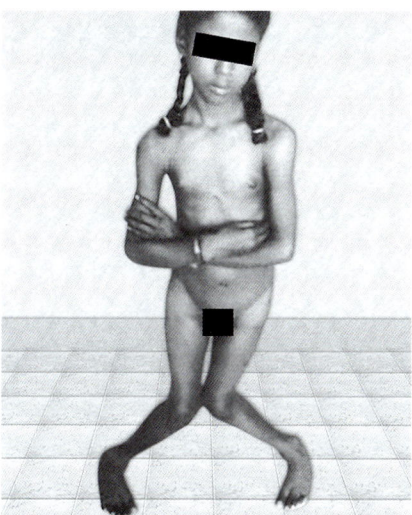

Fig. 13.10: Same patient (**Fig. 13.8**) in squatting position. Note disappearance of genu valgum which indicates the seat of deformity at the lower femur.

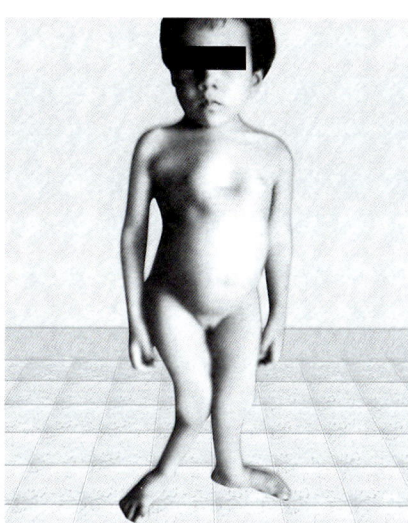

Fig. 13.12: Bilateral rachitic genu valgum, valgus collapse in ankle region and early toe-in deformities of the feet. Note the associated deformity (pectus excavatum-opposite to pectus carinatum) in the chest wall. Management should be more or less on the lines as noted under **Figure 13.11**. However, the chest wall problem will persist.

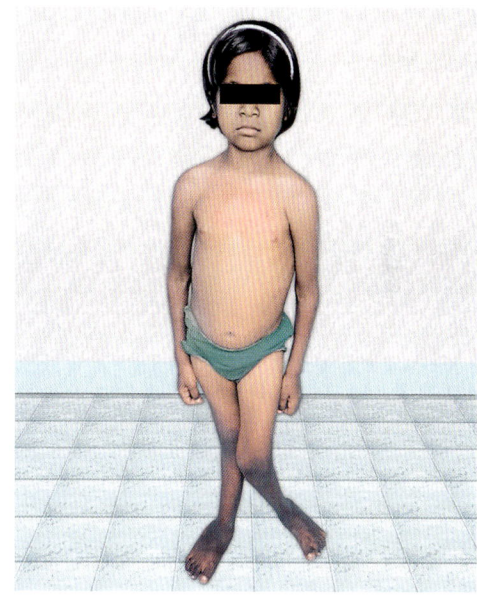

Fig. 13.11: Rachitic bilateral genu valgum (advanced) with varus and toe-in deformities of the feet (developed to catch the centre of gravity as far as possible, while standing and walking). Genu valgum can be corrected by supracondylar femoral osteotomy. The varus and toe-in deformities should get variably reduced after correction of genu valgum. For residual foot deformities, suitable ortholic should be used; however, corrective surgery may be needed for the residual deformity.

Fig. 13.13: Bilateral genu valgum in renal rickets. The girl is 16 years old without any secondary sexual character.

After that age, genu valgum improves and should come to normal of about 7° before the age of 6–8 years.

The physiological genu varum or valgum are bilateral.

An increased intercondylar distance at the knee with the feet placed together denotes bow leg deformity or genu valgum. Most of the infants are bow legged due to the combined effects of femoral torsion and tibial bowing.

Causes of genu valgum (also of **genu varum**):
- Congenital—incidence of genu valgum is less than genu varum (**Fig. 13.28**)
- Acquired:
  - Idiopathic—quite common
  - Metabolic, e.g.
    - Rachitic quite common in under-developed and developing countries.
  - Developmental disorders, e.g.
    - Dyschondroplasia, Osteogenesis imperfecta.
  - Deficiency disease, e.g. scurvy
  - Paralytic, e.g. poliomyelitis, cerebral palsy
  - Traumatic

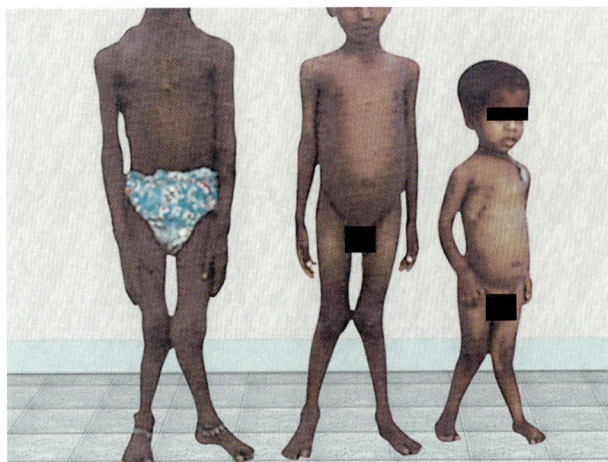

Fig. 13.14: Rachitic bilateral genu valgum in the all three children in a family [brothers (2) and sister (1)].

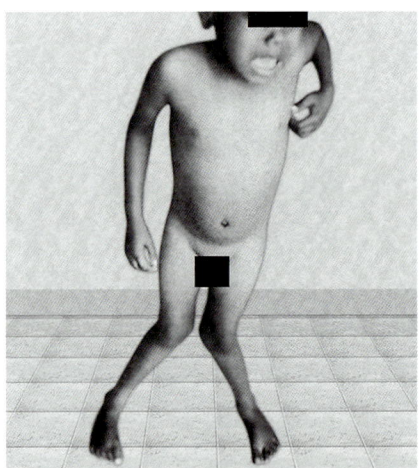

Fig. 13.16: Bilateral idiopathic genu valgum with developing of early toe-in.

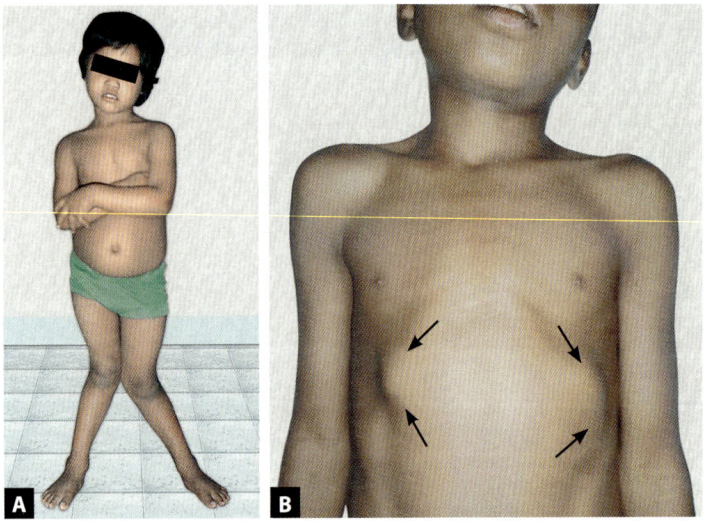

Figs. 13.15A and B: (A) Idiopathic bilateral genu valgum. (B) Harrison's sulcus. Harrison's sulcus or Harrison groove develops at the lower end of the rib cage in young children/infants with abnormally weak bones (e.g., in rickets due to defective minaralisation of bone) or chronic respiratory disease (e.g., in asthma). The lower chest is drawing, due to attachment of diaphragm, with flaring of the rib margin and rachitic rosary. The prominent knobs of bone at the costochondral joints in rickets. patients.

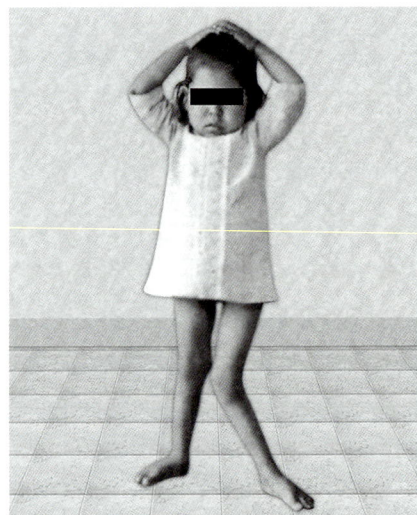

Fig. 13.17: Genu valgum on left side following chronic osteomyelitis of lower end of femur and damage of outer portion of growth epiphysis. Note also the lengthening of femur (due to osteomyelitis).

- Physeal injuries of lower femoral or upper tibial growth zones (due to damage and/or premature fusion of lateral half can produce genu valgum, while that of medial half can produce genu varum). In adults, malunion of lateral/medial condylar fracture may lead to genu valgum/varum, respectively.
- Infective
    - Acute osteomyelitis/septic arthritis may lead to over stimulation of growth plate, such as in low grade infection in juxta-epiphyseo-metaphyseal region (affection of medial half will lead to genu valgum **(Fig. 13.17)** while that of lateral half to genu varum **(Fig. 13.29)**
    - Severe infection damaging the lateral femoral/tibial growth plate and/or condyle leads to genu valgum while damage of medial growth plate and/or condyle of femur/tibia leads to genu varum
    - Chronic infection, e.g. syphilitic sequelae, Charcot's arthropathy.
- Haemorrhagic disease, e.g. in haemophilia
- Degenerative, e.g. unicompartmental or disproportionate degenerative arthritis of knee can lead to angular deformity, i.e. the more affection of medial

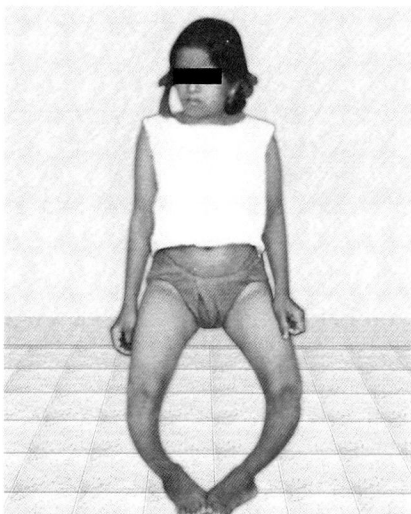

Fig. 13.18: Bilateral rachitic genu varum (bow knee).

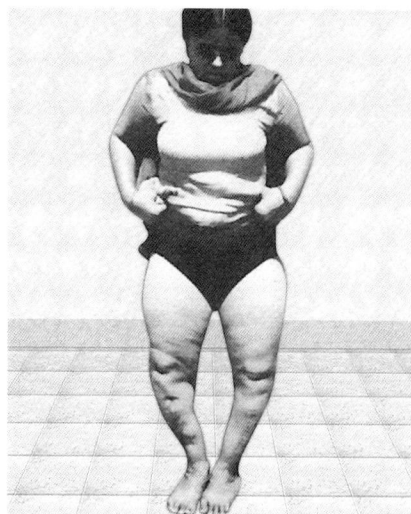

Fig. 13.20: Same patient **(Fig. 13.18)** after 14 years of surgical correction. Note the early recurrence of bowing of knees. Gaining of weight has added to recurrence of bowing. Patient did not come earlier for follow-up.

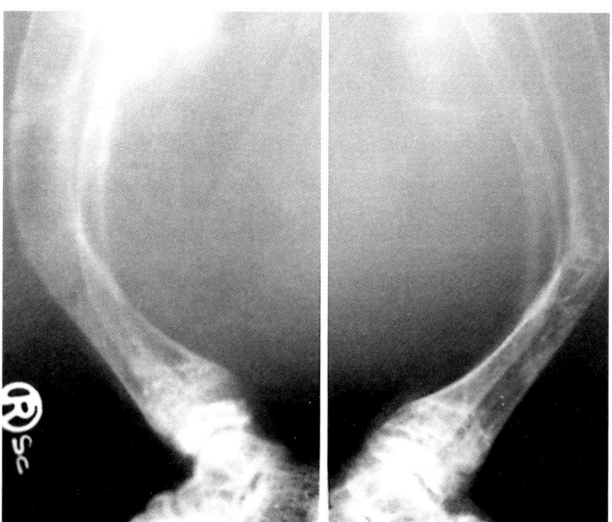

Fig. 13.19: X-ray of same patient **(Fig. 13.18)**.

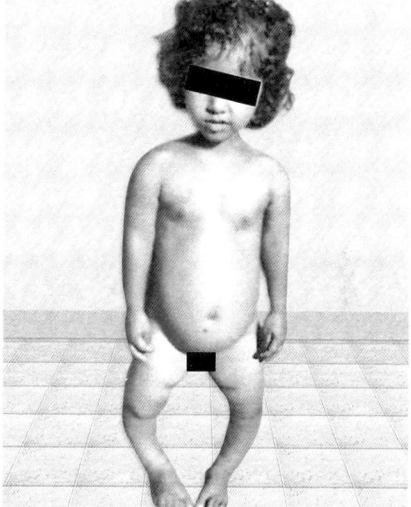

Fig. 13.21: Idiopathic bilateral genu varum.

compartment leads to genu varum and that of lateral compartment to genu valgum. However, classic osteoarthritis of knee has a varus deformity **(Fig. 13.30)**.
- Collagen diseases—Rheumatoid arthritis can produce genu valgum or varum or bizarre deformities according to the portion affected/damaged. However, classic rheumatoid knee remains in more of valgus
- Neoplastic—Deformity is according to the portion damaged.

Before assessing the genu valgum or varum, the birth history and developmental milestones should be noted including the age at which the child stood first and walked first. Check the height centile and the laterality of the deformity (bilateral or unilateral).

A normal child standing with feet together should have ankles and knees that just touch. In genu valgum (knock knee) there is increased intermalleolar distance.

Idiopathic genu valgum persisting after the age of 6 years usually do not resolve spontaneously. At this age, if the intermalleolar distance remains more than 10 cm it should be corrected either by retarding/arresting the growth by stapling across the medial side of distal femoral/or proximal tibial epiphysis until malalignment has been corrected; or corrective osteotomy at the femoral supracondylar level/ or tibial infracondylar level/or both according to the site of deformity. Since most of the valgus deformities occur due to fault in distal portion of femur, they should be corrected by performing distal femoral osteotomy. However, if the seat of

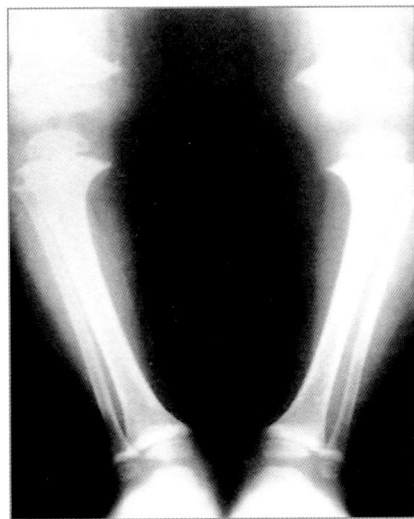

Fig. 13.22: X-ray picture of idiopathic genu varum.

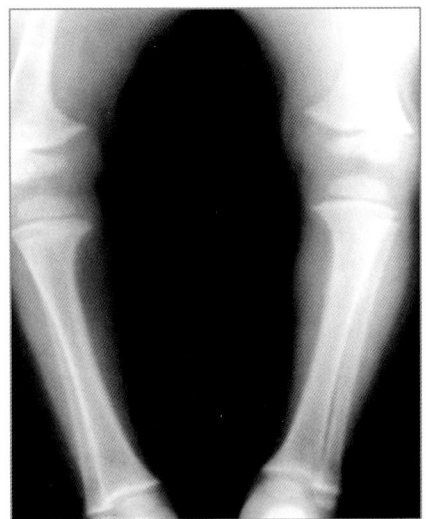

Fig. 13.24: X-ray AP view of both knees and legs of same patient (**Fig. 13.23**).

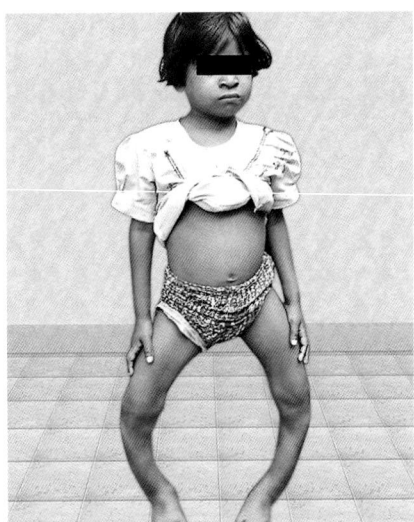

Fig. 13.23: Bilateral rachitic genu varum (bow knee + bow leg).

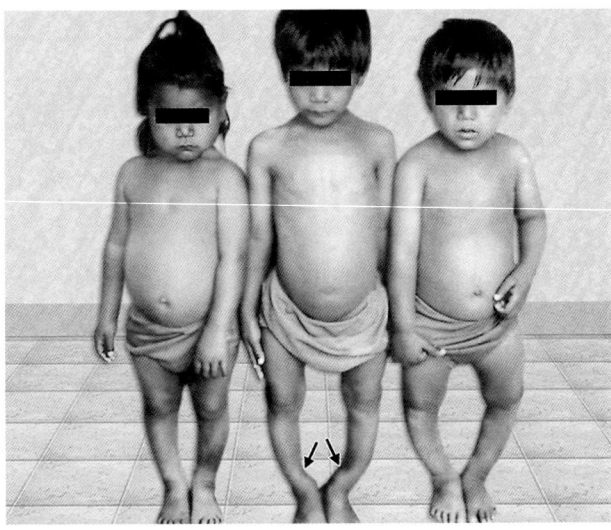

Fig. 13.25: Rachitic bow leg and bow knee in three brother and sisters (less in left one). The seat of bowing of legs in rickets is mainly in the lower third as shown by arrows in the child standing in the middle.

valgus deformity is at the proximal tibia it should be corrected by proximal tibial varus osteotomy.

How to Assess Valgum or Varum

Patient sits at the edge of the couch with both legs extended. In neutral position of the limb, hold the ankles from behind. Try to approximate both malleoli so that they just touch each other. Normally, they must touch before the inner surfaces of the knees come together, rather, there should be an average 0.5 cm gap between the medial surfaces of the two knees. If the gap is more, the deformity will be genu varum (bow knee). This is measured and expressed roughly as finger breadth (better to be measured in centimeters) between the medial surfaces of the knees. For unilateral varus, the distance between the centre of the medial surface of the affected medial condyle and central plumb line of body is measured.

If the medial surfaces of the two knees touch each other before the medial malleoli can be brought together, the deformity will be called genu valgum (knock knee). Measure the distance between the two malleoli while medial surfaces of knee just touch each other, (do not force or cross the knee). This valgum deformity is expressed by finger breadths as the intermalleolar distance, or is measured in centimeters. In unilateral valgus deformity, the deviation of the medial malleolus from central plumb line will be measured.

Genu valgum and genu varum may be due to pathology in the lower femur (mostly lead to genu valgum) and/or upper

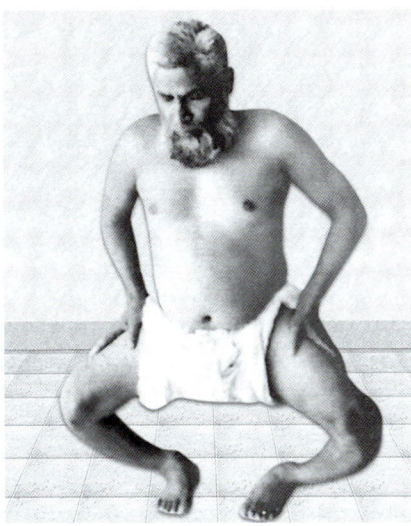

Fig. 13.26: Photograph of advanced rachitic genu varum (bow knee + bow leg) (patient is standing). Note the secondary adaptive changes at ankles and feet.

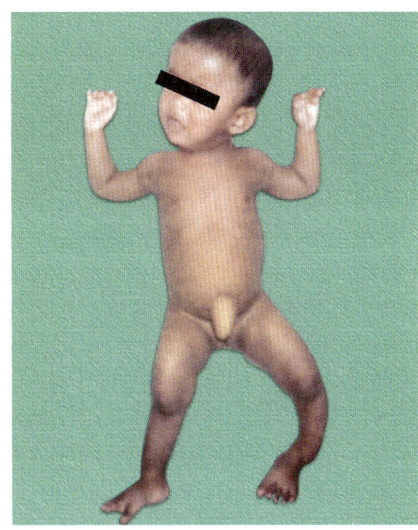

Fig. 13.28: Congenital bow knee and leg and exomphalos.

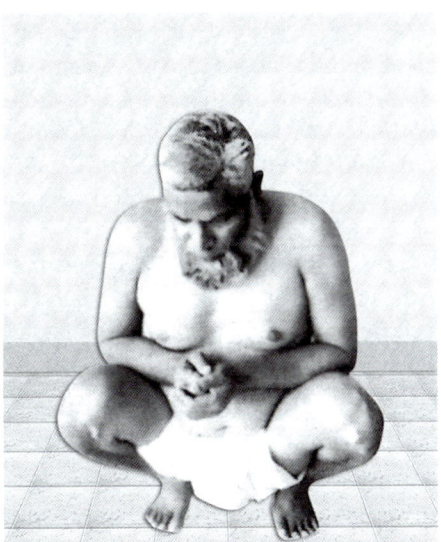

Fig. 13.27: Same patient **(Fig. 13.26)** in squatting position—genu varum apparently disappeared, indicating seat of deformity both at upper tibia and lower femur.

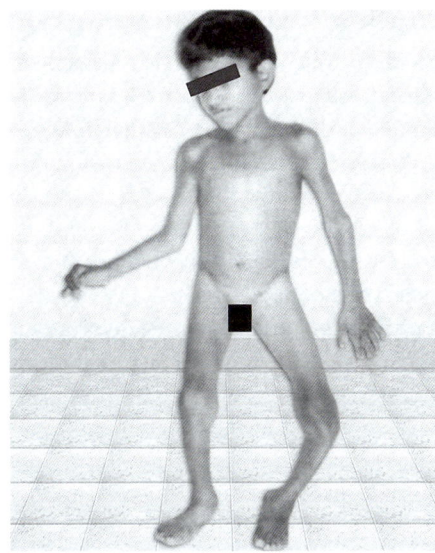

Fig. 13.29: Marked genu varum on left side following old multifocal (left knee, left shoulder and right knee) septic arthritis. There is lengthening of left femur and shortening of left leg bones both due to osteomyelitis.

tibia (usually lead to genu varum). The contribution of each of the components can be assessed, by asking the patient to sit in squatting position **(Figs. 13.8 and 13.10)**. If the deformity completely disappears, the total fault lies in the lower femur. If it disappears partially or does not disappear—the fault will be in both components.

Fallacies of Genu Varum
- Bow leg
- Anteversion of femoral neck.

Bow leg: Genu varum (bow-knee) can be confused with bow leg since the effect appears to be the same. However, genu varum is a deformity at the knee, while in bow leg, bones are at fault by producing an inwards concavity. Bow leg can be due to various causes: (i) Normally during infancy, (ii) congenital, (iii) idiopathic, (iv) traumatic—malunited fracture, (v) rachitic—bowing is at about distal third junction **(refer Figs. 2.12B and 2.25)**, (vi) syphilitic—sabre tibia **(refer Fig. 2.10)**, (vii) Paget's disease **(Fig. 2.47C)**, (viii) pseudoarthrosis of tibia **(Fig. 2.2)**, (ix) degenerative arthrosis of knee joints—varus collapse (leads to genu varum, bow knee rather than bow leg) **(Figs. 13.30 and 13.31)**, (x) osteogenesis imperfecta **(Figs. 1.18 and 1.19)**, (xi) dyschondroplasia, (xii) *Blount's disease*—infantile tibia vara

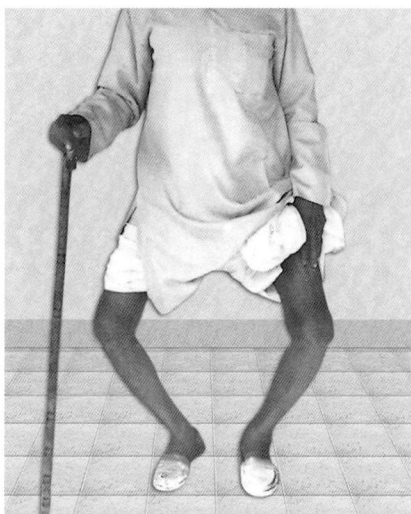

Fig. 13.30: Bow knees (due to varus collapse in osteoarthrosis of knees). It should be managed by high tibial osteotomy; if it fails – total knee replacement can be done after explaining the merits and demerits of TKR, especially in Indian patients with floor sitting culture.

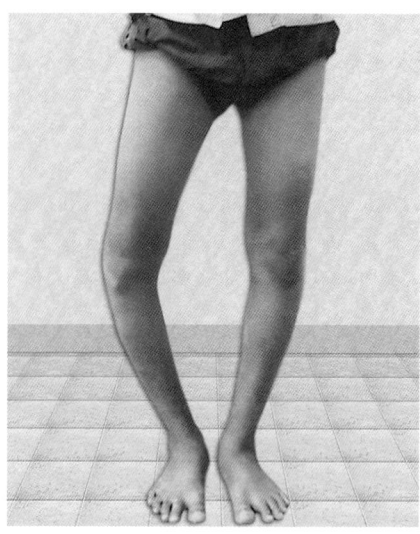

Fig. 13.31: Osteoarthritis knee with varus collapse of right knee. It is common manifestation in osteoarthritis of knee due to affection of medial compartment. It should be managed by high tibial osteotomy or unicompartmental replacement.

first described by Erlacher in 1922, is well known as Blount disease after (classic description in 1937 by WP Blount as a developmental condition of the proximal tibia involving the epiphysis, physis and metaphysis as a rare condition mostly seen in black heavy weight children who walk early. Due to irregularity of growth in the medial tibial epiphysis, there is tibia vara). Mild cases may resolve but the progressive deformity leads to a poor gait.

The natural history of the bow-leg deformity in children has not been clearly understood. The physiological bowing, which is almost always bilateral, usually resolute spontaneously. However, a small number remains in varus, which slowly progresses as pathological genu varum *(infantile tibia vara)*. Infantile form of tibia vara is bilateral and symmetrical in about 60% of affected children and is difficult to differentiate from physiological bowing. If bow-leg deformity does not resolute by the age of 4 years, corrective osteotomy should be considered.

Bow leg can be differentiated from genu varum by the following method:

Drop a plumb line from the mid-inguinal point. In genu varum, the knee lies outward to this line, whereas in bow leg this line passes through almost the centre of the knee joint.

The *'Cover up test'* (Davis et al. 2000) is a simple test to differentiate tibia vara from genu varum (which may be self-limiting and physiological) with very high rate of sensitivity (even 100%).

Method: The child lies supine with hips and knees fully extended and the patellae pointing to the ceiling. The examiner's hand is then aligned perpendicular to the long axis of thigh and placed over the middle third of tibia in such a way that the proximal 1/4th of the leg is exposed. Then the alignment of the exposed proximal segment of the leg is assessed in relation to the thigh segment. If the proximal segment of the leg is in equivocal valgus, neutral or varus alignment in relation to the thigh, the test is positive, and if the proximal segment of the leg is clearly in valgus alignment, the test is negative.

The children, with *tibia vara* have a *positive 'cover up test'*, while the children with *physiological genu varum* have *negative 'cover up test'*. The resolution of physiological bowing can be assessed by this test regularly on each follow-up.

Blount disease can be managed by proper bracing in younger children (2–5 years), however, osteotomy in proximal tibia is required in progressive deformity and in grown-ups.

Anteversion of femoral neck: Femoral anteversion may be defined as the angle of the femoral neck in relation to the femoral shaft in the coronal plane. The angle between the plane of femoral neck and femoral transcondylar plane is about 40° (10°–60°) at birth, and decreases to 10–20° at the maturity. Persistence of increased femoral anteversion leads to internal rotation of the whole leg.

Clinically, the range of internal rotation of the extended hips will be greater than the external rotation.

In the opposite deformity, i.e. femoral retroversion there will be preponderance of external rotation over the internal rotation.

Femoral retroversion usually gets corrected automatically by the age of 3 years. However, it may persist due to faulty sitting and sleeping postures.

Anteversion of femoral neck can produce the apparent effect of genu varum. While the patient lies supine, the patella is made to face upwards. If in this position genu varum disappears, it indicates anteversion of the femoral neck.

Genu recurvatum deformity: In standing position, a normal knee is straight, i.e. in zero degree vertical pendulum position. In genu recurvatum, it buckles back, i.e. popliteal fossa becomes convex (instead of it being normally concave, because the knee gets recurved in the opposite direction, which is normally not possible) **(Figs. 13.32 to 13.36 and 13.38)**. For all practical purposes, it can be measured from zero degree of extension. However, allowance must be given for the normally possible hyperextension of the knee in certain individuals (in which case the other knee will also be the same). It can be measured in the weight bearing position of the limb from the lateral side. The long axis of thigh (tip of trochanter to centre of the lateral surface of lateral femoral condyle) and the long axis of the leg (tip of head of fibula to lateral mid-point of ankle, i.e. tip of lateral malleolus) (for all practical purposes) should be more or less in same line. In genu recurvatum, the long axis of the leg will drift anteriorly and will make an angle with the thigh axis at the knee level **(Fig. 13.35)**. The superoinferior angles made at the point of cut of two axis (which will be equal) will be *angle of genu recurvatum*.

Inspection

Inspect both knees simultaneously from the front, the sides and from behind **(Fig. 13.1, *See* Page 371)**.

From the front (Fig. 13.1A): Mark the normal contour, i.e. quadriceps prominence/bulge; position, shape and size of patella; patellar ligament; supra and infrapatellar fossae; anterolateral and anteromedial tibial flares; tibial tubercle and shin of tibia. Any skin changes, swelling and sinus, if present, should be examined as in the Chapter 1: Introduction.

From the side (Fig. 13.1B): Watch for normal contour, i.e. vastus lateralis bulge, tight sloping of iliotibial band, bulge of biceps femoris, fibular neck depression and normal bulge of the leg. Any abnormal shift and/or prominence of fibular head must be noted.

From behind (Fig. 13.1C): Usually, pathology in and around the knee manifests with some degree of flexion of the knee joint. In that case, ask the patient to comfortably extend the knee joint without altering the position of the hip and spine. Mark the residual angle of flexion at the knee joint. It is better to express or measure the amount of flexion from zero position of extension. Note the contour of back of thigh, suprapopliteal slope, popliteal fossa flanked on both sides by the prominent hamstrings (biceps femoris on the outer side, accentuated by the iliotibial band; and semimembranosus and semitendinosus on the medial side accentuated by the gracilis and more anteriorly by the sartorius). In the lower part of the floor of the popliteal fossa and upper part of the leg, the gradual bulge produced by the popliteus, gastrocnemius and soleus muscles, in that order,

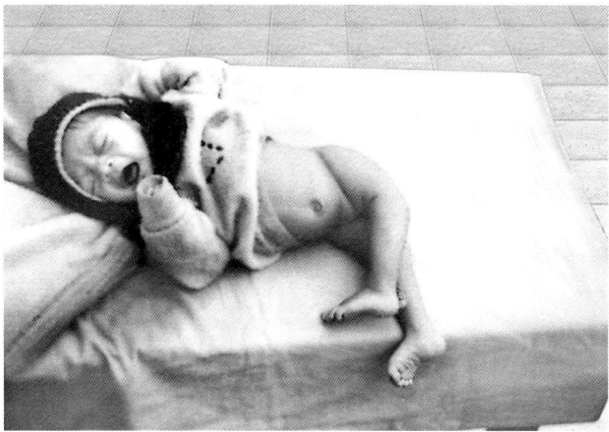

Fig. 13.32: Bilateral congenital quadriceps contracture producing genu recurvatum; congenital genu recurvatum; congenital dislocation of knee. Management of such condition is by gradual stretching – cautions padded plaster wedge correction – For the resistant deformity surgery is indicated—capsular release and quadriceps lengthening; however, in all cases serial cast correction and mini-open tenotomy and capsulotomy for the resistant problems should be tried first cases, if required.

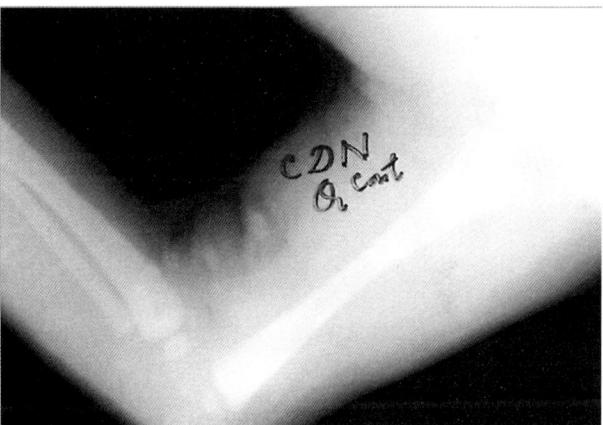

Fig. 13.33: X-ray of congenital quadriceps contracture leading to congenital dislocation of knee. Management as in **Figure 13.32**.

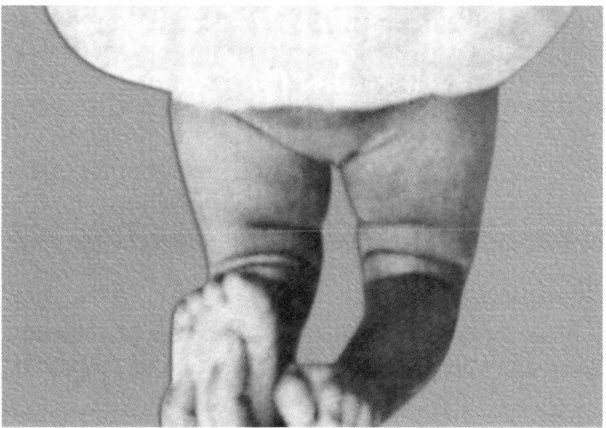

Fig. 13.34: Bilateral congenital genu recurvatum due to congenital quadriceps contracture (congenital dislocation of knee). Management as in **Figure 13.32**.

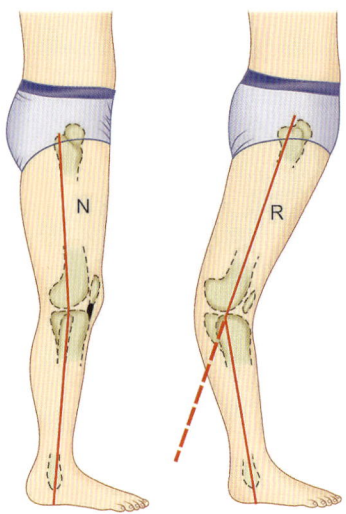

Fig. 13.35: The axis of leg and thigh are cutting much posteriorly rather than having an anterior inclination in a normal limb. N = normal, R = genu recurvatum.

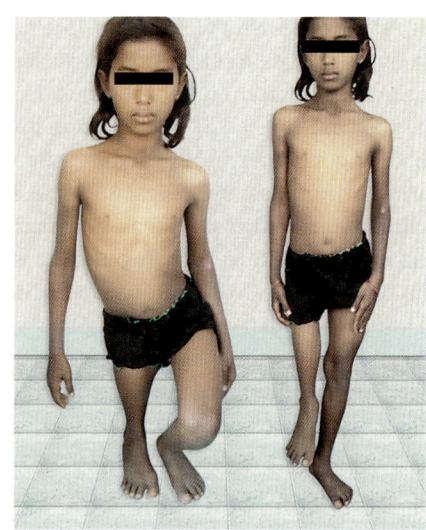

Fig. 13.37: Congenital absence of right knee producing short right lower limb, which can be lengthened by limb (equalisation) lengthening procedures (such as by Ilizarov method).

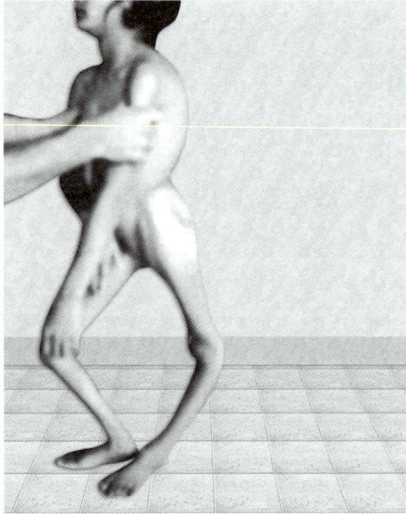

Fig. 13.36: Unilateral (left) genu recurvatum following polio-paralysis, which can be managed by suitable orthotic and surgery on soft tissues or bone or both. Even though fully functional normal knee will not be possible; however, cosmetically functional knee can be achieved to variable extent.

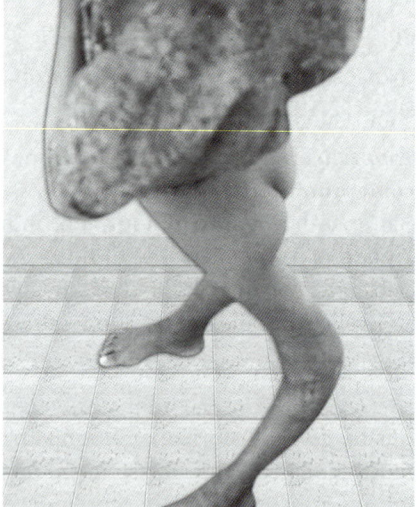

Fig. 13.38: Bilateral genu recurvatum (polio-paralysis) which can be managed by suitable orthotics and surgery on soft tissues or bones or both and cosmetically functional knees can be achieved to variable extent.

is marked. Look for any varicosity, any pulsation or any other abnormality. Any collection in the knee joint or pathology of the posterior part of knee presents with obliteration of the popliteal fossa.

Asses for any spasm and/or contracture of hamstrings and measure the popliteal angle **(Fig. 13.3A on Page 373)**.

Baker's Cyst (Also see Page 389)

Baker's cyst (a synovial pouch communicating with the knee joint usually through a flap-valve mechanism) appears as the median posterior swelling in the popliteal fossa. Semimembranosus cyst occurs on the more medial side.

Palpation

This should be done from anterior aspect, sides and back (as in inspection).

- *Superficial palpation:* Note the temperature, skin surface, sensitivity and elasticity of skin, any subcutaneous adhesions, pliability of subcutaneous layer and any superficial tenderness. If there is any swelling or sinus, these should be examined, as in Chapter 1: Introduction

- *Deep palpation*: Concentrate mainly on palpating the (1) Structures surrounding the joint, i.e. soft tissues, (2) Bony components of the joint, (3) Joint line and articular surfaces as far as possible.

Palpation of Soft Tissue

Palpate muscles, tendons, ligaments, capsule, synovial tissue, peripheral nerves and blood vessels in the vicinity.

Muscles and tendons: Note the tone, texture, pliability of *quadriceps muscle, quadriceps tendon and ligamentum patellae* up to its attachment to tibial tuberosity, and the continuity of *quadriceps apparatus.* On the two sides, palpate *vastus medialis* bulge up to adductor tubercle anteromedially, and *vastus lateralis* merging into quadriceps expansion anterolaterally. Posterolaterally, palpate the *iliotibial band*, specially from the point of view of its tightness, and behind it, the *biceps femoris* up to its attachment into the fibular head region. On the posteromedial aspect, the *semimembranosus* and *semitendinosus* should be assessed by asking the patient to flex the knee against resistance.

Palpate the *quadriceps expansion* on both sides of the patella and ligamentum patellae. Suprapatellar bulge may be due to synovial thickening and/or fluid. *Synovial thickening,* if present *(doughy or boggy or earthworms-in-a-bag feel)* may be palpated in the infrapatellar and suprapatellar fossae. Palpate on both sides to ascertain the continuity, thickening and any tenderness of the collateral ligaments. Palpate for some irregular or regular bony mass at the upper attachment of medial collateral ligament *(Pellegrini Stieda disease).* It occurs due to calcification in the avulsed femoral attachment of medial collateral ligament. Radiologically it may be thin elongated shadow due to raising of periosteum (stable type) or massive new bone formation (evolution type). Posteriorly, it is difficult to feel any synovial thickening because it lies quite deep. In the popliteal fossa, especially palpate the popliteal artery pulsation, any glandular enlargement or any cyst *(Morrant Baker's cyst). Lateral popliteal nerve* should be palpated by rolling it against the neck of the fibula and note for any tenderness, thickening or beading.

Anserine tendinopathy: In tendinopathy of the insertion of the sartorius, rectus femoris and semitendinosus muscles, possibly associated with bursitis, the patient complains of pain on the anteromedial aspect of upper leg and that region is tender.

Thumb nail test: Anterior knee pain oftenly occurs after falling on the ground on knee or after hurt against any hard object. Such trauma usually leads to irritation of subcutaneous sensory nerves (e.g. Infrapatellar branch of saphenous nerve) resulting in neuroma like pain. Striking the skin with thumb nail, elicits focal pain. Similarly, focal pain can be elicited in case of tendinitis, tendinosis of quadriceps or ligamentum patellae.

Palpation of the Joint Line

The knee joint line (both on the lateral and medial side) should be palpated for its sharpness, any tenderness, presence of any cyst (usually attached to the meniscus) or synovial thickening. Sometimes the torn part of the meniscus may be felt as a firm, tender, irregular mass. Sometimes tenderness in the medial joint line may be confusing as it can occur both in meniscal and patellar pathology. Upper tibiofibular joint should also be palpated for any capsular and/or synovial thickening and tenderness (at times tuberculosis or any of the synovial neoplasms have been seen to specifically arise in this area). The capsule of the knee joint is mostly blended with the quadriceps expansion, collateral and other enforcing ligaments, hence palpation of the above mentioned structures will amount to palpation of the capsule in that zone.

Palpation of the articular surfaces: Most of the articular surfaces are not palpable. However, the margins can be well palpated and thus can provide an idea about any existing pathology.

Bony Palpation

It should be done on both the non-articular, as well as the articular parts of the participating bones. Note for normal congruity, presence of any abnormal knob like or irregular swellings and any tenderness, starting from the patella, medial femoral condyle, medial tibial condyle, lateral femoral condyle, lateral tibial condyle, fibular head and neck and tibial tuberosity.

Patella: Extend the supported knee and ask the patient to relax the quadriceps. Now, holding the patella from one side, push it to the other side. Maintaining this position, your opposite index finger can palpate the articular surface to a variable extent. Reverse the direction of push and repeat the palpation on the other side of the articular surface **(Fig. 13.39)**.

For evaluating the *patellar tendinitis* (Jumper's knee) deep fibres of patellar tendon and inferior pole of the patella should be palpated—which are tender. This palpation is facilitated by depressing the superior pole of the patella with the thumb and index finger to elevate the inferior pole.

Assess the patellar mobility and passive patellar tilt. Reduced patellar mobility, a zero or negative passive patellar tilt or superior or inferior glide less than 2 cm confirm the diagnosis of "Infrapatellar Contracture Syndrome" (Characterised by significant loss of movement and reduced patellar mobility after operation or trauma). Try to determine whether the problem is predominantly suprapatellar or infra- and peripatellar.

Femoral condyles: Anteroinferolateral and anteroinferomedial portion of the articular surfaces of the femur can

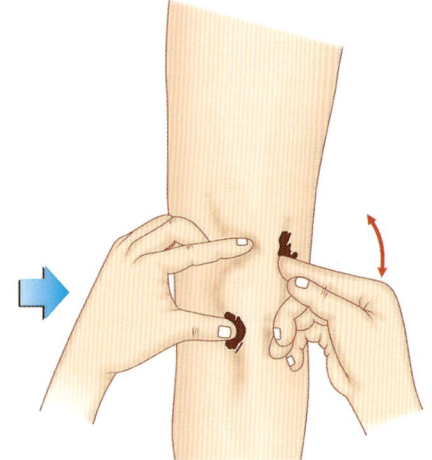

Fig. 13.39: Palpation of under surface of patella (articular surface).

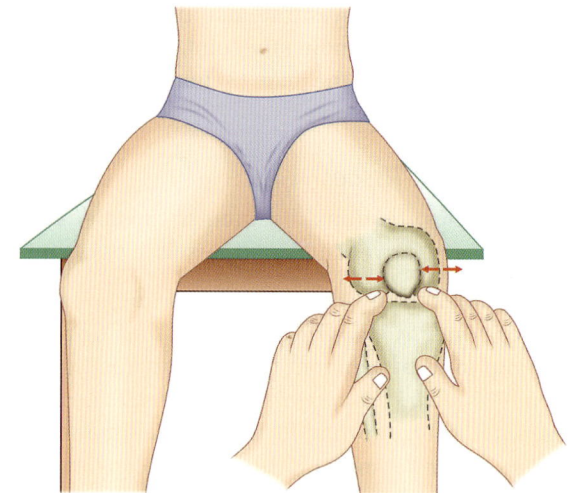

Fig. 13.41: Palpation of accessible articular surface of tibial condyles.

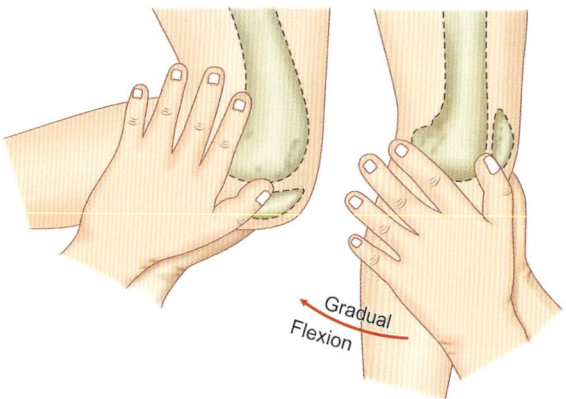

Fig. 13.40: Palpation of accessible articular surface of femoral condyles.

be palpated while gradually flexing the knee to the fullest possible extent **(Fig. 13.40)**.

Tibial condyle: Articular surfaces of the tibial condyles can usually be palpated anterolaterally and anteromedially in 90° flexed position of the knee. Insinuate the index fingers on both sides of the ligamentum patellae. With side to side rolling movements, any irregularity and tenderness of the articular surfaces can be palpated to some extent **(Fig. 13.41)**.

Ascertaining the Presence of Fluid in the Joint

Anatomically, the knee being a composite joint has many crevices and folds, which can conceal varying amounts of fluid before it is manifested. Presence of little amount of fluid manifests as obliteration of the infrapatellar fossae. Usually, fluid in the knee accumulates in the suprapatellar pouch which is lax and accommodative. Thus, if the amount of fluid is more, the suprapatellar swelling becomes tense and presents the look of a shiny, ballooned-up knee. At this stage,

or even earlier, synovial swelling must be differentiated from swelling due to fluid in the joint.

Features of Synovial Swelling

- The feel of synovial swelling is usually doughy or earth-worms-filled-in bag
- Usually, it is warm
- There can be pseudofluctuation, i.e. fluctuation in only one axis
- The edge of the synovial swelling can be palpated and rolled under the fingers
- The swelling cannot be squeezed out to another compartment of the knee joint
- Transillumination will be negative in synovial thickening.

Tests for Fluid in Joint

- *If the quantity of fluid is minimal in the joint:* The symmetry of the medial knee region is affected as compared to other side.
  To evaluate the minimal fluid (effusion) in the knee joint the **"Patellar bulge test"** is quite useful.
  Method: The patient lies supine with knee supported in 10° flexion with relaxed quadriceps muscle. The examiner with the help of his palm milks the potential effusion from the medial side of knee to the suprapatellar or lateral compartment. A reverse similar manoeuvre is then performed on the lateral side. If rapid filling of medial patellar fossa occurs, the *bulge test is positive.*
- *If quantity of fluid is small*: The infrapatellar fossae appear comparatively full. Now compress the infrapatellar fossae. The fluid will be initially displaced, but slowly refills the area after the release of pressure
- *If fluid is localized only in the suprapatellar pouch* **(Fig. 13.42)**: Extend the knee as far as practicable. Fix the patella up and posteriorly towards femur by pressing the

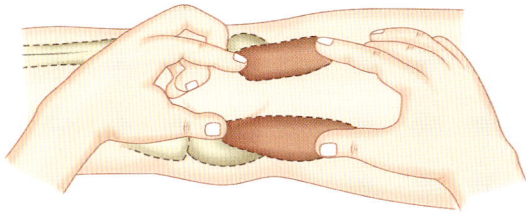

Fig. 13.42: Eliciting (testing) fluctuation in suprapatellar pouch (when fluid is less).

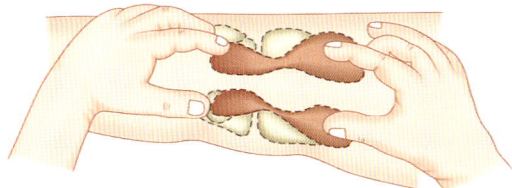

Fig. 13.43: Eliciting (testing) cross-fluctuation from suprapatellar pouch to infrapatellar fossae.

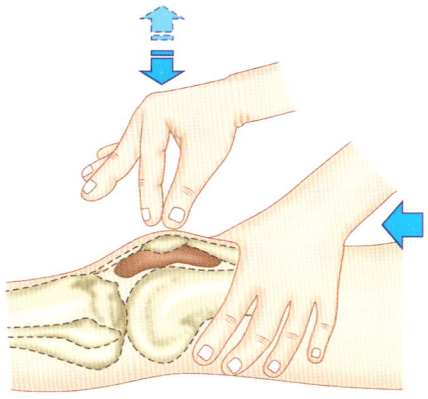

Fig. 13.44: Demonstration of patellar tap.

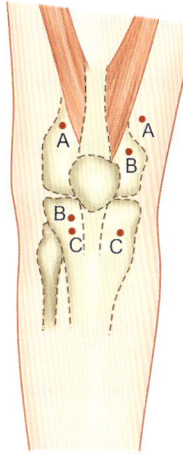

Fig. 13.45: Sites of transillumination. A to A = across suprapatellar pouch, C to C = across infrapatellar fossae, B to B = suprapatellar infrapatellar fossae.

little and ring fingers over it. Now hold the lower part of the swelling with the thumb and index finger of the same hand. Pressing with the thumb and index finger of opposite hand over superior part of swelling, elicit cross-fluctuation.
- *If fluid is moderate*: Elicit cross-fluctuation across under surface of patella **(Fig. 13.43)**, i.e. put the thumb and index finger of one hand on both sides of the ligamentum patellae at infrapatellar fossae. Pushing the fluid by the thumb and index finger of the opposite hand placed over the suprapatellar pouch region, elicit cross-fluctuation.
- *Patellar tap (patellar ballottement or floating patella)*: It cannot be elicited if there is little fluid. It further cannot be elicited if there is massive amount of fluid. It can only be elicited when there is enough of fluid, without it being in much tension. In such a condition the patella floats anteriorly.
Method **(Fig. 13.44)**: Knee should be extended. Now squeeze the suprapatellar pouch region towards the knee by the widely separated first web of the hand. Put the conjoint tips of the thumb and index finger of the opposite hand over the anterior surface of the patella. Give a gentle jerk posteriorly. The articular surface of the patella, displacing the fluid underneath, taps over the anterior articular surface of the femur and immediately comes back (rebounds) to its position thus producing the characteristic 'tap'—*patellar ballottement sign*.

Transillumination

Depending upon the clarity of fluid, transillumination can be positive to a varying extent **(Figs. 13.45 and 13.46)**.

Method: It can be done across the two sides of the suprapatellar pouch. If the fluid is much more, it can be demonstrated across the under surface of the patella, and from the suprapatellar pouch to the infrapatellar fossae. Thirdly, it can also be demonstrated across the two sides of the infrapatellar fossae. It is better to demonstrate this in a dark room. However, it can be done in an ordinary examination room too. Take a black foldable sheet or X-ray plate, and fold it in a tube form. Put its one end firmly adapted over the skin surface, illuminate from the contralateral side and visualise the glow through the upper end of the dark folded tube. This transillumination test is of much value in differentiating synovial swelling (negative) from fluid in joint (positive) and also in clinically ascertaining nature of the fluid—in serous collection the glow will be bright, whereas in haemorrhagic collection there will be no glow.

Patellofemoral joint remains at risk in osteoarthritis. When a person tries to rise from the squatting position the forces acting on the back of patella are six times the body weight. Although the articular cartilage on the back of patella is the thickest in the human being, in many patients the patellofemoral joint surface may still wear through to the bone. In this stage of the disease (Patello-femoral

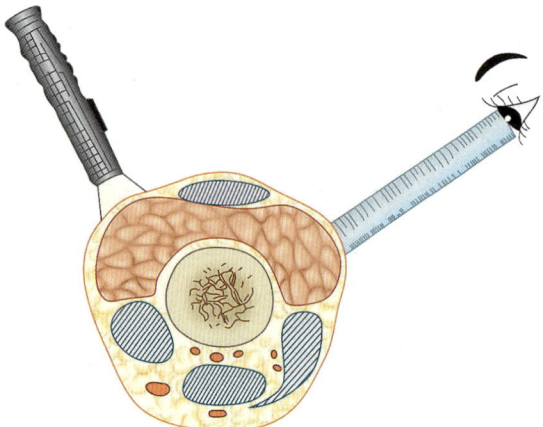

Fig. 13.46: Method of transillumination test.

osteoarthritis), the patients usually complain of pain in squatting or climbing.

Patellofemoral Compression Test

This test is useful in evaluating the damage of the retropatellar surface, such as in patellofemoral joint degeneration. While the patient's knee remains in flexion, the examiner compresses the patella against the femoral condyles. The patient is then asked to extend the knee forcefully. With contraction of quadriceps, the patella moves proximally on the femur. If the retropatellar surface is damaged, the patient will feel pain. Similarly, in *Clark's test* when the patient contracts the quadriceps muscle while the examiner holds the patella down, he/she complains of pain particularly in patellofemoral osteoarthritis.

Cystic Swellings Around Knee

Smaller localized collections can be confused with different cystic swellings, (the bursitis is most frequent) mainly the bursae around knee.

Bursae are closed synovial sacs which act like a buffer and function to reduce friction between surfaces. They lie between skin and bone, or tendon and tendon or tendon and bone. The synovium of bursae may become pathological due to trauma, infection, metabolic disease, neoplasm or occupational strains.

Bursae around knee are numerous, however, most constant ones are as follows which are of more clinical and surgical importance.
Anteriorly placed bursae are:
- *Suprapatellar bursa* is upper extension of suprapatellar synovial pouch and lies between the qadriceps tendon and femur. Although it functions like bursa, it is not a bursa in true sense
- *Prepatellar bursa* lies between skin and lower part of patella. It is also called *Housemaid's knee*—a swelling of knee caused especially by too much kneeling on the floor, e.g. by a housemaid for cleaning and soabing the floor. In prepatellar bursitis, the swelling tends to be localised anteriorly over the patella and pain increases in flexing the knee **(Figs. 13.47A and B)**
- *Superficial infrapatellar bursa* is small and lies between skin and patellar tendon. Its bursitis (disease) affects people with continual mechanical strain and monotone movements of patella. Repeated long-lasting stress leads to inflammation with thickening of the bursal wall and ultimately ending in calcification. It can be prevented by avoiding unnecessary kneeling and/or using padding to cushion the knees
- *Deep infrapatellar bursa (Clergyman's knee)* lies in between the ligamentum patellae and anterior surface of tibia. Clergyman (Christian priest) is more likely to develop swelling (and even inflammation) in his bursa due to frequent and prolonged sitting in kneel-down position **(Fig. 13.47C)**.

Laterally
- *Biceps bursa*—lies between biceps tendon and fibular collateral ligament
- *Posterolaterally lie two bursae:* (1) between popliteus tendon and lateral condyle of femur, (2) between popliteus tendon and fibular collateral ligament
- One bursa lies between lateral head of gastrocnemius and the capsule of knee joint
- Cyst of the lateral meniscus—It is a congenital cyst that usually presents posterior to lateral collateral ligament as transverse fluctuant swelling. Flexing the knee accentuates the swelling. Patient may complain of pain in the cyst region.

Medially
- The *pes anserine (goose foot)* or *bursa anserinus* lies superficially on the medial side of the knee between the aponeurosis of the hamstrings insertion and the medial collateral ligament, approximately 4–5 cm below the anteromedial joint line. Patients complain of pain, worse with activity on anteromedial aspect of knee. This bursitis is a common cause of medial knee pain and is frequently mistaken for the osteoarthritis of knee. It is frequently seen in patients with multiple osteochondromatosis
- A bursa lies between medial head of gastrocnemius and the tendon of semimembranosus
- A bursa lies beneath the tendon of semimembranosus
- Bursa/bursae are located beneath the tibial collateral ligament in relation to meniscus and capsule
- *Cyst of medial meniscus* may be mistaken as bursa. It is a developmental anomaly of the medial meniscus. It is felt along the medial joint line as oval or transversely elongated fluctuant cystic swelling either anterior or posterior to the medial collateral ligament. It becomes prominent on flexing the knee joint. Patient usually complains of dull pain, on prolonged standing, in the cyst region
- Besides these, there may be several unimportant bursae, which are not of much clinical importance.

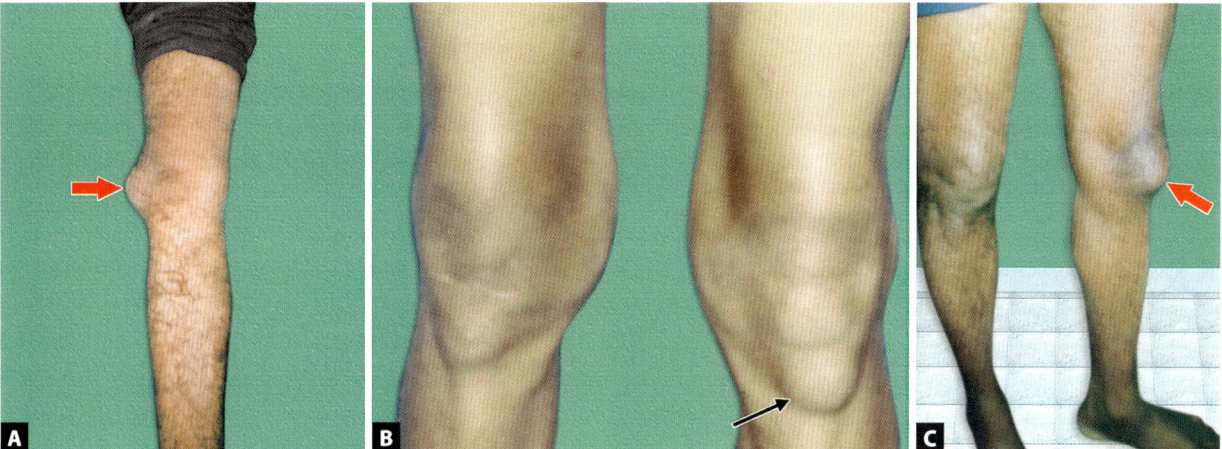

Figs. 13.47A to C: (A) Prepatellar bursitis (housemaid's knee); (B) Non-inflamed infrapatellar bursa in left knee; (C) Infrapatellar bursitis (inflamed) alongwith mild effusion in left suprapatellar pouch **(Clergyman's knee)**. Bursal swelling should be aspirated; aspirated matter should be put to culture. Inflamed bursae should be treated by suitable antibiotic and rest in knee support. Recurrence of bursitis is not uncommon. Recurred bursitis should be excised.

Posteriorly
1. *Morrant Baker's cyst:* In the year 1877, Baker described it in association with tuberculosis. It is a distended bursa in the popliteal fossa. It is a midline synovial herniation (not confirmed), which usually presents as an oval, fluctuant swelling in the intermuscular to subcutaneous planes in the popliteal fossa as popliteal cyst. It is also supposed to be a distension of popliteal bursa—most commonly the gastrocnemio-semimembranosus bursa. Commonly the bursa between the semimembranosus tendon and the medial head of gastrocnemius gives rise to the Baker cyst. It communicates with the joint through an opening in the posteromedial aspect of the joint capsule with a transverse valvular slit-like opening surrounded by capsular folds. This slit allows only unidirectional flow, i.e., from the joint into the cyst. It affects all ages The incidence is higher in children, in whom most of the cysts are asymptomatic. The cysts in the adults are mostly symptomatic with underlying intraarticular pathologies like meniscal tears (common), osteoarthritis, chondral lesions, cruciate ligament tears, chronic inflammatory conditions, rheumatoid arthritis etc., Basically, the cyst appears as a pressure diverticulum of the synovial sac protruding through the posterior joint capsule of the knee. The patient may complain of dull pain. The cyst is best seen in the popliteal fossa when the patient stands. The swelling may be translucent. Large cyst may compress the popliteal vessels. If the popliteal artery is compressed, forced extension of knee or forceful dorsiflexion of foot may obliterate the pulsation in the foot. Treating the symptomatic baker cyst by excision alone is more likely to recur. Arthroscopic management has advantage of simultaneous dealing with the intraarticular pathologies besides minimum soft tissue damage and operative scar.

- *Semimembranosus bursa* (most common)—lies posteromedially between the medial head of gastrocnemius and the musculotendinous mass of the semimembranosus
- *Popliteal aneurysm* can also be confused as a cystic swelling, however it pulsates. Haemangioma may be confused with cystic swelling. It presents as a painful tender, warm soft vascular swelling. Usually on X-ray multiple calcified spots area detected.

■ MOVEMENTS (TABLE 13.2)

Before ascertaining the movement, the power of the following muscles should be tested individually and graded according to MRC scale: quadriceps, biceps femoris, semitendinosus, semimembranosus, iliotibial tract, gastrocnemius, gracilis and sartorius.

Normal Range

From zero position of full extension of the knee, flexion is possible till the upper part of back of the leg touches the lower part of the back of thigh (varies according to musculature and fat; average 120°–130°, however, the normal range of movement can be accepted from 10° of hyperextension to 140° of flexion). With the knee in about 90° flexion, some amount of adduction and abduction as well as lateral and medial rotation (medial more than lateral) elements can also be demonstrated passively in a normal limb. Even in normal flexion 8–12° of rotational movements can occur throughout the entire arc. However, they are not important.

Note for any *"arthrofibrosis" (milder form of joint stiffness in knee* manifested by any symptomatic loss of extension or flexion of knee compared with the opposite normal knee, especially loss of knee extension of more than 10° and knee flexion less than 125°).

TABLE 13.2: Normal knee movements.

Movement	Range of movement	Axis of movement	Prime movers	Nerve supply	Accessory muscles	Limiting factors
1. Flexion	0° to 120°-130° (may be 10° hyper-extension to 140° of flexion)	The axis, around which the movement occurs, is not fixed, but shifts upward and forward during extension of the leg on the thigh, and backward and downward during flexion	• Biceps femoris • Semitendinosus • Semimembranosus	L4, 5, S1,2,3 -do- -do-	Popliteus Sartorius Gracilis Gastrocnemius	• Tension of extensors of knee • Contact of upper calf with posterior part of lower thigh
2. Extension	From full flexion to 0°, i.e. 120°-130° to 0°	The flexion and extension are not as those of a true hinge joint	Quadriceps femoris	L2, 3, 4	Some assistance from tensor fascia latae	• Tension of oblique popliteal, cruciate and collateral ligaments of knee • Tension of flexors of knee
3. Medial rotation of flexed leg	Few degrees		Popliteus Semimembranosus Semitendinosus	L4, 5, S1,2,3 L4, 5, S1,2,3	Sartorius Gracilis	• Position of knee and type of rotation reverses in flexion and extension depending upon whether the foot is on the ground or off the ground • Tightness of the opposite group of muscles
4. Lateral rotation of the flexed leg	Few degrees					
5. Accessory movement	• A wider range of rotations and anteroposterior gliding in semi-flexed position—by passive movement • Limited abduction and adduction in slightly flexed knee • Distraction of tibia on femur on strong traction • Locking of knee in full extension by popliteus					

STIFFNESS IN KNEE: Patient complains of stiffness of knee usually after any injury or after any inflammatory or infective lesion. Post operative stiffness is also common. Congenital contracture of quadriceps is also common.

Management mainly consists of physiotherapy.

Residual stiffness requires surgical management like arthrolysis, tendon surgery. Quadriceps tightness is managed by quadricepsplasty like Thompson`s quadricepsplasty (which may have problems like extension lag and wound dehiscens). Modified Judet`s quadricepsplasty with stepwise release appears to be better procedure with lesser complications.

The cause of Quadriceps contracture may be congenital or acquired. Congenital causes are arthrogryposis multiplex congenita, congenital genu recurvatum, spina bifida

Acquired causes are – prolonged plaster immobilization, repeated intramuscular injections in quadriceps. Gunn (1964) was first to establish direct association between repeated intramuscular injections into quadriceps and its fibrosis contracture. Adhesion of quadriceps to bone following fractures especially open fractures, uncared (for mobilising) post operative adhesion, adhesions in chronic osteomyelitis, improper care of quadriceps injury leading to adhesion to femur.

Limitation of flexion at knee can be due to *quadriceps tightness* (e.g. after above-knee plaster cast, reduction of neglected overridden femoral shaft fracture, etc.); *quadriceps contracture* (e.g. congenital contracture, which may be so much contracted as to produce recurvatum); *quadriceps adhesion* (e.g. after surgery in anterior thigh region, chronic osteomyelitis of femur).

Quadriceps tightness may lead to patellar malalignment. Quadriceps tightness can be assessed by placing the patient prone on the table and passively bringing the heels towards the buttocks. Normally, the heels should touch the buttocks. If the quadriceps will be tight, the springing resistance will be felt and the distance of the resisted heel from the buttock will be in the direct proportion of the contracture.

Start from zero position of knee, i.e. fully extended knee. If the patient cannot extend and you also cannot make him extend to zero position, this indicates a *"fixed flexion deformity"*. If the patient cannot extend beyond a certain range but you can help him to achieve zero degree position, this indicates *"quadriceps lag"*. Fixed flexion deformity is to be measured from zero degree position to the position of the leg from where it cannot be extended. Beyond the position of fixed flexion deformity, ask the patient to flex the knee as far as practicable by himself. This will be *"active free flexion"*.

Beyond this, assist further possible flexion by holding the lower part of the patient's leg. The range of motion gained by this method will be that of *"passive free flexion"*. If the leg still has not flexed up to full range, the deficit will be the *"limitation of terminal flexion"*.

If the joint is not ankylosed, description of the movement should be recorded under following headings:
- *Quadriceps lag*—if any (or extension lag)
- *Fixed flexion deformity*
- *Free active flexion*
- *Free passive flexion*
- *Range of utility or activity* (free active flexion)
- *Range of possibility* (= free active flexion + free passive flexion). This should be modified accordingly if there is fixed flexion deformity
- *Limitation of terminal flexion*—i.e. from end of free passive flexion to full flexion (as in normal knee)
- *Critical arc*—The range of 0°–90° at the knee is the most useful range. If the patient has got this range of useful motion, one should be very cautious in performing any surgery, at least for improving on the range. *0°–30° motion at the knee is critical arc* required for walking
- *Abnormal movements* (in lateral and anteroposterior plane): it can be elicited in the presence of: (i) repeated collection of fluid in the joint; (ii) lax ligaments (congenital or acquired); (iii) neuropathic changes, e.g. Charcot's arthropathy **(Figs. 13.48B and 13.49)**
- *Charcot neuroarthropathy* is a progressive and destructive inflammatory process with typical findings of regional osteopenia, osseous destruction, extra-osseous debris, periarticular fracturing and/or joint disruption. Diabetes is the most common cause of peripheral neuropathy, and thus charcot neuroarthropathy. The bony breakdown can be subdivided into three subtypes: fracture pattern, dislocation pattern, and combined fracture-dislocation pattern (Cates et al. 2022).

Absence of proprioceptive sensation and/or pain in a joint leads to less or loss of integrity of joint. Repeated injuries produce successive three stages of articular damage—swelling, joint degeneration, and new bone formation. In initial stage, erythema and swelling are the only findings. The disease progresses manifesting hypermobility, traumatic osteophyte formation and subluxation leading to painless deformities, crepitus on movements and instability. Clinical conditions leading to Charcot arthropathy are tabes dorsalis (mostly in knee, hip, ankle), diabetes mellitus (mid foot joints), syringomyelia (upper limb joints) and leprosy. *The triad of swelling, instability and absence of pain are mostly suggestive of Charcot joint.* The affected joints become boggy, swollen, non-tender, with painless excessive movements in abnormal direction. Charcot described this condition in 1868 affecting the knees of tabes dorsalis patients with bizarre destruction, instability and indolent swelling of the joint

- *Abnormal sounds during movement*—While the knee is being moved, actively or passively, place your hand over the knee and try to feel and hear any abnormal sound.

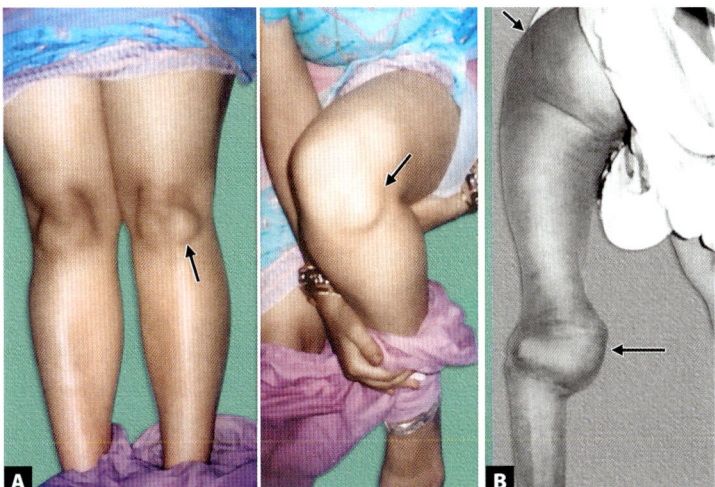

Figs. 13.48A and B: (A) Cyst of lateral meniscus cysts of lateral meniscus should be aspirated with or without corticoid infiltration (injection). Recurred such cysts may be excised out; (B) **Charcot's arthropathy of ipsilateral knee and hip.** Charcot (1892) considered two forms of tabetic arthropathy – benign form which completely disappears; malignant form which proceeds to complete disorganization of joint; (B) Charcot's disease of joint (tabetic arthropathy a neuropathic joint), though has been regarded exclusively of syphilitic origin (more in females), however, it frequently occurs in cases of tabes dorsalis, syringomyelia and even non-specific conditions like prolonged steroid therapy, rheumatoid arthritis, chronic liver disease etc. There is rapid destruction of articular cartilage, under lying bone, intraarticular ligaments. The joint becomes insensitive and gets progressively disorganised. The knee joint is often affected. It should be managed by excision arthrodesis. The failure rate of fusion is common. Proper bracing of joint can help in improving stability of joint.

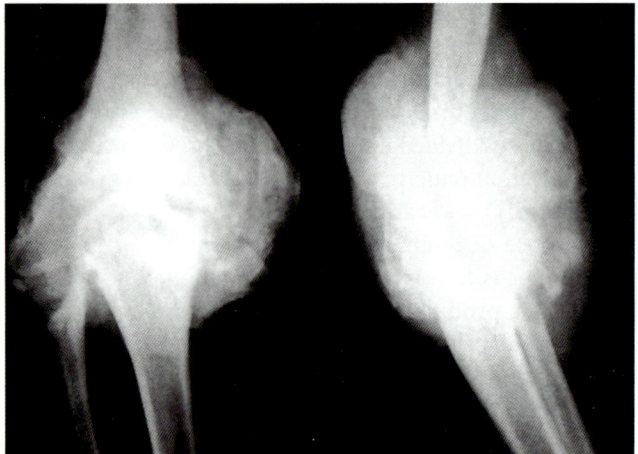

Fig. 13.49: X-ray picture of Charcot's arthropathy of knee of **Figure. 13.48B**.

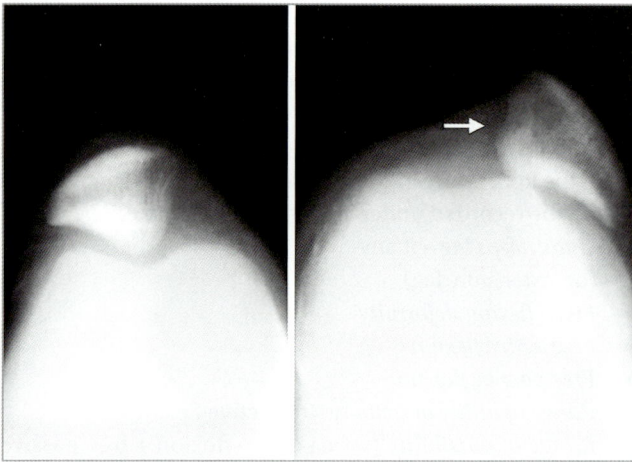

Fig. 13.51: Radiograph showing habitual dislocation left patella.

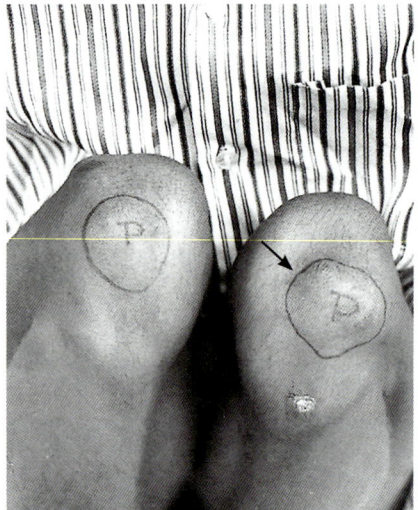

Fig. 13.50: Habitual dislocation left patella.

- *Fine crepitations* in a young girl suggests chondromalacia patellae; Coarse crepitations occur in degenerative arthrosis and neuropathic joint; while a click denotes meniscal tear or cyst
- A *thud* especially on anterolateral aspect indicates discoid lateral meniscus. *Discoid meniscus*—an anatomic variation—is usually seen in lateral compartment remaining either asymptomatic or producing mechanical symptoms. Its exact cause is not known. Probably, it is due to failure of an embryological sequence of degeneration of the centre of meniscus
- If with flexion-extension of the knee, a snap is felt while the patella slips out laterally and then relocates back, it denotes *habitual dislocation* (**Figs. 13.50 and 13.51**).

Patients who walk with flexed knees develop a cephalad displacement of the patella (patella alta). In older patients this may lead to degenerative changes in articular cartilage.

MEASUREMENTS

- Linear measurement (*see* **Fig. 13.37**)
- Circumferential measurement.

Linear Measurement

To ascertain the limb length disparity, linear measurement should be done in the same way as in hip examination, i.e. apparent length measurement and true length measurements (total and segmental lengths).

Circumferential Measurement

It is done—(i) to ascertain any shrinkage or swelling at knee level, (ii) to ascertain wasting and swelling of thigh and leg at their mid levels.

Measurement of genu valgum and genu varum: As described earlier in this chapter (Page 376).

ASSESSMENT OF INTEGRITY OF THE QUADRICEPS APPARATUS

The *quadriceps apparatus* is most important for controlling the knee. It consists of—(i) quadriceps muscles, (ii) quadriceps tendon, (iii) patella, (iv) medial and lateral quadriceps expansions (retinaculum), (v) patellofemoral and patellotibial ligaments, (vi) ligamentum patellae, and (vii) tibial tuberosity. *Biomechanically the resulting forces traversing the quadriceps tendon, patella and ligamentum patellae usually exceed five times of body weight.*

Any of these parts are likely to be affected due to direct or indirect violence (**Fig. 13.52**). Quadriceps muscle tear and avulsion of the patella are well known injuries in athletes. In fracture patella, perhaps the consideration of tear of the quadriceps apparatus as a whole, is much more important than the fracture of patella itself, specially from the treatment and functional recovery point of view.

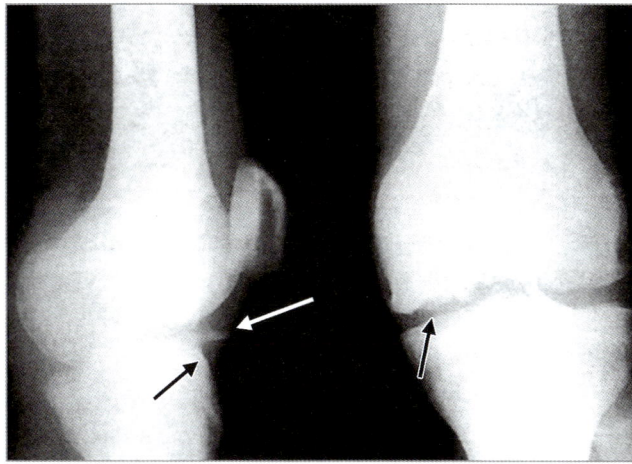

Fig. 13.58: Osteochondritis dissecans. Note (in the lateral view) the anterior ejection of separated dissecans portion.

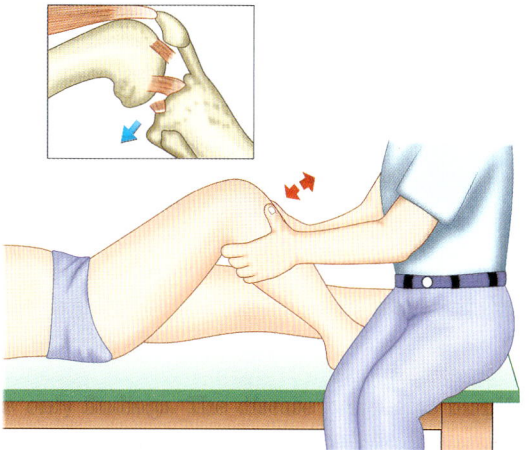

Fig. 13.59: Drawer test.

the patient's planted foot. Pass your hands behind the knee to confirm the relaxation of hamstring muscles. Then also confirm that upper end of tibia is not sagging posteriorly due to laxity of posterior cruciate ligament (which if present will give a false anterior drawer sign positivity). Then hold the upper end of the leg firmly with both hands and glide it both backwards *(posterior drawer)* and forwards *(anterior drawer)* over femoral condyles. It will glide more posteriorly as compared to normal if posterior cruciate is torn or lax. If the drawer sign is inconclusive, and the medial side of the joint opens up more with valgus stress applied on the extended knee, it strongly suggests *posterior cruciate tear*. Sometimes it is difficult to assess if the upper end of tibia is abnormally gliding too much anteriorly or too much posteriorly. However, the following test may help in such situation. Both knees are placed in the position for testing for posterior drawer test and examiner's each thumb is placed at anteromedial joint line on either side. Normally, there should be 1 cm anterior step-off of the medial tibial plateau in relation to medial femoral condyle. Loss of this step off indicates a torn posterior cruciate ligament.

Quadriceps Active Test (After Miller 111 and Azar in Campbell's Operative Orthopaedic, vol-3. 12th. ed pp 2088). In 90° bent knee with adequately supported thigh and relaxed lower limb the patellar ligament moves little posteriorly. The attempt of contraction of quadriceps in such situation does not lead to any anterior shift of upper end of tibia. But in case of posterior cruciate tear, the upper end of tibia sags posteriorly leading to the patellar ligament directed anteriorly. Then attempt of contraction of quadriceps muscle results in anterior shift of upper end of tibia by 2 mm or more.

If the medial side of the joint opens up markedly (across both medial and lateral compartments of the knee) in both extension and flexion, it indicates *tear of both cruciates* (after Muller, W 1983).

The ***anterior drawer test*** should be done in three positions of rotation. First in neutral rotation, then in 30 degrees of external rotation, and lastly in 30 degrees of internal rotation (but, in this position, the posterior cruciate becomes tight enough to affect the otherwise positive anterior drawer test result). The amount of gliding of upper end of tibia should be noted in each position of rotation and compared with the normal knee.

If gliding anteriorly of tibia is 6–8 mm more than normal side, it indicates torn anterior cruciate ligament.

Slocum test: This test is done to assess the integrity of the posteromedial corner of anterior cruciate ligament. In this test, anterior drawer test is done in external rotation and is compared with the same test done with foot in neutral position. The displacement should decrease when the test is done with the knee in external rotation; however, where it does not decrease it indicates (variable) injury of the posteromedial corner of anterior cruciate ligament. (After Miller MD, Dempsey IJ – 2021).

■ KNEE INSTABILITY

In the acute stage, patient is usually in agony. Thus, it would perhaps not be proper to subject that knee to various clinical tests only to satisfy the academic needs. However, wherever possible (acute patients may be put under general anaesthesia for performing the tests), the individual tests must be done for assessing integrity of the various structures.

Traumatic disruption of knee ligaments often lead to complex multiplane instabilities. Their proper understanding and restoration of normal mechanics of knee are of paramount importance especially in sports medicine. Depending upon the direction of displacement of tibia in relation to femur, the knee instability has been simply considered as medial, lateral, anterior, posterior and rotary, however, complex multiplane instabilities have not been considered in this. Considering the need of proper restoration of the stability of knee, especially in Sports Medicine, the committee on Research and Education of American Orthopaedic Society for Sports Medicine has suggested a classification of Knee

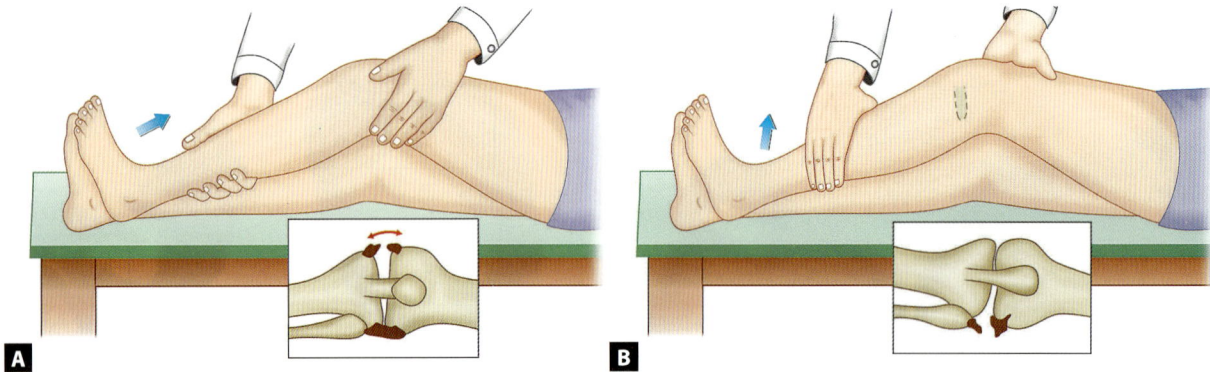

Figs. 13.60A and B: Stress test for collateral ligaments: A = for medial collateral, B = for lateral collateral.

Joint Instability resulting from ligament injury considering the direction of tibial displacement and when possible, structural deficits. Classification has been in three major groups (with subgroupings): One-plane instability (simple or straight), Rotary instability, and Combined instability.

Test for Integrity of the Collateral Ligaments

Flex the knee to about 30° (to make the collaterals maximally tense) and apply valgus stress by holding the lower part of leg. If the inner side of the joint opens more as compared to the normal side, it indicates *medial collateral ligament tear*, which can be felt as well. Reverse the hands and stress for testing the *lateral collateral ligament integrity*, which is comparatively less frequently torn as compared to the medial collateral ligament **(Figs. 13.60A and B)**. However, comparatively more opening of the joint on varus stress, applied both in flexion and extension, indicates disruption of lateral stabilising structures as well as insufficiency of posterior cruciate ligament (Hughston 1969).

Tests for Anterior Cruciate Integrity (Fig. 13.61)

Anterior cruciate tear occurs due to high impact injury where the tibia is driven anterior in relation to the femur.

In acutely painful knee, it will be very difficult and sometimes even not possible to perform anterior drawer test in 90° flexed position of knee (as is done in standard way). In such situation, some degree of anterior gliding of tibia on the femur may be detected well in comparatively extended position of knee when the "doorstop" effect of posterior horn of menisci is neutralised (Miller and Azar in Campbell's Operative Orthopaedics 12th ed. 2013, p.2087).

Lachman test is perhaps the most sensitive test to elicit anterior cruciate disruption. Flex the knee by 10°, keeping the lower thigh fixed with one hand. Hold the upper end of the leg by other hand and try to glide the tibia over the femur anteriorly. The tibia will sublux anteriorly with a tendency to rotate internally *(Lachman's sign)*. Increasing the flexion to 30°, the tibia will be autolocated back *(jerk test)*, indicating integrity of the medial collateral ligament. Thus, it signifies

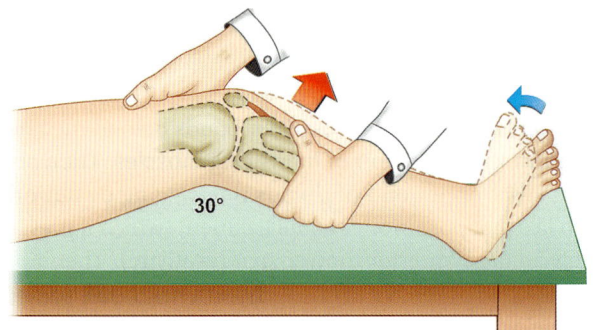

Fig. 13.61: Testing for anterior cruciate integrity—Lachman test.

isolated *anterior cruciate avulsion, laxity or tear*. If tibia can be subluxed anteriorly without any tendency of rotation, when the knee is flexed more than 30° (up to 90°), it indicates *inadequacy of the anterior cruciate, along with the tear of the medial collateral ligament.*

Anterior drawer sign cannot be a conclusive test for isolated anterior cruciate tear. In 90° bent position of knee, anterior gliding of upper end of tibia by 5 mm can be possible in a normal knee. If it is 6–8 mm greater than the opposite normal knee, then it indicates anterior cruciate tear, along with medial collateral ligament tear or laxity.

Sometimes there may be discrepancy between the Lachman test and anterior drawer test. This has been explained by the differential injury of the anteromedial and posterolateral bundles of the anterior cruciate ligament.

Broadly, Lachman test is an anterior drawer test with the knee in 30° of flexion. It tests anterior cruciate ligament integrity, with an emphasis on the posterolateral bundle. However, Lachman test is more specific than the anterior drawer test.

A negative Lachman test indicates an intact posterolateral bundle, whereas a positive anterior drawer test indicates the disrupted anteromedial bundle.

The **"pivot shift test"** of Galway and Macintosh is done to confirm the anterior cruciate ligament injury **(Figs. 13.62A to C)**.

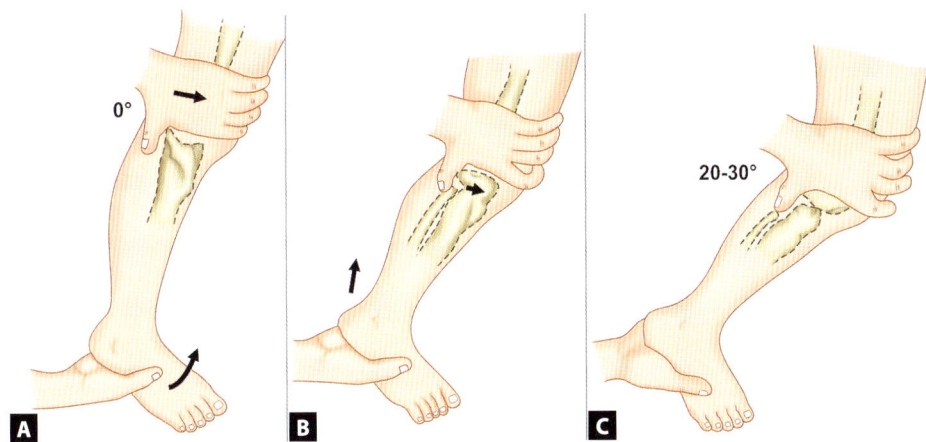

Figs. 13.62A to C: Pivot shift test of Galway and Macintosh to confirm anterior cruciate ligament injury (after Oh and Pitman 2004).

Method

The patient lies supine. The knee to be examined is fully extended. The examiner holds the lower end of thigh from the outer side by his left hand with fully abducted thumb placed over the posterolateral aspect of the head of fibula. By his right hand, holding the hindfoot of patient from the sole side, the examiner internally rotates the leg while his left hand produces valgus stress at knee **(Fig. 13.62A)**. Keeping both manoeuvres in action, the knee is gradually flexed and the examiner's left hand thumb pressing over the head of fibula attempts to sublux the upper end of tibia forward **(Fig. 13.62B)**. If there will be disruption of anterior cruciate ligament a 'clunk' of reduction will be felt at the anterolateral corner of the proximal tibia in the first 20°–30° of flexion **(Fig. 13.62C)**. The patient may also feel anterior subluxation (gliding) of tibia.

Rotational Stress Tests (Test for Menisci)

They are mainly directed towards diagnosing tear of the menisci. Though no clinical sign is of diagnostic accuracy, rotational stresses in which the menisci are subjected to stretching and/or squeezing, can lead us to suspect meniscus tear, if present. The meniscus is usually torn when the femur suddenly rotates medially while the knee remains flexed and the foot and leg are firmly fixed by bearing weight.

McMurray's Test—Method (Fig. 13.63)

The patient lies supine with his hip flexed 90° and knee fully flexed. Hold the knee with one hand from the dorsal aspect in such a way that the thumb is on the lateral, and other fingers are on the medial aspect. With the other hand, hold the heel and ankle. Fixing the knee by one hand, and while gradually pulling, externally rotating and abducting the leg as far as practicable by other hand, extend the knee. The patient feels sharp pain on the medial side of the joint line and

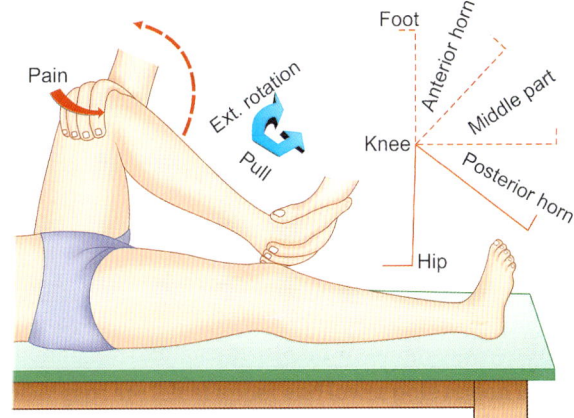

Fig. 13.63: Rotational stress test—McMurray's test.

the examiner feels a click on about the same site while the pulling position is maintained. In flexing and extending the knee in quick successions, every time the knee is extended, the patient will feel pain. This will be a positive *stress test for medial meniscus tear*. In this manoeuvre, *eliciting the painful click in the initial range of extension indicates posterior horn tear, while in the middle range it indicates injury of the middle part. For anterior horn injury,* one has to give more stress on eliciting tenderness at the medial side of ligamentum patellae and then to go for eliciting the painful click. In testing for lateral meniscus tear, other manoeuvres remaining the same, the hand holding the heel and ankle, will pull, internally rotate and abduct the leg as far as practicable. However, this test is not always positive.

Apley's Test (Distraction Test and Grinding Test)

In the light of monumental works on the knee joint, this test has very limited value, specially in acute cases. However, in late cases, quick assessment can be done before proceeding further for confirmation.

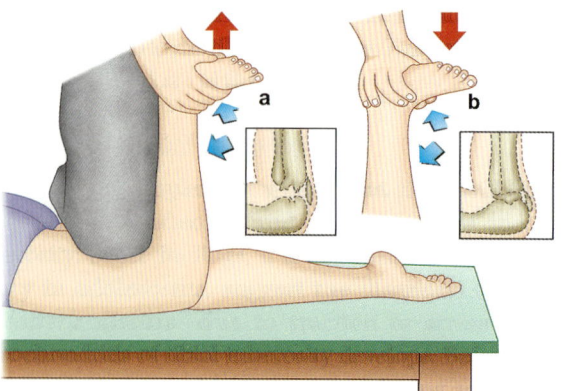

Fig. 13.64: Apley's test: a = distraction test, b = grinding test.

Method (Fig. 13.64)

Initially, patient lies prone, firmly planting his thigh on the couch. Bend the knee 90°, press the patient's thigh with your bent knee and hold the ankle and foot region firmly with your both hands. Now distract the leg upwards and rotate it internally and externally. If there is collateral ligament injury, the patient will complain of pain at the particular site. Then compress the leg downwards and repeat the rotatory motions. In case of semilunar cartilage tear, the patient complains of pain over the corresponding site.

Squat Test (After Sisk, 1980)

For quick assessment of meniscal tear, ask the patient to squat fully and rotate the leg and foot alternately, internally and externally to full extent. If there is pain in the joint line on the lateral side on squatting with internally rotated leg, it suggests lateral meniscus tear; while pain located medially in the joint line on external rotation of leg indicates tear of the medial meniscus.

Childress Duck-Waddle Test

This is a strenuous test, however it can be well performed on athletes. The patient is asked to squat and waddle on the toes while swinging from side to side. If the posterior horn of the meniscus is torn, complete flexion of knee cannot be achieved, and the patient's manoeuvre initiates pain and/or clicking in the posteromedial aspect of the joint.

Wilson's Test

Osteochondritis dissecans can be vaguely represented by local tenderness on the surface of the femoral condyle (especially the medial). However, this can be clinically confirmed by *Wilson's test*. Here the knee is flexed to 90°, internally rotated, then it is gradually extended. Patient will complain of pain, the moment the raw areas come in contact, which gets immediately relieved if the knee is rotated externally.

'Q' Angle

The predisposition of a patella for subluxation can be roughly assessed by determining the 'Q' angle. Due to the anatomical alignment of femur, its valgus inclination and the origin of the quadriceps muscles, the line of pull of patellar movement is never direct, rather it is guided by the Quadriceps (Q) angle. *The quadriceps angle (Q angle) is a measure of the patella's tendency to move laterally when the quadriceps muscles are contracted.* This angle is formed by intersection of a line joining the tibial tuberosity to the centre of the patella and another line joining the centre of the patella to the anterior superior iliac spine. *The normal 'Q' angle is 12° for females and 15° for males. If this angle is more than 15°, it denotes susceptibility of patella for recurrent subluxation.* This angle is increased in patients with a lateralised tibial tuberosity, but it can be false normally when the patella is laterally displaced. Although increased Q angles are associated with genu valgum (valgus knee), some of the highest angles are found in patients who have even genu varum associated with proximal tibial torsion.

Friction Test

In extended position of the knee, the patella is pressed and glided up and down over the femoral articular surface. With affection of the central portion of the articular surface of the patella, painful grating can be felt (e.g. *in chondromalacia patella; degenerative arthrosis*).

Apprehension Sign

In *patellar malalignment* as the knee is extended while a laterally directed pressure is applied to this patella, the patient becomes apprehensive, which reflects extreme malalignment of patella.

Apprehension Test

In recurrent subluxation or dislocation of patella, any attempt of passively subluxing the patella in slightly flexed position of the knee is resisted by the patient.

Loose Bodies in the Knee Joint (Joint Mice)

In such cases, there will be history of moving of an object in the joint and/or occasional sense of "giving way" of the joints; there may be history of intermittent pain in the joint with recurrent effusions or locking. Loose body may be seen and/or palpated.

Causes of Loose Bodies

- *Non-traumatic:* (i) Osteoarthrosis—detached osteophyte, (ii) Sequestrated osteochondritis dissecans, (iii) Synovial chondromatosis, (iv) Fibrinous organisation of haemarthrosis (haemophilia), (v) Rheumatoid arthritis, (vi) Tuberculous arthritis.

- *Traumatic:* (i) Organised haemarthrosis, (ii) Organised snapped synovial fringes, (iii) Detached flakes of articular cartilage, (iv) Loose fragment from intra-articular fractures (condylar and fracture patella), (v) Loose fragment of torn semilunar cartilage, (vi) Foreign bodies.

Auscultation

As usual, auscultation is of importance in case of vascular osseous swellings and in fulminating malignancy. In the back of the knee, sometimes popliteal artery aneurysm and arteriovenous fistula do occur, where one can hear a systolic bruit. The lower end of femur and upper end of tibia are most common sites for osteosarcomas. In telangiectatic variety of this growth, systolic bruit can be heard. In case of early chondromalacia patellae, fine crepitations can be appreciated if the stethoscope bell is kept on the joint while the knee is moved.

■ INVESTIGATIONS FOR KNEE PATHOLOGY

- General—as in the Chapter 1: Introduction
- Local—
  - Plain X-ray—(a) Anteroposterior, (b) Lateral, (c) Oblique, (d) Sky line (tangential), (e) Stress radiography
  - CT scan (Tomography)
  - Aspiration and aspiration biopsy
  - Arthrography
  - Arthroscopy
  - Cine radiography
  - Arthrotomy
  - Radioscintigraphy
  - Arteriography
  - MRI

How to Take X-ray Projections

Weight Bearing Position

Patient stands with equal full weight distribution on both legs keeping knees in symmetrical position (AP view).

Lateral View

In 30° flexed position and relaxed (lying down) position of knee.

Oblique View

Oblique view (Internal and external oblique) in relaxed extended position of knee.

Tangential View (Skyline or Sunrise View or Merchant view)

Skyline view is taken to see the: (a) patellofemoral articular relation **(Figs. 13.65A and B)**, (b) to assess the development of femoral condyles in relation to patella (of special importance in recurrent dislocation of patella), (c) osteochondral fractures of patella and femoral condyle.

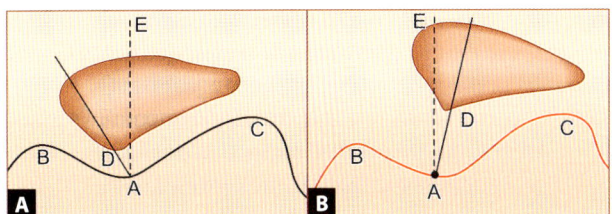

Figs. 13.65A and B: Line drawing of 30° tangential radiograph of the patella with knee flexed by 45°: (A) Normal knee; (B) Knee with subluxation and tilt.

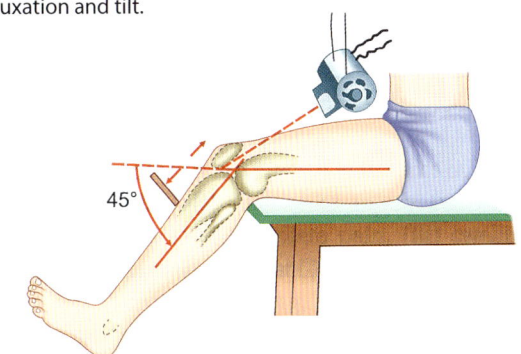

Fig. 13.66: Skyline or sunrise view projection to delineate patellofemoral articulation.

Technique: With patient sitting at the edge of the table with 45° flexion at knee, the X-ray plate is kept at a distance of 10 cm from the knee level, perpendicular to the shin of tibia. The beam is projected from the superior aspect of the patella, striking the plate at 90° **(Fig. 13.66)** Or the patient lies supine with the knee flexed over sand bags or pillows and the film supported along the femur. The beam is centred to the patella with the tube tilted 15° to the lower leg.

Although tangential views are more commonly taken at 45° or 60° of flexion of knee, Merchant radiograph has emerged as the standard as it allows for imaging of the trochlea at 30° of flexion.

Tunnel View

It is taken mainly to display osteochondritis dissecans, the intercondylar notch, and the loose bodies. The patient kneels on the affected side with the film placed under the knee. A sand bag supports the ankle. The patient then leans forward so that the femur is approximately 45° to the table. The beam is centred to the knee joint at right angle to the lower leg.

Stress X-ray

If possible it should be done under anaesthesia in acute cases. However, in chronic cases it can be done as such.

Method: For anteroposterior stress, patient sits on the edge of X-ray table at one end with knee flexed in 30° position with plate kept on the outer side of the joint, the examiner pulls the upper end of tibia forwards, and pushes it backward alternately as much as possible.

For side to side stress, patient stands with full weight bearing on the affected limb. With the knee in maximum possible valgus and varus strain, alternately, anteroposterior X-ray projection is shot to delineate any ligamentous inadequacy on medial or lateral aspect of the knee.

In anaesthetised or lying down position, strap both approximated thighs together at the lower end. The plate is kept behind the knees. The examiner then forcibly abducts the legs at the knee while X-ray is shot from anterior aspect. This will demonstrate any medial ligamentous inadequacy.

Certain X-ray findings may have some clinical significance (after like: Miller MD, Dempsay IJ. 2021)

- Calcification of proximal medial collateral ligament (Pellegrini-Stieda Disease), it → Signifies old/chronic medial collateral ligament injury.
- Segond fracture (lateral capsular sign → Although not common, it is mostly associated with ACL tear.
- High riding patella in trochlears groove i.e. patella alta → Produces patellar instability
- Low riding patella – Patella baja → Produces arthrofibrosis – which produces chronic stiff knee.
- Lucency in lateral aspect of medial femoral condyle → Indicates association of osteochondritis dissecans
- Widening lateral cupping of knee → Is associated with discoid meniscus

Cine-Radiography

This is usually of value in assessing the gait of the patient with knee pathology, as well as the integrity of the stabilising ligaments. Here, the movie camera is fixed with sliding X-ray tubes along the wall of the X-ray room, from where pictures are taken while the patient walks in a definite pattern.

Tomography

With the help of the pre-adjusted scale attached in the X-ray machine, the X-ray is taken at a measured depth penetration.

Arthroscopy

Arthroscopy, first performed by K Takagi in the year 1918, has now become an essential investigation, especially with the development of sports medicine. It is mostly used in the knee joint. However, it cannot be a substitute for thorough clinical examination.

It is being used to directly visualise the menisci, articular surfaces of patella and femur, joint capsule, cruciate ligaments, loose bodies, and synovium. Therapeutically, it is utilised to remove or suture torn meniscus, to repair/replace anterior cruciate ligament, to fix detached osteochondral surface, in plica syndrome, to take out biopsy material and joint lavage. The findings can also be simultaneously photographed and video-recorded. However, it has its limitations in having *'blind spots'* in its visual field (i.e. posteromedial and posterolateral part of knee and inferior surface of meniscus).

Contraindications to its use: (i) stiff knee, (ii) infected knee, (iii) recent haemarthrosis.

Arthrography

This is a contrast study of the joint space. It can be done either by using a radio-opaque dye directly injected into the joint or injecting air or both (double contrast arthrography). It is valuable in assessing menisci tear, cruciate tear, and presence of any space-occupying lesion. Its special advantage lies in delineating the blind spot areas of arthroscopy. Contraindications are: (i) pyoarthrosis, (ii) haemophilia, (iii) dye allergy.

Detection and interpretation of vibration emission from the locomotor system is a sensitive noninvasive method for the objective study of human joints.

Vibration arthrography is a recent advancement in this technique, especially as a diagnostic aid in diseases of knee and neonatal hip.

Scintigraphy (Nuclear Imaging)

Radioscanning is not of much value as a diagnostic aid in knee pathology. However, it can be of academic usefulness for various neoplasm and for investigating blood supply of a bone (affected by any pathology).

Genucom

By this instrument, precise non-invasive computer-based 3D measurement of total knee stability (for ligaments, patella and knee prosthesis) can be done and analysed.

Arteriography

It is more or less of only academic value, except in vascular lesion related to the posterior part of knee joint. Research workers do utilise this investigation to study rheumatoid pathology and various neoplastic conditions and severe injuries around the knee joint which threaten the vascularity.

KEY DIAGNOSTIC POINTS OF COMMON KNEE PATHOLOGY

Non-Traumatic

- *Congenital conditions* (**Figs. 13.67 to 13.69, 13.81**)
  - Usually associated with other congenital defect
  - Bilateral symmetrical defects
  - History since birth
  - At knee, absence of femoral or tibial high-placed, low-placed, bipartite or absent patella are the usually known congenital defects.
- Metabolic diseases and deficiency states

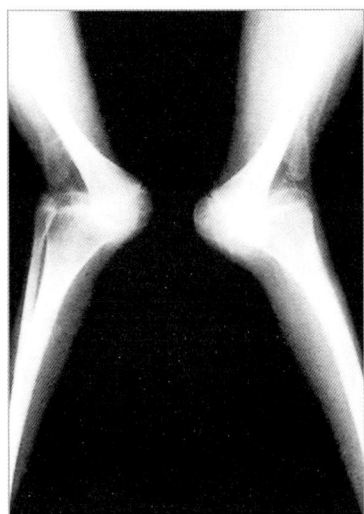

Fig. 13.67: Bilateral congenital posterolateral dislocation of knee. It is extremely difficult to treat such case; In well-equiped setup, very cautions open reduction may be tried, however, after fitting with bilateral HKAFO (hip–knee–ankle–foot orthoses) the patient may be trained to be stable and steping – if upper limbs are supportive.

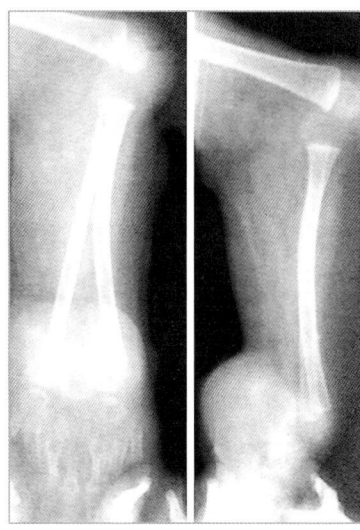

Fig. 13.68: Congenital unilateral posterior dislocation of knee and ankle associated with disorganised ankle and foot – extremely difficult to manage/treat; however, may be made to be stable after prolonged physiotherapy after fitting with modified tailored HKAFO.

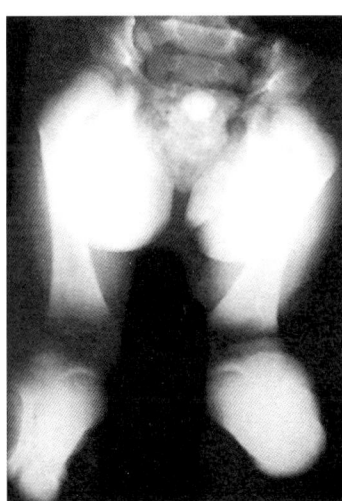

Fig. 13.69: Bilateral congenital absence of lower end of femora and bilateral congenital below knee amputee – such patient should be trained for wheel-chair life.

Rickets occurs due to deficiency of vitamin D or to a defect in its metabolism.

Vitamin D deficiency in childhood before epiphyseal closure leads to inadequate calcification of cartilage and new bone. It can be inferred broadly that deficiency and defect in vitamin D, calcium, and phosphorus metabolism lead to rickets in child and osteomalacia in adult.

Clinical presentation is usually comparatively listless child with flabby look, protruding abdomen, irregular bowels, delayed walking, retardation of growth, deformities.

Usual findings: Poor tone of muscles, delayed closure of fontanelles and cranial sutures, craniotabes, bossing of forehead, thickened and everted look of lips, decaying of teeth, broadening of lower radial epiphysis, pigeon chest, Harrison's sulcus, rachitic rosary **(Fig. 13.15A)**, pot belly, widening of perineum, anterolateral bowing of lower third of femora, bow knee **(Figs. 13.18 to 13.25)**, bow leg (lower third), genu valgum, widening of growing ends of long bones, windswept (tackle) deformity **(Figs. 13.72 to 13.75)**. With the exception of the rosary, all deformities, more or less remain as permanent stigmas of rickets.

X-ray
- *Florid (acute) stage*: Poorly defined and smaller epiphysis (irregular calcified areas); epiphyseal end of metaphysis cup shaped, poorly defined and fraying look; generalised broadening of metaphysis with flared cortices (most marked in wrist and knee regions); widened epiphyseometaphyseal junction; generalised rarefied appearance of bones with less sharply defined trabeculations and cortices; bending of long bones
- *Healing stage*: Epiphysis gets gradually defined, uniformally calcified, larger epiphyseometaphyseal junction gets narrowed with appearance of denser line; gradual narrowing of metaphysis with flattening of cup and reappearance of transverse trabeculations, gradual restoration of normal bony texture
- *Healed stage*: Almost normal epiphysis; denser line at epiphyseometaphyseal junction; legacy of earlier deformities variably persists; normal bony texture.

Scurvy: James Lind discovered its true nature in 1747: It is a deficiency disease due to lack of vitamin C. Acute to subacute presentation, in early childhood (rarely in elderly sailors and soldiers on voyage on sea—'Calamity of soldiers').

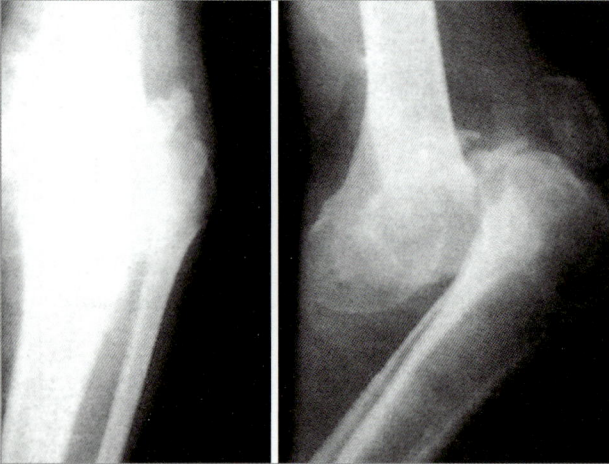

Fig. 13.70: Traumatic neglected (four months) anterior dislocation of knee. No clinical evidence of residual neurovascular damage; should be treated with very cautious open reduction of dislocation – to remain vigilant about neuro-vascular care – guarded prolonged physiotherapy.

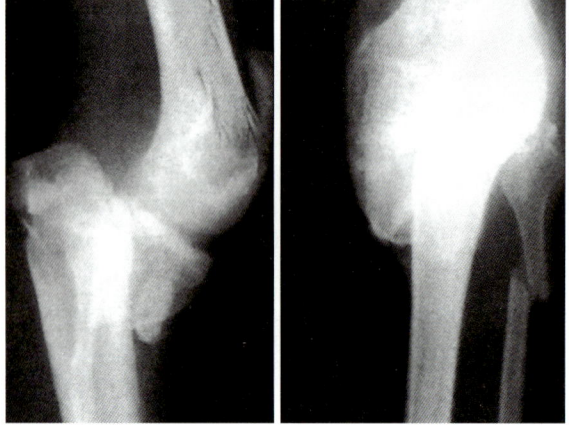

Fig. 13.71: Traumatic neglected (11 weeks) posterior fracture dislocation of knee. No clinical evidence of residual vascular damage, however had partial foot drop; should be treated with very cautious open reduction and fixation of fracture. Movements at knee may remain permanently restricted.

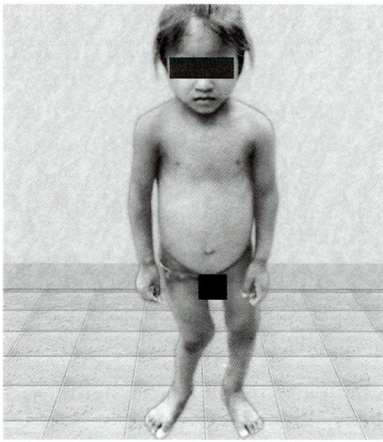

Fig. 13.72: Rachitic windswept deformity in florid stage should be managed by serial plaster cast correction; and vitamin D and calcium.

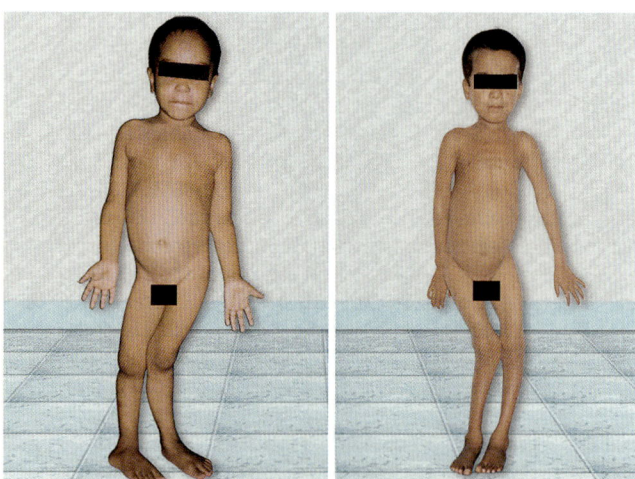

Fig. 13.73: Rachitic windswept deformity towards left in left sided boy and towards right in right sided boy in healing stage; should be managed by serial plaster cast correction along with vitamin D and calcium.

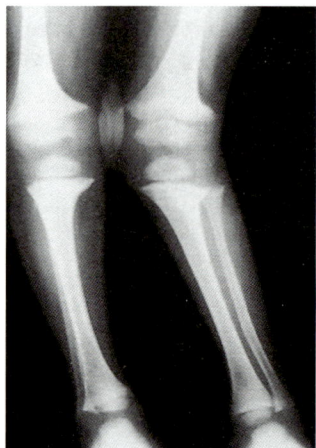

Fig. 13.74: X-ray of rachitic windswept deformity of both legs; should be treated with serial plaster cast correction, along with vitamin D and calcium.

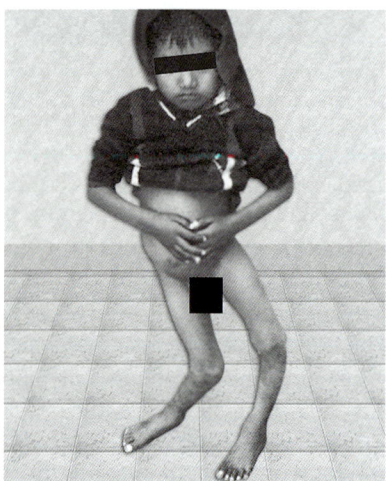

Fig. 13.75: Genu recurvatum tendency of left knee and flexion tendency of right knee with windswept deformity of thighs, knees and legs due to polio-paralysis. May be managed by physiotherapy, orthoses, and surgery.

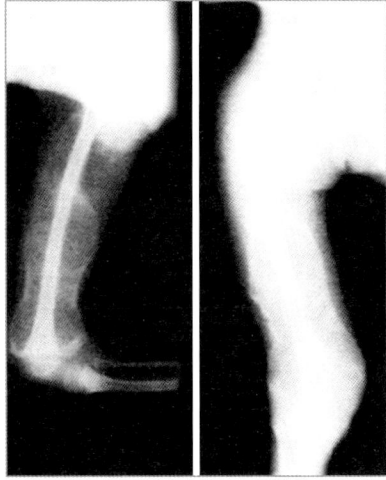

Fig. 13.76: X-ray of scurvy. Note marked subperiosteal haematoma in femur.

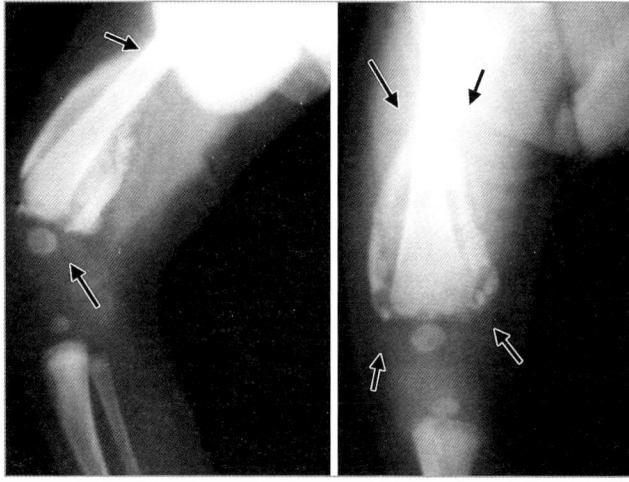

Fig. 13.77: Scurvy—calcification in subperiosteal haematoma in femur.

- Artificially fed infants and children are more likely to develop scurvy, because vitamin C is destroyed by heat in boiling the milk.

  Such infants and children may also develop rickets if the milk has not been supplemented with vitamin D. *The combination of rickets and scurvy is known as "Barton's disease"*
- Epiphyseal fracture separation at the end of long bone
- Markedly tender fixed swelling over bone, especially in thigh, due to subperiosteal haematoma which may get calcified **(Figs. 13.76 and 13.77)**
- Bluish, spongy bleeding gums (specially near upper incisors)
- Mild rise of temperature
- Pseudoparalysis
- Costochondral separation—presenting as sharp protrusion on anterior ends of the ribs—scorbutic rosary (cf. rachitic rosary—rounded)
- Delayed wound healing
- X-ray—*'pencilling' (thinning) of cortex,* marked homogenous rarefaction, subperiosteal or longitudinal bone laying (bone formation). *White line of Frankel,* scurvy line (irregular radio-opaque line caused by calcified cartilage), *Wimberger line*—the dense line encircling the epiphysis *(Ring sign), Pelkan spur*—best seen at the ends of rapidly growing long bones, as a small bony spur mostly on the lateral side of metaphysis near its junction with epiphysis
- The blood ascorbic acid is 0.5 mgm less/dL mL (normal value is 1 mg/dL mL).

Collagen Arthropathy (also see Chapter 3: Joints)

Rheumatoid arthritis: It is usually a polyarthropathy, in which affection of the smaller joints of the hand and wrist (mainly proximal interphalangeal joints, but doubtful/not the distal interphalangeal joints) is typical.

In Monoarticular Affections
- Knee is commonly affected, with mild inflammatory features
- Chronic history, wasting of muscles, fluid in the joint, synovial thickening, joint and bony tenderness
- Gradually, movements get restricted with advancement of disease
- Deformity—usually triple subluxation of knee
- Lymph glands usually not enlarged.

Haemophilia
- May present as acute or chronic haemarthrosis
- Family history
- Haemophilia A and B are X-linked coagulation disorders occurring due to deficiency of factor VIII and factor IX respectively,
- Exclusively in males (X-linked recessive inheritance), except haemophiliac (deficient plasmathromboplastin antecedent-factor XI), which affects both sexes
- Pseudotumour (haemophilic cyst) due to intramuscular or parosteal haemorrhage
- Common joints affected are knee, elbow and ankle
- History of repeated episodes
- Patient pale, history of bleeding from other sites too
- History of prolonged bleeding after any cut
- Flexion deformity, genu varum, genu valgum
- In late cases—degenerative changes; ankylosis of joint (usually fibrous)
- Clotting time increased due to lack of antihaemophilic factor (factor VIII)—haemophilia A (30% cases); lack of Christmas factor (Factor IX)—haemophilia B (15% cases)
- X-ray—distended joint, articular surfaces intact but thinned out. In late cases,—genu valgum or genu varum deformities may be associated due to epiphyseal asymmetry overgrowth, squaring of patella, widening of

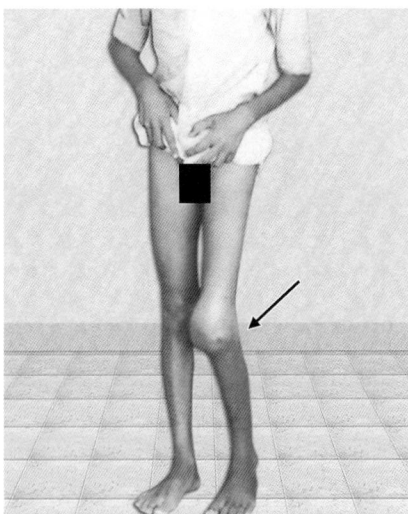

Fig. 13.78: Chronic septic arthritis of knee should be managed by excision of the diseased tissue, suitable antibiotics (according to culture and chemosensitivity) and support of the joint till healing of disease.

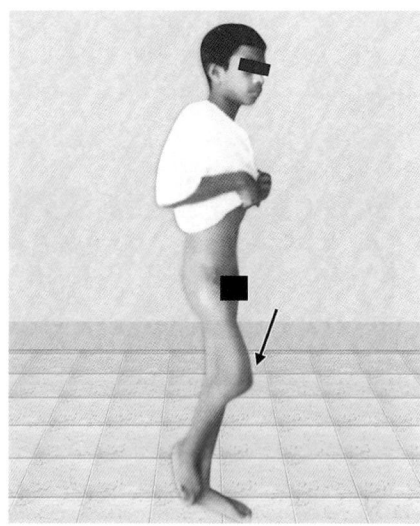

Fig. 13.79: Tuberculosis of knee with sinus with triple deformities—should be managed by excision of the diseased tissues, anti-tuberculous chemotherapy and support to joint, till the heating of the disease.

intercondylar notch of femur. Other nonspecific X-ray signs are bone resorption, osteoporosis, cyst formation, etc.
- Rare disabling or even life-threatening complication may occur like—iliac haemophilic pseudotumour (in femur or pelvis in adults with poor prognosis; in distal part of extremities in children with better prognosis)
- Reasonable elective surgery in patients of classic haemophilia A (factor VIII deficiency), haemophilia A and Christmas disease (factor IX deficiency) or haemophilia B has become possible with availability of factor VIII and factor IX concentrates.

Infective conditions
- *Acute septic arthritis:*
  - Knee commonest site
  - Usually in children
  - Acute onset with constitutional features
  - High fever with rigor
  - Toxic features
  - Femoral or tibial metaphyseal affection
  - Hot inflamed joint
  - Tenderness specially in joint line
  - Fluctuant knee swelling (pus)
  - Inguinal lymph glands enlarged and tender
  - Aspiration of pus clinches the diagnosis
  - Routine haemogram—polymorphonuclear leucocytosis
  - ESR raised mild to moderate
  - Blood culture—positive in limited number of cases
  - Aspiration culture positive in almost all cases
  - X-ray—increased joint space, comparatively homogeneous appearance of area around joint with increased soft tissue shadow, generalised rarefaction, localised varying rarefaction due to destruction in the adjacent bones, depending upon osseous pathology.
- *Chronic septic arthritis* **(Fig. 13.78)**
  - Usually in adults
  - Presence of active (with purulent discharge) or healed sinuses
  - Minimal swelling
  - Usually associated deformities
  - Varying ankylosis
  - Adjacent metaphyseal thickening
  - History of intermittent episodes of flare
  - Inguinal lymph nodes enlarged, firm and may be tender; X-ray—joint space distorted and reduced, areas of destruction, bone formation and sequestration. Aspiration may not be of much value. Aspirated material may be sterile. Routine haemogram not of much value. ESR may be raised.
- *Tuberculosis knee* **(Fig. 13.79)** *Knee is third common site for osteoarticular tuberculosis forming about 10% of skeletal tuberculosis (TB).*

  In children: Synovial swelling (tumour alba—in white-skinned persons), varying flexion deformity, comparatively free movements (as compared to adult affection).
  - Warm, tender, thickened knee
  - Movements painful, specially at extremes
  - Wasting of thigh and calf muscles
  - Triple rather quadruple deformity—in advanced cases
  - Inguinal lymph glands enlarged, usually matted
  - Routine haemogram—varying increase in lymphocyte count, raised ESR
  - Mantoux test positive in varying dilutions

- Aspiration—thin serous/serosanguinous—may be positive for AFB
- ELISA test for tuberculosis mostly positive.

X-ray—Initially increased joint space due to collection, later decrease in joint space when true arthritis supervenes, generalised rarefaction, localised areas of destruction along with cystic areas, varying ankylosis (usually fibrous ankylosis).

In adults:
- Osseous focus more common (in femur, tibia, patella)
- May be synovial swelling
- Warm, swollen joint
- Tenderness along the joint line
- Deformities—usually triple rather quadruple subluxation
- All movements painful and restricted
- May be sinuses of tuberculous nature
- May be shortening of the limb, due to destruction
- Wasting of thigh and calf muscles
- Aspiration—thin, serous or serosanguinous—may be AFB positive.
- Synovial biopsy—chronic lymphocytic infiltration; demonstration of typical Langhan's giant cells and epithelioid cells
- X-ray—reduced joint space, area of subchondral and chondral destruction, generalised rarefaction, varying deformities.

Neoplastic conditions

Benign soft tissue growths:
- These are comparatively rare (e.g. haemangioma, neurofibroma)
- Small swelling
- Deep tenderness
- May be warm if superficial
- Haemangiomas are usually deep seated (mostly intramuscular)
- X-ray—if growth adjacent to bone—may be localised rarefaction or condensation
- *Lipoma arborescens* (tree like) is a very uncommon tumour of synovium, in which there is diffuse replacement of the synovial tissue by mature fat cells, with prominent villous transformation of the synovium.

Presenting soft boggy swelling in the suprapatellar pouch needs to be differentiated from pigmented villonodular synovitis, synovial lipoma, synovial chondromatosis, synovial haemangioma, rheumatoid arthritis, xanthoma, amyloid arthropathy.

Malignant soft tissue growths:
- Usually young adults in thirties
- Synovioma—either in relation to synovial reflection, bursae in relation to tendon, or even penetrating adjacent bone
- Varying size and shape of slowly growing swelling with ill-defined margins
- Warm, tender
- X-ray—combination of bone defects and soft tissue swelling like *snowstorm-appearance*
- Usually eccentrically situated according to site
- Soft to firm in feel.

Benign bony growths: Benign bony growth in relation to bone is rare, except for exostosis which may arise from lower femoral or upper tibial region—as firm to hard, painless knob-like swellings—projecting away from central knee axis. Usually, multiple and associated with deformities. May be pressure symptoms, e.g. foot drop due to pressure on lateral popliteal nerve. May turn malignant.

X-ray—Exostosis usually projects away from the joint axis, and has the medullary cavity continuous with parent medulla.

Giant cell tumour (osteoclastoma):
- Usually in 3rd decade
- Common sites—condylar regions (upper end of tibia, lower end of femur)
- Eccentric, tender, globular swelling
- Feeling of yielding on pressure (demonstration of egg-shell crackling should not be attempted as it may produce fracture of the thin expanded cortex, leading to dissemination of the growth into the surroundings)
- Knee movements fairly preserved for a pretty long time
- Movements only affected due to mechanical obstruction or bursting of tumour into the joint.

X-ray—Expansion of the cortex, trabeculations (leading to soap bubble-appearance), usually delineation of uppermost end of the expanded segment from the normal medullary cavity (if malignancy supervenes, this delineation is usually not marked), may or may not break into the joint. No area of bone formation.

Osteosarcoma:
- The most common sites are the lower end of femur and upper end of tibia
- Fusiform, painful and comparatively huge swelling
- In knee region, perhaps osteosarcoma presents the largest swelling
- All typical features of malignancy
- Pathological fractures
- Aspiration—bloody fluid
- Active movements of knee usually affected due to pain and mechanical reasons, but passive movements are relatively free.

X-ray—Soft tissue shadow, areas of bone destruction and bone formation, sunray spicules, Codman's triangle formation, corticomedullary delineation not lost.

Degenerative Arthrosis (Fig. 13.80) or Osteoarthros or, Osteoarthritis

- Primary osteoarthritis affects the knee more frequently than any other joint
- By far it is most prevalent form of arthritis. In squatters (as in Asian-Indian culture) about 45% people over 60 years, age suffer from osteoarthritis of knee. Women are worst affected than men. WHO estimates that 10% of men and 18% of women past age 60 have osteoarthritis
- Chronic history—symptoms coming on just after rest, amelioration after mild to moderate activities. May again increase with prolonged activities
- Coarse crepitations felt over joint with movements
- Knee osteoarthritis has basically two components—tibiofemoral arthritis and patellofemoral arthritis. However, about 10-15% of patients suffering from knee arthritis have isolated patellofemoral joint arthritis, which typically occur in younger age group
- Osteoarthritis usually affects the medial part of knee joint. 80% of body weight is carried through the medial half of the knee joint. Thus, logically this compartment worns out first. The medial joint space narrows and knee slides into varus
- Patients with osteoarthritis of knee have thicker Achilles tendon AND a correlation exists between knee OA severity and Achilles tendon thickness the treatment of knee OA should not base only on the findings of knee joint but rather on considering the entire lower limb as one kinematic chain
- Hence from very beginning treatment should focus on alleviating loads from degenerated medial compartment of knee and along with should also address the loads at the ankle joint (Elbaz et al. 2017). The footwear with outer heel-sole raised (usually by 1/6" in adults) serves this purpose
- Varus (common)/valgus collapse of knee
- Basically the articular cartilage thins, cracks, and breaks away, often leaving the subchondral bone roughened and thickened. The joints are disfigured with various deformities
- Occasionally, painful or painless soft (or, cystic), mildly warm and tender swelling of the knee—specially localised in suprapatellar area. Patient may present with soft cystic swelling of knee – hydrops knee
- Patellofemoral compression test is positive
- In later stages—limitation of movements; in advanced cases deformities may occur.

In advanced degenerative arthrosis of knee, there is loss of extension of knee, which may affect lumbar lordosis and

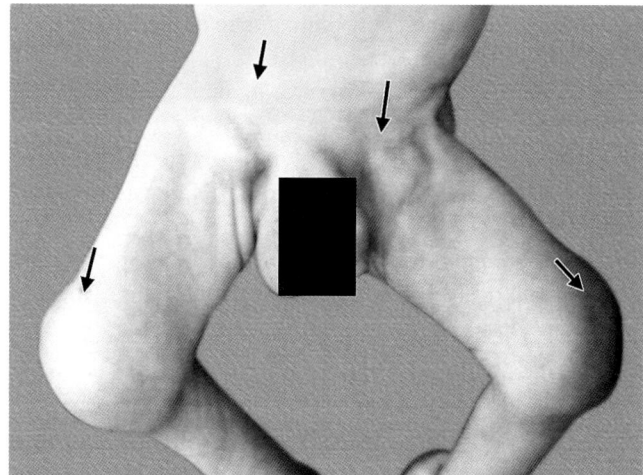

Fig. 13.81: Congenital syphilis (affection of joints and lymph glands).

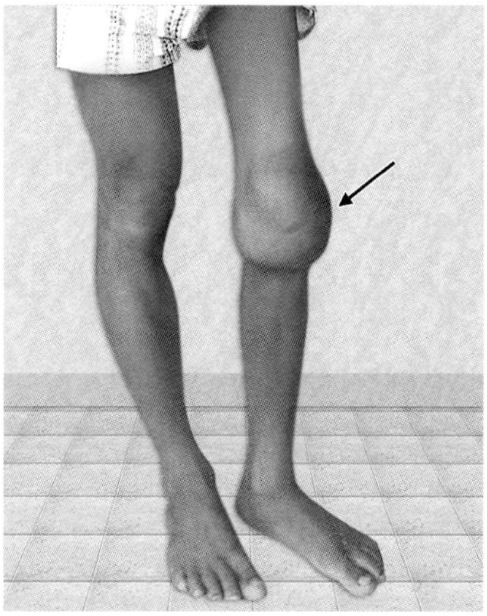

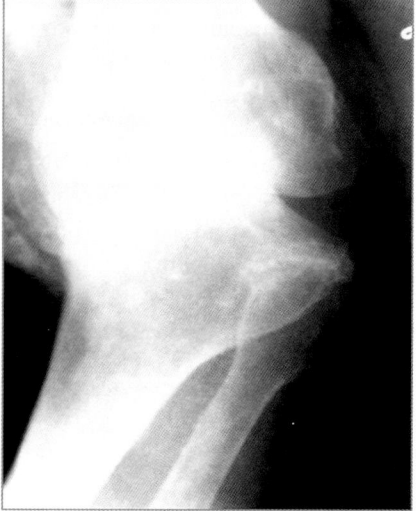

Fig. 13.80: Hydrops knee (Degenerative arthrosis). Aspirations of collected fluid, use of knee brace and physiotherapy usually help. For resistant cases synovectomy is required.

Fig. 13.82: Very advanced degenerative arthrosis of knee with marked varus collapse. In such cases total knee replacement in affluent patients and knee arthrodesis in poor and labourer patients should be the treatment.

overall posture—this may be called *"knee-spine syndrome"* (Murata 2003).

X-ray—(i) Condensation of subchondral plates in upper end of tibia depending upon the particular deformity (e.g. under medial plateau in varus collapse) **(Fig. 13.82)**, (ii) Subchondral cystic areas, (iii) Osteophytic formation, especially at condylar margins, (iv) Compartmental collapse of joint space, depending on deformity, (v) Loose bodies may be present.

Osteoarthritis of knee has been variously treated, such as analgesics, NSAIDs, physiotherapy, steroid injections, arthroscopic lavage/debridement, high tibial osteotomy, patellectomy, etc. Now a total knee arthroplasty (TKA) remains the gold standard of treatment (but not in younger patients, nor in squatters). TKA (all polyethylene or metal-backed components), even if not absolutely indicated, is being more performed by the young surgeons in monyed patients, especially in the third world (where squatting is socially more required) – hence overall result is not that encouraging. However, after total knee arthroplasty its long-term results and Patient reported outcome measures should be evaluated regularly on standard scales like Forgotten Joint Score (FJS), Oxford Knee Score (OKS), and Western Ontario and Mcmaster Universities Osteoarthritis Index (WOMAC). The evaluation will indicate if the ultimate goal of TKR (to replicate a natural joint to allow patients to perform most activities of daily living and give high satisfaction rates) has been achieved or not. Patellofemoral joint arthritis, if not responding to non-operative treatment, may be managed by patellofemoral joint replacement. Proximal Fibular Osteotomy (PFO) (a safe, simple and effective procedure) can reduce pain and improve function in medial compartment osteoarthritis of knee, and it may delay or even replace the non-absolutely indicated TKA. PFO combined with arthroscopic debridement, lavage and PRP injection appears to be more effective for medial compartment OA knee. Of course, medial open wedge high tibial osteotomy has been also a successful procedure in medial compartment osteoarthritis with varus deformity of knee. Taking the larger number of patient of osteoarthritis knee, the TKR is proving to be the gold standard. However, on the whole considerations TKR in patients with anteromedial osteoarthritis of knee is associated with higher degree of dissatisfaction. In such patients other treatment options, like unicondylar knee replacement, should be considered. The number of complex primary knee arthroplasty procedures performed is higher in Indian subcontinent, because usually the patient present with advanced deformities.

Calcifying tendinitis of the gastrocnemius, due to deposition of crystals of calcium pyrophosphate dihydrate (CPPD) can mimic the osteoarthritic pain of knee. Patient complains of pain mainly in the back of knee, usually induced by stretching gastrocnemius. There may be tender swelling near the origin of gastrocnemius muscles.

Plain X-ray shows degenerative changes with calcification in posterior aspect of knee with or without calcification of the menisci.

Local (injection) infiltration of lidocaine with steroids usually provides relief and improvement in the range of movements of knee.

In adolescent age group, common causes of non-traumatic disorders of the knee are overuse syndromes, patellofemoral pain and instability, discoid meniscus, and osteochondral lesions, besides the infective lesions and collagen arthropathy.

Traumatic Conditions

Extra-articular

Soft tissue injuries, except disruption of quadriceps apparatus, may manifest as tender swelling of diffused nature. However, one must examine and investigate repeatedly to exclude any intra-articular damage, which if missed, may jeopardise knee functions.

Intra-articular

- *Anterior cruciate avulsion*
  - Mild to moderate swelling of knee joint following injury (haemarthrosis)
  - Tenderness mostly localised over the anterior tibial plateau region
  - Extremes of movement painful
  - Lag of active terminal extension of knee (by about 15°-20°)
  - Posteroanterior stress test positive (Lachman's sign; Drawer test).

X-ray—A triangular flake of bone is seen in between the femoral and tibial condyles in lateral X-ray **(Fig. 13.83)**. In anteroposterior view, fissures in the tibial spine region are noticed. In stress radiography, anteroposterior laxity can be well demonstrated.

Arthroscopy (diagnostic or even therapeutic).

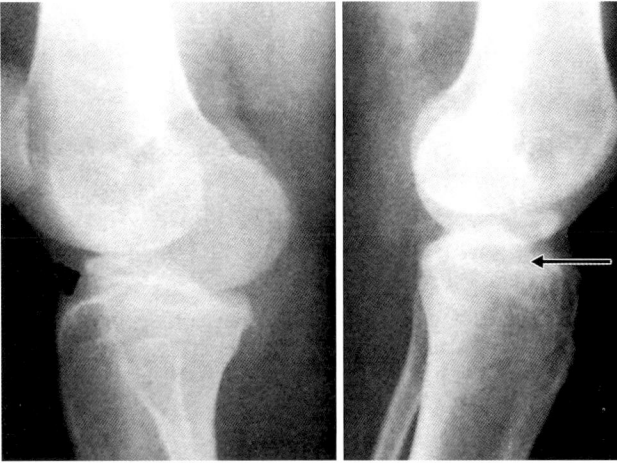

Fig. 13.83: Avulsion of anterior cruciate/fracture of tibial spine—*open fish-mouth appearance.*

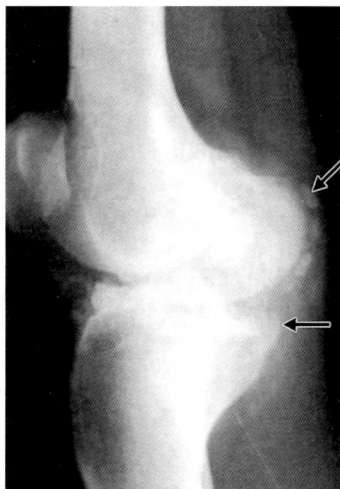

Fig. 13.84: Neglected old case of posterior cruciate avulsion and posterior capsular tear avulsion. Note the calcification along the avulsed capsule.

- *Posterior cruciate avulsion* **(Fig. 13.84)**
  - Posterior cruciate injury usually results from direct violence on the upper end of tibia while the knee remains flexed
  - Features almost comparable to anterior cruciate ligament avulsion except that anteroposterior stress test is positive, i.e. the posterior drawer sign is positive (elicited by pushing the upper end of tibia backward on the femoral condyles with the knee flexed by 90° and foot firmly planted on the couch/bed
  - In complete disruption, a peculiar 'sagging back' of the tibia is observed as compared to the normal side, while the patient is supine with hip flexed at 45° and knee flexed at 90°.
- *Medial meniscus tear*
  - Usually history of rotational strain in weight bearing and partially flexed knee
  - Immediate pain
  - Immediate inability to extend the knee
  - Mild swelling due to haemarthrosis
  - Movements of the knee actively possible, but extreme flexion painful
  - Full range of passive movements possible
  - Rotational stress tests (including Apley's grinding test) positive
  - Maximum tenderness at about a point located in the joint line, in the middle of ligamentum patellae and medial side of the knee joint
  - If there is entrapment of the synovial fringes in between the articular surfaces, tenderness is situated more anteriorly than in meniscal tear
  - Arthroscopy (diagnostic and even therapeutic).
- *Lateral meniscus tear*
  - Almost identical findings except for reversal of point of tenderness and rotational stress tests.

- *Fracture patella* **(see Fig. 13.53)**
  - Incomplete fracture of patella—In crack fracture of anterior surface, except for tenderness localised in that region and mild to moderate swelling, knee may be nearly normal
  - Complete fracture of patella—In an acute case, besides the findings of an acute traumatic knee (swelling, ecchymosis, bruisings, tenderness and all movements painful) other findings are:
    - Gap at the site of fracture can be palpated
    - Quadriceps contraction is not communicated through the fracture
    - Patient can walk (specially in late cases) but with high stepping tendency to clear the ground
    - He may be able to walk on his toes (equinus position) but has difficulty or is unable to walk on his heels.
  - Comminuted fracture of patella—If without any separation of fragments, the presentation is like that of intra-articular condylar fractures. However, quadriceps expansion and integrity of quadriceps apparatus must be assessed fully in such cases.

  X-ray—Confirmatory.
- *Condylar fractures (femoral or tibial)*
  - History of comparatively severe violence
  - Immediate excruciating pain
  - Marked swelling due to haemarthrosis
  - Restriction of movements to a great extent
  - Depending on the position of the fractured fragments, passive laxity of knee, specially in case of tibial condylar fracture
  - Maximum tenderness at that particular condylar end.

  X-ray is confirmatory.
- *Recurrent dislocation of patella or slipping patella* **(Fig. 13.85)**

  Causes of recurrent dislocation or slipping patella may be:
  - abnormally high patella, as may occur after Osgood-Schlatter`s disease
  - congenital causes like due to poor development of lateral femoral condyle; congenital anomalies of patella, malattachment of iliotibial tract, external rotation of tibia
  - Rachitic, traumatic or other causes leading to genu valgum
  - Usually in girls of adolescent age
  - History of recurrent dislocation or subluxation of patella
  - In acute dislocation, the patella is displaced laterally. In recurrent dislocation, this problem frequently occurs. The knee abruptly gives way with pain followed by varied swelling. In between the episodes of dislocations, there is increased lateral mobility of patella

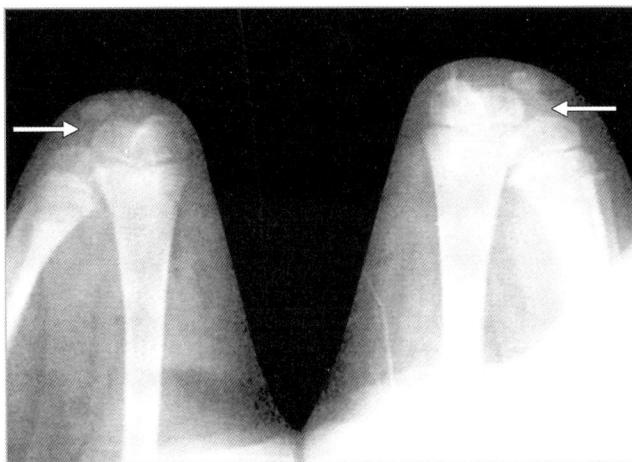

Fig. 13.85: Bilateral recurrent dislocation of patella – Lateral dislocation of patella is most common and important and this type is most liable to become habitual and recurrent or slipping patella.

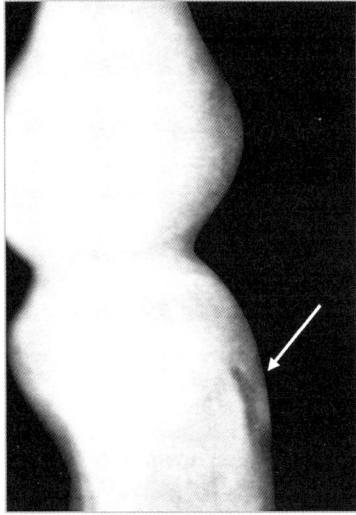

Fig. 13.86: Osgood-Schlatter's disease of tibia.

- Many a time, the patient herself reduces the dislocation/subluxation
- May be associated with genu valgum
- Such episodes are followed by mild to moderate pain and swelling which subside in a few days.
- Gradually quadriceps wasting ensues
- Axial view (skyline view) X-ray to assess patellofemoral congruence—may demonstrate the lateral femoral condylar ridge flattened as compared to the medial.

Acute cases can be easily reduced – preferably under general anaesthesia. Recurrence may be prevented by use of firm bandage or knee-cage, though it proves to be unpractical. Recurrent cases usually need surgical treatment with an aim of realigning the extensor apparatus and stabilization of patella during its functioning. The simple procedure consists of lateral release and reefing of the medial retinaculum to achieve proximal realignment. Distal realignment is achieved by procedures like medial and distal transfer of the tibial tubercle.

Medial patello femoral ligament reconstruction using an autologous hamstring graft with suture anchors usually gives good outcome preventing patellar subluxation or dislocations.

- *Chondromalacia patellae*
  - There is degeneration of articular cartilage of patella
  - Young girl complains of pain deep in the knee, specially behind the patella
  - Pain more in prolonged sitting, getting up and down the stairs with occasional effusion
  - Articular surfaces of patella are tender
  - Anterior surface of medial condyle of femur also tender
  - Rocking the patella in the femoral groove may produce pain with palpable crepitation
  - X-ray—almost normal
  - Arthroscopy (diagnostic and therapeutic).

- *Patellar malalignment (chondromalacia patellae)*
  The word 'chondromalacia' (meaning thereby= soft cartilage) has been correlated to define dry patellar pain (mainly the undersurface) or to refer to cartilage changes anywhere in the knee, has become confusing and controversial, and its features have been encompassed within the broader term "Patellar Malalignment" (Grelsamer 2000). Such patellar pain in adults is mostly due to patellar malalignment (translational or rotational deviation of the patella related to any axis). Patellar malalignment is associated with tightness of the following structures—in order of frequency—the lateral retinaculum, the hamstrings, the iliotibial band, the quadriceps, the hip rotators, and the Achilles tendon. In patellar malalignment, the patient usually complains of a sense of giving way and pain when he gets up from seated position, climbs up stairs or uphill or squats, since these activities exacerbate the abnormal pressure distribution above the patella.

  Pain in patellar region usually comes after prolonged sitting due to venous congestion and stretching of painful tissue—*'prolonged squatting sign'* or *'Movie theatre sign.'* Location of pain should be classically anterior, but it may be medial, lateral or popliteal.

  Once diagnosed and confirmed by MRI or scintigraphy (technetium scanning), the management should be principally stretching of the tight structure and/or braces (to realign the position of patella), and surgery (only for resistant cases).

- *Osgood-Schlatter's disease—tibial tubercle apophysitis (Fig. 13.86)*
  - Osgood in 1903 and Schlatter (1903) first described this condition as the epiphysitis of upper end of tibia in boys.

- Usually adolescents complain of pain in the tibial tuberosity region, specially after strenuous activity. Probably it is a traction (especially repeated) induced inflammation of patellar tendon
- Prominence of tibial tuberosity
- Tenderness on tibial tuberosity, especially while pressing from the lateral side
- Strong contraction of quadriceps causes pain in tibial tuberosity
- X-ray—enlargement with or without fragmentation of tibial tuberosity **(Fig. 13.86)** Osgood-Schlatter's disease
- It has to be differentiated from injury-effect, bone cyst, osteomyelitis, infrapatellar bursitis, some neoplasm
- Management mainly concerns restriction of activities and violent sports
- Physiotherapy
- Injection of corticosteroids
- MRI shows changes suggesting tendinitis of patellar tendon
- Mostly, it is self-limiting by the age of skeletal maturity.

BIBLIOGRAPHY

1. Cates NK, Furmanek J, Dubois KS, et al. Risk factors and outcomes after surgical reconstruction of charcot neuroarthropathy in fracture versus dislocation patterns. J Foot Ankle Surg. 2022;61(2):264-71.
2. Elbaz Avi, Magram-Flohr I, Segal G, et al. Association between knee Osteoarthritis and Functional changes in Ankle joint and Achilles tendon. J Foot Ankle Surg. 2017;56(2):238-41.
3. Grelsamer RP. Patellar malalignment. J Bone Joint Surg. 2000;82A:1638-50.
4. Gunn DR. Contracture of the quadriceps muscle: discussion on the etiology and relationship recurrent dislocation of the patella. J Bone Joint Surg. 1964;46B:492-7.
5. Horstmann HM, Bleck EE. Orthopaedic Management in Cerebral Palsy, 2nd edn, Machkeith Press; 2007.
6. Merchant AC, Mercer RL, Jacobsen RH, Cool CR. Roentgenographic analysis of patellofemoral congruence. J Bone Joint Surg. 1974;56A:1391-6.
7. Miller MD, Dempses IJ. Overview of the knee and lower leg. In: Essential Orthopaedict, Elsevier Inc 2021. Indian Reprint ISBN: 978-81-312-6517-8. pp. 574-85.
8. Oh Young Ho, Pitman MI. Anterior cruciate ligament: Endoscopic reconstruction. In: Atlas of Orthopaedic Surgery by Koval KJ and Zuckerman JD. Philadelphia; Lippincott Williams & Wilkins; 2004 (Reprinted in India in 2005). 260-72.
9. Pandey AK, Pandey S, Pandey P. Results of partial patellectomy. Arch Orthop Trauma Surg. 1991;110(5):246-9.
10. Staheli LI. 'Lower positional deformity in infants, and children: a review. J Pediatr Orthop. 1990;11:559-63.
11. Turek, Samuel L. Orthopaedics, Principles and their Applications. 1984;4:1269-1406.

CHAPTER 14

Ankle Joints

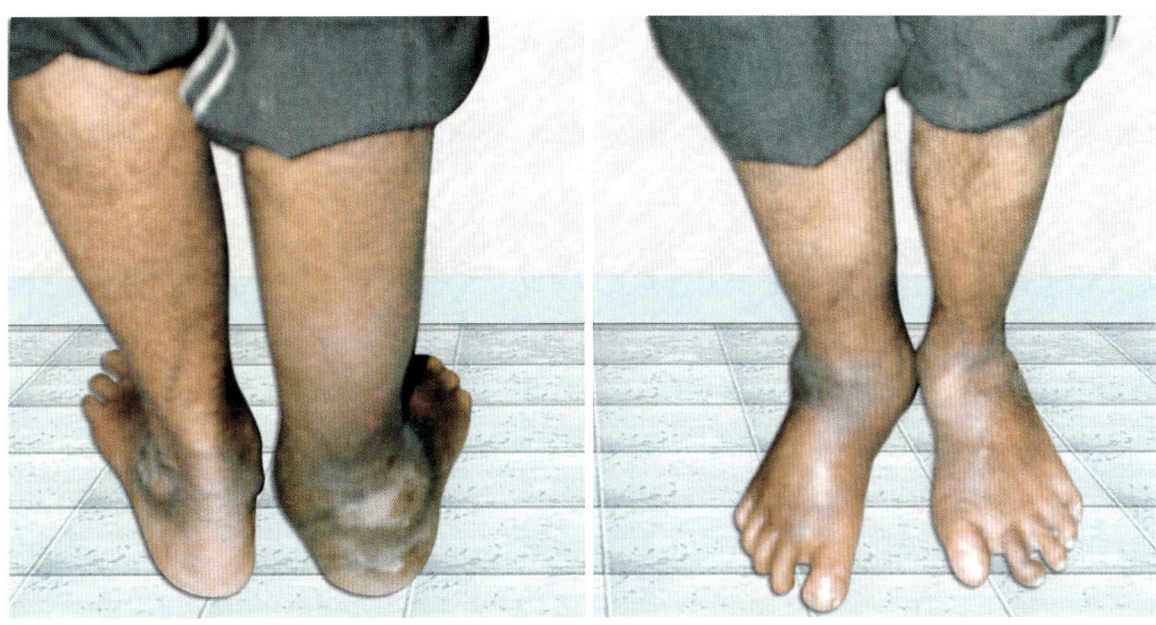

"Peace is not absence of conflict, it is the ability to handle conflict by peaceful means."
—*Ronald Reagan*

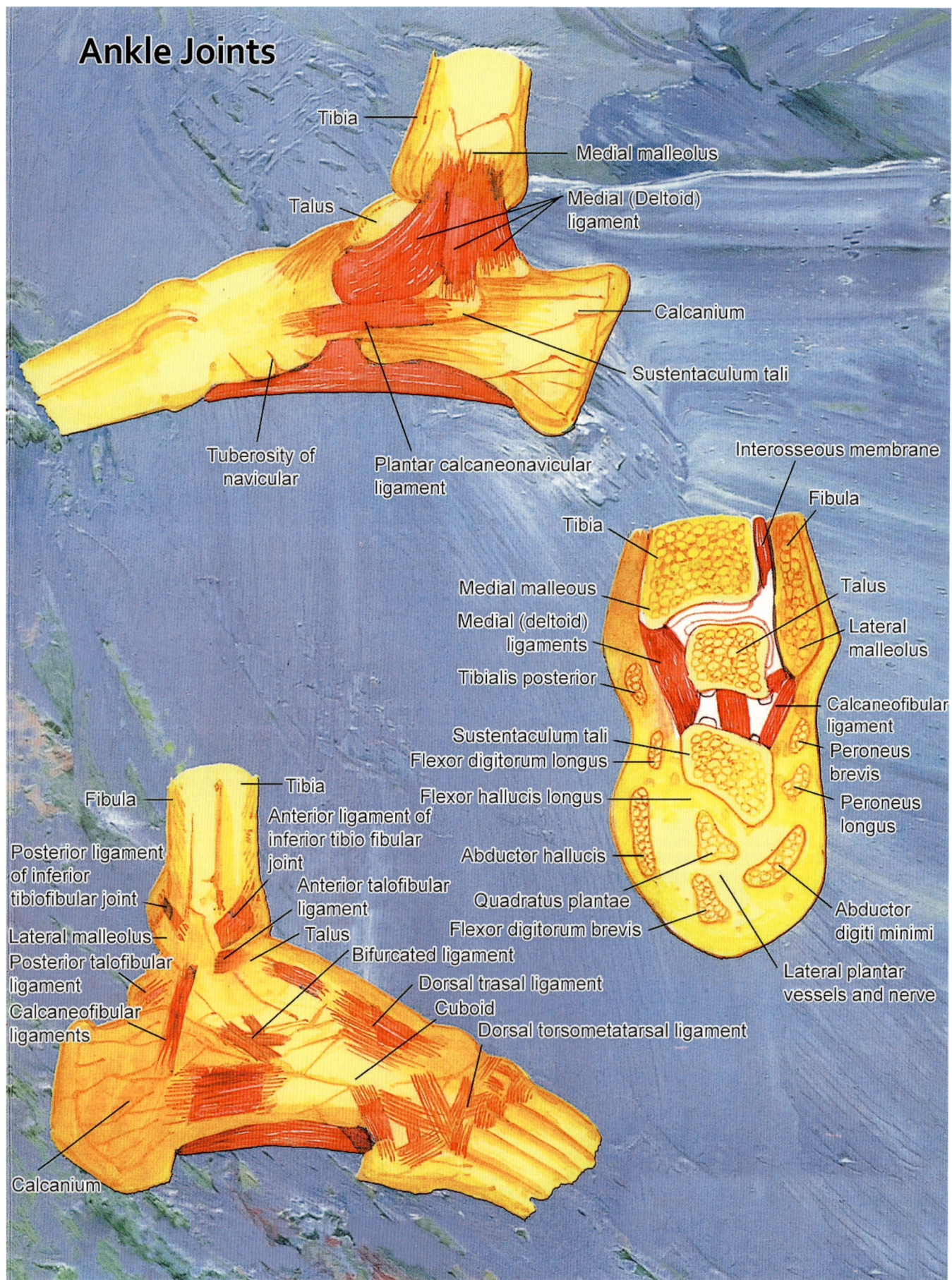

INTRODUCTION

In a biped, each normal ankle assumes the responsibility of transmitting at least 50% of the body weight to the tripod like structure of the foot in such a fashion that the rhythmic gait pattern is not disturbed.

ANATOMICAL CONSIDERATIONS

- Anatomically the ankle joint (a hinge joint) is the articulation of the dome of the talus into the *'ankle mortice.'* The integrity of the ankle mortice is mandatory for normal functioning of the joint.
  - *Ankle mortice is made up of* (a) bony and (b) soft-tissue components.
    - *Bony components are:*
      - Lower articular end of tibia
      - Articular surface on medial aspect of lateral malleolus
      - Articular surface on lateral aspect of medial malleolus.
    - *Soft tissue components are:*
      - Anterior inferior tibiofibular ligament
      - Posterior inferior tibiofibular ligament
      - Interosseous tibiofibular ligament
      - Inferior deep transverse ligament (i.e. the inferior lower and deep portion of the posterior tibiofibular ligament which is a strong thick yellowish band).

    The part of ligaments lying close to the bone have a more or less fibrocartilaginous texture.
- The ankle joint is peculiar in having no muscular coverage on any of the sides
- It has important controlling groups of tendons, almost all around. These are arranged as follows:
  - *Anteriorly:* From medial to lateral:
    - Tendon of tibialis anterior
    - Tendon of extensor hallucis longus
    - Anterior tibial artery and vein
    - Anterior tibial nerve
    - Tendon of extensor digitorum longus
    - Tendon of peroneus tertius.
  - These structures are strapped down by the superior and inferior ('Y'-shaped) extensor retinacula just above and at the ankle level. The extensor retinacula (cruciate crural—'Y'-shaped) is a thick non-complaint extension of the anterior fascia of the leg which restrains the extensor tendons passing in front of ankle and prevents bow stringing. Superior extensor retinaculum lies proximal to the ankle overlying the physis.
  - *On posteromedial aspect:* Below and behind the medial malleolus, the flexor retinaculum straps down the following structures *(from medial to lateral side).*
    - Tendon of tibialis posterior
    - Tendon of flexor digitorum longus
    - Posterior tibial artery and vein
    - Posterior tibial nerve
    - Tendon of flexor hallucis longus.
  - *Posteriorly*, just in the midline, is the stout tendinous mass of triceps surae (tendo-Achilles/tendocalcaneus). In between the posterior capsule of the joint and this tendon lies the slender tendon of plantaris
  - *On the posterolateral aspect* are the peroneus longus and peroneus brevis tendons in the peroneal sheath and they are strapped down by superior and inferior peroneal retinacula.
- The *synovial reflection of the ankle joint is not as complicated as that of the knee, but is intercommunicating with those of the other joints of the foot up to the tarsometatarsal joints.* The synovial swellings can be palpated on anteromedial, anterolateral, posteromedial and posterolateral aspects of the joint. It is not possible to approach the entire synovial reflections through a single incision.

  The tendons around the ankle are surrounded by the synovial sheaths, which are common sites of affection in tuberculosis and rheumatoid arthritis
- *Integrity of the ankle joint depends mainly on collateral ligaments.*
  - The *fan-shaped deltoid ligament is on the medial side.* It is attached superiorly to the tip of the medial malleolus and inferiorly, from in front-backwards, to the tuberosity of navicular, spring ligament, neck of talus, the sustentaculum tali and tubercle and body of talus. Thus, the components of deltoid ligament are the tibionavicular, anterior tibiotalar, tibiocalcaneal (superficial) and posterior tibiotalar (deep) ligaments. The deltoid ligament assists the spring ligament in holding up the head of the talus, and thus helps to maintain the medial longitudinal arch of the foot
  - *On the lateral side, the lateral ligament* consisting of the *three bands of anterior talofibular* (thinnest, flattened and most fragile), *calcaneofibular* (stronger, round and thicker), *and posterior talofibular* (very strong band), is responsible for maintaining a stout check on the ankle joint. Any disruption in these ligaments leads to sprain of the ankle joint. These ligaments are blended with the capsule of the ankle joint.

    Capsule is comparatively loose anteriorly and posteriorly to allow the plantar and dorsi-flexion movements. However, in extreme range of motion they get stretched and behave like check ligaments
  - The *tibiofibular syndesmosis comprises of four ligaments:* the interosseous tibiofibular, anterior and posterior inferior tibiofibular ligament and transverse tibiofibular ligament.
- The ankle forms the fulcrum at which the leg transmits the body weight to the foot. The foot remains in contact with the ground in standing, walking or running. When the foot

is caught either on uneven slope or in a pit hole/ditch, even a little imbalance of the body gets accentuated at the distal end of the long lever arm of leg leading to various fractures along with subluxation or dislocation at the ankle level. These have been grouped together as *"Pott's fracture"*.
- Within the contour of the ankle mortice, the dome of talus is equally vulnerable in the various injuries of the ankle joint. Besides the common sequelae of injuries, the *talus* is also *notorious for undergoing avascular necrosis* because of its comparatively precarious blood supply.

Tibiofibular torsion: The normal degree of tibiofibular rotation should be called as 'version' and the abnormal one as torsion (2 standard deviations from the mean, Staheli 1990). This fixed rotation of tibia is measured as the angle between an imaginary line passing through the tips of the medial and lateral malleoli of the ankle and the polar axis of the proximal articular surface of tibia (Helen et al. 2007).

Blood supply of talus **(Fig. 14.1)**: The *main sources of blood supply to the talus* are:
- Posterior tibial artery
- Anterior tibial artery
- Peroneal artery.

The branches of these arteries are mainly grouped under two headings:
1. Through anterior capsule of ankle joint, blood vessels enter anterosuperior portion of neck of talus
2. The blood vessels coming through the sinus tarsi (tarsal canal) enter from the inferior surface of the neck of talus.

Very few blood vessels enter the posteroinferior portion of the body of talus.
- Head of the talus is supplied by vessels entering:
  - The superior surface of neck
  - The inferolateral surface of neck
- Body of talus is supplied by vessels entering through:
  - The superior surface of neck
  - The anteroinferior surface of neck
  - Medial surface of body
  - Anterolateral surface of body
  - Posterior tubercle.

In any disruption of the anterior capsule of the ankle joint (e.g. fracture dislocation of ankle joint), the blood supply is likely to suffer, resulting in variable avascular necrosis of talus

- The *main blood vessels going to the foot,* i.e. anterior tibial and posterior tibial arteries, are very closely related, anteriorly and posteromedially respectively, to the capsule of the ankle joint. Therefore, major injuries of ankle joint, specially dislocations are likely to press, partially damage or even disrupt the main blood supply, thereby threatening the circulation of the foot
- The skin is very closely disposed over the bony contours almost all around the ankle joint. In dislocation of the ankle joint or similar injuries, the skin gets devitalised due to pressure or overstretch, and may undergo necrosis.

■ METHODOLOGY OF CLINICAL EXAMINATION

History

History taking is as in the *Chapter 1: Introduction*. The main complaints following any trauma or disease in the ankle are pain, swelling, limp, instability and deformity.

General and Systemic Examination

As in the *Chapter 1: Introduction*.

Any affection of the ankle is likely to affect the gait and posture of the patient. Hence, if it is possible, patient should be asked to walk first, as normally as possible, then on the heels and toes alternately. While standing, if possible, note the posture and mode of weight bearing at the affected ankle and foot. Each step of examination must be compared with that of opposite ankle, however, if both are affected, findings should be noted separately.

Footwear should be routinely examined in any affection of ankle and foot (*See* **Fig. 14.31**).

Regional Examination

It should be done from tip of the toes to the hip.

It is always paying to examine the leg as a whole along with the ankle, e.g. even ligamentous disruption at the ankle can be associated with fracture of upper end of the fibula—*Maisonneuve (injury) fracture*.

Effects of Ankle Pathology on Regional Joints

Deformities in and around ankle produce early degenerative changes in it and also affects other joints of foot. Valgus

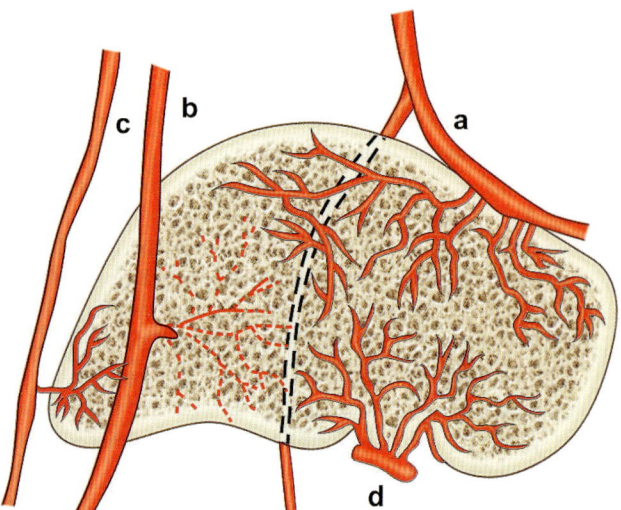

Fig. 14.1: Blood supply of talus. (a = anterior tibial artery; b = posterior tibial artery; c = peroneal artery; d = vessels coming through sinus tarsi).

deformities of ankle lead to secondary varus at subtalar joint and supination of forefoot, and varus deformity on the other hand produces secondary valgus at the subtalar joint and pronation of forefoot.

As already considered while dealing with the knee, various deformities at the knees are likely to affect the ankle, hip and spine and *vice versa.* Further, ankle has to act as a buffer in any affection of the foot and balance weight transmission at the knee. To avoid pain at the ankle due to any pathology, the patient tries to manoeuvre the intrinsics of the foot, which in turn either produce various clawing effects, or fanning out tendency of the toes. When the muscles controlling the smaller joints of the foot are paralysed, the main brunt falls on the ankle. On the other hand, when ankle movements are affected, the smaller joints of the foot try to accommodate as far as practicable, e.g. if plantar flexion at the ankle is lost, either due to any pathology or following arthrodesis, the mid-tarsal, sub-talar and even tarsometatarsal joints provide for varying amount of compensatory workable flexion of the foot.

Except in paralytic conditions (where the overpowering muscles determine the deformities), the ankle has the tendency of postural fixity in the possible position of walking, whereas the smaller joints accommodate to compensate for the loss of ankle movements. Therefore, the overall assessment of the foot and ankle must be done simultaneously.

Varicosities

Blowing out (dilatation with tortuosity) of the venous channels on the medial side of the ankle should be looked for. The integrity of the deeper valves of the veins in the legs and thighs should be tested for. These varicosities may be responsible for pain around the ankle joint. There may be discolouration of the skin, chronic ulcers and sometimes troublesome bleeding from the ulcers.

Oedema Around the Ankle

Ankle is the site of oedematous swelling from various causes, ranging from postural oedema (feet remaining dependent, hanging for longer period), congenital lymphoedema to neoplastic compression. In medical conditions like anaemia, hypoproteinaemia, filariasis, cirrhosis of liver, congestive cardiac failure, nephrotic syndrome, oedema around the ankle and lower leg may be the first sign. Oedema due to posture, pregnancy and pelvic pathology should also be kept in mind. The nature (pitting or non-pitting) and extent of oedema should be noted.

Examination of Lymph Glands

Palpate the lymph glands in the popliteal fossa and inguinal region and also the external iliac group and note their character.

Local Examination

Inspection

Attitude: Typical attitudes (as described in the Chapter 15: Foot) should be looked for **(Figs. 14.2 and 14.3)**.

The attitude of the foot and ankle can also give a clue to the mode of injury and displacement in different types of Pott's fracture.

In most of the pathologies of the ankle, this region is swollen all around. Any swelling of the tendon sheath appears along the long axis of leg and foot beyond the joint level.

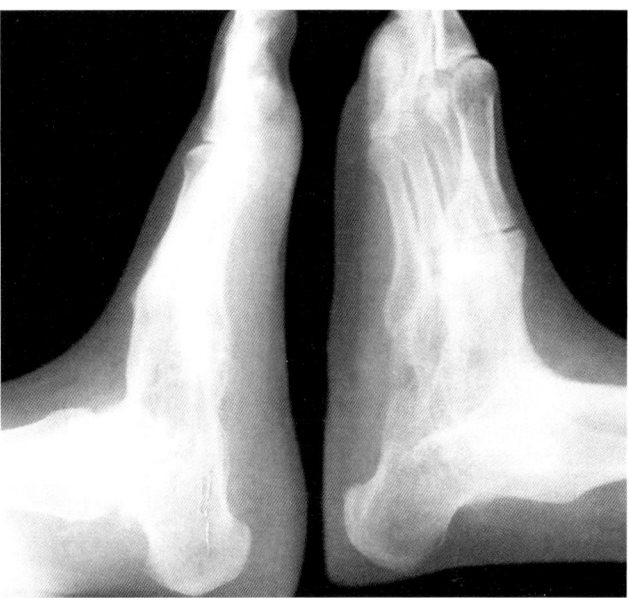

Fig. 14.2: X-ray of congenital solid ankle-feet. Does not require any treatment.

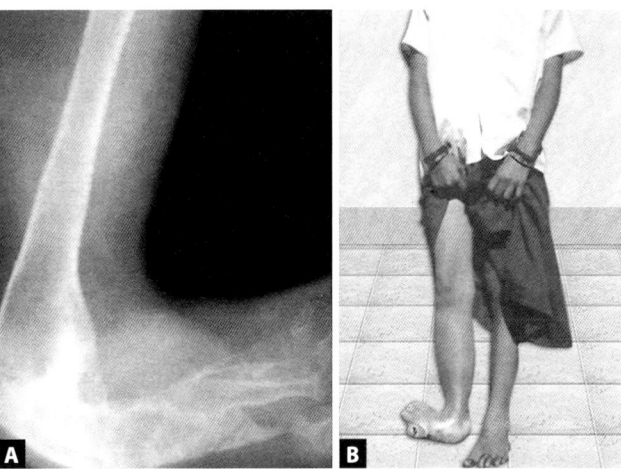

Figs. 14.3A and B: (A) X-ray of leg, ankle and foot of 10 years aged girl with completely fused ankle and foot joints in grossly deformed position due to severely crushed injury at the age of 2 years; (B) Same patient six months after possible correction—in first stage nearly plantigrade foot. The parents not ready for any further surgery.

Keep both ankles and feet in identical position. Inspect systematically from anterior, lateral, posterior and medial sides.

Anteriorly, note the following:
- Relation of the foot to ankle (normal, equinus, calcaneus, valgus and varus)
- Interrelation of the malleoli *(normally the lateral malleolus lies 1 cm below and behind the medial malleolus)* **(Figs. 14.4A and B)**
- Long saphenous vein
- Anterior group of tendons
- Fossae in front of the malleoli (which may be full in swelling of ankle)
- Any abnormal finding, like swelling, sinus, etc.

Laterally, note the following: The tendons of peroneus longus and brevis lie just behind the lateral malleolus. Note if they are prominent. From here, there is a gradual shallow concavity posteriorly up to the fossa on the outer side of the tendo-Achilles (tendo-calcaneus). Note any abnormal finding. Low-lying peroneus muscles bellies, though uncommon and asymptomatic, may produce painful posterolateral ankle impingement pain, which can be treated by surgical excision of low-lying muscle fibers in the peroneal groove.

Posteriorly, note the following:
- Prominence of tendo-Achilles, along with the calf bulk
- Any swelling in relation to tendo-Achilles
- Fossae on both sides of tendo-Achilles
- Pattern, position and size of heel, (broadening or narrowing; tugged up or plantigrade or splashed out; normal, small or large in size).

Medially, note the following: Medial malleolus (its shape, size, placement, prominence—compare with other normal side; surface—smooth, irregular). Tibialis posterior tendon lies just adapted to the posteroinferior margin of the medial malleolus—note if it is prominent. From here, up to the fossa on the medial side of tendo-Achilles, a gradual shallow concavity is maintained. Note any abnormality.

Posterior tibial tendon dysfunction usually occurs in women (40–60 years old). It may be associated with flat foot deformity, obesity, rheumatoid arthritis, etc. Pain and swelling occur along the medial aspect of ankle. Patients cannot stand tip-toe (on their toes) due to pain and/or weakness.

Palpation

- *Superficial (touch):* In superficial palpation, surface and texture of skin, temperature and any superficial tenderness, anaesthesia, hypoaesthesia or paraesthesia is to be noted
- *Deep palpation (feel):* It is not easy to palpate the joint margins of the ankle joint all around. Palpate the malleoli and feel for any thickening, tenderness, and irregularity and also note the relation between two malleoli. Palpate and assess individually the tendons around the ankle joint starting from one side. Note their position and continuity and feel for any thickening. Assess their excursion, power of parent muscle and spasm if any. Note any tenderness, synovial swelling and ganglion along their course. On the posterior side, the presence of a soft to firm swelling in relation to the tendo-Achilles is not uncommon. Usually, it manifests anterior to the tendo-Achilles as *pre-Achilles bursitis (retrocalcaneal bursitis)*—inflammation of bursa between Achilles tendon and calcaneum or posterior to it as *post-Achilles bursitis, or preadventitial Achilles bursitis— pump bump.* Usually, it develops due to rubbing from shoe wear.

Palpate for *anterior tibial arterial pulsation* in between the tendons of extensor hallucis longus and extensor digitorum longus, i.e. at about midway between the malleoli **(Fig. 14.5)**, which may be absent congenitally, or weakly felt.

Palpate for *posterior tibial arterial pulsation* behind the tendon of flexor digitorum longus, i.e. one finger breadth

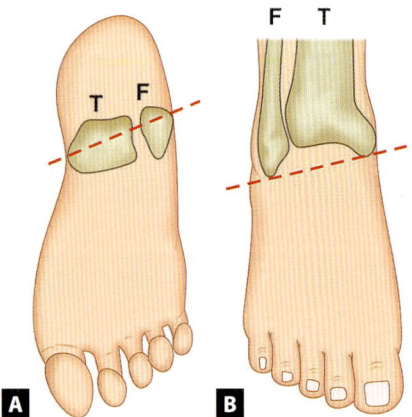

Figs. 14.4A and B: Intermalleolar relation. Note that the tip of lateral malleolus (F-fibula) is distal and posterior to the medial malleolus (T-tibia) in Figure 14.4B.

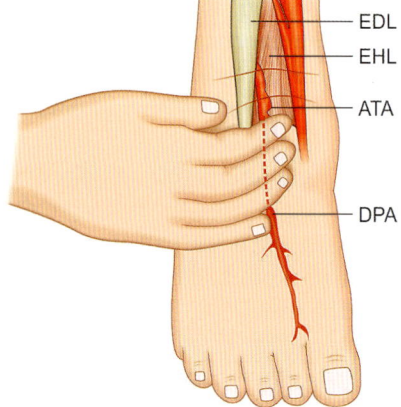

Fig. 14.5: Palpating the anterior tibial artery. (ATA: anterior tibial artery; EHL: extensor hallucis longus; EDL: extensor digitorum longus; DPA: dorsalis pedis artery).

behind the medial malleolus. **(Fig. 14.6)**, which may be congenitally absent or too feeble.

Any synovial swelling or fluid in the ankle joint usually manifests as outpouchings around the ankle, mainly on the posterolateral, posteromedial, anterolateral and anteromedial aspects. Synovial swellings are soft and doughy in feel. It is probably impossible to demonstrate the presence of a small amount of fluid in the ankle joint. In presence of moderate to large amount of fluid, cross-fluctuation can be demonstrated.

Method of demonstration of cross-fluctuation in between the anterolateral and anteromedial swellings **(Fig. 14.7)**; And posterolateral and posteromedial swellings **(Fig. 14.8)**.

Plantar flex the ankle joint as far as practicable. The dorsal tendons form tight longitudinal straps across the ankle joint. Place both index fingers in front of both malleoli. On pressing from one side, the contralateral finger will feel the impulse in presence of fluid in the ankle joint **(Fig. 14.7)**. Similarly, in between the posterolateral and posteromedial pouchings, fluctuation can be demonstrated if the ankle is kept dorsiflexed **(Fig. 14.8)**.

Mode of demonstration of cross-fluctuation in between anterior and posterior swellings **(Fig. 14.9)**.

Ankle should be placed in as much neutral position as possible. The index finger and thumb of one hand are placed anterior to the malleoli. Index finger and thumb of the opposite hand are placed on either side of the tendo-Achilles at slightly lower level. Now, simultaneous pressure by the finger and thumb of one hand propels the fluid to the opposite compartment and, therefore, an impulse is felt by the fingers of the opposite hand.

Due to circuitous disposition of the ankle, transillumination is usually not positive. However, when the amount of fluid is large, the distended joint is so tense that cross-fluctuation may not be demonstrable effectively. Here, transillumination may be positive. Transillumination may also be positive if done from anterolateral to anteromedial

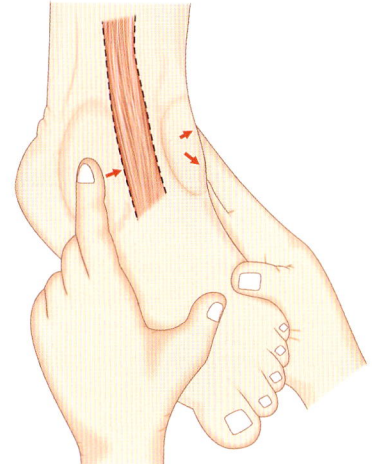

Fig. 14.7: Cross-fluctuation between anterolateral and anteromedial swelling.

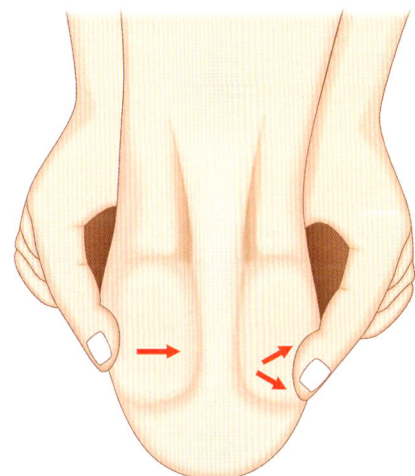

Fig. 14.8: Cross-fluctuation between posteromedial and posterolateral swellings.

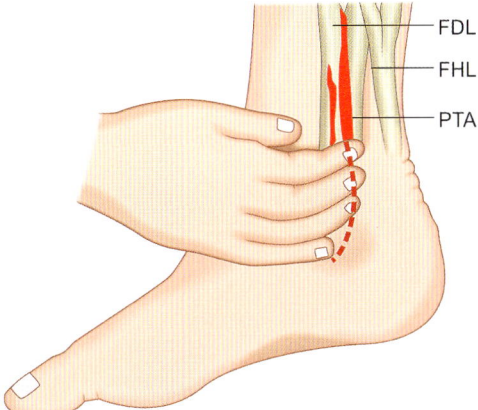

Fig. 14.6: Palpating the posterior tibial artery. (PTA, posterior tibial artery; FDL, flexor digitorum longus; FHL, flexor hallucis longus).

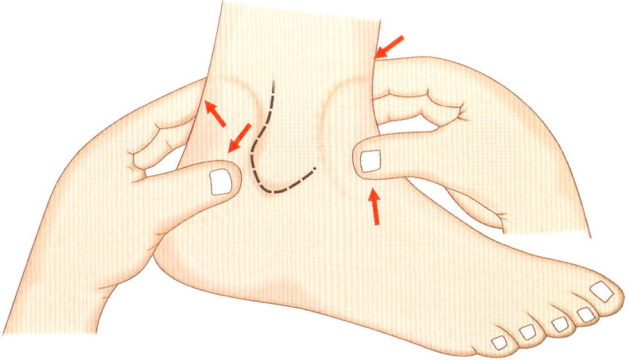

Fig. 14.9: Cross-fluctuation between anterior and posterior pouchings.

or from posterolateral to posteromedial out pouchings (and *vice versa*).

■ MOVEMENTS

Normal movements at the ankle (from 0-position of the ankle, i.e. in right angled position) are:
- *Dorsiflexion (15°–30°):* When the joint is dorsiflexed, the widest anterior part of the talus is wedged tightly between the two malleoli providing sound stability to the joint. Dorsiflexion of foot exerts traction on posterior tibial vein and in case of thrombosis of calf veins, passive dorsiflexion of foot causes pain in the calf—*Homan's sign*
- *Plantar flexion (30°–50°):* In fully plantar flexed position of the ankle, the posterior and narrowest part of the dome of talus articulates with the ankle mortice. In this position, some side-to-side rocking and inversion/eversion of the ankle can be passively demonstrated. Movements should be assessed under different headings, as in the Chapter 1: Introduction. While testing for passive movements at the ankle, stress movements at the ankle should be done to confirm the integrity of the controlling collateral ligaments. Of course, it is better to test dorsiflexion, plantar flexion and stress movements at both ankle joints simultaneously for comparison.

Method

Patient sits on the edge of the bed or examination table keeping his knees bent about 90° and both his legs and feet hanging down the edge of the table. Sitting on one side of the patient, support the lower part of the legs from behind. Patient is then asked to alternately dorsiflex and plantar flex both the ankles simultaneously from the zero position (i.e. foot at 90° to the leg axis). Note the excursion of the hind foot in either direction in both feet (**Fig. 14.10**). Then, holding the mid and fore parts of the foot by another hand, dorsiflex and plantar flex the foot passively, at ankle level, and note the additions possible over the active range.

Assessment for Lateral Collapse of Ankle

The paralytic foot most commonly goes for valgus in various combinations. *Valgus collapse at the ankle* becomes quite apparent when the patient bears weight on that foot (**Figs. 14.11A and B**). Cosmetically, it is ugly and difficult to correct. *It should be assessed separately from valgus at the subtalar joint.*

Method (Fig. 14.12)

Assess the extent of passive valgus at the normal foot under maximum possible stress. In neutral position of the ankle and foot, hold the ankle from dorsum, in between the thumb and index finger. Your first web should firmly grip the dorsum of the talus. Hold the heel, i.e. the body of the calcaneum in between the thumb and index finger of the opposite hand. While the first hand remains firmly static, passively evert and invert the heel as much as possible, using the other hand. This will assess the movements at the subtalar joint. Total valgus of the affected foot, minus the possible valgus at the subtalar

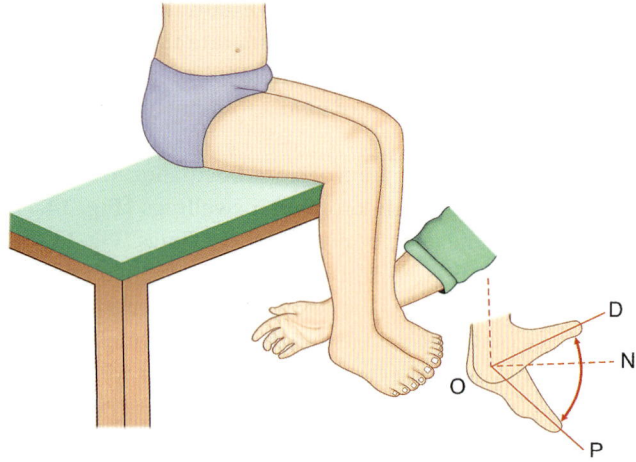

Fig. 14.10: Demonstration of active dorsiflexion and plantar flexion at ankle.

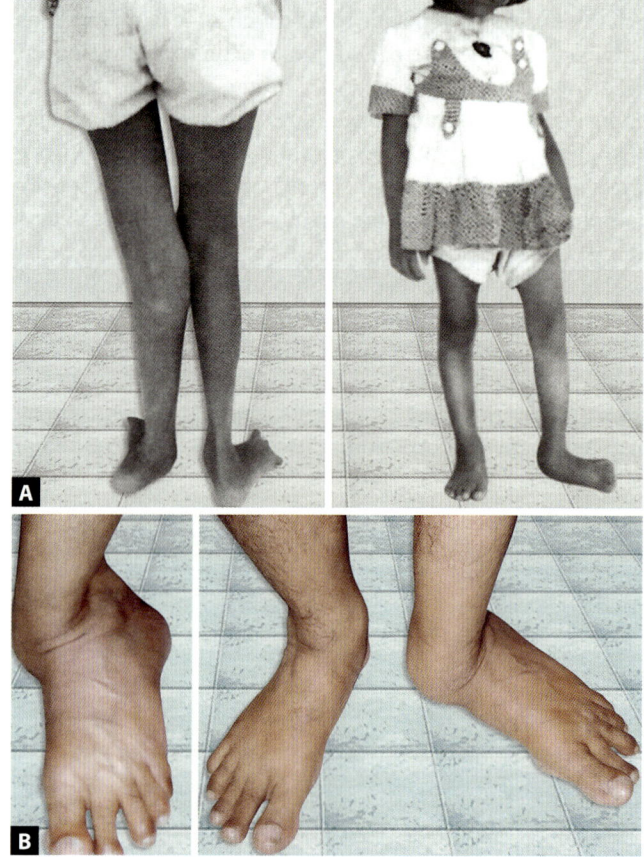

Figs. 14.11A and B: Note the early valgus collapse at ankle besides the valgus at subtalar joint should be treated by 'T' osteotomy of calcaneum and tendon transfer – peroneus longus or even peronei to medial side of foot. In neglected cases or failed cases after surgery—should be treated by arthrodesis of ankle.

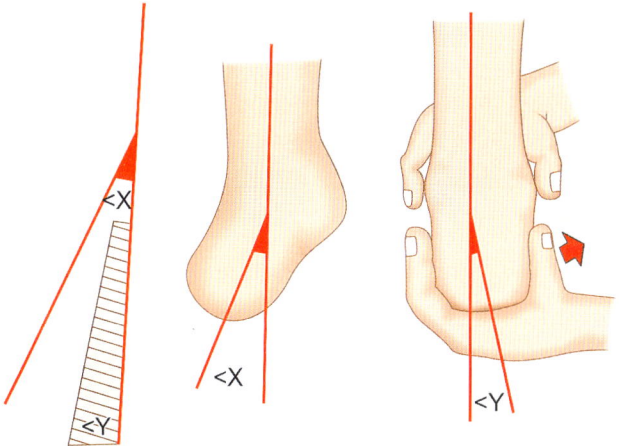

Fig. 14.12: Method of measuring the valgus collapse at the ankle: angle 'Y' denotes the valgus at subtalar joint, angle 'X' denotes total valgus of foot, so X—Y = valgus collapse at ankle.

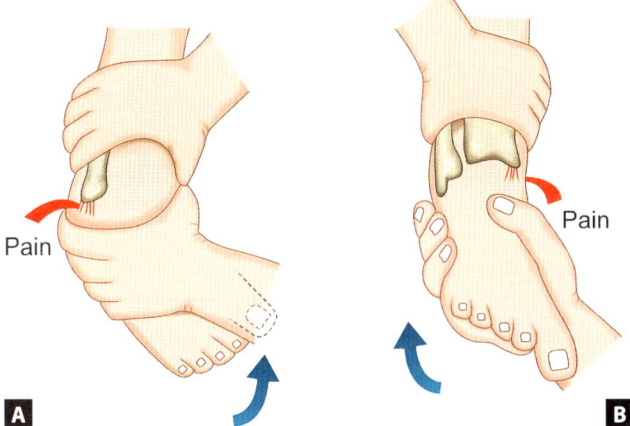

Figs. 14.13A and B: Testing the integrity of (A) lateral and (B) medial collateral ligaments of ankle.

joint will be the valgus collapse at the ankle. Similarly, varus collapse of the ankle (rare condition) can also be assessed. Early stage varies ankle arthritis can usually be treated by the medial open-wedge valgus distal tibial osteotomy for restoring alignment of the hindfoot.

Critical Arc

15° plantar flexion to 15° dorsiflexion (from 0° position, i.e. neutral right-angled position of the foot) *is the critical arc for the ankle.* This is because an average 15° plantar flexion at the ankle is the minimum required for push off phase of the gait. On the other hand, about 15° of dorsiflexion is the minimum required for deceleration to heel strike phase of gait and squatting.

Abnormal Movements

In paralytic and neuropathic ankle and feet and Charcot's arthropathy, abnormal movements are possible. Each type of abnormal movement should be noted separately.

Stress Test (To Assess Integrity of the Controlling Group of Ligaments)

Method (Figs. 14.13A and B)

Place the ankle in neutral position. Hold the lower leg firmly from the front, by one hand. Hold the foot at about the level of the head of talus by the opposite hand. For testing the lateral collateral ligaments **(Fig. 14.13A)**, invert the foot forcibly (within limit of pain tolerance) and note:
- The yield of the foot
- The gap in front of, and beneath and behind the lateral malleolus
- The point of maximum pain
- The range of inversion possible at the ankle.

For testing the integrity of the medial collateral ligament (i.e. deltoid ligament), stress has to be given in the opposite direction. Holding the lower leg in the same position, the foot is everted and the aforesaid points are noted in relation to the medial malleolus **(Fig. 14.13B)**.

Stress tests, for integrity of anterior and posterior ligaments, i.e. capsular reinforcements, are not that important. However, they can be noted as exaggeration of passive dorsiflexion and plantar flexion of the ankle (in laxity or tear of the posterior and anterior capsular reinforcements, respectively).

Anteroposterior Stress Test of Ankle (Brostrom-1965)—Anterior Drawer Sign

The integrity of the capsule and the anterior talofibular ligament (sometimes calcaneofibular ligament as well) can be tested by pulling the heel anteromedially against resistance applied by the other hand over the anterior aspect of the lower leg. *Anterior subluxation of 3 mm of the talus is pathological.*

Special Test

Injury to gastrocnemius and soleus: Both muscles insert into tendo-Achilles. Sudden forceful, dorsiflexion of foot loads both muscles and extension of knee additionally loads the *gastrocnemius.*

Gastrocnemius tear occurs due to sudden forceful ankle (foot) dorsiflexion along with extension of knee. Patient feels sudden pain in about mid-calf region (mainly in posteromedial aspect) especially while walking. The tender palpable defect may be felt in gastrocnemius belly. The power of plantar flexion of ankle diminishes. The ecchymoses usually develops in and below the ruptured region to a variable extent.

Soleus tear may occur due to sudden extreme dorsiflexion of ankle (foot), which produces severe pain and tenderness in the mid-calf region.

Rupture of tendo-Achilles (Figs. 14.14A and B)

Tendo-Achilles formed by a confluence of fibers derived from the gastrocnemius and soleus muscles, is the strongest and second longest (on an average 15 cm long) tendon of the body. It has no true synovial sheath, but it is enveloped by paratenon (a thin membranous tissue). Achilles, the Greek hero, was the son of Peleus and Thetis. When he was a child his mother dipped him in the river Styx by holding his heel to make him invincible in battle. But the heel, by which he was held did not get wet, and so it remained unprotected. Achilles died after receiving an injury in the heel at the siege of Troy.

The *Achilles tendon usually ruptures 2 to 6 cm proximal to its insertion in os calcis,* where the tendon is ischaemic and weaker than normal. It occurs usually in middle aged men as a result of any trivial stumble or a sudden painful snap during walking or negotiating stairs or jumping, or recreational athletic activities.

After rupture dorsiflexion of foot can be done more than normal. Plantar flexion reduces, but never completely even with complete rupture of the tendo-Achilles, since some active plantar flexion is maintained by the combined action of tibialis posterior, long flexors of toes and peroneum longus and brevis.

Test for Rupture of Tendo-Achilles (Figs. 14.15A and B):
Ask the patient to *stand on tip toe. In case of weak tendo-Achilles, there will be a lag in lifting the heel.* In case of partial rupture, the patient will also complain of pain at the site. In complete rupture, the lag will be much more, but standing on tip toe is never completely absent (since some power of plantar flexion exists due to intact tibialis posterior, long flexors of toes, and peroneus longus and brevis). Along with this, *a gap can also be felt at the rupture site* (Fig. 14.14A) in which one can insinuate the examining finger. At both ends of the gap the *rounded ends of the ruptured tendon* can be felt in late cases. In late neglected cases, the ends feel like adder heads.

Thompson's Test (1962)/Simmond's Test (Figs. 14.16A and B):
Patient is asked to lie prone with his feet projecting beyond the examining table. On squeezing the calf muscles transversely, the foot automatically plantar flexes, if tendo-Achilles is intact or even partially torn. However, in complete rupture flexion is not possible, hence there is no movement of the foot. A gap can be felt at the rupture site in the tendon. The distal portion of tendon is thicker and less taut, and the calf muscles are shortened as a visible lump.

X-ray: In true lateral view of ankle and foot, taken in maximum possible plantar flexion, the rugosities at the back of ankle will be lacking; and if taken in maximum dorsiflexion, the soft tissue lining at the back of the ankle will be more or less vertical and close to the bone with marked calcaneus effect of the foot **(Fig. 14.14B)**.

O'Brien's Needle Test:
Tim O'Brien by performing his "needle test" to dynamically assess the integrity of distal 10 cm of tendo-Achilles has reported very reliable results.

Method: The patient lies prone. Under aseptic conditions, a 25 gauge hypodermic needle is pierced through the skin at a point 10 cm above the upper end of calcaneum and just medial to the midline of the calf. The foot is then passively plantar flexed and dorsiflexed. With intact tendo-Achilles, the needle will swivel in a direction opposite to the movement of the foot. Absence of this swivelling indicates complete rupture of the tendo-Achilles.

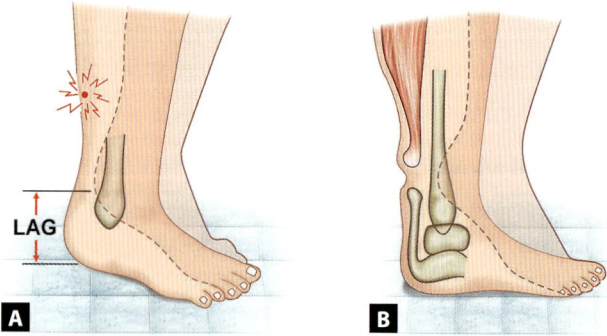

Figs. 14.15A and B: (A) Test for assessing partial rupture of tendo-Achilles; (B) Test for assessing complete rupture of tendo-Achilles.

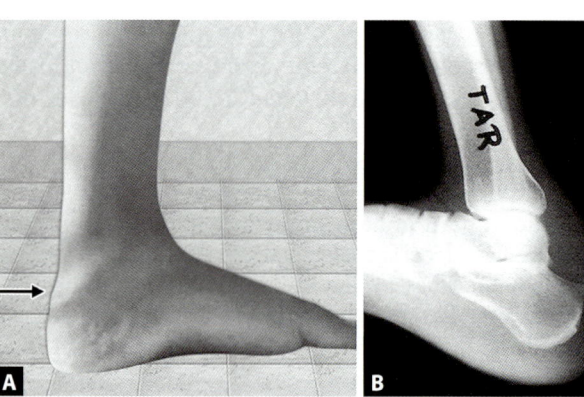

Figs. 14.14A and B: (A) Clinical photograph and (B) X-ray showing complete rupture of tendo-Achilles. It should be operated to repair the tear and reconstruct the gap.

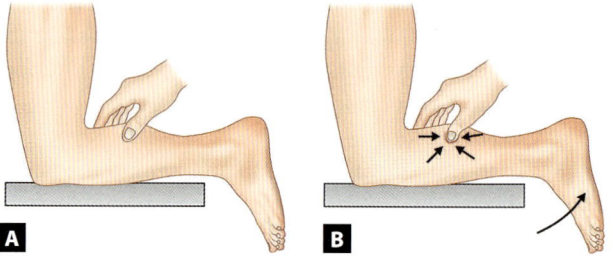

Figs. 14.16A and B: Thompson's test.

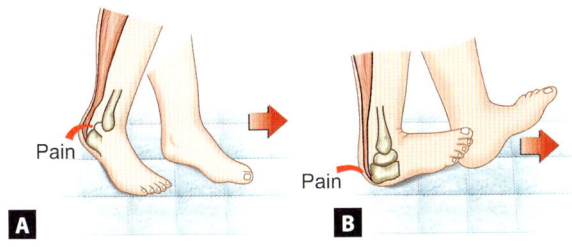

Figs. 14.17A and B: (A) Test for pre-Achilles pathology; (B) Test for post-Achilles pathology.

Test for Pre-Achilles and Post-Achilles Pathologies (Mainly Bursitis) and Achilles Tendinitis (Figs. 17A and B)

The patient is asked to walk on his toes (with the heel off the ground). He will complain of pain in case of pre-Achilles pathology. The patient is then asked to walk on the heel (with the toes off the ground). There will be pain in post-Achilles pathology.

In Achilles tendinitis, pain will be in both mode of walking, but will be more on walking on the toes.

A short tendon or repeated forceful contractions (e.g. in jumping, running, tennis or volleyball playing, etc.) may cause Achilles tendinitis.

Clinical features are: Pain in and around the tendon, which increases after exercises; gradually increasing morning pain and stiffness in the ankle region and heel develop; forceful plantar flexion against resistance aggravates the symptoms; tendon is tender on squeezing.

It may be confused with pre- and post-Achilles bursitis, stress fractures of tibia and fibula, peroneal tendinitis, Achilles tendinopathy.

Management protocol should avoid corticoid infiltration, since it is liable to produce rupture of the tendo-Achilles.

However, in the chronic pain in the retrocalcaneal space, in which if non-operative treatment (such as heel-raise in footwear, NSAIDs, ultrasonic, physiotherapy, hot-cold bath, etc.) fails, endoscopic decompression is feasible and efficient procedure rather than open surgical decompression.

Test for Tendovaginitis of Tibialis Posterior Tendon (Fig. 14.18)

Patient sits with his legs hanging from the edge of the table. Ask him to plantar flex his foot to the maximum and then invert it against resistance. Pain will be complained behind the medial malleolus. At the same site there may be a tender and soft/firm thickening palpable along the tibialis posterior tendon.

Test for Peroneal Spasm (Fig. 14.19)

Patient sits with legs hanging over the edge of the table. Ask him to plantar flex and invert the foot. There will be marked limitations. Forced inversion will lead to pain behind the lateral malleolus.

Shin splints (Anterior leg pain): This problem is mostly faced by young athletes due to poor conditioning for the event, over-exercises/activities, sudden change in the pattern of sport event. Repetitive traction by anterior and posterior tibialis muscles on the edges of the tibia leads to diffuse linear pain along the anterior or medial edge of the mid-shaft or distal one-third of tibia. There is diffuse tenderness along the origin of anterior or posterior tibialis muscles. There may be decrease in the power of dorsiflexors of ankle and foot.

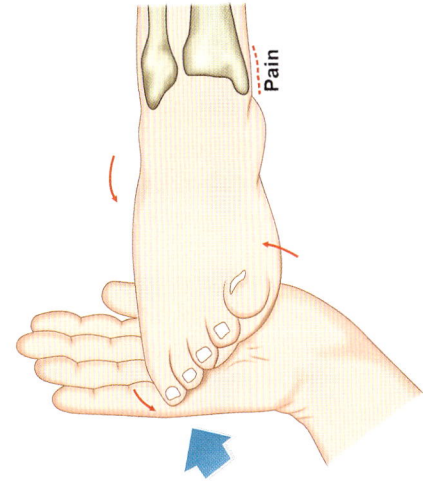

Fig. 14.18: Test for tendovaginitis of tibialis posterior tendon.

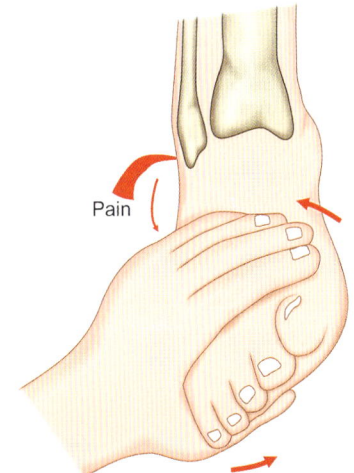

Fig. 14.19: Test for peroneal spasm.

Test to Elicit Anterolateral Synovial Impingement in Ankle (after Molloy et al. 2003)

Chronic pain after inversion sprain of ankle is quite common, of course due to several causes. The synovial hypertrophy and synovial impingement are common differential diagnosis in chronic ankle pain and a feeling of instability. Different modes of radiological imaging (including MRI) are usually not specific for diagnosing soft-tissue impingement in the ankle. However, certain well-performed clinical test can prove to be very useful.

Test to Diagnose Synovial Hypertrophy

For testing at the left ankle the examiner standing at the edge of the examination table, holds the patient's left heel by his right hand in such a way that fingers are placed on the calcaneal tuberosity and thumb over the anterolateral part of ankle (lateral gutter). By his left hand, the examiner grasps the forefoot and plantar flexes the ankle while applying pressure over the lateral gutter by the thumb. If there will be synovial hypertrophy the patient will feel pain due to pressure on it. Thumb is then removed and ankle is dorsiflexed. The extent of dorsiflexion of ankle remains limited as compared to normal side.

To elicit the synovial impingement sign, both the manoeuvres are combined: While maintaining the thumb pressure over the lateral gutter in plantar flexed position of ankle, the foot is dorsiflexed to full extent. In this manoeuvre, the hypertrophied synovium is forced into the ankle joint by the examiner's thumb and is subsequently get impinged between the neck of talus and distal end of tibia in maximum dorsiflexed position. If these combined manoeuvres produce pain or increases the existing pain produced by the thumb pressure on the lateral gutter it indicates *positive ankle impingement sign.* If the pain is not increased, the sign is negative.

While testing for the right ankle, the hands should be reversed.

Arthroscopic debridement of soft tissue impingement is usually very effective treatment.

■ MEASUREMENTS

Linear Measurement

Affection of the ankle as such is comparatively less responsible for producing limb length disparity. However, severe injuries, advanced tuberculous and pyogenic infections, neoplasms and dyschondroplasia in the ankle region are likely to affect the length of the limb. Chronic pyogenic osteomyelitis of lower end of tibia and fibula has been seen to produce limb length disparity (increase in length more frequently than shortening).

Method

Total and segmental measurements of lower limb should be done as in the examination of hip and knee. The distance between the tip of medial malleolus to the sole (along a line dropped vertically from the medial malleolus) indicates roughly the height of talus, calcaneum and heel pad. Affection of any of these can produce disparity in this measurement.

Circumferential Measurement (Fig. 14.20)

It should be done at the level of ankle joint and mid-calf. The first indicates any increase or decrease in girth of the ankle, whereas the latter measures any increase or decrease of the muscular bulk at the mid-calf level.

Oblique Circumferential Measurement (Figs. 14.21A to C)

It should be done across the point of the heel and front of the ankle. In calcaneus deformity, this will be increased, whereas in equinus deformity, it will be decreased.

Auscultation

It is not important, but suspected swelling around the ankle should be auscultated.

Power

The power of the controlling muscles must be tested and charted separately according to MRC scale. Intrinsic muscles of the foot should also be tested, as they are likely to be variably affected in ankle involvements and *vice-versa.*

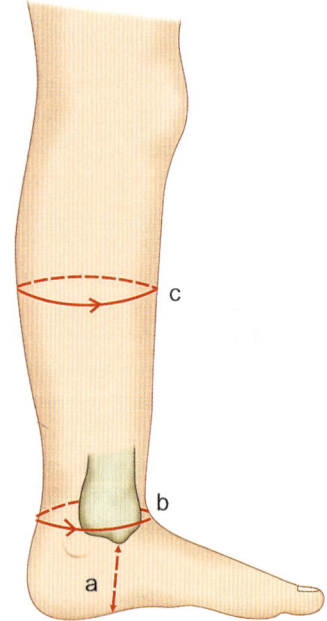

Fig. 14.20: (a) Vertical height of talus + calcaneum + heel pad, (b) Circumferential measurement around ankle, and (c) Circumferential measurement at the mid-calf level.

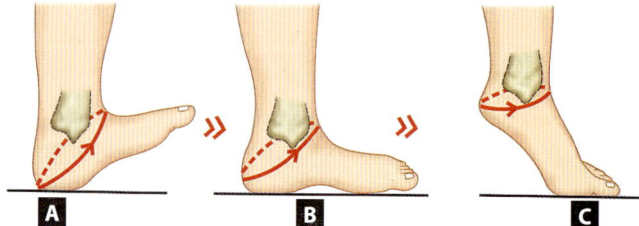

Figs. 14.21A to C: Oblique circumferential measurement across the ankle in (A) calcaneus, (B) normal, (C) equinus positions.

- May be accompanying fracture of the base of the 5th metatarsal
- Stress radiography, putting the feet in maximum possible inversion, should be done to assess the tear of the lateral collateral ligaments of the ankle. In anteroposterior view—there may be avulsion of the tip of the lateral malleolus.
- *In eversion sprain:* Maximum tenderness at the upper attachment of deltoid ligament, i.e. just below and around the tip of the medial malleolus. Swelling is also more in the same region. X-ray may show avulsion of the tip of the medial malleolus.

Anterior impingement syndrome (first described by LH Morris in 1943 and *posterior compression syndrome* (Footballer's ankle—The term coined by TP McMurray in 1950).

Anterior impingement, a common cause of pain and a feeling of instability in ankle is mostly seen in athletes, who overuse their ankle in forced dorsiflexion (leading to recurrent microtrauma—haemorrhage—scarring—new bone formation (spurs) at the anterior aspect of ankle. The clinical "*ankle impingement sign*" is useful in diagnosing this condition. To elicit it, the examiner standing at the edge of the examination table, holds the patients left heel by his right hand in such a way that fingers are placed on the calcaneal tuberosity and the thumb over the anterolateral part of ankle (lateral gutter). By left hand the examiner grasps the forefoot and plantar flexes the ankle, while applying pressure by his right thumb at the lateral gutter, the patient feels pain due to pressure on hypertrophied synovium. The thumb is removed and the foot is dorsiflexed, the range of which is comparatively reduced.

To demonstrate the ankle impingement sign both manoeuvres are combined (as already described on Page 425) anterior impingement syndrome (synovial impingement).

Recurrent subluxation of peroneal tendon (more of peroneus longus) is relatively uncommon sports injury. Acute dislocations of peroneal tendon occur in forceful dorsiflexion of ankle while peroneal muscle is in strong contraction state. Acute injuries can be conservatively managed by cast immobilization. Chronic instability leading to recurrent subluxation/dislocation, which require surgical management like soft tissue repairs, retinaculum reinforcement groove deepening procedure and relocation of tendon, bone block procedure.

Magnetic resonance imaging (kinematic) is imaging modality of choice for the detection of static peroneal tendon

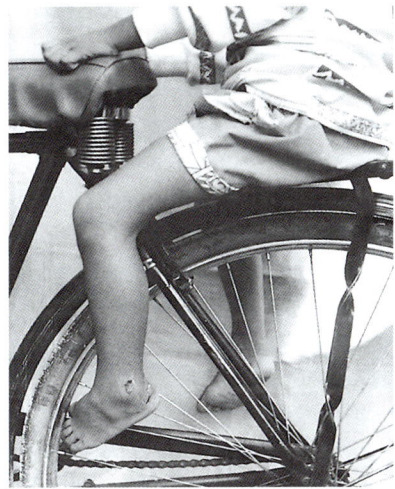

Fig. 14.27: Mechanism of sustaining cycle-spoke injury.

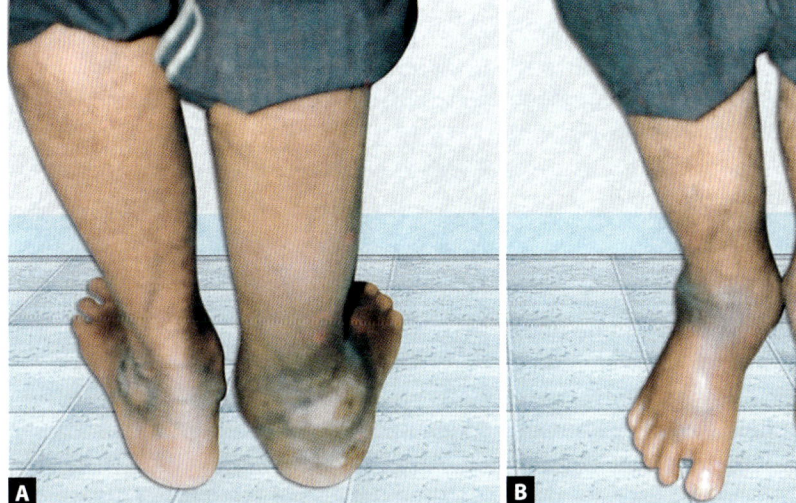

Figs. 14.28A and B: Clinical photographs of cycle-spoke injury in right ankle region in a boy aged 6 years—should be managed by care of soft tissue injury (including debridement-if needed), support (below knee) of leg-ankle foot, antibiotics, usually bony injuries are contusion which heals in rest-support. If there is any more bony injury it should be treated on its merit. If there is any injury to epiphyseal growth plate (clearly visible at first examination or even there is any possibility) the parent's should warned against any possible future deformity.

pathologies like tenosynovitis, tear and tendon subluxation or dislocation.

- *Rheumatoid arthritis:*
  - Gradual onset, usually in females between 20–40 years
  - Usually bilateral affection of the ankle with affections of other joints (especially the smaller joints of the hand) along with typical deformities. In early stage, warm and tender synovial swelling around the ankle, more prominent on anterolateral, anteromedial, posteromedial and posterolateral aspects
  - Swelling may appear along the commonly affected tendons (flexor hallucis longus, tibialis posterior, tibialis anterior and the peronei)
  - Movements are painfully restricted
  - X-ray:
    - Generalised rarefaction and 'pencilling' of the cortex
    - Joint space maintained till late stage which thence gradually reduces
    - In late cases degenerative changes supervene.
- *Crystal arthritis* (*also see* Chapter 3: Joints):
  - Males of about 40 or more are mainly affected
  - Ankle is a common site after the big toe
  - Cartilage, tendon, and bursae are main tissues to be affected
  - History of episodes of attack with inflammatory signs usually coming in small hours of the morning
  - In a typical gouty arthritis affecting the first metatarsophalangeal joint, with or without other joint involvement, search for gouty tophi (on and around the greater toe, thumb, lobule of ear, elbow, etc.)
  - In a typical gout, serum uric acid level is raised
  - In pseudogout—calcium pyrophosphate dihydrate crystals produce chondrocalcinosis usually in the larger joint (symptoms similar to those of gout)
  - In pseudogout, there may be calcification in the menisci of knee
  - In gout (and crystal arthritis), the inadequately processed waste products collect in the synovial fluid triggering painful inflammation
  - Sodium (Na) biurate accumulate primarily in the big toe.
- *Tailor's ankle:* Persons regularly sitting in crossed-leg position, develop adventitious bursae over lateral malleolus, e.g. Hindu priests worshipping–Padmasana, and tailors working while sitting in cross-legged position on the ground; Muslims who offer regular prayers (Namaz) develop Muslim's callus (Pandey S 1988)—two oval callosities on the upper-outer aspect of proximal foot and lateral malleolus.
- *Poliomyelitis:* In poliomyelitis, ankle region can be variously affected. Depending upon the pattern of paralysis, deformities like equinus, calcaneus, varus or valgus individually or in different combinations develop.

There may be simultaneous affections/deformities of the foot, knee or hip, or even other parts of the body.
- History of febrile attack in childhood followed by paralysis which usually improves to varying extent
- Paralysis of lower motor neuron type, which is usually asymmetrical
- No sensory loss.
- *Pigmented Villonodular synovitis:*
  - Most common disorder of synovium
  - Chronic synovitis—ankle affection second to knee.
  - Its localised form was first described by Chassaignac (1852) referring it as a "cancer of tendon sheath".
  - Young adults (usually males)
  - Soft nodular swelling (synovial) with effusion
  - Swelling (rarely ossifies) **(Figs. 14.29 and 14.30)**

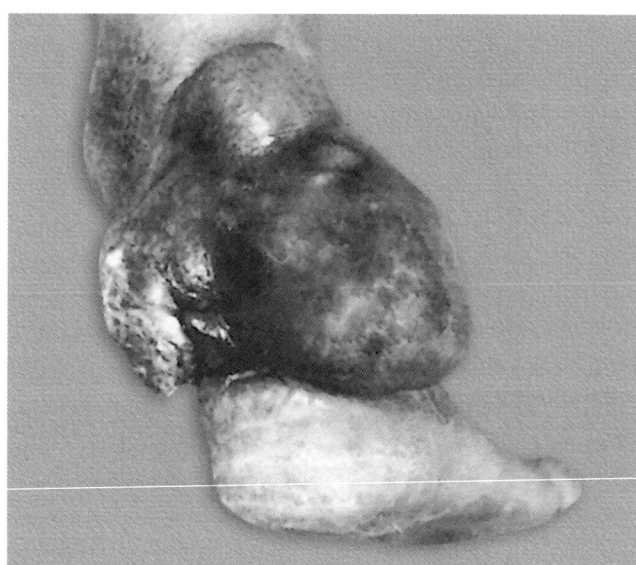

Fig. 14.29: Ossified villonodular synovitis of ankle, very rare presentation (Pandey S 1981). Tumorous like ossified mass should be removed and ankle should be fused.

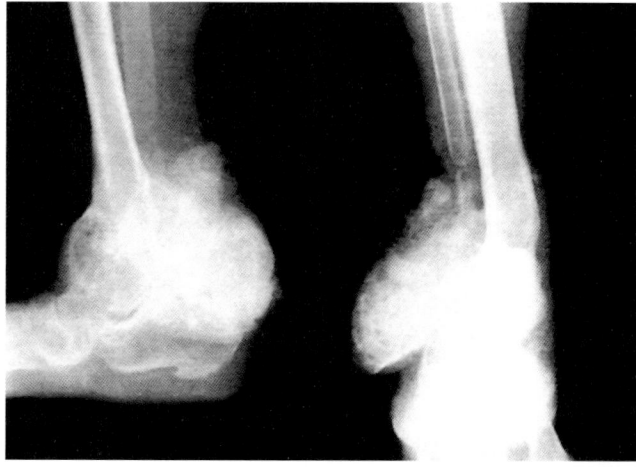

Fig. 14.30: X-ray of the same patient (Fig. 14.28).

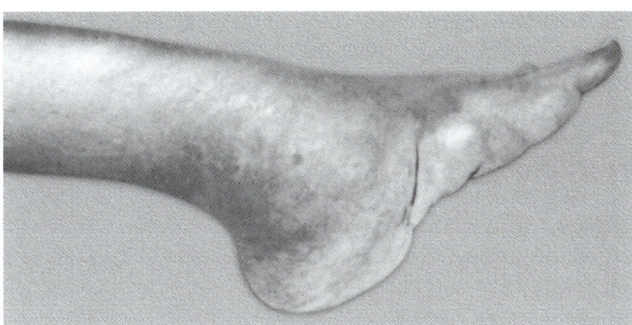

Fig. 14.31: Lymphangioma over ankle, hind foot and lower leg leading to overgrowth of that region.

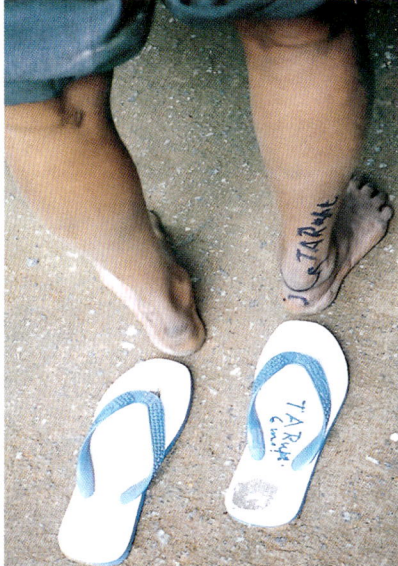

Fig. 14.32: Neglected tendo-Achilles rupture with calcaneus effect—Note the impression on footwear.

- Aspiration of thick orange brown fluid (sterile), containing cholesterol in large amounts—pathognomonic
- May be localised or diffuse form
- Arthroscopy reveals the characteristic picture.
- Total excision as far as possible provides good prognosis.
- Neoplasms:
  - Neoplasms in the ankle region may be of soft tissue [e.g. lymphangioma **(Fig. 14.32)**, synovioma, etc.] or of bony component of ankle (e.g. giant cell tumour of talus (*see* **Fig. 14.19**), Ewing's tumour of talus (*see* **Fig. 14.61**).

NEUROPATHIC (CHARCOT) ARTHROPATHY OF ANKLE

Neuropathic (Charcot) arthropathy of ankle is usually associated with involvement of peritalar joints and becomes a disabling condition characterized by joint instability, deformities, recurrent ulceration and infection. The most common cause is diabetes mellitus (0.08 to 0.13% (Guven et al. 2013), others being polyneuropathy, Hansen's disease, myelomalacia, syphilis, alcoholism, syringomyelia etc. Because of lack of awareness, early cases are misdiagnosed and ultimately end in amputation.

Sidney N Eichenholtz in 1966 defined three stages of chariot arthropathy based on natural history of the condition; stage (I) development; stage (II) coalescence; stage (III) Reconstruction and Reconstitution (reported by Rosenbaum-web search). The philosophy of management of Charcot joint has changed from amputation to limb salvage. Management mainly consists of hind foot arthrodesis using calcaneotibial intramedullary locking nail and bone grafting which provides a stable plantigrade foot for independent ambulation and prevents recurrent ulceration. The primary cause should be treated as needed.

OSTEOARTHRITIS OF ANKLE

Symptomatic osteoarthritis of ankle manifests in 1 to 4% of population mainly in comparatively younger people. Primary idiopathic ankle osteoarthritis occurs in about 7% of cases. Secondary cases are usually occur following trauma in about 70% and following inflammatory arthritis including rheumatoid arthritis and gout in about 12%. (Murphy et al 2017) OA progresses from early damage to diffuse to severe degeneration to deformity since OA ankle affects the younger people, conservative therapies, are recommended in more cases to avoid surgery. Conservative treatment includes symptomatic analgesic, physiotherapy, offloading and restriction of motions with shoe modifications, bracing, orthoses, assistive devices such as canes and crutches. Intraarticular corticoids or platelet rich plasma injections-weekly 4 injections-help in cases in which conservative treatment is not much effective. Use of intraarticular hyaluronic acid-viscosupplementation-appears to be an useful adjunct to conservative treatment. In advanced OA ankle surgery arthrodesis or arthroplasty is recommended—former with lasting painless ankle, with full weight bearing. In several cases minor surgical procedures like curettage and microfracture, retrograde and antegrade drilling, osteochondral fragment/loose body removal, large fragment fixation, abrasion arthroplasty, cartilage or bone transplantation, arthroscopic debridement are also tried before arthroplasty or arthrodesis.

BIBLIOGRAPHY

1. Evelyn PM, Curtin M, Niàll PM et al. prospective evaluation of intra-articular sodium hyaluronate injection in the ankle. J Foot Ankle Surg. 2017;56(2):327-331..
2. Guven MF, Karabiber A, Kaynak G, Ogut T. Conservative and surgical treatment of the chronic charcot foot and ankle. Diabet Foot Ankle. 2013;4

3. Helen M Horstmann and Bleck Eugene E. Orthopaedic Management in Cerebral Palsy, 2nd edn. 2007, Mac Keith Press.
4. Leonard MH. Injuries of the lateral ligaments of the ankle. J Bone Joint Surg. 1949:31A:373.
5. Lettin AWF. Diagnosis and treatment of sprained ankle. Br Med J. 1963;1(5337):1056-60.
6. Molloy S, Solan MC, Bendall SP. Synovial impingement in the ankle. J Bone Joint Surg. 2003;85-B:330-33.
7. Mulfinger GL, Trueta J. The blood supply of the talus. J Bone Joint Surg. 1970;528:160.
8. Pandey S. Muslim's callus. In: B Helal, D Wilson (Eds). The Foot. London: Churchill Livingston; 1998;700-01.
9. Pandey S. Pigmented villonodular synovitis with bone involvement. Arch Orthop Trauma Surg. 1981;98:217.
10. Pandey S. Ewing's tumour of talus. J Bone Joint Surg. 1970;52A:1672-3.
11. Pandey S. Giant cell tumour of the talus Int Surg. 1971;55-3:179-82.
12. Potter TA, Kuhns JG. Rheumatoid tenosynovitis. J Bone Joint Surg. 1958;40A:1230.
13. Rose GK. Ankle injuries. In: Clark JMP (Ed). Modern Trends in Orthopaedics (3rd ed) London: Butterworth; 1962.
14. Rosenbaum AJ, and Dipreta JA. Classification in Brief: Eichen holtz classification of Charcot Arthropathy. Web search.
15. Staheli LT. Lower positional deformity in infants and children: a review. Journal of Pediatric Orthopaedics. 1990;11:559-63.

CHAPTER 15

Foot

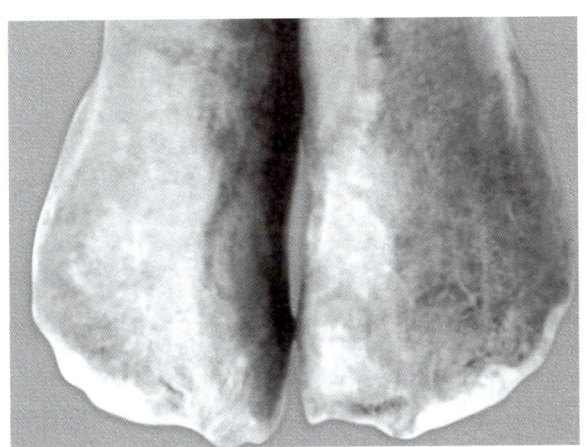 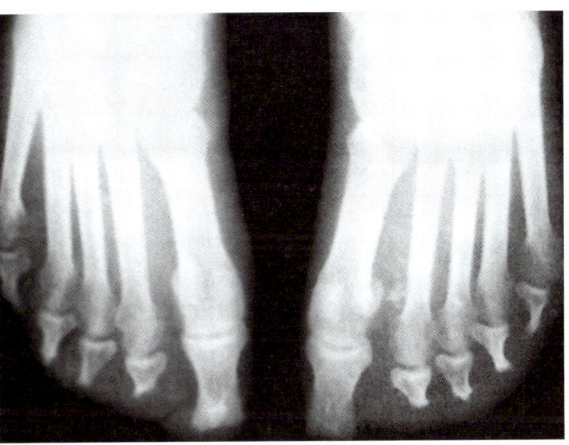

"The highest result of education is tolerance."
—*Hellen Keller*

"If you do not step forward, you will always be in the same place."
"It is the first step that takes all the courage and determination."
—*SP*

"For the most part we have but little pride in our feet, and it is pity that this is so."

—**Wood Jones, 1944**

In "The Language of Love"
As Shakespeare observed:
"There's language in her eye, her cheek, her lip, Nay, her foot speaks; her wanton spirits look out at every joint and motive of her body."

(from Toilus and Cressida)

"You are what your feet are; when your feet hurt, you hurt all over."

■ INTRODUCTION

The *evolution of "foot"*, according to various philogenetic and ontogenetic scales owes to the fins (which contain 5 bony elements–cf foot) of Eusthenopteron—a fish in the Devonian period (about 350 million years ago). Since the mankind evolved as a biped species (about 3 million years ago)—(Leaky and Hay 1979), deformities, injuries and diseases dogged the human foot. The word 'foot' has different names in different languages such as Old English—'fot'; German—'fuss'; Latin—'pes'; 'pedis'; and Greek—'pous', podos'.

In bipeds, the foot, acting as the interface between the lower limb and ground, takes on the important responsibilities of receiving the weight of the whole body and at the same time stabilizing the individual in changing environmental conditions that generate considerable compression and shearing forces. A normal foot must—(i) be plantigrade, (ii) have normal anatomical disposition and physiomechanics, (iii) be resilient with proper springiness to provide a rhythmic normal gait. The average person takes 8,000 to 10,000 steps in a day. The average person walks 2,41,350 kms (150,000 miles) on the feet in lifetime.

The *foot is subtle because it is a sensorial organ*. It is a powerful, adaptive, braking, propulsive structure. Its shape changes continuously and it has great compensatory capabilities. Pathological decompensation occurs only after several years.

The weight bearing area of foot is covered from heel to toes by special thick sensitive skin; which if damaged, its reconstruction becomes very challenging and often requires advanced surgical expertise.

In the foot, the lack of robust soft tissue coverage over the osseous structures makes it vulnerable to trauma and ulceration, that may be a predisposing factor for even osteomyelitis.

There are *over 300 identified foot ailments* ranging from chronic foot strain/discomfort to those that may put the patient's life, limb or mobility at risk. Serious consequences may arise without careful proper examinations, diagnosis and management of the foot and ankle problems. Foot and ankle arthroscopy has become an increasingly used treatment modality.

Foot disorders tend to be progressive, so catching them early can save a lot of grief.

The ankle along with the foot, functionally forms one unit. Hence, while considering the physiomechanics of a normal foot and pathodynamics of any diseased foot, the ankle must also be taken into account.

Feet are said to be the 'mirror' of an individual's health. Sore foot can impair your concentration, make you irritable, and frequently are responsible for pain in the leg, knee, hip and low back. About 80% human being suffer from foot problems. Females suffer four times more than males. About 60–70% of diabetic people suffer from neuritis, the severe ones of which affect lower limbs.

■ ANATOMICAL CONSIDERATIONS

The foot is an Orthopaedic Cinderella. The foot is anatomically complex structure of 28 bones (one-fourth of the bones in body), 33 joints, 57 articulating surfaces, 112 ligaments and 20 muscles. Normal feet are inherently stable and dependant on ligamentous integrity. There are about 2,50,000 sweat glands in a pair of feet. Sweat glands excrete about ½ pint of moisture a day.

Functionally, as well, the foot is complex, designed to withstand the enormous forces transmitted bidirectionally between the body and the ground during walking, running, climbing, going downhill, jumping and dancing. It is strong and at the same time flexible. It is capable to adapt almost to any ground surface.

From biomechanic angle, the anatomical set up of the foot can be considered as a tripod constructed of a series of triangles, each with a base and apex. The overall apex of the tripod is at the tibiotalar joint and its base is constituted of the calcaneum and 1st and 5th metatarsal.

Neuromuscular control, in a rhythmic fashion, is essential to distribute the normal proportion of body-weight through different portions of the foot in changing situations of stance and mobility. The distribution of foot (plantar) pressures has been assessed by different methods right from crude methods like by using clay and plaster of Paris to modern techniques by transducers mats and insole devices. In the normal weight bearing position, each foot carries 50% of the body weight. In turn, the rough distribution of the weight in each foot is represented in **Figure 15.**1.

Taking the unit of weight-bearing as one, the outer four metatarsal heads carry one unit each, the first metatarsal head carries two units and the calcaneal post carries six units of weight. The weight bearing zones of heel and metatarsal heads are protected by the viscoelastic function of the plantar fat pads which are composed of fibrous septae and spaces that are filled with fat cells.

Then this combined unit functions as:

1. *Shock absorber* during increased impact of walking and running;
2. *Lever mechanics for propulsion* of the limb during the gait-cycle;
3. *Support of weight* via foot in bipedal stance.

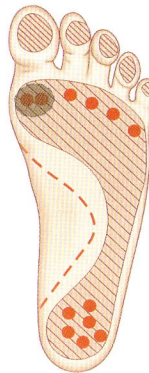

Fig. 15.1: Weight transmission in a plantigrade position. One dot represents one unit.

Though the concept of *"anterior heel"* bearing the load upon the five metatarsal heads is a more or less established fact, however, the depiction of weight bearing has remained controversial. Wulf (1988) believes that in bipodal upright position, the load bearing on the metatarsal heads are as follows, i.e. $4 > 3 > 2$ whereas in monopodal position, it is $1 > 2 = 3 = 4$.

The ratio between medial to lateral border of foot is 1.2:1.

The *length of the foot* in any person represents about 15.176% of his/her stature (i.e. stature in centimeters divided by the foot length is 6.66; i.e. the length of the foot multiplied by 6.66 denotes the stature of the foot owner within a variation of 3 to 8 millimeter).

Arches of the Foot

The function of the longitudinal arches, between the heel and the forefoot and the transverse arch between first and fifth metatarsal heads, is to absorb shock, energy and force and to transmit loading. On the whole, arches play important role in bearing body weight, absorbing ground reaction forces and maintaining balance during weight bearing and or sports activities.

For suppleness of the plantigrade foot, the arches of the foot must be maintained. The structure and function of arch play important role in maintaining balance, bearing body weight and absorbing ground reaction forces. The structure and function of arches may be affected by factors like gender, age and obesity. Women have low-arched feet compared to men. With advancing age arch becomes stiffer and thus older people have stiffer arch than middle aged and younger individuals. The plantar aspect of heel, the anterior transverse arch and the connecting longitudinal anteroposterior arches are the main weight bearing structures.

Sesamoid Bones

Like patellas, sesamoids are articular and buried within the tendons inserted into bone. Sesamoids are formed in separate cartilaginous centers. The word "sesamoid is derived from the Greek word "sesamoeides" which means like sesame or resembling a sesame seed. It is only in the 1970s, that the pathologic anatomy, pathomechanics and clinical syndromes associated with the sesamoids have been elucidated. The sesamoids are firmly attached to each other by a stout thick intersesamoid ligament. Sesamoids often develop from multiple centres of ossification. Like patella, sesamoids suffer from congenital anomalies, interarticular diseases and trauma, (After Jahss MH 1980). The sesamoids of the great toe are a source of symptoms involved in a number of disease processes.

Transverse Arch (Anterior Arch)

The metatarsals and tarsals are arranged with a convex dorsal curve, mainly at the metatarsal heads level, held together by transverse ligament and maintained by transverse and oblique heads of adductor hallucis.

Collapse of this arch may—(i) Press upon the digital nerve (usually the communicating twig between the 3rd and 4th space digital nerves leading to *Morton's metatarsalgia*, (ii) Produce *anterior flat foot.*

Recently, the existence of 'transverse arch' in a normal foot, has fallen in controversies. It is being observed that there is always a longitudinal arch in a normal foot, whereas there is no distal transverse metatarsal arch during the stance phase, i.e. during weight bearing. Rather a transverse arch indicates a possible pathological deformity like cavus and hallux valgus.

Longitudinal Arches

Medial longitudinal arch—formed by the calcaneal tuberosity, talus, navicular, three cuneiforms, inner three metatarsals and corresponding phalanges.

Lateral longitudinal arch—formed by the calcaneal tuberosity, cuboid, outer two metatarsals and corresponding phalanges.

Both these *arches are maintained by*— (i) *Fascia*—plantar aponeurosis, (ii) Ligaments—spring ligament, long plantar ligament, short plantar ligament, (iii) *Tendons*—tibialis posterior, peroneus longus, (iv) *Muscles*—long flexors, intrinsics.

Collapse of these arches result in—*flat foot, valgus foot, spread foot.* Accentuation of these arches (mainly medial)—results in *cavus foot.*

One of the first World Heritage sites in India, the Ajanta caves date back to around 2nd century BCE to 650 CE and consist of the finest masterpieces of 31 Rock CUT CAVE monuments, paintings and sculpture. This bestowed several mechanical and functional principles.

According to the height of the arch, the arch can be divided into a high arch, normal arch and low arch. Based on the flexibility of the arch; the arches can be classified as a flexible arch and stiff arch. It has been observed that the lower arch foot is more likely to be flexible, whereas the high arch foot tends to be stiffer. Women, usually have low-arches feet. Older people usually have stiffer arch. Both low arch and high arch postures have been seen to be associated with plantar fasciitis.

TABLE. 15.1: Broad divisions of foot.

Part	Zone	Contains	Main function	Possible deformities
Hindfoot	Behind the transverse tarsal joints	Talus and calcaneum	Stability	Equinus, calcaneus, varus, valgus
Midfoot	From transverse tarsal joints to tarsometatarsal joints	Navicular, cuboid, medial, intermediate and lateral cuneiforms	Maintenance of longitudinal arches, and springiness of foot	Cavus, planus, rocker-bottom foot
Forefoot	Distal to tarsometatarsal joint	Metatarsals, phalanges, sesamoids	Piano-distribution of weight, Forefoot is quite dynamic zone on which the body leans on and exerts pressure against the support for a longer time than other parts of the foot during the gait cycle	Adduction/abduction of metatarsals, clawing of toes, claw foot, other deformities of toes (e.g. hallux valgus, hallux varus, hammer toe, etc).

For the intricate and finer movements, the foot has multiple smaller joints. These joints have more or less communicating synovial reflections. Hence, any disease starting in one bone or joint is likely to spread and affect the adjoining bones and joints of the foot.

The *skin of the sole* is tough enough to withstand the pressures and pricks of a rough surface and at the same time is sensitive enough to make the person acquainted with the exact condition of the surface. Hence, proper sensation and vascularity of the skin of the sole and subcutaneous pad are of paramount importance for the foot to subserve its proper functions.

Heel pad (Calcaneal fat pad) located beneath the calcaneum is an efficient shock absorber attenuating the peaks of dynamic forces and dampening vibrations. It consists of dense strands of fibrous septa extending from the calcaneal periosteum to the skin (rich in collagen fibres) which form large sealed compartments packed with fat cells.

It is interesting to note that all elephants walk on tip-toe because the back portion of their foot is made of no bone just only fat **(Fig. 15.2)**.

Control of the foot: Besides the long tendons as considered in the chapter on ankle, smaller muscles of foot are no less important as far as finer functions of the foot are concerned.

Anatomico-functionally the foot may broadly be divided into *Hindfoot, Midfoot* and *Forefoot* (**Table. 15.1**).

Ossification of Foot Bones (Fig. 15.3)

Tarsal bones usually ossify from one centre, except for the calcaneus, which has an additional epiphysis for its posterior part. Primary centre for ossification appears as follows:

Talus	6 months IUL	Medial cuneiform	2nd year
Navicular	3rd year	Lateral cuneiform	1st year
Cuboid	9 months IUL	Intermediate cuneiform	3rd year
Calcaneum	5 months IUL		

The epiphysis for the posterior part of calcaneum appears at 6–8 years and unites by the 14th-16th years.

Metatarsal bones: Each metatarsal bone ossifies from two centres, one primary for the shaft and one secondary for the base of the first and for the heads of rest of the metatarsal bones.

Phalanges: Each phalanx ossifies from two centres, a primary one for the shaft, and secondary one for the epiphysis of the base.

Congenital Malformations of the Feet

Congenital disorders can be defined as the defects that can be detected on examination of the neonate. Possible prominent causes of congenital abnormalities include genetic

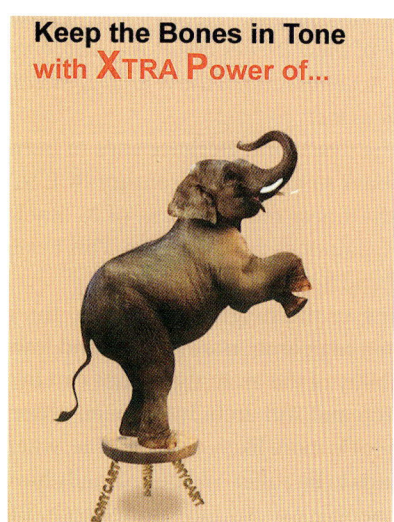

Fig. 15.2: Elephants have no bone in the back portion on foot. They walk on tip-toe absorbing the shock and dynamic forces.

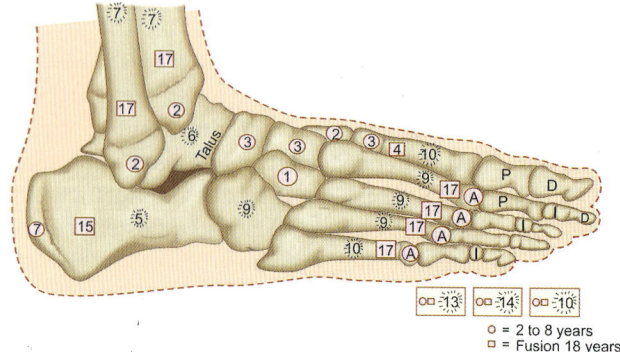

Fig. 15.3: Ossification around the ankle and foot: Dotted circle—primary centre in weeks (IUL), Complete circle—secondary centre in years, Square—fusion in years, P = proximal phalanx, I = intermediate phalanx, D = distal phalanx.

transmission or mutation, maternal illness, maternal drug ingestion, abnormalities of uterine environment, exposure of the pregnant mother to other teratogens, e.g. radiation, etc.
Common congenital disorders of foot are:

- Congenital talipes equinovarus *(club foot)*: Dealt in detail later on (Pages 454–458)
- *Congenital metatarsus adductus.* Dealt in detail on Page 433. See **Fig. 15.39** on Page 447.
- Cleft foot (Partial adactyly; Lobster foot).
  Generally, one or more toes and parts of their metatarsals are absent and the tarsals are abnormal. However, the first and fifth rays are usually present, even though deformity varies in degree and types. The surgical correction (capsulotomies and osteotomies) should improve function and appearance of foot.
- Congenital *elevation of little toe* (the little toe remains hypoplastic and overlies its neighbour, and causes pain due to rubbing in the shoe).
- *Curly toes* (3rd and 4th toes are usually affected, and they get flexed at the distal interphalangeal joint).
- *Syndactyly* usually remain symptom free, unless they are complex syndactyly (when bone is involved with angular deformities causing shoe-fitting problems) **(Fig. 15.4)**.
- *Macrodactyly* **(Fig. 15.12C on Page 439)** (may be due to neurofibromatoses, haemangiomatosis, congenital, lipofibromatosis and congenital vascular anomalies). Here one or more toes or fingers become hypertrophied and significantly larger than other toes or fingers. Surgery can improve the cosmesis and function as required
- *Polydactyly* (accessory digits) **(Fig. 15.5)**. It may be associated with chondroectodermal dysplasia (Ellis-Van Creveld syndrome) in which there are chondrodysplasia, ectodermal dysplasia, polydactyly, congenital heart disease.

Polydactyly of the toes may occur in established genetic syndromes but occurs most commonly as an isolated trait with an autosomal dominant inheritance pattern and variable expressions. The overall incidence is two per 1000 live birth. Polydactyly may be pre-axial or post-axial.

- *Pobble foot* (cf. *Apert's syndrome*, Page 635) (named after Edward Lear's poem about the Pobble, who had no toes). Disarticulation of all the five toes is known as *Pobble operation* (used to be performed for severe clawing of the toes) **(Fig. 15.6)**. It may result following trauma or iatrogenic. It mostly occurs in female and may be bilateral in about 75% of cases.
- *Tarsal coalition* (due to failure of differentiation of mesenchymal mass, there is fusion of tarsal bones.
- *Brachymetatarsia* (congenital shortening of the metatarsal caused by premature closure of the epiphysis) may be associated with brachymetacarpia. Both may have familial history. The fourth ray is mostly involved followed

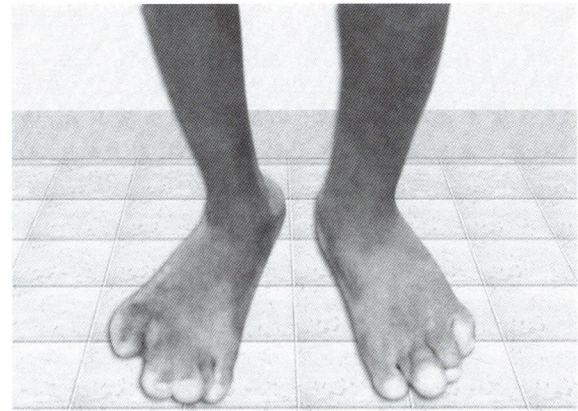

Fig. 15.4: Syndactyly, if desired, the affected toes can be separated by plastic procedure.

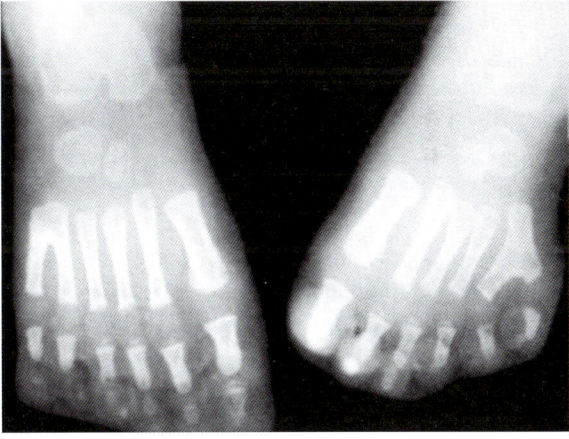

Fig. 15.5: Polydactyly, the extra digit after the 5th one should be removed which improves cosmesis and use of proper footwear.

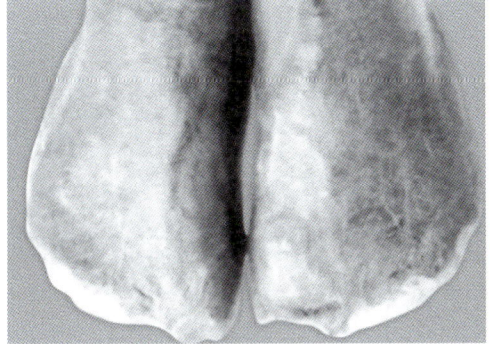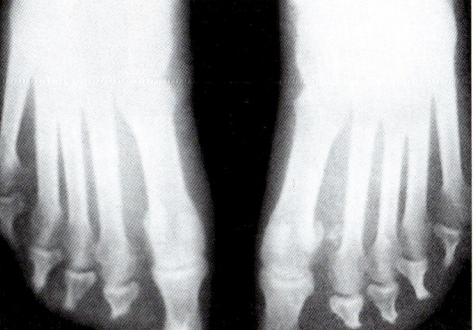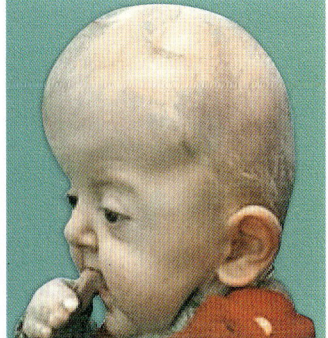

Fig. 15.6: Apert's syndrome (cf. Pobble foot). With constant use of closed footwear, it does not require any treatment.

by first and fifth. Besides the cosmetic complaints, there may be pain around adjacent metatarsal heads while walking. These can be managed by the lengthening of the metatarsals (metacarpals in case of *bradymetacarpia*) even by performing percutaneous osteotomy with a mini-burr and external fixation.

- *Congenital convex pes valgus:* Though described first in 1914 by Henkin, it was named properly by Lamey and Weissman in 1939. The most obvious radiological feature in this deformity is vertical orientation of the talus—*congenital vertical talus.* Talus is also vertically oriented in other conditions, e.g. congenital pes calcaneovalgus and spastic cerebral palsy. In congenital vertical talus (**Figs. 15.7 and 15.8**) there is rocker bottom appearance—due to prominence of the head of talus and equinus of heel (*Also see* Page 446).
- *Rudimentary foot* (**Figs. 15.9A and 15.10**): The leg may also be short with muscular and other soft tissues atrophy (**Fig. 15.10**).

■ DEFORMITIES OF THE FOOT

Any deviation from the anatomical plantigrade foot (**Fig. 15. 11A**) is a deformed foot. The deformities of the foot can be grouped under the following headings. These may exist (a) individually or (b) in various combinations or (c) as complex foot deformities.

Individual Deformities

Equinus Foot (Talepes Equinus Deformity)
(Figs. 15.11B and 15.12A and B)

Equinus deformity is mainly caused by gastrocnemius contracture, which may be:
1. Congenital such as in clubfoot, limb length discrepancy, cerebral palsy, flat foot
2. Secondary condition such as immobilization for trauma or a nonfunctional limb, fibrous gastrocnemius muscle contracture after a direct muscle contusion on the calf (mainly in the football players) in equinus.

In, equinus entire weight is borne by the forefoot, the hindfoot remaining off the ground. The Latin word equinus means horse, which bears weight on the forefoot only. The *equinus deformity may be compensatory to weakness of the quadriceps femoris muscles* and/or the gluteus maximus, and/or *to shortening of that lower limb*. Hence, the power of the quadriceps femoris and gluteus maximus must be assessed and the limb lengths accurately measured, when examining any case with equinus. Toe-walking must be considered before labelling the equinus deformity.

Little equinus is compatible with even strong walking and is much better than even little calcaneus. Before the

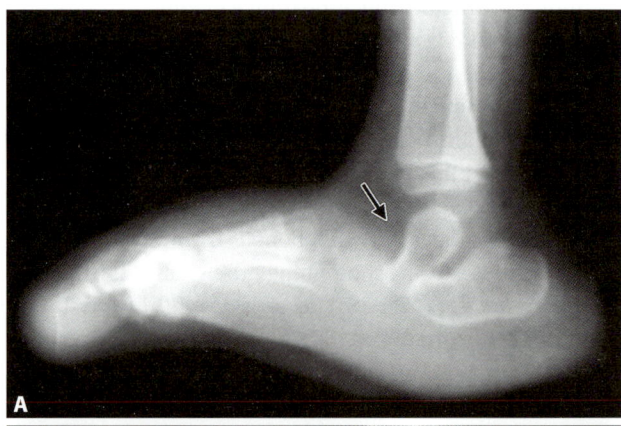
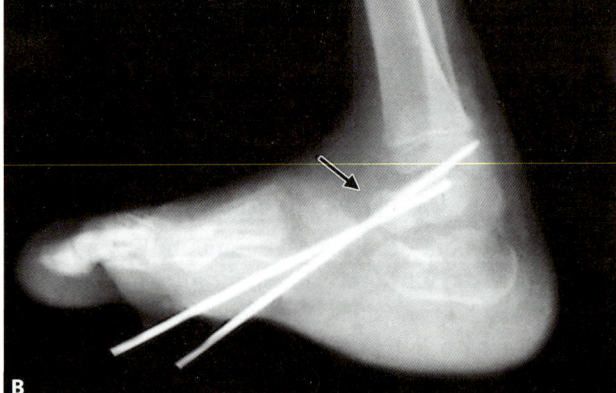
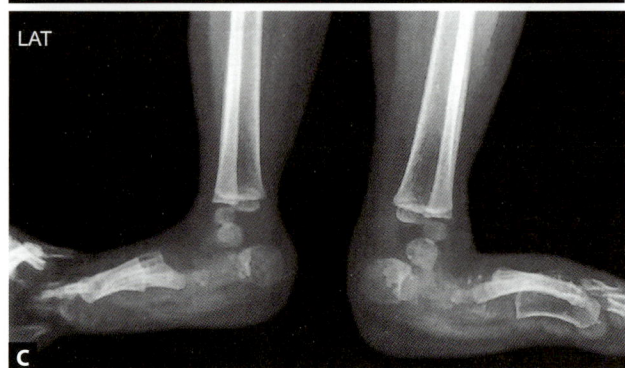

Figs. 15.8A to C: (A and B) X-ray of congenital vertical talus (preoperative and immediate postoperative); (C) Congenital vertical talus very severe degree—Bilateral.

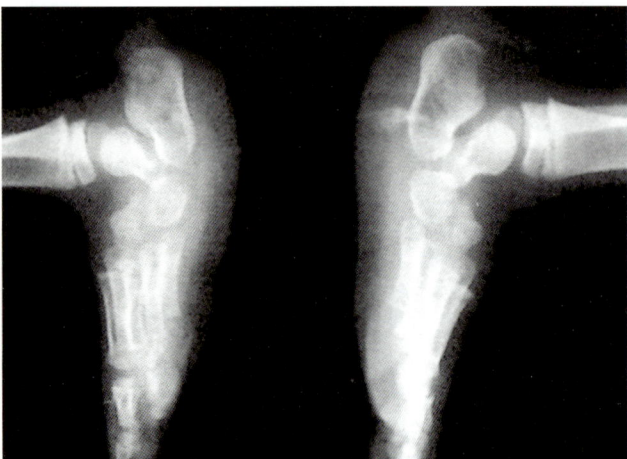

Fig. 15.7: Bilateral congenital vertical talus. To be treated by open reduction and to be maintained by tendon sling.

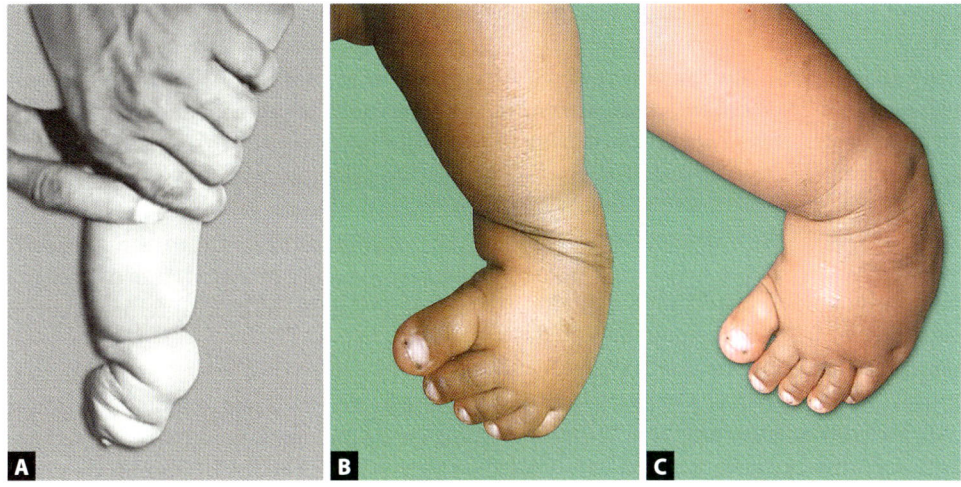

Figs. 15.9A to C: (A) Rudimentary foot with deep skin creases in soft tissues; (B) Congenital metatarsus adductus; (C) Adduction of forefoot to be placed.

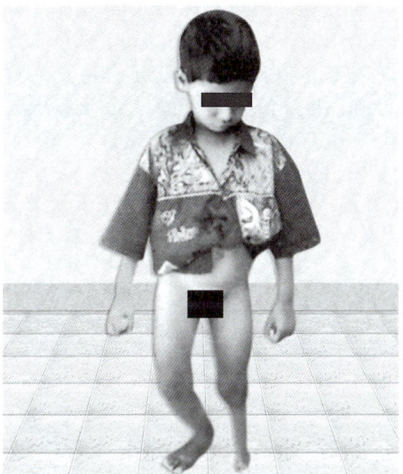

Fig. 15.10: Rudimentary foot and ill-developed leg.

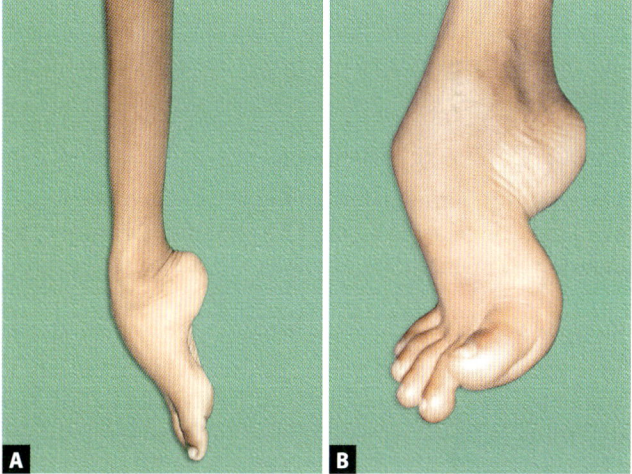

Figs. 15.12A and B: (A) Neglected severe equinocavus—Foot almost in line of leg; (B) Equinocavus (severe) with early claw. To be treated by tendo-Achilles lengthening, posterior capsulotomy, Steindler's fasciectomy and triple arthrodesis

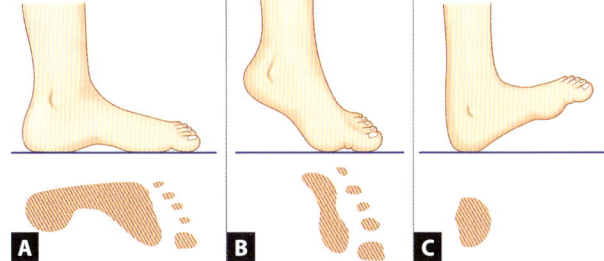

Figs. 15.11A to C: (A) Plantigrade foot with footprint; (B) Equinus foot with footprint; and (C) Calcaneus foot; shaded area below indicates footprint.

equinus develops, the tendo-Achilles starts becoming tighter. *Equinus can be divided into four grades.*

Grade I *Pre-equinus—Tendo-Achilles tightness.* Here patient cannot walk on his heel. He can somehow squat, e.g. by keeping his leg abducted and/or with back markedly bent forward.

Grade II Along with equinus, heel starts becoming smaller with tendency of tilting into varus and mild cavus starts developing.

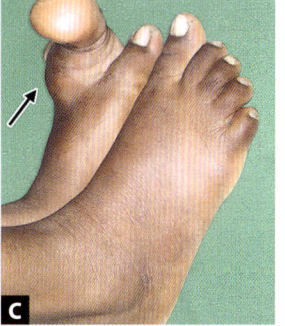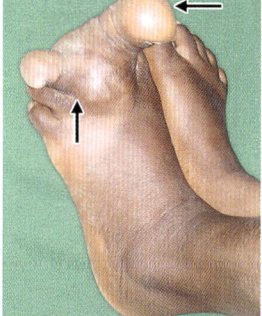

Fig. 15.12C: Macrodactyly. Affected digit should be removed to improve the cosmesis and function and possibility of using normal footwear.

Grade III Heel becomes obviously small with soft skin and cavus accentuates along with splaying of the forefoot. The heel varus also becomes perceptible.

Grade IV   Clawing of the toes also develops along with accentuation of the deformities of grade III.

Equinus deformity may be due to contracture of gastrocnemius and/or soleus. *If the equinus disappears after flexing the knee by 90° or more, it indicates its cause lying in gastrocnemius; if it persists, the cause is in soleus; and if it gets partially corrected the causes are in both. Almost same inferences are drawn after Silfverskiold test for gastrocnemius versus soleus contracture.*

In Silfverskiold test (described in 1923), the patient sits at the edge of the table. With knee extended and affected side foot held in varus, the ankle is dorsiflexed passively and the limitation of dorsiflexion of ankle is noted. The same manoeuvre is repeated with the knee flexed 90°. If the ankle can be easily dorsiflexed when the knee is flexed, it indicates the contracture of gastrocnemius alone.

Calcaneus Foot (Figs. 15.11C, 15.38, 15.78 to 15.81)

Here the weight is borne mainly by the hindfoot. The forefoot may have varying degrees of weight bearing but definitely below normal.

Varus Foot (Figs. 15.13A and B)

The weight is borne mainly on the outer side of the foot in a gradually increasing amount from behind forwards. This deformity is mainly at the hindfoot.

Valgus Foot (Figs. 15.14 to 15.18)

Here weight is mainly borne on the inner side of the foot in gradually increasing amount from before backwards. This deformity is of the hindfoot or of both the forefoot and hindfoot.

Inverted Foot (Fig. 15.23)

As such, inversion qualifies the act of a particular movement (to invert) of the foot mainly occurring at subtalar joint, the persistent effect of which manifests in a particular deformity, i.e. 'varus'. However, when the hindfoot varus gets associated with forefoot adduction alongwith some cavus element at the midfoot it leads to inverted foot **(Figs. 15.22 and 15.23)**. The accentuation of this position will gradually tend to turn the sole towards the sky—*supinated foot* **(Figs. 15.24 to 15.26)**. In these positions, i.e. in inverted and supinated foot, the plantarflexion of the ankle will also co-exist. Thus, supination of foot = varus of heel + cavus at midfoot + adduction of fore foot + plantarflexion at ankle.

Everted Foot (Fig. 15.27)

The eversion qualifies the act of a movement (to evert) occurring mainly at the subtalar joint, the persistent effect of which will result in a deformity, i.e. valgus. When the hindfoot is in valgus, collapsing tendency of medial longitudinal arch and abduction of forefoot lead to the deformity complex, i.e. everted foot **(Fig. 15.27)**. Here the outer part of the sole bears lesser and lesser weight. In the exaggerated situation, the outer part of the sole acquires a tendency to face towards the sky. This is called a *pronated foot*. In these, i.e. everted and pronated foot **(Fig. 15.28)**, some amount of dorsiflexion at the ankle will also co-exist.

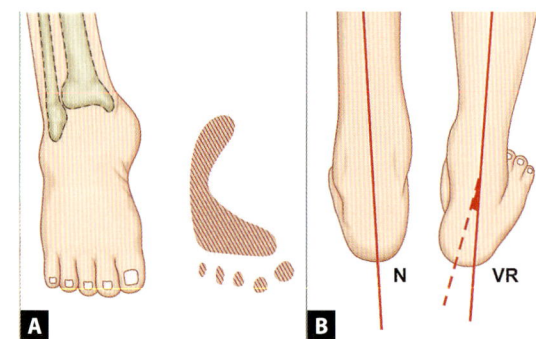

Figs. 15.13A and B: (A) Varus foot from front with footprint; (B) Varus foot from behind. (N: normal; VR: varus)

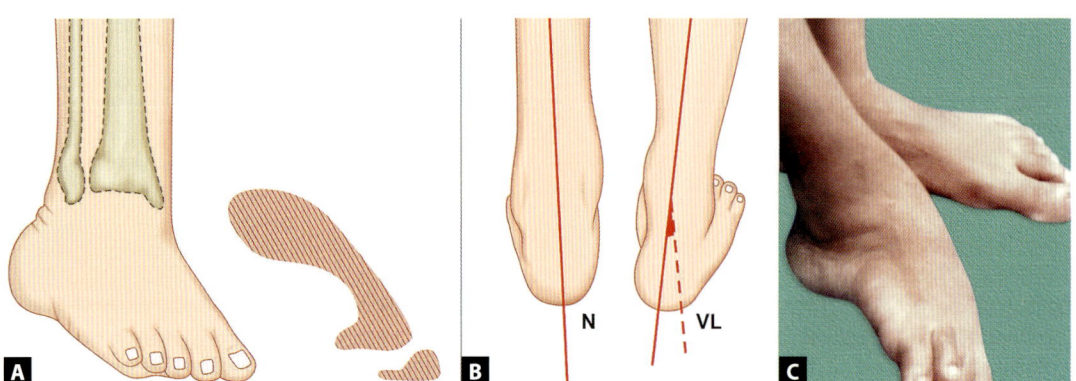

Figs. 15.14A to C: (A) Valgus foot seen from front with footprint; (B) Valgus foot seen from behind; (C) Neglected right pes valgus. (N: normal; VL: valgus. In neglected pes planus, pes valgus, hind foot valgus, posterior tibial tendon dysfunction, lateral column lengthening is a common procedure for correction. LCL was originally described by Evans as an osteotomy from the lateral cortex to medial cortex of calcaneum using a bitrapezoidal graft for inserting at the osteotomy site. He believed that in a true functional foot the medial and lateral columns should be of same length and the lateral column has an enormous influence on the shape and function of foot).

Foot

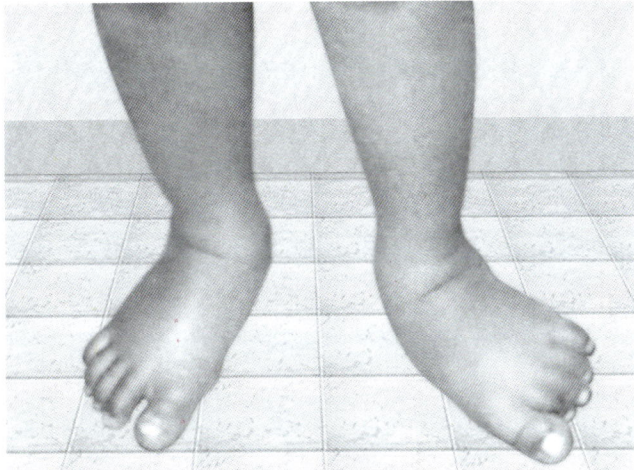

Fig. 15.15: Left foot pes valgus, right foot pes planus in a child.

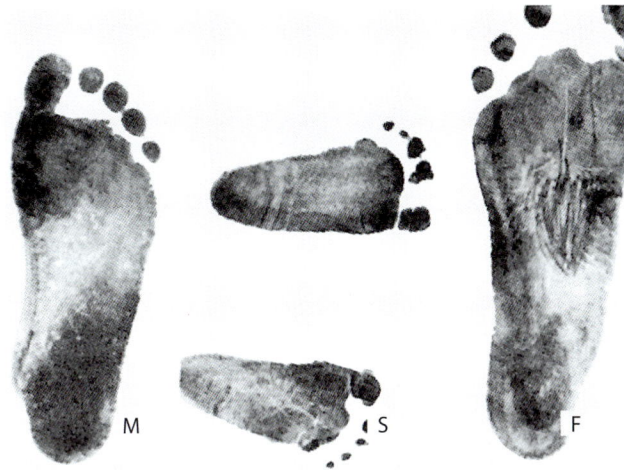

Fig. 15.16: Footprints: On the left of mother (M), on the right of father (F), in the centre of the son (S). Pes planus (flat foot) may be hereditary.

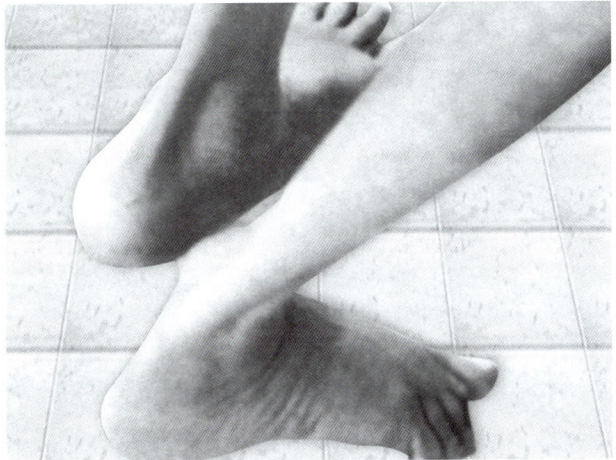

Fig. 15.17: Pes valgus in adult—should be treated by lateral column lengthening of foot or 'T' osteotomy of calcaneum.

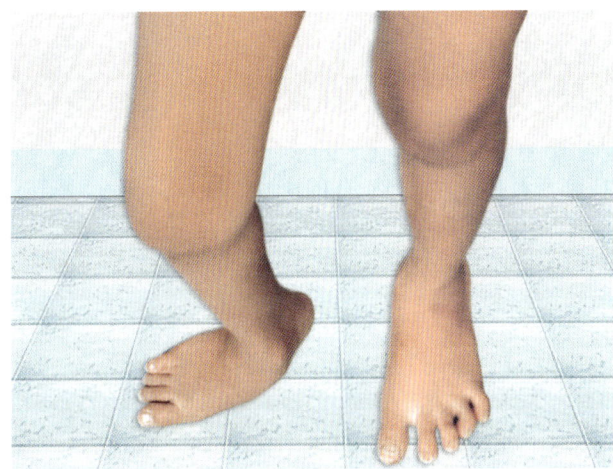

Fig. 15.18: Congenital convex pes valgus.

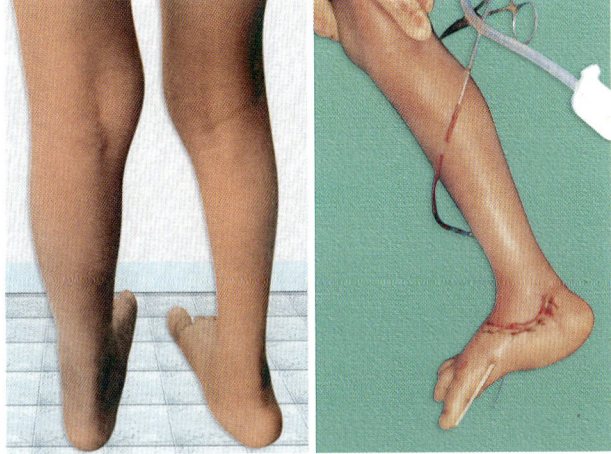

Fig. 15.19: Congenital vertical talus in right foot. On the left is preoperative picture and on the right is immediate postoperative picture. Note that the medial arch has been restored.

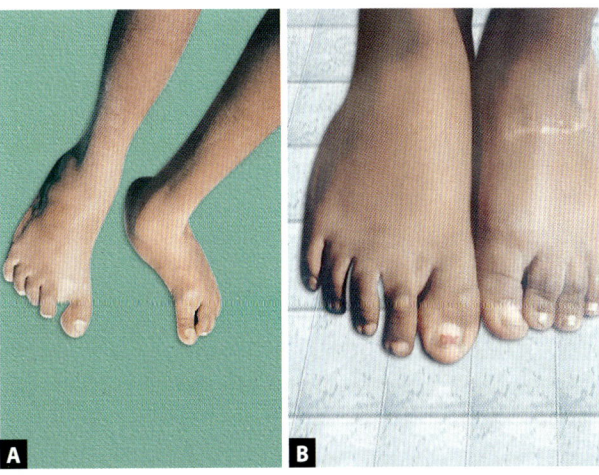

Figs. 15.20A and B: Painful neglected congenital vertical talus (on left side)—Same foot corrected by pantalar arthrodesis (Pandey's long bone's growth preserving arthrodesis technique), albeit size of foot remained smaller.

442 Foot

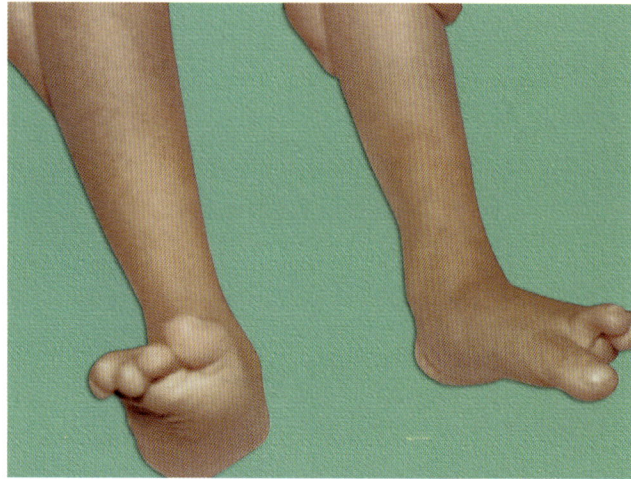

Fig. 15.21: Same foot (**Fig. 15.18**) viewed from the sole side.

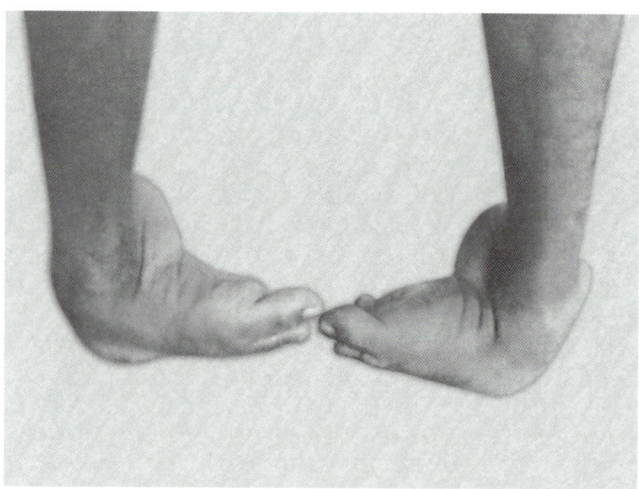

Fig. 15.24: Neglected very severe clubfeet (supinated feet)—viewed from the front.

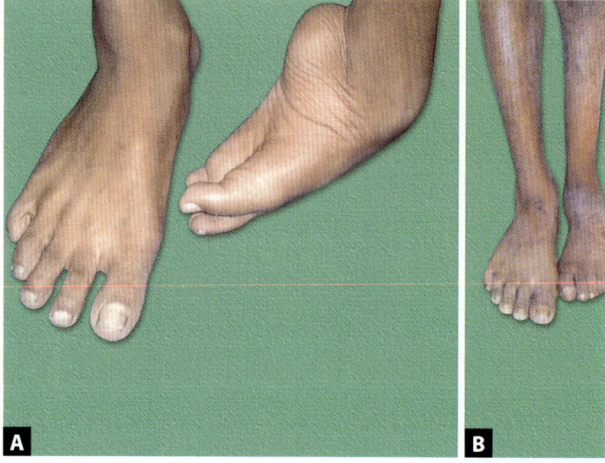

Figs. 15.22A and B: (A) Neglected post injection (in gluteal region) supinated foot deformity managed by surgery (modified triple arthrodesis and tendon transfer); (B) 2 years after operation.

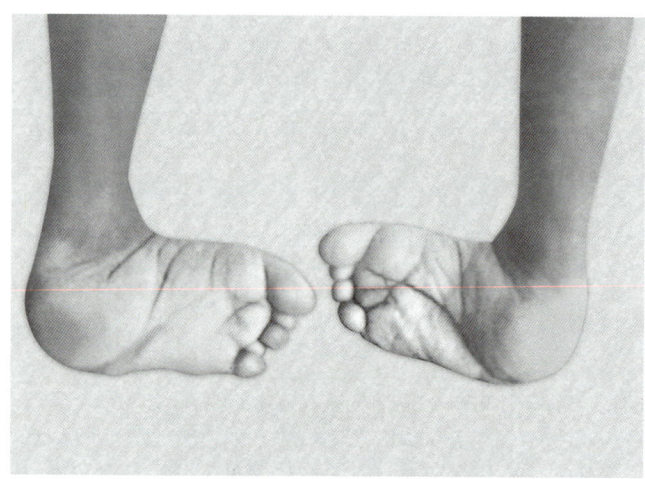

Fig. 15.25: Neglected severe clubfeet (supinated feet)—viewed from the back.

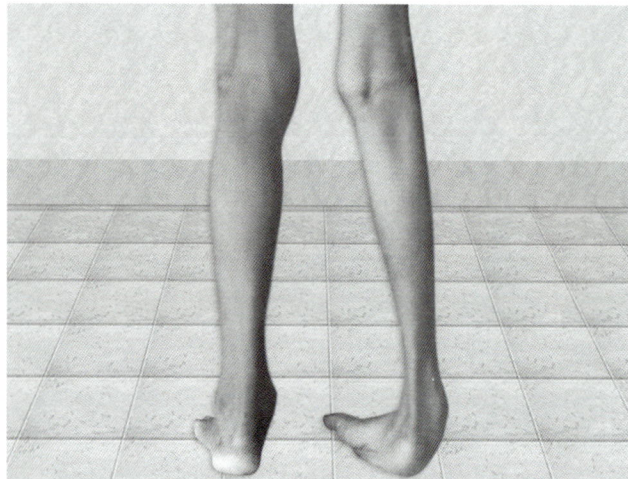

Fig. 15.23: Severe equinocavo-varus foot (inverted foot). Can be corrected by tendo-Achilles lengthening and 'T' osteotomy of calcaneum.

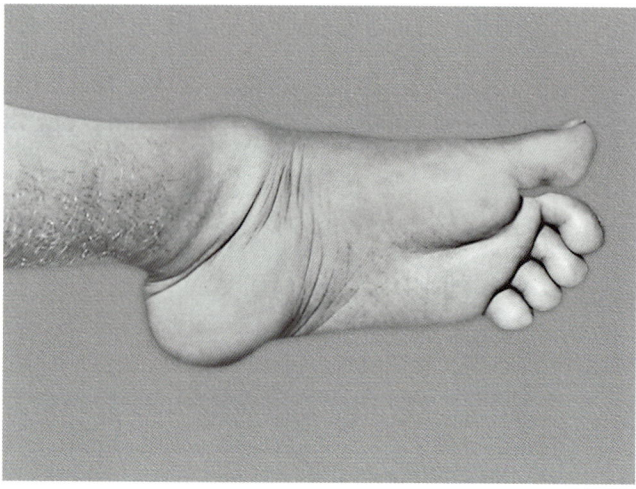

Fig. 15.26: Paralytic (polio-paralysis) supinated foot (cf. **Fig. 15.28**).

Pes Cavus (High-arched or High-dome Foot, Hallowing the Instep) (Figs. 15.29 to 15.31)

A normal foot has a medial longitudinal arch which is higher than the lateral one. When this normal proportion is accentuated, the medial side of the foot tends to assume the shape of a high arch and looks like a cave. Nicholas Andry described such condition in 1741, in which the medial longitudinal arch is abnormally elevated and it does not get corrected on weight bearing. It rarely occurs as a single deformity. It is a common accompaniment of equinovarus, equinus and dorsal subluxation of the metatarsophalangeal joints (claw foot). *Pes cavus can be flexible* (which can be corrected by pushing the first metatarsal head upwards) *or rigid*.

Hyperpronation of Foot

It is a dynamic structural deformity of excessive motion of the talus on the calcaneus. This abnormal motion disturbs

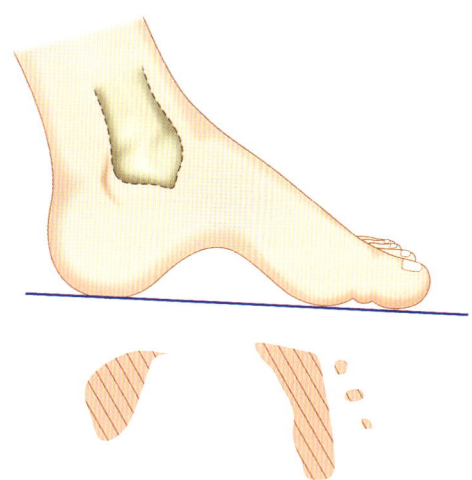
Fig. 15.29: Pes cavus with its footprint (below line drawing figure of foot).

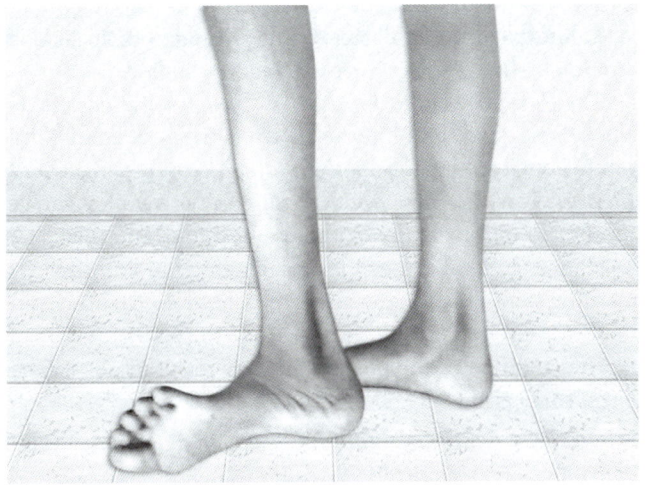
Fig. 15.27: Everted foot. Can be corrected by 'T' osteotomy of calcaneum.

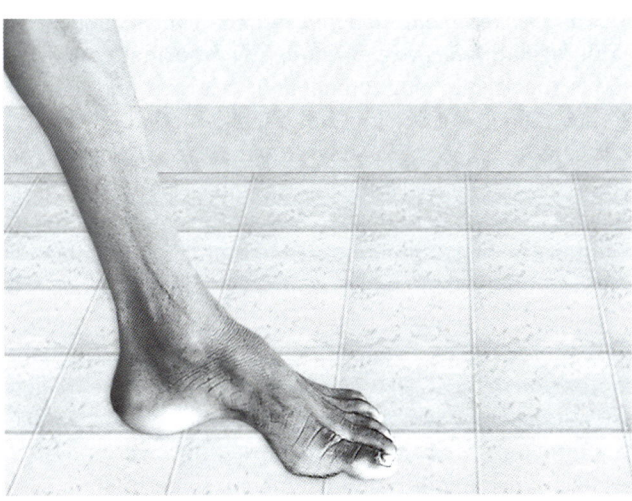
Fig. 15.30: Clinical photograph of pes cavus with tight tendo-Achilles and smaller heel.

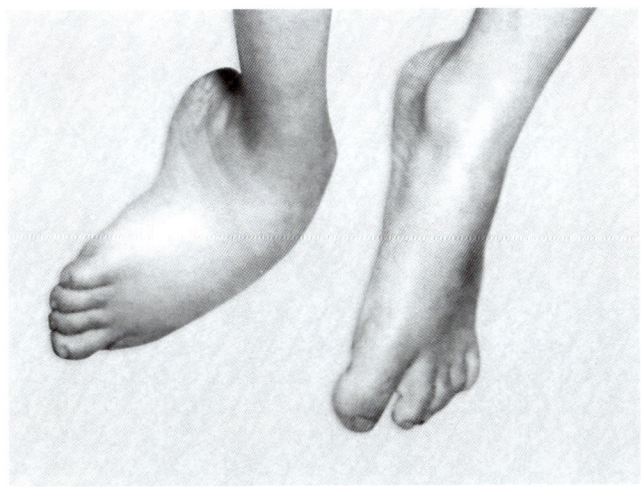
Fig. 15.28: Markedly pronated foot (cf. **Fig. 15.26**).

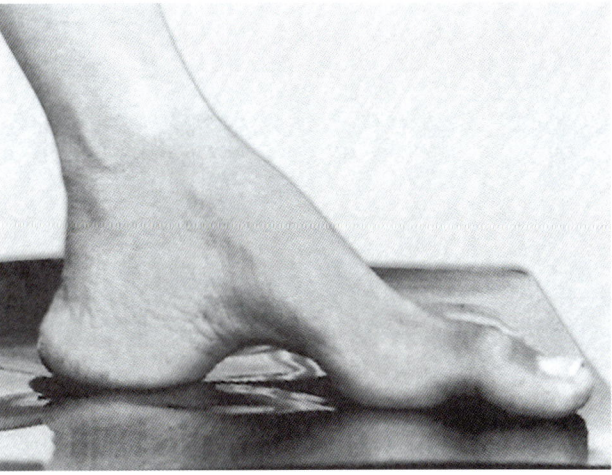
Fig. 15.31: Calcaneocavus foot (note the splashed-out heel).

the physiomechanics and causes obliteration of the sinus tarsi leading to proximal and distal deforming forces that may lead to preventable (by inserting subtalar implant that blocks abnormal and excessive motion of the subtalar joint) pes planus, posterior tibial dysfunction, tarsal tunnel syndrome, plantar fasciitis, calcaneal spurs, Hagelund's deformity, Achilles tendinitis, calcaneal apophysitis, neuroma formation, hallux abducto-valgus, hallux rigidus, hammer toe, sinus tarsi syndrome, etc.

Pes Planus (Flat Foot) (Figs. 15.15, 15.16 and 15.32)

With the collapse of medial longitudinal arch following anatomical abnormalities commonly develop: valgus of heel; mild subluxation of subtalar joint, resulting in medial and plantigrade tilt of talar head, which will appear, foreshortend on standing, dorso-plantar X-ray; eversion of calcaneum at subtalar joint; abduction at talonavicular and calcaneocuboid joints; supination of forefoot in relation to hind foot, placing the first ray in plantigrade position (Inuik et al 2017).

Collapse of medial longitudinal arch (physiological or pathological) *leads to pes planus*. The normal concavity due to the medial longitudinal arch is absent and instead the medial side of the foot bulges as a medial convexity, particularly on weight bearing. In *physiological or paralytic* cases, the *flat foot* is supple and full passive inversion of the foot is possible. Idiopathic flatfoot (pes planovalgus) in children (the most common skeletal disorders in childhood–a multidimensional change in foot) is usually associated with hind foot valgus, decreased longitudinal medial arch, abduction and supination of forefoot, and frequent contraction of the triceps. Flexible flatfoot should be treated when it becomes symptomatic by conservative means like physiotherapy, inlay and foot orthoses, however; majority resolve of itself and the remaining ones can be managed by surgical methods like, lateral column lengthening, sinus tarsi bone-block - ARTHROERESIS, calcaneal osteotomies, tendon releases tendon transfer-with an intention to straighten the arch of foot.

In adults, flat foot commonly develops in sports injuries as a secondary adaptation to lower limb injuries, including medial tibiofemoral cartilage damage, anterior knee pain, and musculoskeletal overuse injury. Features characteristic of flatfoot are: collapse of medial longitudinal arch, external rotation of calcaneum, eversion of anterior foot. Weight bearing X-rays are used to confirm the diagnosis of flat foot on which following measurements are taken: talonavicular coverage angle (TNC) measured on anteroposterior view X-rays, lateral talar-first metatarsal angle (LTM) and calcaneal pitch angle (CP) measured on lateral view X-rays.

In physiological pes planus, almost normal medial arch appears, when the person attempts to walk on the forefoot or when one attempts to push up the first metatarsal head from the plantar surface or when the foot is not bearing weight. There is rarely an identifiable abnormality, if such feet are pain free, mobile and of normal power and strength. Pain in flat foot is usually along the medial border, and is usually caused by overstretching of medial ligaments of foot.

Painful weak or stiff flat feet or the presence of skin lesions should be examined and investigated thoroughly.

The flat foot resulting from the spasm of the peronei is spastic and rigid. It is a protective mechanism against the painful foot resulting from *congenital vertical talus, congenital intertarsal osseous bars, and irritating bed of peronei*. On an attempt to passively invert this type of foot, there will be resistance, and patient will feel pain along the prominently standing peroneus longus and brevis tendons, behind and above the lateral malleolus **(Figs. 15.33 to 15.36)**.

Exaggeration of the pes planus may result in pes valgus **(Figs. 15.15 and 15.17)**.

Test for flexible flat foot: With full weight bearing, if the heel is in valgus position, which changes to varus when child is on tip toe position (bears weight only on fore foot), it indicates flexible flat foot.

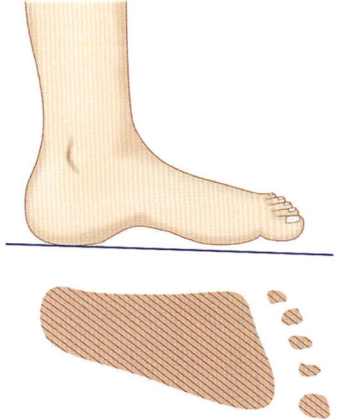

Fig. 15.32: Pes planus (*see* Figure 14—right foot pes planus and left foot pes valgus.

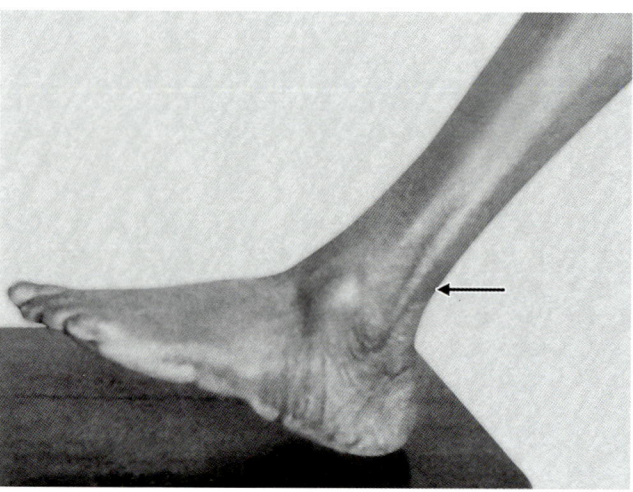

Fig. 15.33: Spastic flat foot. Note the prominent spastic peroneus.

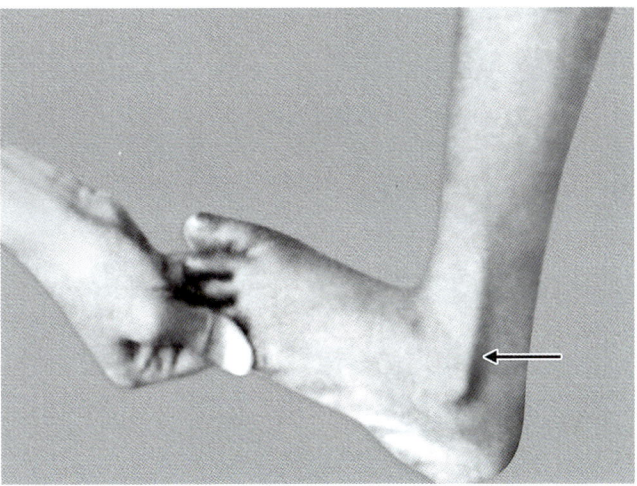

Fig. 15.34: In spasmodic flat foot, any attempt of passively inverting the foot makes the peroneus longus and brevis tendons more and more prominent.

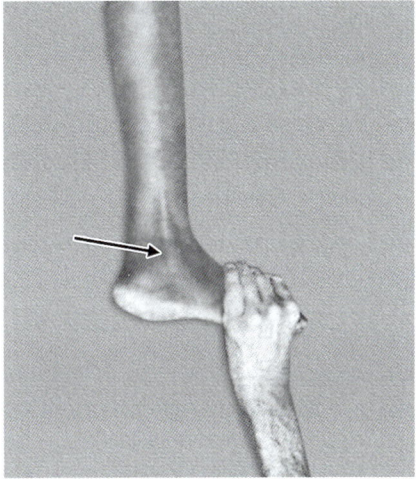

Fig. 15.35: Spastic/rigid flat foot: Note that even with the attempt of forceful inversion, it is not possible to do it and peronei stand prominent resisting the attempt of inverting the foot.

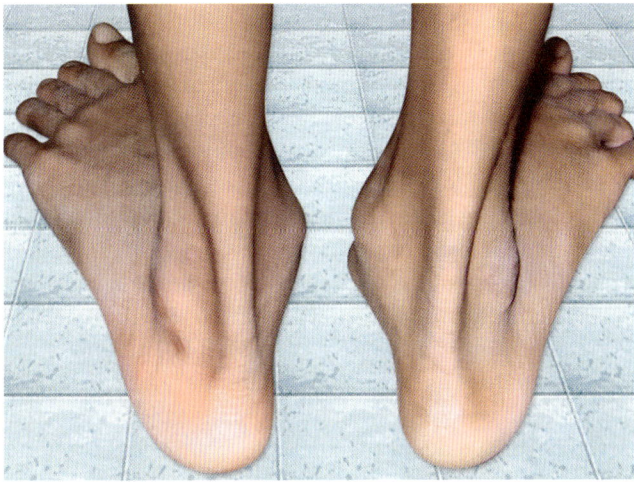

Fig. 15.36: Bilateral spastic pes valgus in adult.

Jack test: Jack's test demonstrates a synchronised activity of the intrinsic and extrinsic musculature and its influence on the physiopathomechanics of the *flaccid flat feet*. It is performed by passively extending the great toe with the patient standing. If the flat foot is due to collapse of the navicular-cuneiform joint, the arch will be restored, the foot tends to be supinated, and there is tendency of external rotation of tibia with inversion of the heel. When these occur, it indicates a *flexible flat foot.*

Chronic stenosing tenosynovitis of peroneal tendon sheath: In this condition, inversion of foot produces pain especially on the posterolateral aspect of ankle and foot along the peroneal tendons. Tender swelling occurs in the sheath of peroneal tendons behind and below the lateral malleolus.

If summarily assessed on functional background, the flat foot may be considered as relaxed flat foot (in which the longitudinal arch is collapsed when weight is borne on the foot); rigid flat foot (caused eventually by tarsal coalition; bony or fibrous ankylosis); spasmodic flat foot (caused by spasmodic contraction of peroneii), transverse flat foot (caused by collapse of transverse arch), stiff flat foot (neglected tibialis posterior tendon dysfunction may lead to stiff flat foot).

Tarsal coalition may lead to varying degrees of fixed hindfoot valgus with some loss of normal longitudinal arch of foot, however, it is not responsible to produce congenital rigid pes planus.

Tibialis posterior tendon (TPT) dysfunction, if neglected can produce stiff flat foot (see Page 462)

Insertional tendinosis of the anterior tibial tendon: Beischer et al. (2009) observed the clinical features of distal anterior tibial tendinosis as nocturnal burning pain in medial midfoot, localised tenderness over the insertion of anterior tibial tendon and often little swelling over the distal part of tendon. They described a clinical test which has 90% sensitivity and 95% specificity, to diagnose this condition as follows: the ankle is plantarflexed, the hindfoot is everted, the midfoot is abducted, and the foot on the whole is pronated to passively stretch the anterior tibial tendon. When the test is positive, the patient will complain of starting of pain or aggravation of already existing pain at the insertion of the anterior tibial tendon. MRI may be done to confirm the diagnosis.

Peroneal tendons disorders: Disorders of peroneal tendons are mainly of three types: (1) Peroneal tendinitis without subluxation of peroneal tendons and with or without attrition or rupture. This type usually occurs in middle-aged sports persons who develop swelling and effusion in peroneal tendon sheath. (2) Peroneal tendinitis with instability of peroneal tendons at the level of superior peroneal retinaculum with or without

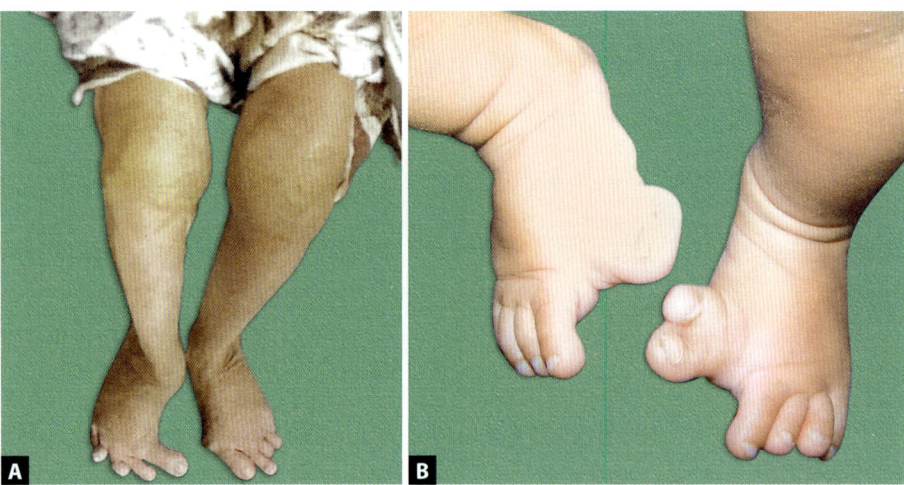

Figs. 15.37A and B: (A) *Windswept deformities of the toes.* Marked adduction of the forefoot led to sickle deformity of the right foot. In left foot, hallux valgus of the great toe has pushed other toes laterally; (B) Bilateral duplication of big toes with hyperplasia and bilateral hallux varus.

rupture of superior peroneal retinaculum. It is often seen in young athletes after acute ankle injuries. They develop chronic lateral ankle instability. (3) Stenosing tenosynovitis of peroneus longus tendon with or without enlarged peroneal tubercle.

Clinical findings of peroneal tendinitis: Palpable fluid in peroneal tendon sheath; crepitation felt in active-passive movements of subtalar joint; in standing position the hindfoot remains in varus or sometimes in valgus; swelling and tenderness at the site of synovitis or rupture. Tenderness may also be at the point where peroneus longus tendon enters the cuboid peroneal groove. Peroneal spasm may develop. Tendons may rupture at musculotendinous junction, or beneath superior peroneal retinaculum or in cuboid tunnel. Peroneal tendon affections may occur after calcaneal fractures. Plain X-ray, USG and MRI are helpful in confirming and localising the pathology. A shallow or convex posterior groove of fibula is likely to be associated with peroneal tendon instability.

Bassett (Quoted by Murphy GA in Campbell's Operative Orthopaedic, 12th Ed, page 3946) described in 1985, about subluxation of the peroneal tendons within the peroneal tendon sheath without subluxation in the posterolateral groove of fibula. When the foot is everted in extension popping or snapping of the peroneal tendons can be noted.

Side car Deformity

Side car deformity of foot: It is relatively uncommon deformity, in which there is chronic lateral dislocation of the subtalar joint. As described in literature it develops secondary to trauma, however it can be acquired and seen in severe longstanding cases of flatfoot and charcot neuropathy. Mostly the soft tissues on the medial side of foot are first affected. It produces progressive disability even upto limb - threatening stage. Management consists of reconstruction by intramedullary nail fixation for tibio - talar - calcaneal (TTC) or tibiocalcaneal fusion along with or without adjunctive procedures like midfoot fusion, talonavicular fusion and posterior muscle group lengthening (Elbert DR 2020).

Congenital Vertical Talus or Congenital Convex Pes Valgus (Congenital Vertical Talus, Rocker-bottom Flat Foot, Congenital Rigid Flat Foot)

It is the most severe malformation of the spectrum of congenital flat foot. The most obvious radiological feature in this deformity is vertical orientation of the talus—congenital vertical talus **(Figs. 15.7 and 15.8)**.

Congenital vertical talus (CVT) is not common condition characterized by a fixed dorsal subluxation/dislocation of the navicular on the talar head and neck leading to a rigid flatfoot deformity. Congenital vertical talus may be associated with numerous neuromuscular disorders, such as cerebral palsy, arthrogryposis, myelomeningocele or may occur as an isolated congenital anomaly. Basic pathology is variable degree of dorsal dislocation of the talonavicular joint. Severe degrees of CVT is obvious even at birth with the presence of a rounded prominence at the medial and plantar surfaces of the foot produced by the abnormal location of the head of talus. The talus is displaced medially and plantarward remaining almost vertical. Calcaneum also remains in variable degree of equinus position (but much less than talus) and gradually is displaced posteriorly with development of foot, and the plantar surface of its anterior part becomes rounded. With weight bearing adaptive changes occur in the tarsals. The talus becomes hourglass-shaped, with its longitudinal axis lying almost nearing same to that of tibia and only about posterior third of its superior articular surface articulates with tibia. In full weight bearing position, the forefoot becomes severely abducted and the heel does not touch the ground. On the dorsum of foot the capsules of joints, ligaments and tendons become contracted. The tibialis posterior, peroneus

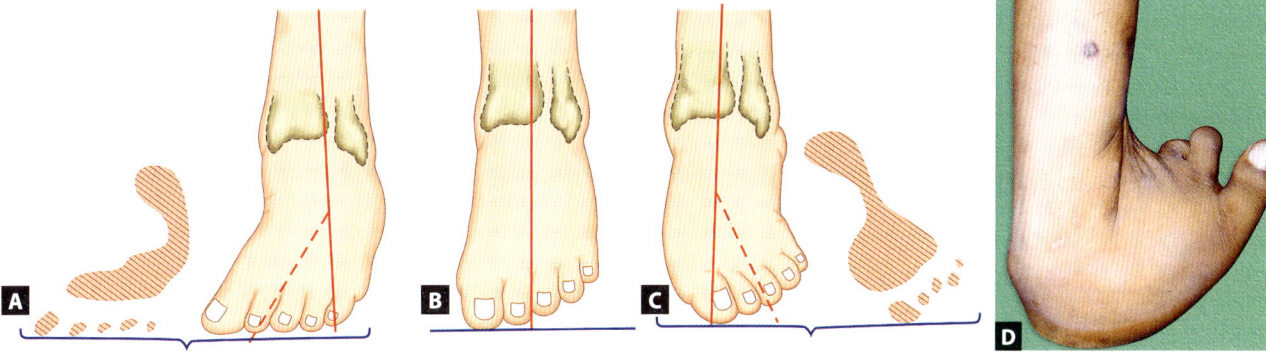

Figs. 15.38A to C: (A) Footprint of adduction of forefoot, (B) Normal alignment of forefoot, (C) Abduction of forefoot with footprint, (D) Dorsiflexion and eversion deformity of foot.

longus and peroneus brevis tendons get translocated anterior to their respective malleoli and even may act as dorsiflexors rather than plantar flexors of foot. Milder form is likely to be missed in standard X-ray, however sonography is helpful in the early diagnosis of CVT in infancy. There is variable equinus at tibio-talar joint. There is abnormal flexion-extension movement between forefoot and hindfoot. The lateral X-ray in maximum dorsiflexion and plantar flexion of foot is mandatory for diagnosis. Classification of vertical talus – congenital vertical talus, has been variously classified like Kumar's, (1982); Coleman and colleagues (1970); Lichtblau's however, Kumar's classification into four groups appears to be more practical.

- *Group I:* Supple feet that resemble calcaneovalgus feet – radiograph needs to make diagnosis
- *Group II:* Children with rigid feet some of which are part of a syndrome
- *Group III:* Vertical talus associated with trisomy 13–15 or 18.
- *Group IV:* Vertical talus associated with neuromuscular problems such as spina bifida (After Dhillon M. congenital vertical talus chapter 299.2 page 2756. JAYPEE Textbook of Orthopaedics &Traumatoly 3rd Ed. 2016.

Mild or even moderate deformities can be managed by percutaneous reduction followed by casting, however severe ones require open reduction.

Adduction of the Forefoot (Pes Adductus, Congenital Metatarsus Adductus or Sickle Foot) (Figs. 15.38A and B—right foot and Figure 15.39)

From the transitional zone of mid to forefoot the foot assumes a tendency of deviation towards the inner side. In a normal neutrally aligned lower limb, a line joining the centre point of the patella to the anterior mid-ankle point, if extended distally, passes through the second toe or the second web (**Fig. 15.38B**). In adduction of the forefoot, this line passes through the toes or webs outer to this axis.

There is adduction of forefoot in relation to midfoot and hindfoot. The exact pathogenesis is not known. Though

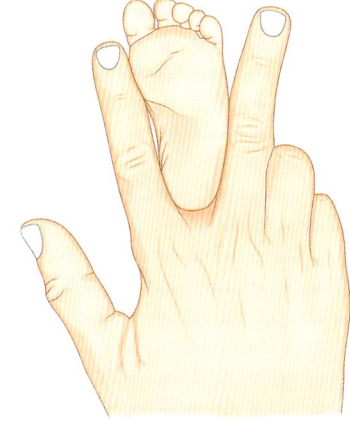

Fig. 15.39: Metatarsus adductus (MTA) can be suspected by performing the "V" test (Alvin & Jeanne 2004).

deformity is present at birth, it is very often diagnosed in the first year of life. Along with adduction there may be varying degree of supination of forefoot, mild heel valgus and internal tibial torsion. It is a common anomaly leading to in-toeing in children. It is usually associated with clubfoot, however it may remain as isolated deformity. In young children, serial stretching and casting may help. In grown up children, surgery (soft tissue or bony or both procedures) is required to correct the deformities, especially when it causes pain, problems in footwear or unacceptable deformity.

Metatarsus adductus is a transverse plane congenital deformity, known as the metatarsals adducted (MA) in a position relative to the longitudinal axis of the lesser tarsus. Metatarsus adductus is commonly seen in patients with hallux valgus deformity which is as acquired first ray multiplanar deformity. The prevalence of MA in HV patients has been reported to be 35% (La Reaux 1987).

Abduction of Forefoot (Pes Abductus) (Figs. 15.38C and 15.39)

From the transitional zone of hind to midfoot the foot deviates to the outer side. Here, the axis (as mentioned in pes abductus) passes inner to the second toe (**Fig. 15.38C**).

Brachymetatarsia (see also Page 438)

Lesser toe deformities: Deformities of lesser toes (such as mallet toe, hammer toe, claw toe or cross-over toe) are not infrequently related to the instability of the metatarsophalangeal joint, especially of the second toe. These deformities are oftenly seen in women of more than 50 years age who use narrow high heeled shoes and in athletes with chronic overuse and hyperextension of the toes and usually have hallux valgus, and degenerative changes in the first metatarsophalangeal joint. Lachman test of metatarsophalangeal joint, done to assess its dorsal-plantar instability, is mostly positive in these cases.

Clawing of the Toes (Figs. 15.42 and 15.43)

There is hyperextension at the metatarsophalangeal joint and plantarflexion at the interphalangeal joints. As a result, the pulps of the toes do not touch the ground even in full flexion of the interphalangeal joints. Passively elevating the depressed metatarsal head further exaggerates the plantarflexion of the toe **(Fig. 15.43)**. *Complete paralysis of both plantar nerves causes a 'pied-en-griffe' deformity.*

Clawfoot/Claw Toe

Clawfoot (originates) develops due to muscular imbalance either due to neuromuscular diseases, wear of the plantar fascia or due to an anatomical defect or faulty length of the first ray.

Clawfoot may be: (a) *Dynamic clawfoot*—it occurs when the first ray suffers from relatively insufficient length in relation to the medial rays an insufficiency which may be anatomical, constitutional or after some surgery, e.g. shortening first metatarsal or proximal phalanx; or arthrodesis of first metatarsophalangeal joint, (b) *Static clawfoot* is the ultimate result of degradation of an external ray in the context of hallux valgus. IPP arthrodesis is part of the treatment of clawfoot to complement certain operations on the tendons or bone.

In claw toe, oftenly a similar deformity is present in all toes. Claw toes have always extension deformity at the *metatarsophalangeal* joint and often have flexion deformity at the distal interphalangeal joint.

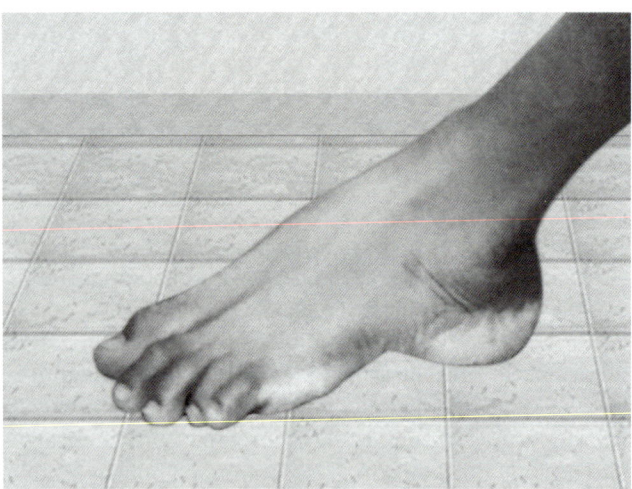

Fig. 15.40: Pes abductus.

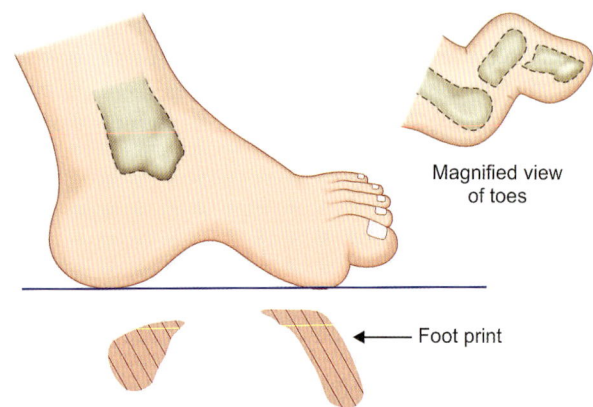

Fig. 15.42: Clawing of toes (line drawing).

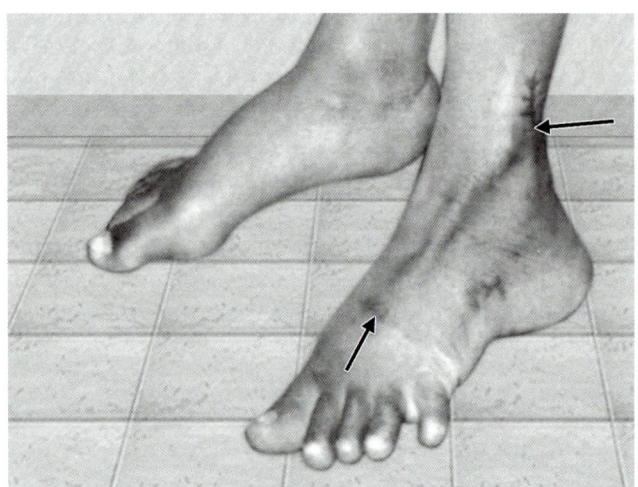

Fig. 15.41: Pes abductus due to overactive transferred peroneus brevis tendon.

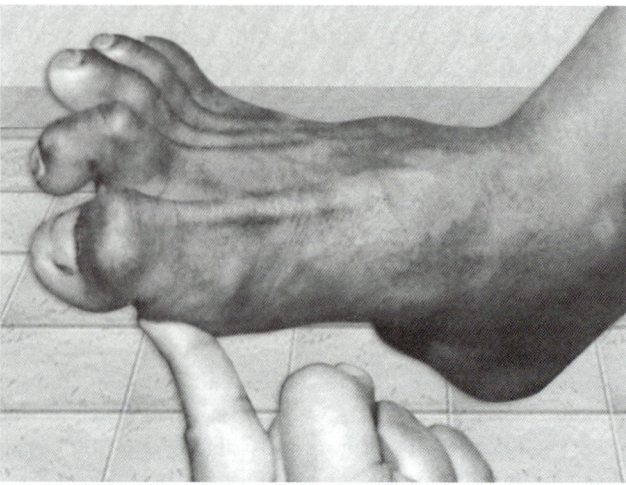

Fig. 15.43: Clawing of toes.

Hammer-Toe Deformity: Flexible or Fixed (Figs. 15.44 to 15.47)

There is acute plantar flexion—flexible or fixed (contracture)—at the proximal interphalangeal joint and flexion or extension at the distal interphalangeal joint (There is no marked change at the metatarsophalangeal joint, however, it may remain fixed in dorsiflexion; some times metatarsal head may be depressed on the plantar surface). A hammer toe may involve either a single or multiple toes, and are usually bilateral. The second toe is the most commonly involved. It often accompanies halux valgus. The wearing of too narrow short shoes causes the long second toe to buckle. *Abnormal extrinsic forces and muscle imbalance lead to the development of a hammer-toe deformity. In hammer toe, patient may complain of pain at three places.* A painful inflamed bursa and/or callus overlies the dorsal prominence of the flexed interphalangeal joint. The tip of the affected toe is broadened and thickened with callus due to excessive pressure—called an end corn. A painfull callus may develop beneath the metatarsal head when the proximal phalanx subluxates dorsally.

Various procedures have been used to correct a hammer-toe deformity, e.g. tendon release, proximal phalangeal condylectomy, proximal interphalangeal joint fusion, partial phalangectomy, etc.

Mallet toe: In mallet toe, which develops mostly in second toe (which is usually the longest toe), the distal interphalangeal joint assumes a flexion position. It may develop alone or in association with hammer toe at the proximal interphalangeal joint. Due to flexed position of the distal interphalangeal joint, the patient complains of problem in using shoes with small or narrow toe box. The deformity is more common in diabetic neuropathy. The toe may develop pain, end corn and even ulcer. Rarely mallet toe, like hammer toe, may be congenital. Combined hammer toe and mallet toe deformities may be associated with large prominent corns, usually, over the

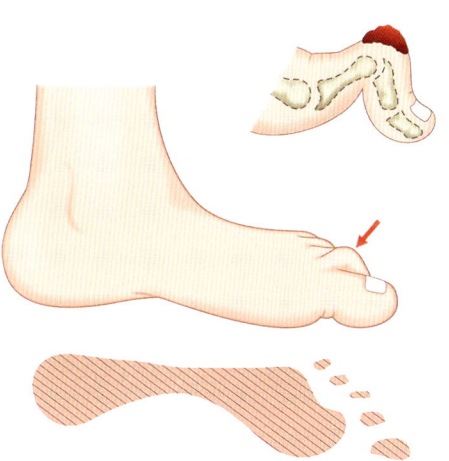

Fig. 15.44: Hammer toes (line drawing).

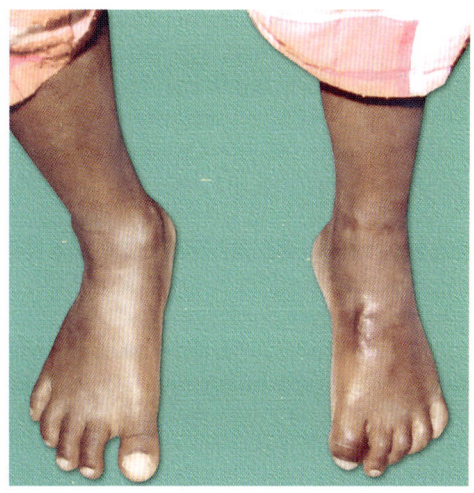

Fig. 15.46: Hammer toes of all left side toes following infection in the left midfoot region.

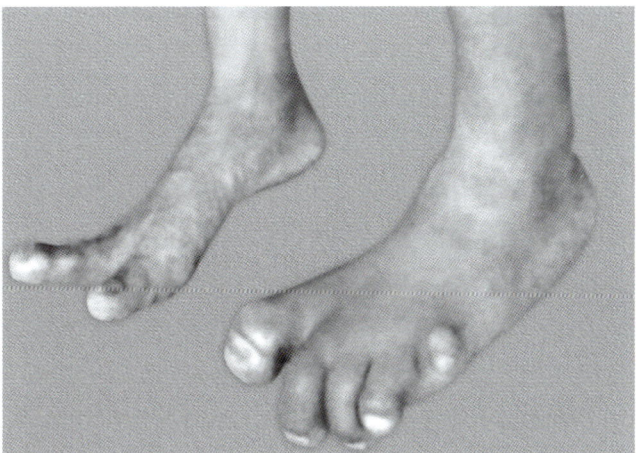

Fig. 15.45: Clinical photograph: left foot showing hammer toe of big toe, 2nd toe with DIP in some flexion, 3rd toe with DIP in flexion, 4th toe going for hammer toe, 5th toe subluxated dorsolaterally with tendency of hammer toe; right foot—macrodactyly of 2nd toe.

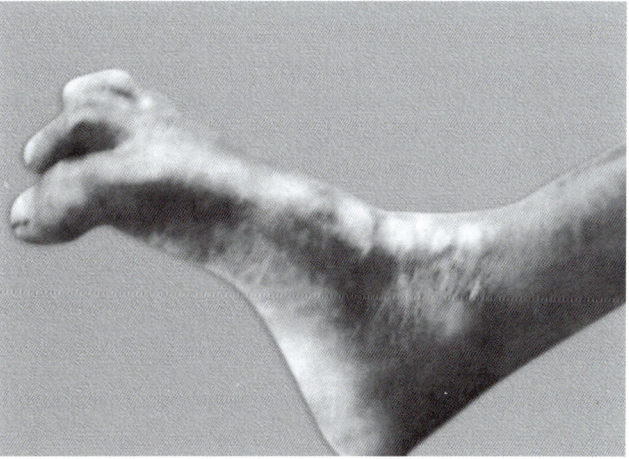

Fig. 15.47: Hammer toe of all the toes.

proximal and distal interphalangeal joints. There is hardly any extension deformity at the metatarsophalangeal joint.

Hallux Valgus Bunion (Figs. 15.48 to 15.52)

Hallux valgus is one of the most common structural foot deformities. Hallux valgus is a complex deformity of big toe (1st ray), however, deformities and symptoms are frequently present in other toes also. The average normal angle between first and second metatarsal is 8°–9°. The first metatarsophalangeal joint is normally set at the valgus angle of 15°–20°. When the angular deviation of hallux is >15 — 20 degree towards the lesser toes with respect to the first metatarsal bone, appearing as a medial bony enlargement of the first metatarsal head, it can be diagnosed as hallux valgus.

The long axis of the great toe deviates outwards at the metatarsophalangeal joint. The superomedial aspect of first metatarsal head, which deviates medially, stands markedly prominent and is usually associated with thickened overlying soft tissues (bunion, callosity). The great toe in turn may push the other toes (second and even the third) laterally (*see* **Fig. 15.37**), and may even override the next toe (**Fig. 22.50**). Sometimes second toe may also override the deviated great toe (**Figs. 15.48, 15.51 and 15.52**) 87% bunions have a metatarsal frontal-plane rotational deformity (Kim Y et al 2015). *Radiologically when the angle between the first metatarsal shaft and the proximal phalanx is greater than 15°, hallux valgus is diagnosed.*

Hallux valgus is one of the most common orthopedic deformities with a prevalence of 23% in adults. (Nix S et al 2010).

It is one of the most common deformities of the toes especially in white population ladies using the narrow toe-box/strapped footwear. The wearing of badly fitting footwear is often blamed for hallux valgus. It is more common in girls. *Adolescent hallux valgus* has a strong family history in about 75% of cases.

Patients usually complain of pain in foot, impaired gait patterns, poor balance, ugly look and sometimes falls in older adults. The symptomatic hallux valgus may respond to special hallux-valgus splint, shoe-insert, or orthotic, however, it needs surgery in most of the cases. More than 730 different surgical approaches have been described to correct hallux valgus deformity like arthrodesis (first described by Clutton HH in 1894 for severe hallux valgus deformities, and also recommended for severe hallux rigidus, rheumatoid arthritis, post traumatic arthritis, gouty arthritis, failed bunion and implant surgeries and neuromuscular conditions), implants, resection arthroplasty, osteotomy of various types. Of all these surgeries, fusion of first metatarso - phalangeal joint proved to be reliable method with patients' lasting satisfaction.

Though about 400 surgical procedures have been described to correct hallux valgus, choice of optimal approach

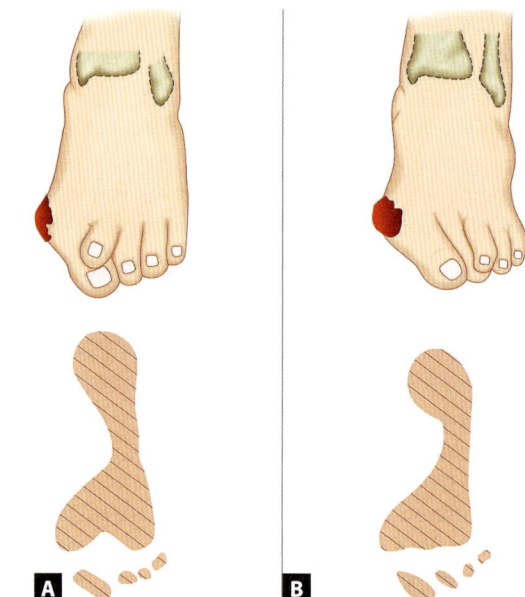

Figs. 15.48A and B: Hallux valgus with footprint: (A) hallux valgus with cross-over 2nd toe, (B) hallux valgus (bunion) with hammer toe of second toe.

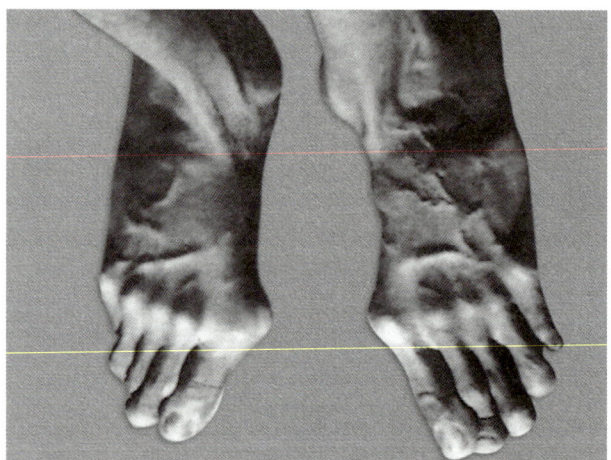

Fig. 15.49: Clinical photograph of bilateral hallux valgus. Right markedly pronounced with bunion and callosity.

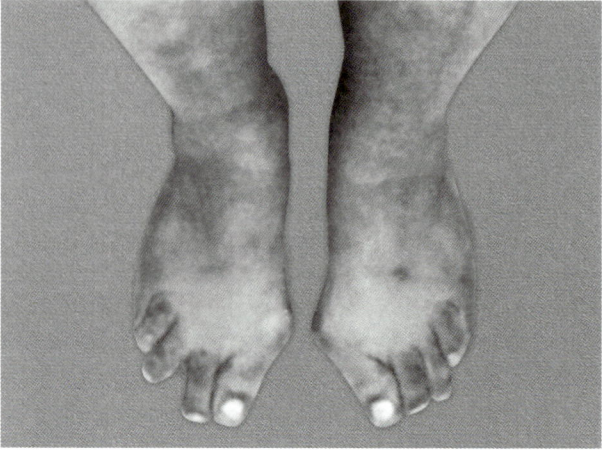

Fig. 15.50: Hallux valgus in both feet. Note that the *deviated big toes are tending to override their corresponding second toe.*

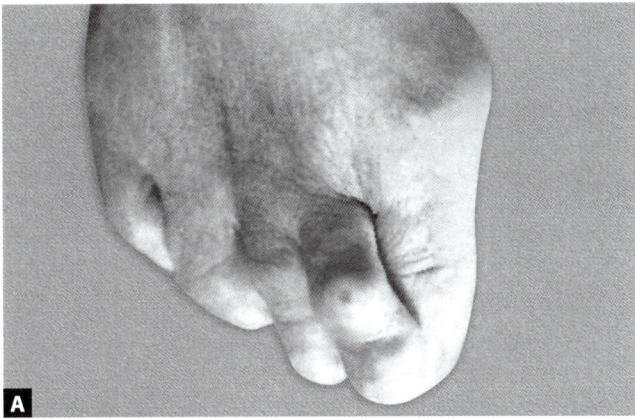

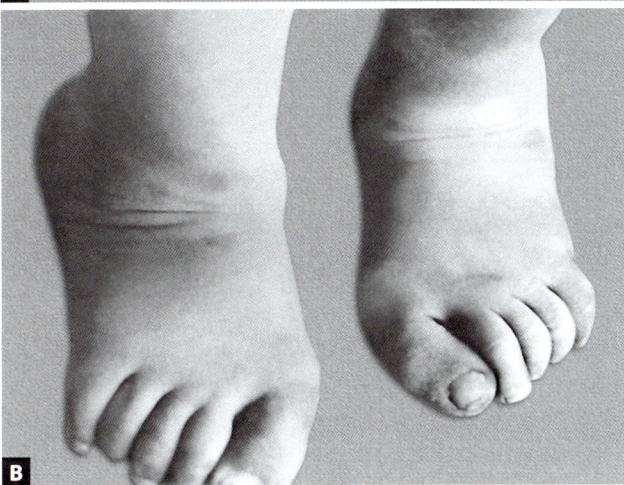

Figs. 15.51A and B: (A) Hallux valgus with tendency of cross-over toe. Note the second toe overriding the deviated first toe; (B) Bilateral congenital hallux valgus.

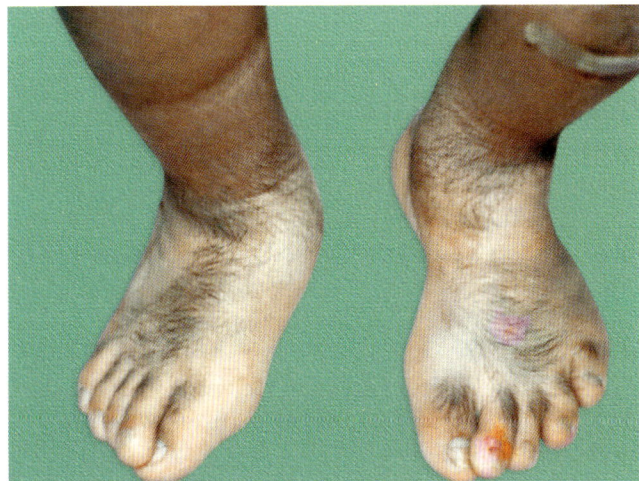

Fig. 15.52: Bilateral congenital hallux valgus with second toe overriding the deviated big toe on each side.

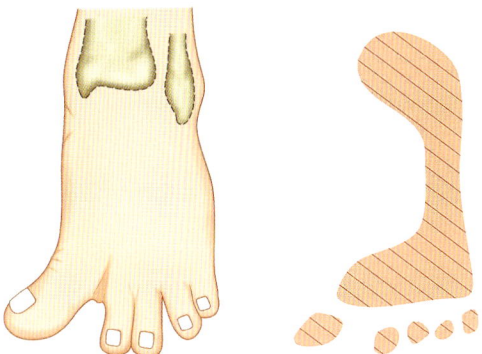

Fig. 15.53: Hallux varus.

scarf osteotomy associated with Weil osteotomies proved to be the standard surgical treatment of advanced hallux valgus. The patients should be thoroughly assessed on a standard scoring system before and after treatment [e.g. American Orthopaedic Foot and Ankle Society Hallux Valgus Score (AOFAS score)]. Disease-specific outcome measures for hallux valgus are the Manchester-Oxford Foot Questionnaire (MOXFQ), the Foot And Ankle Outcome Score (FAOS) and the self-reported foot and ankle score.

Hallux Varus (Figs. 15.53 to 15.55)

Hallux varus is a deformity of the great toe in which there is adduction of the hallux and medial subluxation of the first MTP joint and thus the great toe is angulated medially.

The great toe deviates inwards at the metatarsophalangeal joint. The second toe often follows suit. Typically, congenital hallux varus occurs on one side only and may be associated with other anomaly of toes. Hallux varus also occurs as a complication of hallux valgus surgery (over or malcorrection) in about 2 to 17% due to complete release of the lateral structures of the metatarsophalangeal joint alongwith excessive plication of the medial capsule or excessive resection of medial eminence or excision of fibular sesamoid or release of the lateral head of the flexor hallucis brevis or combinations of two or three of above causes (after Richardson EG 2013). Idiopathic hallux varus is a very rare problem. Lesser hallux varus can be corrected by reversing the soft tissue releases (of what is done for correcting the hallux valgus and temporarily immobilizing the MTP joint with a k-wire for about 8 weeks). In unacceptable/severe/symptomatic cases surgical fusion of great and second toes (surgical syndactyly) is indicated.

Windswept Deformities of the Toes

In rheumatoid arthritis, sometimes there may be windswept deformities of the toes, i.e. valgus deformities of the big toe (followed by others) in one foot and varus in other (*see* Fig. 15.37A).

remains controversial. Recently Minimally Invasive Surgery (MIS) has become popular, because of its reduced surgical trauma to both bone and adjacent soft tissues. However, the

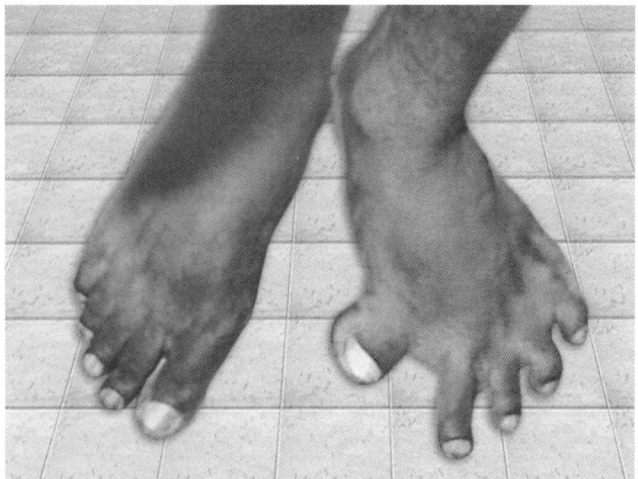

Fig. 15.54: Hallux varus (left) deformity. Other toes of the same (left) foot are also deviating inwards.

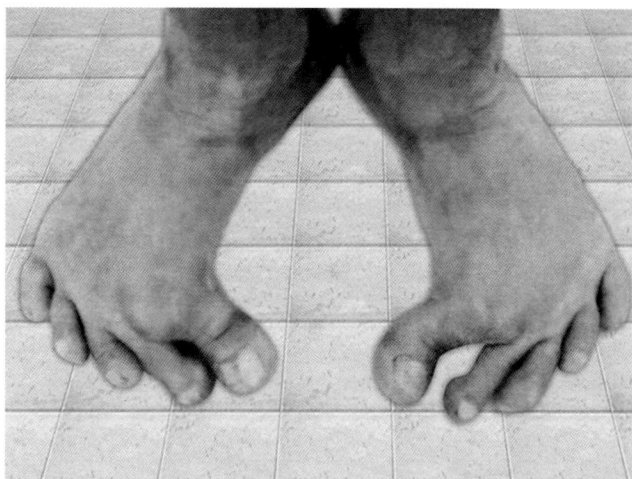

Fig. 15.55: Bilateral hallux varus. Note that all the toes in each foot are going for varus deformities. Note that in hallux varus the big toe is angulated at the metatarsophalangeal joint towards the medial side while in metatarsus primus varus, the angulation occurs in the metatarsal cuneiform joint.

Hallux Rigidus (Synonyms—Hallux Fluxus, Hallux Dolorosus, Dorsal Bunion, Metatarsus Primus Elevatus, Hallux Limitus)

The word 'hallux-rigidus' was coined by Cotterill JM in 1888. It is a disorder characterized by a progressive restriction of the first metatarsophalangeal joint or joint stiffness. Hallux rigidus is basically a degenerative arthritic condition of the first metatarsophalangeal joint characterized by decreased dorsiflexion. It is more common in females over 40 years of age complaining of pain in foot which may be in mild, moderate and severe forms. It has been managed usually by several surgical procedures like cheilectomy, proximal phalangeal osteotomy, drilling or autograft plantation for osteochondral lesions, arthrodesis, arthroplasty, keller osteotomy, metatarsal osteotomy etc. Of the above cheilectomy for grades 1 and 2 disease and arthroplasty or arthrodesis for grades 3 and 4 have been generally accepted. (Nakajima 2022). There is osteoarthritis of 1st metatarsophalangeal (MTP) joint. A prominent osteophyte is usually present on the dorsal aspect of metatarsophalangeal joint. Pain may be complained during walking and climbing. Extension of metatarsophalangeal joint is severely limited. If during the growing period short shoes are regularly used, the metatarsophalangeal joint of the *big toe* becomes *stiff* (hallux rigidus) *due to osteoarthrosis*. However, some degree of movement is generally available, hence the term 'hallux limitus' has been used. This may also result following intra-articular fractures, osteochondritis of the metatarsal head, gout or pseudogout. The role of metatarsus primus elevatus and first ray hypermobility is also being considered to explain the pathoanatomy of hallux rigidus. Severe hallux rigidus and metatarsus primus elevatus problems have been claimed to be solved by first tarsometatarsal realignment arthrodesis with cheilectomy which corrects the deformity and stabilizes the medial column. (Boffeli JJ et al. 2020).

Hallux Limitus

'Hallux limitus' indicates a decrease or a limitation of the range of motion in the metatarsophalangeal joint of the big toe, while 'Hallux-rigidus' indicates the absence of the movements of the big toe. It is often associated with a mechanical block to dorsiflexion caused by periarticular osteophytes with an impingement exostosis of the first metatarsal head against an osteophyte at the base of proximal phalanx.

Duplication Toes

Duplication mostly occurs in big toe, which hinders the use of footwear (*see* **Fig. 15.37B**)

Digitus Quintus Varus

Deviation of long axis of the little toe medially is known as digitus quintus varus (**Fig. 15.56A**) in right foot. However, when the little toe is so much deviated as to override the fourth toe, this is called 'digitus quintus varus superinductus' (**Fig. 15.56B**).

Overriding Toes

Congenital elevation of the little toe with rotation causes the little toe to sit on the top of the fourth toe, which usually results in painful corns.

Early cases may be managed by strapping. In the late presenting cases surgery can realign the soft tissue, especially if symptoms are problematic.

Curly Toes

The fourth and fifth toes are flexed and medially rotated at the distal interphalangeal joint. Usually, it resolves of itself

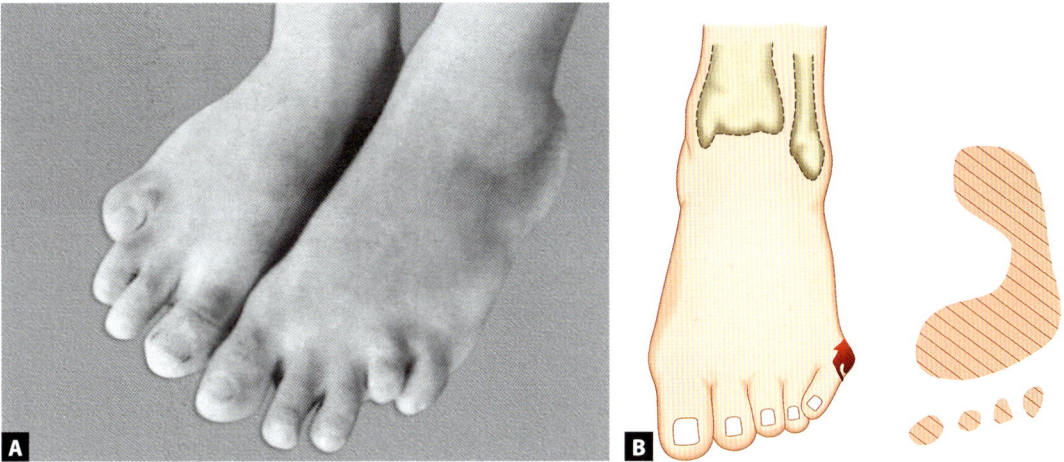

Figs. 15.56A and B: (A) Digitus quintus varus; (B) Digitus quintus varus super inductus.

or remain asymptomatic. It is rare in adults. If it becomes symptomatic, flexor tenotomy usually helps.

Bunionette (Tailor's Bunion)

Bunionette or the lateral prominence of the head of the fifth metatarsal accompanied by a moderate Quintus varus may be seen as an isolated deformity or associated with hallux valgus or as an element of generalised pathology in triangular-shaped foot. The lateral prominence of the head of the fifth metatarsal often called a tailor's bunion, referring to the position in which tailors usually sit on the floor with their legs crossed, is responsible for the painful impingement.

Bunionette can be classified into three types based on whether it exists with an increased intermetatarsal angle, an enlarged fifth metatarsal head or a deformation of the fifth metatarsal like the blade of a sword. It can be managed by resection of the lateral prominent condyle (especially in isolated impingement in elderly patients). However, excellent correction of the painful impingement can be obtained by SCARF osteotomy. It is better in more severe impingement, with a moderately increased intermetatarsal angle. Weil's osteotomy should be a part of the overall treatment of the problems associated with a triangular foot.

Pes Transversus or Spread Foot (Fig. 15.57)

In a normal foot, while weight bearing, the concentration of weight is more on the first and fifth toes (tripod stand concept of foot). Sometimes the third metatarsal head collapses. This can be clinically felt as a bony swelling through the sole in that area. In addition, there is an increase in the breadth of forefoot. The concentration of weight in this area also increases. Such a foot is known as *pes transversus or spread foot.*

Cockup Deformity of Toes (Fig. 15.58)

In elderly diabetics and in patients of posterior tibial nerve neuropathy, a deformity, like the clawing of toes, is produced and is known as cockup deformity.

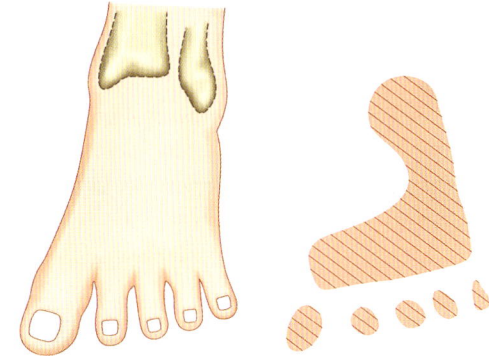

Fig. 15.57: Spread foot (Pes transversus).

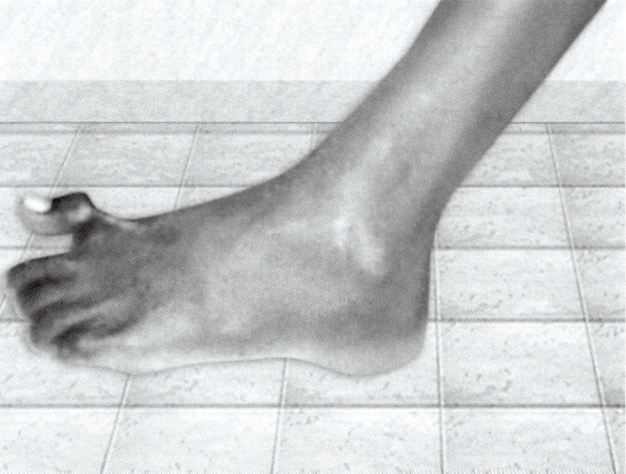

Fig. 15.58: Cockup deformity of big toe.

Skew Foot (Fig. 15.59)

In congenital metatarsus adductovarus or skew foot, there is adduction of distal shafts of metatarsals, inversion of forefoot, eversion and lateral displacement of navicular and calcaneum leading to severe valgus of hindfoot along with adduction of the forefoot and varying degree of cavus. It is

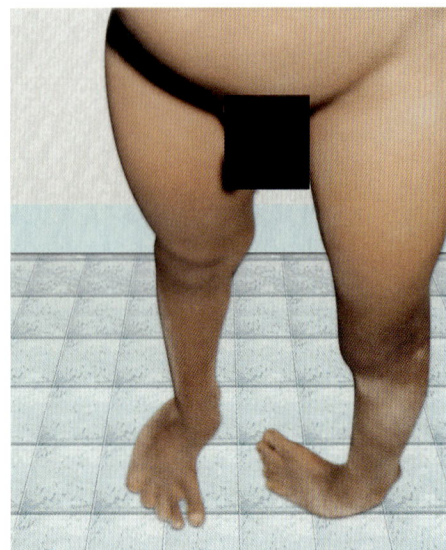

Fig. 15.59: Skew foot on right side and cavovarus deformity of left foot with some equinus.

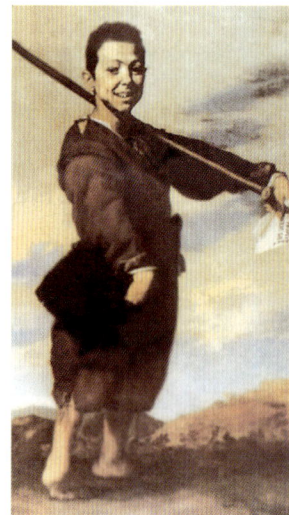

Fig. 15.60: Jusepe de Ribena's "The Clubfoot boy" painted in 1642 in the Louvre museum of Paris.

cosmetically acceptable in the beginning, but with neglect in advancing age the "serpentine or Z-foot" deformity develops consisting of adduction and varus of metatarsals, hallux valgus, calcaneal valgus and cavus leading to ugly gait.

Talus Foot

This is usually a postural moulding defect seen in the neonates. It may be in exaggerated form presenting high arching in midfoot, calcaneus look at hindfoot (heel) and hammer-toe position of the big toe. Such cases require corrective splint.

Common Combinations of Deformities

- Equinus + cavus + varus with or without adduction of the forefoot—Clubfoot (**Figs. 15.60 to 15.62 and 15.63 to 15.75**).
- Varus + cavus + adduction of forefoot with clawing of toes—Hollow foot (**Fig. 15.76**).
- Pes planus + valgus + abduction—Knock flat foot.
- Cavus + valgus—Knock hollow foot.
- Cavus + pes transversus—Hollow spread foot.
- Equinus + cavus—Equino-cavus foot (**Fig. 15.77A**).
- Calcaneus + valgus + cavus—Calcaneo-cavo-valgus (**Figs. 15.78 to 15.81**)

Complex Foot Deformities

Complex foot deformities may be described as a foot with multiplanar deformities with or without shortening of the foot. Such deformities are usually caused by severe trauma, polio-paralysis, neglected or relapsed club foot, burn contractures, chronic osteomyelitis, neuromuscular disease, cerebral palsy, etc. They may be complicated with poor soft tissue coverage, leg-length descrepancies,

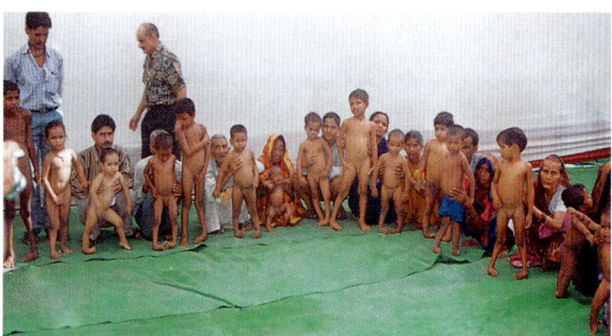

Fig. 15.61: Clubfoot camp.

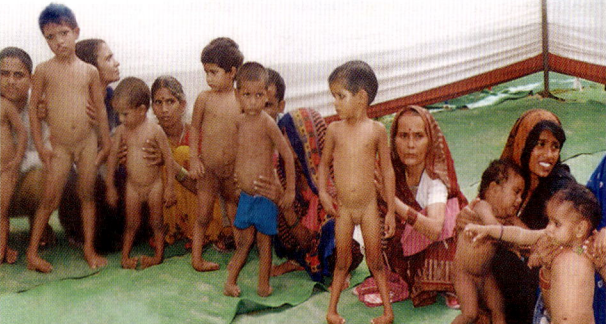

Fig. 15.62: Neglected clubfeet selected for surgery in the temporary camp hospital.

lower leg deformities, chronic extensive bone infections, ununited fractures. Correction of these deformities (e.g. by extensive soft tissue release, osteotomies at various levels, Ilizarov or other external fixators, with or without osteotomies, arthrodesis of the joints, etc.) are likely to have complications like neurovascular injury, soft tissue problems, shortening of foot, etc. The procedure of correction must be chosen carefully after fully explaining the nature of management, possible outcome, limitations, complications, etc.

Foot 455

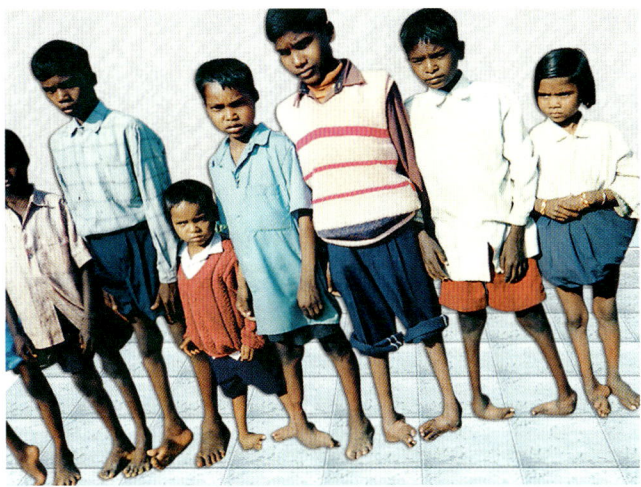

Fig. 15.63: A group of neglected clubfoot patients waiting for mainly bony operative correction.

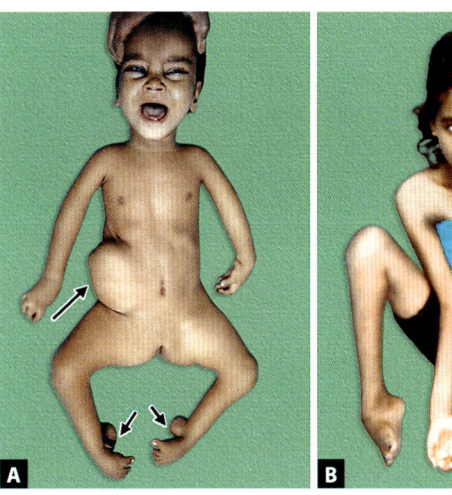

Figs. 15.65A and B: (A) Clubfeet as part of arthrogryposis multiplex congenita alongwith weak abdominal wall which balloons up while child cries; (B) Bilateral clubfoot in myopathy.

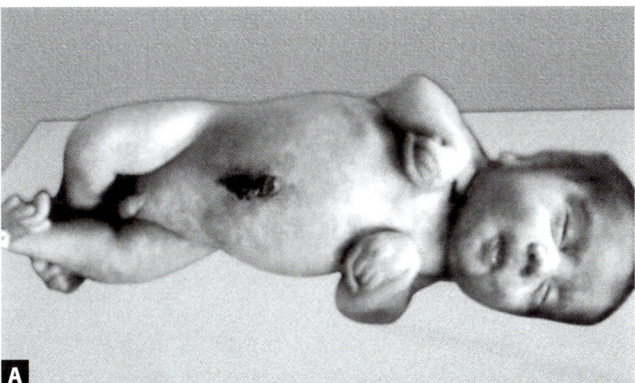

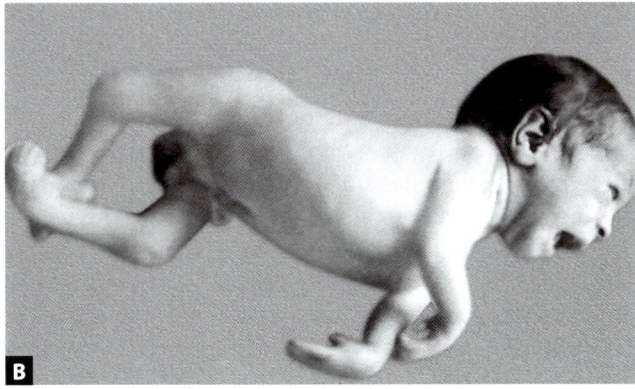

Figs. 15.64A and B: Clubfeet as part of arthrogryposis multiplex congenita. Arthrogryposis word denotes multiple joint contractures present at birth associated with varying degree of muscle weakness. This term was coined by otto in 1841, who described his such patients as human wonder with curved limbs. Stern described this disease as arthrogryposis multiplex congenita.

Types of Forefoot

The type of forefoot varies according to the relation of the first and second toe. *Three common varieties of forefoot have been recognised* (After Debrunner, HU):

1. Egyptian type of forefoot (**Fig. 15.82A**) 1 > 2 > 3 > 4 > 5: The great toe is longer than the 2nd toe, the 2nd toe is

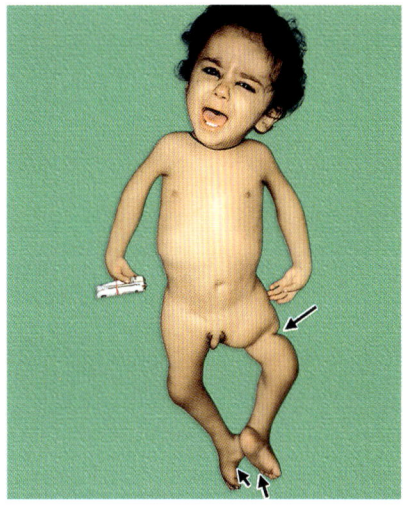

Fig. 15.66: Clubfeet as part of arthrogryposis multiple congenita alongwith congenital constriction band in the left thigh.

longer than the 3rd toe. 3rd longer than the 4th and 4th longer than the 5th.

2. Intermediate rectangular foot/square foot (**Fig. 15.82B**): The great and second toes are equal. However, the 2nd toe may be equal or longer than the 3rd toe. The 3rd toe may be equal or longer than the 4th toe. The 4th toe may be equal or longer than the 5th toe.

3. Grecian (Greek) foot (**Fig. 15.82C**) 1 < 2 > 3 > 4 > 5 (J Lelievre): The great toe is smaller than the 2nd toe. The 2nd toe is bigger than the 3rd toe. The 3rd toe is bigger than the 4th toe. The 4th toe is bigger than the 5th toe.

There can be abnormal congenital or acquired patterns which must be assessed carefully, e.g. in Marfan's syndrome in which the feet and hands are extremely long and thin with great length of the toes and fingers. The big toe is much longer than the rest of the toes and may result in varus or

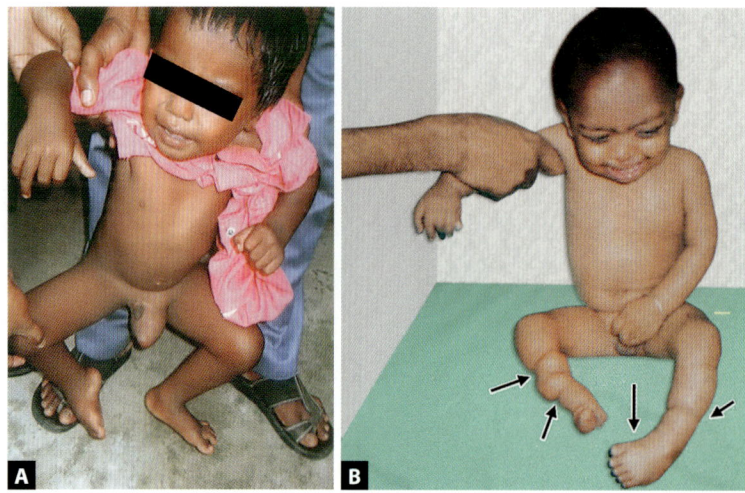

Figs. 15.67A and B: (A) Neglected clubfoot(R) with congenital (left) hernia (ring); (B) Multiple congenital constriction rings in the legs with ill-developed right foot and associated clubfoot on left side.

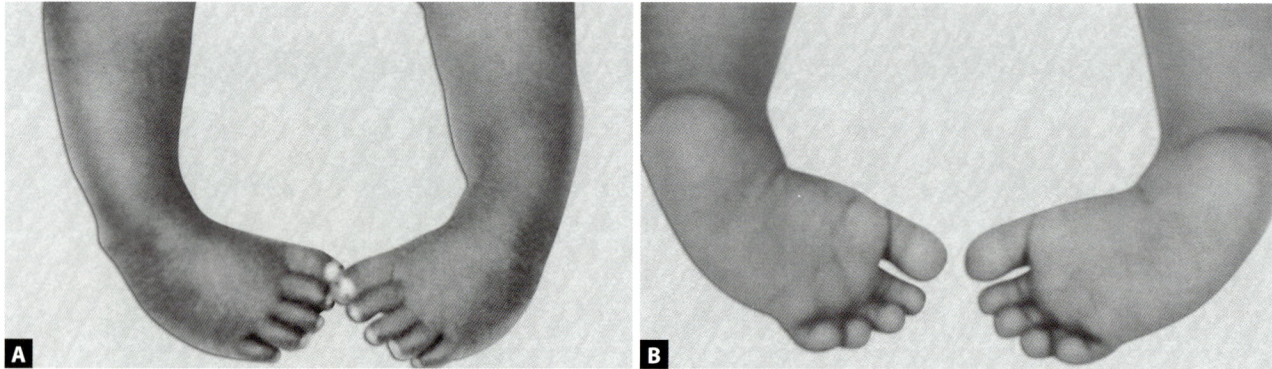

Figs. 15.68A and B: Mild clubfoot.

valgus deformities. The marked laxity of the ligaments produce flat foot.

■ METHODOLOGY OF EXAMINATION

History Taking
(As in the Chapter 1: Introduction)

The main complaints regarding the feet of children are about deformities, while in adults they are mainly regarding pain and swelling. When pain is complained of, enquire about its specific site and relation with standing, walking (distance usually covered before pain starts) and rest. In case of congenital deformities (e.g. club foot), the family history (for such deformities) and obstetrical history (age of mother, drug used during pregnancy, foetal presentation in uterus, mode of delivery, etc.) must be taken in detail.

General and Systemic Examinations
(As in Chapter 1: Introduction)

While the clinical history is taken and analysed, the patient's psychological profile should be assessed.

If the patient can stand and walk, the gait must be noted. The position of the foot in stance phase should be noted with particular emphasis on the weight bearing pattern of different parts of the sole. While examining the gait, ask the patient to walk as his/her normal gait, then on tiptoes (the forefoot), heels, outer border, and inner border of the feet, respectively. This gives an overall impression about the function of the foot. If one is able to walk in the above patterns normally, the foot is most probably normal.

Regional Examination

As usual for the lower limb, i.e. from the lumbosacral region to the tips of the toes.

Local Examination

Prerequisites

- Both feet must be examined simultaneously in identical positions as far as possible.
- Expose up to the ipsilateral hip or till at least above knee level.
- The foot is better examined while the patient is sitting at the edge of the couch.

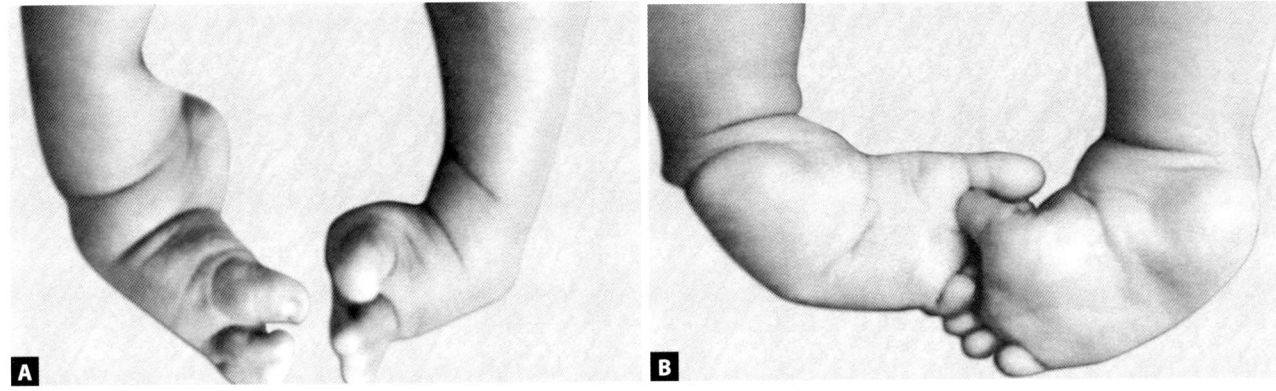

Figs. 15.69A and B: Moderate clubfoot.

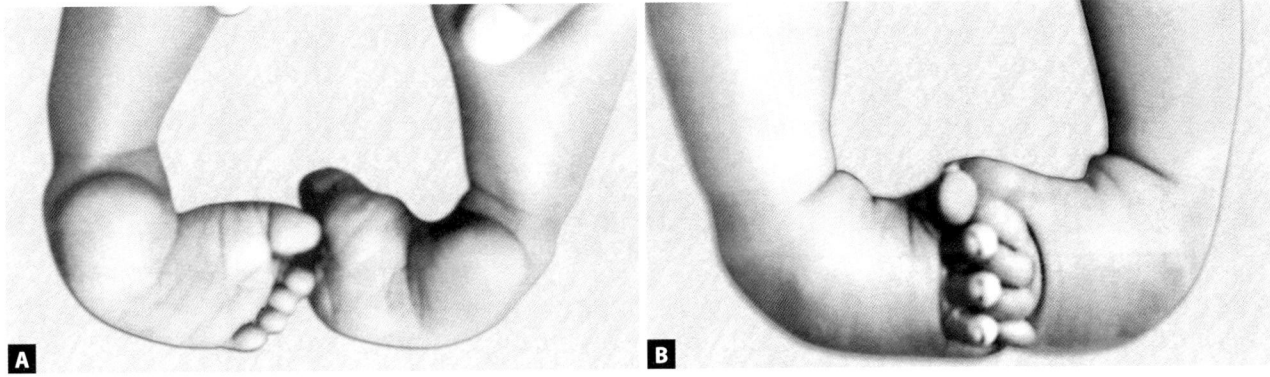

Figs. 15.70A and B: Severe clubfoot.

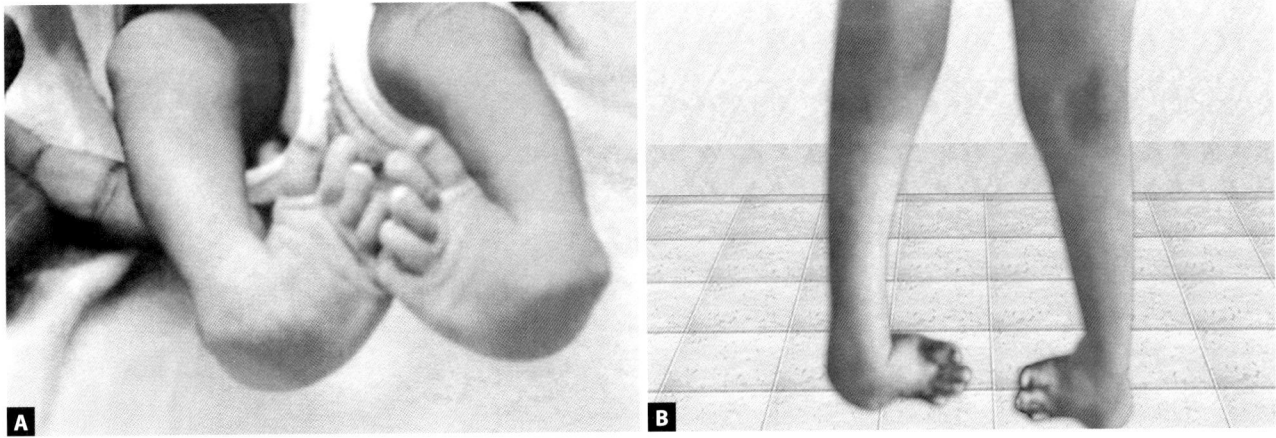

Figs. 15.71A and B: Very severe clubfoot.

- Examination of the footwear, specially the older used one, must also be done. Also enquire about the type and duration of footwear **(Figs. 15.83 to 15.85)** used and condition of ground, where maximum walking is done by the patient.

Attitude

The axial relation of the foot with that of the leg should be noted and compared with the opposite side. The attitude of the foot when the patient is in lying down position should also be noted—this has special importance, particularly when examining a paralytic foot. Note the effect of any foot pathology on the ankle, knee and hip.

Inspection

It should be done from the dorsal and plantar as well as the medial and lateral aspects.

Note the anatomical alignment of the foot and toes, interrelation of toe lengths, any overriding of toes, skin condition, oedema, venous prominences, nail beds, the

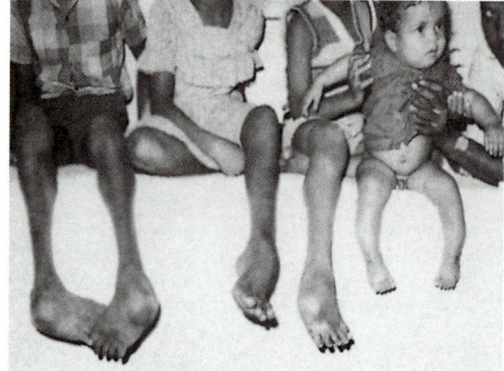

Fig. 15.72: Clubfeet in a family. Father and three children (out of four) have clubfoot.

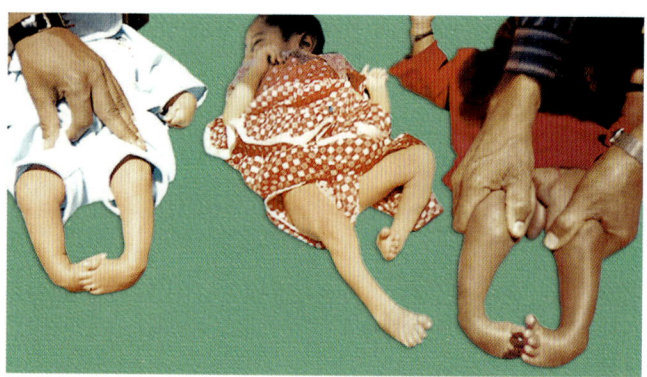

Fig. 15.73: Clubfeet in a family (in three children)—two own brothers and one sister.

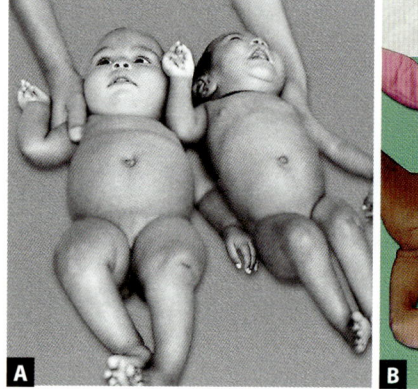
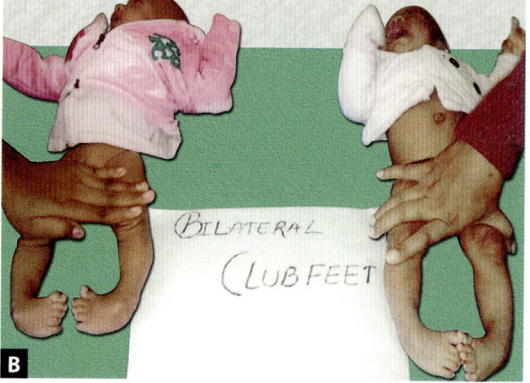

Figs. 15.74A and B: Clubfeet in twins.

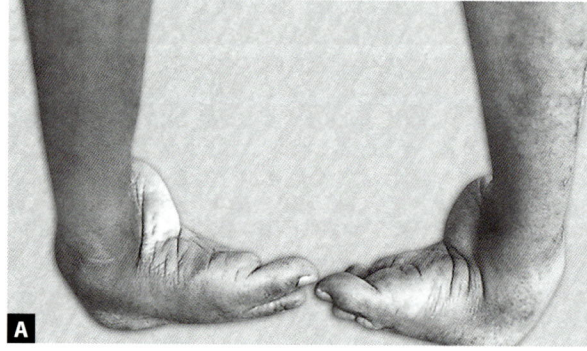
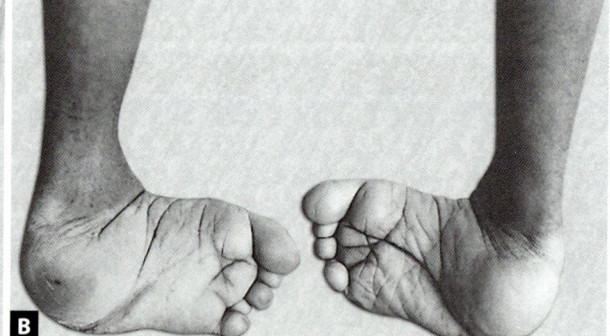

Figs. 15.75A and B: Grossly Neglected very severe clubfeet.

webs and the tips of the toes. Looking from the plantar side, the anatomical disposition, skin condition, presence of any callosities, oedema, corn, shoe bite, trophic ulcer or any other abnormal findings should be noted. Any swelling or sinus in this zone must be examined. For any swelling, examine like any swelling anywhere (Remember, it may be any—even pseudoaneurysm of even dorsalis pedis artery following any old trauma). The foot may be riddled with multiple sinuses specially in the tropics (e.g. in tuberculosis, mycetoma of foot—Madura foot, Kaposi's sarcoma, tropical ulcer). While looking from behind, note the shape and size of the heel, besides the prominence, alignment and continuity of the tendo-Achilles.

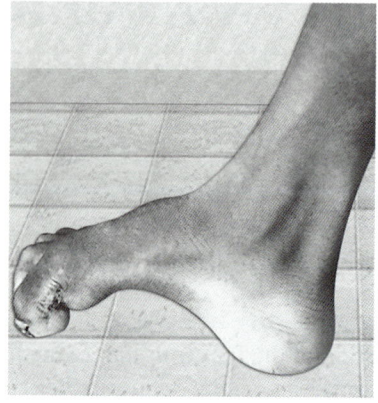

Fig. 15.76: Hollow foot.

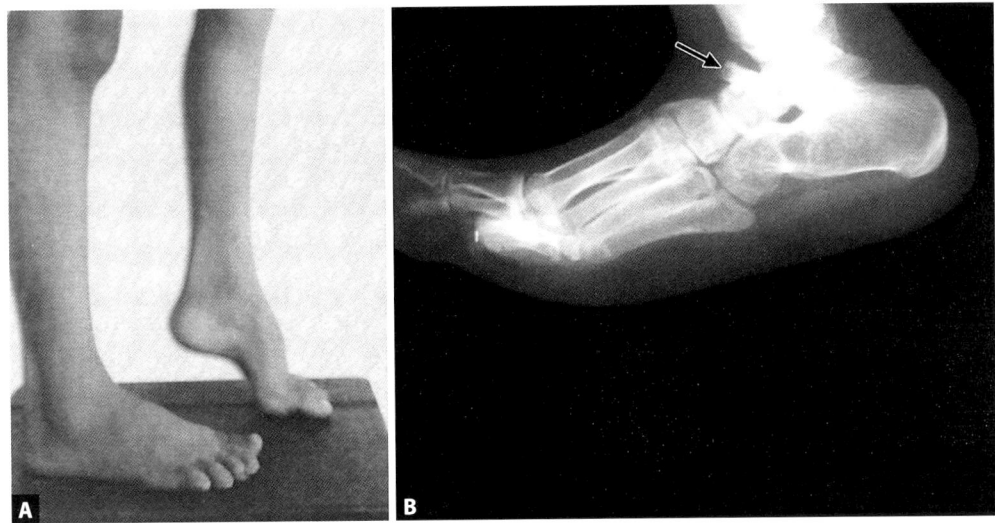

Figs. 15.77A and B: (A) Equinocavus left foot with early clawing; (B) Bony spur from dorsal distal aspect of talus.

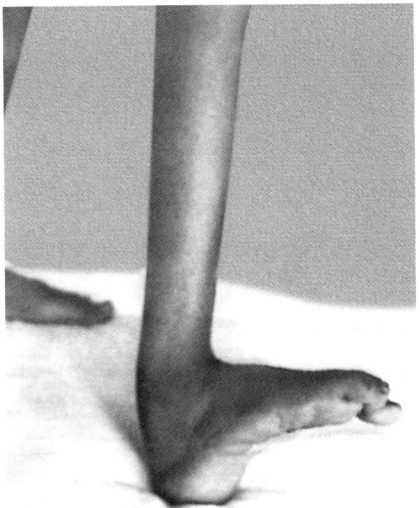

Fig. 15.78: Calcaneovalgus foot.

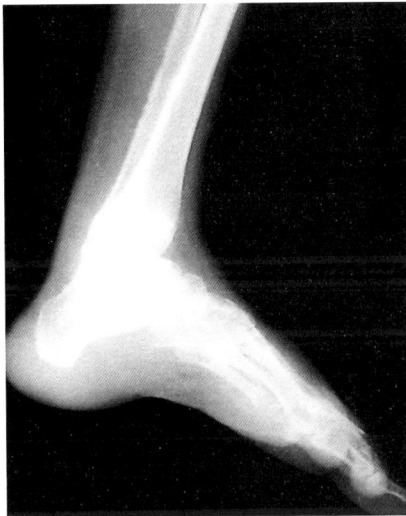

Fig. 15.79: X-ray of calcaneo-cavo-valgus deformity.

Palpation

Superficial Palpation

Feel the skin surface and temperature. Feel for dorsalis pedis, posterior tibial and anterior tibial arterial pulsation. Note must be made of any superficial tenderness or any anaesthesia/paraesthesia/hypoaesthesia, both on the dorsal and plantar aspects of the foot.

Neurosensory Testing (NST) is essential for early detection of neuropathic changes, especially in diabetic foot. NST with the *pressure specific sensory device (PSSD)* is a state-of-the-art non-invasive painless and accurate diagnostic instrument, by which one can carefully measure and evaluate the degree of neuropathy starting at its very early stage.

For *palpating the dorsalis pedis*, gently put two fingers (index and middle finger) over the proximal part of the first intermetatarsal space. For the posterior tibial artery, palpate one finger breadth posteroinferior to the medial malleolus. For the anterior tibial artery, palpate at about the centre of a line with a slight upper convexity joining the two malleoli anteriorly or at about half finger breadth lateral to the extensor hallucis longus tendon at the ankle level.

Deep Palpation

Confirm the anatomical alignment of the bony structures. Palpate the tendons individually. If any abnormal finding like swelling or sinus is present, proceed as given in the Chapter 1: Introduction.

Palpate to elicit deep tenderness with certain common conditions in mind.

- With the index finger, press upwards, backwards and laterally on the medial border of the foot at a point

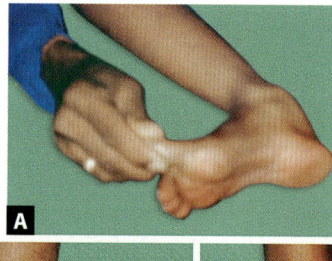

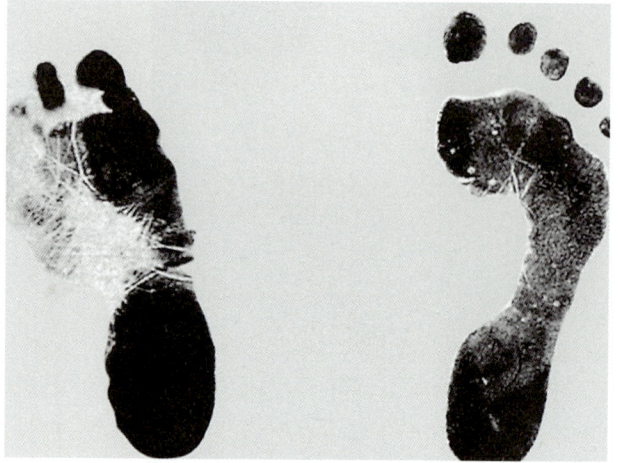

Fig. 15.80: Footprint of calcaneovalgus (left) foot.

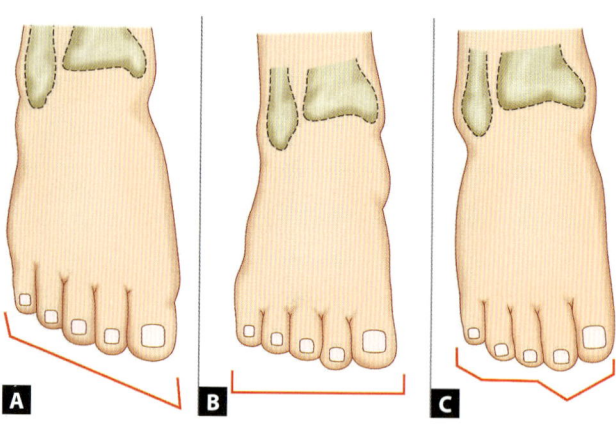

Figs. 15.82A to C: (A) Egyptian foot, (B) Rectangular foot, and (C) Grecian foot.

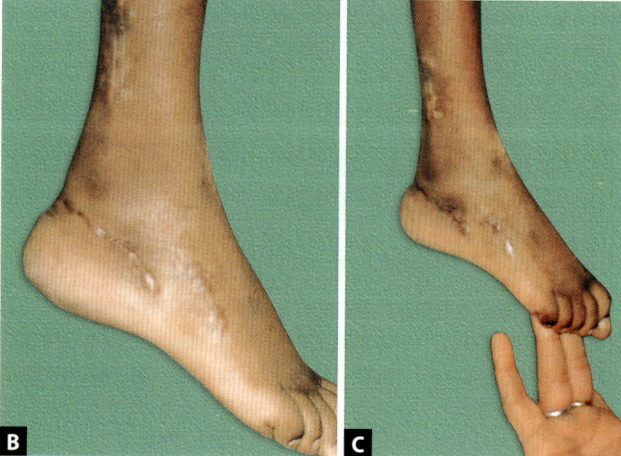

Figs. 15.81A to C: (A) Preoperative photo of calcaneo-cavo-valgus deformity, (B) Postoperative photo after Pandey's calcaneal sling sliding osteotomy, (C) Testing for the power of plantarflexion of ankle against resistance after operative correction.

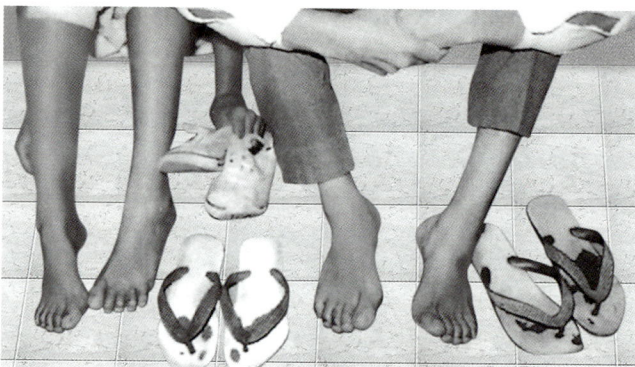

Fig. 15.83: Examination of footwear.

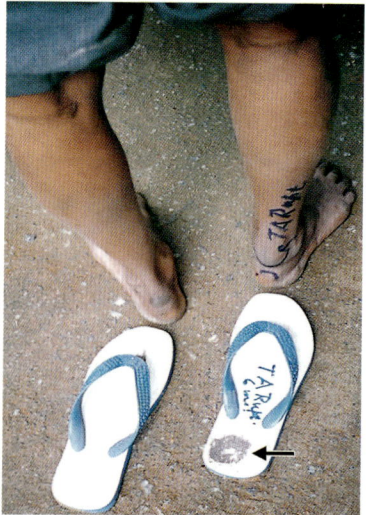

Fig. 15.84: Note the impression on footwear due to calcaneus effect after rupture of tendo-Achilles.

almost a finger breadth behind the drop line from the tip of medial malleolus where the medial arch just starts—tenderness indicates *calcaneal fasciitis*.

Palpate just behind and below the navicular tuberosity—tenderness indicates hyperstretching of the spring ligament *(strained foot)*.

- In athletes, especially footballers, a bony spur may appear on the dorsal distal aspect of talus, which may be painful and tender **(Fig. 15.77B)**.
- With the index finger tip, press upwards from sole in between 3rd and 4th metatarsal head and also on the adjoining proximal area—tenderness indicates *metatarsalgia*. Further confirmation can be taken by squeezing the forefoot which will trigger the original pain of the patient.

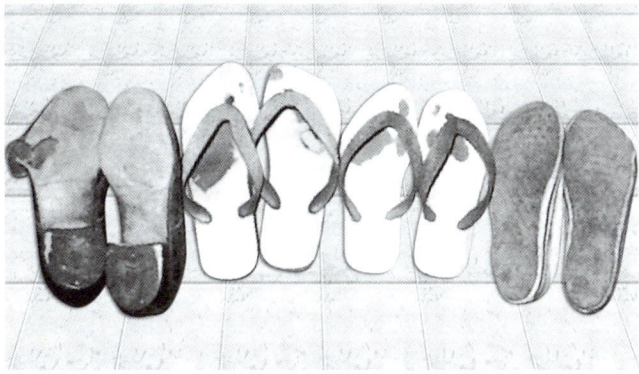

Fig. 15.85: Examination of footwear.

Disorders of Achilles tendon are much frustrating to treat. The Achilles tendon (triceps surae) is formed by the union of two muscle units—the gastrocnemius and soleus.

The gastrocnemius portion effectively plantar-flexes the ankle while the knee is extended, whereas the soleus effectively plantar flexes the ankle while the knee is flexed. Just beyond the calf, the fibres of Achilles tendon gradually rotates by 90° before its insertion into the calcaneal tuberosity and thus the gastrocnemius fibres insert on lateral side and soleus fibres on medial side.

Chronic problems of Achilles tendon are either insertional tendinitis associated with pump bump or Haglund deformity and retrocalcaneal bursitis, or non-insertional tendinosis with or without peritendinitis manifesting 2-6 cm proximal to tendinous insertion (zone of relative avascularity). Patient usually complains of slowly increasing pain and swelling in the insertional zone of Achilles tendon

- Squeeze in between the thumb and index finger, just in front and above the attachment of the tendo-Achilles at the heel—tenderness indicates *pre-Achilles bursitis*, while pain on pressing the posterior aspect of tendo-Achilles, indicates *post-Achilles bursitis*. These can be further confirmed by asking the patient to walk on toes (pain will be complained in case of *pre-Achilles bursitis*) and heels (pain in case of post-Achilles bursitis). In *Achilles tendinitis* (tendinosis) (e.g. in active ankylosing spondylitis and rheumatoid arthritis), pain in heel region will be there both on heel and toe walking, and tendo-Achilles will be tender on side to side squeezing. Thickening and bogginess of the Achilles tendon can be felt. Lateral view X-ray preferably in standing position usually shows calcifield spurs and large posterosuperior process of calcaneal tuberosity.

■ **MOVEMENTS (FIG. 15.86)**

Though the smaller joints of the foot have been anatomically disposed as to produce certain groups of movements, but in normal physiomechanics of the foot, the movements are more

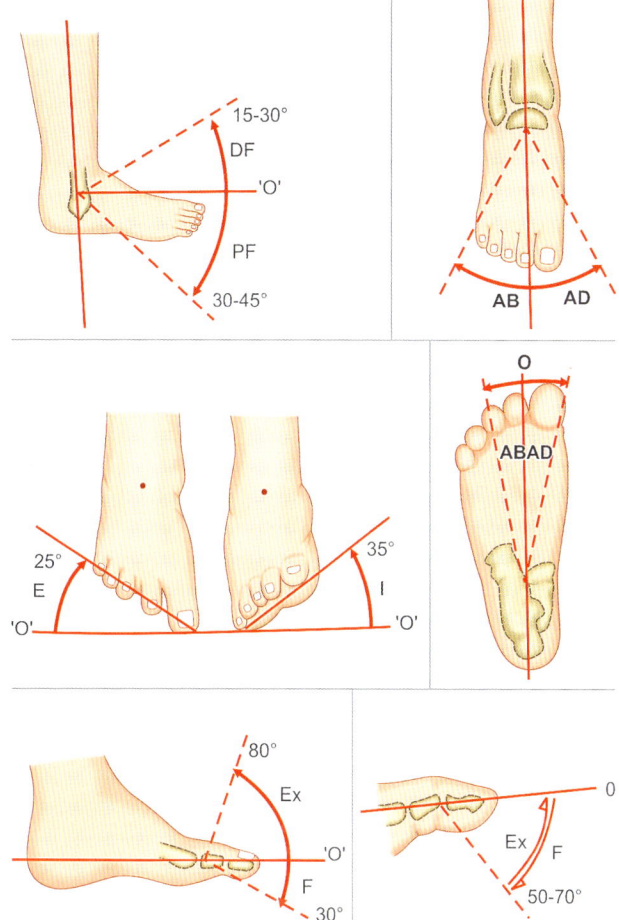

Fig. 15.86: Zero axis and normal range of movements of ankle and foot. (DF: dorsiflexion; PF: plantarflexion; E: eversion; I: inversion; AB: abduction; AD: adduction; Ex: extension; F: flexion)

or less interrelated. However, different sets of movements should be tested at different joints. In assessing any movement, the standard pattern (as given in the Chapter 1 Introduction) should be followed but, it may not be easy to evaluate the movements of the smaller joints of the foot under the desired headings. Enquire and observe for any earlier surgery done on the foot. Subtalar joint arthrodesis is a common procedure done for various indications for both pain and deformity correction.

Method of Eliciting Different Movements and Zero Axis of Ankle and Foot

It is very difficult to test isolated active movements of the foot, hence it is advisable to proceed with accessing the movements passively.

Inversion and Eversion

It can be better tested by making the patient sit on a stool with knee flexed at about 70°. It can be tested also while the patient is lying supine. With one hand, hold the ankle firmly from the dorsum to fix the talus. The other hand holds the body of calcaneum in between the thumb on one side and the index and middle finger on the other. Now try to move the calcaneum on the fixed talus. Turning-in the heel will demonstrate inversion and turning-out eversion at the fulcrum of the subtalar joint. *The axis of these movements lies 45° above the horizontal plane and 16° inner to the long axis of the foot and runs upwards, forwards and medially.*

Adduction and Abduction of the Forefoot (Fig. 15.87)

Hold the hindfoot from the dorsum with one hand, i.e. the first web firmly grips the talus, while the thumb and index finger fix the calcaneum from the two sides. Now with the other hand, hold the forefoot with the thumb on the dorsum and other fingers on the sole. Passively *deviating the forefoot inwards demonstrates adduction and outwards abduction.* The fulcrum is at the midtarsal joints, i.e. the talo-navicular on the inner and the calcaneocuboid on the outer side. The axis of these movements runs from behind forwards, more or less, coinciding along a line joining the centre of the patella, mid ankle point and second web.

Movements of the toes are not as important as those of the fingers of the hand. However, a gross assessment of active plantarflexion and dorsiflexion of the toes (specially of the big toe) should be done. Beyond the active range, the pliability of the joint should be tested by noting the passive range of movement.

Intrinsic Tests

Hitherto the intrinsics of the foot have been neglected in clinical methodology. As discussed earlier, these small but powerful muscles are essential for the springy and rhythmic pattern of gait. Hence, they must be tested as far as practicable. Even if tested as 'group movers' it will be a worthwhile examination.

Closing and fanning out of the webs are produced by the interossei—the *dorsal interossei* being responsible for *fanning out* while *plantar interossei* are for *closing the webs,* the axis being the second metatarsal.

Method **(Fig. 15.88)**: Hold the forefoot just distal to the midtarsal joint level. The *card test* as done for the fingers will suffice here too. Put the card in the particular web to be tested. Ask the patient to grip it between the adjacent toes and judge the strength of the grip.

The lumbricals are difficult to test here individually, since the action of the long and short flexors of the toes are difficult to be neutralized in any particular position. However, a rough estimation can be made of the conjoint action of the lumbricals and the interossei.

Ask the patient to plantarflex the toes at the metatarsophalangeal joints, keeping the interphalangeal joints extended as far as possible. The *lumbricals, along with the interossei are the prime movers for flexing the toes at metatarsophalangeal joint and extending them at the interphalangeal joints.*

Stress Tests

The testing for the exaggerated and passive aforesaid movements will be the stress tests for these joints. These tests are not that important in the foot because the joints are very small and the ligaments of one joint more or less reinforce other joints also. Besides, there are almost two tiers of ligaments holding the main joints.

Dysfunctions of Tibialis Posterior Tendon

The function of tibialis posterior muscle-tendon is plantar flexion, inversion of foot and stabilization of the medial longitudinal arch of foot. These functions of tibialis posterior tendon get variably affected due to chronic tenosynovitis (degenerative or traumatic or following arthritis), rupture of tendon or a distortion in its distal attachments or its bed behind medial malleolus, e.g. in gross malunion of Pott's fracture, etc.). The affection of the functions of tibialis posterior has been described as "Insufficiency of the posterior tibial tendon" or "Tibialis posterior tendon dysfunction (TPT)". It may also develop secondary to an accessory navicular.

Sometimes, in the anamnesis, hyperpronation (or allied) injury occurs leading to the elongation or rupture of the

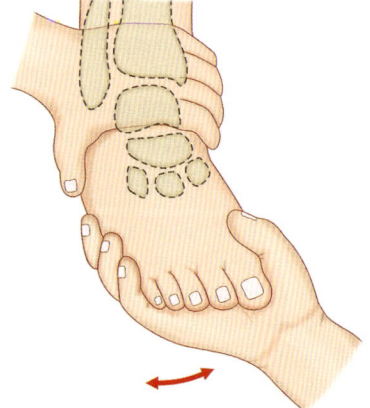

Fig. 15.87: Demonstration of adduction and abduction movements of forefoot.

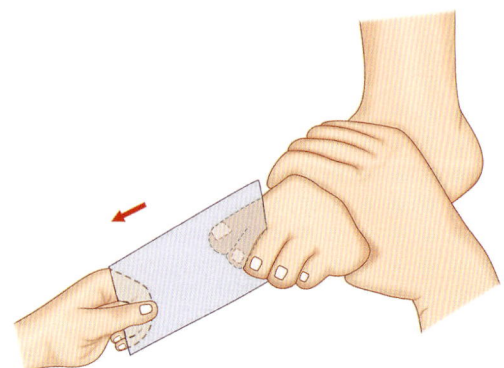

Fig. 15.88: Test for intrinsic muscles—Card test.

talonavicular ligament (spring ligament) resulting in TPT dysfunction. The talar head subluxes downwards, decreasing the medial longitudinal arch.

The blood supply of the tendon below the medial malleolus is poor, hence TPT degeneration is common at this point and below.

Three stages of TPT degeneration have been recognised (Johnson 1982):
- Pretendinitis with low degeneration of the tendon.
  - Flexible hind foot valgus
  - Little retromalleolar pain
  - No static flat problem
- Elongation or partial rupture of the TPT
  - Severe hind foot valgus
  - Rigid hind foot valgus.
- Stiff hind foot valgus
  - Discontinuity of the tendon
  - Lateral (sinus tarsi) pain
  - Subtalar degenerative (arthrosis) arthritis
  - Calcaneocuboid joint degenerative (arthrosis) arthritis.

TPT dysfunction can be clinically assessed by:
- *Metatarsal rise sign*—If the tibia is rotated outwards the head of the first metatarsal is lifted off in contrast to the healthy side.
- *Too many toe sign*—From the back view the positive 'too many toe sign' is typical of the transverse flat foot.

Tibialis posterior pathology (traumatic, degenerative or otherwise) leads to various types of problems, e.g. crippling pain; collapse of medial arch—valgus heel or even pronated foot; limitation of walking, etc. The precise clinical diagnosis of tibialis posterior pathology is perhaps not possible, and it can be only ascertained by exploration. However, CT and MRI scanning can demonstrate different *(three) stages of the pathology*—(i) tendon fissuring followed by tearing; (ii) elongation with scarring; (iii) in some cases separation (Welton and Rose 1993).

Clinically strong suspicion should arise if the patient has (i) crippling pain with marked reduction of walking ability, coming on slowly over sometime or even suddenly, (ii) change in shape of foot, (iii) distortion of the heel counter of shoe, (iv) wasting of calf, (v) loss or less of power of tibialis posterior muscle, (vi) *too many toes sign* (An indicator of forefoot adduction)—the foot when viewed from behind shows "too many toes" laterally (Johnson 1983), (vii) '*Single limb heel rise test*'—when attempting to rise on the ball of the foot with the contralateral foot already raised, the normal foot will assume a stable position, but does not do so when the tibialis posterior is not functioning properly (Johnson 1983), (viii) on *dynamic paedobarograph recording* of the foot/ground pressure, if the tibialis posterior tendon is not functioning properly, the medial longitudinal arch immediately collapses at 'heel off'.

Adult acquired flatfort is a progressive painful disabling deformity usually caused by posterior tibial tendon dysfunction and the progression of the deformity is due to gradual degradation of posterior tibial tendon function. As the posterior tibial tendon degrades it elongates with marked weakness, secondary forefoot abduction and hindfoot valgus. The mainstay of treatment remains the repair/reconstruction of diseased and damaged tibialis posterior tendon by transfer of flexor digitorum longus or flexor hallucis longus tendon or by using the allograft tendon alongwith lateral column lengthening and/or medial displacement calcaneal osteotomy (Dominick DR & Catanzariti 2020).

■ MEASUREMENTS

These measurements are of paramount importance for chiropodists and orthotists.
- *Longitudinal measurements give an idea about the length of the foot.*
  - It should be measured in two axis **(Fig. 15.89)** (OX and OY).
    From the most prominent point on the back of the heel (0) to the tip of the greater toe (X) and from the first point to the tip of fifth toe (Y).
  - The relation of the long lever arm (tip of medial malleolus to tip of the great toe on the inner side, and tip of lateral malleolus to the tip of 5th toe on outer side) and the short lever arm (tip of medial malleolus to the most prominent heel point on medial side, and tip of lateral malleolus to the most prominent heel point on the lateral side) of the foot should be symmetrical on both sides.
- *Circumferential measurement* **(Fig. 15.90)** should be done at three levels.
  - Metatarsal head level (i)
  - Maximum height of the medial arch (ii)
  - Just behind the ankle (iii)
    The third measurement will be more or less the axial circumferential measurement.

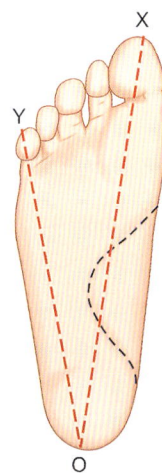

Fig. 15.89: Longitudinal measurement of foot.

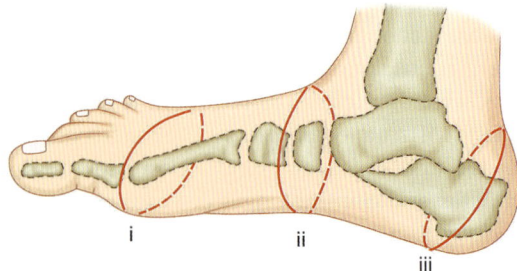

Fig. 15.90: Circumferential measurement of foot: (i) At metatarsal head, (ii) At maximum height of arch, (iii) Just behind the ankle.

- *Vertical measurement:* Any variation in the height of calcaneum and the heel-sole-cushion, will disturb the height of the foot—the distance from the tip of the medial or lateral malleolus to the undersurface of sole at the corresponding margin.

Measurement of Equinus Deformity

Patient lies on the bed on his lateral side (to eliminate gravity). He is asked to dorsiflex the ankle then examiner further dorsiflexes passively as far as possible. Measure the angle between the long axis of the leg (i.e. from midpoint of joint line on medial side of knee to tip of medial malleolus) and long axis of hind foot to midfoot (i.e. from tip of medial malleolus to the head of first metatarsal bone). Subtract 90° from this angle. The remaining will be the 'angle of fixed equinus deformity'.

Measurement of Calcaneus Deformity

Keeping the feet in zero axis of the legs (mid patella, mid ankle, and second web in one line), dorsiflex them passively as far as possible. Normally, in an adult, 15°–30° will be possible. Anything beyond that is due to calcaneus. Measure the total angle of dorsiflexion from 90° position of the ankle. Substract the angle of normal side (if both ankles affected, substract 30°), remainder will be angle of calcaneus deformity, however, for clarity, expression should be of total dorsiflexion from zero position.

Auscultation

If any doubtful swelling exists it should be auscultated.

Examination of the Footwear (Figs. 15.83 to 15.85)

The used footwear should be assessed for:
- Distortion of the shape—indicates underlying rigid deformity of the foot.
- Wrinkling of the footwear (specially of the upper-leather or vamp and around the heel). In persistent toe-in there will be exaggerated wrinkling on distal upper medial aspect of the vamp. In persistent heel varus, deep wrinkles may appear on the inner aspect of the heel.
- Bulging out and thinning (due to pressure) of the vamp (e.g.—in hallux valgus—bulging on the distal medial side; in valgus foot—bulging on the medial side; in inverted foot—excessive bulging on the lateral side)
- Deformation of the sole and the vamp, e.g. in neglected or relapsed or resistant club foot.

Study of the Sole of Footwear

- Bulging out of the sole in any particular direction.
- Pressure erosion of the sole.
- Comparative height of the inner and outer borders (normally there is tendency of wearing off of the sole on the outer side).
- Any pricking point on upper surface of the sole (shoe nail, rough leather margin).
- Hollowing out or scooping tendency at any particular point of the insole (indicative of localised pressure—of great importance in insensitive foot).
- Unused portion on the insole.

INVESTIGATION OF A CASE WITH FOOT PATHOLOGY

Routine Investigations

As in the Chapter 1: Introduction.

Radiological Investigations

- *Superoinferior view*: The patient sits with hip and knee flexed 90°. Ask the patient to firmly press his foot on the plate. The whole span of the foot must be focussed on and the beam centred at the midfoot level.
- *Lateral view*: While the patient lies half-way on the affected side with that lower limb rotated outward, the foot is adjusted until the plantar surface is at right angles to the film. The beam is centered to the middle of the foot. It is better to have a comparative lateral view of both ankles and feet at a time while both ankles and feet have been kept at as far as possible in 90° position between leg and foot (90–90 position) and both soles are closely apposed to each other—then the beam is centered at the midfoot regions.
- *Oblique view*: This is essential to delineate the inter-tarsal relations properly **(Fig. 15.91)**.
  Method: The patient sitting with hip and knee flexed at 90°, the inverted foot is placed, on the plate with the forefoot fanned out. The beam should be focussed vertically on the plate.
- *Oblique view for the hindfoot*: It is also known as axial view for the calcaneum. This view is essential to see the body and posterior part of the calcaneum.
  Method: This can be taken with the patient standing or lying down **(Fig. 15.92)**.
  While the patient is lying down, the plate is placed beneath the heel. The ankle is passively dorsiflexed as far as possible

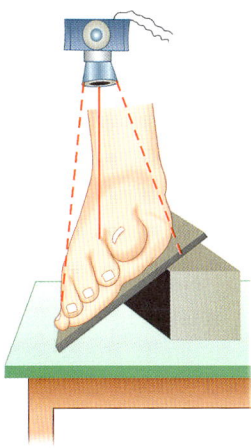

Fig. 15.91: Positioning for inversion oblique view X-ray of mid and forefoot. For eversion oblique views the placement of the block and the board will be reversed.

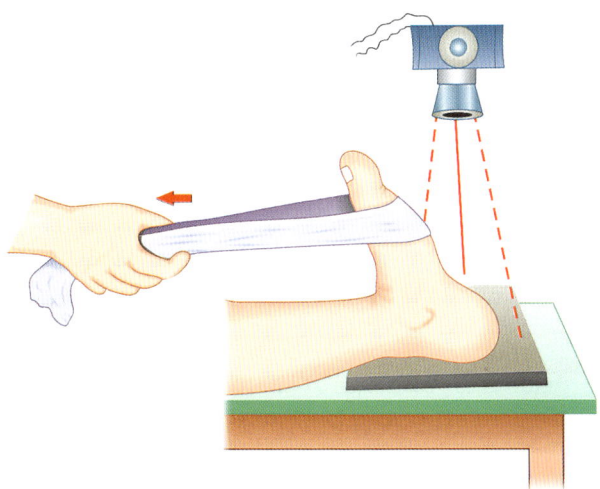

Fig. 15.92: Positioning for axial view of hindfoot (for calcaneum).

using a strap. The beam is focussed on the plantar aspect at the midpoint of the junction of the heel with the midfoot.

Footprint

(Podogram, Ichnogram = imprint of the soles of the feet taken standing)

This is a very useful and cheap method for investigating problems of the foot.

Method: The patient's feet (soles) are uniformly painted with duplicating ink and then he/she is asked to step on a white paper to give his/her footprint, this may be taken as a static imprint of the foot, when it is desired to assess the weight bearing pattern of one foot.

For studying the gait pattern of the patient, dynamic footprints may be taken, where the patient walks with painted (inked) feet on the white papers placed in continuity.

Electrical Recording of Footprints

Different electronically controlled devices have been instituted to study the weight bearing pattern of the foot in static or dynamic phase. This has been used especially for studying gait patterns.

Image Intensifier Radiography and Cine-Radiography

These devices are useful in studying different gait patterns.

Photopodogram

By this method, fine impressions of the skin lines of the sole are obtained on photographic silver bromide paper.

The sole of the foot is coated with concentrated developing solution, and then the foot is carefully put on a silver bromide paper, which is exposed to day-light or lamp light for about 30 seconds. The paper is thereafter removed, fixed and washed.

Podoscopy

A sheet of glass is illuminated from beneath. When the foot is placed on it, the sole of the foot can be observed in a mirror placed below. The area of weight bearing, the overall shape of the foot and the condition of arches can be thus studied.

Arthroscopy

This has in general not been utilised for joints of the foot. However, in very specialised centres, this is being used for diagnostic as well as therapeutic purposes.

The more developed investigations, like computerized radiopodography, podostatiradiography, pressopodostatiradiography, photoscopic studies, televideopodometry, etc. can be utilised to understand the intricate physiomechanics of a normal foot and the pathodynamics of an abnormal foot.

Foetal Surveillance Techniques

These are much helpful for early and accurate diagnosis of malformations (e.g. in spina bifida manifesta and arthrogryposis multiplex congenita).

KEY DIAGNOSTIC POINTS OF COMMON FOOT PATHOLOGY

Assessment of a Case of Clubfoot

[Club means = Heavy tapering stick, knobby or massy at one end] **(Tables 15.2 to 15.4)**

The first description of clubfoot is probably in Indian ancient literature—The "Yajurveda"—in 10th century BC. However, Jusepe de Ribena's *"The clubfoot Boy"* painted in 1642 and now hanging in Louvre Museum in Paris is perhaps the first depiction of clubfoot (though with several controversies regarding the cause of clubfoot like deformity) **(Fig. 15.60)**. Clubfoot is a relatively common birth defect with an incidence ranging from 0.09% in the newborn population to 0.43% when diagnosed antenatally by ultrasound. It is one of the most common congenital orthopaedic conditions. 50% cases are bilateral.

The incidence of clubfoot is maximum (6 to 7 per thousand live births in Maoris and Pacific islanders and perhaps least in Chinese and Japanese population—0.5 per thousand live birth (Chapman et al. 2000). In India, the incidence is probably 1 to 4 per 1000 births in different regions (**Figs. 15.61 to 15.63**).

This has more value in determining the prognosis and the line of management rather than diagnosing the disease, which is quite obvious from the very beginning. Besides general assessment depending upon the clinical grades certain important aspects must be looked into.

NB: Certain MUSTS in an examination of a club foot.
- Search for evidences of spina bifida (manifesta or occulta) in the lower part of the spine/back **(Table 15.3)**
- Look for other congenital deformities in bone and joints such as in knees, hips and upper limbs; and cleft palate; and in soft tissue—cleft lip, congenital hernia, exomphalos.
- Congenital malformation of the vital organs, e.g. heart, liver, lung, etc. should be excluded.
- Test for sensation in the foot (specially the sole).

Aetiologically Clubfoot (Equinovarus deformity) Grouping

Equinovarus deformity can be divided into two broad groups **(Table 15.2)**

Congenital
- Postural (Persistent foetal position)
  - Foot can be manipulated back to normal position.
- Idiopathic (Typical or Atypical)
  - Foot cannot be manipulated back to normal position
  - (Mild-Gr I; Moderate-Gr II; Severe-Gr III; Very severe-Gr I— *see* **Table 15.4**).
- Complicated
  - Arthrogryposis multiplex congenita
  - Myogenic (imperfect muscle development)
  - Neurogenic (e.g. in spina bifida)
  - Osteogenic (e.g. with absent tibia).

Clubfoot may be inherited (**Figs. 15.72 to 15.74**); also occurs with few genetically inherited conditions, e.g. diastrophic dwarfism, Freeman-Sheldon syndrome, Down syndrome, Streeter's syndrome, Nagar syndrome, Tethered Cord syndrome.

Equinovarus/clubfoot deformities associated with meningomyelocele (Figs. 15.105, 15.104, 15.106, 15.108) are mostly teratologic in nature. The deformities are mostly rigid and resistant to treat and further have rate of recurrence. Initially they should be managed by serial manipulations and well padded cautious (due to sensory issue to avoid pressure sores) casting, however surgeries are required for resistant and recurred deformities.

Acquired
- Paralytic (poliomyelitis, Guillain-Barre paralysis, cerebral palsy, myopathy)
- Inflammatory (post-infective contracture of calf muscles)
- Traumatic (injury in leg or ankle or foot, compartment syndrome—Volkmann's ischaemic contracture—VIC)
- Neoplastic (in calf or foot; intraspinal)
- Tumours
- Diastematomyelia
- Charcot-Marie-Tooth disease.

TABLE 15.2: Clinical differences between congenital and acquired equinovarus (clubfoot) deformities.

Congenital	Acquired
1. History since birth	1. Deformity appears after birth
2. Usually bilateral (about > 50%)	2. Usually unilateral
3. These types more common in boys	3. Not such preference (sexwise)
4. Set pattern of deformity, i.e. equinovarus with adduction of forefoot and cavus	4. Usually only equinovarus
5. Congenital groove mostly present	5. Not present
6. Heel looks smaller and tugged up	6. Heel almost maintains its shape and size except in severe and neglected cases
7. Look of calf—in severe and very severe type— looks more or less cylindrical	7. Configuration of calf usually maintained, but may be atrophied
8. Feel of calf usually tough	8. Calf is usually supple
9. In severe and very severe type, subcutaneous tissue of foot has tight and adherent feel on posteroinferomedial aspect and atrophied on dorsolateral aspect	9. Except in neglected cases, sub-cutaneous tissue feels softer more or less on all aspects
10. May be associated with other congenital deformities	10. Associated paralytic deformity in same leg and/or other leg and/or other part of body
11. Neurological examination—normal	11. Motor and/or sensory deficit

In arthrogryposis multiplex congenita **(Fig. 15.64)**, club foot exists along with flexion and adduction at hip (may be congenital dislocation of hip), congenital contracture of quadriceps, extension at elbow, adduction and medial rotation at shoulder, etc. in various combinations.

Late cases of clubfoot can be divided into:
- Resistant (certain elements of the deformity resist correction)
- Relapsed (certain elements of the deformity recur due to several reasons including that of genetic defects stored in memory)
- Neglected clubfeet are those which have not been taken up for treatment within 9 months **(Fig. 15.62)**.

The idiopathic congenital clubfoot can be differentiated from acquired specially the poliotics on the points mentioned in the Table 15.2.

Now clubfoot can be diagnosed by ultrasound of the foetus in more than 60% of cases. The earliest week of gestation in which the clubfoot can be diagnosed with degree of confidence is the 12th and the latest is the 32nd. Ultrasound can be performed transabdominal scan (TAS) or transvaginal scan (TVS). TVS gives better visualisation of the foetus. Modern high-resolution TVS provides better detection of skeletal anomalies upto four weeks earlier than TAS ultrasound. The latest three-dimensional ultrasonographic equipment should further improve the rate of detection of clubfoot and other anomalies.

Based on the age of prenatal ultrasonographic detection the clubfeet have been grouped into three types, though with several falacies (e.g. lack of enough experience in detecting the deformity earlier; false positivity, etc.):

1. *Early clubfoot:* Detected from 12th week of gestation to 17th week by TVS ultrasonography. Forty-five per cent of children with idiopathic clubfoot at birth were included in this group.
2. *Late onset clubfoot:* Detected between the 18th and 24th weeks of gestation and 45% of the children born with clubfoot and detected prenatally belong to this group.
3. *Very late-onset clubfoot:* Detected between 25th and 32nd week of gestation. Ten per cent of children born with clubfoot belong to this group.

TABLE 15.3: Clinical differences between idiopathic clubfoot and clubfoot associated with spina bifida.

Idiopathic clubfoot	*Clubfoot with spina bifida*
1. Present since birth	1. Usually appears later (usually after 2 years of age)
2. Cause not known	2. Neurogenic, due to paresis/paralysis of the roots controlling the muscles on the dorsolateral aspect of the leg and foot
3. Sensation intact	3. Affected
4. Trophic ulcers—not present	—
5. Associated congenital deformity may be present in other joints	5. Usually other joints remain free
6. Management to be started at the earliest	6. Wait and watch for the progress of the deformities
7. Deformities are fixed from beginning	7. Deformities are usually not fixed till late

TABLE 15.4: Clinical grades of idiopathic clubfoot.

Clinical parameters	Grades of clubfoot			
	1	2	3	4
	Mild (Fig. 15.68)	Moderate (Fig. 15.69)	Severe (Fig. 15.70)	Very severe (Fig. 15.71)
Look of foot, ankle and leg	Almost normal	Crowding tendency on postero-inferomedial aspects and stretching tendency on dorsolateral aspects	Features more marked than in 'Moderate' clubfoot with tougher appearance	'Club' like appearance
Skin condition	Normal	Almost normal in other regions but with variable atrophy of subcutaneous fat on the dorsolateral aspect; tendency of developing creases on the posteromedial and less on inferomedial aspect	Stretched on superolateral aspect, crowded skin creases on posteromedial aspect. Congenital grooves on the inferomedial aspect of the foot and rarely in the lower leg. Thin callosities on the dorso-lateral aspect	Atrophied skin on dorsolateral aspect of foot congenital groove always present in inferomedial aspect of foot and lower leg, thick callosities

Contd...

Contd...

Clinical parameters	Grades of clubfoot			
	1 Mild (Fig. 15.68)	2 Moderate (Fig. 15.69)	3 Severe (Fig. 15.70)	4 Very severe (Fig. 15.71)
Stretchability of the deformity	Fully correctable on passive stretching	75% at present down to 50% correctable on passive stretching	Correctable by 50% at present down to 25% on passive stretching	Less than 25% correctable, on passive stretching
Effect of stretching on vascularity	No effect	Blanching of the toes after 75-50% correction.	Blanching of the toes after 50-25% correction	Blanching of toes after less than 25% correction on passive stretching
Heel	Almost normal	Comparatively smaller; mild heel valgus	Small, moderate heel varus	Small, severe heel varus
Look/Shape of calf	Normal	Almost normal	Tendency to become tapering and cylindrical	Almost cylindrical (peg like)
Feel of foot	Almost normal resilient	Nearly normal, Nearly resilient	Tough	Rigid
Feel of calf muscles	Normal	Almost normal	Firm	Markedly firm, and presents the feel of fixity (tough)
Treatment	Manipulative massage, strapping, POP casting and maintenance with orthotics	Manipulative massage, serial strapping, serial plaster cast, maintenance orthotics. For resistant cases—posteroinferomedial soft tissue release	• Trial of serial plaster casting. Several of these type require soft tissue release, • External fixator • Bony operation may be required after 2½ years in resistant, relapsed and neglected cases	• Soft tissue release, maintenance with orthotics, regular stretching and physiotherapy—even then recurrence is common • External fixator • Combined soft tissue release and bony operation
Prognosis (on overall assessment) (% are approximately on broad analysis)	Excellent in most of cases (95%) Few—good (5%)	Excellent in majority (80%) in rest cases—good (20%)	• Few—excellent 20% • Mostly good—65% • Few fair—13% • Very few—poor 2%	• Hardly excellent—10% • Good—40% • Fair—35% • Poor—15%
Curvature of lateral border of foot	Mild curvature which is smooth and uniform	Moderate convexity more marked in forefoot	More convexity mainly in mid and forefeet	Acute convexity from hind to forefoot

NB: For neglected, resistant and relapsed clubfoot presenting beyond 3 years of age, bony operations are usually needed for satisfactory correction. These can also be corrected by external fixators (like JESS: Ilizarov apparatus)

Atypical idiopathic Clubfoot (Turco): It is nothing different at birth from the typical clubfoot. The main difference is that it responds quite differently to the treatment schedules (operative or nonoperative), results being unpredictable. In such cases conservative management should be preferred, since early surgery usually result in a grotesque, overcorrected severe flat-foot

Corns (Helomata and Clavi)

Corns are localised callosities over bony prominences of foot and occasionally of the fingers. They occur due to friction and pressure. *Corn consists of a central hyperkeratotic spike projecting downwards towards the dermis and forming a hard 'core' on the surface, surrounded by an area of semi-opaque thickening of horny layer.* The pressure of the core on the nerve causes exquisite pain which is worse in high humidity. In diabetes or after faulty paring, it may get infected.

Clinically, corns are hard or soft—both result from pressure by unyielding structures. Hard corns usually develop over the dorsolateral aspect of the proximal interphalangeal joint of fifth toe or as plantar corn (heloma durum and clavus durus). A rare lesion is the neurovascular corn, which is usually located beneath the first and fifth metatarsal head and is very painful.

Soft corns are usually interdigital and are more persistent hyperkeratotic lesion mostly between 4th and 5th digital interspace usually as kissing lesions. There may be underlying bony spur. Removal of cause, ring pad, shoe-padding, metatarsal bar may be useful. Salicylic acid application and cautious paring may help. Any underlying bony spur should be removed.

TABLE 15.5: Types of callosities.

Type of callosity	Site	Cause	Presentation	Management
Orthopaedic callosities	Sole, beneath metatarsal heads	Structural abnormality of foot; unsuitable footwear; abnormal gait; trophic disorders	Abnormal look, tenderness, fissuring	Treat underlying cause; callosity softened by salicylic acid and gently pared away; regular supervision of susceptible region, chiropodist care
Callosities due to repeated pressure, appliances, and wears	Sites of straps of calipers; front of lower thigh in hand to knee gait	Repeated pressure in calipers; Ill-fitting trusses		
Occupational callosities	Sites affected are according to occupation, e.g. Muslim callus on forehead and upper outer aspect of foot (**Fig. 15.93**)	Repeated pressure at particular site (e.g. in Muslim prayer positions)		
Callosities due to habits and tick	Gnaw-warts on fingers, back of hands	Regular biting habit of certain child or mentally ill person		

TABLE 15.6: Differentiation between wart and callosity of foot.

	Wart	Callosity
Cause	Infection with human DNA papilloma virus	Thickening of the skin at the points of excessive pressure
Common sites	More in the forepart of the sole	Beneath the heads of the metatarsals. Also on the dorsum of the foot, e.g. in clubfoot, hammer toe, etc.
Basic pathology	Lesions are intraepidermal, dry, friable papillomatous projections	Hyperkeratinisation
Tenderness	Marked	May be tender
Surface	Mosaic like	Thickened, smooth surface
Relation to surrounding skin	Can be clearly demarcated from the surrounding skin	Blends with the surrounding skin

Injection of silicon fluid underneath the corn (silicon prosthesis) can cure many corns.

Callosities

Callosities are circumscribed plaques of hyperkeratosis induced by intermittent trauma. They can be usually of four types according to the causative factors (**Tables 15.5, 15.6** and **Fig. 15.93**).

Causes of Pain in the Heel (Painful Heel) (As shown in Fig. 15.95)

Heel pain is the fastest growing and most challenging foot problem in the community, growing popularity of sports activities being one prominent cause of it. Crawford (2003) has estimated that one out of every ten persons suffer from heel pain.

Osteomalacia, obesity, rheumatoid arthritis, ankylosing spondylitis, prolonged standing, diabetes, faulty footwear, protozoal and helminthic infections of gut can also produce pain in the heel. Pain in calcaneum is called *calcaneodynia*.

Plantar fasciitis is a common and often disabling condition. Its aetiology is multifactorial although a degenerative process with inflammatory reaction, microscopic tears and cystic degeneration in the origin of plantar fascia and the flexor digitorum brevis like the changes in tendinous origin of the extensor carpi radialis brevis in 'tennis elbow'—in fact plantar fasciitis has been also called as 'tennis heel', and fibrosis may play an important role. A calcaneal bone spur is evident in 50–60% of patients with painful heel. The entrapment of first branch of lateral plantar nerve to abductor digiti minimi may cause painful heel syndrome.

It is variously treated like—stretching, cryotherapy, heel cushion pads and inserts, corticosteroid injection and immobilization. Patients resistant to conservative treatment may need surgical interventions like endoscopic or open plantar fascia release or heal spur resection. However, the recalcitrant plantar fasciitis may also be successfully managed by applying repeated extracorporeal shockwave

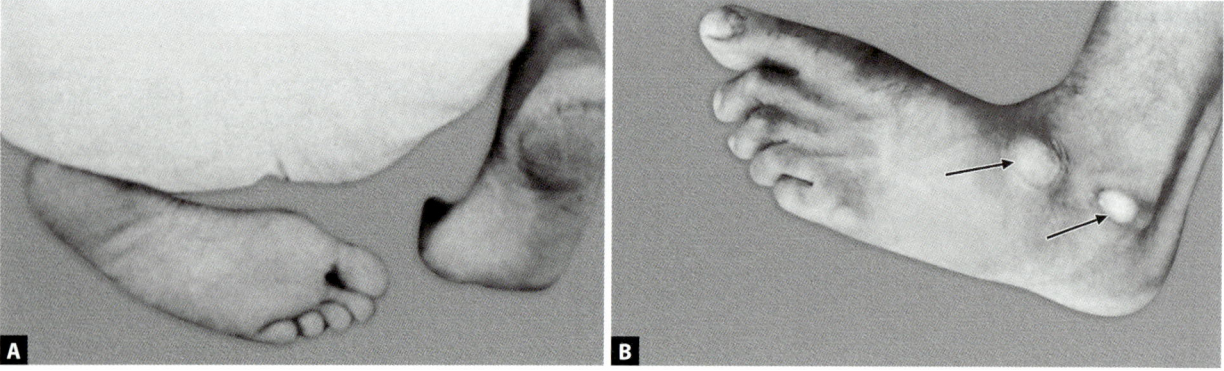

Figs. 15.93A and B: (A) Prayer-position of feet by Muslim's which leads to the formation of Muslim's callus; (B) Muslim's callus. Note the typical Muslim's callus (Pandey S 1988)

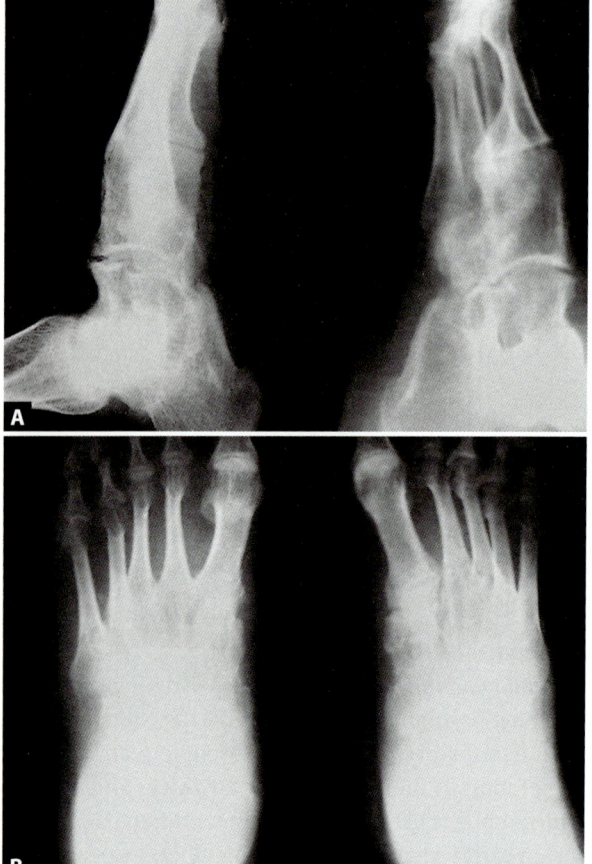

Figs. 15.94A and B: Congenital solid midfoot region, i.e. there is no joint in between the cuneiforms and cuboid and also the tarso-metatarsal joints.

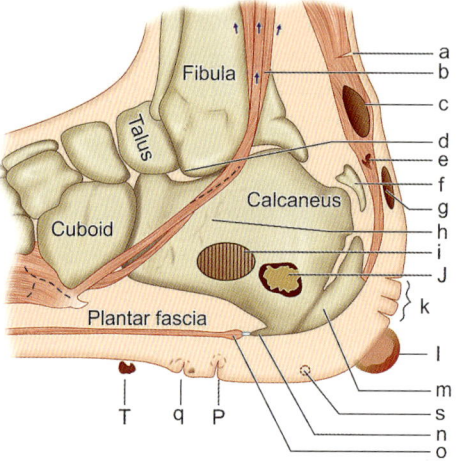

Fig. 15.95: Painful heel: a = partial rupture of tendo-Achilles, b = peroneal spasm, c = xanthoma, d = sub-talar arthritis, e = Achilles tendinitis/tendinosis, f = pre-Achilles bursitis, g = post-Achilles bursitis (retrocalcaneal bursitis, pump bump, Haglund deformity). Any of the above (e,f,g) pathological entities may be an isolated cause of posterior heel pain; when all three occur together—they comprise **'Haglund's triad'**. Haglund's syndrome/disease/deformity can be safely and effectively treated by endoscopic resection (better by two portal technique) endoscopic calcaneoplasty is an effective minimally invasive treatment option, especially when there is failure of conservative treatment. h = fracture calcaneum including calcaneal stress fracture, i = neoplasm of calcaneum, j = cyst/tuberculosis of calcaneum, k = fissures, l = melanoma, m = traction or stress injuries induced osteochondritis of posterior calcaneal apophysis— calcaneal apophysitis—(Sever's disease—**Fig. 15.142**), n = calcaneal spur, o = plantar fasciitis, p = thorn prick (Figs. 15.98 and 15.99), q = corn, r = wart, s = infection/inflammation of heel pad (calcaneal fat pad).

therapy (ESWT—3X2000 impulses) with relatively high energy flux densities (0.25 mJ/mm^2) that can be tolerated without local anaesthesia. (Gollwitzer et al. 2007) (Ref. Gollwitzer Hg, Diehl P, Korff AV, et al. Extracorporeal shockwave therapy for chronic painful heel syndrome: A prospective, double blind, randomized trial assessing the efficacy of a new electromagnetic shock wave device. The Jr of Foot Ankle Surgery. 2007, 46-5:348-357).

Plantar Fasciitis (Calcaneal fasciitis; calcaneal spur syndrome): The presence of calcaneal spur probably has hardly any role in the cause or treatment. Plantar fasciitis is an acute/subacute inflammation of the plantar fascia which extends from undersurface of calcaneum to metatarsal heads. This fascia is often the continuation of the fibres from the tendo-Achilles attachment in the calcaneum. Anatomically, it is a thick band of fibrous tissue arising from the medial tuberosity of calcaneum and spreading like a fan across the sole to insert on the proximal phalanges of toes. Repeated

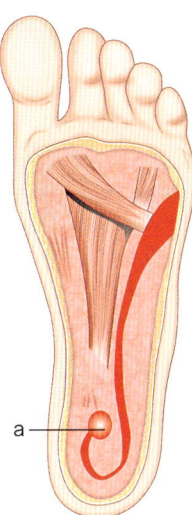

Fig. 15.96: Line drawing showing site of maximum tenderness (a) in calcaneal fasciitis/calcaneal spur syndrome.

excessive unusual or prolonged weight-bearing leads to microtrauma and inflammation of plantar fascia mainly at its attachment on calcaneus.

Patient complains of pain in the region under the calcaneum which becomes worst on putting the heel on the floor as the first step after getting out of bed in the morning, and it eases with gradual steps. However, dull pain persists and variably increases with footwear, prolonged standing, prolonged walking, change in posture. First step pain of morning is diagnostic.

Tenderness is along the plantar fascia, but is maximum medially at the calcaneal insertion of fascia **(Fig. 15.96)**. It can be easily located when the fascia is under tension by dorsiflexing the big toe.

Management is mainly by providing softly-padded heel top and raising the arch with insole (to reduce tension on the fascia); NSAIDs; reducing weight, ultrasound; calf stretching and exercises to develop the intrinsics of the foot; friction therapy; iontophoresis, microwave, laser, extracorporeal shockwave therapy, dry needling local corticoid infiltration, local injection of platelet rich plasma, injection of botulinum toxin etc. Of the conservative modalities, the combined treatment by extracorporeal shock wave therapy and dry needling has been found to provide relief in shorter period, while the patients continue the activities of daily living with very few complications. Further the combinations of these techniques provide a curative effect on the pain parameters. (Bagcier & Yilmaz 2020). However in about 15% of patients, conservative treatment does not help much and such condition is known as intractable plantar fasciitis, which may require surgery like plantar fasciotomy, neurotomy, neurolysis, calcaneal spur resection, calcaneal decompression. However, surgery is also not always helpful.

Plantar fasciitis, is a degenerative disease of the plantar fascia. The main cause of plantar fasciitis is abnormal biomechanics of foot. When the plantar fascia is subjected to forces exceeding its physiological limits, the repeated long-term overload triggers an inflammatory process which gradually leads to degeneration and fibrosis.

Pain is believed to be caused by microtears of metatarsal fascia, causing repeated microdamage, secondary microtears of plantar fascia and microbleeding, which results in local aseptic inflammatory reaction. As the disease progresses the contracture of plantar fascia causes continuous traction on its calcaneal attachment. To increase the strength of the abraded area more calcium salt is deposited and the bony attachment is ossified forming a calcaneal spur (Tang Y et al 2020).

Calcaneal spurs are not the cause of plantar pain, however, they can aggravate the painful symptoms of plantar fasciitis.

Currently, arthroscopic surgery is the primary treatment for plantar fasciitis; the endoscopic treatment of plantar fasciitis using the lateral double incisions via the suprafascial approach has good clinical results (Tang Y et al 2020).

In most (almost 80%) of the patients symptoms eventually resolute with conservative treatment. However, in a small group of patients mechanical perturbations (equinus, aponeurotic thickening, loss of tissue elasticity) and increased hydrostatic tissue pressures reduce vascular flow and initiate degenerate process, which is called as *refractory plantar fasciosis*. (Rushing CJ et al 2020). They treated their patients with bipolar radiofrequency controlled ablation alongwith platelet-rich plasma injection. In majority of patients they found highly satisfactory results, which can be favourably compared to the long term outcomes reported for plantar fasciotomy.

In heel pad pain: Sharp pain, aching or stiffness in the heel region is very common ailment. There is often a more rapid onset of a dull bruise-like pain over the heel fat pad, which is not altered by fascia stretching (dorsiflexing the big toe) and can be precipitated by even mild trauma to the heel. It settles with rest and padding.

Heel pad pain may be severe and too much tender when there is infection or inflammation, which is compartmentalized by the fibrous bands leading to increased tissue pressure and intense pain. Weight bearing augments the pain very much. Ankle region may also be swollen.

Causes of Pain in Midfoot

Pain in midfoot region may be due to injuries, infections, and neoplasm, conditions like pes planus, accessory navicular and osteochondrosis of navicular—(KÖhler's disease). KÖhler's disease was originally described by KÖhler in 1908, of not definitely known cause—may be due to mechanical compression or avascular necrosis. It is self-limiting condition. Cast immobilisation produce quicker resolution of symptoms like pain and disability. Congenital coalition of the tarsals leading to spastic flat foot, midfoot syndrome **(Fig. 15.94)** (Complete congenital fusion of navicular, cuneiforms, cuboid and almost all tarsometatarsal joints; becomes symptomatic by adulthood with stiffness of foot and dull pain after walking some distance) may cause pain in the midfoot.

Causes of Pain in the Forefoot

- *Metatarsalgia*
  - March fracture—stress fracture usually occurs in the neck of second metatarsal; history of unusual amount of walking; tender swelling on the dorsum of the foot, at the site of fracture.
  - *Morton's metatarsalgia (Interdigital neuroma):* Durlarkar was the first to describe interdigital neuroma in 1845, but Thomas G Morton was the first to report this condition in 1876 as a peculiar and painful affection of the fourth metatarsophalangeal articulation. Since then it has been known as Morton's neuroma/Morton's disease/Morton's metatarsalgia.

  Patient usually a lady in her 5th decade complains of pain in forefoot localised mostly in 3–4 interspace followed by 2–3 interspace followed by other interspaces, that worsens with weight bearing. Local tenderness is in the web space and may be paraesthesia in adjacent toes. Compressing or squeezing the intermetatarsal space or hyperextending the metatarsophalangeal and interphalangeal joints triggers the pain.

  X-ray is usually non-contributory. Ultrasound scan (with a 5–10 MHZ broadband linear array transducer) carried out in the transverse and longitudinal plane on the plantar surface of the foot at the level of the metatarsal head, gives about 98% of sensitivity and positive predictive value. CT and MRI can also be of diagnostic value. In MRI, a well-defined ovoid, hypo-echoic area in the intermetatarsal region represents a neuroma. Final treatment is the excision of neuroma, of course shoe-inserts, NSAIDs and physiotherapy should be tried first. If conservative treatment fails, careful operative excision of the involved interdigital nerve should be done at the proximal region of surgical incision to minimize the risk of formation of a symptomatic stump neuroma. The operated patients should be cautioned that due to surgical procedure there will be permanent numbness in the affected lesser toes.

  - *Dropped transverse arch (anterior flat foot)* is a common cause of pain in the forefoot. Less or loss of normal *transverse metatarsal arch* extending from the first to fifth metatarsal heads produces abnormal weight bearing on the 2nd to 4th metatarsal heads which are usually insufficiently padded. Patient complains of pain in the region of metatarsal heads. Here there is broadening of the forefoot, callosities beneath the metatarsal heads and weakness in raising the metatarsal heads. Pressure on callosities reproduce the pain.

- *Freiberg's disease:* Osteochondritis of the distal epiphyses (metatarsal head, *usually of the 2nd metatarsal*), occurs in adolescent or adult males (**Figs. 15.97A and B**) it is a rare chronic progressive condition characterized by avascular necrosis of the lesser metatarsal heads, that results in pain and loss of normal function of the metatarsophalangeal joint of foot. Kenny et al (2017) have cautioned that this diagnosis should be considered in any presentation of metatarsalgia in a patient who has received either long-term or short–term steroid therapy. Radiographic finding were typical of various stages of metatarsal head necrosis and articular depression. Its exact cause is not known. AH Freiberg, in 1914, described six infractions (incomplete non-displaced fracture) of 2nd metatarsal head in young adult females considering it as a sequel of acute trauma.

There is osteonecrosis of subchondral cancellous bone followed by a reparative process. Varying distortion of

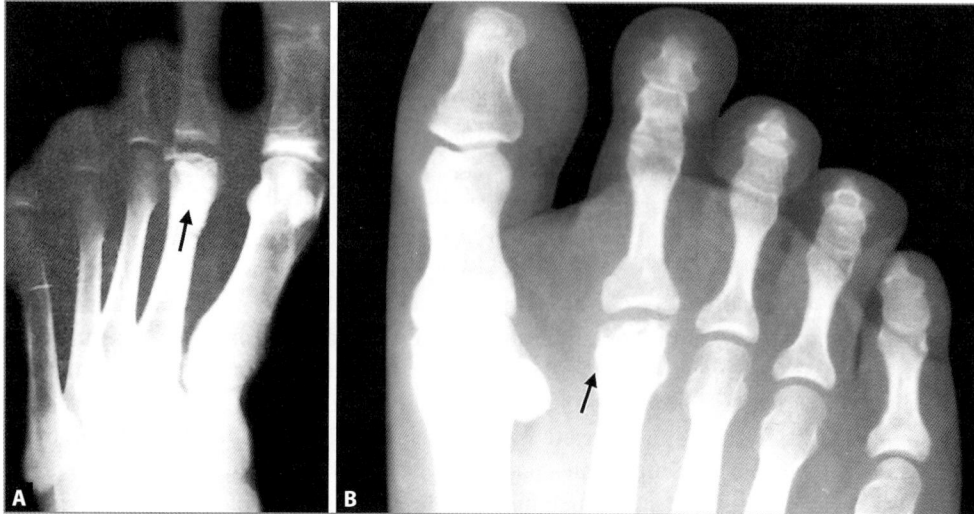

Figs. 15.97A and B: (A) Freiberg's disease showing dense, deformed and enlarged 2nd metatarsal head with osteoarthritic changes in the metatarsophalangeal joint on left foot; (B) Freiberg's disease in 2nd metatarsal head in right foot.

metatarsal head and widening (thickening) of adjacent metatarsal shaft with or without synovitis occurs. Pain in the affected zone on weight bearing, varying tenderness with or without swelling are presenting features. The incidence is highest amongst adolescent females the second metatarsal is the most commonly affected, followed by third. Smillie (1967) described a classification of Freiberg's disease based upon intraoperative appearance of effected metatarsal heads.

Majority of the patients should be managed with a forefoot offloading insole conservatively [modified activities, semirigid orthoses, metatarsal arch support (bar) analgesic (if needed)]. Failed cases may need surgery (such as joint debridement, remodelling of metatarsal head, and even second and third Weil's osteotomy etc.

- *Fractures of metatarsals including metatarsal stress fracture: Metatarsal stress fractures* usually develop due to repetitive stress applied to the bone which does not have the structural strength to stand it, e.g in excessive amount of walking, running, jogging, prolonged route marching (by army recruits—justifying its name as march fracture). Dull pain develops gradually in forefoot. Muscle cramps may appear. Movement of corresponding toe is painful. Standing or walking on tiptoe is painful. Slight tender swelling may appear at the painful site—few centimeters proximal to metatarsal head. Initially X-ray looks normal, however, radio-isotope scan shows increased uptake in quite early stage. Later on X-ray shows periosteal bone formation all around the stress fracture site.
- Infection of metatarsal—mainly in bare-foot walker due to thorn-prick **(Figs. 15.98 and 15.99)**

Plantar Plate Pathology: The plantar plate is a thick fibrocartilage tissue intracapsular structure composed mainly type 1 collagen 20 mm (L-long) × 16 mm (W-wide) × 2-5 mm (thick) located at the ball of the foot—first discussed in 1980s. It usually causes pain and deformity in the forefoot due to inflammation, attenuation and rupture of plantar plate. This condition is also described by the terms such as metatarsalgia, pre-dislocation syndrome, lesser metatarsophalangeal joint instability, crossover toe deformity. It occurs mostly in second MTPJ in women over 50 years of age. In rheumatoid arthritis it tends to manifest in 4th and 5th MTPS. Other deformities may co-exist like hallux abducto valgus, hallux rigidus, hallux varus.

Plantar plate is in direct contact with the lesser metatarsal heads during gait and functions as the primary static stabilizer of lesser MTPJs. Any biomechanical abnormality leading to overload of lesser metatarsals may lead to plantar plate deterioration which leads to MTPJ instability with rupture of plantar plate and dorsal displacement of proximal phalanx, the dynamic stability of intrinsic and extrinsic musculature providing stability of lesser MTPJs is impaired. Clinically, patient complains of pain and discomfort about the metatarsal heads. There may be pain in plantar sulcus and swelling at MTPJ. Physical examination like

(1) Kelikian pushup test, manual loading of plantar plate by applying direct pressure on the metatarsal heads produce pain.

(2) Lachman drawer maneuver—consists applying vertical stress to the proximal phalanx with one hand while stabilizing the metatarsal of involve MTPJ with the other hand – greater 2 mm of dorsal displacement is significant;

(3) Paper pull - out test—A thin strip of paper is placed beneath the pulp of plantarflexed testing toe – there will be decreased strength in plantarflexion of involved toe

High resolution dynamic ultrasound is more sensitive than MRI to diagnose the plantar plate disease.

Treatment: In acute injuries – shoe modification, ice, foot elevation anti-inflammatory drugs, taping.

In chronic cases – surgery with plantar or dorsal linear incision approach – to excision repair of plate. A Weil

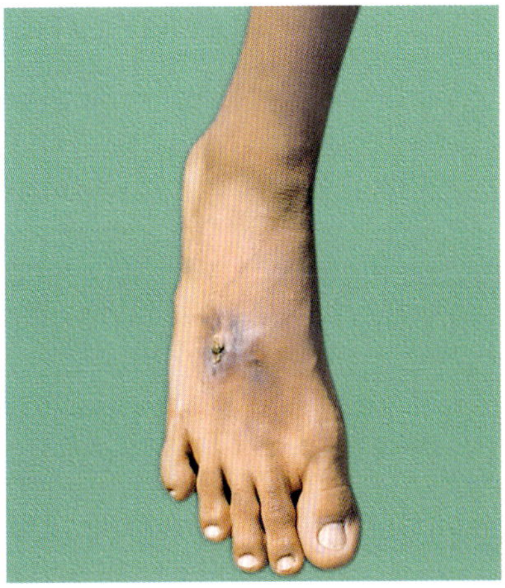

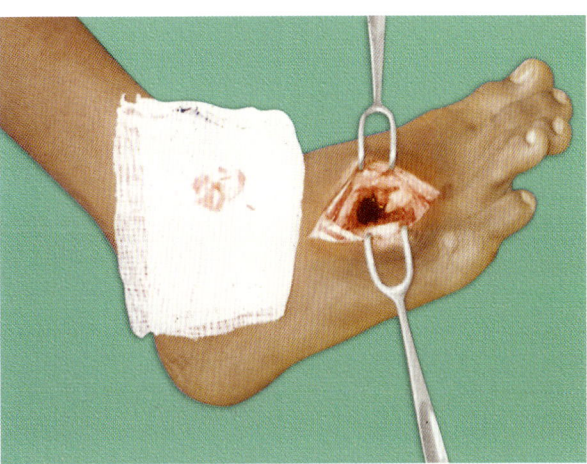

Fig. 15.98: Persistent infection and chronic osteomyelitis of 3rd and 4th metatarsals following thorn prick through sole.

Fig. 15.99: Intraoperative photograph—thorn pieces removed (on the gauze piece).

metatarsal shortening osteotomy with plantar plate repair usually produce successful result.
Ref. Maier Michael, Pham Peter, Kreplick A, Ringwood. M...Plantar plate pathology: A review article. Texas Sports Medicine Institute, USA. (google search).

- *Gouty arthritis:* Middle-aged men, complain of acute onset of pain with or without burning sensation usually in the region of 1st metatarsophalangeal joint (in pseudogout, the ankle is more affected).
  - Symptoms usually precipitate in the small hours of the morning
  - Local inflammatory features
  - Other joints, like ankle, knee, elbow, small joints of hands and feet may be affected
  - Serum uric acid level raised
  - In chronic cases, gouty tophi occur on big toe **(Figs. 15.100 and 15.101)** pinna of ear, fingers, elbow, etc.
  - Aspirate from joint, tophi, ligaments, etc. may show presence of sodium borate salt (cf. in *pseudogout—calcium pyrophosphate crystals*).

Causes of Ulcers in the Soles

- Trophic ulcer—Hansen's disease **(Figs. 15.102 to 15.105)**, sciatic or medial popliteal nerve palsy, spina bifida **(Figs. 15.106 to 15.111),** paraplegia (traumatic).
- Diabetic ulcers—20% or even more hospitalised diabetic patients are admitted for the foot problems, mainly the infections ranging from simple superficial cellulitis to chronic osteomyelitis, persistent ulcers and even gangrene.
  - *Thorn prick ulcer:* These usually manifests after months or even years. The patient complains of chronic dull ache/pain in mid and or forefoot region with or without swelling with mild inflammatory

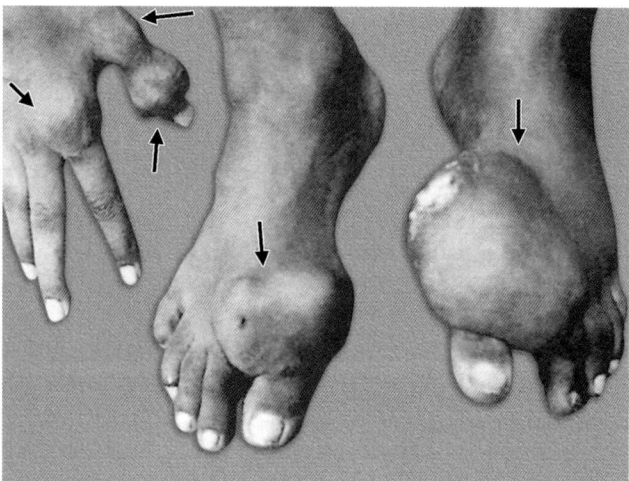

Fig. 15.100: Typical gouty tophi on both 1st metatarsophalangeal joint of both feet and also on the right thumb and base of index finger.

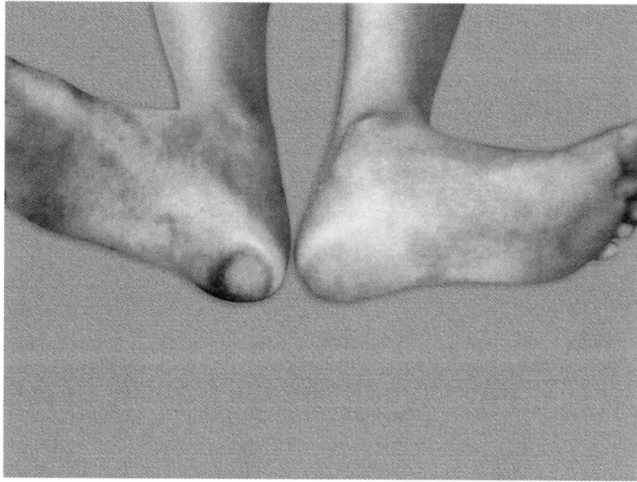

Fig. 15.102: Pre-ulcerative appearance of trophic ulceration in the both of heels due to Hansen's disease.

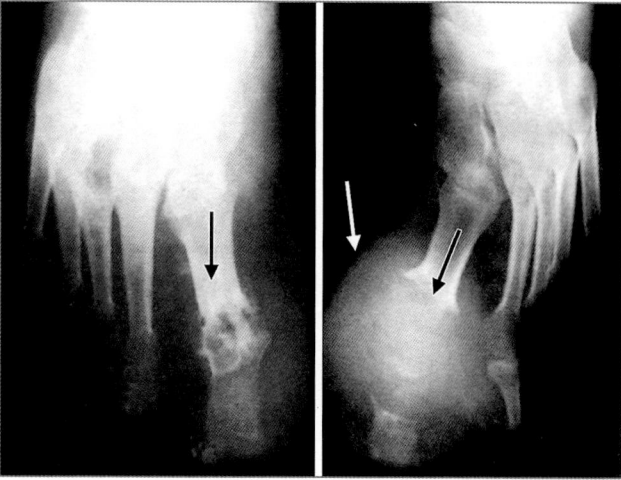

Fig. 15.101: X-ray photograph of same patient (**Fig. 15.100**). Note the destruction in the first metatarsophalangeal zones due to deposit of urate crystals.

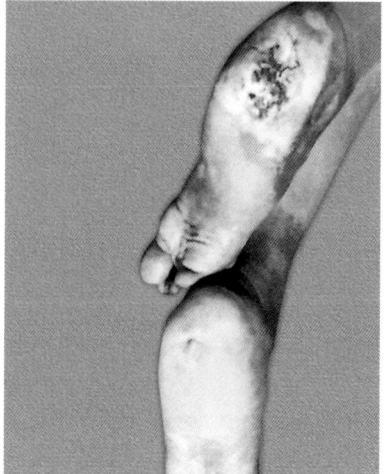

Fig. 15.103: Trophic ulcers (Hansen's disease)—on left heel healed; on right still very active.

feature. Radiologically, reactionary bone formation, and in advanced cases even cavity and sequestrum, may be seen. On exploration, the broken piece of thorn is usually found within the infected tissue (**Figs. 15.98 and 15.99**).
- Ulcers of vascular origin—Buerger's disease
- Arteriosclerotic ulcers
- Neurosyphilitic ulcer
- Infective—Actinomycotic (Madura foot) (**Figs. 15.112A to 15.114**), pyogenic (**Fig. 15.115**)
- Post-traumatic
- Post-burn
- Neoplastic, e.g. melanoma of calcaneum (**Fig. 15.146**)
- Giant cell tumour of calcaneum (**Fig. 15.145**).

Tuberculosis of Foot
(Figs. 15.117, 15.118 and Fig. 15.112B)

- Mostly affects tarsals (talus and calcaneum) and subtalar, midtarsal, intertarsal zones
- Chronic gradually increasing pain and mild to moderate swelling (may even fluctuate) on the dorsal aspect of foot
- Tuberculous sinuses (usually more than one with indrawn, puckered margin, discoloured surrounding, serosanguinous or thin straw coloured discharge)
- Tenderness at affected bones and joints
- Regional lymph glands may be enlarged and matted.

Certain Rare But Interesting Conditions

- Ainhum (**Fig. 15.119**)
- Xanthomatosis (**Fig. 15.120**)
- *Hyperplasia of foot* (**Fig. 15.116**)
- *Ewing's sarcoma of talus* (**Fig. 15.122**)
- *Haemangiosarcoma of foot* (**Figs. 15.123 and 15.124**)
- Filarial elephantiasis—tortoise foot (**Fig. 15.125**)
- Jiggers infection (**Fig. 15.126**)
- Cold fire burn (**Fig. 15.127**).

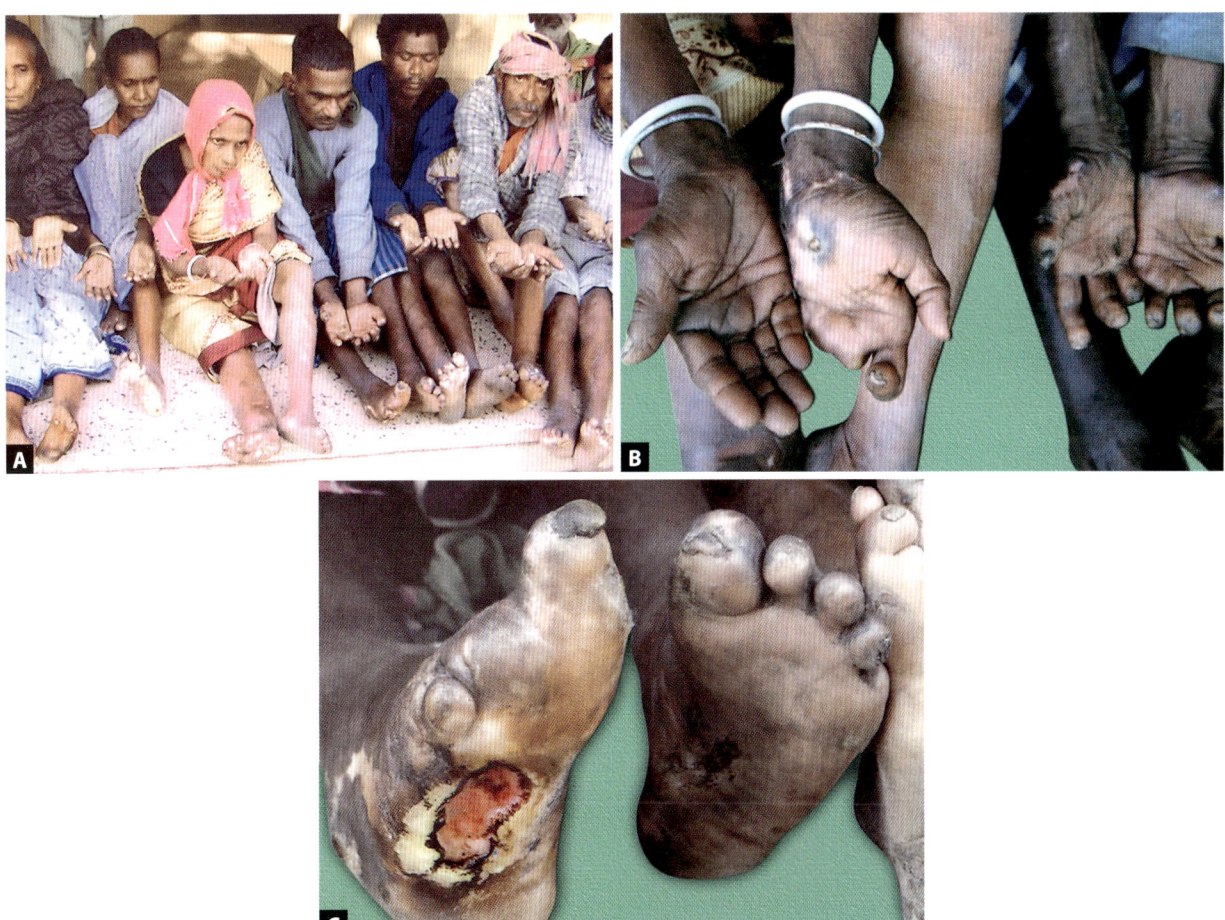

Figs. 15.104A to C: Foot and hand affections in leprosy: Leprosy is a chronic infectious disease caused by *Mycobacterium leprae*. It mainly involves the skin, respiratory mucosa and peripheral nervous system. It continues to be a public health problem, mainly in developing countries. Neuropathic changes lead to ulceration and destruction in feet and hands. Though earliest described in Asia in about 6th century BC Dr Gerhard Henrik Armauer Hansen of Norway discovered its causative organism – *M. leprae* in 1873. Early diagnosis of leprosy depends on high suspicion index, skin lesions, sensory loss, thickened peripheral nerves, and detection of AFB in skin or nasal smear.

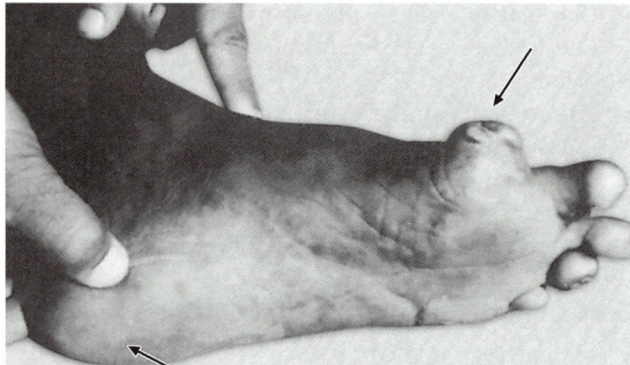

Fig. 15.105: Trophic ulcer in heel and destroyed and fallen off big toe due to Hansen's disease.

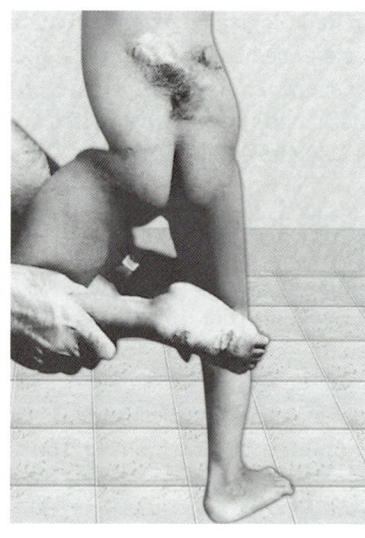

Fig. 15.108: Neglected equino-varus deformity with trophic ulcer on the dorsum of foot due to spina bifida.

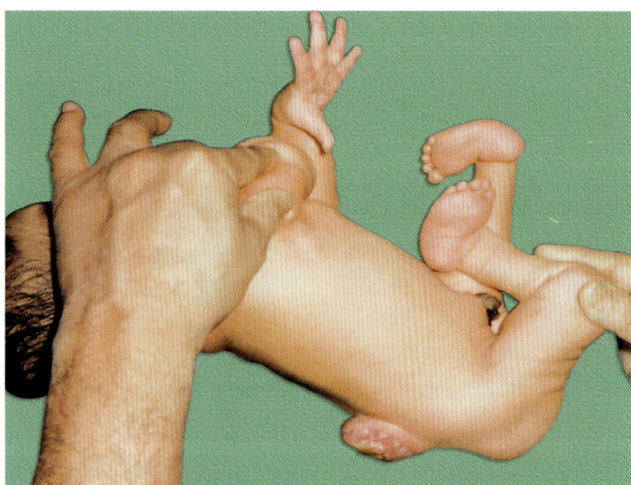

Fig. 15.106: Spina bifida manifesta with clubfeet.

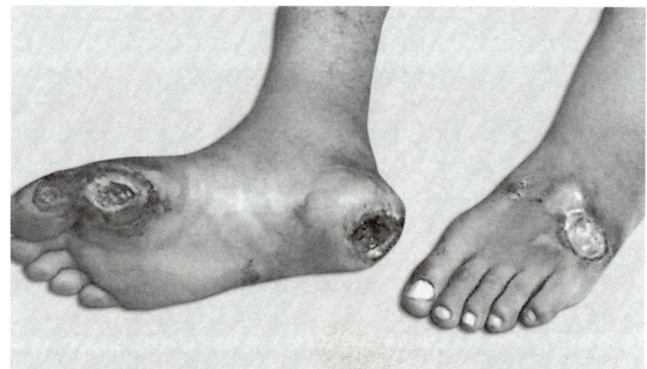

Fig. 15.109: Trophic ulceration on both desensitised feet due to spina bifida.

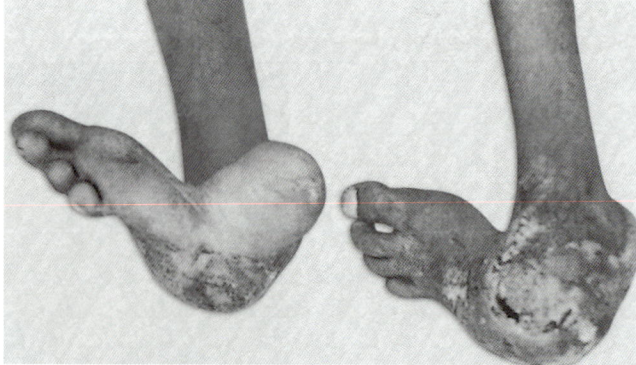

Fig. 15.110: Neglected severe equino-cavo-varus deformities with extensive ulcerations associated with spina bifida.

Disorders of Toenail
(Figs. 15.128 to 15.133)

Nails are exoskeleton. The normal nail complex consists of nail plate, nail bed, and immediately surrounding soft tissue including skin. Their disorders include congenital affections to neoplasm.

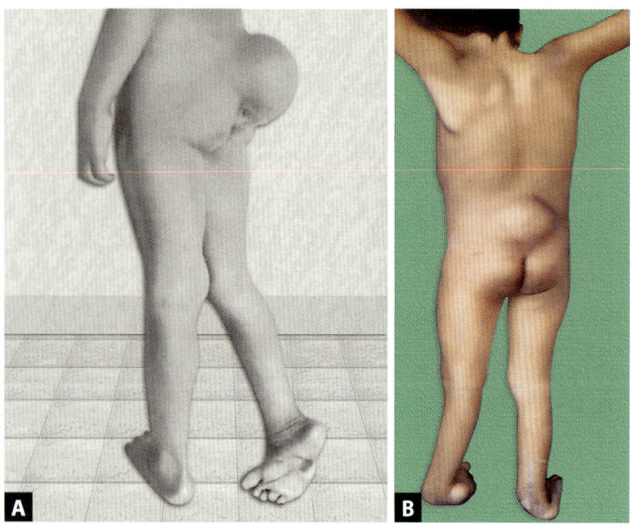

Figs. 15.107A and B: (A) Neglected equino-cavo-varus deformity of right foot with ulceration on the dorsum of foot associated with spina bifida manifesta; (B) Neglected equino-cavo-varus deformity of left foot with spina bifida occulta.

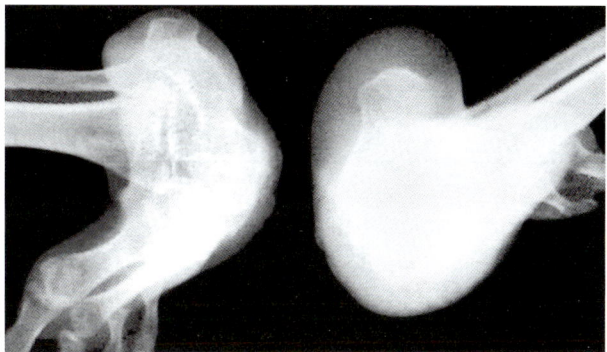

Fig. 15.111: X-ray of the same patient (**Fig. 15.110**).

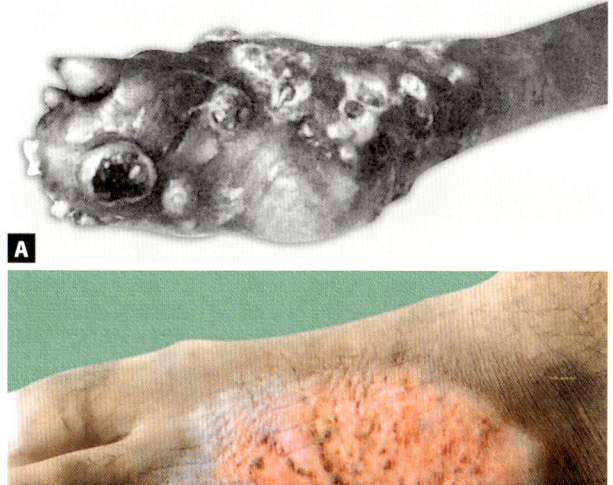

Figs. 15.112A and B: (A) Advanced Madura foot. V Carter (1860) established the fungal aetiology and proposed the term 'mycetoma'; (B) Tuberculous ulcer of dorsum of foot.

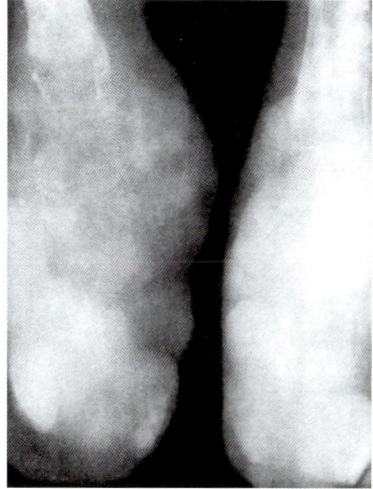

Fig. 15.113: X-ray of the same patient (**Fig. 15.112A**). See also **Fig. 7.25, 7.26,** AND comments written under the figures.

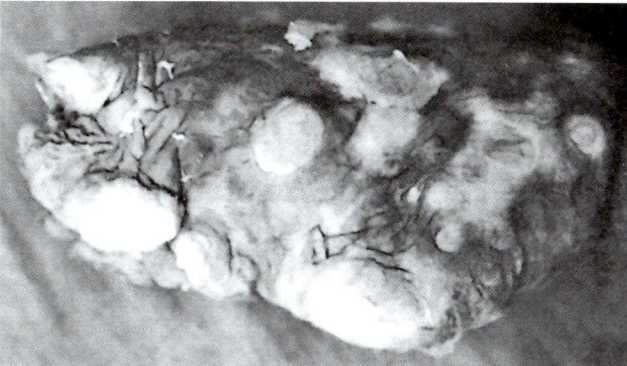

Fig. 15.114: Amputated foot ridden with extensive Madura foot ulcers. The name Madura foot comes from its high incidence around Madurai (a city in South India). The term mycetoma, an uncommon chronic infective disease of skin and subcutaneous tissue – characterized by triad of tumefaction, draining sinuses and presence of colonial grains in the exudates, was proposed by V Carter, who established (1860) the fungal aetiology of this disease. The foot is the most commonly affected site (about 70%), the disease is very common around Madurai (south India) hence the synonym "Madura Foot" (Figs.15.112A, 15.113, 15.114). Hand is next commonly affected (Figs. 7.25, 7.26). Infection is caused by true fungi in 40% of cases when it is called as eumycetoma; and by filamentous bacteria (in 60% of cases) of actinomycetes order and then it is known as actinomycetoma. Since the etiological organisms are different in two – groups, the treatment – mainly the drugs are different i.e. antifungal in eumycetoma and antibiotics in actinomycetoma.

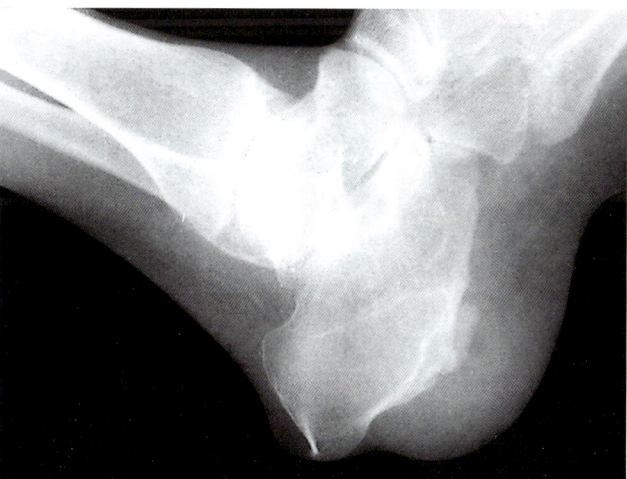

Fig. 15.115: Chronic pyogenic osteomyelitis calcaneum following thorn prick.

Common affections are traumatic (usually blunt crush).

Acute infections are usually sub or paraungal. Chronic infections are usually fungal in origin.

Acute infections are extremely painful and usually require surgery. Chronic infections are extremely difficult to eradicate.

Onychocryptosis or Ingrowing of toenail (embedded toenail) that is a common podiatric problem the term

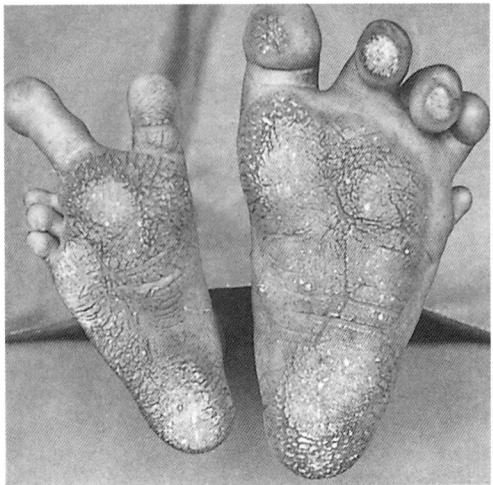

Fig. 15.116: Hyperplasia of foot. Note the sole aspect of hyperplastic foot with hyperkeratosis.

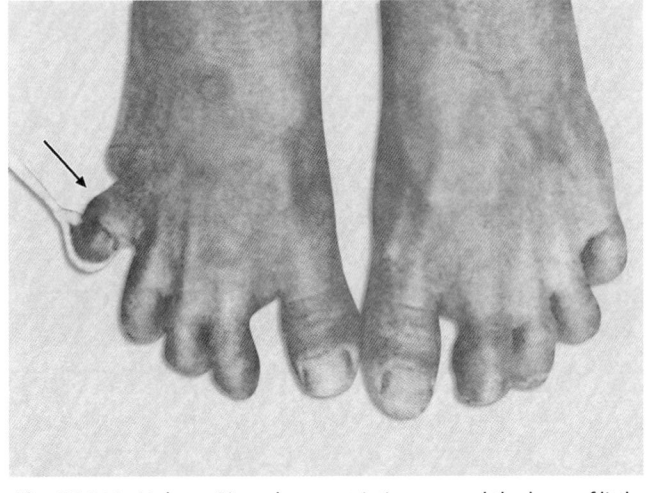

Fig. 15.119: Ainhum. Note the constriction around the base of little toe beyond which the toe is advancing for gangrene.

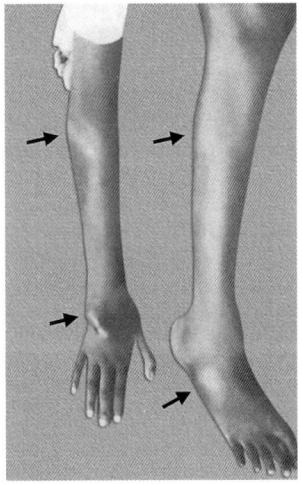

Fig. 15.117: A lady aged 27 with multi-focal tuberculosis (right elbow, hand; right upper tibiofibular joint and right foot).

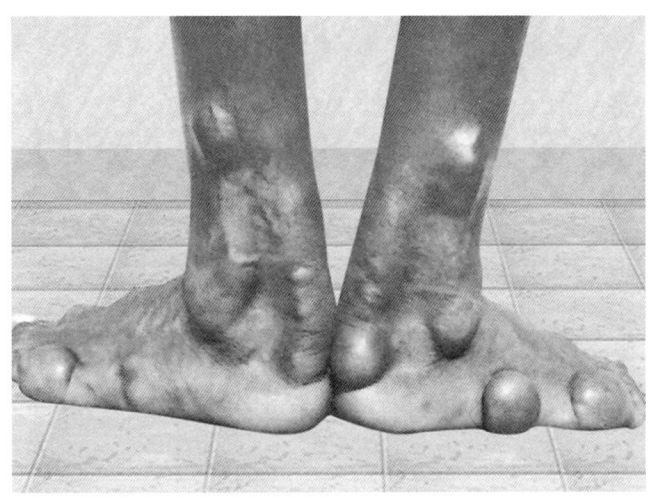

Fig. 15.120: Multiple xanthomatous swellings over both feet and around ankles.

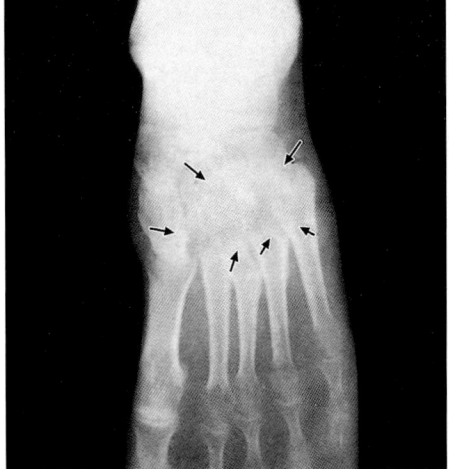

Fig. 15.118: X-ray photograph of her foot lesion (Fig. 15.127) (photo taken on reverse film).

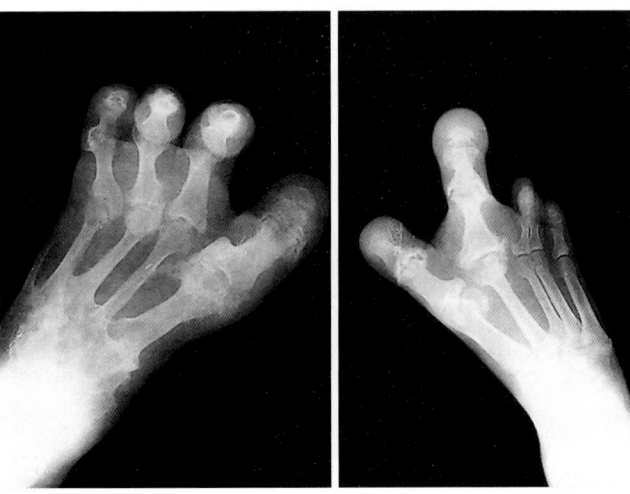

Fig. 15.121: X-ray of hyperplasia of both feet. Note the giant development of short long bones.

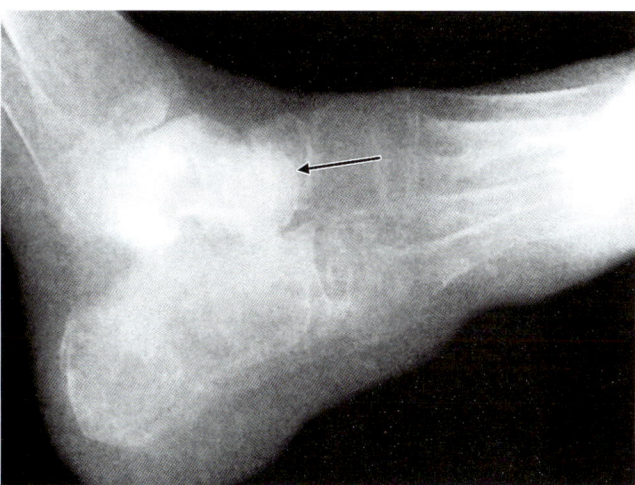

Fig. 15.122: Ewing's sarcoma of talus which may be misdiagnosed as avascular necrosis.

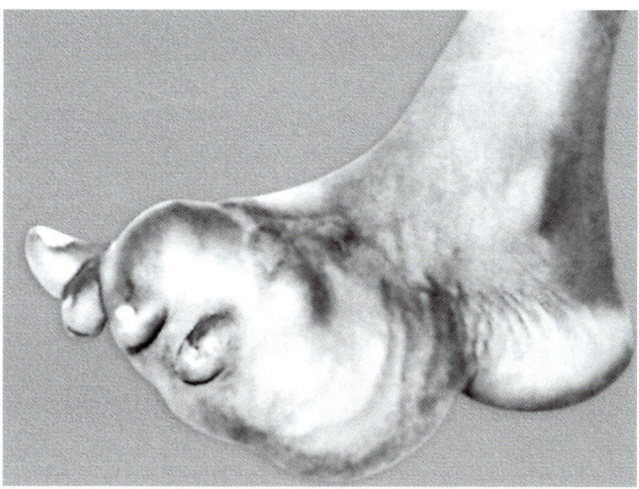

Fig. 15.123: Haemangiosarcoma of foot.

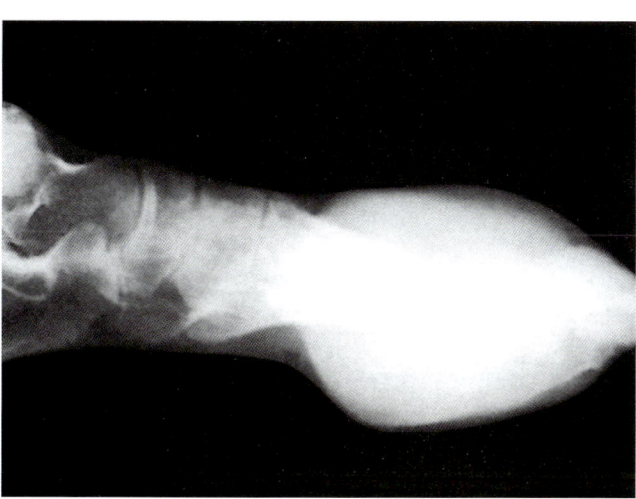

Fig. 15.124: X-ray of the same foot (**Fig. 15.123**).

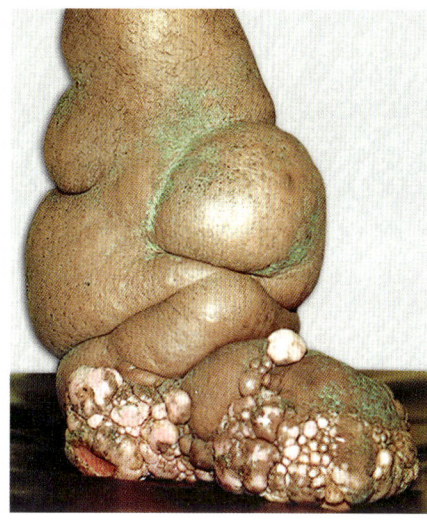

Fig. 15.125: Filarial elephantiasis with lobulations, nodulations, fissures and ulcerations. Tortoise foot (the sole is not affected in elephantiasis).

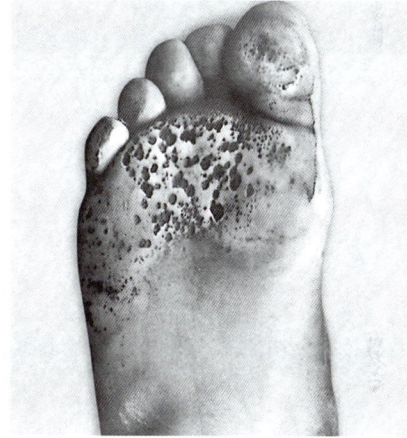

Fig. 15.126: Jiggers infection (by Tunga penetrans in the sole of foot).

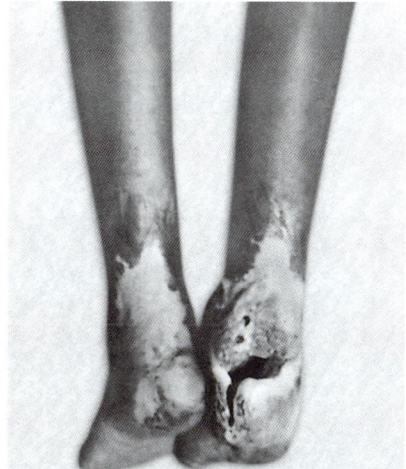

Fig. 15.127: Cold fire burn effects on the back of heels (After continuous heating the feet in winters). The burning charcoal is kept in an earthenware, which is kept beneath the cord – woven cot in the heel - foot region. The person feels better due to slow heating, however gradual burning of soft tissues occur.

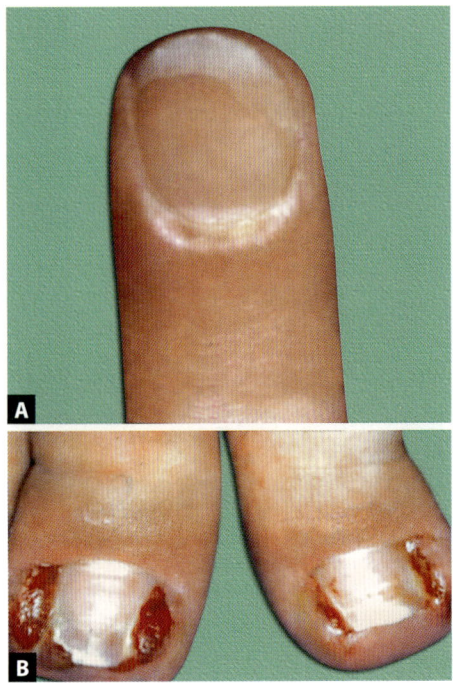

Figs. 15.128A and B: (A) Acute paronychia with painful, bright red swelling due to pus behind the cuticle, (B) Acute paronychia due to ingrowing toenails.

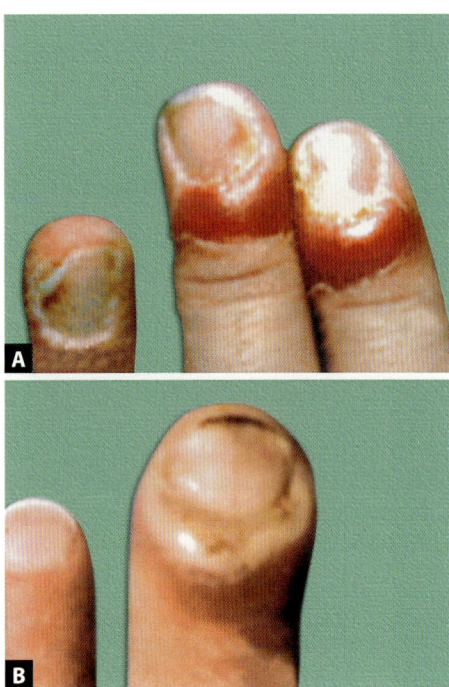

Figs. 15.129A and B: (A) Extremely tender paronychial infection with blood tinged pus, (B) Acute suppurative paronychia requiring immediate incision and drainage.

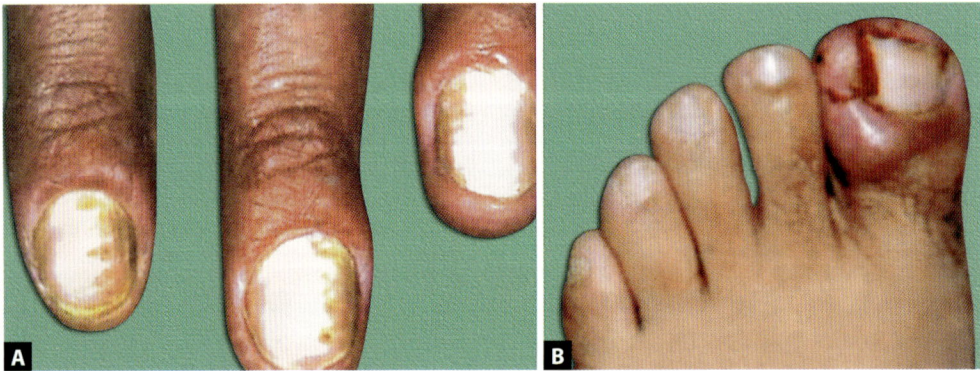

Figs. 15.130A and B: (A) Mild chronic paronychia, (B) Severe acute paronychia of the left hallux.

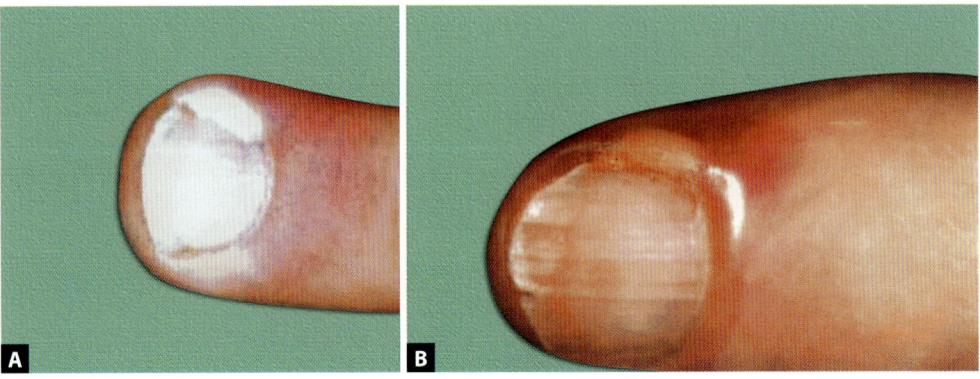

Figs. 15.131A and B: (A) Acute paronychia due to nail biting, (B) Acute paronychia of the thumb.

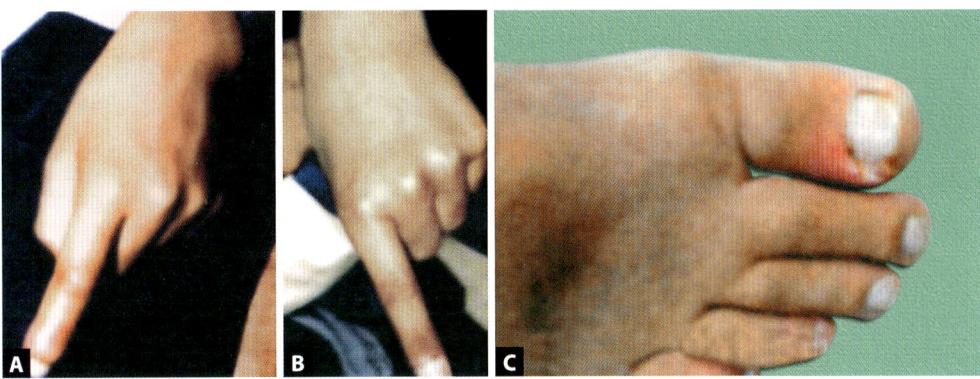

Figs. 15.132A to C: Acute paronychia: (A) Before treatment, (B) After treatment, (C) Acute paronychia due to arterial insufficiency.

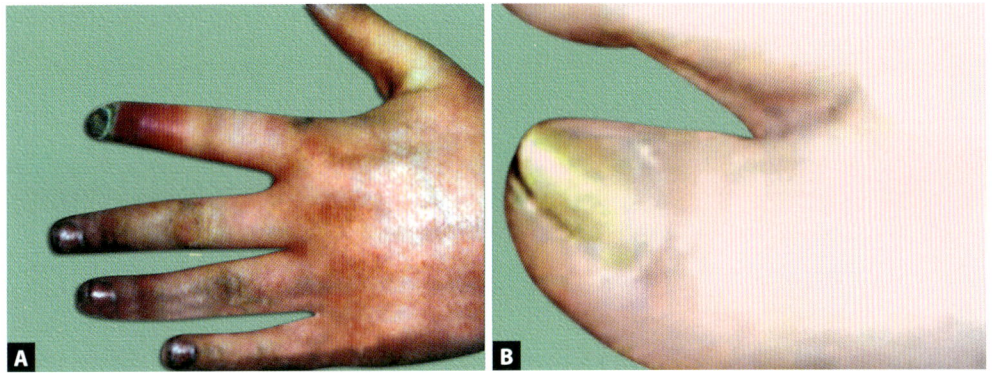

Figs. 15.133A and B: (A) Acute paronychia of the index finger with oedema of the finger and cellulitis, (B) Acute paronychia due to pincer nails.

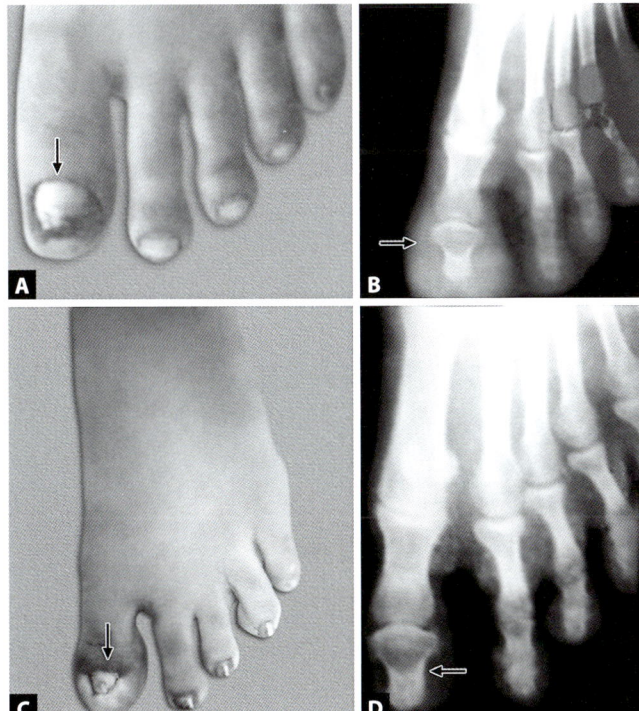

Figs. 15.134A to D: Ingrowing nail of big toe. Clinical photographs—Pre- (A) and (C) postoperative. X-ray of same patient—Pre- (B) and postoperative (D).

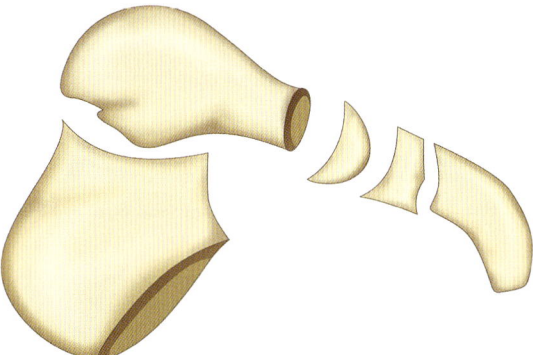

Fig. 15.135: Bound foot deformity (Chinese foot binding).

onychocryptosis comprises of two greek words – 'onyx' (meaning nail) and 'kryptos' (meaning hidden) – (James et al 2006) of the big toe (**Figs. 15.128 to 15.134B**) may be familial. It can result from using tight shoes with crowded toe-box. Lateral nail-fold is commonly affected. Patients with fleshy nail folds and thin nail plates are more vulnerable. Patient presents with buried tender side margins of the nail with frequent/recurrent features of inflammation/infection with or without discharge of thick beads of pus. On the whole, the term ingrown is misleading.

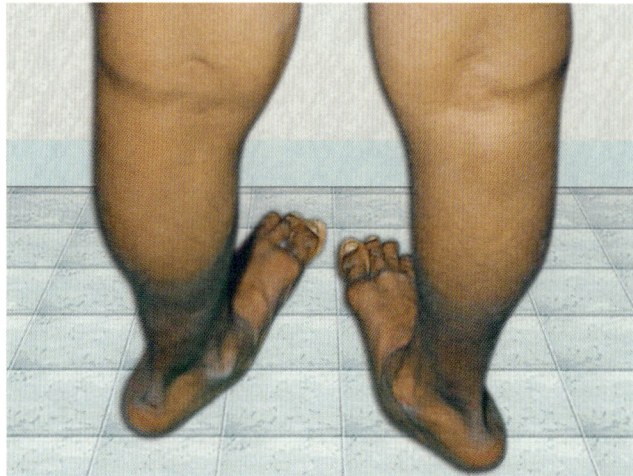

Fig. 15.136: Pes valgus on the left and congenital convex pes valgus on the right—viewed from back.

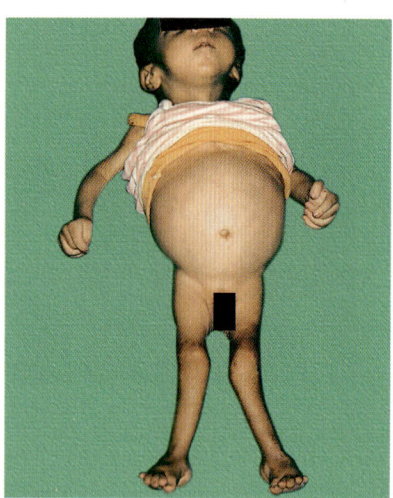

Fig. 15.139: Rickets with bilateral *metatarsus adductus* with tendency of 2nd and 3rd toes overriding the medially deviated big toes of both feet.

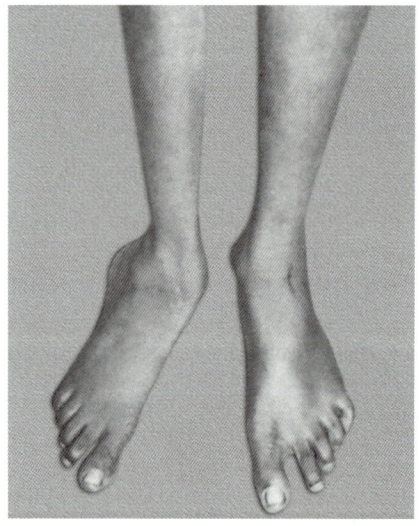

Fig. 15.137: Paralytic valgus collapse at right ankle.

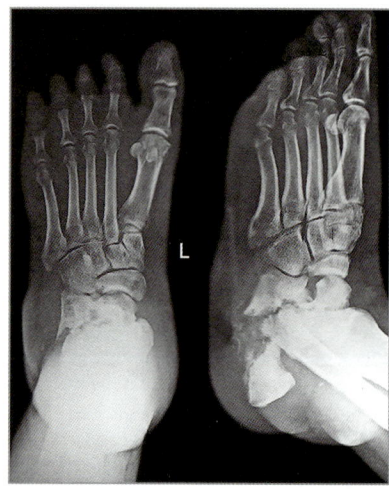

Fig. 15.140: Diabetic neuropathy—pathological fracture of calcaneus.

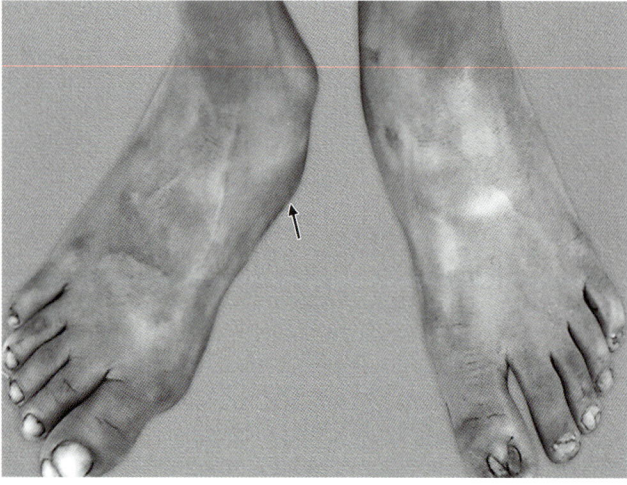

Fig. 15.138: Accessory navicular on right side producing pes valgus.

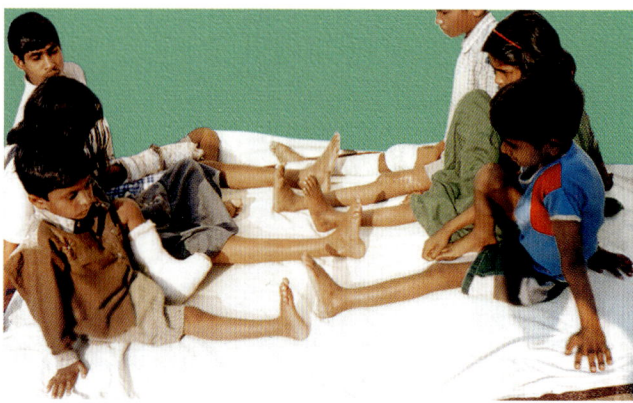

Fig. 15.141: After correction of various foot deformities, such as equino-cavo-varus, calcaneocavovalgus, rigid cavus, claw foot, etc.

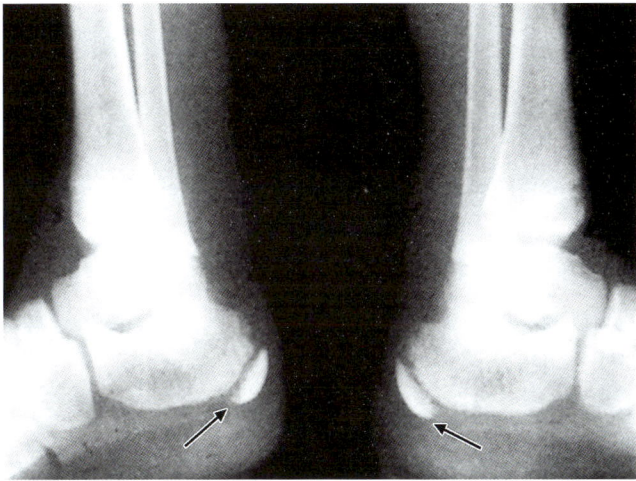

Fig. 15.142: Calcaneal apophysitis (Sever's disease).

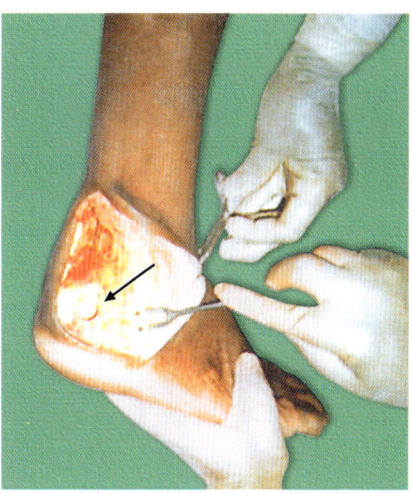

Fig. 15.144: Transoperative picture of the patient of **Figure 15.143** showing the sequestrum sitting at the mouth of hole in osteomyelitic calcaneum.

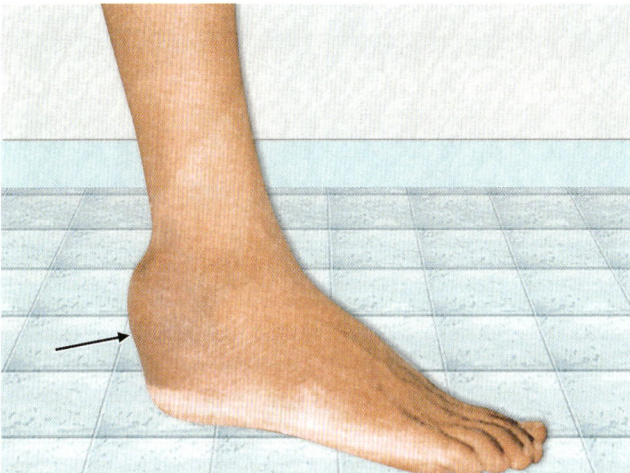

Fig. 15.143: Osteomyelitis of calcaneum with collection of pus.

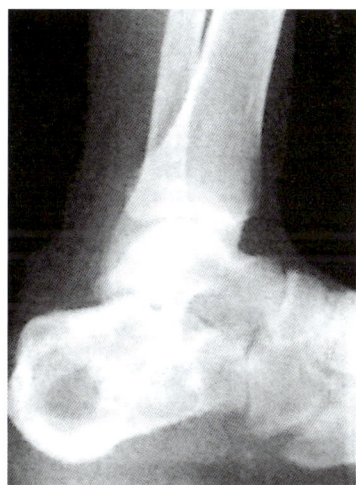

Fig. 15.145: Giant cell tumour of calcaneum.

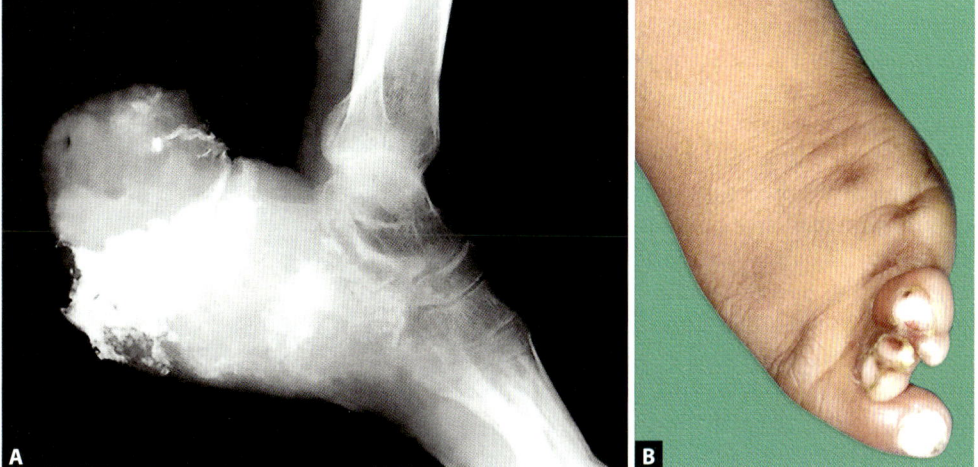

Figs. 15.146A and B: (A) X-ray of advanced malignant melanoma of calcaneum; (B) Congenitally fused almost all outer four toes (rays). So long there is no demanding problem in footwear it can be accepted.

484 Foot

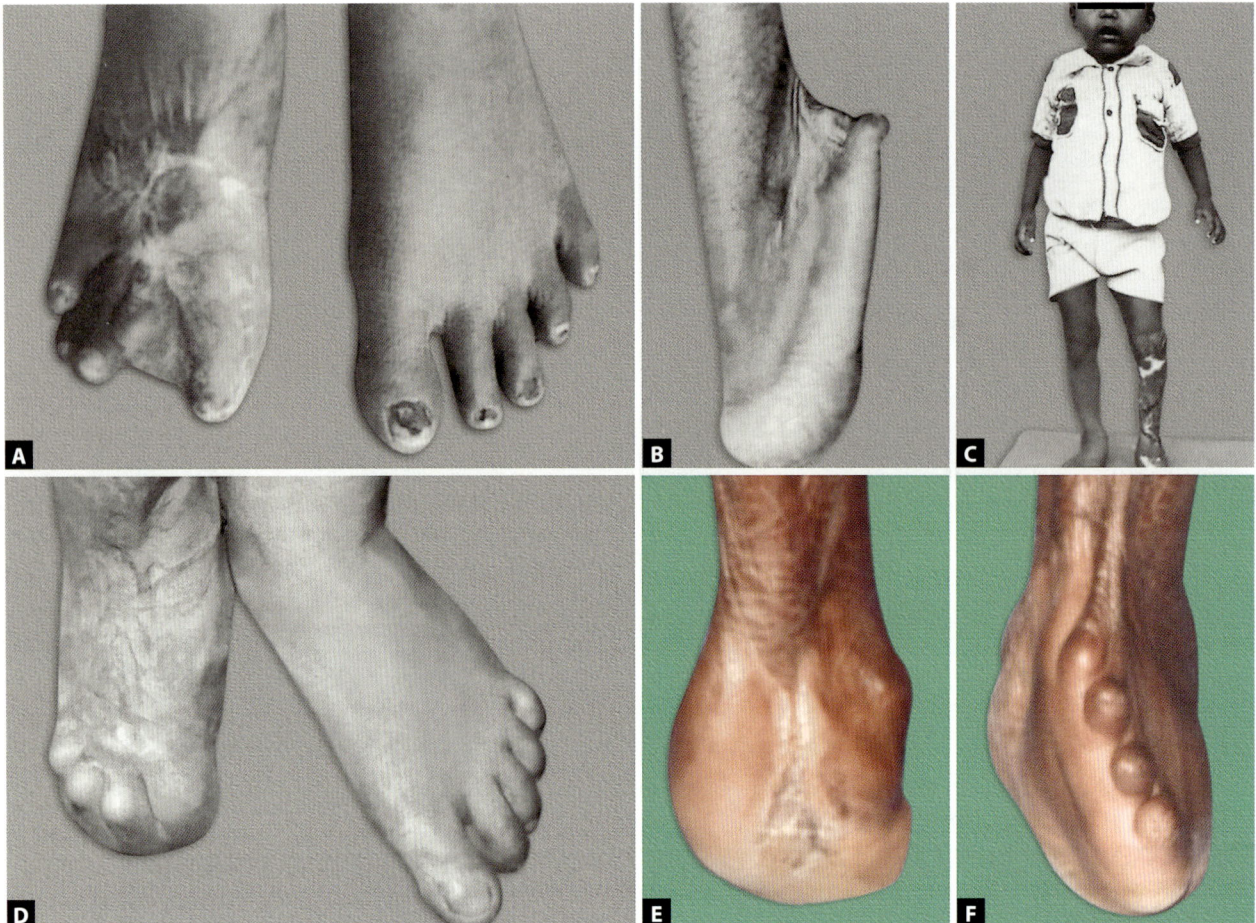

Figs. 15.147A to F: The post-burn contractures of the foot usually produce varied deformities of the foot, toes and ankle. Besides the cosmetic affections, they can produce problems in the overall use of the foot and footwear. Besides orthopaedic care, the plastic surgery is mostly needed in such cases.

Paronychia is the infection (which is subcuticular and under eponychium) around (and may be under) the nail. The affected digit is usually acutely inflamed at the distal end, painful and markedly tender.

Onychogryphosis is the thickened and crooked (may be curly) overgrowth of toenail.

The big toe of an elderly bedridden people is more vulnerable.

Subungal exostosis was probably first described by Dupuytren in 1847, hence it is also called Dupuytren's exostosis. It predominantly affects the young female (10 to 25 years of age) and female male ratio is 2 : 1. Though attention is drawn mostly after trauma (unestablished traumatic origin) it may be congenital. The exostosis (radiologically opaque), extending from the dorsum of the phalanx towards the nail bed, elevates the nail causing discomfort and pain. Oblique view X-ray, especially the magnified one, helps in locating the lesion. Gradually, fibrous reaction may develop around it and the lesion may become verrucous and ulcerate. It can be confused with subungal wart, pyogenic granuloma, malignant melanoma and squamous cell carcinoma. Surgical excision is the treatment of choice.

Glomus Tumour

It presents as a peculiar painful, exquisitely tender mass underneath the nail giving a faint-bluish hue, otherwise the nail looks normal. The mass (glomus tumour) consists of proliferated normal capsular-neural glomus apparatus. Removal of mass along with the overlying portion of nail plate is the treatment of choice. However, corticosteroid (depo-medrol 12.5 mgm) injection to and around the mass at 15 days intervals has been found to subside the symptoms—2 to 3 injections.

Accessory Ossicles

The accessory ossicles of the foot are developmental in origin and are inconstant, independent, well-defined bones with regular margins in an otherwise normally developed foot. They may be symptomatic in themselves or may be misinterpreted as a fracture (which may create medicolegal problems). The accessory ossicles can be visualised on:

- *Medial aspect:* (i) Os trigonum, (ii) Os subtentaculi, (iii) accessory navicular, (iv) Os supranaviculare, (v) Os intercuneiform; (vi) Os intermetatarseum
- *Lateral aspect:* (vii) Os calcaneus secundarius, (viii) Os peroneum, (ix) Os vesalianum, (x) Os infranaviculare, (xi) Os accessorium supracalcaneum, (xii) Os subcalcis
- *Superior aspect:* Above noted Nos (i), (iii), (iv), (v), (vi), (vii), (viii), (ix) are seen.
- *In anteroposterior view of ankle:* (xiii) Os subfibulare, (xiv) Os subtibiale, and (xv) Intercalary bone.

BOUND FOOT DEFORMITY

In China, between the age of 3 and 7, the feet are bound in stout iron boots to make it short and to give them the shape which is thought to be erotic. The deformities complex consist of cavus foot + flexion contractures of the toes. Hibb's angle on average remains about 75° and Meary angle 128° **(Fig. 15.135)**. The cause of the deformities can easily be levelled as iatrogenic. Historically, in ancient Chinese culture, the shortened high arched feet were considered to be synonymous with being born into nobility (Berg EE1995). This system continued till 20th century.

FOOT INVOLVEMENT IN RHEUMATOID ARTHRITIS

Foot is involved in 80 to 90% patients of rheumatoid arthritis. The affection is mainly in forefoot. The pathomechanical features of rheumatoid foot deformities mainly consists of distension of capsule, stretching of ligaments, erosion of metatarsal heads, and dislocation of metatarsophalangeal joints. The great toe usually undergoes valgus deviation with pronation. The plantar plate and fat pad get stretched dorsally and loose their capacity of shock absorption.

In the advanced stage the lesser toes develop clawing deformity. The weight-bearing capacity of first ray gets gradually lost which leads to development of metatarsalgia and callus formation.

DIABETIC FOOT

With increase of diabetes mellitus in epidemic proportions worldwide, its the most common and serious complication—the foot infection **(Fig. 15.148)** and ulceration—are also on increase. About 15% of all diabetic patients develop foot ulcers at some point in their lifetime. Unless properly evaluated and managed, there is a greater risk of lower extremity amputation. Diabetic foot ulcers are variously managed according to facilities and expertise available and the stage of advancement of ulcer. However total contact casting (TCC) appears to be more practical and effective. Overlapping factors contribute to foot ulcerations, such as peripheral neuropathy, altered or complete loss of sensation, ischaemia, vasomotor neuropathy, poor vision, limited joint mobility, consequences of cardiovascular and cerebrovascular diseases, etc. However, accidental trauma and ill-fitting footwear are common precipitating factors.

Diabetic foot syndrome is a serious complication of diabetes and is most common causes of nontraumatic lower extremity amputation.

The prevalence of amputation is expected to increase as the incidence of diabetes is worsening in the present days and number of diabetes patients is expected to rise in the coming years.

When attempts to preserve an infected or ischaemic limb (in diabetes the foot and ankle regions are mainly affected) prove to be futile, below knee amputation can preserve the life and workable function. Once hospitalized with diabetic foot infection usually about 50% of patients require some level of lower - extremity amputation (Johnson MJ 2022).

The staged approach to below knee amputation has been found to be an effective method of reducing complications and achieving successful closure of the amputation stump. In this staged approach, the first amputation is a transtibial or guillotine amputation, which is performed as a drainage amputation a few days before the actual below - knee amputation with closure. Ankle disarticulation at the tibiotalar interface (without tibial and fibular osteotomy) may also be used as a first stage operation to help faster and proper healing of actual below knee amputation stump when it is performed for unsalvageable limb. (Carroll PJ 2020).

Diabetic foot ulcers have been variously classified, however, Wagner-Meggitt classification is most practical

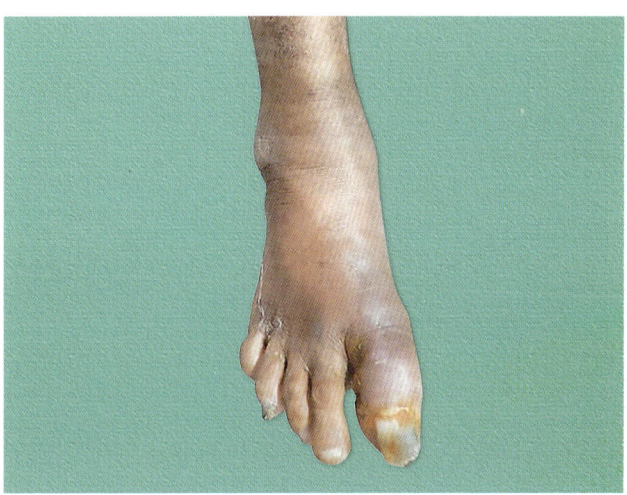

Fig. 15.148: Diabatic foot infection (Early stage).

system in grading ulcers, which helps in the prediction of healing and the possibility of amputation in a simple way.

Classification of Diabetic Foot Ulcers

Classification by ulcer depth and gangrene tissue (Wagner-Meggitt)	
Grade 1	Partial skin thickness
Grade 2	Full skin thickness
Grade 3	Underlying tissues involved (fascia, ligaments, tendons)
Grade 4	Grade 3 + abscess or osteomyelitis
Grade 5	Grade 4 + necrotic tissues
Grade 6	Gangrenous tissues found

Diabetic foot ulcers are generally polymicrobial, however, most common isolated organisms are aerobic gram-positive bacteria, mainly *Staphylococcus aureus* and β-hemolytic streptococci. In deep infections, gram-negative bacteria, such as *E. coli*, *proteus* spp; *klebsiella* spp, methicillin resistant *S. aureus* (MRSA) are also found. Management of diabetic foot infection (D F1) should be multimodal, such as controlling hyperglycaemia, targeted antibiotics especially against (MRSA), local wound management, correction of vascular insufficiency, and adequate surgical drainage and debridement.

Patients must be educated about proper good quality of foot care, self- examination, proper washing of feet, proper footwear without socks and regular podiatry check- up. The treatment of diabetic foot syndromes should involve multidisciplinary teams which include general, vascular, orthopaedic, surgeons; neurologist; cardiologist; nephrologist; microbiologist; radiologist; ophthalmologist; dietitian; physiotherapist; diabetes and podology nurses; shoemaker.

Flowchart 1

DIABETIC FOOT DISORDERS

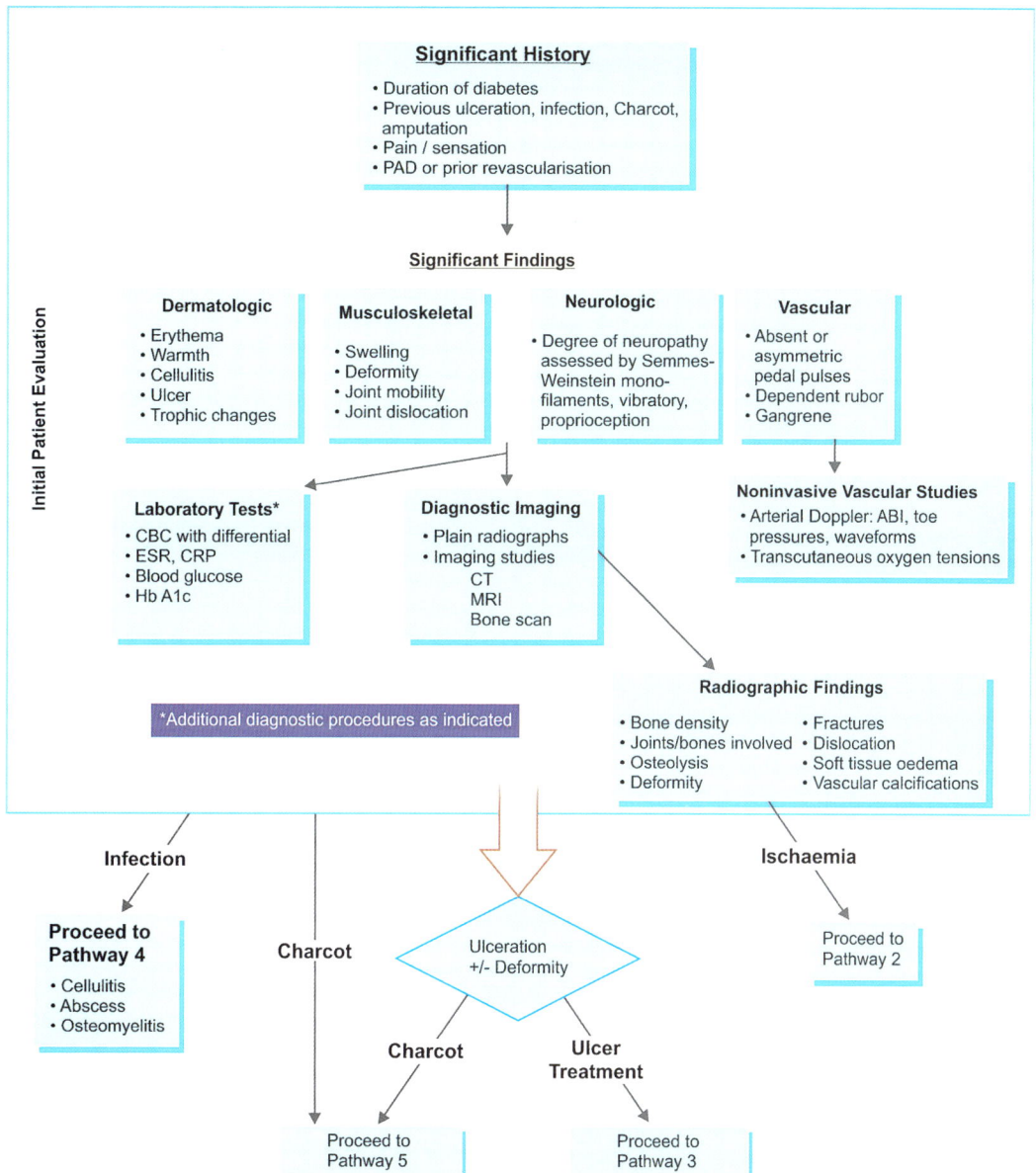

Courtesy: Dr Robert G Frykberg, Chief Podiatry, Carl T Hayder, VA Medical Centre, Phoenix.

Flowchart 2

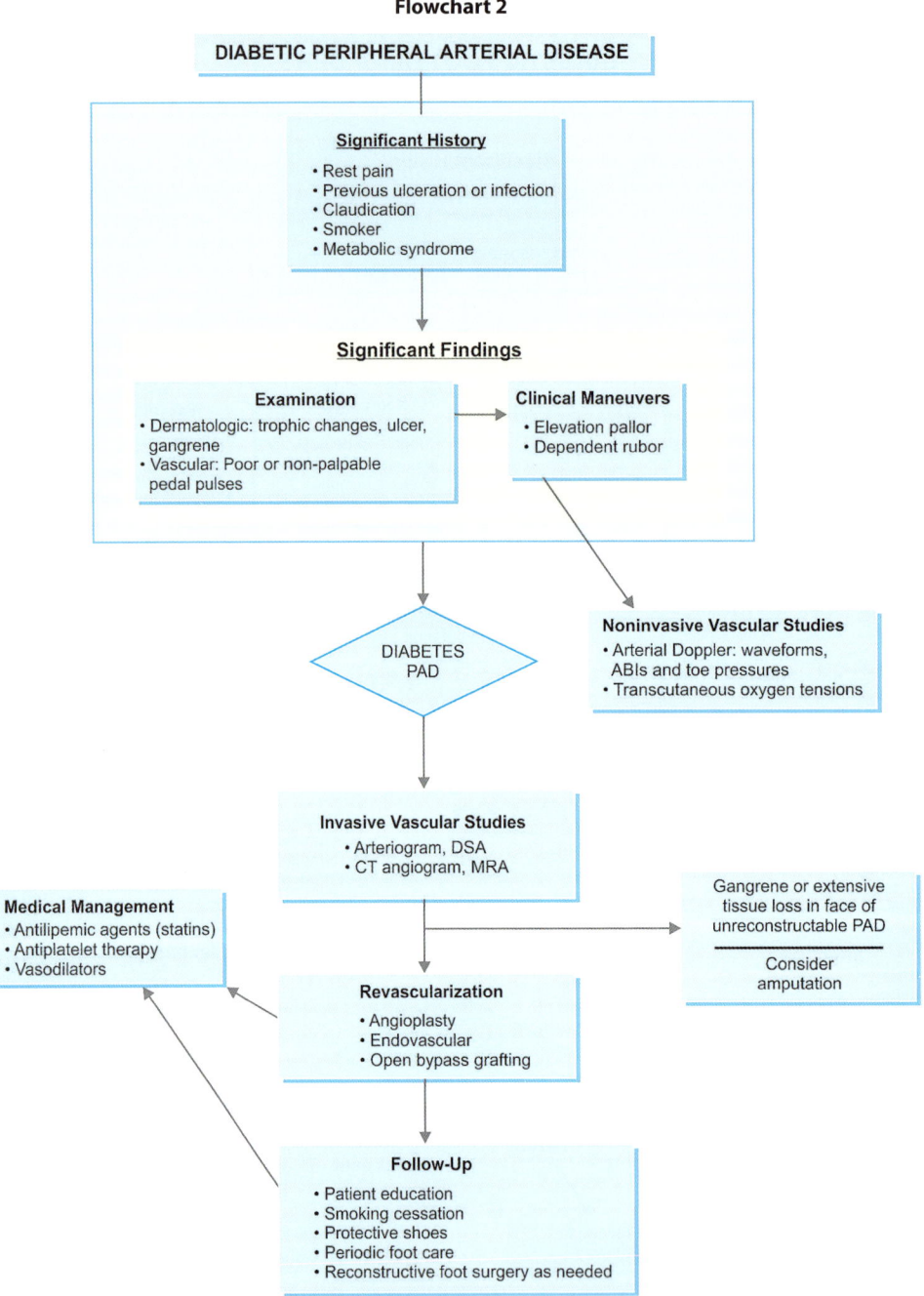

Courtesy: Dr Robert G Frykberg, Chief Podiatry, Carl T Hayder, VA Medical Centre, Phoenix.

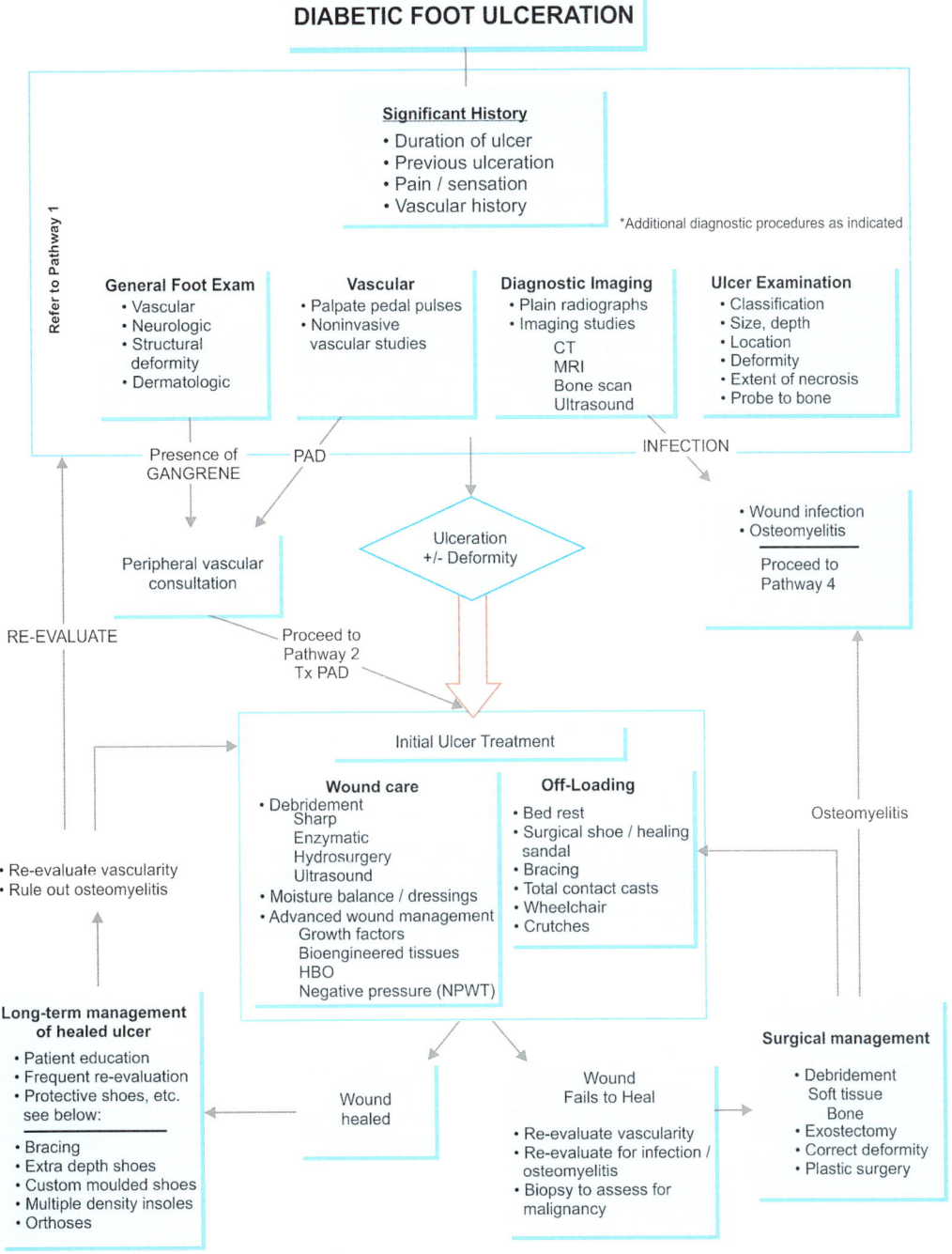

Flowchart 3: DIABETIC FOOT ULCERATION

Courtesy: Dr Robert G Frykberg, Chief Podiatry, Carl T Hayder, VA Medical Centre, Phoenix.

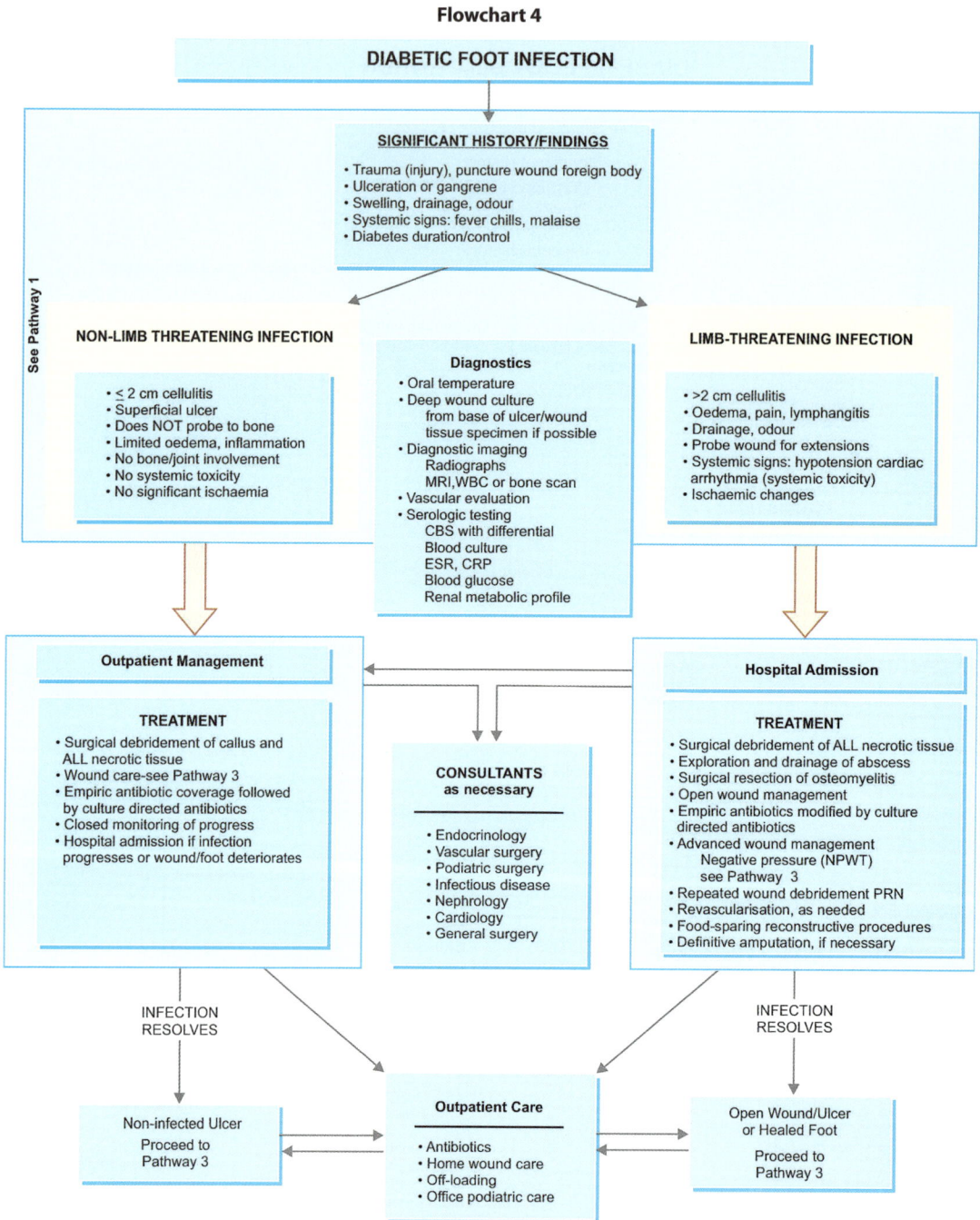

Courtesy: Dr Robert G Frykberg, Chief Podiatry, Carl T Hayder, VA Medical Centre, Phoenix.

Foot 491

Flowchart 5

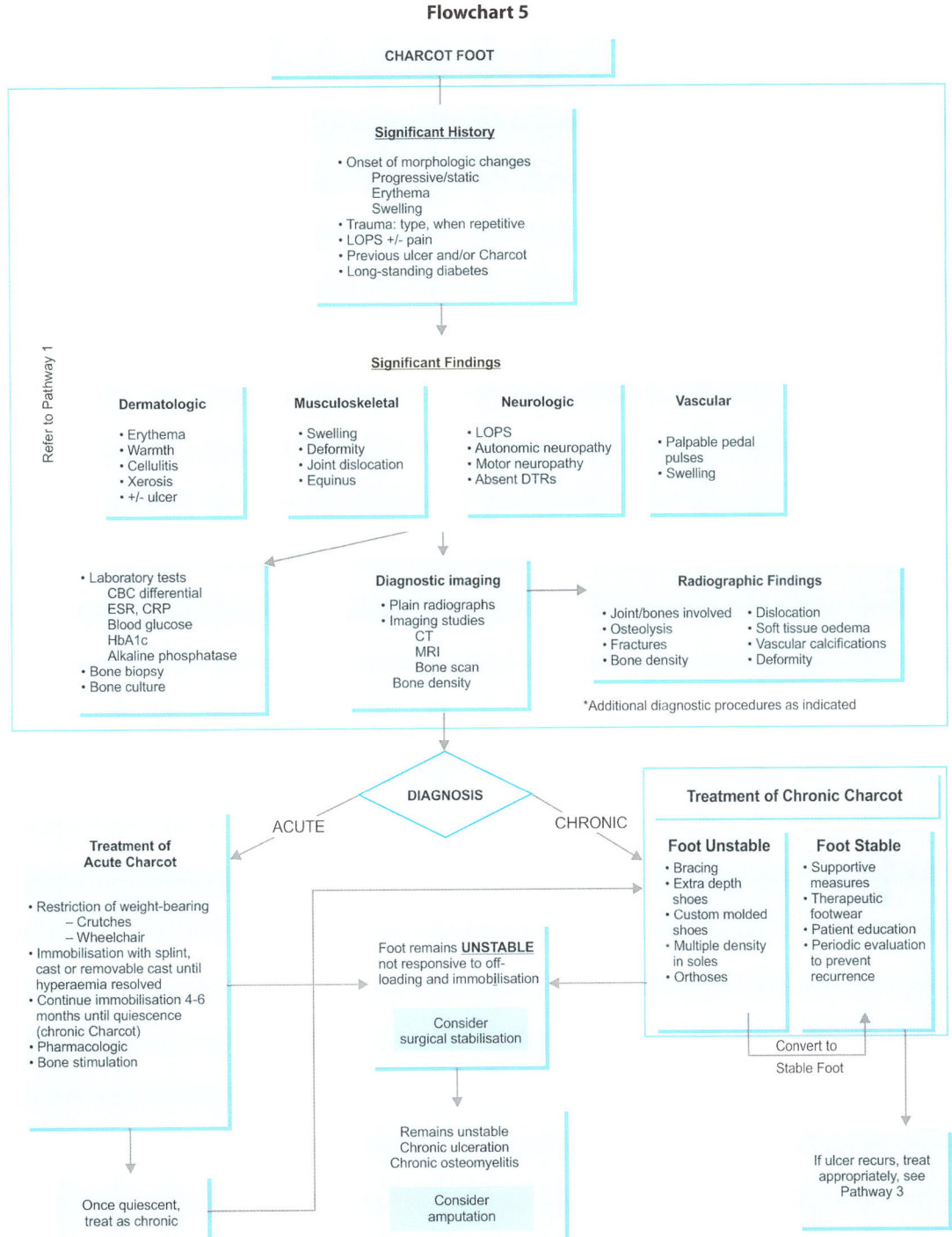

Courtesy: Dr Robert G Frykberg, Chief Podiatry, Carl T Hayder, VA Medical Centre, Phoenix.

Flowchart 6

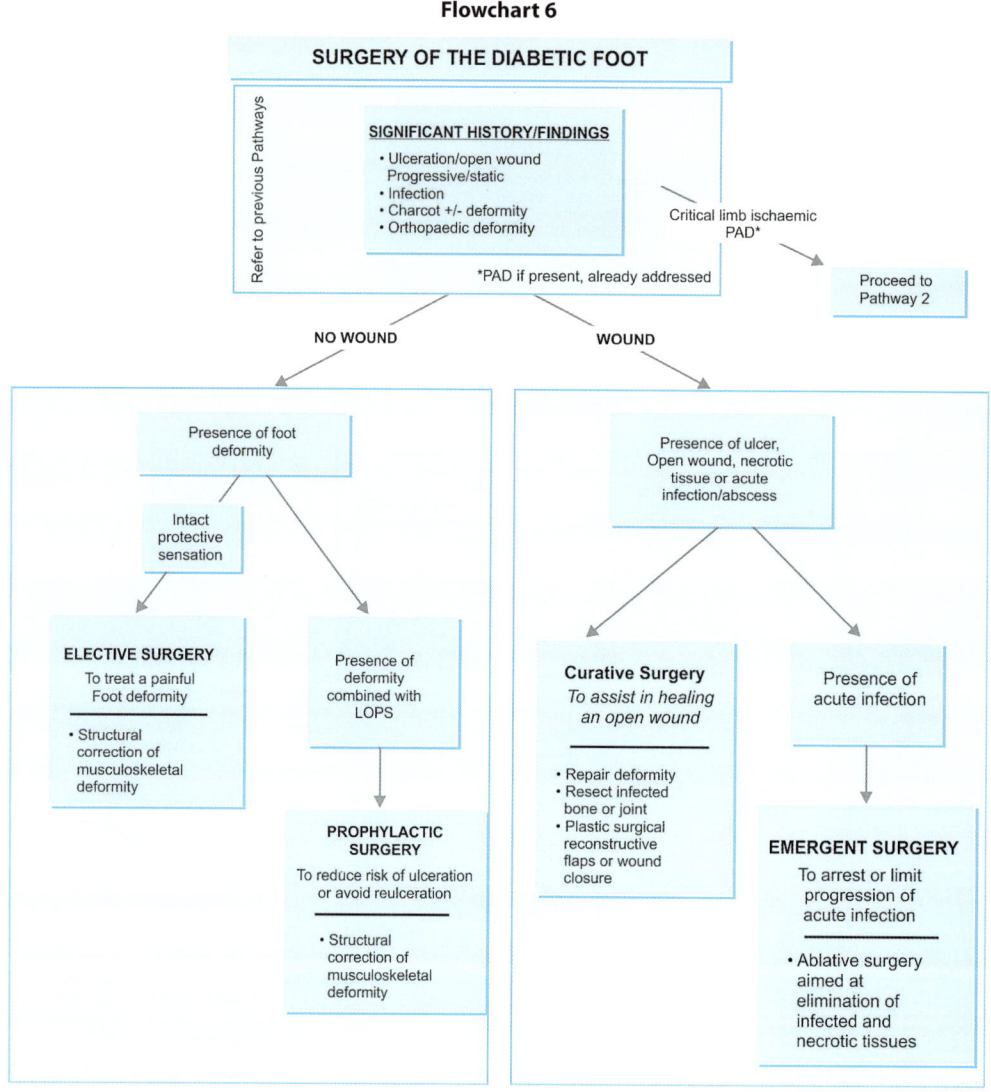

Courtesy: Dr Robert G Frykberg, Chief Podiatry, Carl T Hayder, VA Medical Centre, Phoenix.

Diabetic Foot Evaluation

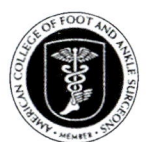

Patient: _____

Chart # _____ Age: _____

Date: _____

Medications:

Type 1
Type 2
Rx - Insulin
   - Incretin
   - Oral Hypoglycemic
   - Diet

Diabetes duration _____

Attending MD _____

Height _____ Weight _____

BP _____ HbA1C _____

History of:
- Foot Ulcer _____
- Infection _____
- Amputation _____
- Revascularization _____
- Renal Disease
- CAD _____
- Stroke _____
- Tobacco _____
- Alcohol _____

- Paresthesia/Tingling
- Numbness
- Burning
- Sharp Pain
- Night Pain
- Muscle Weakness
- Gait Difficulties
- Claudication

  toes
  plantar
  feet to above ankle
    ... to below knee
  night
  daily
  occasionally

  wheelchair
  walker
  cane
  brace
  foot orthosis
  MDI

Shoes _____

Skin:
- Turgor _____
- Color _____
- Temperature _____
- Texture _____

Lesions
- Fissures _____
- Corns _____
- Calluses _____
- Ulcers _____
- Nails _____

Musculoskeletal
- Joint Flexibility _____
- Deformities or Sites of High Pressure _____
- Gait assessment _____

/// Mark areas of callus, ulcer or pre-ulcer, erythema, swelling, tenderness or deformity

Courtesy: American College of Foot and Ankle Surgeons.

Neurologic Exam

Sensory - Semmes-Weinstein Monofilament
Ability to detect 5.07 or 10 gm Monofilament: + or −

Deep Tendon Reflexes (+Present; −Absent)

	Right	Left
Patella	_____	_____
Achilles	_____	_____

Right   Left

Vascular Exam

Pulses:	Right	Left	Pulse Exam
Dorsalis Pedis	0 +1 +2 +3	0 +1 +2 +3	0 absent
Posterior Tibial	0 +1 +2 +3	0 +1 +2 +3	+1 diminished
			+2 normal
			+3 bounding

	Right		Left	
Elevation Pallor	Absent	Present	Absent	Present
Dependent Rubor	Absent	Present	Absent	Present
Capillary Filling Time	<1 1-3 >3		<1 1-3 >3	
Oedema	Absent		_____	

Risk Status

0   No sensory Neuropathy, No PAD,
    Negative Hx of Foot Ulcer
I   Neuropathy (LOPS), No PAD, No Deformity
II Sensory Neuropathy + PAD &/or
    Foot Deformity
III Previous Foot Ulcer or Amputation
    — Prior Ulceration &/or Amputation
    — Charcot Deformity - Location
    _____
    _____

Examiner: _____

Date: _____

Recommended Management:

Periodic Foot Care
Extra Depth shoes
Multiple Density Insoles (MDI), Orthotics
Bracing
Vascular Testing: Doppler
Consultation:
Other: Diabetic Education
_____
_____
_____
_____
_____
_____
_____

Courtesy: American College of Foot and Ankle Surgeons.

BIBLIOGRAPHY

1. Bagcier F, Yilmaz. The impact of extracorporeal shock wave therapy and dry needling combination on pain and functionality in the patients diagnosed with plantar fasciitis. J Foot Ankle Surg. 2020;59:689-93.
2. Balkin SW. Arch Derm. 1975;111:1143.
3. Beischer AD, Beamond BM, Jowett AJL, O'Sullivan R. Distal tendinosis of the tibialis anterior tendon. Foot Ankle Int. 2009; 30:1053.
4. Bergg EE. Chinese foot binding. Orthop Nurs. 1995;14:66-8.
5. Boffeli TJ, Collier RC, Thompson JC, et al. Cheilectomy combined with first tarsometatarsal joint arthrodesis for surgical treatment of midstage hallux rigidus complicated by medial column insufficiency: Prospective evaluation of outcomes. J Foot Ankle Surg. 2020;59:829-34.
6. Carroll PJ, Ragothaman K, Mayer A et al. Ankle Disarticulation: An underutilized approach to staged below knee amputation – case series and Surgical technique. J Foot Ankle Surg. 2020;59:869-2.
7. Clutton HH. The treatment of hallux valgus. St. Thomas Hosp. Gaz. 1894;22:1-12.
8. Crawford F, Thomson C. Intervention for treating plantar heel pain. Cochrane Database Syst Rev. 2003;3:CD000416.
9. Dominick DR, Catanzariti AR. Posteriortibial tendon allograft reconstruction for stage II adult acquired flatfoot: a case series. J Foot Ankle Surg. 2020;59:821-5.
10. Durlacker L. Treatise Corn, bunions and the disease of nails and the general management of the feet. London, Simplin Marshall; 1845;25.
11. Elbert DR, Langan TM, Burns PR. Surgical treatment and management for chronic dislocated subtalar joint. J Foot Ankle Surg. 2020;59:379-84.
12. Freiberg AH.Infraction of the second metatarsal bone, a typical injury. Surg Gynecol Obstet. 1914;19:191-3.
13. Gollwalzer HG, Diehl P, Korff AV et al. Extracorporeal shockwave therapy for chronic painful heel syndrome: A Prospective, Double Blind, Randomized Trial Assessing the Efficacy of a New Electromagnetic Shock Wave Device. J Foot Ankle Surg. 2007;46(5):348-57.
14. Inui K, Ikoma K, Imaik et al. Examination of the correlation between Foot morphology measurements using pedography and radiographic measurements. J Foot Ankle Surg. 2017;56: 298-303.
15. Jack EA. Naviculocuneiform fusion in the treatment of flat foot. J Bone Joint Surg. 1955;35-B:75-81.
16. Jahss MH. The Sesamoids of the Hallux. 64 East 86 th St. New York NY;10028.
17. James WD, Berger T, Elston D. Diseases of the skin appendages. Andrews' Diseases of the skin. Clinical Dermatology, 10th edition. Philadelphia. PA: Elsevier/Saunders; 2006. pp. 749-93.
18. John P, Shami SK. Comment on the published paper—subungal exostosis presenting as an ingrowing nail. Edited by Paul AS, et al. The Foot. 1992;2:117.
19. Johnson KA. Tibialis posterior tendon rupture. Clin Orthop. 1983;177:140-147.
20. Johnson MJ, Wukich DK, Nakonezny PA, et al. (2022). The impact of hospitalization for diabetic foot infection on health-related quality of life: Utilizing PROMIS. J Foot Ankle Surg. 61(2022) 227-32.
21. Kenny L, Purushothaman B, Teasdale R et al. Atypical presentation of acute Freiberg disease. J Foot Ankle Surg. 2017;56;385-9.
22. Keret D, Ezra E, Lokiec, et al. Efficacy of prenatal ultrasonography in confirmed clubfoot. J Bone Joint Surg. 2002;84-B: 1015-19.
23. Kim Y, Kim JS, Young KW, et al. Foot Ankle Int. 2015:36;944-52.
24. La Reaux RL, Lee BR. Metatarsus adductus and hallux abducts valgus; their correlation. J Foot Surg. 1987;26:304-8.
25. Leaking M, Hay R. Pliocene foot prints in the Laetopil beds at Lactoli, Northern Tawzania Nature. 1979;278.
26. Luger EJ, Nissan M, Karpf A, et al. Pattern of weight distribution under the metatarsal heads. J Bone Joint Surg. 1999;81-B:199-202.
27. Morton TG. Peculiar and painful affection of the Fourth metatarso-phalangeal articulation. Am J Med Sci. 1876;71:37.
28. Nakajima K. Sliding oblique metatarsal osteotomy fixated with k-coire without cheilectomy for Hallux rigidus. J Foot Ankle Surg. 2022;61(2):279-85.
29. Nix S, Smith M, Vicenzino B. Prevalence of hallux valgus in general population: a systematic review and meta-analysis. J. Foot Ankle Res. 2010;3-21.
30. Pandey AK, Pandey S. Calcaneal osteotomy and tendon sling for the management of calcaneus deformity. J Bone Joint Surg. 1989;71-A:1192-98.
31. Pandey S, Jha SS, Pandey AK. 'T' osteotomy of the calcaneum. International Orthopaedics (SICOT). 1980;4:219-24.
32. Pandey S. 'Infections and Infestations'. In: Helal B, Rowley DI, Gracchiolo III A et al (Eds). The Surgery of Disorders of the Foot and Ankle. London; Martin Dunitz. 1996;630-51.
33. Pandey S. Tropical Diseases. In Helal B, Wilson D (Eds) 'The Foot' London: Churchill Livingston. 1988;642-702.
34. Pandey S: Ewing's sarcoma of talus. Jr of Bone Joint Surg. 1970;52A:1672-73.
35. Richardson EG. Disorders of the hallux. IN Cambell's Operative. Orthopaedics, 12th ed. Elsevier-mosby Philadelphia; 2013. pp.3805-3906.
36. Rook, DS Wilkinson, FJG Ebling. Oxford, London: Blackwell Scientific Publication. 1979;485-87.
37. Rushing CJ, Rathnayake VR, oxios AJ, et al. Patient-perceived recovery and outcomes after Bipolar radiofrequency controlled ablation with Platelet-Rich-Plasma injection for Refractory Pantar Fasciosis. J Foot Ankle Surg. 2020;59:673-8.
38. Simons GW (Ed). The clubfoot—The present and a view of the Future. New York; Springer Verlag. 1993.
39. Smillie IS. Treatment of Freiberg's infraction. Proc R Soc Med. 1967;60(1);29-31.
40. Tang Y, Deng P, Wang G, Yao Y, Luo Z. The clinical efficacy of two endoscopic surgical approaches for intractable plantar fasciitis. J Foot Ankle Surg. 2020;59:280-5.
41. Welton EA, Rose GK. Posterior tibial tendon pathology: The foot at risk and its treatment by os calcis osteotomy. The Foot. 1993;3:168-174.
42. Wilkinson DS. Cutaneous reaction to mechanical and thermal injury. In: Arthur (Ed): Textbook of Dermatology (3ed). 1979.

CHAPTER 16

Peripheral Nerve Injuries

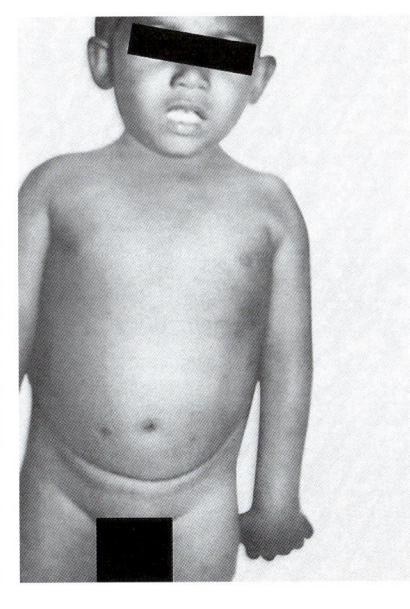
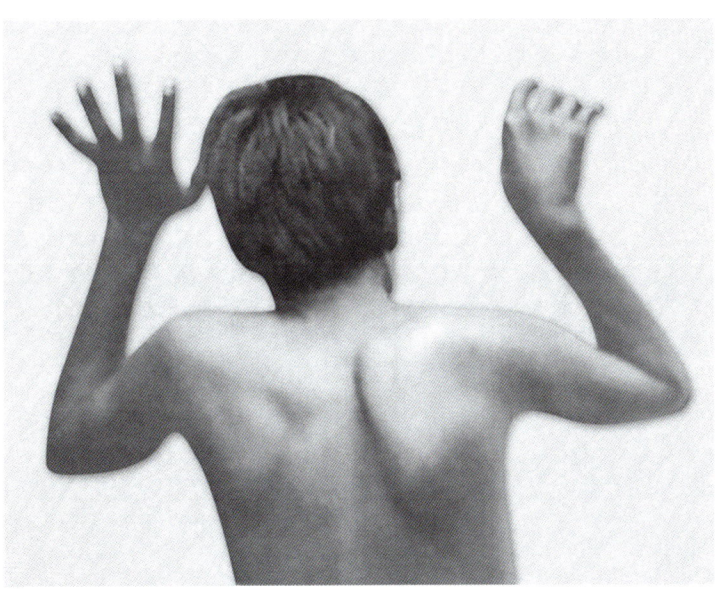

"Life is a mixture of unsolved problems, ambiguous victories and amorphous defeats."
—*APJ Abdul Kalam*

Peripheral Nerve Injuries

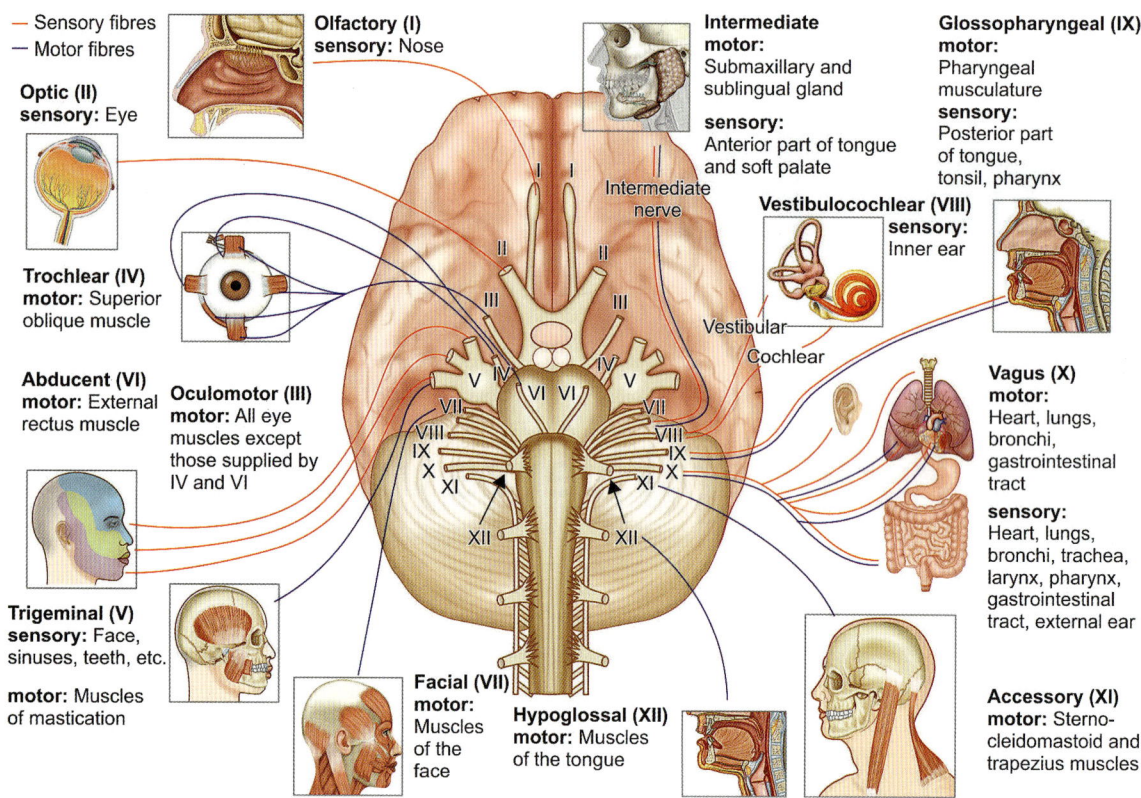

Fig. 16.1

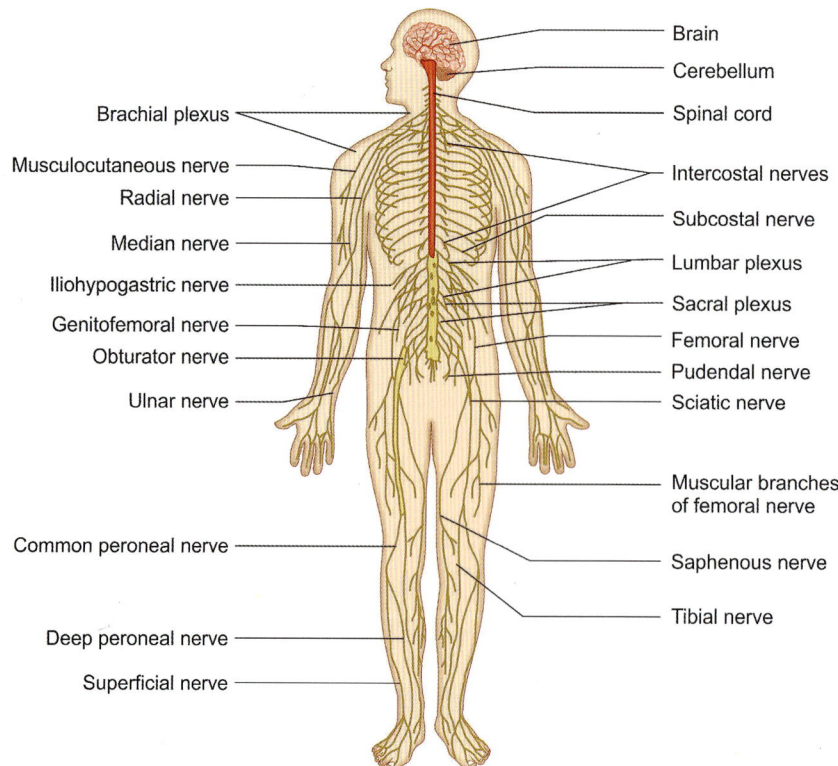

Fig. 16.2

'People seem to have difficulty accepting that a 75-year-old individual has 75-year-old neurons'
—*Pasko Rakic 1985*

Broad assessment of integrity of cranial nerves appears essential before proceeding for assessing the peripheral nerves. There are 12 pairs of cranial nerves designated as Roman numbers I to XII according to their position in brain from forebrain to brain stem. They emerge from brain and pass through respective foramina in the base of skull to supply their designated areas **(Table 16.1)**.

TABLE 16.1: Broad assessment of cranial nerves (See also Fig. 16.1).

Name and number of cranial nerve	Main area of supply	How to test the integrity of nerve
• Olfactory nerve (CN I)	• Olfactory mucosa of upper third nasal septum; superior nasal concha severe injuries affecting the nerve produce anosmia (loss of smell)	• Inspect nostrils patency, any swelling, any discharge. Ask the person to close the eyes and tell about the odour of few familiar objects placed below his nostrils to smell like that of onion, coffee, peppermint, etc.
• Optic nerve (CN II). It is the nerve of sight distributed to the eyeball. It is prolongation of brain substance	• It concerns the vision and vision apparatus like retina, optic chiasm, tract, etc.	• The optic nerve oftenly undergoes (suffers) optic neuritis or papilloedema due to intracranial lesions like new growth, increased intracranial pressure. Ophthalmic examination by ophthalmologist should be done
• Oculomotor nerve (CN III). It is a motor nerve with its nucleus lying in posterior midbrain. It supplies extrinsic eye muscles: superior rectus, inferior rectus, medial rectus, levator palpebrae, superioris and inferior oblique	All muscles of eye except superior oblique and lateral rectus	Complete paralysis of oculomotor nerve leads to ptosis, lateral strabismus, dilatation of pupil, loss of power of accommodation, diplopia and slight prominence of eyeball
• Trochlear nerve (CN IV)	• It is a motor nerve to supply superior oblique muscle	• When this nerve is paralysed, the patient is unable to turn the eye downwards and laterally due to loss of function of superior oblique muscle
• Trigeminal nerve (CN V)	• It is a mixed nerve: sensory root receives supply from superficial and deep structures of face and head, teeth, mouth nasal cavity. Motor roots supply the muscles of mastication	• A lesion affecting whole of trigeminal nerve leads to anesthesia of corresponding anterior half of scalp, face (expect a small area near angle of mandible, cornea and conjunctiva; and mucous membrane of nose, mouth and anterior half of tongue. Pain referred to various branches of trigeminal nerve is very frequent. • Ask the person to close the eyes and test for pain, touch, and temperature in face region • Ask the person to clench in the teeth and palpate the bulk of temporal and masseter muscles • Note any malalignment of incisors when the mouth is opened.
• Abducent nerve (CN VI). It is a motor nerve to supply lateral rectus muscle of eyeball	• It may be involved in fractures of base of skull. Its paralysis produces medial or convergent squint. Diplopia develops	

• Facial nerve (CN VII)
• Facial nerve palsy (Bell's palsy) is usually unilateral. It may be
  – Peripheral due to lesion of facial nerve
  – Nuclear—due to damage of facial nucleus
  – Central, cerebral or supranuclear due to brain injury affecting the fibres passing from cortex to facial nucleus or injury involving face-area in cerebral cortex
  – Entrapment of the sural nerve is most often caused by fascial thickening at the site where the nerve becomes superficial to the gastrocnemius, called the superficial sural aponeurosis. A patient with sural nerve entrapment will present with sensory changes in the area the nerve innervates.
	It is a mixed nerve:
	• Motor fibres supply scalp, face, aurelia, buccinator, platysma, stapedius, stylohyoideus, and posterior belly of diagastric
	• Sensory fibres are carried from behind the ear, ear canal, and taste organs on anterior 2/3rd of tongue
	• Its chorda tympani nerve branch carry the autonomic fibres to supply submandibular and sublingual salivary glands
		For tasting motor functions: Look for any spasm and/or paralysis of facial muscles leading to any deformity in face, which can be delineated in palpebral fissure, nasolabial fold and corner angles of mouth. To test the motor power of facial muscle, ask the person to : Wrinkle the forehead, elevate the eyebrow, show the teeth, to look up; to close the eyes tightly; to show the teeth; to whistle (by lips), to blow out the cheek, to smile. If there is any asymmetry or weakness—determine if the paralysis/paresis is of LMN or UMN
		For sensory assessment: Assess the tasting sensation on anterior 2/3rd of tongue by putting sugar (sweet receptors are located on the tip of tongue), salt, vinegar, etc. Touch sensation should be tested by touching different parts of anterior 2/3rd of tongue

Contd...

Contd...

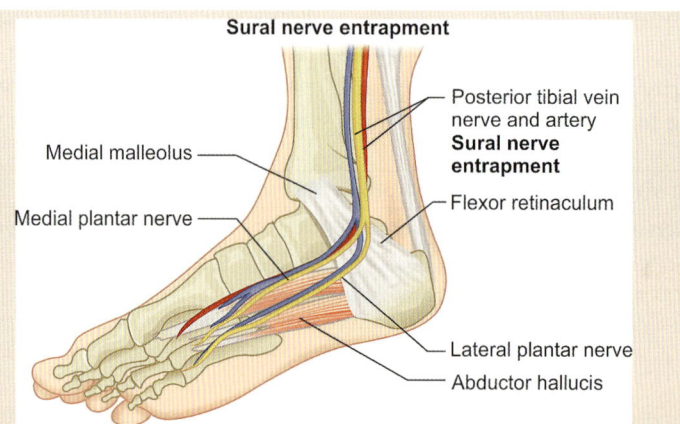

Name and number of cranial nerve	Main area of supply	How to test the integrity of nerve
• Vestibular nerve (CN VIII) Stato-acoustic nerve	• It consists of 2 sensory nerves: (i) The cochlear nerve supplies the organ of Corti (ii) Vestibular nerve consists of sensory endings for the semicircular ducts. The VIII CN is frequently injured along with facial nerve in fracture of middle cranial fossa. Tumours of cerebellopontine angle involve VIII and VII cranial nerves	• For assessment of cochlear portion, tests for hearing are done • For vestibular portion look for any nystagmus and perform labyrinthine tests
• Glosso-pharyngeal nerve (CN IX)	It is a mixed nerve: • Motor fibres travel through both the glossopharyngeal and vagus nerves to innervate the muscles of pharynx • Sensory fibres are carried for pain, touch and temperature from mucosa of pharynx, fauces and palatine tonsil. The nerve of taste for the posterior third of tongue is also carried through autonomic fibres	• It is tested with vagus nerve
• Vagus nerve (CN X)	It is a mixed nerve carrying the motor, sensory and autonomic fibres to and from the neck, thorax and abdomen. After exiting from skull in the jugular fossa, it gives branches in different regions: • In cervical region, its branches are the pharyngeal, superior laryngeal, recurrent laryngeal and superior cardiac nerves • In thorax, the branches are inferior cardiac, anterior and posterior bronchioles and oesophageal nerves • In abdomen, its main branches are gastric nerve, hepatic nerve, and celiac and superior mesenteric ganglion	• Assessment of glossopharyngeal and vagus nerves concerns the examination of pharynx and larynx. Assess the quality of voice and if any change in voice. • Paralysis of both sides adductor muscles of larynx is common which may be functional as well. The voice is reduced to whisper, but the power of coughing is preserved
• Accessory nerve (CN XI)	• It is motor nerve to supply trapezius and sternocleidomastoid muscle. Its functions may be affected with the central changes, or, in fractures involving the jugular foramen. In neck region, it may involved by inflamed lymph nodes	• Ask the patient to shrug up the shoulder to test power of trapezius. • Ask the patient to lean towards the wall and push the wall with palms with arms extended. Note for any winging of scapula. • Ask the patient to turn the chin to one side against the resistance of your hand to test the power of sternocleidomastoid muscle
• Hypoglossal nerve (CN XII)	• It is the motor nerve to supply the tongue. This nerve is affected in injury on the side of neck or by diseases like gumma or new growth of the base of skull	• Look for any wasting and fasciculation in the tongue • Ask the person to protrude the tongue outside mouth as far as possible in midline. If one side of tongue is paralysed, it will deviate towards the weak side • To test the strength of tongue muscle ask the person to press the tongue against the cheek while resistance given by examiner's hand from outside. Lingual speech is tested by asking the patient to repeat "La, La, La, ..."

INTRODUCTION

The peripheral nerves are formed from the spinal nerves which emerge in 31 pairs (8 cervical, 12 thoracic, 5 lumbars, 5 sacrals and 1 coccygeal), representing each segment of the spinal cord. These spinal nerve roots either branch directly or through a network (plexus) as the peripheral nerves.

Peripheral nerve affections usually leave legacies, sometimes quite disabling to the patient and even affecting his ADL (activities of daily living). Though peripheral nerves are mixed nerves, but the main disabling factor is the residual motor weakness. However, complete sensory loss is none the less disabling.

Though, several advances have been made in the field of management of peripheral nerve injuries such as microsurgical technique, interfascicular nerve grafting, etc, the earlier observations and suggestions made by pioneers in this field, like Seddon, Sunderland and Woodhall are still very much relevant.

Modern research works in this field, like use of pharmacological agents, immune system modulation enhancing factors, and entubulations chambers still lack clinical authentication.

ANATOMICAL CONSIDERATIONS

A typical mixed spinal nerve has three distinct components—motor, sensory and sympathetic. Each nerve fibre or axon, myelinated or unmyelinated, has a direct extension from a dorsal root ganglion cell (sensory), an anterior horn cell (motor) or a postganglionic sympathetic nerve cell.

The main nerves in the upper limb are ulnar, median and radial. In the lower limbs, the sciatic and its two main branches, lateral and medial popliteal nerves, are the main motor nerves. The femoral nerve is less important.

All these nerves have more or less the same anatomical structure. The main structural and functional unit of a peripheral nerve is the axis cylinder. This is surrounded by myelin sheath, which in turn is surrounded by a fine *neurolemma sheath (Schwann's cell sheath)*. This forms a nerve fibre. Multiple nerve fibres are loosely connected together by a fine network of collagen—*endoneurium,* which contains fine vascular and lymphatic capillaries. These together form a nerve bundle or fasciculi which is surrounded by an epithelial layer—the *perineurium*. Multiple bundles are bound together by a fibrous sheath—the *epineurium* in which run the main blood vessels and lymphatics of the nerve.

Except for the ulnar nerve behind the medial epicondyle and lateral popliteal nerve winding around the neck of the fibula, the rest of the peripheral nerves are well protected.

In their course, most of the peripheral nerves have to pass through some myofascial or fibro-osseous tunnels where they are likely to be entrapped in certain pathologies of the surrounding tissues—*entrapment neuropathy* **(Fig. 16.3) (Table 16.2)**.

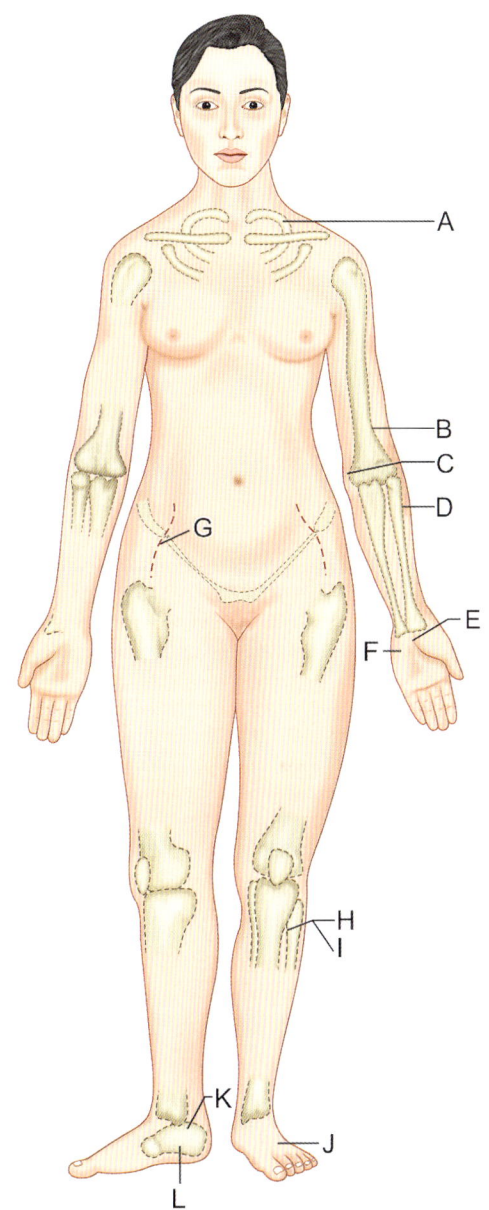

Fig. 16.3: Sites of common entrapment neuropathy: A—thoracic inlet, B—radial nerve, C—ulnar nerve, D—posterior interosseous nerve (supinator tunnel), E—carpal tunnel, F—Guyon's canal, G—lateral cutaneous nerve of the thigh (meralgia paraesthetica), H—common peroneal nerve (lateral popliteal nerve), I—deep peroneal nerve (anterior tibial nerve), J—Morton's metatarsalgia, K—posterior tibial nerve (tarsal tunnel syndrome), L—medial calcaneal branch of posterior tibial nerve, M—sural nerve entrapment.

TABLE 16.2: Common entrapment neuropathies.

Nerve	Site
• Ulnar nerve	• In between the medial epicondyle and the Osborne's ligament—a tight fibrous band forming an arch joining the origin of the two heads of the flexor carpi ulnaris—Elbow tunnel syndrome or cubital tunnel syndrome or ulnar tunnel syndrome. In this tight myofascial-osseous tunnel, the ulnar nerve becomes vulnerable to injury • Beyond the ulnar groove, the ulnar nerve passes between the superficial flexors and deep flexors of the forearm where it is liable to be stretched and compressed during vigorous muscular activities and then may produce features of ulnar nerve entrapment neuropathy • At the hook of the hamate (Guyon's canal—pisiform hamate tunnel). F Guyon (1861) described a fibro-osseous tunnel in the proximal medial aspect of palm. It is bounded by the pisiform medially and proximally, and the hook of the hamate laterally, and posteriorly by the transverse ligament. JR Hunt was the first to describe ulnar nerve entrapment at this site

• Median nerve	• Median nerve entrapment/compression can occur at three places:
	  1. Pronator teres syndrome is most proximal
	  2. Anterior interosseous syndrome in proximal forearm
	  3. Carpal tunnel syndrome at the most distal end of forearm and in front of wrist (in the carpal tunnel)
	• A double crush syndrome, though controversial, may exist when carpal tunnel syndrome coexist with degenerative cervical spinal disease (cervical spondylosis)

• Anterior Interosseous Nerve Compression Syndrome (AINCS). AIN entrapment was first described by JW Goodfellow in 1965. Palsy of anterior interosseous nerve was first described by Tinel J in 1918 under the title "Dissociated paralysis of the median nerve". Anterior interosseous nerve is the largest branch of median nerve. Arising 5–8 cm distal to the level of lateral epicondyle, it runs between superficial and deep heads of pronator teres, thence on anterior interosseous membrane and terminates in the capsule of wrist. It contains only motor fibres and supplies flexor pollicis longus and flexor digitorum profundus to index (occasionally to middle finger) and pronator quadratus	The incidence is less than 1% of all compression syndromes in upper limb Causes of AIN palsy; mostly entrapment. It occurs mainly due to compression by tendinous origin of different muscles (e.g. deep head of pronator teres, flexor digitorum sublimis slip to middle finger); aberrant radial artery; thrombosis may be dissociated with neuralgic amyotrophy, isolated neuritis or traumatic The typical manifestation of palsy is the inability to make (form) an 'O' with the index finger and thumb due to paralysis of FPL and FDPI when patient is not able to flex the interphalangeal joint of thumb and the distal interphalangeal joint of index finger *Management:* For AIN compression syndrome, decompression is the remedy. For other causes 'wait and watch' should be followed, however, it is difficult to differentiate between these two
• Radial nerve	• At about the junction of the lower fourth and upper three-fourth of the arm where it enters from posterior to anterior compartment
• Posterior interosseous nerve	• Where it passes through the supinator muscle from anterior to posterior compartment in the upper forearm
• Thoracic inlet syndrome (Scalene syndrome; cervical rib syndrome)	• A vice like action compresses the brachial plexus and subclavian artery
• Sciatic nerve—compression sciatic neuropathy; Piriformis syndrome (*See* Page 240 in the chapter on Spine)	
• Lateral popliteal nerve	• Lateral popliteal compartment (at the neck of fibula)

Contd...

Contd...

Nerve	Site
• Peroneal nerve entrapment or fibular tunnel syndrome	• The nerve is compressed under the fibrous arch in the region of the bifurcation of the nerve into its deep and superficial branches
• Medial calcaneal branch of posterior tibial nerve	• At anteroinferomedial aspect of the calcaneum
• Posterior tibial nerve (Tarsal tunnel syndrome)	• Posterior tibial nerve gets compressed in the fibro-osseous tunnel formed between the medial malleolus and flexor retinaculum
Meralgia paresthetica is a neurological disorder characterized by paresthesia and numbness in the anterolateral cutaneous area of thigh due to compression or dysfunction of Lateral cutaneous nerve of thigh (Meralgia paraesthetica)—It is a pure sensory nerve – a branch of the upper lumber roots ($L_2 - L_3$). Bernhardt was the first person to describes it as meralgia paraesthetica in 1895. Currently it is known as syndrome of various causes and manifestations.	• Beneath the anterior superior iliac spine and the outer end of the inguinal ligament or directly compressed by tight fitting restraints or work belts. It frequently occurs in the setting of obesity or pregnancy. Patient complains of numbness in the outer part of thigh. Avoidance of known pressing causes usually helps. In persistant cases anaesthetic blocks, pulsed radiofrequency ablation, spinal cord block
• Morton's metatarsalgia	• Due to regular, intermittent pressure on 3rd or 4th digital branch of the medial plantar nerve, a granuloma develops at the level of the metatarsal neck, causing plantar hyperaesthesia of 3rd and 4th toes, mainly in females
• Suprascapular nerve entrapment described by Koppel and Thompson (1963)	• Can occur in throwing athlete who complains of pain in shoulder region, confusing with tendinitis, rotator cuff tear, cervical disc disease. Diagnosis is usually after excluding other causes. Important finding is weakness/atrophy of infraspinatus, Suprascapular nerve, arising from upper trunk of brachial plexus, is a mixed nerve – motor to supraspinatus and infraspinatus; sensory to coracohumeral & coracoacromial ligaments, subacromial bursa, acromioclavicular & glenohumeral joints.
• Compression of lateral antebrachial cutaneous nerve (LACN). LACN is the terminal sensory branch of the musculocutaneous nerve continuing mainly the fibres from C5 and C6 roots. It was first described by Narasanagi, in 1972 and later by Hale in 1976 as "hand-bag paraesthesia"	There is a high risk of compression at two sites: 1. When it enters the coracobrachialis muscle—compression here is aggravated by abduction and external rotation of shoulder—produces both motor and sensory disorders 2. Where it emerges from the lateral side of the biceps tendon, before piercing the deep fascia during rotatory (pronation-supination) movements of the forearm with the elbow extended—produce purely sensory symptoms *Symptoms:* Complain of pain over lateral aspect of lower arm and elbow; ill-defined dysesthesia on the lateral aspect of forearm *Sign:* A zone of maximum tenderness on the anterolateral aspect of lower arm about 2–4 cm above the elbow crease, where firm pressure also distributes the pain over the lateral aspect of upper forearm. Pronating the forearm with the extended elbow aggravates the symptoms *Differential diagnosis:* Confusion can occur with lateral epicondylitis, cervical spondylosis, median nerve compression, entrapment of superficial sensory branch of the radial nerve. Electrodiagnostic test may help. Local anaesthetic infiltration may be of value in confirming the diagnosis *Treatment:* Initial conservative—POP immobilisation in 90° flexed elbow; NSAIDs; local corticoid + anaesthetic infiltration. If it fails, operative decompression

ETIOLOGY

Causes of Peripheral Nerve Injuries

- Trauma
  - Mechanical
    - Direct as for example—cut by sharp object (knife, glass), blunt trauma, fracture ends, bony ends (e.g. in dislocations); gunshot injury
    - Indirect
      - Stretch/traction injury, e.g. Brachial palsy (Erb's palsy)
      - Entrapment neuropathy.
  - Thermal
  - Chemical.
- Infective pathology, e.g. Hansen's disease
- Metabolic disease
- Collagen diseases
- Damage by toxins
  - Endogenous
  - Exogenous.
- Malignant conditions
  - Of the nerve itself
  - Entrapment in or damage by malignant conditions in the surrounding tissues.

The peripheral nerves are commonly affected due to injuries. The nerve injuries have been classified by Seddon (1943). Later on Sunderland (1951) suggested another classification, which is more practical, readily applicable clinically and helpful in determining the prognosis (Sunderland's classification at the bottom of **Table 16.3**).

TABLE 16.3: Gross differentiation of Seddon's three types of nerve injuries (After Seddon 1943).

	Neuropraxia	*Axonotmesis*	*Neurotmesis*
1	**2**	**3**	**4**
Definition	• Shock of the peripheral nerve suspending the physiological conduction (Nerve concussion or transient nerve lesion)	• Damage/section of axons, sheath remaining intact	• Complete damage/section of the nerve, i.e. axon and its sheath
Pathology	• Local demyelination of the nerve fibres. No Wallerian degeneration axis cylinders are intact	• Axons distal to site of damage degenerate • Wallerian degeneration occurs	• Axons distal to damage degenerate Wallerian degeneration occurs • Neuroma at distal end of the proximal segment, palpable after 8 weeks • Glioma at the proximal end of distal segment, palpable after 8 weeks
Etiology	• Pressure over the nerve, mild stretch	• Prolonged, marked pressure • Moderate to severe stretch • Entrapment in surrounding fibrosis • Friction neuritis • Injection neuritis	• Cut injuries • Avulsion injuries
Depth of paralysis	• Mild, mainly motor palsy, may be varying temporary sensory loss	• Moderate to severe (mostly severe) • Motor, sensory, vasomotor, pilomotor and sudomotor	• Always severe • Motor, sensory, vasomotor, pilomotor, and sudomotor
Electrical excitability	• Normal (both galvanic and faradic)	• Altered (only responding to long duration stimuli) • Reaction of degeneration	• Altered (only responding to long duration stimuli) • Reaction of degeneration
Nerve conduction	• Possible	• Ceases	• Ceases
Recovery	• Complete	• Evident in 6–8 weeks may be complete	• Never complete (complete recovery only possible after proper surgical anastomosis)
Usual time taken for recovery	• Days to weeks	• Months to year—at the rate of 1–3 mm a day (1 inch/month or 1 foot/year)	• After surgical repair—months to year (the rate more sluggish than axonotmesis) (In closed injuries, difficult to differentiate from axonotmesis in first three months)

Treatment	• Wait and watch,
	• Splintage of paralysed parts in functional position
		• Splintage
		• Wait and watch
		• If no recovery in three months,
		  – Exploration
		  – Neurolysis
		  – Resection and anastomosis
		  – Nerve grafting
			• Exploration; Neurolysis
			• Primary suturing
			• Secondary suturing followed by splintage
			• Nerve grafting
			• Reconstructive procedures
			  – Tendon transposition
			  – Bone shortening
			  – Joint stabilisation

Note:
I. Neuropraxia and axonotmesis commonly occur due to same injury. When pressure is relieved from the involved segment of nerve, two periods of recovery typically occur. Neuropraxia recovers early—in hours to weeks—then according to axonal regrowth second phase of recovery occurs in weeks to months.
II. Sunderland (1951) has classified the nerve injuries into five degrees depending upon the depth of the damage; damage of myelin sheath; damage of myelin sheath and axon; further damage of endoneurium; further damage of perineurium; and complete division of nerve trunk.

SUNDERLAND'S CLASSIFICATION OF NERVE INJURIES (1951)

First degree: No anatomical disruption. Only physiological
Second degree: Only axon disrupted, sheath intact
Third degree: Axon + Schwann's cell sheath + endoneurium disruption. Intact perineurium
May be neuroma in continuity. Prolonged uncertain recovery
Fourth degree: Axon + Schwann's cell sheath + endoneurium + part of perineurium:
Part of epineurium, though intact in continuity, but almost no recovery
Fifth degree: Complete section

CORRESPONDING SEDDON'S CLASSIFICATION OF NERVE INJURIES

Neuropraxia
Axonotmesis

Axonotmesis (+)

Neurotmesis
Neurotmesis

METHODOLOGY

History Taking

General and systemic examinations to be done as in Chapter 1: Introduction.

Assessment/Investigations of Peripheral Nerve Injury

Following any nerve injury, patients mostly complain about the effects of motor power loss of the muscles supplied by that nerve, followed by the problems concerning sensory loss.

Pain from nerve injury is usually burning in character and is along the concerned dermatome.

Injury/damage of the important peripheral nerves can be excluded as follows:

In upper limb: If the person can make a firm first and fully extend the thumb and fingers—the motor power of median, ulnar and radial nerves is intact.

Normal sensibility to pinprick in the tips of fingers exclude damage of median (specially in the tip of index finger) and ulnar nerve (specially in the tip of little finger).

In the lower limb: If the person can walk firmly on toes and heels—the motor power of sciatic nerve is intact. If he/she can extend the knee fully and firmly—the motor power of femoral nerve is intact.

Following severe injuries in the body, it is difficult to diagnose the damage of any main particular peripheral nerve, however, quick assessment can be done to a fair extent as follows, albeit there may be sometimes confusion.

Main finding	Inference
Loss of pain perception in the tip of little finger	Damage of ulnar nerve
Loss of pain perception in the tip of index finger	Damage of median nerve
Inability to extend the thumb fully	Damage of radial nerve
Loss of pain perception in the sole of foot	Damage of tibial (medial popliteal) or sciatic nerve
Inability to extend the ankle-foot or great toe	Damage of peroneal/lateral popliteal or sciatic nerve

FEATURES OF DIFFERENT NERVE AFFECTIONS OF UPPER LIMB (ALSO SEE FIG. 16.2)

Brachial plexus is formed by union of anterior rami of C5, C6, C7, C8, T1. C5 usually receives some fibres from C4 and T1 usually receives some fibres from T2. Each root receives its sympathetic portion via a grey ramus (cervical roots receive from one of the cervical sympathetic ganglion, and T1 from its own sympathetic ganglion).

Brachial Plexus
(*Upper Type—Erb-Duchenne* C5,6)
(*see* **Figs. 16.4 to 16.6**)

- First clinically described by William Smellie in 1768/1779
- First anatomical description by Danyau in 1851
- Duchenne in 1872 attributed the injury to traction on the arm. He introduced the term obstetric paralysis
- Erb in 1874—wrote a monograph on brachial plexus injuries. He reported his experiments on electrical stimulation of the brachial plexus.

Muscles Supplied

Deltoid, teres minor, supraspinatus, infraspinatus, clavicular head of pectoralis major, biceps, brachioradialis, supinator, brachialis.

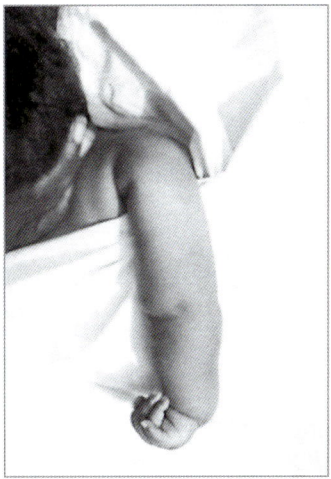

Fig. 16.4: Erb's palsy at birth (Policeman's tip position). If the child is brought at the very early age (rather in neo – natal period) – the paralysed upper limb should be fitted on shoulder – abduction splint (i.e. palm to sun splint) – usually it recovers.

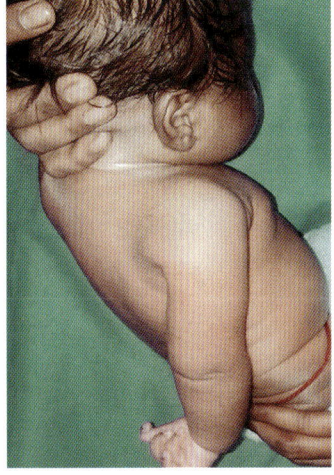

Fig. 16.5: Erb's palsy in 2 weeks—neonate: neglected one.

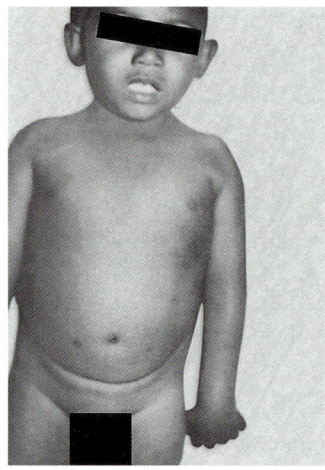

Fig. 16.6: Patient of neglected Erb's palsy showing typical deformity. Note the wasting of the shoulder muscles. Typical Policeman's tip position—Though it is late presenting case, still the limb should be supported on the shoulder – abduction splint till the expert neurosurgeon decides for any definite surgical intervention.

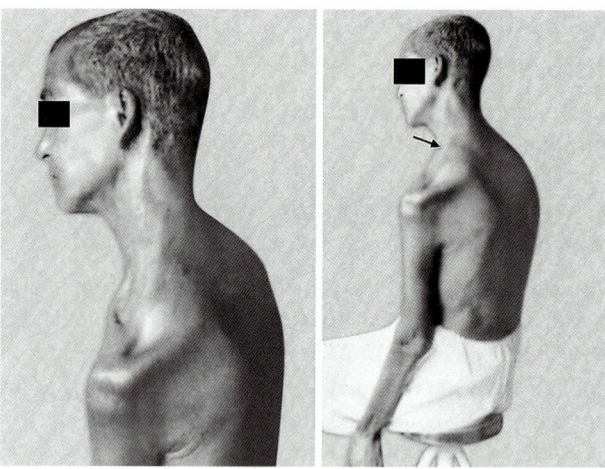

Fig. 16.7: Complete brachial plexus palsy—following a stab injury in the supraclavicular region (arrow showing the site of stab).

Sensory Area

May be some sensory loss on outer aspect of arm and forearm.

Vasomotor Effect

Nil.

Mode of Injury

- Obstetrical palsy
- Obstetrical brachial plexus lesion (OBPL)
- Traction injury
- Vehicular accidents
- Fall on shoulder point
- Fire arm injury
- Stab injury (**Fig. 16.7**).

Presentation

Typical policeman tip position, i.e. arm internally rotated, adducted, elbow extended, forearm mild pronated, wrist in flexion and flexion of the fingers (**Figs. 16.4 to 16.6**).

Neglected OBPL develop secondary shoulder deformities, e.g. abnormal humeral retroversion (declination), deformed glenoid, alteration in glenoid version, subluxation of humeral head—and thus a complex deformity of glenohumeral joint.

Neglected brachial plexus birth palsy also usually develop internal rotation contractures leading to glenoid deformities (flat glenoids, biconcave glenoids, pseudoglenoids) with or without posterior subluxation or dislocation of the glenohumeral joint, which are severely advanced by the age of two years. It should be investigated early by imaging. MRI can be done from the early age; and CT after five years of age.

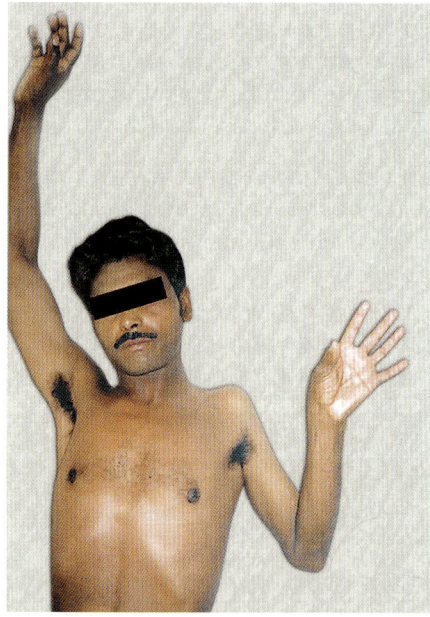

Fig. 16.8: Complete paralysis of left shoulder abductor. Patient not able to abduct the shoulder.

Arthrography helps to visualise the skeletally immature glenohumeral joint.

Currently available choices of management are: microsurgical nerve reconstruction in infants; secondary reconstruction with tendon transfers or osteotomy (e.g. humeral derotation osteotomy).

Tests

Ask the patient to abduct the shoulder, flex the elbow—it will not be possible. To assess shoulder congruity in chronic obstetrical brachial plexus palsy (OBPP) (**Fig. 16.8**). Plane X-ray, arthrography, CT, MRI and ultra-sonography with posterior approach are useful.

Prognosis
Varying; may recover to workable extent.

Treatment
The basis of management of brachial plexus injuries should be conservative and expectant one, since a significant number of patients recover usefully.

Wait and watch, use splintage for all flail joints (shoulder abduction—palm to sun splint). All these joints should be put through a range of motion daily. Most children show spontaneous recovery with little deficit. If no recovery—exploration, neurolysis, primary suturing of the nerve, nerve graft, nerve transfer muscle/tendon transfer as necessary.

Brachial Plexus
(*Lower Type-Klumpke's Paralysis* C8, T1)

Klumpke in 1885 described the paralyses of the lower roots brachial plexus. He highlighted the involvement of the sympathetic fibres in this paralysis.

Muscles Supplied
Intrinsic muscles of the hand, flexion and extension of fingers are controlled by lower trunk.

Sensory Area
Ulnar side of forearm and hand and a narrow strip over arm.

Vasomotor Effect
Horner's syndrome (*see* below).

Mode of Injury
As in Brachial Plexus upper type (vide supra).

Presentation
Claw hand, i.e. metacarpophalangeal joints hyperextended and interphalangeal joints flexed. If oculopupillary paralysis occurs due to affection of 1st thoracic nerve before its communication with white ramus—**Horner's syndrome** develops—It usually results by the lesion that destroys sympathetic preganglionic neurons in the upper thoracic spinal cord lesion that interrupts the cervical sympathetic chain or which damages the lower brain stem in the region of reticular formation. **Horner's syndrome** may occur with ipsilateral mediastinal tumour. In this syndrome ipsilateral apparent enophthalmos, partial ptosis, contraction of pupil with absence of dilatation on shading the eye or on instillation of cocaine, loss of ciliospinal reflex and often absence of sweating on corresponding half of face and neck develop. If damage of sympathetics occur in early life pigmentation of iris may be affected.

Tests
Ask the patient to extend the fingers fully and then make a firm fist. He/she will not be able to do.

Prognosis
Usually bad.

Treatment
Wait and watch. For intrinsic minus claw hand use knuckle-bender splint. If no recovery—exploration, neurolysis, primary suturing, nerve graft, nerve transfer as necessary.

Circumflex Humeral or Axillary Nerve C5, 6

Muscles Supplied
Deltoid, teres minor.

Sensory Area
A small area on the lateral side of upper arm overlying the insertion of the deltoid *(regimental badge area)*.

Vasomotor Effect
Nothing significant.

Mode of Injury
Dislocation of shoulder, fracture of neck of humerus, fracture-dislocation of shoulder.
- Infective neuritis
- Operations on shoulder and upper arm.
- Injection palsy.

Presentation
Inability in actively abducting the shoulder. (Sometimes with the help of supraspinatus and rotation of scapula, full abduction can be possible).

Tests
The patient is asked to abduct the shoulder, while the examiner observes and palpates the deltoid for any contraction.

Prognosis
Variable recovery.

Treatment
Wait and watch.
- Splint (shoulder abduction splint)
- Neurolysis
- Nerve repair
- Tendon transfer (Trapezius)
- Arthrodesis of shoulder.

Brachial Plexus
(whole arm or mixed type C5,6, 7, 8, T1)
(*see* Fig. 16.7)

Muscles Supplied

Complete paralysis of all muscles of arm, forearm and hand.

Sensory Area

Part of arm, whole of forearm and hand.

Vasomotor Effect

May be present. Oculopupillary paralysis may occur.

Mode of Injury
- Pancoast tumour
- Hypercallus in fracture clavicle
- Aneurysm of subclavian artery.

Presentation

Presentation varies according to roots involved.

Tests

As in Erb's paralysis and Klumpke's paralysis.

Prognosis

Constantly bad, especially in neglected cases.

Treatment

Wait and watch; shoulder abduction (palm to sun splint) splint to be used. There may be variable recovery. If no useful recovery—exploration, neurolysis, primary suturing of nerve, nerve graft, nerve transfer as may be necessary.

Nerve to Serratus Anterior C5, 6
(long thoracic nerve) **(Figs. 16.9 to 16.11)**

Muscles Supplied

Serratus anterior.

Sensory Area

Not significant.

Vasomotor Effect

Not significant.

Mode of Injury

Root avulsion, root pressure, iatrogenic.

Presentation

Winging of scapula **(Figs. 16.9 to 16.11)**.

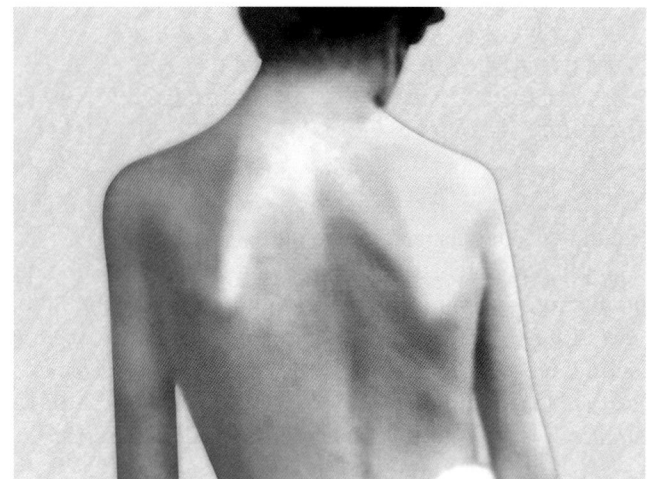

Fig. 16.9: Typical bilateral winging of the scapula due to marked weakness of serratus anterior (a patient of myopathy).

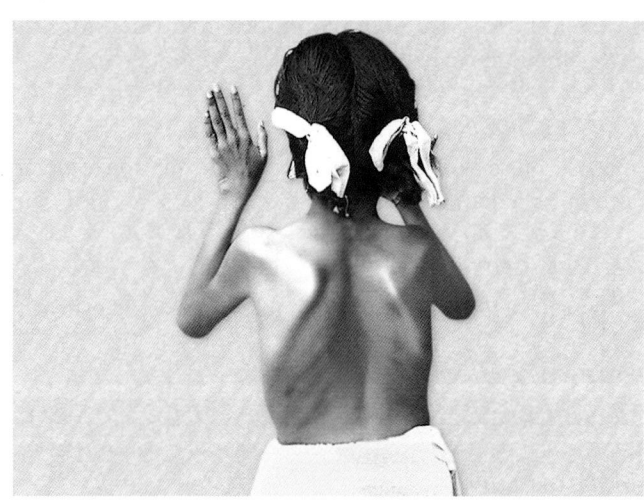

Fig. 16.10: Pressing against the wall the winging of scapula becomes more prominent.

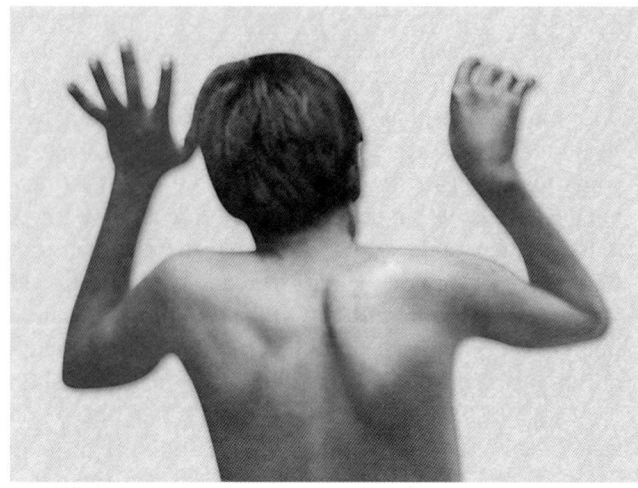

Fig. 16.11: Winging right scapula due to traumatic serratus anterior paralysis.

Tests

Ask the patient to press with hands against the wall.

The medial border of scapula on affected side stands prominent (wings out).

Prognosis

Usually recovery is not satisfactory. Persistent winging of scapula can be improved by surgery like osteoplexy.

Treatment

Wait and watch, tendon transfer (teres major, pectoralis major)—Osteoplexy (Fix medial border of scapula to vertebra).

Median Nerve C6, 7, 8, T1

Median nerve is formed by the union of medial and lateral cords of brachial plexus.

In 15% of limbs, there may be a Marin-Gruber anastomosis between ulnar and median or anterior interosseous nerves.

Median nerve is injured in about 15% of patients of skeletal and nerve injuries in upper extremity.

Muscles Supplied

In forearm—pronator teres, palmaris longus, flexor digitorum superficialis, flexor carpi radialis, flexor digitorum profundus (lateral half), flexor pollicis longus, pronator quadratus. In hand—abductor pollicis brevis, opponens pollicis, flexor pollicis brevis (partly), Ist and IInd lumbricals.

Sensory Area

In both high and low lesions—Palmar side—radial 3 fingers, corresponding part of palm. Dorsal side—terminal phalanges of thumb and 2 fingers. Autonomous supplies zone: dorsal and palmar surfaces of the distal phalanges of index and middle fingers

Vasomotor Effect

- Causalgia (irritative syndrome of varying degree) is a common development
- Trophic disturbances specially in terminal phalanx of index finger.

Mode of Injury

- *Injury:* Supracondylar fracture, penetrating and glass cut injuries.
- *Entrapment neuropathy:*
  - **Carpal tunnel syndrome;** VIC
  - **Disease:** Leprosy.

Presentation

- Ape thumb
- While the patient raises his arm with palm facing forwards, he is asked to make a fist, the index finger stands outstretched while the other fingers go for serial flexion (Benediction attitude, Preacher's hand)
- Trophic changes, ulceration on tip of index finger.
- Wasting of thenar muscles
- In lesion above the wrist
  - Loss of pronation of forearm, flexion of wrist, flexion of index and middle fingers, flexion and opposition of thumb
  - Lesion near wrist: Loss of opposition of thumb.

Tests

1. Ask the patient to clasp both hands—the index finger of the affected hand remains extended due to loss of power in flexor digitorum profundus and superficialis of the index finger, which flex the interphalangeal joints **(Fig. 16.12)** other fingers can be flexed by the intact medial half of flexor digitorum profundus (supplied by the ulnar nerve).

   The above two tests indicate lesion near about the cubital fossa.

2. Ask the patient to make a tight fist—index finger remains extended **(Fig. 16.13)**.
3. Ask the patient to oppose the thumb to the ring finger. This opposition and flexion of terminal phalanx is lost.
4. While the dorsum of the patient's hand rests on the table, put the ulnar border of your fisted hand with extended index finger over the proximal part of his palm. Ask the patient to touch your index finger by the radial border of his thumb—this will not be possible due to paralysis

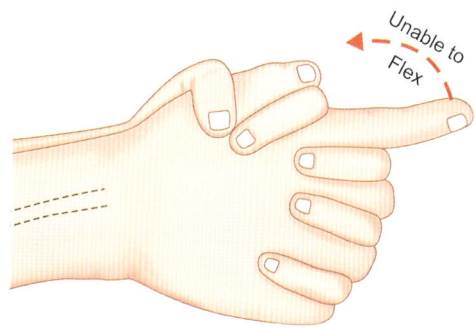

Fig. 16.12: Method of demonstration of Oschner's clasp test.

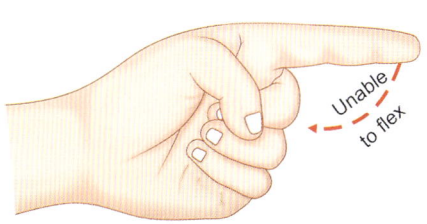

Fig. 16.13: Test for median nerve injury.

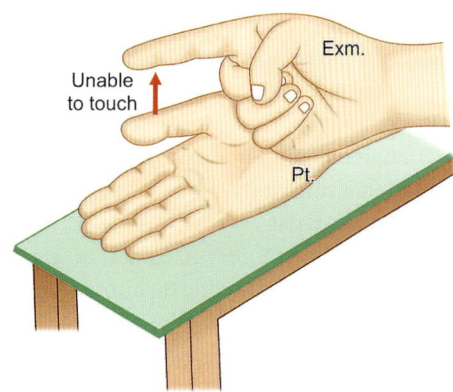

Fig. 16.14: Testing for abductor pollicis brevis muscle in median nerve injury.

of abductor pollicis brevis innervated exclusively by the median nerve (most important) **(Fig. 16.14)**.

Another test is 'Pen test', in which while the patient rests his hand on the table with palm facing the ceiling, a pen is held over his thumb and he is asked to touch the pen with the tip of his thumb. It will not be possible due to weakness of abductor pollicis brevis.

Besides special tests, individual muscle should be tested, e.g. (i) Flexor pollicis longus—while the PIP is kept steady, the patient is asked to flex the terminal phalanx against resistance. (ii) Flexor carpi radialis—Ask the patient to flex the wrist, it deviates to ulnar side due to unopposed action of flexor carpi ulnaris (due to weakness of flexor carpi radialis).

Further flexor carpi radialis tendon does not stand prominent nor it can be felt taut on attempting to flex the wrist against resistance.

Another test for abductor pollicis brevis is by Wartenberg Oriental Prayer position. In this position, the person extends and adducts the four fingers of each hand with thumbs extended; both hands are kept side by side in same plane and raised in front of face with tips of thumbs and index fingers touching each other (PRANAM Position)—weakness of abductor pollicis brevis prevents full range of abduction of thumb which cannot be brought in the same tip-to-tip position to normal thumb.

Kiloh-Nevin sign: To test terminal function of the digits against resistance, ask the patient to form an "O" with the tips of the thumb and index finger. It is not possible due AIN palsy.

In anterior interosseous nerve (AIN) deficit (syndrome), fine pinch posture is abnormal. The index finger becomes extended at the distal interphalangeal joint, as it makes contact with the pulp of the thumb, which also gets hyperextended at the interphalangeal joint, due to weakness of flexor digitorum profundus and flexor pollicis longus muscle respectively (supplied by anterior interosseous nerve).

Prognosis
Bad.

Treatment
- Wait and watch
- Neurolysis
- Nerve pedicle graft
- Nerve cable graft
- Reconstruction specially for opponens of the thumb.

Ulnar Nerve C8T1

- It emerges from the medial cord of brachial plexus
- Ulnar nerve is injured in about 30% of patients of skeletal and nerve injuries in upper extremity.

Muscles Supplied
- In forearm—ulnar half of flexor digitorum profundus, flexor carpi ulnaris.
- In hand—palmaris brevis, flexor digiti minimi, abductor digiti minimi, opponens digiti minimi, all interossei, IInd, IIIrd and IVth lumbricals, adductor pollicis, flexor pollicis brevis (part).

Sensory Area
- Ulnar one finger—palmar and dorsal aspects, corresponding part of palm and dorsum of hand.
- *Autonomous supply:* Dorsal and palmar aspect of middle and distal phalanges of little finger.

Vasomotor Effect

Insignificant: Trophic changes over the desensitized part of tip of little finger.

Mode of Injury
- Injury:
  - At the elbow
    - Medial epicondylar fractures, supracondylar fractures, fracture-dislocation of elbow
    - Stretch tardy ulnar palsy following ununited lateral condylar fracture.
- At the wrist:
  - Glass cut
  - Penetrating injury.
- *Entrapment:* behind the medial epicondyle or immediately distal to it between two heads of flexor carpi ulnaris.
- Entrapment in muscles of hypothenar eminence.
- *Disease:* Hansen's neuropathy.

Presentation
- Ulnar claw hand (*see* **Figs. 7.32 to 7.35 and Fig. 16.15**)

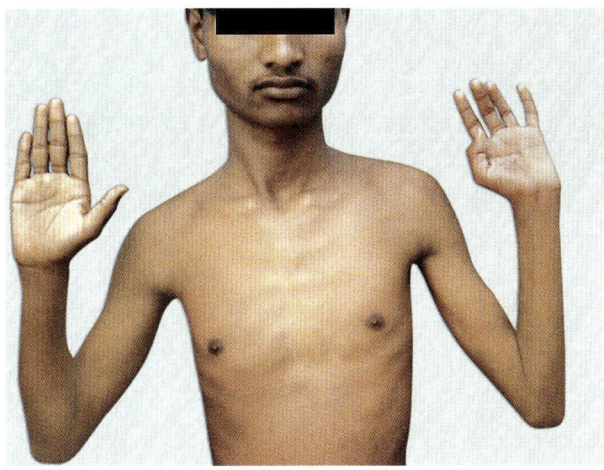

Fig. 16.15: Early ulnar claw developing in left hand due to Hansen's neuropathy.

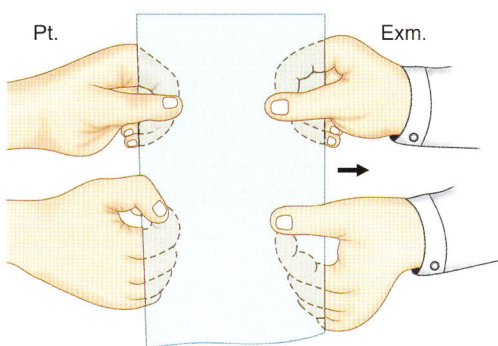

Fig. 16.16: Method of demonstration of Froment's sign for ulnar nerve injury. Note the patient's right thumb acutely flexed to grip the newspaper.

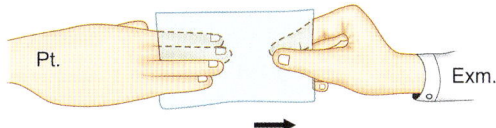

Fig. 16.17: Card test to assess the power of interossei for ulnar nerve injury.

- Flattening of the palm. Shrunken inter-metacarpal spaces and back of first web.
  i. **In lesions at elbow**, flexor carpi ulnaris is also involved resulting in loss of flexion and ulnar deviation at wrist, while in wrist lesions it is spared.
  ii. **In high ulnar palsy,** action of ulnar half of flexor digitorum profundus is lost. So the terminal interphalangeal joints are not flexed **(ulnar paradox)**.
- **Ulnar nerve compression at elbow** (e.g. **cubital tunnel syndrome; tardy ulnar nerve palsy**): one of the earliest diagnostic sign is interosseous atrophy, disturbed sensation in the 4th and 5th fingers, inability to separate the fingers.
- Even gentle pressure on the cubital tunnel reproduces the pain.
- Nerve conduction studies show slowing of the ulnar nerve conduction velocity as it crosses the elbow.

Ulnar nerve compression at the wrist:
- **Usually both superficial and deep branches are affected simultaneously**. Compression of superficial branch causes sensory disturbances, e.g. burning sensations in 4th and 5th digits.
- Compression of deep branch causes motor loss, e.g. weakness in abduction of little finger and thumb and decreased pinch **(Fig. 16.18)**.

Pressure in the Guyon's canal (pisiform-hamate tunnel) causes distal pain if the sensory branches are affected. **Ulnar dominance and median dominance:** At times, the ulnar and median nerve supplies intermingle, hence even if there is complete damage of one nerve its effect is not complete due to its intermingled supply. To confirm it, inject xylocaine in the median nerve (in case of ulnar nerve damage and vice versa). If the paralytic effect becomes complete, then the confused picture was due to aberrant supply.

Tests

1. Froment's sign **(Fig. 16.16)**. Ask the patient to hold a newspaper between his thumb and other fingers, while you pull it firmly away.
   Normally, the distal phalanx of the thumb is extended when holding the newspaper firmly. On the affected side, the distal phalanx of the patient's thumb become markedly flexed and the newspaper is held by the very tip of the thumb, due to paralysis of adductor pollicis and intrinsics.
2. Card test—Put the card in between the fingers and ask the patient to hold it firmly between the fingers. In ulnar nerve affection, the hold will be very loose or not possible **(Fig. 16.17)**.

In ulnar nerve damage certain individual muscle can be tested, e.g. for:
- *Flexor carpi ulnaris:* Ask the patient to keep the dorsum of the hand flat on the table and to palmar flex the wrist, in flexor carpi ulnaris weakness. The hand deviates radialwards.
- *Abductor digiti minimi:* With the hand position same as in flexor carpi ulnaris test ask the patient to abduct the little finger—it will not be possible if abductor digit minimi is paralysed.
  Further while palmar flexing the wrist apply resistance over the distal part of palm and fingers, the tendon of flexor carpi ulnaris does not stand prominent, as it does normally.

Egawa's test: It is done to test the power of dorsal interosseous of middle finger. Ask the patient to put the hand on the table

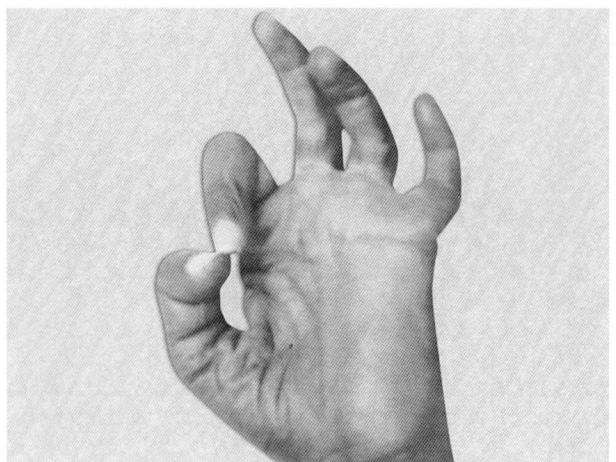

Fig. 16.18: Decreased pinch in ulnar nerve damage.

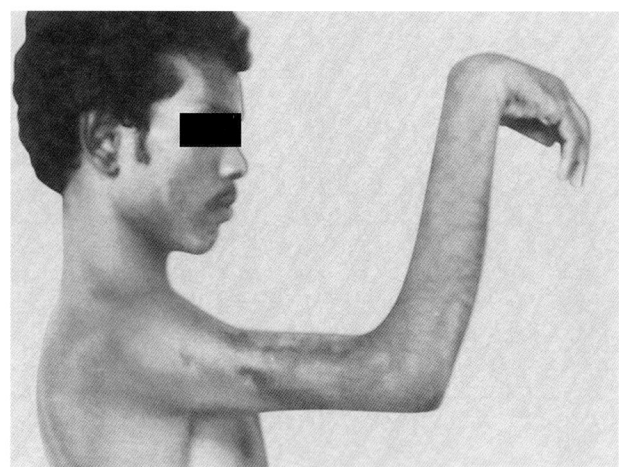

Fig. 16.19: Typical complete wrist drop following open fracture of humerus.

with palmar surface down and the fingers straight. Now ask to move the middle finger on either side. Patient will not be able to do it if interossei of middle finger are affected.

Prognosis
- Variable, usually bad.

Treatment
- Wait and watch
- Neurolysis
- Nerve pedicle graft
- Nerve cable graft
  - Treat primary cause if any
  - Decompression
  - Anterior transposition
  - Medial epicondylectomy
  - Reconstructive surgery for ulnar claw-hand.

Radial Nerve C5, 6, 7, 8 T1
- It is direct continuation of the posterior cord of brachial plexus.
- It is most commonly injured nerve in upper extremity.

Muscles Supplied
- **In arm**—Triceps, anconeus, brachio-radialis, extensor carpi radialis longus, extensor carpi radialis brevis, brachialis (lateral half).
- **In forearm**—Supinator, extensor pollicis longus, extensor pollicis brevis, extensor indicis, extensor digitorum, extensor digiti minimi, extensor carpi ulnaris, abductor pollicis longus.
- **In posterior interosseous nerve** (deep branch of radial nerve) affection the muscles supplied by radial nerve in arm are spared. Hence there will be only **partial wrist drop.**

Sensory Area
- Back of the thumb and 2½ of radial side fingers (except terminal phalanges) and corresponding area on the dorsum of the hand.
- Autonomous supply: stamp shaped area on dorsum of 1st web.

Vasomotor Effect
Insignificant.

Mode of Injury
- *Injury:* In axilla and arm:
- Axillary crutch palsy; pressure in spiral groove—against any hard object, e.g. Saturday night palsy, operation table palsy, fracture of shaft of humerus; Penetrating injury; Elbow region.
- Supracondylar fracture; fracture head and neck of radius; iatrogenic (excision of head of radius), VIC Entrapment: At the junction of lower 1/4 of arm where posterior interosseous nerve passes through supinator.
- Disease: Chronic lead poisoning, leprosy may cause partial wrist drop **(Fig. 16.20).**

Presentation

Wrist drop **(Figs. 16.19 and 16.20)**
In radial nerve compression in elbow region, if the superficial radial nerve is involved, there will be pain and sensory disturbances in the area of distribution. If deep branch is involved, there may be pain in the lateral epicondylar region. The nerve trunk is tender near the proximal portion of extensor muscle origin. Extension of fingers increases the pain. Since the extensor carpi radialis brevis tendon inserts at the base of third metacarpal and it helps in stabilising the wrist during extension of middle finger, elevation of this finger against resistance with elbow extended produces the typical pain.

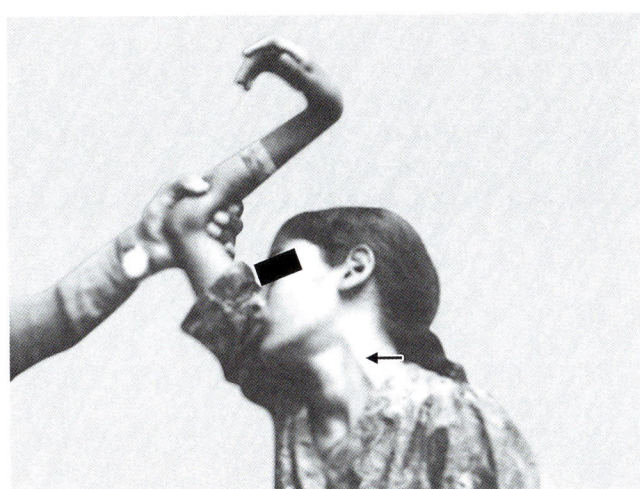

Fig. 16.20: Wrist drop due to Hansen's disease. Note the thickened nerve on left sternomastoid and posterior auricular nerve.

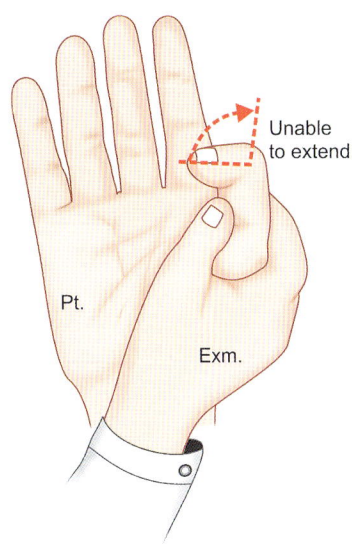

Fig. 16.22: Testing the power of the extensor pollicis longus—lost in radial nerve injury.

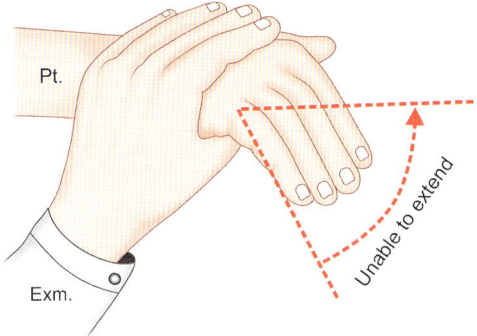

Fig. 16.21: Testing for the extensors of the fingers of metacarpophalangeal joint (In radial nerve injury, patient is unable to extend the fingers of metacarpophalangeal joints).

Tests

1. Support the head of the metacarpals and ask the patient to extend the fingers at metacarpophalangeal joints— not possible **(Fig. 16.21)**.
2. Hold the thumb at its root—ask the patient to extend terminal phalanx of thumb—not possible **(Fig. 16.22)**.
3. In above elbow radial nerve injury total wrist drop develops **(Fig. 16.19)**.
   In below elbow injuries (i.e. posterior interosseous nerve injury) partial wrist drop occurs in which partial dorsiflexion with radial deviation of wrist is possible due to spared extensor carpi radialis longus.
4. Flex the elbow at 90° with forearm in midprone position. Ask the patient to flex elbow further. Brachioradialis will not stand prominent as in normal cases.
5. Ask the patient to take the flexed elbow over the head and then extend the elbow—it will not be possible with paralysed triceps **(Fig. 16.23)**.

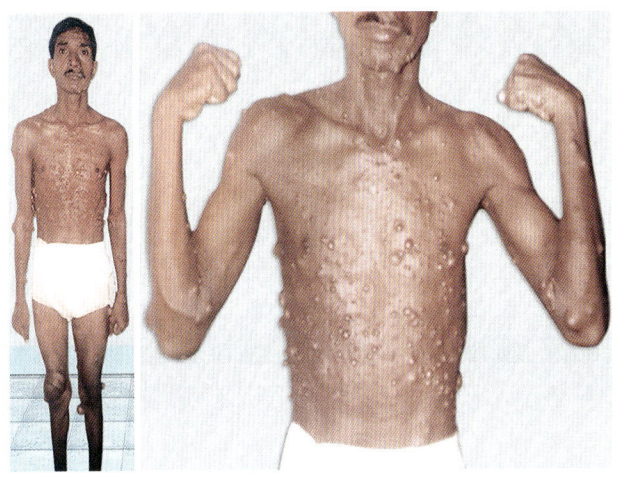

Fig. 16.23: (Also see Fig. 17.94A). Extensive multiple neurofibromatosis Neurofibroma is a rare tumor, which also occurs along the trunks of peripheral nerves. It is composed of masses of fibrous and fatty tissue which is intimately mixed with the nerve fasciculi and axons. It is rather impossible to dissect out this tumor from the parent nerve. It hardly occurs singly. It mostly occurs as part of the syndrome of neurofibromatosis. It should be left as such, unless there is any evidence of malignancy like rapid growth, increasing local temperature and pain with confirmation by histopathology and then it should be treated by wide excision.

Prognosis

Comparatively good

Treatment

- Treat the primary cause
- Wait and watch
- Splintage for wrist drop by cock-up splint
- Neurolysis

Peripheral Nerve Injuries

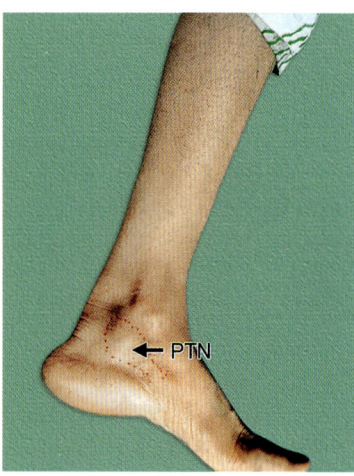

Fig. 16.24: Neurofibroma of posterior tibial nerve.

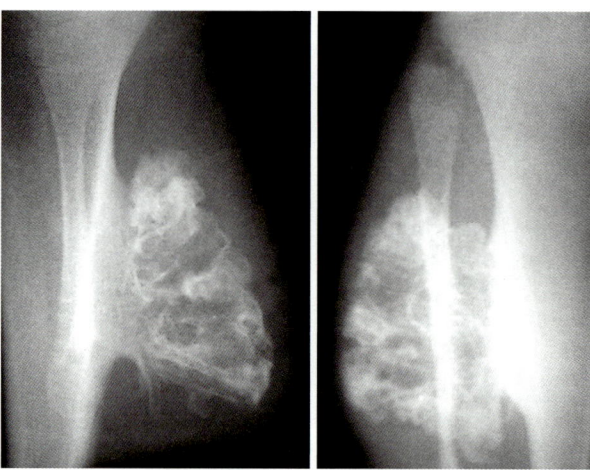

Fig. 16.25: Exostosis from upper end of fibula producing pressure over lateral popliteal nerve.

- Primary suture
- Secondary suture
- Resection anastomosis
- Reconstructive procedure for wrist drop.
- **Jone's triple tendon transfer**
- Stabilization of wrist.

Sciatic Nerve L4, 5 and S1, 2, 3

Muscles Supplied

Hamstrings and all muscles of leg and foot.

Sensory Area

Outer 3/4 to 4/5 of leg anteriorly and posteriorly, and whole of the foot.

Vasomotor Effect

- Trophic ulcers specially beneath balls of 1st and 4th metatarsals and calcaneum
  - Causalgia.

Mode of Injury

Injury to sciatic nerve in:
- Fracture dislocation of hip
- Fracture acetabulum
- Posterior dislocation of hip
- Iatrogenic—In surgery done through posterior approach of the hip
- Penetrating injury, e.g. in gunshot injury of thigh or buttock
- Injection paralysis—following IM injection in buttock region which may unknowingly damage the sciatic nerve (*see* **Figs. 16.27A and B**).

Presentation

- Foot drop to flail foot
- Clawing of toes
- Trophic ulcers
- Features of lower lumbar (L5 or S1) compressive radiculopathy in which usually multiple segments are involved (cf. in disc herniation usually one segment is involved).

Tests

Ask the patient to dorsiflex the ankle and toes—not possible. In flail foot no active movement possible.

In straight leg raising, there will be limitation (mainly in traumatic and compression neuropathy).

Differentiation from lumbar radiculopathy (e.g. disc prolapse): straight leg raising is done just short of discomfort. In this position, pain caused by sciatic neuropathy is increased by internal rotation of hip, and relieved by its external rotation (this is not in lumbar radiculopathy).

Prognosis

Variable

Treatment

- Treat the primary cause
- Wait and watch
- Neurolysis
- Stabilization operations of the foot
- Protective orthotics.

Common Peroneal Nerve or Lateral Popliteal Nerve L 4, 5, S, 1, 2

At or just below the neck of fibula, it divides into two branches: The superficial and deep peroneal nerves.

Muscles Supplied

Tibialis anterior, extensor hallucis longus, extensor digitorum longus, peroneus tertius, peroneus longus, peroneus brevis.

Sensory Area

Outer 3/4 of dorsal aspect of leg and medial half of dorsum of foot.

Vasomotor Effect

Insignificant.

Mode of Injury and Affection of Nerve

- *Injury:* Fracture head and neck of fibula, fracture tibial condyles.
- Penetrating or cut injuries. Iatrogenic. Pressure by neoplasm of underlying bone, e.g. giant cell tumour, exostosis **(Fig. 16.25)**.
- Entrapment at the neck of fibula.
- In anterior tibial compartment syndrome.
- *Disease:* Hansen's neuropathy **(Fig. 16.26)**.

Presentation

Foot drop: In traumatic condition of nerve, the patient may complain of pain in the lateral aspect of the leg and foot.

Tests

- Ask the patient to dorsiflex the ankle and toes—not possible. Ask the patient to stand on heel— not possible.
- Ask the patient to evert the foot—not possible.
- Pressure over the nerve may cause local and referred (along the sensory distribution) pain.

Prognosis

Variable.

Treatment

- Treat the primary cause
- Wait and watch
- Decompression
- Neurolysis
- Orthotics with dorsi flexion assist of foot
- Tendon transfer (tibialis posterior—tendon transfer to 3rd or 4th ray of foot)
- Stabilisation of foot; (Lambrinudi's or modified triple arthrodesis).

Tibial Nerve or Medial Popliteal Nerve
L4, 5 S 1, 2, 3

Muscles Supplied

Gastrocnemius, soleus, tibialis posterior, flexor digitorum longus, flexor hallucis longus, intrinsics of the foot.

Sensory Area

Sole of the foot.

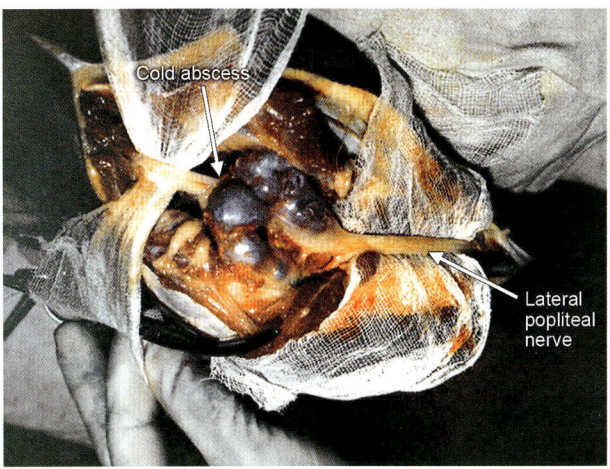

Fig. 16.26: Hansen's cold abscess in lateral popliteal nerve—Management should be removal of abscess material, neurolysis of nerve, to treat Hansen`s disease (MDT regimen), support to affected part (such as special footwear/splint for feet drop, etc.)

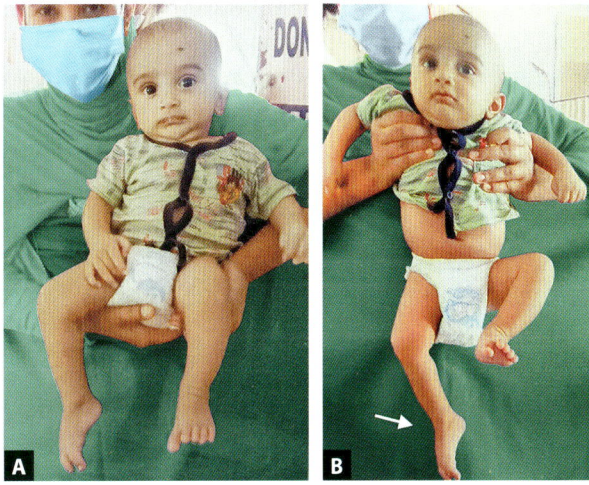

Figs. 16.27A and B: Post injection (in gluteal region) right foot drop (A); After injection in gluteal region Rt foot drop (B).

Vasomotor Effect

- Causalgia (Silas Weil Mitchell described Causalgia in 1864).
- Trophic ulceration.

Mode of Injury

- *Injury:* Penetrating injuries, open fractures
- *Entrapment:* Posterior compartment syndrome.

Presentation

- Clawing of toes
- Calcaneus and/or valgus foot.
- Foot drop **(Figures 16.27A and B)**.

Tests

- Ask the patient to stand on the toes—not possible.
- Ask the patient to plantar flex the ankle and toes—not possible.

Prognosis

Not good.

Treatment
- Treat the primary cause
- Decompression
- Orthotics—for calcaneus deformity
- Tendon transfer
- Correction of clawing
- Stabilisation of ankle and foot.

Posterior Tibial Nerve Compression (Tarsal Tunnel Syndrome)

Compression involvement of posterior tibial nerve occurs due to tenosynovitis; venous engorgement; Hansen's neuritis; sustained valgus deformity of foot, neoplasms **(Fig. 16.24)**.

Presentation

Patient usually presents with burning pain in sole; retrograde pain along medial popliteal nerve even up to the buttock; clawing of toes (decreased flexion at MPJs and extension of IPJs).

Tests

Palpation of nerve on posterior region of medial malleolus causes pain in sensory distribution of the nerve.

Treatment
- Treat the cause
- Release of flexor retinaculum to decompress the nerve; explore the area of abductor hallucis.

Lateral Cutaneous Nerve of the Thigh

It is a sensory nerve.

Sensory Area

Lateral part of front of thigh

Mode of Injury

Entrapment (meralgia paraesthetica) Meralgia paraesthetica is characterized by altered sensation and pain (±) on the anterolateral aspect of thigh purely in the distribution of sensory lateral cutaneous nerve of thigh, produced due to some entrapment/pressure on the nerve.

Presentation

Pain along distribution.

Tests

Hypoaesthesia.

Prognosis

Variable.

Treatment
- Local xylocaine and corticosteroid injection
- Decompression
- Section of nerve.

Femoral Nerve (L 2, 3, 4)

It is formed by union of posterior divisions of L2, L3, and L4 roots.

Muscles Supplied

Quadriceps, pectineus, sartorius.

Sensory Area

Front of middle and lower thigh.

Vasomotor Effect

Insignificant.

Mode of Injury
- Pressure by or entrapment in intrapelvic neoplasm
- Stab or gunshot injury in upper thigh.

Presentation

Disturbed gait.

Tests
- While lying down ask the patient to extend the knee from flexed position—not possible
- Loss of knee jerk.

Prognosis

Poor.

Treatment
- Treat the primary cause
- Wait and watch
- Quadriceps reinforcement (Hamstring to quadriceps transfer).

Obturator Nerve

Muscles Supplied

Adductors of thigh.

Sensory Area

Sensory fibres to hip joint; small area on the lower medial aspect of thigh.

Mode of Injury

Pelvic injury, entrapment: compression or irritation of obturator nerve initially leads to obturator neuritis, causing pain on the medial aspect of thigh.

Presentation

Atrophy or spasm or weakness of adductor muscles. Absence of adductor reflex.

Tests

While lying down supine, ask the patient to abduct the thigh and then adduct it—it will be deficient.

Prognosis

Poor.

Treatment

Wait and watch, exploration, decompression if required.

Martin-Gruber anastomosis is an anomaly. In few patients, there may be crosslinks among the three peripheral nerve of the upper limb. In this anomaly, the motor nerve fibres, normally entirely carried in the ulnar nerve, enter the ulnar nerve from the median nerve via the branches in the forearm. In this condition, the dysfunction or disruption of the ulnar nerve above the level of anastomosis may not result in motor loss of muscles in the hand typically supplied by the ulnar nerve.

Vulnerable Anatomical Sites for Peripheral Nerve Damage in the Upper Limb:

Brachial Plexus: Roots coming out of intervertebral foramina may be avulsed. Upper roots at the Erb's point: lower roots in supraclavicular lesions, posterior triangle of neck.

Axillary Nerve: Underneath the deltoid, around the surgical neck of the humerus.

Median Nerve:
1. Infront of the lower end of the humerus, e.g. supracondylar fracture; after exit between two heads of pronator teres, e.g. Volkmann's ischaemic contracture.
2. In the carpal tunnel.

Ulnar Nerve: Behind the medial epicondyle and beneath the Osborne's ligament (epicondylar tunnel); above the wrist joint where it lies superficial to the flexor retinaculum; in proximal hypothenar region where it lies lateral to the pisiform bone—Guyon's tunnel.

Radial Nerve: In the base of the axilla, e.g. in crutch palsy; spiral groove, e.g. in fracture shaft of humerus; while piercing lateral intermuscular septum; in front of elbow capsule.

Posterior Interosseous Nerve: While passing through the supinator around the neck of the radius.

Vulnerable Anatomical Sites for Peripheral Nerve Damage in Lower Limbs

Sciatic Nerve: Behind the hip capsule, e.g. in fracture and/or dislocation of hip.

Lateral Popliteal Nerve: Around the neck of the fibula.

Lateral Cutaneous Nerve of Thigh: Behind the outer end of the inguinal ligament, near anterior superior iliac spine.

Femoral Nerve: During its intrapelvic course at the base of Scarpa's triangle.

Clinical Examination

Inspection

Note any typical attitude and any abnormal finding in the area supplied by the concerned nerve.

Palpation

Besides palpating on usual lines, feel for the texture and pliability of subcutaneous tissues and muscles supplied by the concerned nerve.

Palpation of the nerve
- If there is tenderness on pressure along the course of the nerve, it indicates irritational stage of the nerve, which is present in an incomplete lesion, or inflammation of the nerve. Feel for texture, girth, uniformity, pliability, any beading, any thickening, etc. of the nerve **(Fig. 16.26)**.
- In the course of a nerve, where complete division of nerve is expected, feeling of a neuroma (a firm, tender, nodular mass at the distal end of the proximal segment) and a glioma (a firm, almost non-tender, fibrous mass at the proximal end of the distal segment) almost confirms the diagnosis.
- Tinel's sign (Jules Tinel, 1917).

The *importance of Tinel's sign* ***is in determining:***
- Whether a nerve is interrupted
- Whether a nerve is in process of regeneration
- Rate of regeneration
- Whether a nerve suture has succeeded or failed. However, even in incomplete regeneration this sign may be positive.

Method of eliciting Tinel's sign: Press the nerve gently or percuss about 2.5 cm below the site of lesion or nerve suture. If young axis cylinders are present, the patient will feel a sensation of "pins and needles" *(formication)* for a few seconds, along the course of the nerve. According to the progress of regeneration of the axis cylinder, the site of formication also advances. Tap along the course of the nerve, starting from the periphery. The moment the level of regeneration is reached, pain and/or tingling will be felt along the course of the nerve.

Assessment of the Muscle Power According to 'MRC' Scale

(*Also See* Chapter 1: Introduction, Page 31)

In peripheral nerve injury, all motor functions distal to the level of injury get abolished. The muscles supplied by that nerve distal to the injured level, are paralysed, become atonic and get wasted. Spontaneous fibrillations may become evident by 2–4 weeks. With proper regeneration of the nerve, variable muscle-power recovers. The extent of recovery can be assessed clinically by grip meter, pinch meter, evaluation of endurance, speed of movement and individual muscle power and function.

Elicitation of Reflexes

See Chapter 8: Spine. **Tables 8.6** (Page 248) and **8.7** (Pages 250).

Mapping out the Deficits in Sensations

Vide line drawing with different zone mapping on Page 216 of Spine chapter.

Vasomotor Assessment

Sweat test: Using iodine/starch, this can be done to map out the anaesthetic areas as dry and devoid of sweating.

Guttman's test: Quinizarin powder turns purple when it comes in contact with sweat.

Skin and Nails

Nails, working like claws of animals for scratching protects the fingertips and help in tactile sensation, precise touch and to some extent for defense.

Note the condition of the skin supplied by the affected nerve. Specially look for the: (i) texture, any discolouration, (ii) presence/absence of normal skin folds, and rugosities, (iii) atrophic changes, (iv) trophic ulcerations, (v) condition of nail bed, and (vi) condition of finger/toe tips.

The condition of the followings should be noted about the nail.

Paronychium (skin on the sides of nail; Hyponychium (skin at distal part of nail); eponychium (skin which covers nail fold proximal to the nail); nailbed (soft tissue beneath the nail plate).

Perionychium (It includes paronychium, hyponychium, eponychium, nail bed and nail fold);

Nail fold (The most proximal part of the perionychium consisting of the dorsal roof, which helps the shine on the nail and the ventral floor formed by the germinal matrix).

Investigations

Electrodiagnosis

These provide more or less quantitative assessment of the nerve deficit. The important ones are:
- Motor nerve conduction test
- Strength duration curves
- Electromyography.

However, 'Nerve stimulation' and 'Nerve action potential recording' have also been suggested (Seddon, 1972).

- *Motor nerve conduction test*: Basis of the test—ability of the nerve to transmit an electrical impulse.
  Method: First, calculate the approximate threshold of the current strength required to cause a muscular contraction, by stimulating the nerve on the sound side. The stimulating electrode is then applied on the affected nerve, distal to the possible site of lesion. **If a current strength twice as great as the calculated threshold fails to produce a muscular contraction, nerve conduction is absent.** *Slow rate of conduction suggests damage to the nerve.* The site of an incomplete lesion can also be located by this test. So long the stimulating electrode lies distal to the lesion, the conductivity is good, but this nerve conductivity is markedly reduced or even absent when the stimulating electrode is placed proximal to the lesion.

- *Strength duration curve:* Basis—depending upon the excitability of the nerve and muscle, a graph is prepared by plotting the minimum voltage required for the muscle to contract, against duration of the stimulus in milliseconds. The status of a muscle as regards innervation, denervation or reinnervation can be indicated by these curves.
  If the voltage is kept constant, a normal muscle will respond to an electrical stimulus given for a duration of 300 milliseconds to less than a millisecond, even down to 0.1 milliseconds. The strength-duration curve obtained for such a muscle has been named as **'nerve-curve'**, since the stimulation becomes effective through the motor nerve of that muscle.
  In a *completely denervated muscle*, a low voltage stimulus can only be effective if the electrical stimulus is given much longer, e.g. 100 milliseconds or more. The curve for such a muscle is called **'muscle-curve'**, since muscular contraction has been obtained from direct stimulation of the muscle fibres. The *partly innervated muscle is characterised by superimposition of the two basic curves (nerve and muscle curves)* producing an upward kink in the plotted graph.

- *Nerve conduction monitor* is a noninvasive diagnostic aid, which can effectively perform motor and sensory latency testing in the upper and lower extremity. It can be of much use for testing the peripheral neuropathies such as carpal tunnel syndrome. Immediate printed test results are obtained which can be corelated to standard electrodiagnostic testing.

- *Repetitive stimulation* studies for the evaluation of the neuromuscular junction (e.g. in myasthenia gravis).

- *Somatosensory evoked potentials* are used to evaluate conduction within the spinal cord and brain.

- *Electromyography:* EMG (needle EMG—when needle is used; surface EMG—when surface electrodes are used) helps in analyzing the neural control mechanism of muscle (the motor unit). The anatomical structures involved in forming the motor functional unit of the peripheral nervous system, i.e. **the motor unit consists of motor neuron situated in the anterior horn of spinal cord, its axon, the neuromuscular junction, and the muscle fibres.** Basis—the electrical changes going on in a muscle are suitably amplified and assessed in the form of sound patterns or recorded in the form of tracings. While a normal muscle is electrically silent at rest, partially/completely denervated muscle shows spontaneous fibrillatory contraction of individual fibres *(fibrillation potential)*. Comparing with the standard wave forms and sound patterns in various disorders, the electromyographic record is studied. This investigation can accurately determine the site of the lesion, i.e. anterior horn cells, peripheral nerves or muscles.

Innervation ratio: There are variable number of terminal axons and muscle fibres for each efferent motor axon. Depending upon the specific requirement of control, the ratio may be quite low or extremely high. Because of more force required in plantar flexion of ankle, the innervation ratio of the gastrocnemius can be as high as 1:2000, conversely, the innervation ratio of the extraocular muscle is typically 1:3 for the fine control required for binocular vision.

Biopsy

Biopsy of the affected muscle may help in differentiating whether the effect is of denervation or of ischaemia. *The ischaemic muscle shows sudden infarction with early fibrosis, whereas, in denervation, gradual diffuse atrophy is followed by late fibrosis.*

Silas Weill Mitchell (the father of modern Neurology) described *causalgia* (derived from *Greek* word – '*Klaus*' which means fire + '*Algos*' which mean pain) in 1864

■ BIBLIOGRAPHY

1. Bernhardt M. Uber isoliert in gebiete nervus eutaneus femoris extrenus vorkommende paresthesia. Neural centralbl. 1895; 14:242
2. Dialiana ZH, Roulot E, Viet DL. Surgical treatment of compression of the lateral antebrachial cutaneous nerve. J Bone Joint Surg. 2000;82-b:420-3.
3. Eversmann WW Jr. Entrapment and compression neuropathies. In: Greep DP (Ed). Operative Hand Surg, 3rd edn. New York: Churchill Livingstone. 1993;1341-85.
4. Fearn CBDA, Goodfellow JW. Anterior interosseous nerve palsy. J Bone Joint Surg (Br). 1965;47-B:91-3.
5. Gelberman RH, Eaton R, Urbanik JR. Peripheral nerve compression. J Bone Joint Surg. 1993;75A:1854-78.
6. Hale BR. Handbag paraesthesia. Lancet. 1976;2:470.
7. Koppel HP, Thompson WAL. Peripheral entrapment neuropathies. Baltimore: Williams and Wilkins. 1963; 131-42.
8. Narasanagi SS. Compression of lateral cutaneous nerve of forearm. Neurol India. 1972;20:224-5.
9. Pearl ML, Edgerton BW. Glenoid deformity secondary to brachial plexus birth palsy. J Bone Joint Surg. 1998;80A: 659-67.
10. Rakic P. Limits of neurogenesis in primates. Science, 1985;227: 1054-6.
11. Tienel J. Nerve Wounds. Wilkam Wood, New York, 1918;183-5.

CHAPTER 17

Bone Tumours

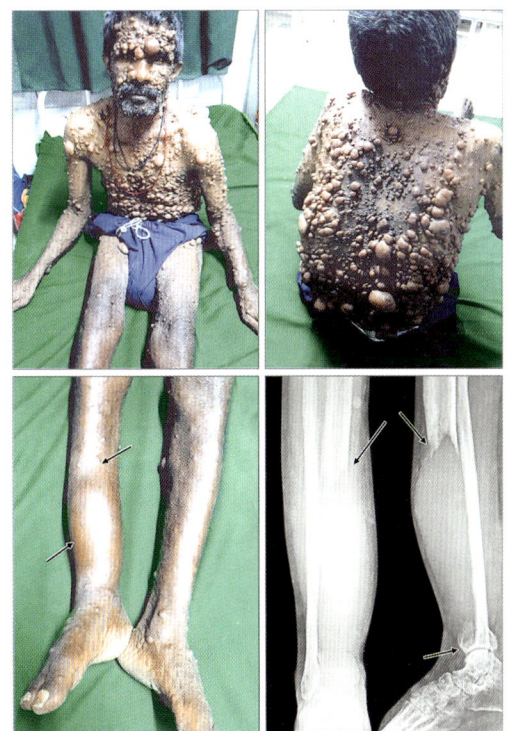

"Surviving is important, thriving is elegant"
—*Maya Angelou*
"Success is not final, failure is not fatal. It is courage to continue that counts."
—*Winston Churchill*
"Learning, and Earning—are never final nor perfect."
—*SP*

INTRODUCTION

"World's oldest cancer arose in a dog 11,000 years ago. The genome of the transmissible dog cancer still harbours the genetic variants of the individual dog that first gave rise to the cancer 11,000 years ago"

PTI (HT)

Literally, any tumour means swelling, and its examination implies all norms of examining a swelling but while examining a tumour, a few points deserve special considerations.

Tumours are usually of unknown cause, non-inflammatory and develop independent of and unrestrained by normal laws of growth and morphogenesis.

Except for vague cases of growths which are confined to the marrow, most of the tumours manifest obviously and there is hardly any doubt in making up our mind that one is proceeding to examine a tumour. The problem which remains is that of assessing the type, nature and extent of the growth.

History of modern cancer treatment goes back to about 200 years, even though cancer is as old as humankind.

'Cancer care' is the new buzz word in the field of medicine involving multidisciplinary care and inputs from the allied specialties. Although musculoskeletal oncology is starting to enjoy its moment is the sun, to echo Robert frost "we have promises to keep, and miles to go before we sleep" Quoted by Ajay pare 2018.

PRIMARY AND SECONDARY BONE TUMOUR

Bone tumors account only about 02% of the benign and malignant tumors of body.

A *primary tumour* always originates due to hyperactivity of the pluripotent neoplastic cells (not as a result of secondary implantation). It is almost always solitary, except in extremely rare conditions like multiple exostosis, multiple myelomatosis, skip lesion in osteosarcoma (*see* **Fig. 17.14**).

A *secondary tumour* is mostly a malignant neoplasm, occurring as a result of implantation of neoplastic cells, in bone or soft tissue, coming from a primary malignant growth (of soft tissue or bone), and may occur at one or several sites. The primary may be manifest or occult.

The *usual primary sites are prostate, breast, bronchus, thyroid, kidney, stomach, adrenals and skin.* Usual manifestations are *complications of neoplasm*, for instance *pathological fracture and paraplegia*, besides *pain, swelling, anaemia* and *cachexia* (*see* **Figs. 17.80, 17.81, 17.84, 17.85, 17.86 and 17.95**).

Benign tumours are comparatively less harmful, except for the cosmetic deformity and the mechanical pressure effects. However, *features suggestive of a transition to a malignant stage* must be thoroughly enquired and looked into. *These features are:*

- Sudden rapid growth
- Appearance of pain in a swelling, which was painless earlier
- Evidence of increased vascularity (venous prominence)
- Warm overlying skin surface
- Clinically invasive nature, e.g. lack of clear demarcation, comparatively warm
- Regional lymph gland enlargement of neoplastic nature (i.e. hard but not tender)
- Above all, affection of the general health of the patient (cachexia, anaemia).

Benign tumours are generally slow growing and rarely metastasize. However, a few are biologically more aggressive locally and may occasionally metastasize.

According to the behaviour of the benign tumours *Enneking has classified the benign tumours.*

- **Pseudotumours (including iatrogenic—a surgeon's legacy), such as 'textiloma'**

Any embedded foreign body, invites granulomatous reaction around it. *Textiloma is defined as a tumour composed of cotton matrix surrounded by granulomatous reaction* (Mboti et al. 2001). Similarly, *Glossy fibroma* (from Latin '*Gossypium*'—cotton and from kiswahili 'born'—place of concealment) is an iatrogenic legacy mass caused by retained sponge (Rajagopal and Martin 2002).

Textiloma may present as an acute exudative lesion or delayed tumoural lesion. The exudative pathology results in sepsis and ultimately as a sinus or fistula. The tumoural lesion manifests late as swelling which may be of benign look and feel. Radiologically, it casts a soft tissue shadow. Right from the beginning, it is essential to boost up the morale of the patients suffering from malignancy. While examining a tumour, one must be very gentle. This is essential not only on compassionate grounds, but also due to the fact that while roughly examining a malignant neoplasm, one can produce disastrous consequences like pathological (micro or macro) fractures, and local and/or distant dissemination of the growth. Features of malignancy are usually so obvious that they do not require much handling. Passing the hand gently over and around the growth can acceptably delineate the extent, dimension and relations of the growth. Through advances in diagnostic imaging, histological evaluation, staging procedures, operative strategies, *adjuvant (postoperative) and neoadjuvant (chemotherapy* also in preoperative setting) chemotherapies, there appears to have a great future in managing the various skeletal neoplastic growths. Therefore, it is imperative that a very careful and gentle assessment of the neoplasm be done, specially with regard to its relations with surrounding soft tissues and adjoining joints.

While examining a benign neoplasm, all possible mechanical pressure effects must be searched for. Even with the slightest doubt of malignancy, the possible sites of metastasis must be sought for. Unfortunately, the *pulmonary bed, working as a filter for circulating neoplastic cells, is a common site for implantation of metastatic tissues.* Hence, thorough examination of the pulmonary system is essential. Then, various possible osseous foci (e.g. vertebral column, skull, ribs, pelvis, femora and so on) should be looked for.

In certain neoplasms like multiple myelomatosis, there may not be any obvious swelling anywhere. The only manifestations may be general systemic features, vague generalised pain, progressive anaemia or other complications like renal failures and paraplegia.

Understanding the genetic predisposition of certain sarcomas, newer diagnostic modalities and path breaking novel treatment regimens offer renewed hopes in the field of cancer care.

- **Carcinoma and sarcoma**
  - *Carcinomas are malignant tumours arising from epithelial or endothelial tissues*
  - *Sarcomas are tumours arising from mesoblastic tissues.* Sarcomas of bone and soft tissue are uncommon malignant lesions, characterised by a diversity (variegated) in presentation and biological behaviour.
- **Post-irradiation neoplasms**

Irradiation therapy was a very popular treatment till the sixth to early seventh decade of 20th century, but it is getting unpopular because of the advent of more promising chemotherapeutic agents and irradiation hazards. In certain situations like benign giant cell tumour and ankylosing spondylitis, therapeutic irradiation has been blamed for malignant transformations.

- The intent of cancer therapy may be curative or palliative depending on the disease and patient characteristics.
- The incidence of cancers in all age groups combined together is increasing, from 182.3 per 100,000 in 2012 to 197.9 per 100,000 in 2018 globally.

Classification of Bone Tumours (Tables 17.1 to 17.4: Tables also contain the salient diagnostic features, gross pathological and radiological findings and broad outlines of possible management)

A lot of controversy exists regarding the classification and nomenclature of bone tumours, probably because of disagreement between the clinicians, radiologists and pathologists. The controversy regarding the cell origin of different tumours, varying behaviour of certain tumours and confusing histopathological changes in different fields of same tumour also complicate the issue. However, in the year 1972, a World Health Organization sponsored meeting of radiologists, pathologists and clinicians agreed to classify

TABLE 17.1: Classification of primary bone tumours (Based on WHO classification (1972) (Ackermann, Sison and Schajowicz).

Cell of origin	Benign	Intermediate or indeterminate	Malignant	Tumour like lesions
Osteoblasts	• Osteoma • Osteoblastoma • Osteoid osteoma (Described by Jaffe in 1935 — Jaffe tumour). It represents 10–12% of the benign bone tumours, of which 2 to 15% cases involve the foot and ankle.		• Osteosarcoma • Juxta-cortical osteosarcoma (Parosteal osteosarcoma)	• Solitary bone cyst (Unicameral bone cyst) • Aneurysmal bone cyst • Juxta-articular bone cyst (Intraosseous ganglion)
Chondroblasts	• Chondroma • Chondroblastoma • Osteochondroma (**see Figs. 17.18 and 17.19**) (The most common benign tumour) • Chondromyxoid fibroma		Chondrosarcoma is malignant tumor of cartilage producing cells–chondroblasts. It is most common sarcoma of bone of persons over 20 years of age. WHO (2002) classifies malignant cartilaginous tumors as: Chondrosarcoma — Primary / Secondary Juxtacortical chondrosarcoma Dedifferentiated chondrosarcoma Mesenchymal chondrosarcoma Clear cell chondrosarcoma	• Non-ossifying fibroma (Metaphyseal fibroma) (**see Figs. 17.20 and 17.30**) • Fibrous dysplasia • Eosinophilic granuloma (mostly in patients of <10 years age) • Brown's tumour of hyperparathyroidism. In hyperparathyroidism, rarely the skeletal changes (such as diffuse mineralisation) become markedly focal and produce "brown tumour", which resembles a typical giant cell tumour
Osteoclasts	• Osteoclastoma (Giant cell tumour) (Locally malignant)		• Malignant osteoclastoma (Giant cell tumour)	
Medullary tumours			• Ewing's sarcoma • Reticulum cell sarcoma • Multiple myeloma	• Hodgkin's disease • Lymphosarcoma • Neurofibrosarcoma

Contd...

Contd...

Cell of origin	Benign	Intermediate or indeterminate	Malignant	Tumour like lesions
Vascular tumours	• Haemangioma (see Figs. 17.23, 17.24A and B, 17.49)	• Haemangiopericytoma • Hemangioendothelioma (see Figs. 17.50 to 17.52)	• Angiosarcoma of hand can develop with regular contact with polyvinyl chloride (pipes and cement) • Haemangiosarcoma (see Figs. 17.28)	
Fibrous tissue	• Desmoplastic fibroma		• Fibrosarcoma including myofibrosarcoma (see Figs. 17.5, 17.6 and 17.8)	
*Adipose tissue	Lipoma (Fig. 9.2)		• Liposarcoma	
*Nerve tissue	• Neurofibroma—Neurofibromatosis – 1 (NF–1) (see Figs. 9.3, 16.23, 17.25 and 17.94) • Neurofibrosarcoma (autosomal dominant inheritance) • Neurilemmoma	NF-1 is one of the most common single gene disorders in humans. Patients with NF-1 may present with wide variety of clinical manifestations. About 50% of patients with NF-1 develop severe orthopaedic complications. Spinal deformity (e.g. dystrophic form of scoliosis) is the most common musculoskeletal manifestation of NF-1	• Neurofibrosarcoma	
*Lymphatics **Inclusion tissue	• Lymphangioma (see Figs. 17.91A and B)	Admantinoma (derived (see Fig. 17.46) from Greek word adamantinos, meaning very hard) is a rare primary low grade malignant biphasic (epithelial and osteofibrous components) bone tumor predominantly located in mid portion of tibia usually in 25 to 35 years of age more in men. This lesion was first described by Maier in 1900. Fischer named "Admantinoma" because of its characteristic resemblance to adamantinoma of jaw (ameloblastoma). Its incidence is 0.4% of all bone tumors. Surgery (wide excision and reconstruction using autograft or allograft) is main stay of treatment.	Lymphomas; (see Fig. 17.47) Chordoma (from notochordal remnants in the sacral region, coccyx and sella turcica of the skull). Primarily a midline tumour of adults. Males are affected two times more. MRI provides excellent delineation. Surgical resection with wide margins, albeit it is more likely to cause neurological deficit	
Synovium	Synovioma (see Fig. 17.79)	Synovioma	Synovial sarcoma	

Striated muscles cells—rhabdomyoscarcoma (see Figs. 17.48 and 17.58)
Common in head and neck of infant and adult—making 20% of all soft tissues sarcoma. Histologically characterised by gaint rhabdomyoblast.
Myelocyte of skin—myeloma (see Figs. 17. 74 to 17.78).

1. *These (*) marked growths have not been included in classification but it appears logical to include them.
   Secondary bone tumours—Primary from breast, prostate, bronchus, thyroid, kidney, stomach, adrenals, and skin.
   Note To facilitate the selection of surgical procedure and comparing the results of different modes of managing malignant musculoskeletal lesions, Enneking et al. (1980) suggested staging of these lesions basing upon physical, radiological, radioisotopic and histopathological examinations. The system suggested by them is as follows:

IA	—	Low-grade intracompartmental (lesion confined to a single anatomical compartment)
IB	—	Low-grade extracompartmental (lesion extends beyond a single compartment)
IIA	—	High-grade intracompartmental
IIB	—	High-grade extracompartmental
III	—	Lesions (low- or high-grades, intra- or extracompartmental) with regional or distant metastasis

   A local procedure with dissection carried out through normal tissue
   Amputation at proper level
   Radical excision with removal of all normal tissues of the involved compartments

2. **WHO classification system,** as modified by Enzinger and Weiss, recognises 82 distinct benign and malignant soft tissue lesions and tumours of 10 major histogenic types, which can arise in the distant part of leg (besides other regions).
3. **Neurofibroma,** though not an osseous tumour but neurofibromatosis (the word introduced by von Recklinghausen in 1882) is frequently associated with skeletal anomalies. Telesius was credited by von Recklinghausen with having given the first adequate description of the fibroma molluscum in 1793 (see Fig. 17.25).
4. **Fibroma of tendon sheath** (first described by Geschickter and Copeland in 1949) is slow growing fibrous nodule frequently adjoining a tendon sheath with a predilection for occurring on the fingers and hands usually in middle-aged persons. It may also originate from the synovial membrane of a joint. Microscopically-there is proliferation of uniform plumpy bland fibroblastic/myofibroblastic cells (with elongated cells) arranged in short intersecting bundles. Treatment consists of marginal excision, however, with possible recurrence.

TABLE 17.2: Table showing diagnostic features of important benign bone tumours.

	Osteoma	Osteochondroma	Osteoid osteoma	Osteoblastoma
1	2	3	4	5
1. Synonyms	A true osteoma is ivory exostosis (*see* **Figs. 17.10, 17.12, 17.13 and 17.34**)–a benign slow growing tumor arising mainly in the membranous bones of skull and face	Familial exostoses (*see* **Fig. 17.14**). Multiple hereditary exostoses (autosomal dominant inheritance), Diaphyseal aclasis, Biotrophic osteoma (*see* **Figs. 17.7A and B**) (osteoid) Metaphyseal aclasia (*see* **Fig. 17.22**), Exostosis (single or multiple). Common benign tumor. Generally single affecting long bones in an immature skeleton and deform them (*see* **Figs. 17.9A and B, 17.11, 17.29, 17.18, 17.19, 17.17, 17.67A to C**)	• Osteoid osteoma is a benign skeletal tumor first described by Bergstrand in 1930. In 1935, Jaffe, accurately described this entity and coined the term "osteoid osteoma"– hence named as Jaffe's tumour; for pain relief aspirin suits, hence Aspirin tumour. It is a small benign painful bony tumour • It represents 12% of benign bone tumours • A benign cortical-based osteoblastic neoplasm of only a few millimeter in diameter characterised by an osteoid-rich nidus in a highly vascular connective tissue stroma, surrounded by sclerotic bone. • Etiology is unknown. It is a self limiting disease process, which mature spontaneously over several years. In maturation, the nidus gradually calcifies, then ossifies and finally blends into the surrounding sclerotic bone (*see* **Figs. 17.10A and B**)	Giant osteoid osteoma; osteogenic fibroma of bone
2. Cell of origin	Osteoblast	Chondroblast, arise from growth cartilage cells (*see* **Figs. 17.11, 17.21**)	Views of origin: • Jaffe (1935)—a slow growing neoplasm • Infective origin of self-limiting nature (because of sclerosed bony shell, characteristic location, in some cases organisms cultured) • A vascular lesion • Embryonic rest • Hamartoma	Osteoblast
3. Age, sex	Starts in childhood, manifests in adults	Occurs during adolescence, never after epiphyseal fusion. Equal in both sexes	Usually males (5–40 years)	Any age group usually less than 30 years, male more than females (2:1)
4. Bones affected	Membranous bones—cranial bones, orbit, nasal bones, external auditory meatus, mandible	Bones of cartilage origin. Most Common at the extremities of long bones—lower end of femur, upper end of tibia, upper end of femur. Frequently from epiphysis of flat bones—scapula, innominate. Arise from growth cartilage cells (*see* **Figs. 17.17A and B**)	Any bone (except skull) predominantly in bones of lower extremities, e.g. tibia, femur (>50% of cases), humerus, vertebrae	Rare tumour. In vertebrae, limb bones, e.g. femur
5. Clinical presentation	Hard, immovable, small, sessile, single, slowly growing, smooth surface, may be nodular, growing within may cause pressure on the brain	• Usually pedunculated with bulbar extremity projecting towards diaphysis away from epiphyseal plate and is capped by a detached fragment of epiphyseal cartilage • Comparative broadening of metaphysis due to base of growth. With cessation of growth the cartilaginous cap shrinks even up to degenerative disappearance	Usually pain (dull ache) at night, relieved by salicylates, may be a tender swelling if superficially located in tibia. May be limp (in lower limb affection). If near joint—effusion, stiffness, contracture. Tumours at times are non-progressive and self- limiting	Pain and tenderness. Vertebral involvement may cause weakness and paraesthesia of lower limb

Contd...

Contd...

		Osteoma	Osteochondroma	Osteoid osteoma	Osteoblastoma
1		2	3	4	5
6.	Pathology	Tumour usually composed of bony tissue as dense and hard as ivory	• Grows till fusion of adjacent epiphysis, summit often covered by adventitious bursa • When fully developed, the marrow of the shaft is continuous with that of exostosis (see Fig. 17.12) • May be familial. Symptoms—cosmetic, pressure effect, local pressure upon nerves (lateral popliteal), vessels, e.g. in popliteal fossa • May turn malignant (chondrosarcoma, osteosarcoma) • When fully developed, growth consists of shell of compact bone enclosing cancellous tissue with a cap of cartilage • Cut section—central core of cancellous tissue continuous with medullary canal of parent bone, containing a central blood vessel with branching up to tip of the growth	• Lesions very vascular with numerous nerve fibres • Histology—an inner region of vascular granulation tissue containing osteoblasts, outside with calcification and osteoid formation surrounded by trabecular formation of bone (see Figs. 17.13A and B)	• Cuts with gritty sensation, vascular • Histology—fairly regular orientation of new bone formation with trabeculation • Osteogenic cells having look of malignancy. Predominantly osteoid and primitive bone trabeculae, giant cells; distinct and uniform stromal cell, which rarely show mitotic figures (cf. GCT)
7.	Investigation Mainly X-ray	Sessile rounded densely opaque shadow (see Figs. 17.34A to C)	Pedunculated or sessile outpouching of the trabeculated corticocancellous bone from the metaphysis. Size of growth comparatively smaller than felt clinically (due to cartilaginous cap)	In X-ray, central radiolucent nidus surrounded by a zone of sclerosed bone, further surrounded by normal adjoining bone; On CT and scintigraphic findings—"double density sign"; on MRI—marrow oedema with periosseous oedema and well seen nidus Page number = 515. The goal of imaging is the visualization of the nidus which is usually intermediate signal intensity on T1- weighted images and intermediate to high signal intensity on T2 weighted images.	Circumscribed expanding osteolytic lesion with some radio-opaque mottling
8.	Complications	Mainly cosmetic problems Very rarely early intracranial pressure symptoms	General—cosmetic, stunted growth; Local—turn malignant (osteochondrosarcoma or chondrosarcoma** (see Fig. 17.41) • Pressure/stretch neurovascular complication (lateral popliteal nerve) • Fracture	• Radicular irritation • Psychic depression • Entrapment neuropathy (e.g. posterior interosseous neuropathy following osteoid osteoma of upper end of ulna • Its malignant transformation is not known, albeit transformation into osteoblastoma (osteogenic fibroma of bone) have been reported	May turn to malignant growth
9.	Differential diagnosis	Foreign body (bullet, etc.)	Mimicking the histological findings of osteochondroma – rarely 'dysplasia epiphyseal (see Fig. 17.23) is dysplasia epiphysealis hemimelica' may occur. It is of unknown etiology and consists of an abnormal osteocartilaginous growth at the epiphysis, usually hemimelic. It produces pain and deformation of child's affected/nearby joint.	• Brodie's abscess • Sclerosing non-suppurative osteomyelitis of Garre—A chronic disease of unknown origin (may be infection by low-grade anaerobic bacteria in which bone is thickened and distended but without abscess or sequestrum • Patients usually children /young adults, complain chronic intermittent dull pain and tender swelling. The lesion mimics osteoid osteoma and Paget's disease	• Osteoid osteoma • Osteogenic sarcoma • Giant cell tumour

Contd...

Contd...

	Osteoma	Osteochondroma	Osteoid osteoma	Osteoblastoma
1	2	3	4	5
			No treatment is reliably helpful Fenestration of sclerotic bone and broad-range antibiotic may help • Non-ossifying fibroma • Syphilitic osteitis • Osteogenic sarcoma • Chronic osteomyelitis with annular sequestrum (e.g. pin tract infection)	
10. Treatment	• For pressure symptoms or cosmetic reasons • Excision with normal bone margin	Excision with wide base for cosmetic improvement, any pressure symptoms, and the slightest doubt of malignancy (sudden increase in growth rate, warm, pain)	• Surgical options: Removal of nidus is most effective cure excision with surrounding bone; removal of roof of nidus and curettage • CT-guided core drill excision; • Radiofrequency ablation—ILP* • Intraoperative isotopic identification of osteoid osteoma is highly reliable and it allows precise localisation which helps in optimal resection • Injection of ethanol • Symptomatic: Salicylate or NSAID for pain	Resection cures; Curettage with bone grafting; Radiotherapy for inaccessible lesions, e.g. vertebrae

NB
* **Percutaneous interstitial laser photocoagulation** (ILP-first described in 1983 by Bown SG). In this technique, the tumour tissue is destroyed by direct heating using low-power laser light energy delivered by thin (400 mm) optic fibres radiofrequency electrode introduced through the cannula of the biopsy needle and electrode connected to a radio- frequency generator. A temperature of 100° celsius is applied for 3 minutes. If needed this cycle is repeated once more. The principle of radiofrequency ablation (RFA) is to induce thermal coagulation in the lesion and to cook the lesion to death. Cure rate by RFA is 80–90%. Little complication like thermal burns and procedural pain may occur.
** **Chondrosarcoma,** the second most common form of primary bone cancer primarily affects the cartilaginous cells. It is the most common sarcoma of bone accounting for about 25% of bone sarcomas and occurring typically in adults between 30 and 60 years. The distinction between a well-differentiated chondrosarcoma and an enchondroma can be difficult. Adequate surgical excision is the most important treatment of conventional chondrosarcoma, as there is no effective adjuvant treatment, like chemotherapy and radiotherapy. With complete excision of the tumour with a wide margin, chondrosarcoma is a surgically curable condition (*see* **Figs. 17.59A to C and 17.83**).
*** CHONDROBLASTOMA is a rare primary benign cartilaginous tumor accounting for about 1% of all benign tumors. It mostly occurs at the epiphyseal region of immature long bones. Though benign, it metastasises to lung in 2% of cases. Histologically it is marked by the presence of chondroblasts arranged in chicken wire pattern with the presence of multinucleated giant cell and mononuclear stromal cells. Chondroblastomas are treated by curettage and bone grafting or cementation. Recently radio frequency ablation of the tumor is also being done with promising results, albeit local recurrence may occur. (Narhari et al. 2018) the tumor can be aggressive as: Benign chondroblastoma with lung metastasis or malignant chondroblastoma or malignant transformation of benign chondroblastoma

bone tumours on the basis of histological typing. At the same time, certain facts presented in the classification of 'bone registry' cannot be denied.

Staging is the process of classifying a tumour, specially a malignant tumour with respect to its degree of differentiation as well as its local and distant extent, in order to estimate the prognosis and to compare between groups of patients.

Staging is done on the basis of clinical findings, imaging and histopathological studies, basically to guide, the operative procedure, goal of treatment (curative or palliative), the extent of excision, the perceived efficacy of adjuvant therapy, prognostise the ultimate outcome.

The *first staging system was developed by League of Nation based on TNM system* (T = extent of primary tumour; N = presence or absence of nodal metastasis; M = distant metastasis). At present, the most commonly used system of staging of the malignant soft-tissue tumours is that of American Joint Committee on Cancer. However, the Musculoskeletal Tumour Society adopted a staging system, as described by Enneking et al. (1980, 1983) for both benign and malignant bone tumours. This system has been more or less agreed upon by AJCC with minor adaptations for malignant bone tumours.

■ METHODOLOGY

History Taking

In history taking, the following points should be noted in detail:
- Onset of symptoms in chronological order
- Duration of each symptom: The usual symptoms of bone tumours are:
  • Symptoms due to primary growth

- *Local symptoms*: Swelling, pain, affections of joint movement to varying extent, wasting of adjoining muscles, ulcers.
- *Constitutional symptoms*: Occasionally, constitutional symptoms like fever, weakness, loss of weight, anorexia, progressive anaemia.
- *Pressure symptoms:* Like weakness in the distal parts and other symptoms due to pressure on vital parts and neurovascular structures.
- Symptoms due to Metastatic Lesions
    - Common complaints due to secondaries in lungs are—cough, haemoptysis, and pain chest.
    - Secondaries from primaries of the secreting glands (e.g. thyroid, adrenals, salivary, pituitary) may induce the manifestations of hyperfunctional effects of primary glandular secretions.
    - Sometimes, the patients primarily present with severe complications, e.g. paraplegia due to secondary deposits without any obvious complaints regarding the primary tumours.
- Rate of growth
- Fluctuations in symptoms with/without any treatment, e.g. lessening or exaggeration of swelling and/or pain
- Treatment given and its results—Usually, the modes of treatment tried are:
    - Indigenous medicines, local applications, radiotherapy (doses, period and sittings of applications), chemotherapy (drugs used, doses and duration) and surgical treatment (for biopsy or ablation)
    - The details of the treatment should be noted as far as possible.
- Family history may not be of that significance in the examination but with the proven role of genetic transmission in certain cases of neoplasms (familial or diaphyseal aclasis, neuroblastoma, etc.), the detail family history should be taken **(Figs. 17.1 to 17.4)**.
- Occupation of the patient, specially with reference to radiation exposure, regular use of certain chemicals, inhalation of certain obnoxious vapours, exposure to any irritant—physical, chemical or others, should be noted. Certain relations of these irritating substances with neoplastic growths have been proved, e.g. radium responsible for osteogenic sarcoma, coal tar as a carcinogen, etc.
- Of these multiple benign growths as in **Figures 17.1 to 17.4** perhaps only those require treatment (as far as possible total excision) which show complications like any feature of malignancy; starts growing rapidly/fast; becomes painful; shows inflammatory feature; presses upon the adjoining nerve/blood vessel; becomes cosmetically unacceptable

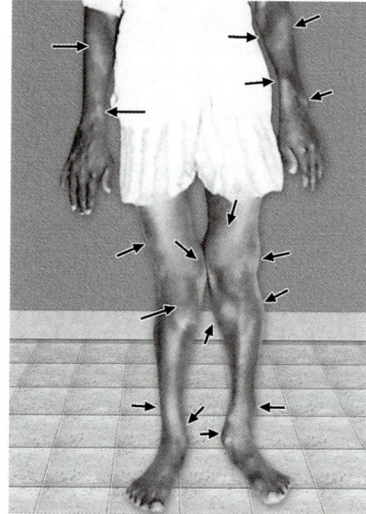

Fig. 17.2: Multiple exostosis.

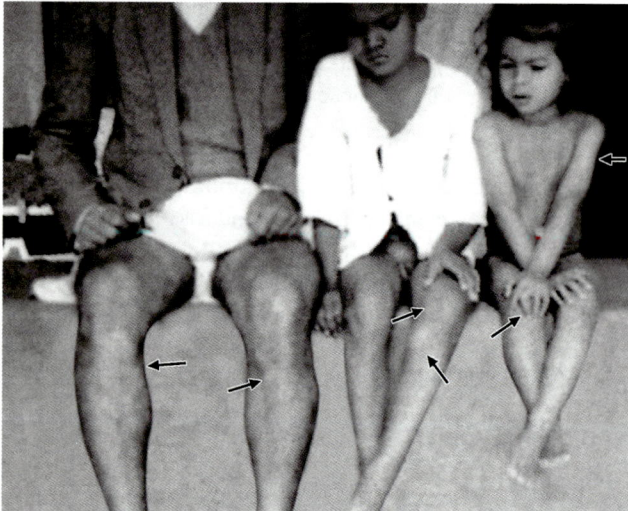

Fig. 17.1: Familial exostosis (multiple osteochondroma). Father having exostosis in both upper tibiae and other places; first son having exostosis in left upper tibia, left lower femur and ribs; second son having exostosis in left upper humerus, left middle finger, right upper tibia and ribs.

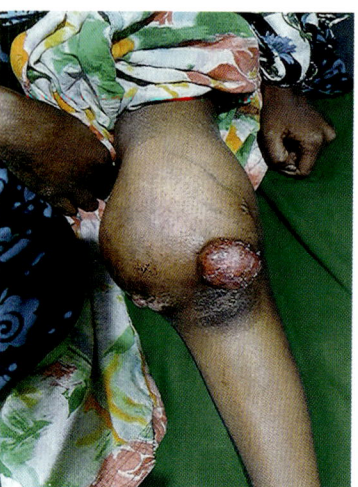

Fig. 17.3: Osteosarcoma from upper region of femur.

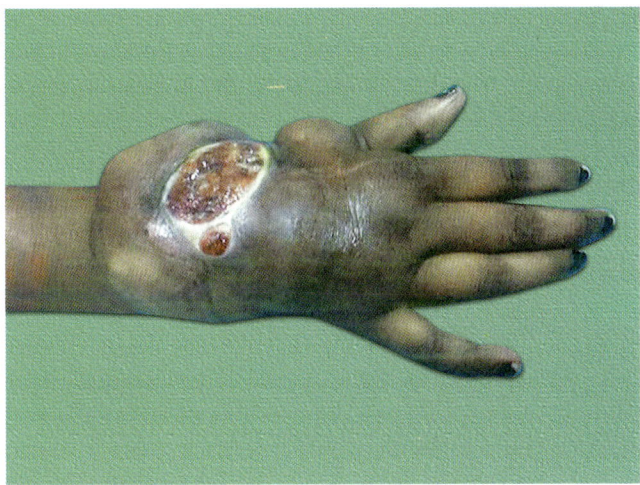

Fig. 17.4: Sarcoma from lower end of radius.
Courtesy: Dr PK Raina and Dr Anamika Kumari.

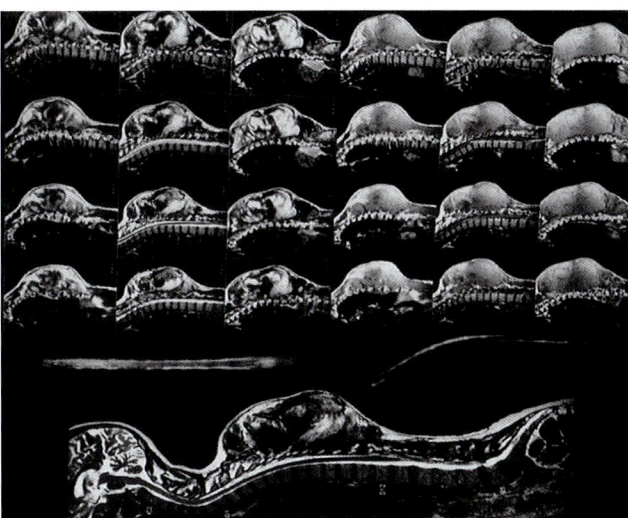

Fig. 17.6: MRI of patient of Figure 17.5 – Myofibrosarcoma showing intrathoracic extension.
Courtesy: Dr PK Raina and Dr Anamika Kumari.

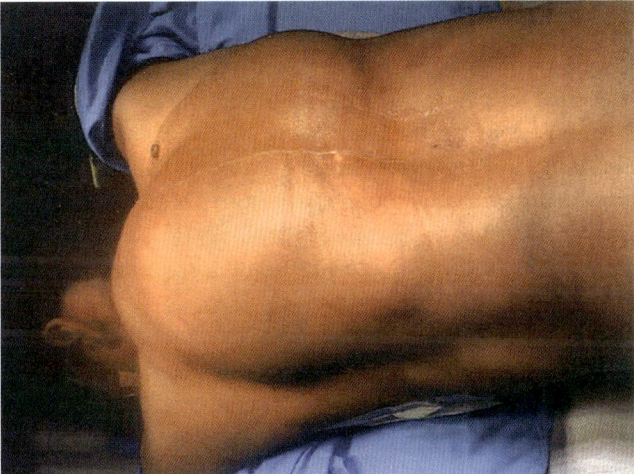

Fig. 17.5: Myofibrosarcoma from back. From bilateral erector spinae.
Courtesy: Dr PK Raina and Dr Anamika Kumari.

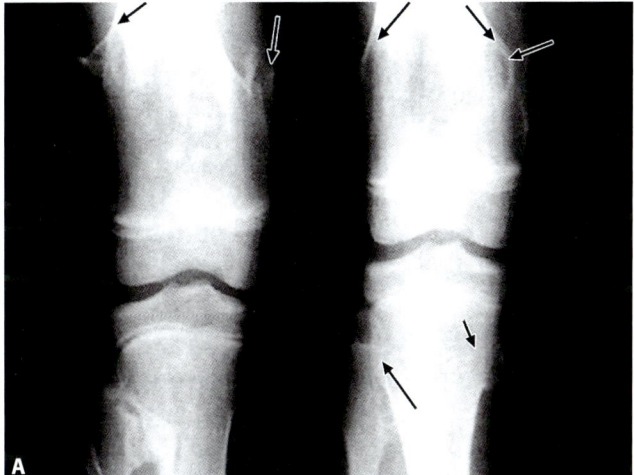
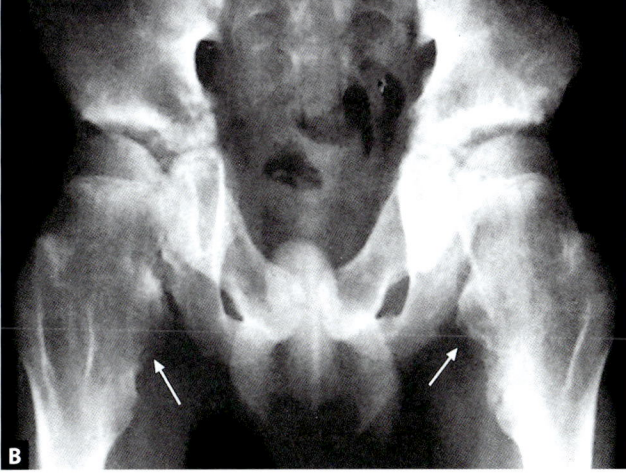

Figs. 17.7A and B: Metaphyseal aclasis.

Examination

General Examination

The early stages may not be of much significance, but in long standing cases of malignant tumours, general effects of cachexia and anaemia may be obvious. The effects of tumour on general behaviour, attitude, gait, posture and functional abilities of the patient should be noted clearly. Any obvious deformity (e.g. in multiple exostosis, chondroma, etc.), should be noted. As a general rule, the hand should be passed from the skull down to the face, chest, pelvis, spine and limbs, in any case of suspected neoplasm. Sometimes, various swellings in the skull or pelvis may be masked by hair and undergarments.

Systemic Examination

As a routine, respiratory system, cardiovascular system, abdomen and urogenital system should be examined. Whenever indicated, examination of the central nervous system and endocrinal assessment should be done.

Local Examination

Swelling must be categorically and systemically examined.

Bone Tumours

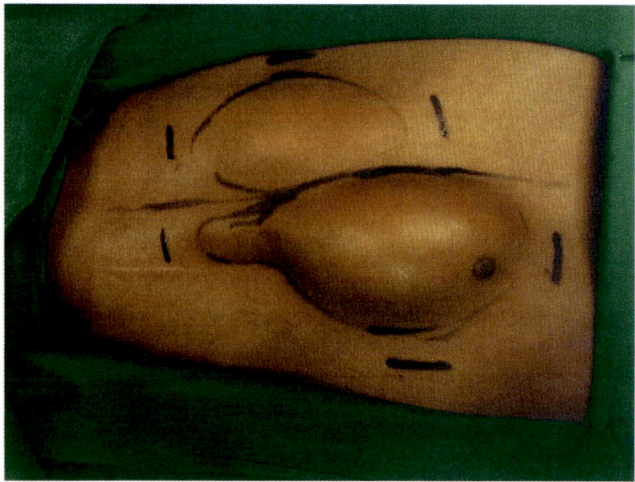

Fig. 17.8: Myofibrosarcoma from back.

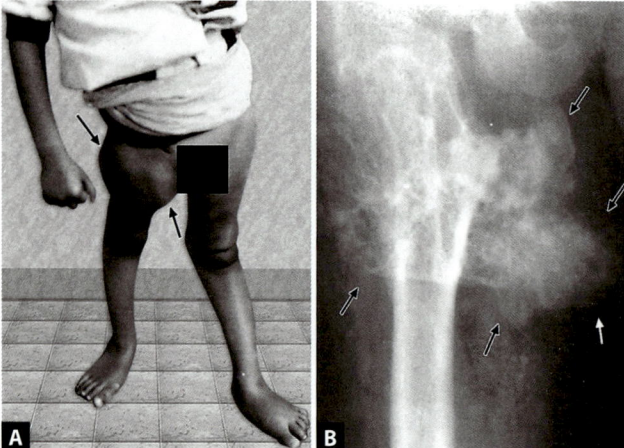

Figs. 17.9A and B: Osteochondroma upper end of femur.

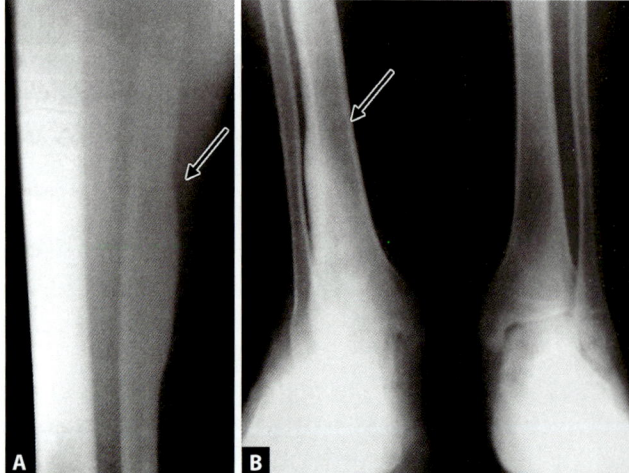

Figs. 17.10A and B: (A) X-ray picture showing osteoid osteoma from fibula; (B) X-ray picture showing osteoid osteoma from right tibia.

Inspection

Look for site, size, shape, extent, direction of growth, engorgement of veins, skin condition, any pulsation, stretching of overlying soft tissue, any scar or ulcer, any movement of the swelling with movement of the limb or part, encroachment of the swelling over adjoining joints and muscle wasting in relation to the swelling.

Palpation

Superficial palpation (touch): Temperature, pliability of skin and superficial tissue, hyperaesthesia, or analgesia or anaesthesia, superficial tenderness, surface of the swelling, and confirmation of the findings of inspection.

Deep palpation (feel): Assess surface of the swelling, extent, margin, deep tenderness, consistency of different areas, fixity of the tumour to superficial tissue, deeper tissues and the underlying bone. The adjoining joint should also be palpated specially because the joints may be affected directly or mechanically. The movements of the adjoining joints must be noted clearly. While palpating, if one gets obvious crepitus or yielding it should be noted. But one should not attempt to demonstrate any crepitus (e.g. egg shell crackling in giant cell tumour). Crackling is due to fracture of thinned out bony shell. In an attempt to demonstrate this crackling repeatedly, the chances of producing further pathological fractures of the thinned out cortical shell increases. This is very likely to disseminate the neoplastic tissues into the surrounding soft tissues and/or distantly.

Examination of the regional lymph glands is mandatory. Almost all malignant neoplasms have glandular disseminations. The nature of the glandular enlargement should be noted categorically.

Examination for any skip lesions: Usually, it is a radiopathological diagnosis. However, in rare instances, there may be other palpable swellings in the same bone. The intervening bone may appear clinically normal. This 'skip-lesion' (as in osteosarcoma), is probably due to medullary spread and implantation of neoplastic tissue at that site. However, multifocal neoplasms have also been reported.

Sometimes unusual manifestations, such as ONCO-GENIC RICKETS, have to be explored. Rickets may be associated with small benign mesenchymal tumors, found in skin, subcutaneous tissue, nasopharynx bone, para nasal sinuses, sole, palm etc., and which are difficult to locate

Auscultation

This ritual should not be forgotten while examining the neoplasm. In highly vascular tumours (e.g. telangiectatic osteosarcoma, or even any secondaries with high vascularity), systolic bruit may be heard.

Examination of the possible sites for secondaries, specially the lungs, liver, spine, skull, pelvis, ribs, orbital region and other long bones is mandatory.

Search for complications: Possible complication must be kept in mind and search must be made for pressure effects, pathological fractures, paraplegia, hormonal manifestations, etc.

Investigations

- Routine haemogram
- Routine urine examination
- Plain X-ray, in different views, is still the gold standard for arriving at diagnosis of the bone tumours
  Points to look for in the X-rays:
  - Disproportionate increase in soft tissue shadow
  - Breach in the continuity of the cortex or any other obvious pathological fracture
  - Amount of destruction
  - Evidence of new bone formation and its appearance
  - Any reactionary bone formation (e.g. subperiosteal longitudinal bone laying)
  - Corticomedullary delineation (sharp or lost)
  - Any evidence of expansion of the cortex
  - Obvious infiltration into joints
  - Skip lesions.
- Tomography
- Contrast radiography
- Angiography
- *Scintigraphy*—Radioactive isotope studies. Radioactive isotopes are being utilised for localising the neoplastic tissue. Technetium-99m, Strontium 85, Fluorine 18, Strontium 87m, Phosphorus 32, Calcium 45, Iodine 131 and gold have been used for various neoplastic conditions. The results of these investigations are of much help in ruling out any secondaries (which may not be obvious otherwise).
  SPECT scans remain the mainstay in oncology, e.g. for detecting the presence of skeletal involvement
- Computerised axial tomography. A CT scan of chest at the initial stage itself can help in detection of disseminated diseases
- Nuclear magnetic resonance (NMR/MRI). Because of its excellent soft tissue contrast, its sensitivity to bone marrow and soft tissue oedema, and its multiple imaging planes provide valuable informations about musculoskeletal tumours.
  MRI is highly suitable for follow-up examinations in cancer patients due to its ability to visualize the whole body with high contrast and without ionizing irradiation
- Cytological examination—Confirmation can only be obtained by histopathological examination. The material for this examination can be obtained by—closed (FNAC and core needle biopsy) or open (incisional) method. Biopsy should be regarded as the final diagnostic procedure. Biopsy should be performed by or under the direct supervision of the treating surgeon.

- Fine needle aspiration cytology (FNAC)
- Core needle biopsy
- Ultrasound and/or CT or even MRI-guided needle biopsy
- Open biopsy.

A biopsy should be planned as carefully as the definitive procedure regardless of whether a needle biopsy or an open biopsy is taken. The biopsy track must be taken as contaminated with tumour cells. To decide the biopsy track is a crucial decision, because it needs to be excised en-block with the tumour.

While taking biopsy from bone, the defect created in bone should be as round as possible which helps in minimizing the stress concentration and thus avoids to a greater extent the possibility of pathological fracture.

Fine needle aspiration cytology: It is an almost painless outdoor or ward procedure with a very high rate of accuracy (97–98%) with the added advantage of obtaining a result within a few hours. In this, a fine needle (18, 20 or 22 bore) is passed into the suspected tissue and negative pressure is created and maintained in the syringe. The needle is then passed in 3–5 different directions through the same entry. After completing the aspiration, the pressure in the syringe is equalised, and the needle is withdrawn. Contents of the needle are then expressed on a glass slide, smeared and fixed immediately with cytofix. It is then stained for study for Papanicolaou or Haematoxyline. With comparatively more accurate result of core needle biopsy, the use of FNAC is being undermined, specially in bone and soft tissue sarcomas, since only few cells are supposed to be inadequate for making a specific diagnosis and conducting ancillary studies.

Core needle biopsy: Percutaneous core needle biopsy is a better, safe, and approximately accurate method for diagnosis of bone tumours. It is performed by a small stab using a wide bore needle (like Jamshidi needle) and multiple cores are taken from the representative part of tumour. It can be quickly done under local anaesthesia. For children a short general anesthesia may be required. There is minimal soft tissue trauma and less contamination of normal tissue by the tumour cells around the tract of needle (which is easily excisable during the limb salvage surgery). It can be done under image guidance (like CT, MRI, or USG), which augments its efficacy and accuracy. It is very suitable for deep and difficult areas like spine and pelvis. In a thick smear, the nature of the cells can be studied. This may be almost of confirmatory value (e.g. by sternal puncture in multiple myeloma). In case of bone tumor with a soft tissue component, the biopsy specimen can be obtained from the soft-tissue component by a Tru-Cut needle-biopsy system.

Open biopsy: Open biopsy, of course, can be authentic but a word of caution is due before embarking on it. As far as the medicolegal aspect is concerned open biopsy can confirm the diagnosis and one must not embark on ablation surgery without confirmation of the diagnosis. But when one thinks of primary resection of neoplasm followed by a possible reconstruction, open biopsy may come in the way. Not only it does damage to the area of operative exposure, but also carries the grave risk of dissemination of neoplastic tissues to the surrounding area. This dissemination may nullify the basic benefit of primary resection, and recurrence of the growth becomes almost a rule rather than an exception. However, the evolution of multiagent chemotherapy provides a comparatively safer umbrella for this procedure. Still, this issue is not that easy and it should be left entirely on the discretion of the surgeon whether or not he should decide to go in for an open biopsy before embarking on primary resection and reconstruction procedures. A thorough gentle clinical examination, supplemented by various investigations can often give very helpful clues in circumventing this tricky problem. However, open biopsy has the major advantage of obtaining adequate amount of tissue for histopathology and ancillary studies like immunohistocytochemistry (IHC) and genetic studies.

Immunohistochemistry is process in which cell-specific antigens /proteins on the cell surface are identified using antibodies, the tagging of which is identified using a color reaction, radioisotopes or immunofluorescence.

Peroperative frozen section study is worthwhile. Depending upon the report about the nature of the growth, the surgeon may proceed for definitive surgery.

- Tetracycline staining studies
- Various biochemical tests:
  - Serum acid phosphatase
  - Serum alkaline phosphatase.
- Renal function tests
- Paper chromatography
- Electrophoresis of serum for various protein components
- Proton emission tomography (PET)
  PET—High resolution and high sensitivity 3D PET detector system provide excellent image quality with lower dose requirements
- The diagnostic limitations of individual PET and CT procedures in oncology are now eliminated by a revolutionary hybrid new PET/CT imaging technology
- Tumour embolisation.

One of the most important factors which affects the outcomes of orthopedic tumor surgeries is surgical planning and its efficient execution. Surgical planning has a vital role, be it limb salvage or limb sacrifice surgery. In the recent years it has evolved for two dimensional images, through 3D images and virtual-3D models to life size 3D printed models. Advances in image processing have led to the clinical use of RP technology, giving the surgeon a realistic physical medals of the anatomy upon which he will operate (Verma Tarun and Maini Lalit 2019)

Navigation in Musculoskeletal Oncology: (Morris GV et al. 2018)

The role of navigation is to facilitate adequate surgical margins and safe resections defined by a reduction in avoidable functional impairment. Preoperative imaging in the form of MRI, CT, and positron emission tomography-CT is performed to assess tumor placement, size, proximity to vital structures and extent of intraosseous disease. The location and involvement of vital structures then determine whether tumor resection with limb salvage is possible or whether amputation is the safest procedure. These image modalities can be fused to form a three dimensional (3D) representation of the pelvis and tumor. (Morris GV et al. 2018)

The navigation in musculoskeletal oncology has following *advantages*:
1. Optimal surgical margins and therefore reduced local recurrence
2. Perceived reduction in operative time.
3. Beneficial in complex pelvic or periarticular resections.
4. More accurate tumor resection and allograft implantation.

Disadvantages of navigation system are (a) Cost of equipment (b) Increase setup time (c) Learning curve (Morris GV et al 2018)

Benign tumours are generally slow growing and rarely metastasise. Some are biologically more aggressive locally and may occasionally metastasise.
Based on Enneking's classification of benign bone tumours, benign tumours are classified as follows:

Stage	Definition	Behaviour	Example
1.	Latent (Stage 1) remains intracapsular, asymptomatic and never metastasises	Remains static or heals spontaneously	Non-ossifying fibroma
2.	Active (Stage 2) remains intracapsular, but actively growing, often symptomatic and rarely metastasises	Progressive growth but limited by natural barriers	Aneurysmal bone cyst
3.	Locally aggressive (Stage 3) often breaks through its capsule and extends into an adjacent compartment. Rarely may metastasises	Progressive growth but not limited by natural barriers	Giant cell tumour

Staging Systems for Malignant Bone Tumours (Based on Lichtenstein L 1972) (Tables 17.3A and 17.3B)

STAGING SYSTEM FOR MUSCULOSKELETAL NEOPLASMS:

Purpose:
1. To provide prognostic information
2. To plan possible treatment strategies
3. To provide comparison of results in similar cohorts of patients
   Two commonly followed staging systems are:
   (a) The common staging system is the simpler musculoskeletal tumor society (MSTS) staging system is devised by Enneking.
   (b) Tumor lymph nodes metastasis (TNM) staging system, as advocated by the union for International Cancer Control (VICE)or American Joint Committee on cancer, is based on histological grade, tumor size, presence or absence of regional lymph nodes and distant metastases.

A. Enneking system is for staging malignant musculoskeletal tumours. It is based on the histological grade of tumours, its local extent and the presence or absence of metastasis.

TABLE 17.3A: Enneking system for staging malignant musculoskeletal tumours.

Stage	Grade	Site	Metastasis	Notable features
1A	Low	Intracompartmental	None	Well differentiated
				Few mitoses
1B	Low	Extracompartmental	None	Only moderate cytological atypnia
				Low risk of metastasis
11A	High	Intracompartmental	None	Poorly differentiated
11B	High	Extracompartmental	None	High mitotic rate
				High cell to matrix ratio
111	Any	Any		Regional or distant metastasis regardless of size and grade

B. American Joint Committee on Cancer (AJCC) for staging bone sarcomas (based on Klein and Siegal, 2006) AJCC system for bone sarcomas is based on tumour grade size, presence and location of metastasis.

TABLE 17.3B: AJCC system for staging bone sarcomas.

Stage	Grade	Size	Metastasis
IA	Low	<8 cm	None
IB	Low	>8 cm	None
IIA	High	<8 cm	None
IIB	High	>8 cm	None
III	Any	Any	Skip metastasis
IVA	Any	Any	Pulmonary metastasis
IVB	Any	Any	Non-pulmonary metastasis—These patients have worse prognosis than those with only pulmonary metastases

A Precise Note on Treatment of Bone Tumors

Overall treatment options for cancer are divided into four types: chemotherapy, radiotherapy, surgery, and targeted therapy. Few patients need combination treatment.

Earliest detection of cancer provides high chances of cure.

In chemotherapy, patients are treated with anticancer medicines, prescribed by a medical oncologist, to be given intravenously or orally (in from of capsule or pills). The drugs used in chemotherapy are to destroy the quickly dividing cancer cells by ending their ability to grow and divide. As the side effects of the chemotherapy drugs, other quickly dividing cells in the body such as in the bone marrow, lining of mouth and intestine, and the hour follicles are likely to be affected leading to lowering the blood cells count, fatigue risk of infections, mouth sores, nausea, vomiting,

534 Bone Tumours

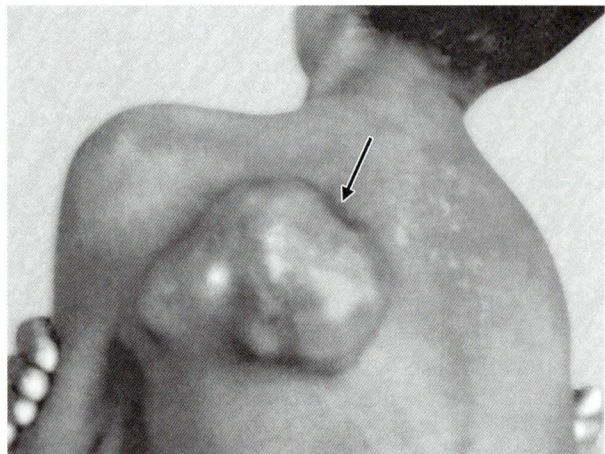

Fig. 17.11: Osteochondroma of scapula producing mechanical disability in lying down. Removal of growth along with the underlying scapula should solve his problem.

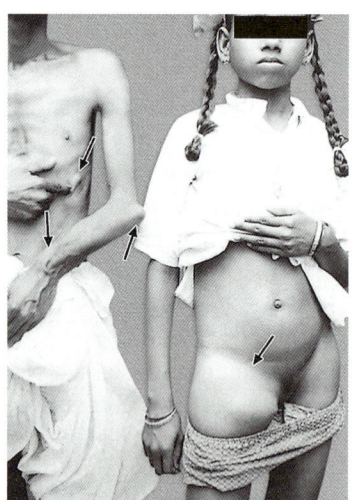

Fig. 17.14: Father and daughter with multiple exostosis.

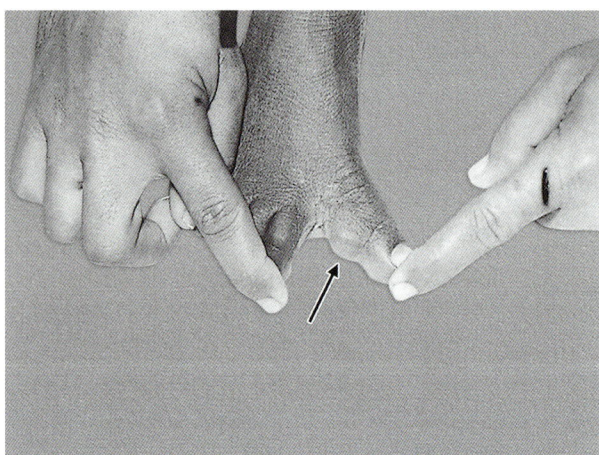

Fig. 17.12: Exostosis from proximal phalanx of big toe.

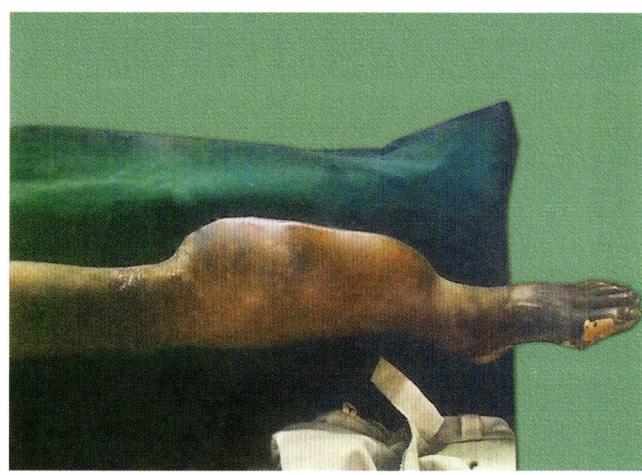

Fig. 17.15: Ewing sarcoma from lower part of tibia.

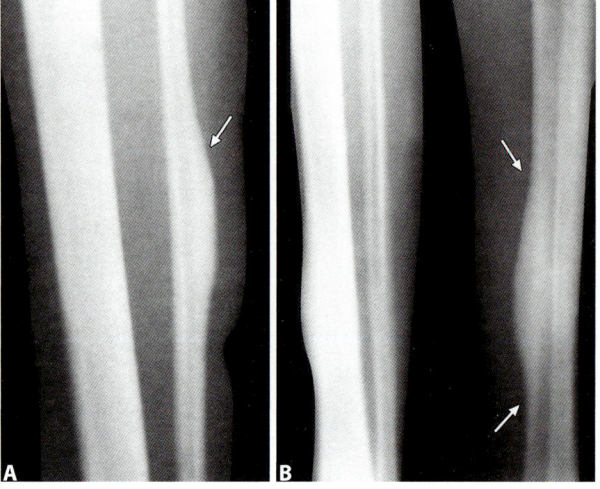

Figs. 17.13A and B: Osteoid osteoma from fibula (A) and tibia (B).

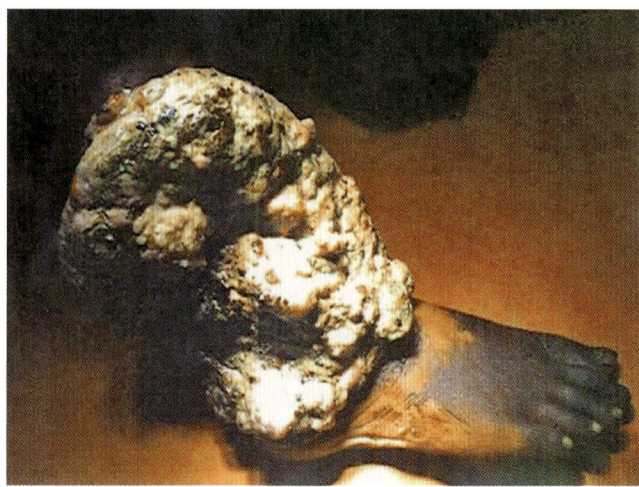

Fig. 17.16: Ewings sarcoma from lower tibia.
Courtesy: Dr PK Raina.

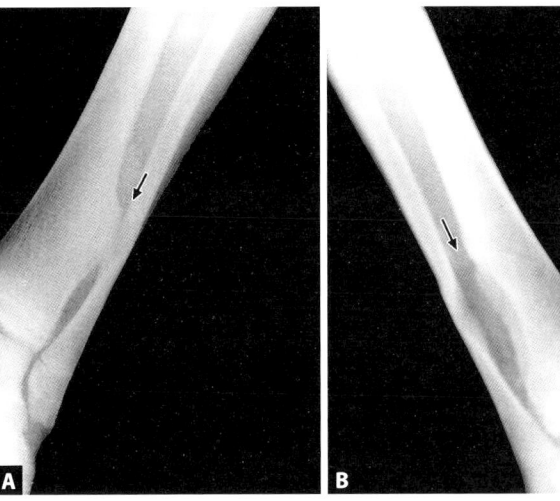
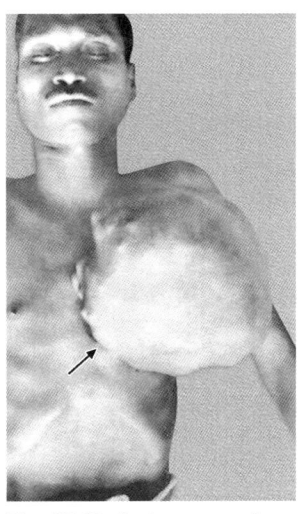
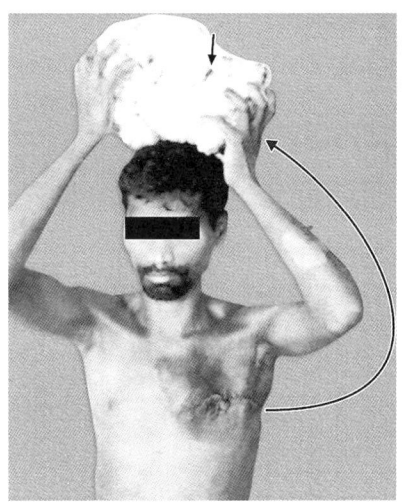

Figs. 17.17A and B: On right side (A) Exostosis/osteochondroma from lower end of tibia producing pressure on neurovascular bundle with more of neurological symptom); on left X-ray picture (B) After total excision of the growth—symptoms completely relieved.

Fig. 17.18: A giant osteochondroma from left second rib.

Fig. 17.19: Same patient (**Fig. 17.18**) with the growth weighing 9.5 kg on his head after its removal. Note the cut end of rib which is being pointed by the patient's left ringfinger. After removal of the growth, he became a happy cultivator.

loss of appetite, diarrhoea, numbness and tingling in hands and feet, and loss of hairs. These side effects go away after chemo-cycles are finished. Chemotherapy regimen consists of specific number of cycles given over a set period of time. Chemotherapy can be given before surgery (sometimes along with radiation therapy) to shrink a tumor it is known as ***neoadjuvant therapy***. Chemotherapy given, after surgery, to kill any cancer cells that might have been left behind, is called ***adjuvant therapy***. Chemotherapy given along with radiation therapy to kill the cancer cells that can't be removed by surgery because the cancer has grown into in to nearby important structures is called ***concurrent therapy***. Chemotherapy can be the main treatment (sometimes along with radiation therapy) for more advanced cancers and also in people who are not fit for oncosurgery. Chemo is often not recommended for patients in poor health.

Recent advances: (in radiotherapy).
Proton beam Therapy can treat tumors with high precision and safely.

In treatment of cancer, conventional radiation therapy is commonly used where X-rays deliver a high dose of radiation as they pass through and exit the body. The therapy treats tumors effectively, however it causes damage of the surrounding healthy tissues to such an extent that the patient may develop radiation-induced secondary cancers later in life.

In proton beam therapy the single beam therapy can treat tumors with high accuracy, precision and safety without any risk of exposure to unwanted radiation. Proton therapy can treat a wide range of tumors.

Proton therapy uses ionizing radiation. Protons are positively charged subatomic particles which attack the DNA of cancer calls and destroy them.

It has a finite range in tissues. When protons are delivered to the tissues, they go up to certain distance in the tissue, depending upon the imaging imparted to it in the beginning. They can be made to stop exactly where the tumor is located; and the surrounding tissues get very little radiation, unlike the X rays, most of which are delivered in the surrounding tissues before they hit the targeted tumor. Proton therapy can confine the radiation dose to the tumor with no exit door.

Proton therapy is particularly useful in treatment of cancers of spinal cord, base of skull, optic nerve preventing the complications like hearing, cognitive and visual impairments. It is very much suited for paediatrics tumor like medulloblastoma of brain. Its newer forms like pencil beam scanning are very exciting. They are ideally suited for treating various pediatric cancers, some types of brain tumors, and head neck, pelvic cancers and when patients require second time radiation.

(Based on article entitled "Beam of hope" by Mini P. Thomas: The week -2017 Oct. 29:14-15)

Targeted therapy is a new type of pharmacological therapy in which medicines target growth factors in the tumor leading to slowing the growth of cancer (mainly meant for lung cancer). This therapy does not much harm to the healthy calls.

TABLE 17.4: Diagnostic features of important (malignant) bone tumours. Primary malignant bone tumours account for less than 0.2% of all malignancies + metastatic tumours soft tissue sarcomas account for about 1% of all malignancies. On broader inclusions osteosarcoma is being observed as the second most common primary malignant bone tumour after multiple myeloma. The most common malignant bone tumours are osteosarcoma, ewings sarcoma (both generally occur in children and adolescents)and Chondrosarcoma (frequent in adults and elderly) **(Figs. 17.15, 17.16).**

	Primary osteosarcoma	Ewing's sarcoma*	Multiple myeloma	Giant cell tumour (Primary malignant bone tumors account for less than 0.2% of all malignancies +metastatic tumors)	Secondary growth (Metastatic tumours)
1	2	3	4	5	6
1. Synonyms	Osteogenic sarcoma is a systemic disease. Its incidence is 0.2% of all malignant tumours. However, it is the most common primary malignant tumour of bone accounting for about 35% of all primary malignant bone tumours (Fletcher et al.). It is a primary malignant mesenchymal bone tumour in which the malignant tumour cells directly from the osteoid or bone or both Soft tissue sarcomas account for about 1% of all malignancies on broader inclusions osteosarcoma is being observed as the second most common primary malignant bone tumor alter multiple myeloma **(Figs.17.3, 17.37, 17.38, 17.42, 17.43, 17.45, 17.53 to 17.57, 17.60 to 17.65).**	Ewing (1928) described; Endothelial myeloma, perithelioma, undifferentiated round cell sarcoma Ewing's sarcoma bone tumour arises from marrow stem cells and is one of the round cell tumor. Ewing's Sarcoma is second (first being osteosarcoma) most common primary malignant bone tumor; slight male predominance and higher incidence in the Caucasian population It is part of a spectrum of neoplastic diseases- Ewing's Sarcoma family of tumors, which includes extraosseous Ewing's Sarcoma, peripheral primitive neuroectodermal tumor, malignant small- cell tumors of the thoracopulmonary region and atypical Ewing's sarcoma	Plasma cell myeloma; Myelomatosis; Multiple myelomatosis; Monoclonal gammopathy; Plasmacytoma **(see Figs. 17.71 to 17.73A and B, 17.82, 17.86, 17.92 and 17.94)** (solitary). It is not a rare disease and accounts for about 1% of all cancer patients in United States. Incidence is four times higher in western people than Asian ones.	Giant cell tumor of bone was first described by sir Astley cooper in 1818. Giant cell tumor (GCT) Osteoclastoma; represents 5% of neoplasms of bone (Mayo clinic series) and 20% of all primary bone tumors in southeast Asian regions. Usually GCT was classified as benign lesion along with nonossifying fibroma, osteitis fibrosa cystica, chondromyxoid fibroma, aneurysmal bone cyst, chondroblastoma. It stems from neuroepithelial cells which have the ability to differentiate into various mesenchymal cells and metastasise to distant locations. Coley and Higinbotham (1936) stated that about 15% GCT become malignant and they could present with pulmonary metastasis **(Figs. 17.26, 17.27, 17.31, 17.32, 17.33, 17.35, 17.36, 17.39, 17.40, 17.43).**	• Metastatic growth. It is a catastrophic complication for most patients of cancer • Metastatic tumours are the most common malignant lesions seen in bone—seen about 40 times more than all other primary malignant bone tumour combined **(Figs. 17.80, 17.81, 17.84, 17.85, 17.86, 17.95)**
2. Age	Predilection for 2nd decade though may occur at any age	mainly in adolescents peak in 10-24 years of age.	Above 40 years	After fusion of growth plate. 3rd–4th decade	Usually elderly age group
3. Sex	Most common in males than females	More common in males **(Figs. 17.15, 17.16, 17.66A and B and 17.68 to 17.70)**	More common in males	Almost equal/or little more in females	Sex—Depending upon the nature of primary

Contd...

Bone Tumours

	Primary osteosarcoma	Ewing's sarcoma*	Multiple myeloma	Giant cell tumour (Primary malignant bone tumours account for less than 0.2% of all malignancies + metastatic tumors)	Secondary growth (Metastatic tumours)
1	2	3	4	5	6
4. Cell of origin and causative factors	Osteoblast • Exact cause not known • Defects in RB and p53 genes play important role in the process • Radiation may be causative factor • It close to the joint of a matured bone	Controversial— Possibilities: • Reticulum cells of marrow • Endothelial elements in marrow (Ewing) • Secondary from adrenal neuroblastoma (Willis) • A variant of reticulum cell sarcoma • On the whole, it is the most common malignant bone tumour with multicentric origin	• Neoplastic proliferation of cells which normally produce gamma globulins • Plasma cell Production occurs in red marrow • Multiple myeloma is a malignancy of plasma cell uncontrolled proliferation leading to excessive production of monoclonal immunoglobulins. • It is most common (>40% of primary bone cancers) primary malignant tumour of bone	Osteoclast	• Cells of parent tumour • Skeletal metastasis may be presenting feature with unknown primary tumour in about 50% of patients
5. Most common sites in bone	Metaphysis (91%)	• Diaphysis • Most common malignant tumour of long bones and flat bone–pelvis, chest, wall, spine.	• Grow over whole extent of mature bone • Of the primary malignant bone tumours, multiple myeloma is the most common	Eccentrically located in epiphyseal or epiphyseo-metaphyseal area of long bones. Mostly, it occurs as solitary lesion; very rarely may be synchronously or metachronously multicentric	Usually bone containing the red marrow are the sites of secondaries. In long bones, upper metaphyseal ends and proximal part of diaphysis are more affected than distal part bones
6. Bones affected	Lower femur, upper tibia, upper humerus, radius, ulna. Scapula, small bones (very rare). Almost 50% occur around the knee	Long bones—tibia, femur, pelvis, fibula, humerus, clavicle, also short bones, e.g. calcaneum, talus	Usually, flat bone containing red marrow—sternum, ribs, vertebrae, skull, pelvis. Long bones, extremely rare distal to knee and elbow Spine is most common	50% about the knee (upper end of tibia, lower end of femur), lower end of radius, (Third most common site of affection and 1% of which metastasise upper end of fibula, lower end of tibia, vertebrae	a. Bones affected— vertebra, pelvis, cervicotrochanter region of femur, ribs, skull, humerus, (almost negligible in below knee and below elbow bones) b. Soft tissues affected— lung, liver, lymph gland, spleen, skin, etc. Metastatic destruction of bone reduces its load-bearing capacity. Initially, there is trabecular disruption and microfractures and subsequently loss of bony integrity

	Primary osteosarcoma	Ewing's sarcoma*	Multiple myeloma	Giant cell tumour (Primary malignant bone tumors account for less than 0.2% of all malignancies +metastatic tumors)	Secondary growth (Metastatic tumours)
1	2	3	4	5	6
7. Clinical presentation —general and —local	• Pain, followed by swelling • Rapidly growing, later on cachexia, anaemia and symptoms due to mechanical pressure	Features mimic subacute osteomyelitis—pain, fever, mild swelling, pathological fracture	Generalised slowly increasing pain, weakness, progressive unexplained anaemia, pathological fracture, paraplegia, renal dysfunction	• Swelling, followed by mild pain, tumour tissue prevented from entering the joint space by even thinned out articular cartilage, but may affect joint movements mechanically • May be pathological fracture	Usually manifests as complications like pathological fracture, paraplegia (Medullary compression due to vertebral metastasis may present in 5% of patients with skeletal metastasis) pressure symptoms besides pain, pallor and cachexia Symptoms due to hypercalcaemia, which is present in 10% of patients with skeletal metastasis
8. Salient features	Warm, fusiform swelling with variegated feel, highly vascular, near by joint free except in affections due to mechanical reasons, pathological fractures, features of metastasis. Swelling tender (more at margin)	Fusiform, warm, firm, mildly tender, diaphyseal swelling	Rarely presents as mild swelling, e.g. in clavicle, upper end of the femur and rib. Generalised tenderness specially of the flat bones, e.g. rib, sternum, pelvis, scapula, etc.	Eccentric swelling, hard to firm in feel, slightly warm, nearby joint may be affected, egg-shell crackling. GCT is notorious for its locally aggressive behavior and tendency to recur.	• Usually, comparatively less warm than primary tumour • Diffuse swelling, no respect for joint
9. Vascularity	Mostly high, even may be pulsating, e.g. in malignant bone aneurysm	Moderate to severe	Mild to moderate	Low grade, except when it turns frankly malignant, when vascularity increases proportionately	Vascularity depends upon nature of primary growth but comparatively less
10. Regional lymph nodes	Occasionally enlarged	Moderately to severely enlarged	May or may not be enlarged.	May be enlarged but in very few cases (about 7%)	Regional gland usually involved
11. Possible sites of metastasis	Lung (diffuse bronchitis, cough, fever, haemoptysis)	Lungs, skull, other bones	• Dissemination to different bones is controversial • Perhaps never settles in lung • May block the renal tubules by protein casts	All growths expand locally Frankly malignant ones may metastasise to lung in 1 to 2% patients with good prognosis although 25% of patients die from the disease (Sung HW 1980)	Itself a metastatic tumour

	Primary osteosarcoma	Ewing's sarcoma*	Multiple myeloma	Giant cell tumour (Primary malignant bone tumors account for less than 0.2% of all malignancies +metastatic tumors)	Secondary growth (Metastatic tumours)
1	2	3	4	5	6
12. Investigations general	• Nothing significant; ESR raised • Molecular biology of cells helps to improve the chemotherapy agents • Biopsy—which confirms the diagnosis, reveals specific type and grade of tumour,—should be done at treating centre by the chief of treating team or under his/her guidance and presence • It must be done after imaging investigations	Leucocytosis even with moderate increase in polymorphonuclear count, confusing picture with subacute osteomyelitis	• Normocytic and normochromic anaemia, microcytic and hypochromic anaemia when there is bleeding, haemoglobin level is lowered, ESR is raised; increased total serum protein • Routine examination of urine—30% cases may show Bence Jones protein; albuminuria and casts because of renal involvement • Bone marrow aspirate must be examined and it should be supplemented by examination of M-protein in plasma and in urine Hypercalcaemia and elevated serum creatinine levels are important complication in multiple myeloma	Nothing significant	Macrocytic hypochromic anaemia, ESR raised
13. Imaging-investigations: • X-ray provides the best clue; • MRI delineates the local extent; • Thorax CT to detect lung metastasis • Tc 99 bone scan to detect bone metastasis	• X-ray shows: Increased soft tissue shadow, sun-ray spicules, Codman's reactive triangle, corticomedullary delineation maintained, evidence of bone destruction and bone formation, respect to joint,—no penetration into joint • MRI, CT (chest and local lesion) and PET (positron emission tomography) help to decide surgical decisions and extent of surgical excision	In X-ray: Expansion of diaphyseal medulla (destructive enlargement) by cystic destruction, onion-peel appearance, mainly due to reactionary sub-periosteal bone formation	In X-ray: Round punched out clear cut areas in a number of bones without any surrounding reactive sclerosis	• In X-ray: Cortical expansion, growth traversed with multiple septae giving soap-bubble appearance; may be breach in the thinned out cortex; about 25% may break into joint. Usually expanded growth margin is sharply demarcated from normal marrow but with malignant transformation this sharpness is not obvious and thin septae area also less visible giving a homogenous ground glass appearance • In MRI, usually the lesion is dark on T1-weighted images, and bright on T2-weighted images	• In X-ray: Irregular, distorted lytic lesions (see Figs. 17.80A and B) except secondaries from prostate or scirrhous carcinoma of breast, stomach, etc. • Skeletal metastasis can be lytic (increased resorption of bone), sclerotic (increased production of bone) and permeative (multiple small lytic destruction in cortical bone) • The prostatic cancer normally causes sclerotic metastasis, whereas breast cancer normally gives rise to lytic metastasis • In a lytic lesion, at least half of the trabecular structure must be destroyed before it can be detected in plane X-ray

	Primary osteosarcoma	Ewing's sarcoma*	Multiple myeloma	Giant cell tumour (Primary malignant bone tumors account for less than 0.2% of all malignancies +metastatic tumors)	Secondary growth (Metastatic tumours)
1	2	3	4	5	6
14. Naked eye appearance	Greyish white tumour which does not transgress the cartilage of epiphysis. In mature bones, it extends up to the end, but does not penetrate the articular cartilage; variegated appearance, soft, fleshy, vascular with areas of haemorrhage and necrosis	Greyish-white, firm from outside	Soft grey tumour of marrow, multiple circumscribed areas of destruction of marrow, pure rarefying lesion, no new bone formation, later marrow cavity filled with tumour tissue	Tumour is encapsulated, firm to hard in feel except when soft tissue is invaded, where it may even be soft	Irregular variably nodular surface with firm to soft or cystic feel
15. Cut section	Cuts with gritty or variegated feel, greyish-white, variegated look or cut section presents fleshy to sinusoidal appearance	Cuts with soft feel—resembling cutting of brain tissue; or very soft cake; areas of necrosis and haemorrhage with cyst formation; necrotic lamellae (cf. osteomyelitis)	Presents localised or multiple honey-combed appearance In one variety known as chloroma, cut surface turns green (due to a pigment), which gradually fades off	Cuts with gritty sensation Multiloculated maroon-coloured cut surface	Cuts with gritty sensation, cut surfaces present look mimicking the primary growth
16. Histological examination a. Dominant cells (mostly seen in peripheral zone)	Most frequently seen cells are small spindle-shaped with hyperchromatic nuclei Pleomorphism—cells may be polyhexoid, round, cuboidal or columnar, variously arranged in—band, pallisade, columns; multinucleated giant cells, even osteoclast type of cells	Markedly cellular, almost no intercellular substance, Cells—round or polyhedral, uniform cytoplasm, indistinct in appearance (cellular monotony), arranged in cords or sheets, may be arranged around central blood vessels/spaces giving angioendotheliomatous appearance—pseudorosette (cf. in true rosette, cells are arranged around central core of neurofibrils), nuclei—prominent and round	Cellular tumour. Plasma cells with abundant cytoplasm, and eccentrically placed nucleus, i.e. typical cart-wheel nucleus, with abnormal features (no perinuclear halo, and polychrome methylene blue stain negative)	Histological grading (I, II, and III) of not much value unless, biopsy material obtained from different sites. Dominant cells—oval-shaped stromal cells containing small, elongated darkly stained nucleus; stroma cells may manifest features of malignancy Osteoclastomatous giant cells with multiple centrally placed nuclei—usually 40–60, may be even 100 in number (cf. In tuberculosis—in Langhans giant cell, nuclei are peripherally arranged, about 20 in numbers; in foreign body giant cell—usually less than 15 centrally placed variously sized nuclei)	Similar to parent growth

Contd...

	Primary osteosarcoma	Ewing's sarcoma*	Multiple myeloma	Giant cell tumour (Primary malignant bone tumors account for less than 0.2% of all malignancies +metastatic tumors)	Secondary growth (Metastatic tumours)
1	2	3	4	5	6
b. Matrix	In osteosclerotic type—extensive irregular new osteoid and bone with few stromal cell. In osteolytic type—blood containing spaces without endothelial lining lying in anaplastic stromal and necrotic cystic areas. Usually scanty may be myxomatous, cartilaginous, osteoid, fibromatous	Almost no matrix	Almost no matrix	Scanty, fibrous tissue	
c. Vascular pattern	Blood vessels are numerous and thin walled, may be lined with cells	—	—	Mild or moderate	
17. Special features if any	—	Rosette arrangement—pseudorosette are common, osteoclasts never found	—	—	
18. Mode of metastasis	• Direct to surrounding soft tissues • Along medullary canal • Lymphatics • Blood vessels—emboli • Skip metastasis—direct along the medullary canal • Distant metastasis to lungs, other bones or even to soft tissues to other region, e.g. chest wall	Direct along medullary canal, Via lymphatics—lymph nodes; Via blood vessels—to other bones (skull, vertebrae, ribs), lung	Through blood vessels principally to other bones; to internal organs like liver, spleen, pulmonary metastasis only in 1–2% almost **never to lungs**	Direct to surrounding tissue, also through blood vessels, lymphatics; pulmonary metastasis only in 1–2% with good prognosis, although up to 25% of patients die from the disease (Sung et al 1982)	—
19. Radiosensitivity	Radioresistant in average doses, may respond to higher doses	Highly radiosensitive, but reappears soon after	With irradiation tumour responds markedly but reappears	Moderately sensitive	As primary tumour
20. Complication	Huge growth, pathological fracture, metastasis, malignant cachexia	Distant metastasis, cachexia, pathological fracture	Anaemia, bacterial infection, paraplegia, pathological fracture, renal damage, amyloidosis in 10% cases	Joint affection, frank malignant transformation, (about 10%), pathological fracture	Pathological fracture, pressure symptoms

Contd...

	Primary osteosarcoma	Ewing's sarcoma*	Multiple myeloma	Giant cell tumour (Primary malignant bone tumors account for less than 0.2% of all malignancies +metastatic tumours)	Secondary growth (Metastatic tumours)
1	2	3	4	5	6
21. Chemotherapeutic sensitivity & allied treatment if any. With cisplatin, Adriamycin, Ifosfamide chemotherapy (PAI regimen) overall survival in pediatric osteosarcoma patients appears good, however, disease free survival even for localized disease calls for much improvement in overall treatment and alternative chemotherapy regimens.	Definite role[1] Multiagent chemotherapy—methotrexate in high doses, doxorubicin and cisplatin. More recent protocols include Iphosphamide with or without etoposide[2]	Successful regimen have used combinations of vincristine, actinomycin D, doxorubicin and cyclophosphamide Iphosphamide, etoposide	Chemotherapy by melphalan (alone or with prednisolone) and cyclophosphamide has increased survival rate. Chemotherapy with Bortezomib, steroid and cyclophosphamide has further increased survival rate	Nothing specific. Zalendronic acid affects osteoclasts and stromal cells in GCT and thereby reduces recurrence rate. It accelerates fibrosis and calcification, thus providing better marginalization for extended curettage Kundo et al. 2018	As primary growth
22. Special investigation	As in Chapter 1: Introduction Alkaline phosphatase—raised	As in chapter on Introduction To distinguish from reticulum cell sarcoma—PAS positive diastase soluble glycogen granules in cytoplasm of cells of Ewing's sarcoma	• Serum calcium raised, hyperproteinaemia (serum protein rising to 10 g/liter, or higher). Distorted serum electrophoretic pattern with marked inversion of albumin/globulin ratio. Demonstration of monoclonal paraproteinaemia • Low/normal alkaline phosphatase in spite of bony destruction • In 5% of cases—Bence Jones protein in urine (this is also seen in leucaemia, skeletal carcinomatosis, nephritis). Red cells—rouleaux formation in blood and in marrow • ESR high	Acid phosphatase raised Receptor activator nuclear kappB ligand (RANKL) expression is generally high in GCT-B-III (is known to have higher risk of local recurrence and pulmonary metastasis Sung et al 1982) which correlates with aggressiveness of the disease. Thus RANKL may be one of the reliable prognostic markers in predicting risk of local recurrence in GCT-B-III BUT not lung metastasis (Ghani et al. 2018)	Estimation of acid phosphatase or alkaline phosphatase. Increased acid phosphatase usually seen in secondaries from prostate

	Primary osteosarcoma	Ewing's sarcoma*	Multiple myeloma	Giant cell tumour (Primary malignant bone tumors account for less than 0.2% of all malignancies +metastatic tumors)	Secondary growth (Metastatic tumours)
1	2	3	4	5	6
23. Survival rate (more than 5 years)	• Patients with localised osteosarcoma with adequate chemotherapy—50-76% • Patients with metastatic lesions—excision of primary tumour + wedge resection of lung lesions + chemotherapy— 20-40%. Overall cure rate is 55-70% • Multimodal intensive chemotherapy adjuvant regimens provide disease-free survival rates to approximately 60-80% in non metastatic localised tumour. (The rate in early 20th century was <20%) • Improved attention to the long term care of sarcoma patients will allow them to survive and thrive despite the aggressiveness of their treatment protocols (Weiss & Zimel 2018)	Multimodal therapy (Intensive combination of chemotherapy + radiotherapy) of non-pelvic Ewing's sarcoma —50-70%. 5% survival rates—about 70% in those with localized disease and 33% in those with overt metastasis.	Variable (2-10 years). Bad prognostic features: Raised serum protein more than 10 g/L; Bence Jones proteinuria; Involvement of vertebrae, kidney; severe anaemia; severe reversal of AG ratio with timely aggressive treatment may be even more than 60%. In vast majority of cases, death occurs within 3 to 5 years.	Improved attention to the long term care of sarcoma patients with allows them to survive and thrive despite the aggressiveness of their treatment protocols. (Weiss & Zimel 2018) Of all the malignancies of the bone, this has the best prognosis	Depending upon nature of primary growth but usually less than 10%
24. Differential diagnosis	• Among the primary and secondary malignant bone tumours • Subacute and chronic osteomyelitis; synovioma	• Neuroblastoma (vanillylmandelic acid in urine— VMA) • Reticulum cell sarcoma (silver stain positive reticular fibres)	Unexplained anaemias; Polycystic disease of bone in elderly; senile osteoporosis; secondary carcinoma	Earlier cystic lesions of bones; lesions containing tumour giant cell (**Fig. 17.90**): • **Aneurysmal bone** cyst–It was first described and named in 1942 by Jaffe and Lichtenstein It affects the metaphysis of long bones (and posterior elements of vertebrae) of children and adolescents, more in males. It is an osteolytic, blood filled, expansile, sponge like tumor containing numerous giant calls, and present eccentrically in the metaphysis. Fluid levels are often seen due to previous hemorrhage. MRI is usually diagnostic. Radio logically a centrally or eccentrically lytic lesion without matrix and a thin shell of reactive periosteal bone.	

1	Primary osteosarcoma	Ewing's sarcoma*	Multiple myeloma	Giant cell tumour (Primary malignant bone tumors account for less than 0.2% of all malignancies +metastatic tumors)	Secondary growth (Metastatic tumours)
2	2	3	4	5	6
25. Surgery Limb saving surgery (LSS) is feasible in majority of pediatric osteosarcoma, albeit local recurrence may occur in variable cases. After resection of the tumors affected bone re-construction can be done by autograft (e.g. nonvascular-ized or vascularized fibular graft); using a composite of an allograft and prosthesis; sequential controlled bone transportation by Ilizarov technique; Recently, interest is increasing in using the patient's own tumor bone and replacing it after it has been sterilized by autoclaving, or microwave or pas-teurizing, or liquid nitrogen or extracorporeal radiotherapy.	• Disarticulation • Amputation (being favoured based upon concept of tumour immunity) • Resection with reconstruction/endoprosthesis calcium sulphate pellets • Resection of metastatic lesion (lobectomy in lung) • Limb preservation (limb salvage). Limb salvage consists of successful to safe margin resection of a tumour and reconstruction of a viable functional extremity. Improvements in prosthesis (light weight, strong, inert material, modular prosthesis) help limb salvage. Limb salvage surgery with end prosthesis reconstruction around the knee provide good functional outcome both objectively and subjectively, as observed by the symmetrical gait pattern and significant correlation with musculoskeletal score. (Sigh VA et al 2018)	• Radiotherapy followed by resection and reconstruction in very early case (still prognosis poor) • Postoperative radiotherapy is debatable. In surgical excision the adequacy of surgical margins and the amount of chemotherapy induced necrosis should be the parameters to decide to add post-operative radiotherapy.	Only for complications, e.g. for pathological fractures; paraplegia	• **Solitary Bone Cyst** – (also called simple or unicameral bone cyst). It usually occurs in the metaphysial region of humerus and femur of children (1st s 2nd decade) as osteolytic expansile lesion containing serous or serosanguinous fluid, and causing thinning of cortex, which may lead to fracture. • **Eosinophilic granuloma** It is multisystem disease occurring in second and third decades, affecting the epiphyses in the long bones and geographical lesions in skull and spine • **Fibrousdysplasia(seeFigs. 17.20AtoC)** It may be monostotic or polyostotic. Long bones, pelvis and skull are usually affected. Classically it presents as a ground glass medullary lesion, however, cortical blisters may be seem Thorough curettage with/without filling with acrylic cement (polymethyl-methacrylate-PMMA) or bone grafting or calcium sulphate pellets. Recurrence is about 30% within 2 years. Excision of growth with or without reconstruction (e. g. For GCT of distal end of radius en block excision and reconstruction with ipsilateral fibular graft vascularize or nor vascularized) and centralization of ulna or fusion of the neighbouring joint or endoprosthetic replacement. • Amputation • Cryosurgery (curettage + liquid nitrogen cryotherapy)	Total excision with/ without reconstruction and replacement can prolong comparatively comfortable life under cover of radiotherapy, hormonal therapy and chemotherapy

Contd...

Bone Tumours

	Primary osteosarcoma	Ewing's sarcoma*	Multiple myeloma	Giant cell tumour (Primary malignant bone tumors account for less than 0.2% of all malignancies +metastatic tumors)	Secondary growth (Metastatic tumours)
1	2	3	4	5	6
	observed that the combined use of a vascularised fibular graft and allograft is of value as a limb salvage procedure for intercalary, reconstruction after resection of bone tumours around the knee, especially in skeletally immature patients				
26. Radiotherapy	—Only for inaccessible or inoperable lesion. To be given in higher doses	Tumour almost dissolves with radiotherapy but recurrence is the rule	Mainly palliative	Only for inaccessible region and unoperable lesions, e.g. vertebrae	Depending upon nature of primary tumour
27. Possible ideal treatment	Neoadjuvant (preoperative induction of chemotherapy) multiagent chemotherapy with limb preservation surgery	Trials of multimodal therapy consisting of intensive combination of chemotherapy and radiotherapy	Chemotherapy, palliative irradiation	Excision and reconstruction	Treatment of the primary growth, radiotherapy for secondaries, and suitable chemotherapy
28. Any genetic relation—The genetic basis for some tumors can't be denied, if one considers the increased incidence of bone sarcomas in patients with hereditary retinoblastoma. Or patients with Li-fraumeni syndrome. The genetic basis of these tumors is based on the concept of oncogenes, tumor suppressor genes and mutation.	• Price (1958) (**Figs. 17.22 and 17.29**) noted significant similarity between osteochondroma and osteogenic sarcoma regarding male predominance, peak incidence between 15–20 years, and anatomical distribution • This is of interest because of hereditary background shown by osteochondroma	Nothing particular	Nothing particular	Nothing particular	In recent years, there has been significant improvement in the prognosis of patients with bone metastasis, mainly due to advances in chemotherapy and hormonal treatment Postoperative radiotherapy should be considered in all cases once initial wound healing occurs after reconstructive surgery

Primary osteosarcoma	Ewing's sarcoma*	Multiple myeloma	Giant cell tumour (Primary malignant bone tumors account for less than 0.2% of all malignancies +metastatic tumors)	Secondary growth (Metastatic tumours)
2	3	4	5	6
29. Subclassification (based on WHO classification 2013) (based on WHO				

Aetiological:
1. Primary osteosarcoma, which can be of following types:
(a) intramedullary/central high grade (most common)—subtyped as:
  – Osteoblastic (50%)
  – Chondroblastic (25%)
  – Fibroblastic (25%)
(b) Surface osteosarcomas (3–6% of all osteosarcomas)—subtyped as:
  – Parosteal (least malignant followed by periosteal and high-grade surface osteosarcoma. It can be treated by surgical excision without neo-adjuvant chemotherapy unlike high-grade lesion and even periosteal one)
  – Periosteal
  – Adequate removal of tumor is more predictive for the outcome of surgery than the use of adjuvants.
  – High-grade surface
(c) Small cell
(d) Telangiectatic (purely lytic lesion)
(e) Low-grade central
2 Secondary osteosarcoma on:
• Paget's disease
• Osteochondroma
			Campanacci radiological grading of giant cell tumors
			
			| Grade
				Radiological Finding

---	---
I	Well defined border of a thin rim of mature bone
II	Bony cortex is intact Well-defined margins
III	Radiopaque cortical rim absent Fuzzy borders.		Secondary tumors can be subdivided into: • Metastatic tumours • Tumours developing by contiguous spread of adjacent soft tissue tumours. • Malignant transformation of preexisting benign tumours.

Contd...

	Primary osteosarcoma	Ewing's sarcoma*	Multiple myeloma	Giant cell tumour (Primary malignant bone tumors account for less than 0.2% of all malignancies +metastatic tumors)	Secondary growth (Metastatic tumours)
1	2	3	4	5	6
30. Immuno-therapy	• Chronic osteomyelitis • Post-irradiation osteosarcoma in ankylosing spondylitis • Immunological approach for managing lethal metastasis is still in experimental stage • Osteosarcoma has been shown to possess specific tumour associated antigens				

The *primary soft-tissue sarcomas* are a rare heterogeneous group of tumors arising in connective tissues embryologically derived from the mesenchyme, and there are many their subtypes arising from cartilage, muscle, blood vessels, nerves and fat. They are best managed by multidisciplinary teams in specialist sarcoma referral centers (Ante D et al 2018. Their morbidity and mortality rates have significantly reduced due to advances in diagnostic modalities, adjuvant therapies and surgical techniques.

* **Ewing's Family of Tumours:** Ewing's family of tumours comprises a spectrum with Ewing's tumour as an undifferentiated form at one end and Primitive Neuroectodermal Tumours (PNET) at the differentiated end. At the time of diagnosis these tumours are often micrometastatic. Without chemotherapy long-term result was poor with a 5-year survival rate less than 20%. With the multimodality treatment (chemotherapy, surgery, and radiotherapy) the overall long-term survival now approaches to 60–80% or even more.

Note:
1. **Use of multiagent chemotherapy** has substantially improved the outcome, however, more than 30% of the tumour cells still appear to be resistant to current chemotherapy regimen. Chemotherapy remains the chief factor in obtaining local control, in improving the survival and curing the patients.
2. **COSS (German-Austrian Swiss Cooperative Osteosarcoma Study Group) protocols** include doxorubicin high dose of methotrexate (MTX), Cyclophosphamide, and additionally in different combinations bleomycin, dactinomycin, vincristine, cisplatin and iphosphambil. It is claimed to be more effective.

After discontinuation of chemotherapy DXA (dual-energy X-ray absorptiometry) measurement should be performed, and in case of lower BMD, antiosteoporotic treatment should be instituted.

Note:
*Irradiated autograft prosthesis composites reduces the complications of ECIR (Extra Corporeal irradiation of the resected specimen and reimplantation), helps in achieving predictable healing at the site of osteotomy and gives good functional results. It may be a good alternative to limb-salvage surgery, especially in countries (such as Asian) where it is difficult to obtain allograft. In skeletally immature patients, the irradiated autologous proximal femoral bone combined with distal femoral replacement may prove useful.

Limb salvage in tumour surgery includes resection-arthrodesis with autografts or allografts; resection-reconstruction; resection-endoprosthetic replacement; rotation plasty; bone transport technique, e.g. by Ilizarov method, and arthroplasty using allografts.

On the whole **limb-salvage procedure** is relatively safe in osteosarcoma treated by neoadjuvant chemotherapy. However, they should only be performed in institutions, where there is adequate provision to accurately assess the margins of surgical excision and the histological response to chemotherapy. If the margins are inadequate and the histological response to chemotherapy is poor, immediate amputation at proper level should be the choice. The 'surgical margin' is the least adequate margin (for excision) of the whole specimen. These margins may be (1) *'radical'* (if all the bone and muscles involved are removed as one block); (2) *'wide'* (if the lesion, its reactive zone, and a surrounding cuff of normal tissue are removed as a single block); (3) *'marginal'* (if the plane of dissection leaves microscopic disease at the margin of the wound; (4) *'intralesional'* (if the dissection passes within the lesion) (Bucci G et al. 2002).

Preservation surgery must be preceded by neoadjuvant chemotherapy, which not only serves as the immediate treatment of tumour micrometastasis, but also has the ability to shrink the primary tumour. This can make tumour margin more definable and simplify the surgery.

Caffeine potentiated chemotherapy is highly effective by virtue of its DNA-repair-inhibiting effects.

Note: Giant Cell Tumour of tendon sheath [Synonyms: nodular tenosynovitis, localised villonodular synovitis, fibrous histiocytoma of the synovium, GCT-TS] is a solitary benign Slow growing soft tissue tumour—presenting as a localised tumour arising from the complex of the tendon sheath, or soft tissue e.g. paratenon periarticular soft tissues of small joints of hands and feet. The lesions contain fibroblasts, macrophages, including collections of foamy macrophages and scattered macrophages, polykaryons and deposits of haemosiderin. GCT-TS is differentiated from pigmented villonodular synovitis, which usually arises from the synovial membrane of a joint. Localized tenosynovial giant cell tumor (TSGST) was described by Chassaignac in 1852, as nodular swelling in flexor tendon of finger. Dater Jaffe et al, first coined the term pigmented villonodular synovitis in 1941 a condition with affects synovial membrane of joints, tendon sheaths or bursae. A diffuse type tenosynovial giant call tumor is also known as an extra articular form of pigmented villonodular synovitis. GCT-TS occurs most commonly in the fingers (about 75%) and less so in the ankle and foot. In about 20% of cases there may be history of trauma. Plane X-ray, CT, MRI help in detecting the suspected lesions. The lesion presents as a slow growing painless firm mass. There may be about 10% associated bony involvement. Total excision should be the treatment since there may be recurrence in about 25% of incompletely excised tumours.

In 2013, the WHO defined tenosynovial giant cell tumor (TGCT). After unification of giant cell tumor of tendon sheath and pigmented villnodular synovitis (PVNS), as a benign monoarticular disease arising from the synovial lining of joints, bursae or tendon sheath in predominantly young adults. (Quoted by Mast boom MJL et al 2019)

Few Cystic Lesions of Bone deserve attention as neoplasms; such as:

Name	Age & sex	Common sites	Clinical presentation	X-ray/Image appearances	Histology	Broad lines of treatment
Aneurysmal bone cyst (ABC) Exact cause not known Probably it results from local circulatory disturbance leading to increased venous pressure and local haemorrahage. ABCs are locally aggressive lesions which are notorious to recur.	• 1st and 2nd decade • Comparatively more in females	• Proximal part of humerus • Distal region of femur • Proximal part of tibia • Spine-mainly in posterior elements (Management is difficult as it involves resection and reconstruction of involved portion.	• Pain dull in character • Vague swelling • Local tenderness • Pathological fracture	• Eccentrically expanded lytic lesion • The cortical shell visible • MRI shows fluid-fluid level	• Haemorrhagic cavernous space • Fibroblastic septae • Haemosiderin laden macrophages • Multinucleated giant cells • Histiocytes	• Extended curettage and filling with bone graft substitute. Detail radiological evaluation is mandatory for meticulous planning of surgery • In extensive lesion and pelvic lesions preoperative embolization facilitates by reducing tumor vascularity. Local adjuvant therapy decreases the chances of recurrence • Radiation therapy for recurrent inoperable and inaccessible ones
Unicameral bone cyst • Exact cause not known • May be a focal defect in metaphyseal remodelling which blocks interstitial fluid drainage	Ist and 2nd decade, more in males	Proximal part of humerus • Proximal region of femur	• Mostly asymptomatic or dull ache • Pathological fracture	• Concentrically expanded intact cortex with central lytic lesion	Cyst filled with pale straw coloured fluid lining of cyst is thin fibrovascular	• Wait and watch as it may heal itself • Aspiration of cyst • Intracystic injection of steroids, bone marrow, bone graft substitute
Intraosseous ganglion cyst • Probably these are intraosseous extension of overlying soft tissue ganglia	Usually middle-aged men	Ends of long bones—mainly distal end of tibia; lower end of femur, upper end of tibia	Local dull pain	In X-ray and MRI-unilocular or multilocular well-defined lytic lesion with sclerotic bone margin		If symptomatic, the overlying soft tissue ganglion to be excised and bony lesion to be curetted
Epidermoid cyst of bone resemble inclusion cysts of skin		Mostly in skull bones; Phalanges of fingers (usually traumatic		Rarefied lesion surrounded by sclerotic bone	Cysts filled with keratinous material and lined with flattened squamous epithelium	

Note: After Robert KH Jr & Patrick C Toy—In Campbell's Operative Orthopaedics, 12th Ed. Elsevier/mosby; 2013.P862.
In onco surgery wide exposures is essential which can be achieved by S-incision **(Fig. 17.93)**.

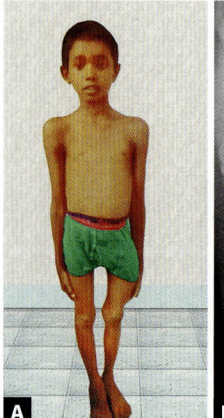 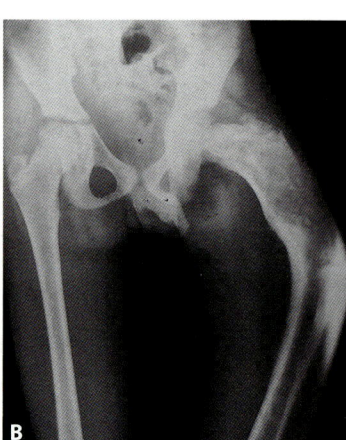 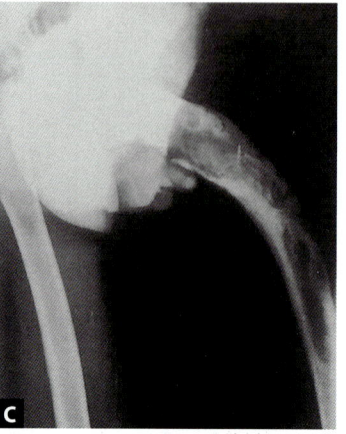 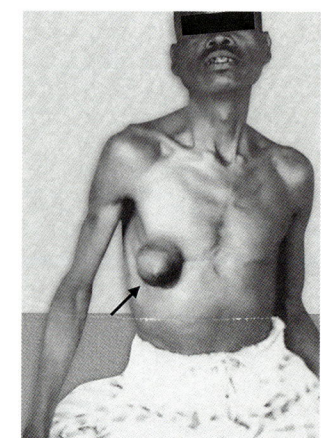

Figs. 17.20A to C: Fibrous dysplasia—pathological fracture malunion—Bowling thigh.

Fig. 17.21: A ball like osteochondrosarcoma from ninth rib.

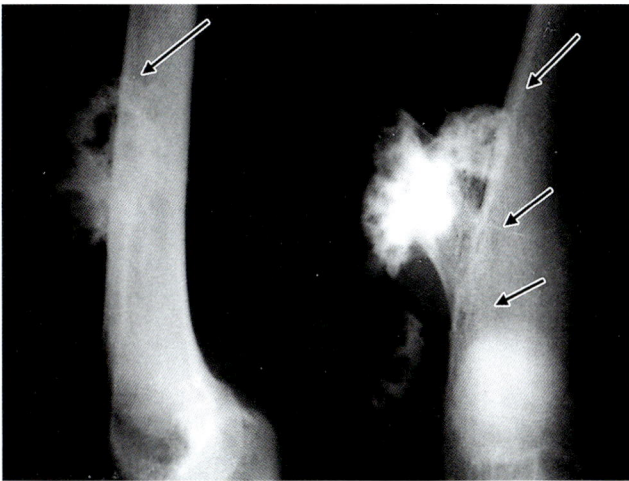

Fig. 17.22: Solitary exostosis (osteochondroma) from lower diaphysis of femur.

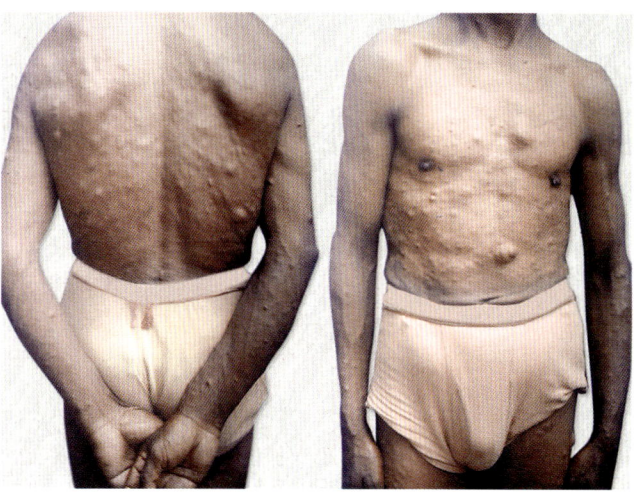

Fig. 17.25: Extensive multiple neurofibromatosis.

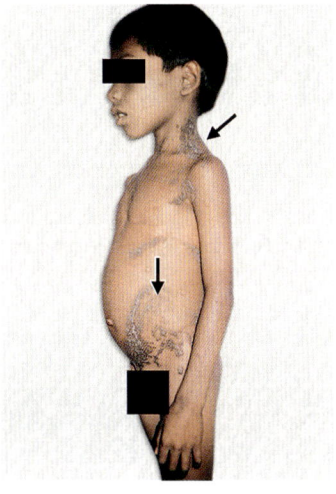

Fig. 17.23: Haemangiomatous streaks and discolouring patches on left side of body from neck to thigh.

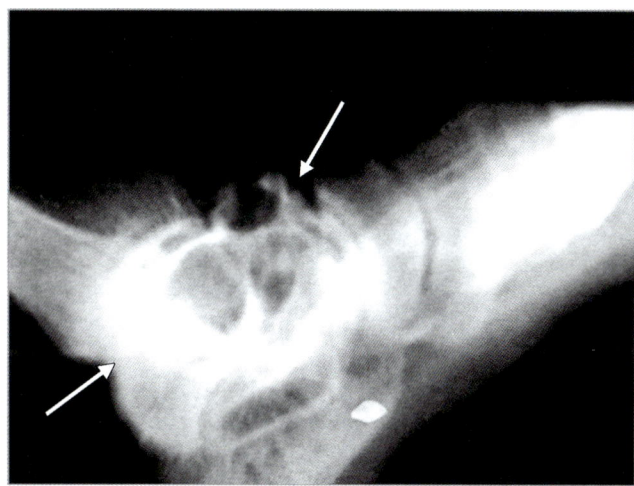

Fig. 17.26: Giant cell tumour in talus.

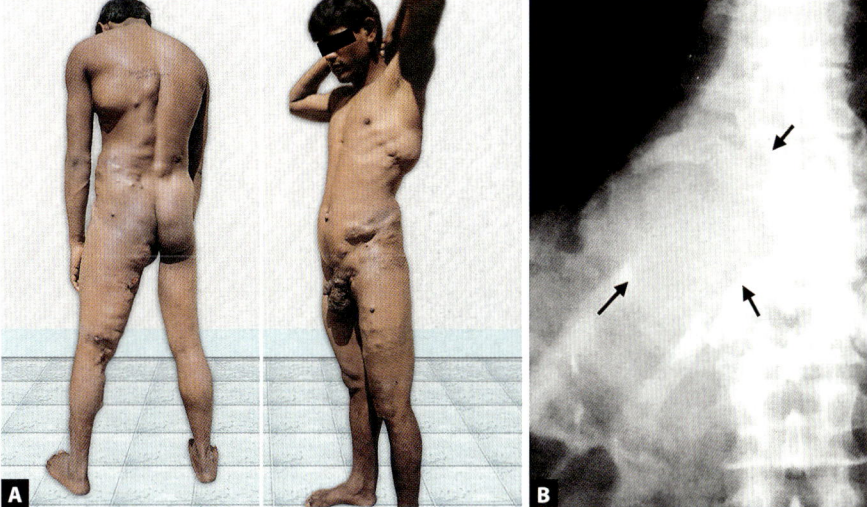

Figs. 17.24A and B: (A) Extensive large vessels haemangioma; (B) Haemangioma of vertebrae extending into the ribs.

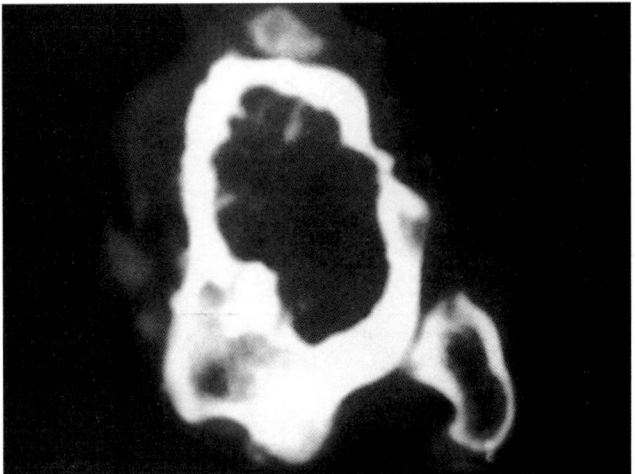

Fig. 17.27: CT scan of the same patient (**Fig. 17.26**) with giant cell tumour of the talus.

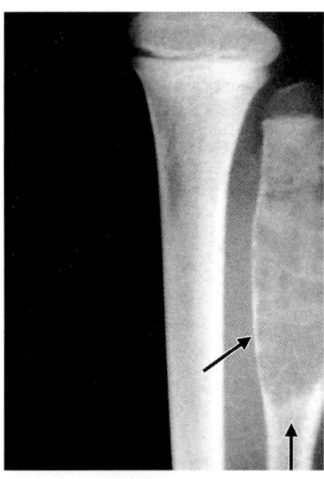

Fig. 17.30: Fibrous dysplasia from upper end of fibula.

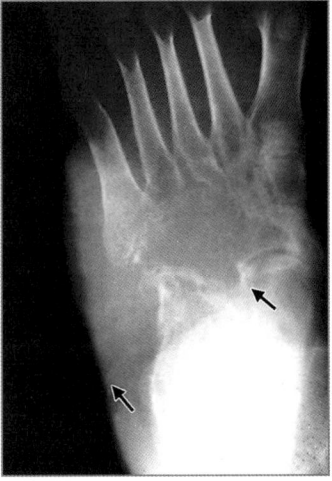

Fig. 17.28: Haemangiosarcoma mainly affecting the cuneiforms and cuboid.

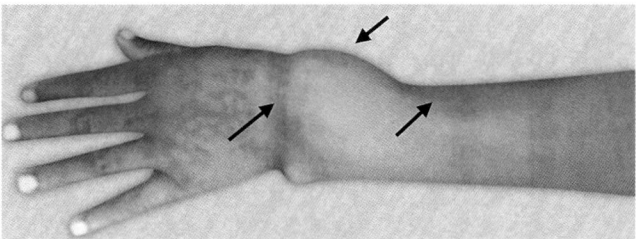

Fig. 17.31: Typical giant cell tumour of lower end of radius—eccentric growth.

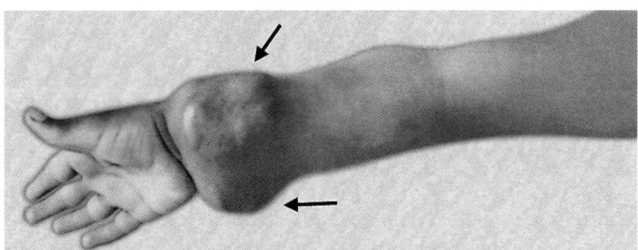

Fig. 17.32: A malignant giant cell tumour from lower end of radius, which also involved lower end of ulna.

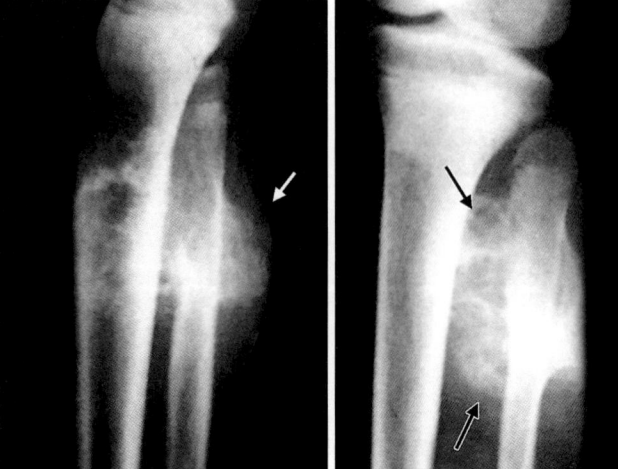

Fig. 17.29: Solitary exostosis (osteochondroma) from upper end of fibula producing mechanical pressure leading to paralysis of lateral popliteal nerve. Effective Treatment of such tumors (and lesions as in **Figure 17.30 and 17.44**) is proximal fibulectomy, however, one must be very cautious about the lateral popliteal nerve and trifurcation of popliteal artery as posterior tibial, anterior tibial and peroneal arteries.

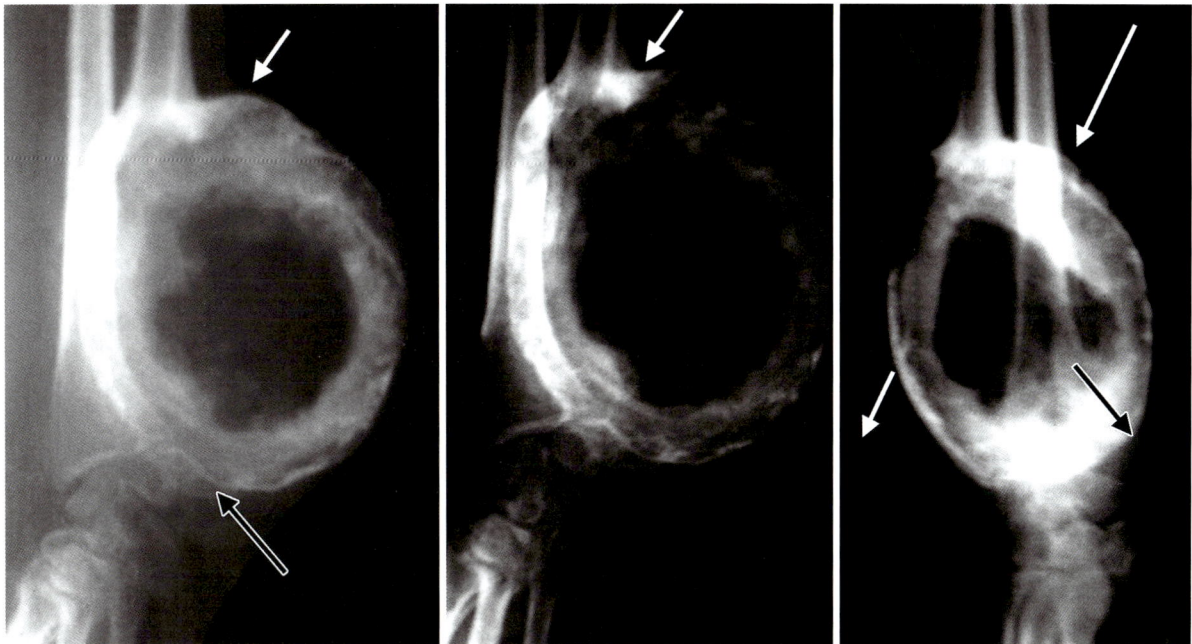

Fig. 17.33: X-ray of wrist region showing peculiarly presenting giant cell tumour from lower end of radius.

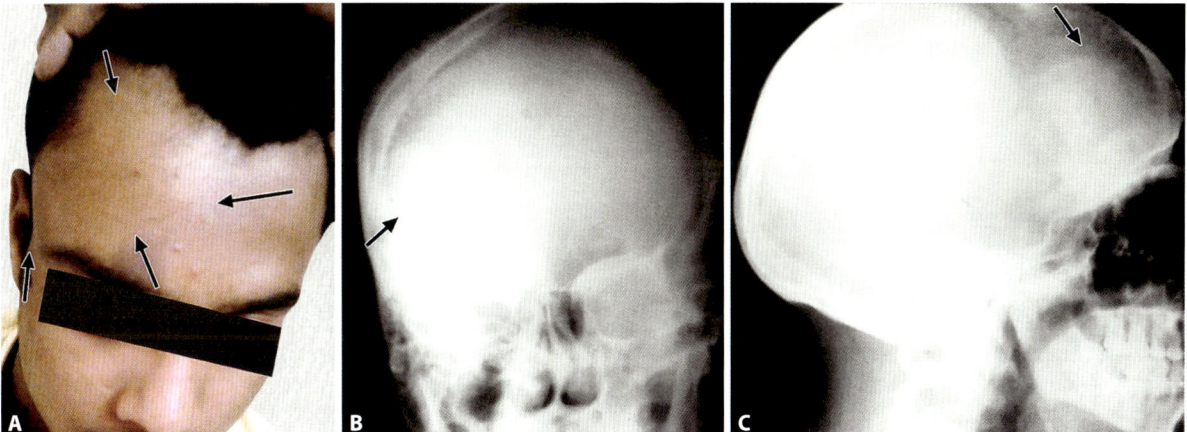

Figs. 17.34A to C: (A) Osteoid osteoma in frontal bone; (B) AP view X-ray of skull; (C) Lateral view X-ray of same patient **(Fig. 17.34A)**.

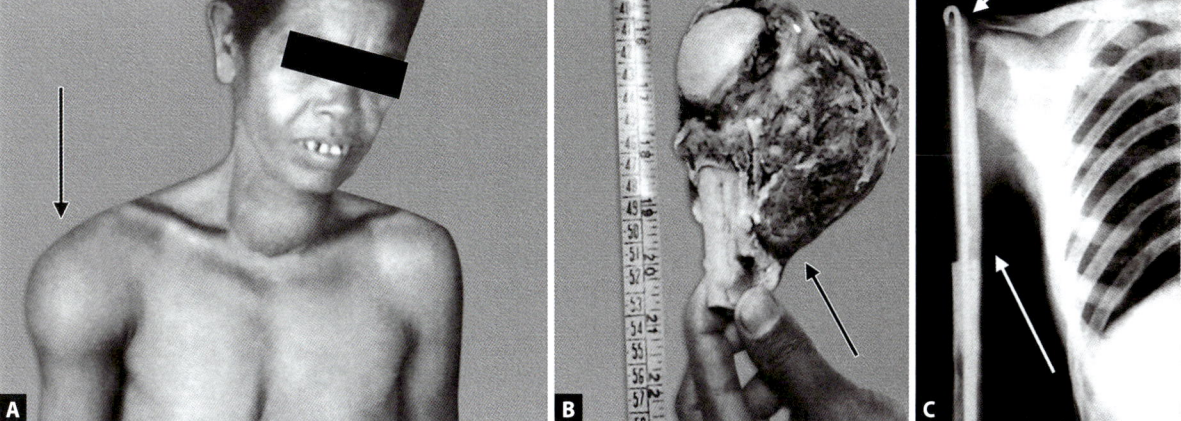

Figs. 17.35A to C: (A) Malignant giant cell tumour from upper end of humerus; (B) The growth was totally excised with the upper 2/5th of humerus; and (C) The deficiency of the humerus was reconstructed by the ipsilateral fibula.

552 Bone Tumours

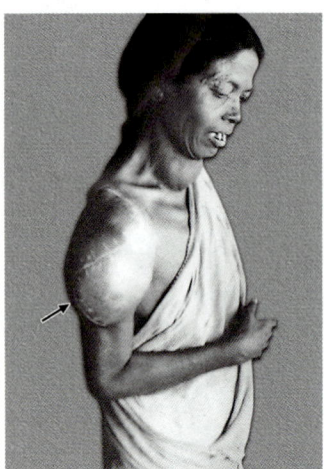

Fig. 17.36: Recurrence of tumour after 27 months of operative excision (same patient—**Figs. 17.35A to C**).

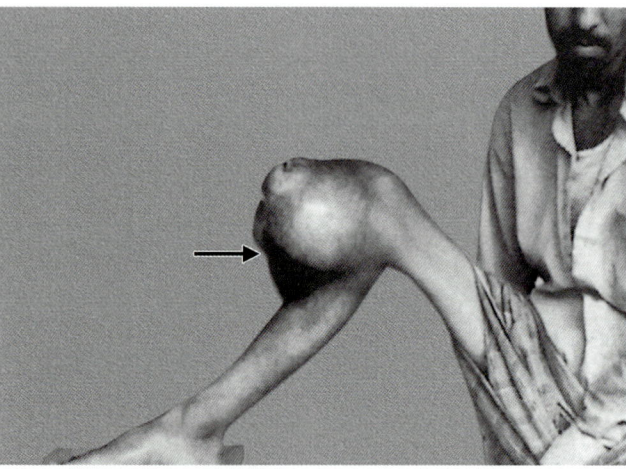

Fig. 17.39: Huge giant cell tumour from upper end of tibia producing triple deformity of knee joint. Indigenous cauterisation produced ulcers over the growth.

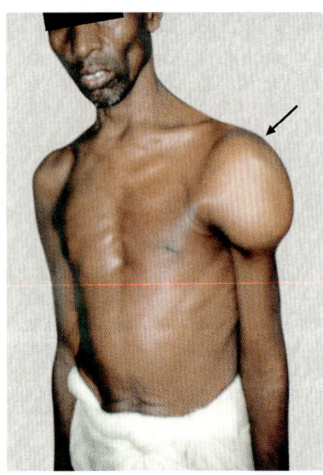

Fig. 17.37: Osteogenic sarcoma from upper end of humerus infiltrating in soft tissues around shoulder.

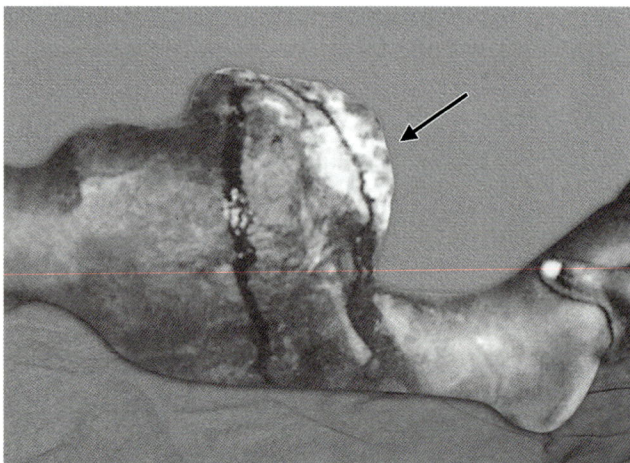

Fig. 17.40: Fungating huge malignant giant cell tumour from upper end of tibia; history of some local chemical application.

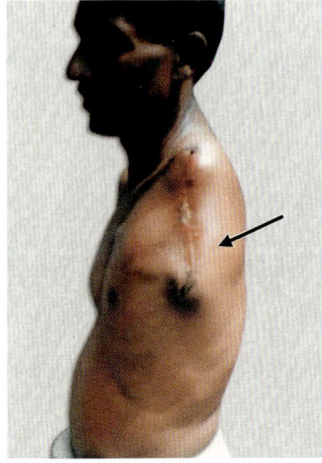

Fig. 17.38: Same patient (**Fig. 17.37**) after 4 years of neoadjuvant chemotherapy and almost fore-quarter amputation.

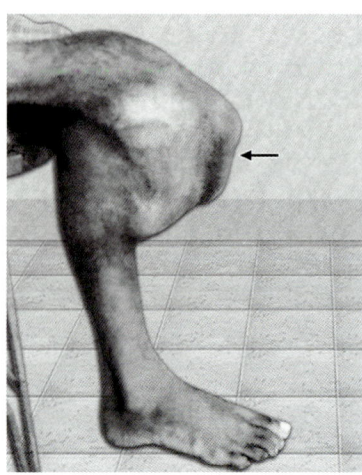

Fig. 17.41: Chondrosarcoma arising from solitary exostosis from upper end of tibia.

Bone Tumours

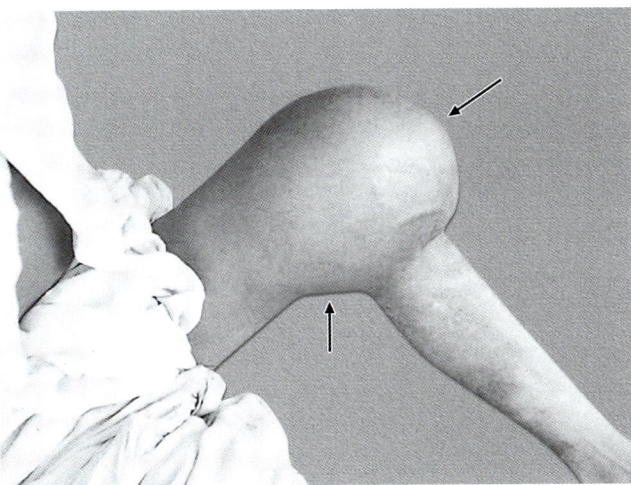

Fig. 17.42: Osteosarcoma from lower end of femur.

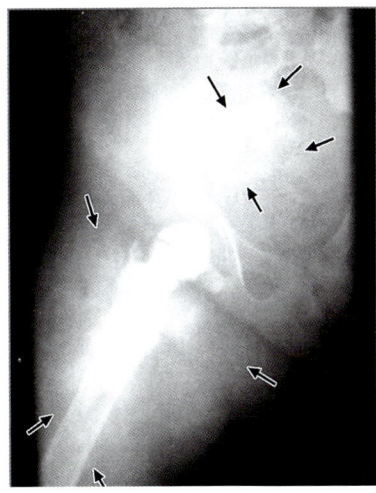

Fig. 17.43: Huge osteogenic sarcoma affecting upper region of femur and ipsilateral pelvis.

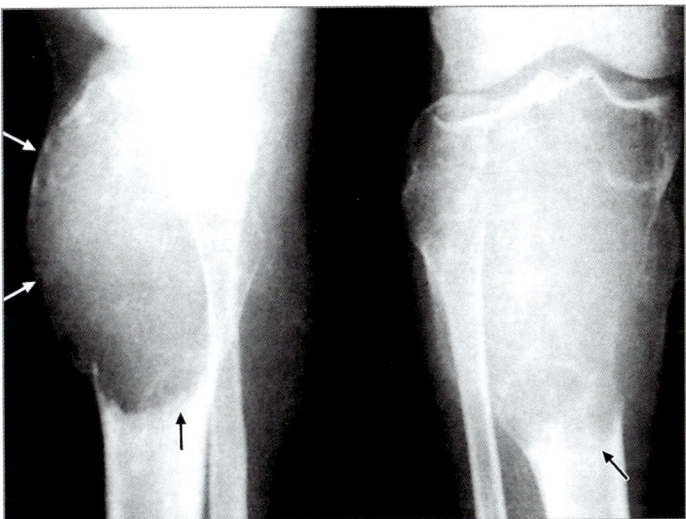

Fig. 17.44: Invasive giant cell tumour from upper end of tibia with pathological fracture.

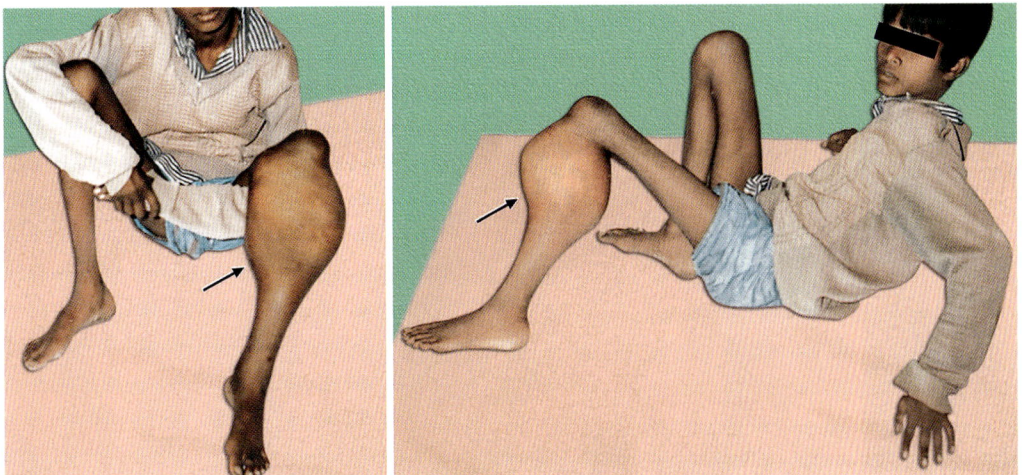

Fig. 17.45: Osteosarcoma upper end of tibia. Note that knee joint is not involved.

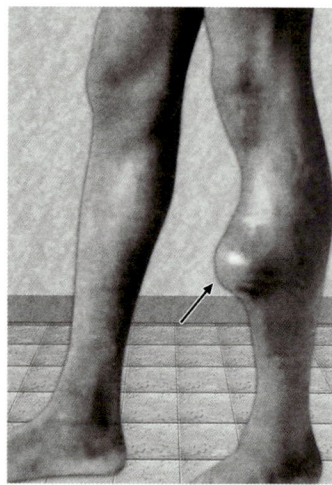

Fig. 17.46: Adamantinoma of tibia, a rare tumour from inclusion tissues—Treatment is wide resection and possible reconstruction or amputation.

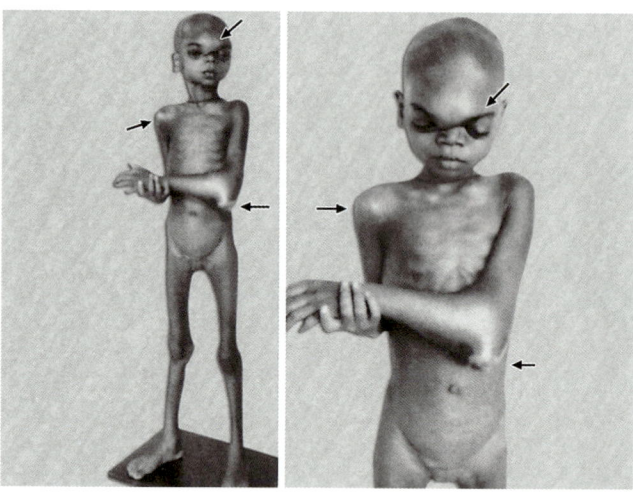

Figs. 17.47: Multifocal lymphoma affecting skull, clavicle, elbow region, right ankle. One at elbow ulcerated due to some indigenous application.

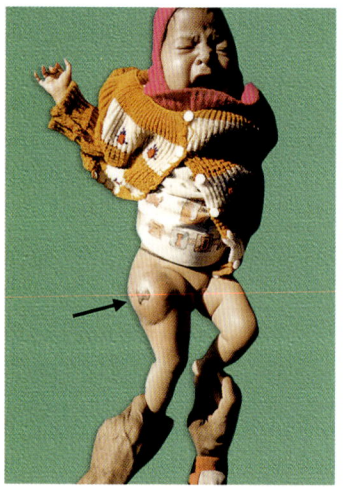

Fig. 17.48: Rhabdomyosarcoma right tibia thigh.

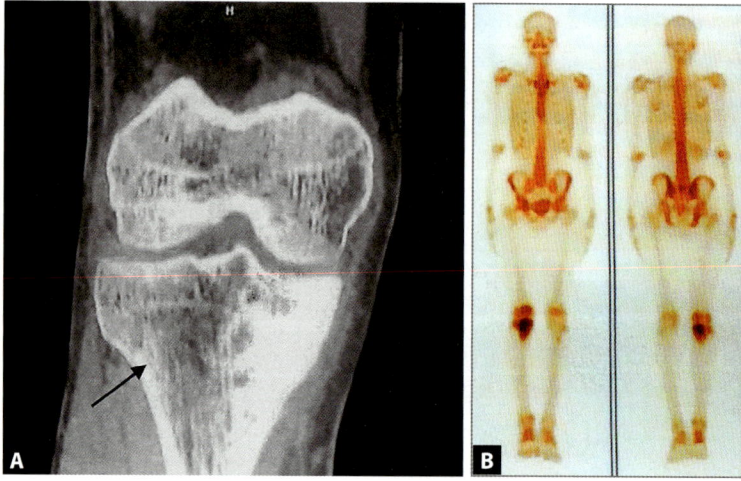

Figs. 17.48A and B: Rhabdomyosarcoma from (right) medial condyle of right tibia. (A) AP X-ray; (B) Scintigraphy.

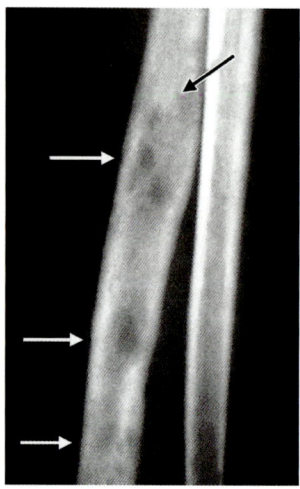

Fig. 17.49: Osseous haemangioma.

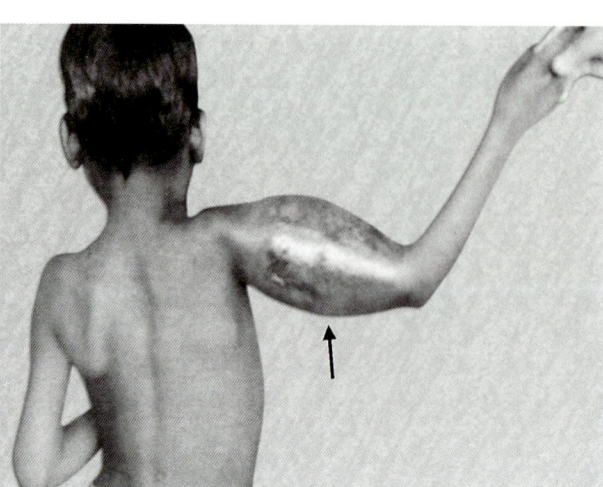

Fig. 17.50: Haemangioendothelioma of humerus (back view).

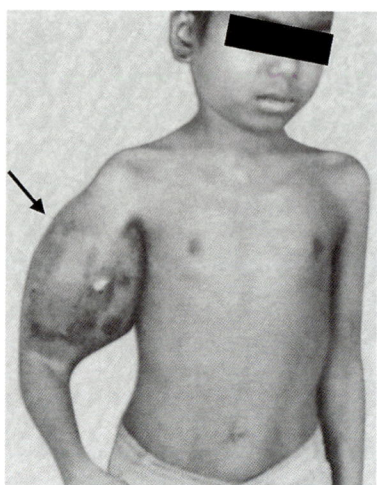

Fig. 17.51: Haemangioendothelioma of humerus (front view).

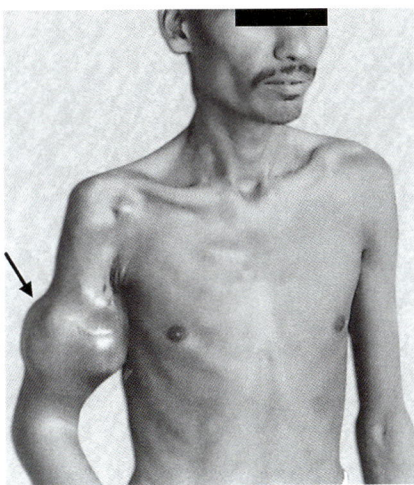

Fig. 17.52: Haemangioendothelioma from humerus.

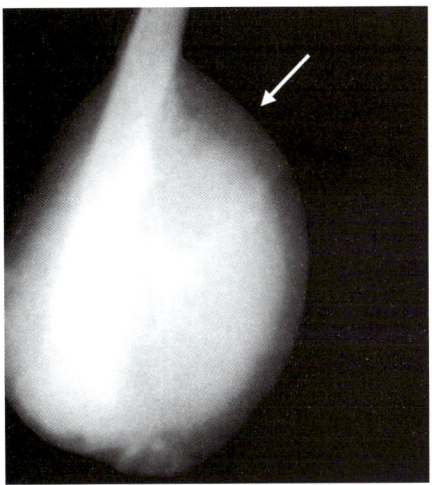

Fig. 17.54: X-ray of same patient (**Fig. 17.53**). Osteosarcoma of lower end of femur.

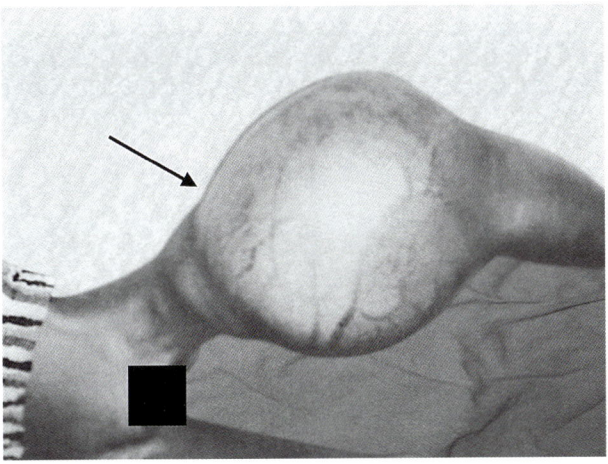

Fig. 17.53: Osteosarcoma of lower end of femur in a boy aged 5 years. Note size of growth and vascular prominence.

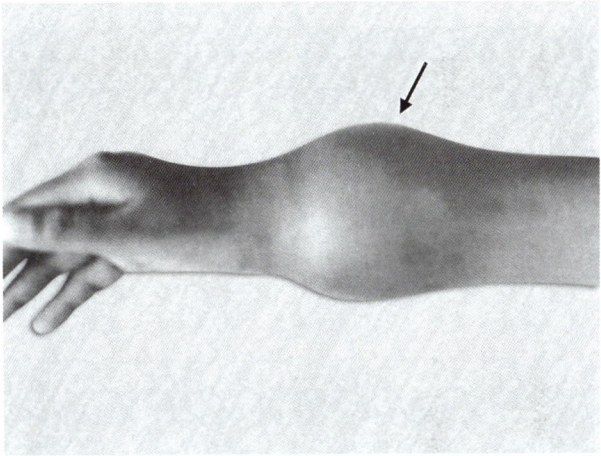

Fig. 17.55: Osteosarcoma of lower end of radius—note the fusiform growth (cf. giant cell tumour with eccentric growth).

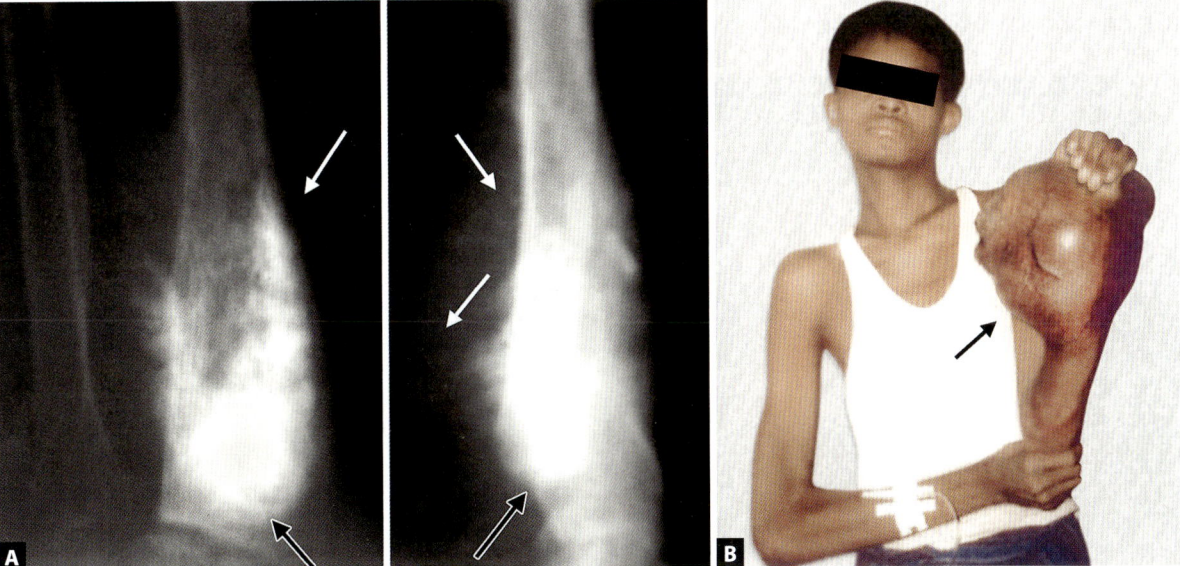

Figs. 17.56A and B: Osteosarcoma from lower end of radius—(A) X-ray showing typical picture of osteosarcoma; (B) Clinical photograph of same patient.

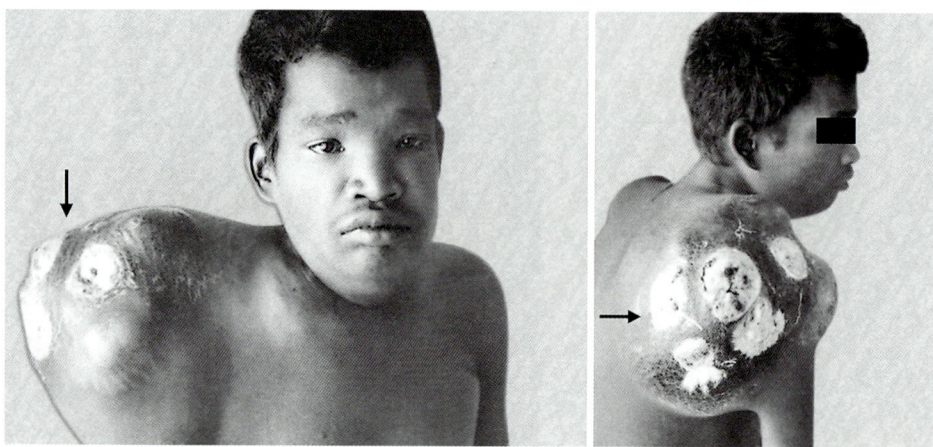

Figs. 17.57: Osteosarcoma from scapula with fungations due to indigenous applications.

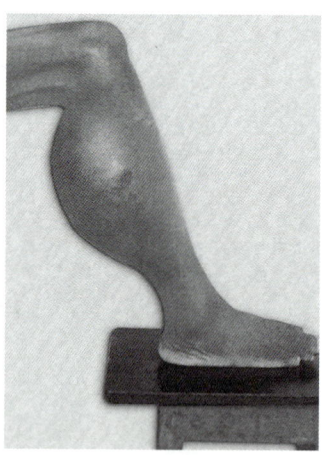

Fig. 17.58: Huge soft tissue growth from upper calf (rhabdomyosarcoma) mimicking osteosarcoma of fibula.

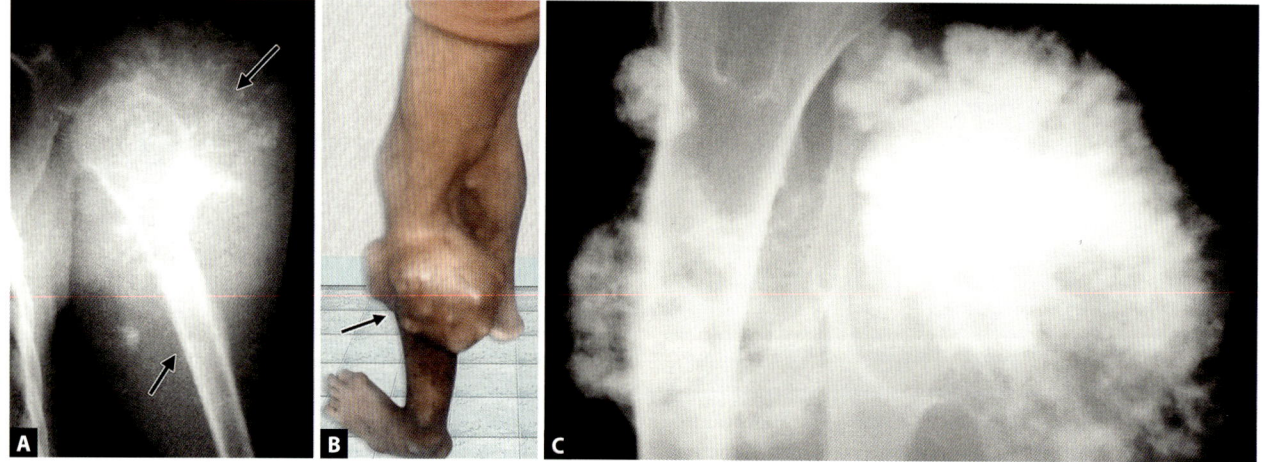

Figs. 17.59A to C: (A) Chondrosarcoma from upper end of humerus; (B) Osteochondroma from fibula turned to chondrosarcoma; (C) X-ray picture of patient of **Figure 17.59B.**

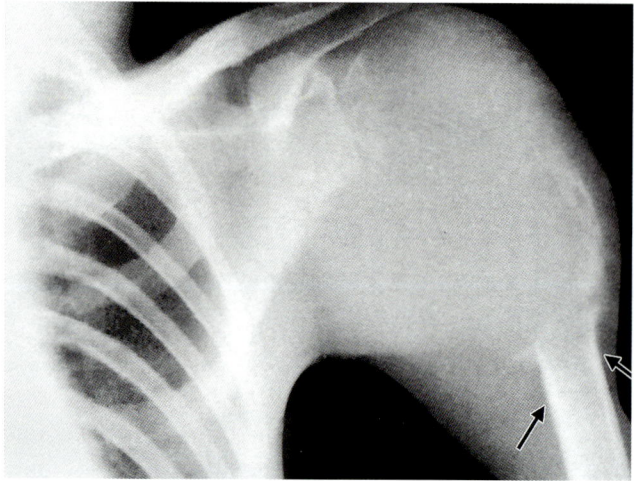

Fig. 17.60: Osteosarcoma from upper end of humerus.

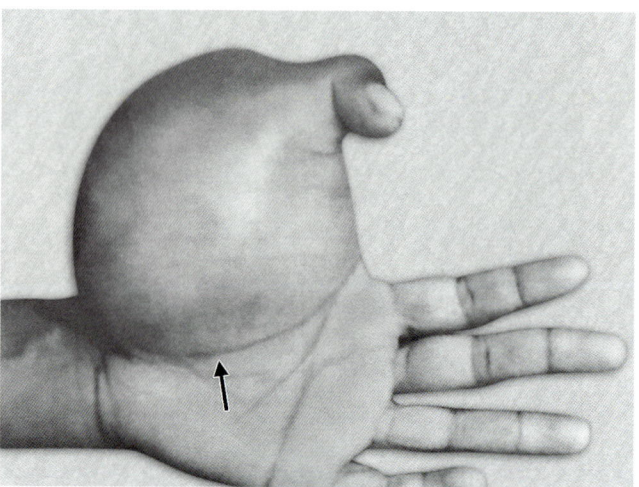

Fig. 17.61: Clinical photograph (palmar aspect)—Osteosarcoma from first metacarpal.

Bone Tumours

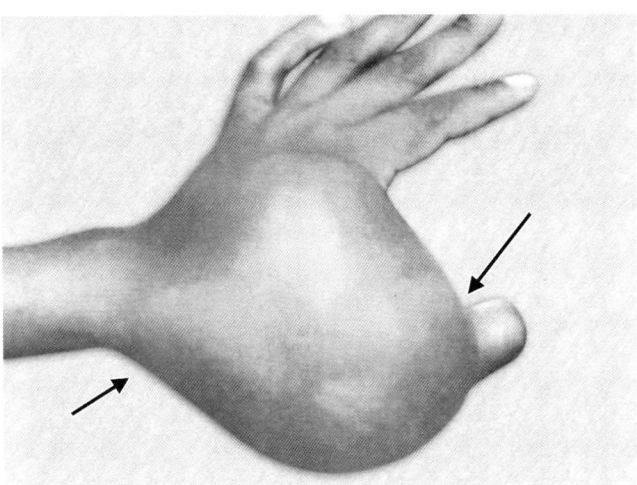

Fig. 17.62: Clinical photograph (dorsal aspect)—Osteosarcoma from first metacarpal (same patient as in **Figure 17.61**).

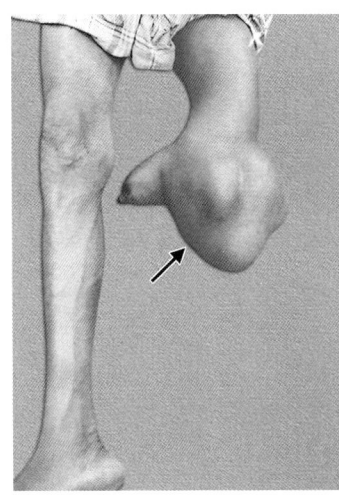

Fig. 17.65: Osteosarcoma in rudimentary knee-leg foot.

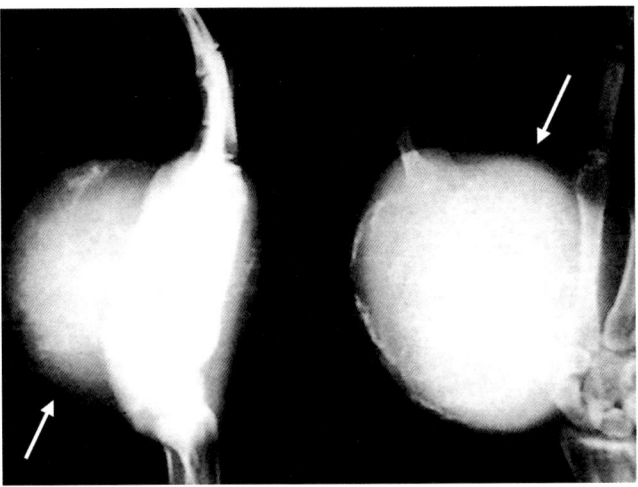

Fig. 17.63: X-ray of same patient (**Figs. 17.61 and 17.62**).

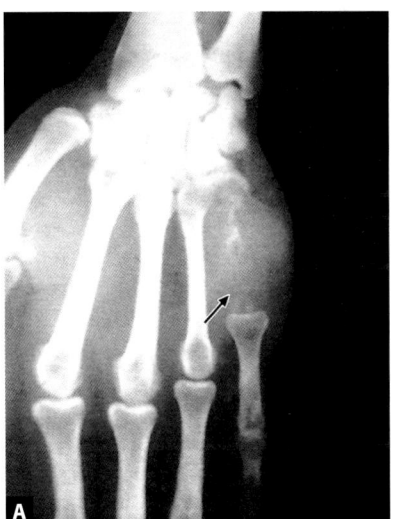

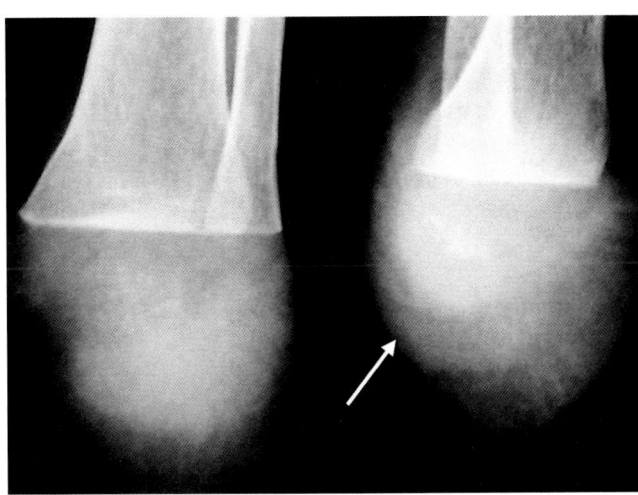

Fig. 17.64: Osteosarcoma in Syme's amputation stump.

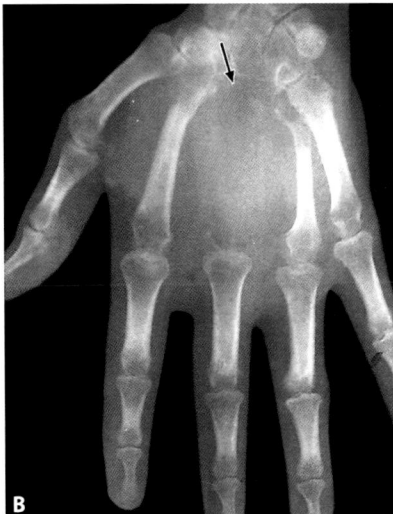

Figs. 17.66A and B: (A) Ewing's sarcoma from fifth metacarpal; (B) Ewing's sarcoma from third metacarpal.

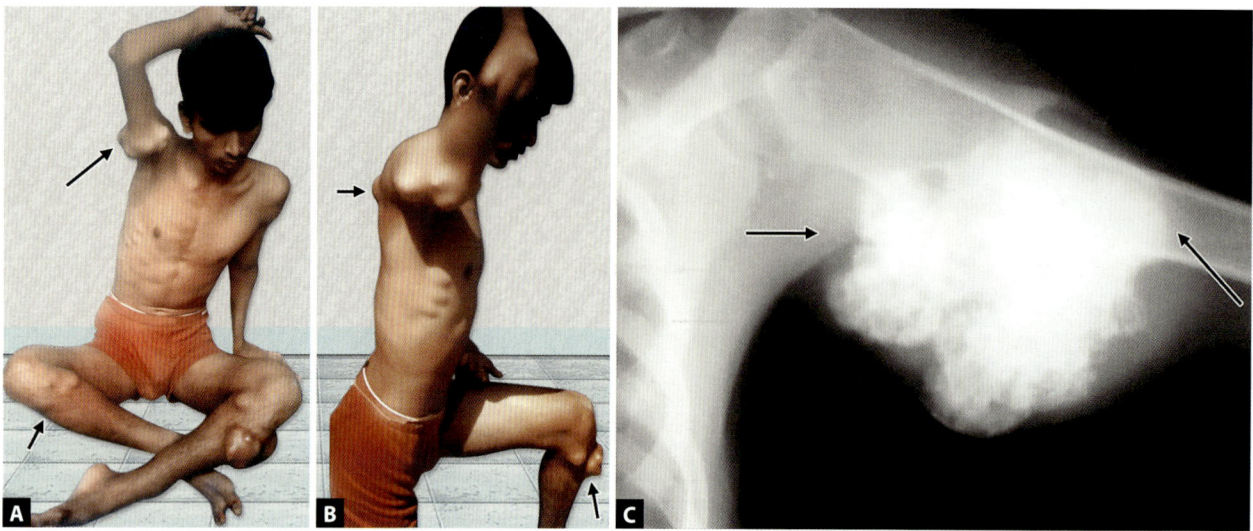

Figs. 17.67A to C: Multiple osteochondroma from upper medial aspect of right humerus, and left tibia. They should be carefully removed to relieve the mechanical discomfort.

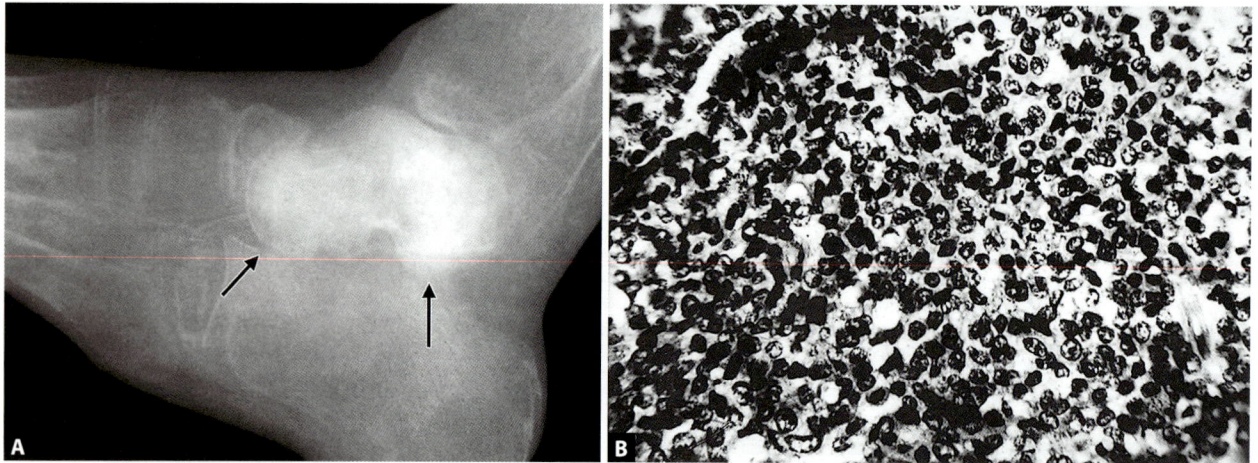

Figs. 17.68A and B: (A) Ewing's sarcoma of talus; (B) Histopathology of Ewing's sarcoma of talus.

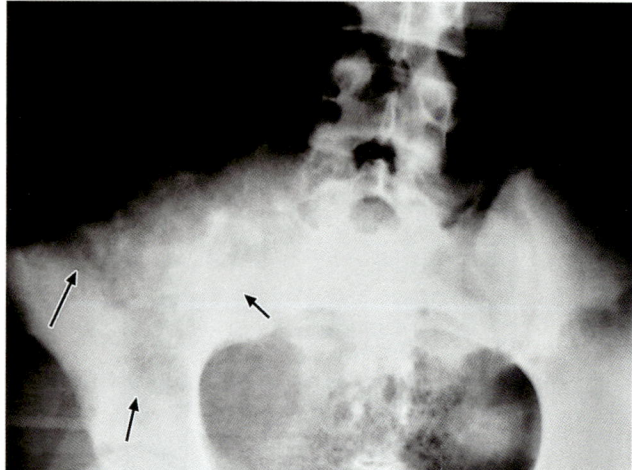

Fig. 17.69: Ewing's sarcoma affecting ileum.

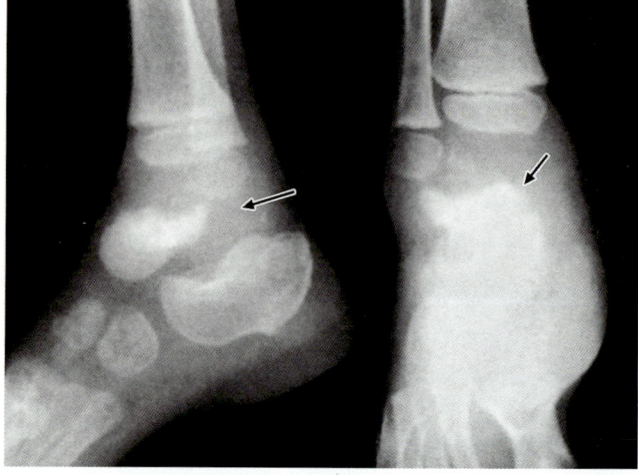

Fig. 17.70: Pyogenic arthritis of ankle with osteomyelitis of talus (Compare with **Figures 17.68A and B**); Osteomyelitis may be confused with Ewing's sarcoma (such as in **Figures 17.68A and B**).

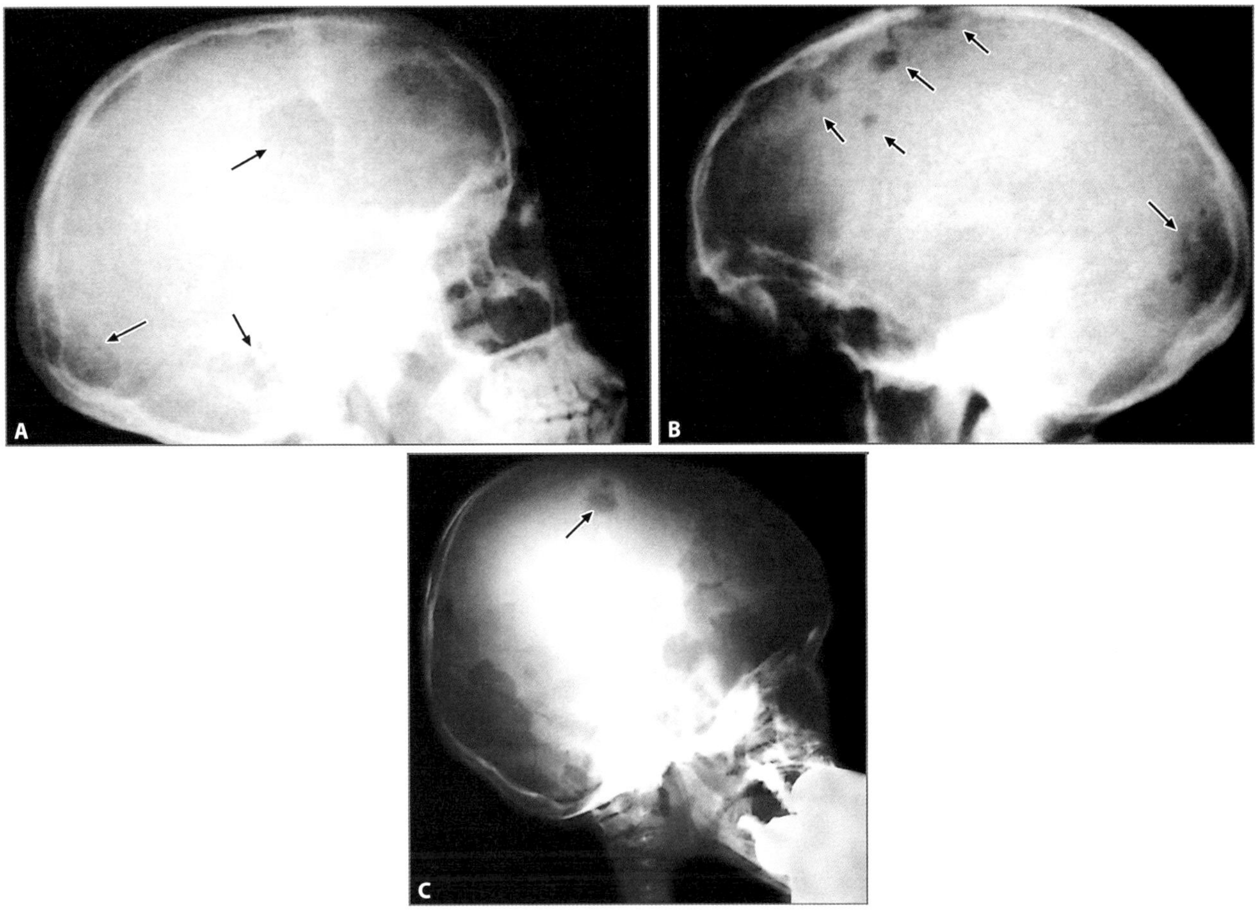

Figs. 17.71A to C: Multiple myeloma in skull.

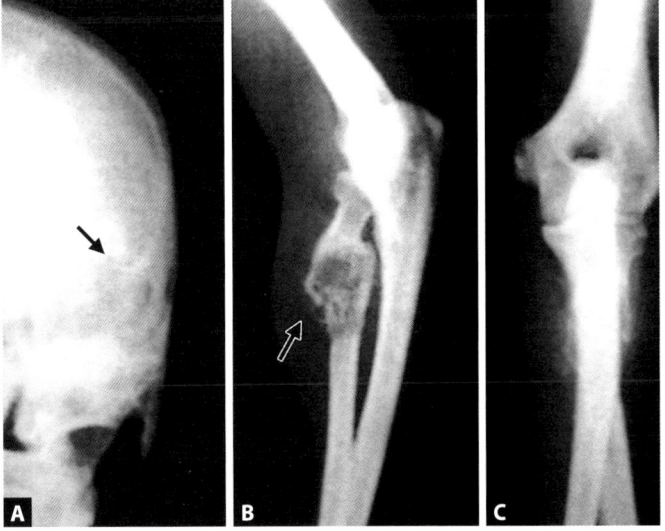

Figs. 17.72A to C: Multiple myeloma in upper end of radial shaft (B and C) with pathological fracture and lesions also in skull (A).

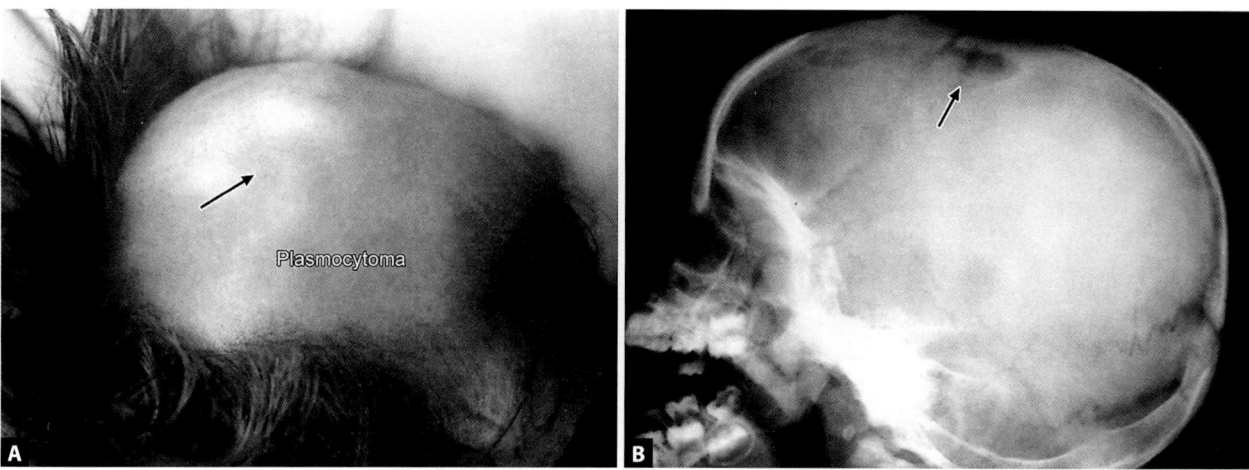

Figs. 17.73A and B: Plasmacytoma in skull (A) Clinical photograph; (B) X-ray of same patient.

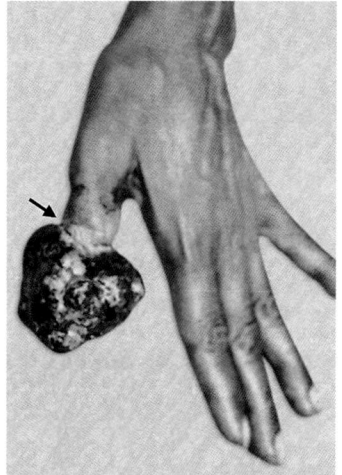

Fig. 17.74: Melanoma of thumb.

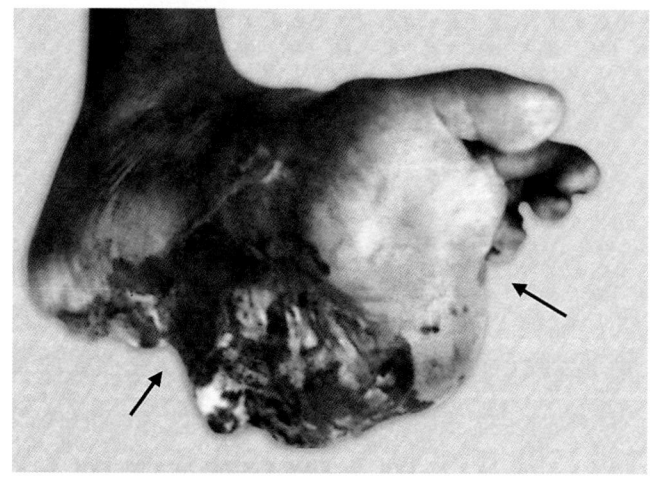

Fig. 17.76: Melanoma of sole.

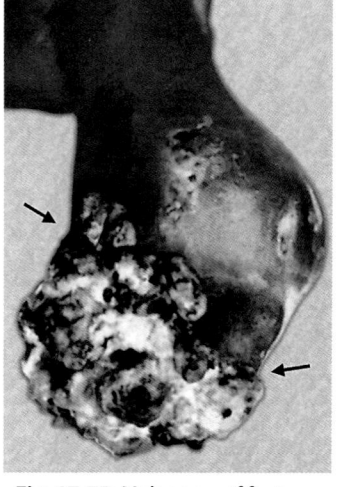

Fig. 17.75: Melanoma of foot.

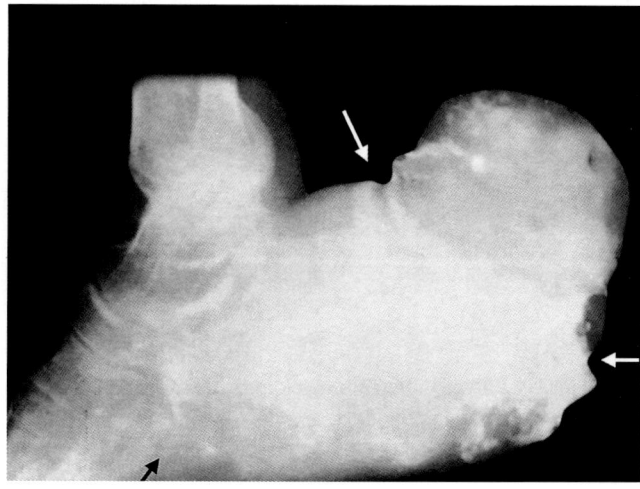

Fig. 17.77: Melanoma of heel (calcaneum).

Bone Tumours

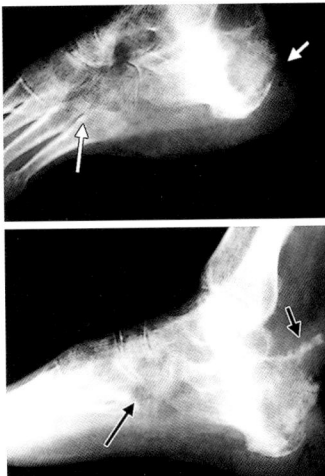

Fig. 17.78: Melanoma of calcaneum and midfoot region.

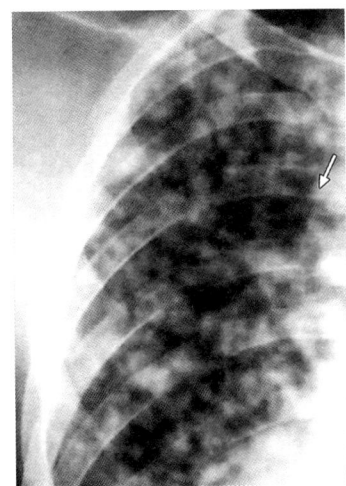

Fig. 17.81: Carcinomatous lung.

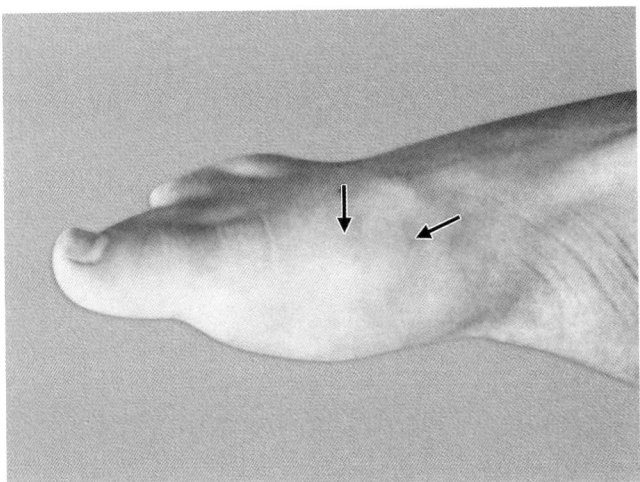

Fig. 17.79: Synovioma from tibialis anterior tendon sheath.

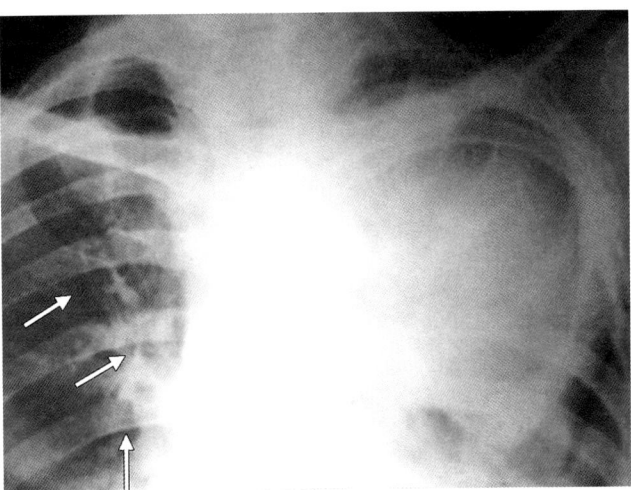

Fig. 17.82: Multiple myeloma destroying fifth rib with malignant mass in the lung as well (affecting lung directly).

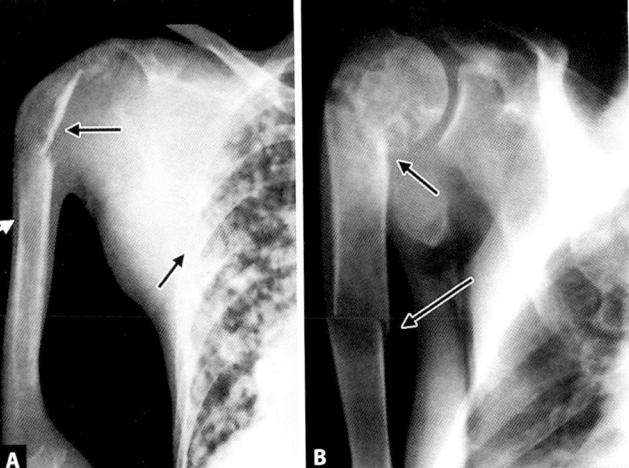

Figs. 17.80A and B: (A) Metastatic carcinoma in upper end of humerus (with pathological fracture) and carcinomatosis lung; (B) Multiple myeloma with pathological fractures at two places in right humerus.

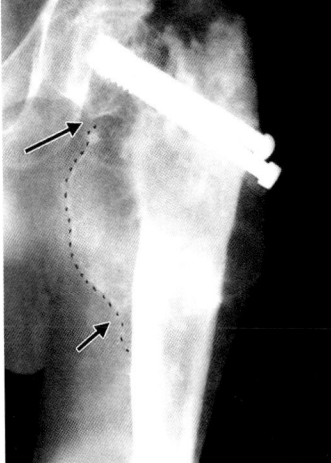

Fig. 17.83: Chondrosarcoma affecting upper end of femur and neck with pathological fracture—fixed with screws Chondrosarcoma is the most common primitive bone cancer that occurs in adults after the age of 50 years. It usually affects the long bones like femur, tibia, humerus.

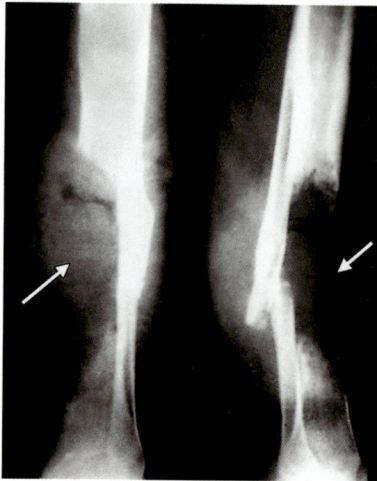

Fig. 17.84: Marjolin ulcer in leg producing destruction of tibia.

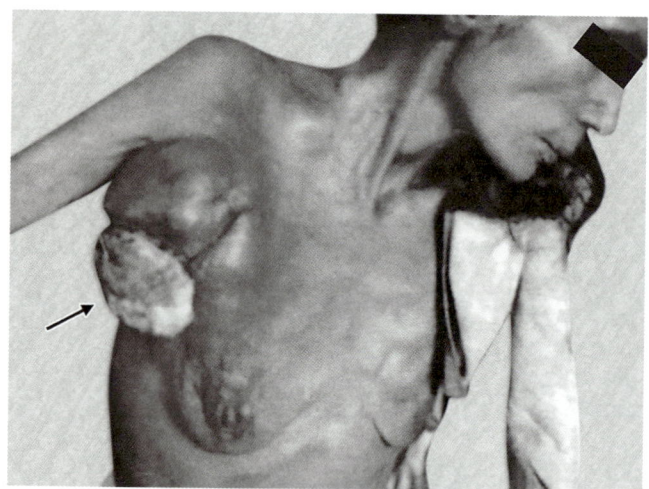

Fig. 17.85: Fungating carcinoma from axillary gland.

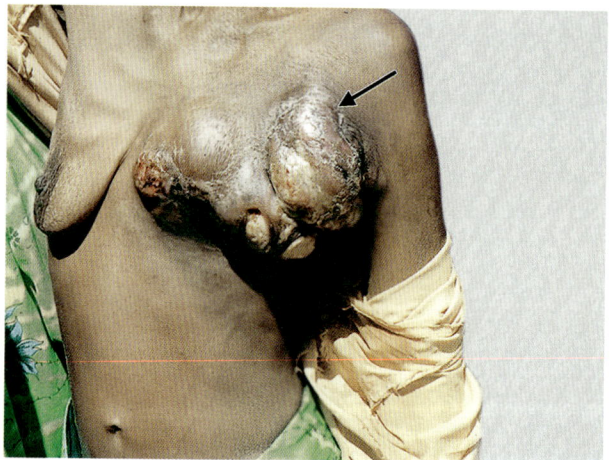

Fig. 17.86: Advanced CA breast with involvement of chest wall and deeper.

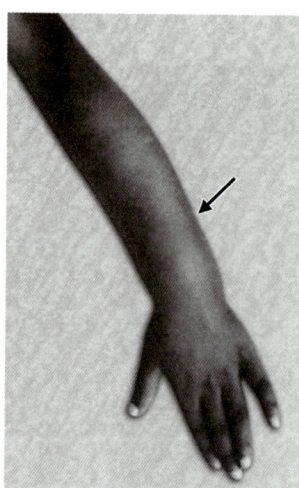
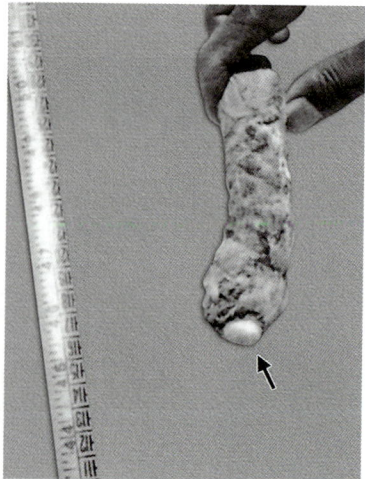

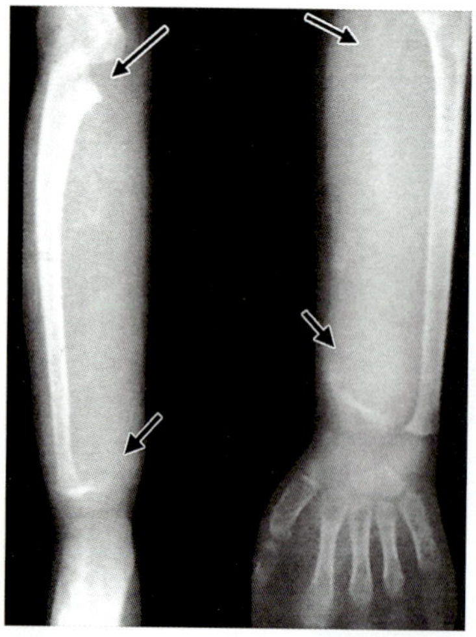

Bone dissolving disease in a boy aged 6 years (Gorham-Stout syndrome).
In syndrome chapter 24, alphabetically arranged Gorham-Stout syndrome **(Figs. 17.87 to 17.89)**

Fig. 17.87: Note the swelling of the forearm.

Fig. 17.88: X-ray of same patient **(Fig. 17.87)**. Note almost complete dissolution of radius, except little bone at the lower end.

Fig. 17.89: Specimen; of the totally removed radius (and reconstructed with ipsilateral mid-shaft of fibula) which histologically showed markedly vascularised fibrous tissue.

Bone Tumours

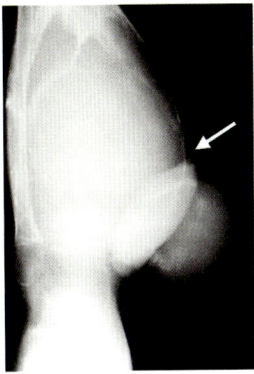

Fig. 17.90: Malignant aneurysmal bone cyst.

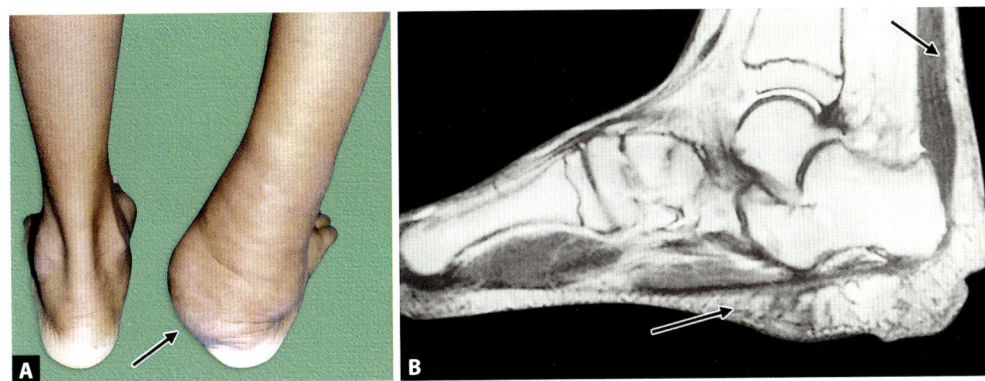

Figs. 17.91A and B: Lymphangioma in ankle-heel region (A) Clinical photo, (B) MRI of same region.

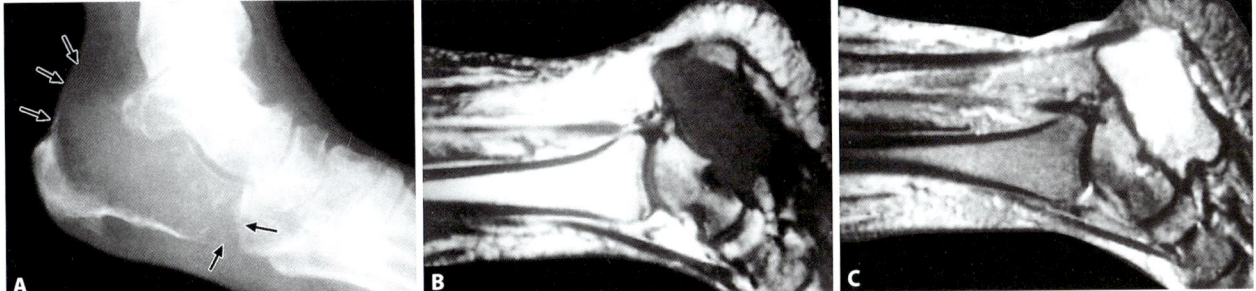

Figs. 17.92A to C: (A) Lateral X-ray showing expansile destructive lesion of calcaneum; (B and C) MRI—T$_1$ and T$_2$ weighted sagittal images of ankle and foot showing soft tissue mass replacing the marrow fat of calcaneum. There is extension of lesion into talocalcaneal joint—Plasmocytoma of calcaneum (*Courtesy:* Dr MS Dhillon.)

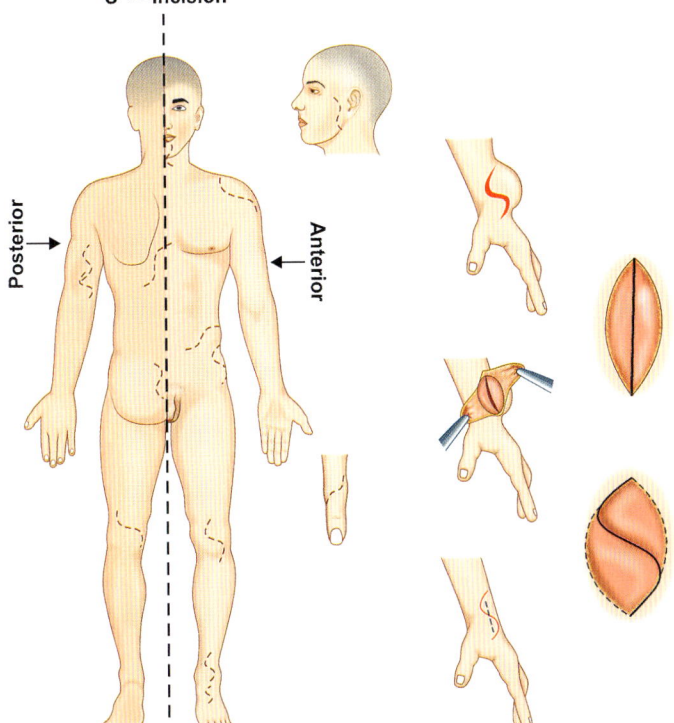

Fig. 17.93: In tumour surgery 'Pandey's 'S' type incisions facilitates non-strained easy wide approach to the growth.

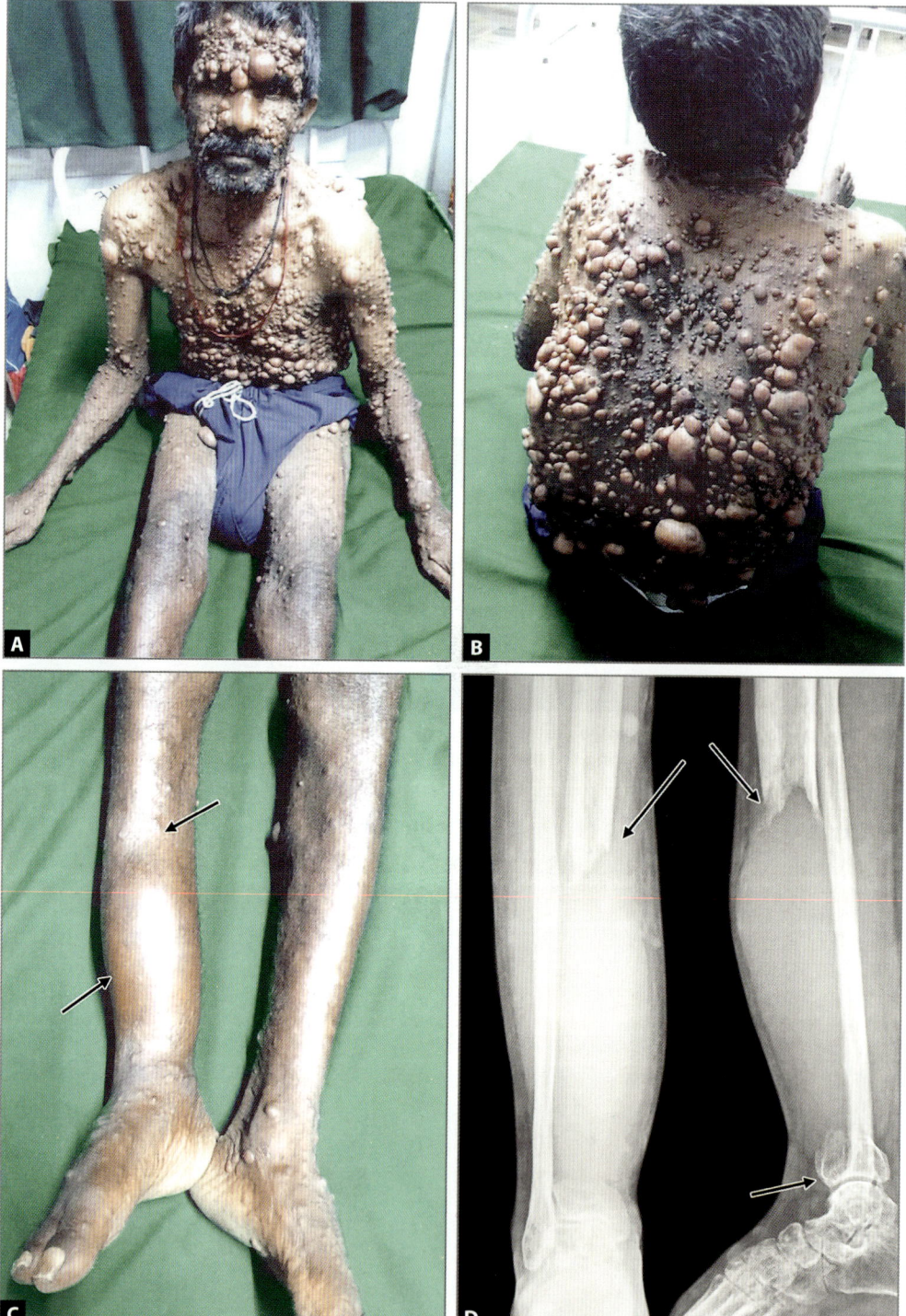

Figs. 17.94A to D: Multiple neurofibromatosis (also *see* **Fig. 16.23**) with solitary osseous plasmacytoma of this right tibia originates from plasma cells of bone and soft tissues anywhere in body.
Courtesy: Dr PK Raina and Dr Anamika Kumari. Neurofibroma is a rare tumor, which also occurs along the trunks of peripheral nerves. It is composed of masses of fibrous and fatty tissue which is intimately mixed with the nerve fasciculi and axons. It is rather impossible to dissect out this tumor from the parent nerve. It hardly occurs singly. It mostly occurs as part of the syndrome of neurofibromatosis. It should be left as such, unless there is may evidence of malignancy like rapid growth, increasing local temperature and pain with confirmation by histopathology¬ and then it should be treated by wide excision.

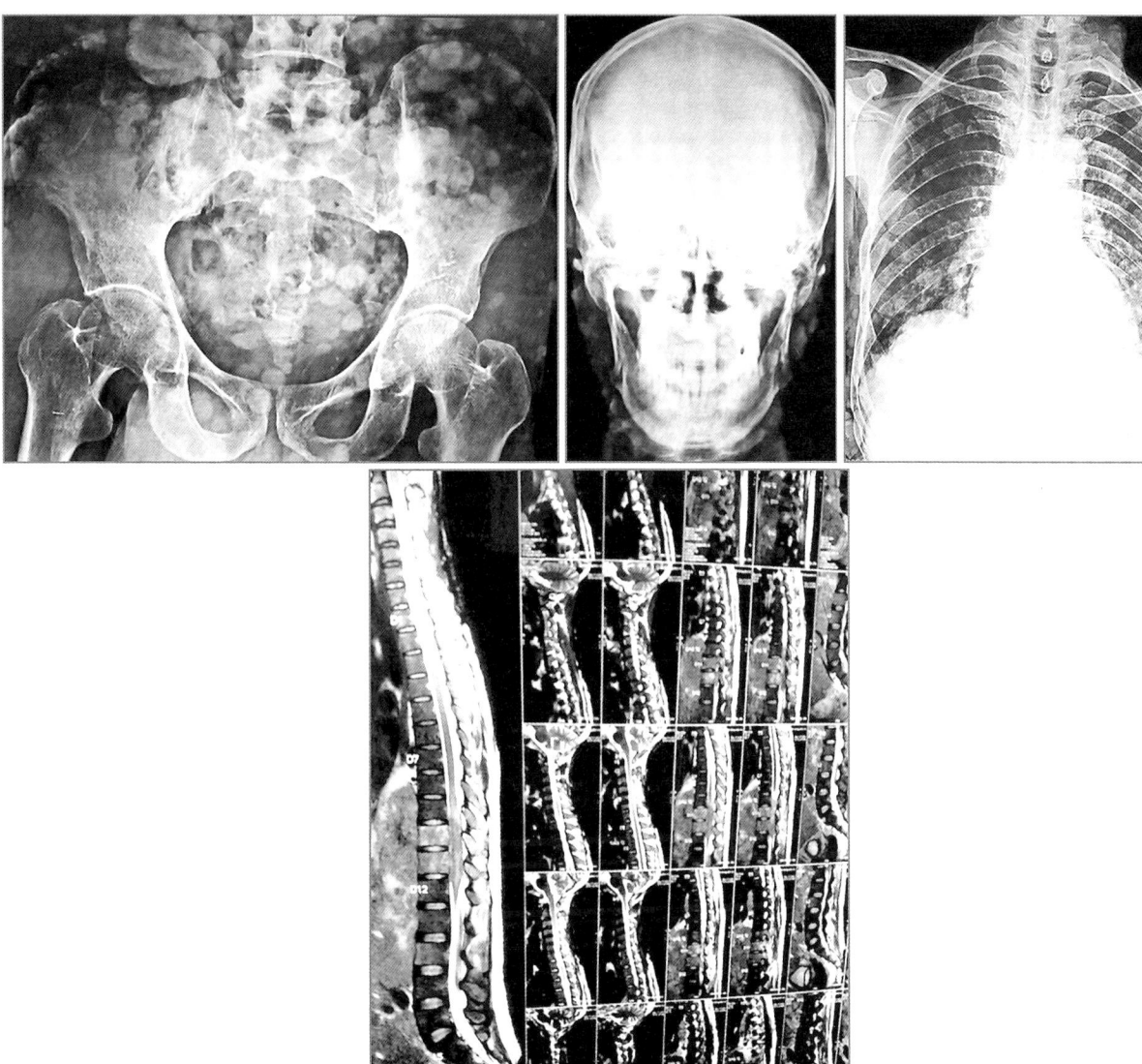

Fig. 17.95: Young male 34 years with testicular tumour—nonseminomatous germ cell tumour with retroperitoneal lymph glands with secondary to bones—mainly spine producing compression paraplegia.
Courtesy: Dr PK Raina and Dr Anamika kumari.

■ BIBLIOGRAPHY

1. Abed YY, Beltrami G, Campanacci DA et al. Biological reconstruction after resection of bone tumours around the knee. J Bone Joint Surg (Br). 2009;91(B):1366-72.
2. American Joint Committee on Cancer Bone. In: Feming ID, Copper J, Henson DE, et al. (Eds). AJCC Cancer Staging Manual (5 Edn) Philadelphia: Lippincott-Raven, 1997;143-7.
3. Ante Domagoj, Vodanovich, Peter FM, Choong : Soft-tissue Sarcomas. Indian Journal of Orthopedics vd. 52.2018: pp. 35-44.
4. Ante D, Vodanovich, peter FM, Choong: soft–tissue Sarcoma. Indian J Orthop. 2018;52(1):35-44.
5. Bacci G, Ferravi S, Lari S, et al. Osteosarcoma of the limb. J Bone Joint Surg (Br). 2002;84(B):88-92.
6. Based on-Pathology of Bone Tumors by Joshis, Panchwagh In Textbook of Orthopaedics & Trauma by kulkarnigs, Babhulkars. 3rd ed . JAYPEE, New Delhi: pp. 638.
7. Chen WM, Chen TH, Huang CK, et al. Treatment of malignant bone tumours by extracorporeally irradiated autograft-prosthetic composite arthroplasty. J Bone Joint Surg. 2002; 84-B:1156-61.
8. Enneking WF, Spanier SS, Goodman MA. A system for the surgical staging of musculoskeletal sarcoma. Clin Orthop. 1980;153:106.
9. Enneking WF. Staging musculoskeletal tumors. In: WF Enneking (Ed): Musculoskeletal Tumor Surg. New York: Churchill Livingstone; 1983.pp.87-8.
10. Fletcher CDM, Bridge JA, Hogendoom PCW, Mertens F, (Eds). World Health organization, classification of tumours: Pathology and genetics of tumours of soft tissue and bone. Lyon: IARC Press; 2013.
11. Galasko CSB. Diagnosis of skeletal metastasis and assessment of response to treatment. Clin Orthop. 1995;312:64-5.
12. Ghani AG, Wan WF, Ismail, salleh Md S Md, Yahaya S, Muhamad Z, Fitri S. The values of Receptor Activator Nuclear

kappa B Ligand expression in stage III giant cell tumor of the Bone: Indian J Orthop. 2018;52(1):31-34.
13. Kundu ZS, Sen R, Dhiman A, Sharma P, Siwach R, Rana P. Effect of Intravenous Zoledronic acid on Histopathology and Recurrence after extended Curettage in giant cell Tumours of Bone : A comparative prospective study: Indian J Orthop. 2018;52(1);45-50.
14. Lichtenstein L. Bone tumours, 4th edn. St. Louis: Mosby; 1972.
15. Mastboom MJL, Staals EL, Verspoor FGM et al. Surgical treatment of localized-type Tenosynovial giant cell tumors of large joints. J Bone Joint Surg AM. 2019;101:1309-18.
16. Morris GV, Jonathan D, Stevenson, Evans S, Parry MC, Jeys L. Navigation in Musculoskeletal Oncology: An Overview. Indian J Orthop. 2018;52(1):22-30.
17. Narhari P, Haseeb A, Lee S, Singh VA. Spontaneous Conventional Osteosarcoma Transformation of a Chondroblastoma: A case Report. Indian J Orthop. 2018;52(1):87-90.
18. Pandey S. Ewing's sarcoma of the third metacarpal. Int Surg. 1972;57:984-5.
19. Pandey S. Ewing's tumour of talus. J Bone Joint Surg. 1970;52-A: 1672-3.
20. Pandey S. Giant cell tumour of talus. Int Surg. 1971;55-3:179-82.
21. Pandey S. Giant chondromas arising from the ribs. J Bone Joint Surg. 1975;57B:519-25.
22. Pandey S. Intraosseous haemangioma. Abst Book SICOT, Japan: Kyoto; 1978.
23. Pandey S, Pandey AK. Osseous haemangiomas. Arch Orthop Traumat Surg. 1981;99:23-8.
24. Pandey S. Pulsatile skeletal metastasis from thyroid carcinoma. Int Surg. 1970;53(1):62-4.
25. Pandey S. Voluminous osteochondroma of the second rib. Int Surg. 1971;56(6):419-21.
26. Pandey S. 'S' Incision-Clinical Orthopaedics.
27. Puri Ajay. Musculoskeletal Oncology: Finding its place in the sun! guest editorial. Indian J Orthop. 2018;52(1):1-2.
28. Quoted by Vyas A, Patni P et al : Retrospective Analysis of giant cell Tumor Lower end Radius Treated with Enblock excision and Translocation of ulna. Indian J Orthop. 2018;52(1):10-14.
29. Rosenthal DI, Hornicek FJ, Wolf MW, et al. Percutaneous radio-frequency coagulation of osteoid osteoma compared with operative treatment. J Bone Joint Surg (Am). 1998;80(A): 15-21.
30. Singh VA, Heng CW, Yasin NF.: gaint Analysis in Patients with wide resection and Endoprosthesis Replcement Around the knee. Indian J Orthop. 2018;52(1):65-72.
31. Sung HW, DP kuo, chai YB, Liu CC, SM li. Giant-cell tumor of bone: Analysis of two hundred and eight cases in Chinese patient. J Bone Joint Surg Am. 1982;64:755-61.
32. Verma Tarun & Maini Lalit 2019: 3D printing in orthopedic oncology: techniques, our experience and review of literature IOACON 2019 Abstract book, Kolkata 2019, p. 120
33. Vijayans S, Bartlett, Robert Lee, et al. Use of irradiated autologous bone in joint sparing endoprosthetic femoral replacement tumour surgery. Indian J Orthop. 2011;45:161-7.
34. Vyas A, Patni P, Saini N, Sharma R, Arora V, gupta SP. Retrospective Analysis of giant cell Tumor Lower End Radius Treated with En bloc excision and Translocation of Ulna – Indian Orthop: 2018;52(1):10-14.
35. Weiss KR, Zimel MN: Considerations for the Long Term Treatment of PedIATRIC Sarcomd Survivors. Indian Orthop. 2018;52(1):77-80.

CHAPTER 18

Mandible and Temporomandibular Joint

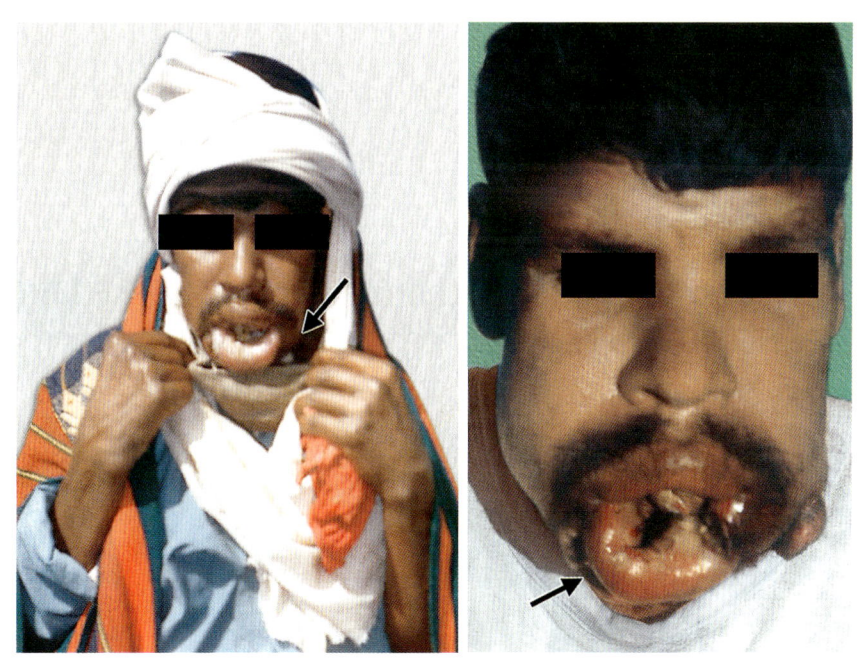

*"You may not control all the events that happen to you,
but you can decide not to be reduced by them".*
—*Maya Angelou*

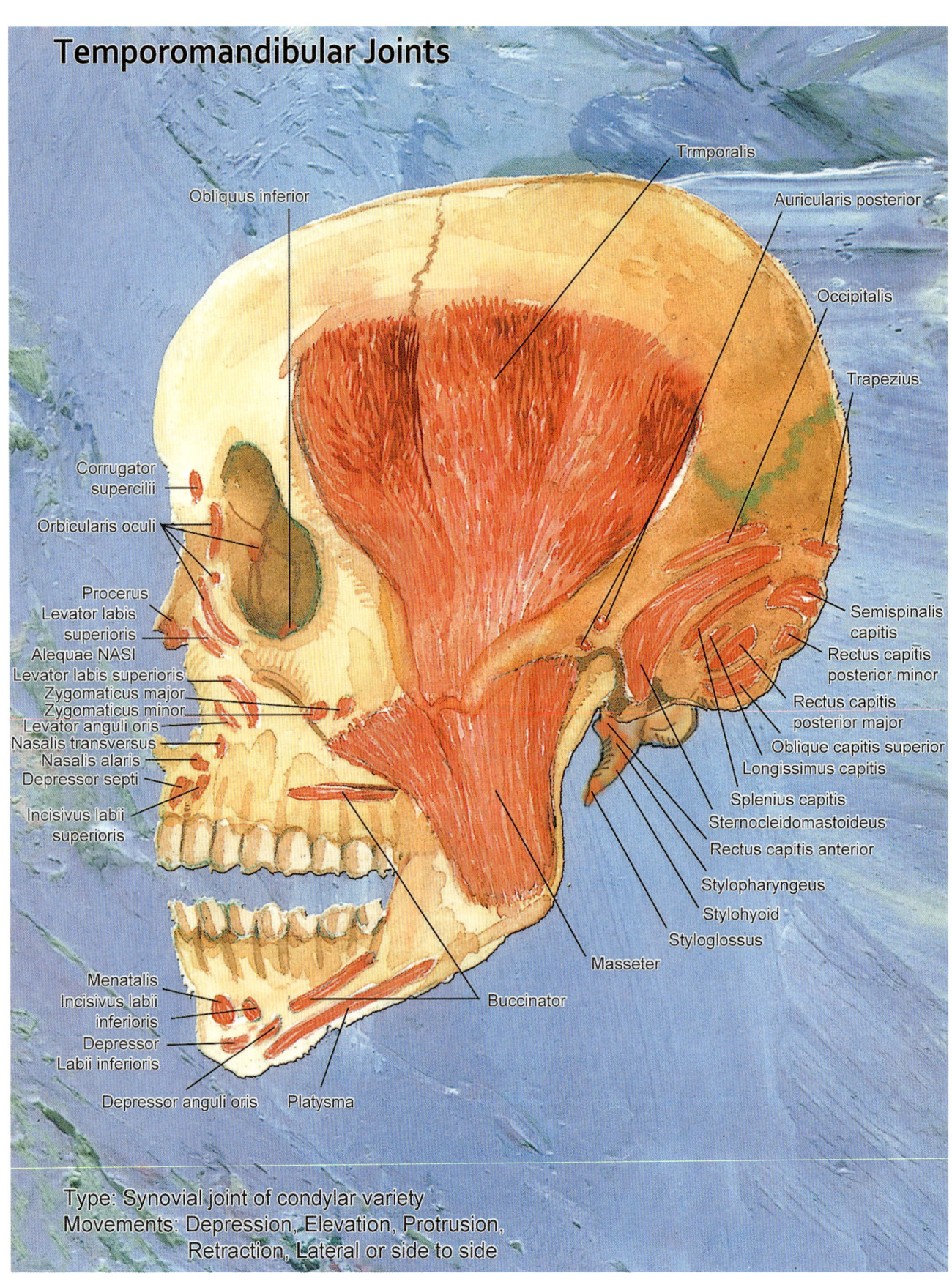

INTRODUCTION

Ideally, the temporomandibular joint should fall in the domain of an orthopaedic and facio-maxillary surgeons. However, an orthopaedic surgeon primarily comes in the picture for managing traumatic, congenital, and other acquired pathologies of the temporomandibular joint.

ANATOMICAL CONSIDERATIONS

- The temporomandibular joint is the articulation between the articular tubercle and the anterior portion of the mandibular fossa of the temporal bone above and the condyle of the mandible below. A fibrous articular disc divides the joint into an upper and a lower part. As such the condyle and disc move together during retraction and protraction of the mandible. *Derangement of this articular disc may result in clicking and pain on jaw movements* (e.g. in various trauma, over-grinding)
- The disposition of the temporomandibular joint (a condylar joint) is such that the condyloid process of the mandible is at a disadvantageous position. In fact, when the mouth is open, the mandibular condyles sit almost on the watershed, i.e. articular eminences. In this mechanically disadvantageous position, any sudden violence (even muscular spasm or yawning) may thrust one or both condyles into the infratemporal fossa
- The mandible at the temporomandibular joint remains almost suspended through muscular and facial attachments. Though the joints are quite small, the joint space more or less always remains maintained due to the passive distractive force of gravity. Still, *ankylosis is perhaps the most common pathology, which involves this joint*. Of course, in most of the cases, the causes are in the soft tissues in and around the joint
- Both temporomandibular joints act in harmony, forming together a bicondylar arrangement. Therefore, affection of one joint is bound to affect the function of the other
- The main function of the temporomandibular joint is for mastication. Secondarily, they help in articulation, phonation, and certain facial expressions.

Muscles of mastication—Main muscles are: (i) Temporalis, (ii) Masseter, (iii) Lateral pterygoids, (iv) Medial pterygoids. Assisted by: (i) Digastric, (ii) Mylohyoid, (iii) Omohyoid, (iv) Stylohyoid, (v) Sternohyoid, (vi) Thyrohyoid.

Ossification of Mandible

Mandible is ossified in dense membranous tissue. Each half develops from one centre appearing at the 6th week of intrauterine life. The mandible is the second bone to ossify in the body, first being clavicle.

Anatomical Landmark of Temporomandibular Joint

Just in front of and slightly above the tragus, the transverse slit of the temporomandibular joint can be felt. Put your index fingertip over this slit and ask the patient to open and close the mouth repeatedly. Movements of the condyloid process of mandible can be felt under the fingertip.

METHODOLOGY

History

Besides taking history in the usual way, few important points to be enquired about are—(i) Biting any hard/tough stuff, (ii) Malocclusion, (iii) Any history of discharge (blood-tinged, serous, black grain and/or pus) from gums or buccal region, (iv) Any discharge from ear, (v) History of infection (intra/periarticular) in that region, (vi) Past history of tetanus with prolonged illness.

General and Systemic Examinations

As in the Chapter 1: Introduction (special reference to speech, swallowing, dribbling of saliva).

Regional Examination

Regional examination includes examination of cranial nerves, cervical spine, different groups of cervical lymph nodes, examination of the throat (naso-oropharynx) and examination of the ear (external auditory meatus may be fractured in temporomandibular injury; middle ear infection can cause pain and ankylosis of the joint).

Local Examination

Attitude

Certain peculiar attitudes of the lower jaw can indicate certain pathologies at the temporomandibular joint.

Certain Fixed Attitudes

- A retracted or small chin with shrunken lower cheeks, assuming more or less a triangular shape with an imaginary line joining temporomandibular joints, indicates *micrognathia* (hypoplasia); congenital bilateral ankylosis of temporomandibular joint; symmetrically underdeveloped chin can be associated with cleft palate and breathing problems (Pierre Robin syndrome); *Agnathia* (absence of mandible); *Prognathism* (hyperplasia of mandible)—commonly symmetrical and manifests in late childhood—chin and lip protruded with dental malocclusion
- Asymmetric shape of mandible, more or less in one half, with chin deviated to one side indicates unilateral

temporomandibular ankylosis (a very rare congenital condition)
- Protracted chin with massive body of mandible, thick and extruded lower lip, broad lower jaw, wider lower face, more or less quadrangular shape of lower jaw (lantern jaw)—indicates *acromegalic jaw* (hyperpituitarism). In acromegaly, the hands enlarge due to overgrowth of bone and soft tissues, stimulated by excess of growth hormone, usually from an adenoma of anterior pituitary gland. When such problem occurs before the epiphyseal closure, the skeletal system grows in well proportionate manner resulting gigantism. When growth occurs after epiphyseal closure, it results in acromegaly in which the hands, feet, face, head and soft tissues are thickened
- Partially opened up mouth, protracted chin, lower lip at a level distal to that of the upper, patient unable to close the mouth, difficulty in speaking clearly, any passive attempt of closing mouth causing marked pain at temporomandibular joints—indicates bilateral dislocation of temporomandibular joints
- Mouth partially opened up, more on the opposite side, chin deviated to the opposite side, angle of mandible at a higher level on the side of affection; difficulty in articulation, passive attempts at closure causing pain in the affected temporomandibular joint indicates unilateral dislocation of the temporomandibular joint
- Post-burn contractures at the neck cause pulling down of the lower jaw with or without subluxation at the temporomandibular joints. Facial burn contractures affect the facial symmetry and may lead to ankylosis of the temporomandibular joint. The attitude of the chin, rather the lower jaw, will vary as a whole according to the contracture.

Inspection

Look for the symmetry of the zygomatic processes. At the posteroinferior end of the zygomatic process, a shallow depression is seen. This should be symmetrical on both sides. Any fullness in this area may be due to some pathology of the temporomandibular joint or overlying tissues. Fullness below this region is due to parotid affection. The parotid swellings may also encroach below and behind the lobules of the ears.

Any abnormality in the skin condition, shape and size of mandible and any swelling in its relations should be noted. Certain peculiar attitudes of the lower jaw (as described earlier) usually indicates some pathology at the temporomandibular joint.

Large glandular enlargements in posterior digastric fossa or behind the ear, if present, may be obvious on inspection.

Inspection through Buccal Cavity

- Look for the *number and inter-dental relations of the teeth* on the lower jaw and their interrelations with their counterparts on the upper jaw. In case of fracture—displacement of the jaw bones may be obvious. The disturbed relation in the level of the teeth is an important finding
- Ask the patient to *clench the teeth*—normally the teeth should sit on their counterparts. Note any asymmetry in the relations of the teeth
- Look at the relations of the teeth and gums. Any obvious space occupying lesion in gingivolabial fold should be clearly noted. Along with, also note its surface, vascularity, size, shape, relation to the corresponding tooth (present or missing)
- Any *obvious infection* in any tooth should be noted
- Look at the *buccal mucosa*. Normally, it should look pink with a slight bluish tinge here and there due to venous channels. In the posterior part of the oral cavity, the mucosa gives an impression of its more firm adherent relation as mucoperiosteum. Note for any change in colour and texture of the mucosa and periosteum.

In a very rare condition which may be called *'pale mucosal fibrosis,'* the mucosa becomes pale and tightly adherent to the underlying surface. The same pathology also spreads over the tonsillar pillars. Consequently, there is gradual extra-articular *ankylosis* of the *temporomandibular joint*. We have seen only five cases and all were females in their twenties/thirties.

Look for the symmetry of the tonsillar folds, tonsils, oropharynx, tongue, salivary ducts and sublingual surfaces and note any abnormality in the form of swelling, adhesions, puckering, discolouration, sinuses and abnormal discharge.

All fractures involving the teeth are compound within the mouth due to rupture of firmly attached mucoperiosteum. Subperiosteal haematoma, due to fracture of body of mandible, may present as a soft or cystic swelling in the floor of the mouth.

Palpation

Superficial Palpation

Feel for texture, temperature and sensation of skin (affection of inferior dental nerve, usually in fracture of mandible, disturbs the sensation of lower lip).

Deep Palpation

Temporomandibular joint can be palpated easily from outside than from inside. Both joints must be palpated simultaneously.

Method (Fig. 18.1): Stand behind the patient who is sitting on a stool, keeping her head erect as far as possible. With both thumbs, support the back of the head while both ring fingers gently rest at the angle of the mandibles to appreciate movements of the lower jaw, the tips of index fingers being kept in front of the tragus. The patient is asked to gently open

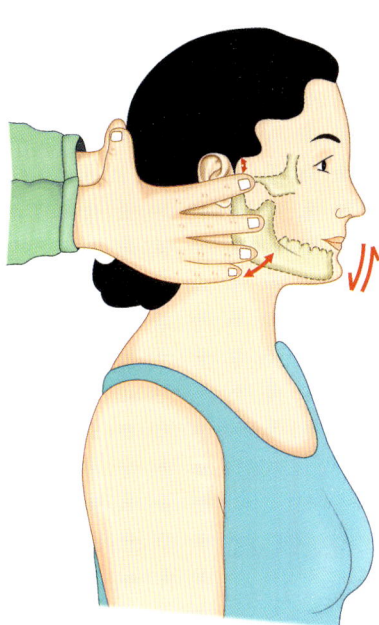

Fig. 18.1: Method of palpation of temporomandibular joint.

and close the mouth. Your index fingers will appreciate the movements of the condyloid processes of the mandible with each movement of the jaw. Note the excursion of the movements by:
- Appreciation of going down of jaw on your ring finger
- Looking from the front, see the approximate gap created at the angles of the mouth. In the midline note the maximum extent of opening up of the mouth by fingers-width assessment. Accurate measurement for prognostic value should be done by a graduated scale or graduated mouth blocks.

The joint is felt as a transverse slit running anteroposteriorly below the posterior end of the zygomatic process. Note the shape, size, regularity and any abnormal swelling or tenderness of the condyloid process.

Palpating the joint from the buccal cavity is neither easy nor much informative. However, putting one index finger through the mouth cavity along the line joining the angle of mouth to the tragus, and the other outside in front of the tragus, one can appreciate movements at the joint (only limited assessment is possible since the patient cannot close the mouth fully).

From inside, also palpate the gum, gingivolabial fold, palate, mucosa, sublingual region, salivary ducts and floor of the mouth, and note any abnormality.

Note pliability of the mucosa, any tenderness, any firm to hard structure in the salivary ducts (stone) and enlargement of salivary glands (usually submandibular). Count the teeth and note any distortion, infection, or impaction of the tooth, specially in the molar region.

In case of trauma, palpate the mandible through the submandibular region for its contour, shape, size, any tenderness, crepitus, swelling, irregularity, and displacement of the fracture.

In case of any scar or sinus, palpate as in the Chapter 1: Introduction.

■ MOVEMENTS (TABLE 18.1)

Anatomically, movements of the temporomandibular joint may be described as depression, elevation, protrusion, retraction and lateral rotating movements. The actual physiomechanics, though, is not that simple, functional mandibular movements are actually the resultant of complex rhythmic movements of the aforesaid types. However, clinical assessment must be for individual anatomical movements.

■ INVESTIGATIONS

- *X-ray is the main investigation (Fig. 18.2).* For mandible posteroanterior, lateral, oblique and inferosuperior views are helpful. For temporomandibular joints lateral, oblique and 35° fronto-occipital views are useful. However, tomography may be very useful
- Aspiration from the distended temporo-mandibular joint may be useful to know and examine the nature of collection.

The introduction of rotograph plus panoramic dental X-ray is proving much useful in delineating the topography, health and any abnormal finding of the teeth and jaw bones **(Fig. 18.3)**.

■ KEY DIAGNOSTIC POINTS

Key diagnostic points of common pathologies of the mandible, temporomandibular joints, and swellings of the jaw.

Disease

Congenital

Absence of lower jaw (agnathia).
- Hypoplasia or deficient development of lower jaw (micrognathia)
- Hyperplasia or over development of lower jaw (prognathism)
- Asymmetric development of lower jaw
- Congenital ankylosis of temporomandibular joint (ankylosis develops during ossification of Schmidts parietal bone and is a rather rare condition).

Ankylosis of Jaw (Fig. 18.4)

There is fusion of the condyle with glenoid fossa by either fibrous or bony tissue.
- Congenital ankylosis—Leads to deficient development of lower jaw
- Acquired ankylosis—Usually follows:

Mandible and Temporomandibular Joint

TABLE 18.1: Movements of temporomandibular joint.

Movement	Physiomechanics	Muscles involved in movement	Nerve supply
Depression	When the mouth is open, head of mandible first rotates, then glides downwards and forwards with the lower surface of the articular disc	• Lateral pterygoids assisted by digastric • Omohyoids • Mylohyoids	• Mandibular division of trigeminal nerve • Trigeminal and facial nerve • Hypoglossal nerve • Trigeminal nerve
Elevation	In closure of the mouth, the head of the mandible glides upwards and backwards along with the articular disc back into the temporal fossa	• Temporalis • Masseter • Medial pterygoids of both sides	Mandibular division of trigeminal nerve
Protrusion	Jaw remaining occluded, the lower teeth are drawn forward over the upper	Lateral and medial pterygoids	Mandibular division of trigeminal nerve
Retraction	Mandible is drawn backwards from protrusion to the position of rest	• Temporalis assisted by middle and deep parts of Masseter • Digastric • Geniohyoids	• Mandibular division of trigeminal nerve • Trigeminal and facial nerve • Hypoglossal nerve
Rotatory movements	In grinding or chewing, the head of one side along with the corresponding disc glides forwards, rotates around a vertical axis and then glides backwards rotating in an opposite direction as the head of the opposite side comes forwards in its turn	Medial and lateral pterygoids of each side acting alternately	Mandibular division of trigeminal nerve

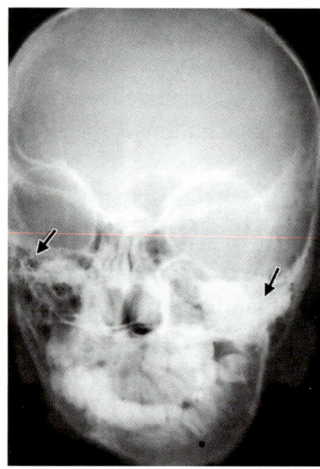

Fig. 18.2: Bilateral temporomandibular joint ankylosis with facial asymmetry.

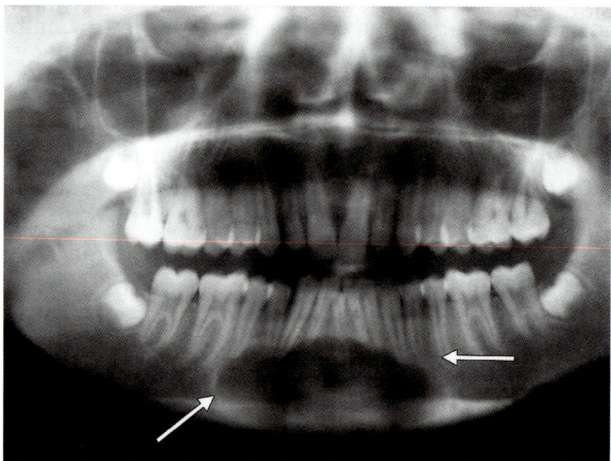

Fig. 18.3: Rotograph plus panoramic dental X-ray showing solitary cyst in the mandible.

- Inflammatory lesions, e.g. septic arthritis, osteomyelitis, mumps, measles, scarlet fever, enteric fever, tetanus, rheumatic fever, otitis media, mastoiditis, parotitis, caries teeth, parotid stones, cancrum oris
- Collagen arthropathy, e.g. rheumatoid arthritis, ankylosing spondylitis
- Traumatic—fractures of condyles, neck, ramus of mandible; subluxation, dislocation; fracture-dislocation; even strains and sprains have been seen to cause ankylosis to some extent
- Neoplastic—malignant neoplasm of buccal region, buccal cavity, cheek, parotid gland, gums, jaw and ear may lead to ankylosis of jaw
- Miscellaneous—pale mucosal fibrosis, hysterical.

Ankylosis can otherwise be classified as:
- *Unilateral* (often marked by asymmetry of face with the chin deviated to the side of ankylosis).
- *Bilateral*—congenital or acquired ankylosis in childhood leads to symmetrically retarded growth of the jaw. Inability to open the mouth results in bad oral hygiene and foul smell.

Diseases Affecting the Temporomandibular Joint
- *Infective:*
  - Following open injuries
  - Through haematogenous route (e.g. in rheumatic fever, tonsillitis, influenza)
  - Spread from surrounding tissues (e.g. otitis media, osteomyelitis of mandibular process, parotid abscess).

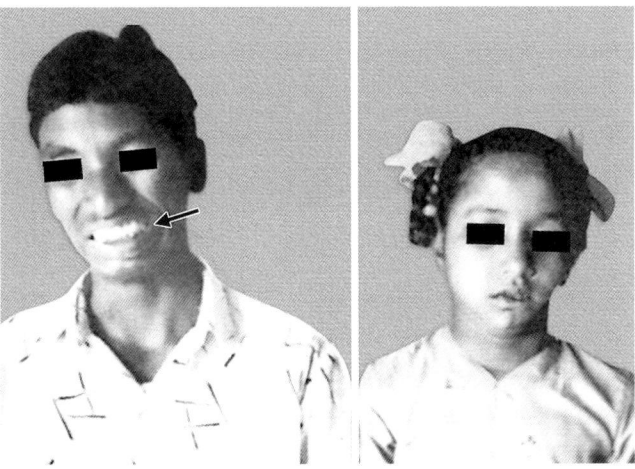

Fig. 18.4: Ankylosis of jaw: On the left—acquired type; on the right—congenital—Note the lesser development of left sided jaw (mandible).

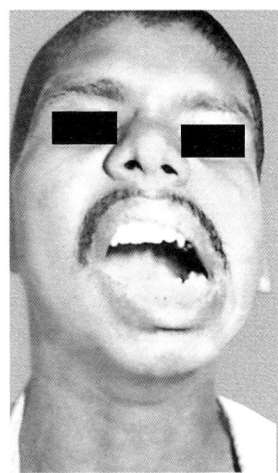

Fig. 18.5: Anterior dislocation of left temporomandibular joint.

- *Arthrosis*—following:
  - Involution
  - Developmental defects of jaws
  - Malocclusion of the teeth
  - Reduced occlusion of teeth
  - Improper prosthetic management following excisional surgery
  - Collagen arthropathy.

In arthrosis, symptoms are—
- Articular—pain, crackling and clicking in the joint.
- Regional—pain, feeling of obstruction in nose and ears, tinnitus, glossalgia, pain in face and eyes, dryness of mouth, hearing defects, headache, etc.

People suffering from chronic migraines are fairly more (about three times more) likely to suffer from severe temporomandibular disorders causing joint pain, reduced movements of jaw, clicking or popping of temporomandibular joint and radiating pain in face and neck. The diseases of temporomandibular joint may increase the frequency and severity of migraine attacks.

Traumatic Conditions

Dislocation

- Dislocation of temporomandibular joint can occur in any direction **(Figs. 18.16A and B)**.
- Most common is anterior dislocation (in which mouth remains open and cannot be closed) **(Fig. 18.5)**.
- Very rarely posterior dislocation occurs. Here, following a direct blow on the lower jaw, the condyles rest against the mastoid process after fracturing the auditory meatus or slipping underneath it. In this condition, it becomes impossible to open the mouth.
- *Lateral dislocation:* The condyle is displaced lateral to the zygomatic process. This is encountered in fracture of the mandible. The chin is displaced in the direction of the fracture. The mouth is easily opened.
- *Habitual mandibular dislocation:* Patients, usually ladies in late teens and twenties, complain of click and slipping of the temporomandibular joints; they can voluntarily repeatedly reproduce and reduce subluxation/dislocation of the joints.

Subluxation of the Temporomandibular Joint

- Traumatic
- Habitual subluxation is more common—The patient manages herself to produce and reduce the subluxation. The symptoms are annoying discomfort in temporomandibular joint, with or without clicking of the joint.

Fracture of the Mandible

For all practical purposes, *fractures of the jaw are potentially infected open fractures,* having communication with the (dirty) oral cavity.

Any part of the body, angle, ramus or neck of mandible may sustain a fracture. Fractures of mandible are classified according to the site of fractures as follow: Fractures of body; Fractures of angle; Fractures of condyle; Fractures of coronoid; Fractures of ramus; Fractures of symphysis; Fractures of parasymphyseal region; Dentoalveolar fractures.

Besides thorough clinical examination, various views of X-rays of mandible and face help in localising and classifying the fracture of mandible. Usual view of X-ray taken are: Posteroanterior; Intraoral periapical; right and left. Temporomandibular joints are, in fact, two along with their articular ligaments and masticatory muscles, form craniomandibular joints. The articular disc, consisting of nonvascularized and noninnervated dense fibrous tissue, divides the joint into upper and lower compartments.

TABLE 18.2: Swelling of the jaw.

Type of swelling	Site	Presenting features	X-ray findings
1	2	3	4
1. Inflammatory swellings **(Fig. 18.6)**	• Anywhere, but common are alveolar abscess, gum abscess, tooth-gum infection, osteomyelitis, tuberculosis, actinomycosis, submandibular salivary gland infection with or without stone in duct **(Fig. 18.11)** • Acute osteomyelitis is rare, seen mostly in infants as a complication of scarlet fever and measles • Subacute osteomyelitis is common and occurs due to infections in and around the tooth and open fractures. Chronic osteomyelitis affects mandible **(Fig. 18.7)** following infections of tooth, open fractures, irradiation and chemical necrosis (phosphorus poisoning), Mucoperiosteum of gum	• Varying constitutional features • Local tenderness, pain, swelling, with or without fluctuation • Thickening of the bone. • Sinuses • Earlier difficulty in opening mouth due to spasm, later on ankylosis of jaw (if neglected)	If bone is involved, areas of destruction, may be new bone formation, bone abscess shadow, sequestrum **(Fig. 18.7)**
2. Epulis word is derived from the Greek επ (on top of) and gum Epulis (Swelling arising from gum) classified as:			Soft tissue shadow; if bone is involved, areas of rarefaction or destruction
i. Congenital	Like fibrous epulis of older people, it occurs as a pink swelling on the gums in relation to unerupted incisor teeth		
ii. Fibrous Pregnancy epulis or pregnancy tumours	• Slow growing regular fibrous growth • Arise at sites of local irritation, usually as an enlargement of an interdental papilla • In pregnant women, insignificant deposit of calcium causes irritation and hormonal changes in pregnancy	Soft, pink, vascular, rapidly enlarging lumps appear on the gums	
iii. Myelomatous	Purple looking swelling, osteoclastomatous feel, expansile nature	Foul smell, salivation	
iv. Granulomatous	Granular mass around an infected tooth	Caries tooth, foul smell, salivation	
v. Carcinomatous **(Figs. 18.8 and 18.12 to 18.15)**	Epithelioma, fungating margin	Arising from the gum, having firm ulcer, irregular surfaces, everted margin, bleeding, tenderness	
vi. Sarcomatous	Rapidly growing, firm, vascular, tender swelling from the gum		
3. Odontomes (Swelling usually arising from tooth germs. The epithelial debris left out in the process of development of enamel of tooth are supposed to be the site of origin of odontomes) Classification of odontomes:	A tumour arising from any tissue taking part in the development of a tooth		
I. Epithelial odontomes:	Cysts of eruption—bluish swellings of the gum, occurring where deciduous or permanent teeth are to erupt		
i. Dental cyst **(Fig. 18.9)**	Usually upper jaw, arises from the root of normally erupted but chronically infected tooth	Expansion of bony cortex, leading to thinness or even pathological fractures. It contains clear watery fluid with sparkling cholesterol crystals. Under finger pressure yielding tendency of cystic wall—may even be fluctuant	Expansion of the cortex with a clear cavity in relation to the root of a tooth

Contd...

Contd...

Type of swelling	Site	Presenting features	X-ray findings
1	2	3	4
ii. Dentigerous cyst (Follicular odontomes) **(Fig. 18.10)**— the most common type of odontogenic cyst (20% of all jaw cysts)	More common in mandible. Associated with unerupted permanent tooth. No relation with infected caries tooth occurs mainly in relation to 3rd molar or 3rd maxillary canines.	• Any age but common in teens (second and third decade) • Expanded cystic wall occupies floor of the mouth	Evidence of tooth in the cyst. Removal of cyst and extraction of unerupted tooth prevent recurrence on the whole prognosis - good
iii. Adamantinoma— (Cusaic 1827) (Akin to osteoclastomatous lesion)	Lower jaw mostly affected near about angle of mandible, rarely in maxilla upwards	Most common in the age of 40 or more in females, slow growing. Can occur 11 years upwards	Expansion of cortex, multiple septae, soap bubble appearance
Synonyms: Carcinoma of tooth-germ residue	Multilocular hard to firm swelling (may even burst in the mouth and get infected)	Swelling more obvious from cheek side than from mouth, egg shell crackling may be elicited	
Ameloblastoma (formerly known as adamantinoma and clinical features are same)	Difficult to differentiate from osteoclastoma clinically or even histopathologically	• Has been known to metastasise to bones, lung. Locally invasive within medullary bone and soft tissues; not radiosensitive. • Excision with 1 cm margin and substitution by iliac crest graft	Cluster of small cysts in the centre of the lesion

Eve's disease
II. Connective tissue odontomes:
  i. Fibrous odontomes—
  ii. Cementoma—
  iii. Osseous odontomes—
	• Usually in rachitic children, more or less features of dentigerous cyst, but here the cyst is small and with a dense fibrous wall
	• Occurs as a mass of cement in nodular form in relation to the root of an erupted tooth
	• Bone deposition in the wall of a fibrous odontomes		

III. Composite odontomes:
  i. Radicular odontomes—
  ii. Compound follicular odontome—
	• A very rare tumour, developing in connection with tooth fang
	• A number of ill-formed teeth are produced due to disordered activity in the cells of dental papilla
	• Other conditions like—extra cups and roots, dichotomy (two or more teeth developing as one), enamel nodule and extra-denticle have also been described as composite odontomes		

4. Neoplastic conditions:
  I. Benign—
  II. Locally malignant— Osteoclastoma (GCT)
	• (i) solitary cyst (ii) fibroma (iii) chondroma (iv) osteoma—may occur in the jaw
	• Difficult to differentiate from adamantinoma, may develop centrally in the jaw
	• Jaw may be affected by xanthomatosis, osteitis fibrosa cystica, Paget's disease		

III. Malignant—
  i. Sarcoma
  ii. Carcinoma
  iii. Melanoma
  iv. Metastatic carcinoma
	• Usually from the antrum
	• Maxilla is usually involved secondarily from the palate
	• Mandible is commonly involved in advanced carcinoma of tongue or the floor of mouth or from secondarily involved cervical/submandibular lymph glands		

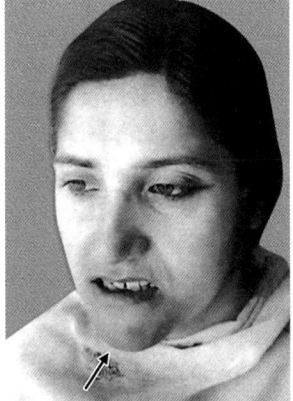

Fig. 18.6: Subacute osteomyelitis of lower jaw due to periapical abscess.

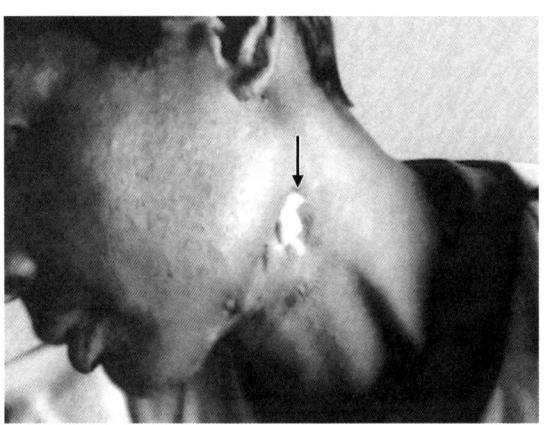

Fig. 18.7: Chronic osteomyelitis of mandible with a sequestrum ejecting through the sinus.

576 Mandible and Temporomandibular Joint

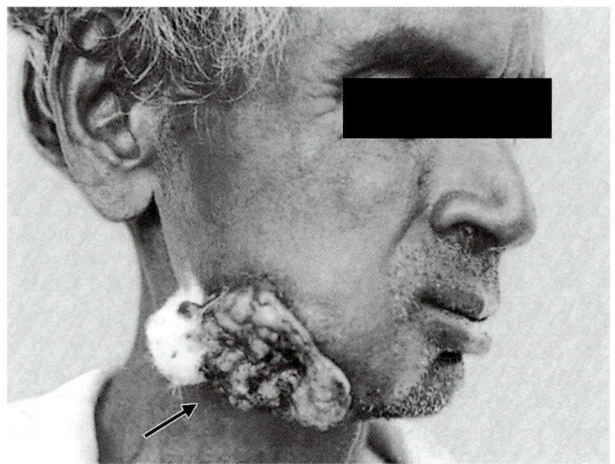

Fig. 18.8: Carcinomatous epulis fungated out after biopsy.

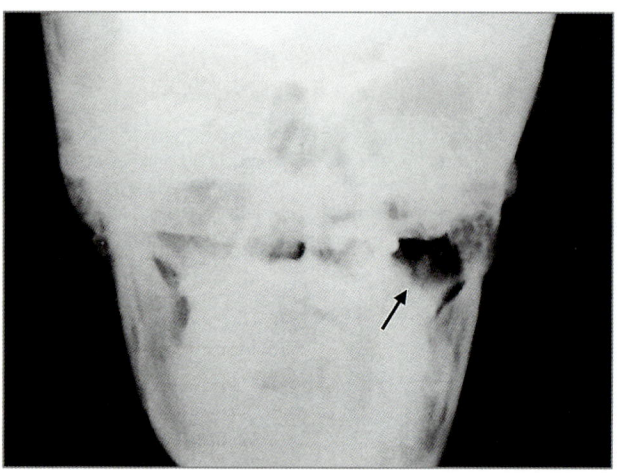

Fig. 18.9: Dental cyst.

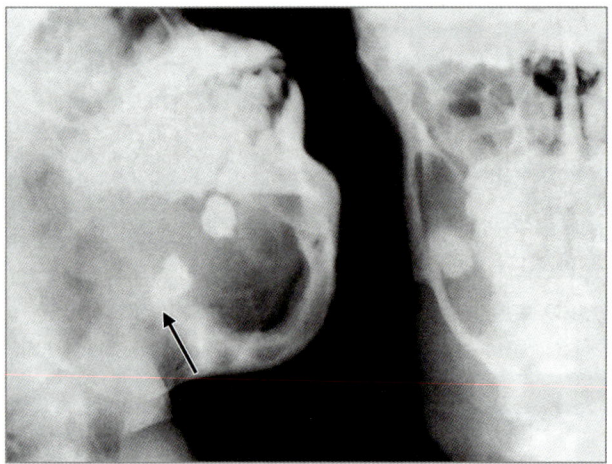

Fig. 18.10: Dentigerous cyst in the mandible.

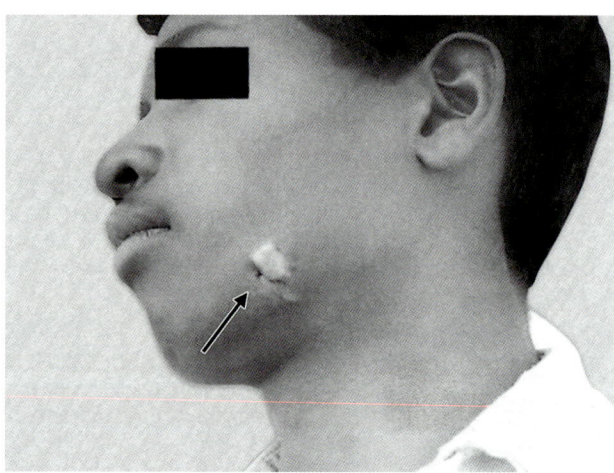

Fig. 18.11: Chronic osteomyelitis mandible following caries tooth.

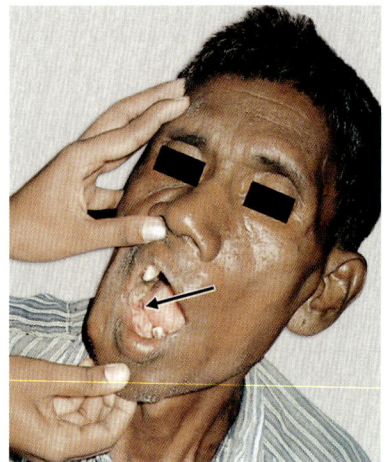

Fig. 18.12: Carcinoma jaw—carcinomatous epulis.

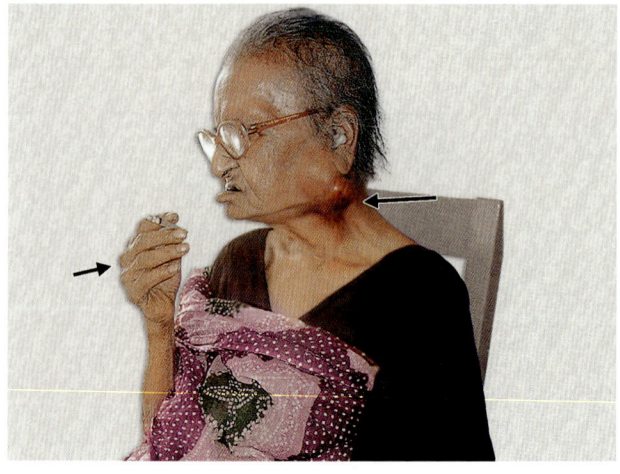

Fig. 18.13: Advanced carcinoma jaw originating from buccal region fungating through mandible and affecting the glands. She has been smoking regularly (Note 'bidi'—in her hand).

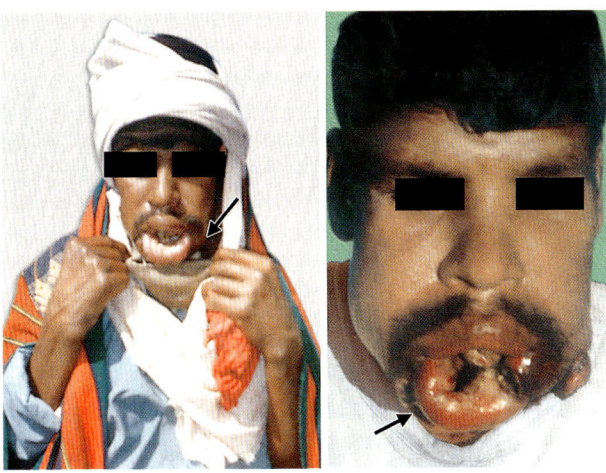

Fig. 18.14: Advanced carcinoma of jaw—typical site after tobacco chewing.

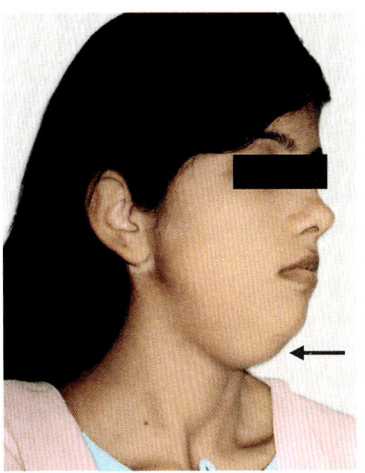

Fig. 18.15: Submental cyst.

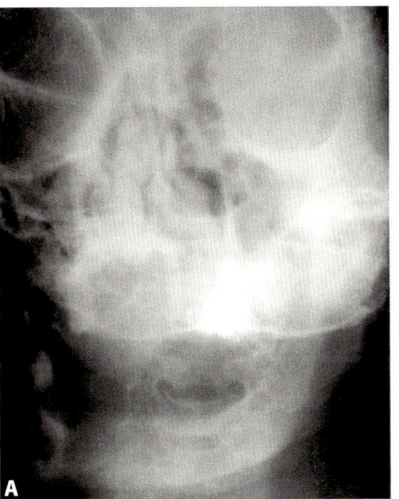
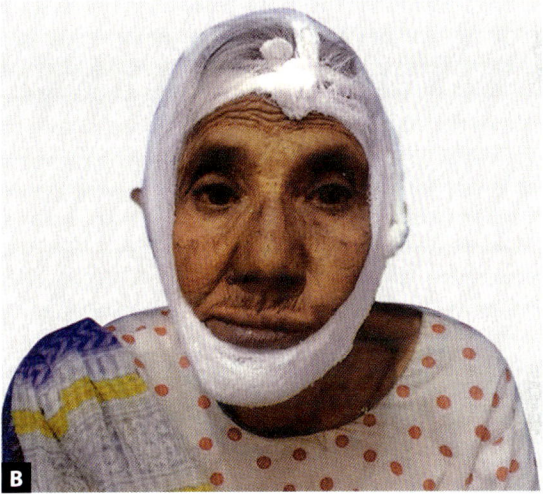

Figs. 18.16A and B: Temporomandibular joint dislocation in a 80 years old lady with only three teeth left in her jaws. On the left (A) is her X-ray, on the right (B) post reduction clinical picture with securing bandage. Reduction was difficult, since joint appeared unusually locked. After 4 weeks she is using her jaw freely.

Fractures up to the body and angle are usually displaced, which becomes obvious by the displacement in the teeth level. Patient complains of pain, swelling and restricted movements of the mandible and difficulty in articulation. Gentle and cautious palpation through the submandibular region can provide the clue regarding the site of fracture. Bilateral fractures may lead to serious complications, like—drooping of the jaw, swelling of the tongue, oedema of the glottis or even endanger the patency of the airway. There will also be disruption in the teeth level.

The pressure of teeth provides almost accurate guide for aligning the fractured fragments of mandible. However, fractures in geriatric edentulous patients and pediatric patients with deciduous or mixed dentition present various difficulties in treating their mandibular fractures.

Swellings of the Jaw (see Table 18.2)

As such, any osseous or soft tissue swelling, right from inflammatory to neoplastic, may arise in the jaws. However, there are a few swellings which are peculiarly localised only to the jaw and deserve separate consideration.

■ BIBLIOGRAPHY

1. Cusack JW. Report of the amputations of portions of the lower jaw. Cusaic: Dublin Hosp Rep. 1827;4:1-38.

CHAPTER 19

Gross Examination of Head Injury

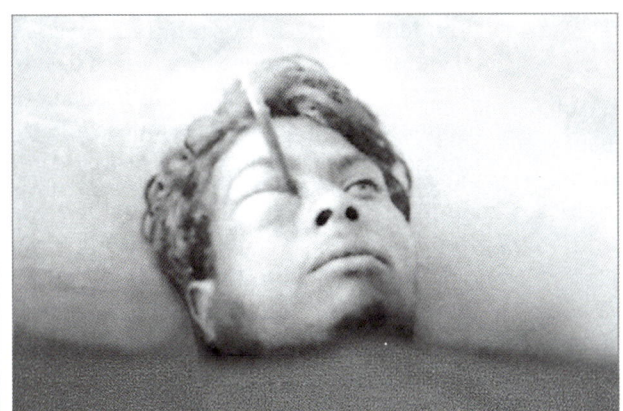
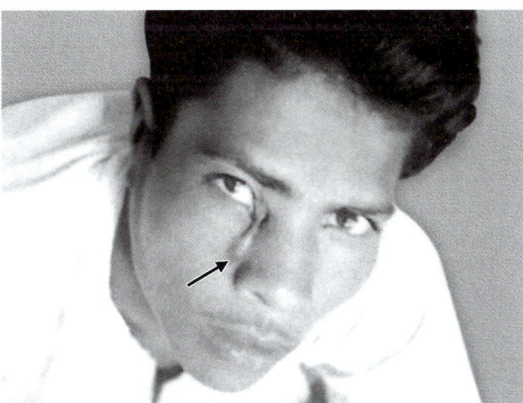

Four basic factors involved in successful outcomes: good setting, positive thinking, visualizing, and believing.
—*APJ Abdul Kalam*

Head injury is one of the most common injuries in accidents especially the road traffic accidents by motorcyclists. However, the use of crash helmet and legislation concerning head protection and body constraint for traffic and sporting events have definite effect in reducing the incidence. In case of polytrauma, head injury is a frequent occurrence; however, fortunately about 80% of the patients of head injury fall under the category of mild head injury.

Remember small lesions can make large impairments and large lesions small impairments.

With the highly advanced diagnostic and therapeutic aids (angiography, ultrasonography, CAT scanning, stereoscopic examination, MRI, 3-D and 4-D NMR with isotopic labelling) being used in managing head injuries, it has become further imperative to suspect and diagnose head injuries at the earliest. The aphorism of Hippocrate's— *"No head injury is so slight that it should be neglected, or so severe that life should be despaired of"* is a moral and duty bound incentive for any clinician confronted with this injury.

Head injury is often an accompaniment of multiple injuries—as occurs commonly in road traffic accidents, fall from height, industrial accidents, sports injuries, etc. Here again, the orthopaedic surgeon, being the team leader of the 'accident services', owes the responsibility of seeking the help of a neurosurgeon at the earliest in managing this injury.

In assessment of head injuries, three points are significant: (1) Clinical course is not always classical and a free interval does not exclude subdural haematoma; (2) 25% of patients with skull fracture with diminishing consciousness have chance of having an intracranial haematoma; (3) CAT scan is the most important diagnostic mean to assess the head injury, over which the treatment protocol can be based.

In any head injury, the *first assessment is of A, B, C* (A = Airway, B = Breathing, C = Circulation). The real assessment **(Tables 19.1 to 19.5)** must begin only after the above are attended to. Following that, a quick general assessment of the patient should be made regarding *level of consciousness* (comatose, semiconscious, stuporose, delirious, irritable, confused), however, he may not be unconscious initially; patency of airway; any other obvious vital injury (severe chest injury, severe abdominal injury; injury to neck or groin (especially penetrating injury); pulse; respiration; blood pressure; pupillary condition; temperature (on both halves of the body); bladder condition (wetting of bed), if bladder is full—catheterise and collect sample of urine for examination; smell coming from mouth (alcoholic, uraemic, diabetic); scalp (any obvious bruising, haematoma, cut, lacerations; bony depression, deformity, etc), bleeding (or leak of CSF or very rarely brain matter) through—nose, ear and mouth. CSF leak through nostrils (rhinorrhoea) or through external auditory meatus (otorrhoea) is usually mixed with blood. If a drop of it is dropped on a sheet it produces the double ring of blood and CSF. Further the clotting of this blood is delayed due to the presence of CSF. Note for any neck rigidity (may be due to meningeal irritation in subarachnoid haemorrhage) and also look for evidence of Jacksonian fits. Then neurological examination should be done in detail if the condition of the patient permits. Following this a quick but thorough systemic examination should be done.

Make a note of each finding. *Frequent repeated and thorough examinations at short regular intervals (half to two hourly) is mandatory.*

Patient is usually brought unconscious or comatosed. Coma is a state of prolonged unconsciousness. It results from serious disruption of the functions of brain, which impairs the reticular activating system to the extent that consciousness is lost. Whenever possible, take a detailed history from the attendants and/or the patient (if conscious) regarding:

- Mode of injury, circumstances and time of accident, use of a crash helmet
- Immediate status after injury (transient unconsciousness, vomiting, continued unconsciousness). Transient unconsciousness should be differentiated from 'syncope' [(Gr synkopi, fainting) i.e. a transient loss of consciouness due to inadequate blood flow to the brain]
- Intake of alcohol
- Known history of diabetes, epilepsy, renal failure, any addiction (i.e. opium or any drug, etc.)
- If patient can respond, the initial history should be taken for the followings: **A**-allergies (e.g. to drugs, etc. like penicillin); **M**edicine taken regularly (e.g. steroids, hypotensives, antidiabetics, anticoagulants, etc.); **P**ast-illness; **L**ast meal taken, **E**vents of accident (AMPLE).

Certain attitudes and postures provide clues in the assessment of head injuries, e.g. Lying flaccid with the mouth relaxed and angle of mouth sagging denotes a serious condition. *Decerebrate posturing,* whether unilateral or bilateral, is of grave prognostic significance, since it usually signifies severe and most likely, irreversible midbrain damage. If patient is curled up on his side and resents interference, it indicates *cerebral irritation,* which is a favourable sign in head injury.

Besides examinations on general principles, certain factors deserve special mention.

- *Pupil:* Size and equality of the pupils are of more importance than the reaction to light.
  The pupil may be fixed and dilated immediately after injury due to direct involvement of the oculomotor nerve in case of fracture of the anterior cranial fossa. It is of particular importance when the patient is not in deep coma
- *Ciliospinal reflex:* This reflex (minor pupillary dilatation of both eyes on painful stimuli) signifies integrity of the sympathetic pathway and thus the midbrain. This reflex is usually more marked in comatose state

- *Oculocephalic reflex* (Doll's eye phenomenon): On rapid rotation of the patient's head, the eyeball moves away from the direction in which the head is turned. Proprioceptive impulses transmitted from the neck muscles to the longitudinal fascicle are responsible for this reflex, which denotes severe brain damage
- *Oculovestibular* (Caloric) *reflex:* Integrity of the brainstem function can be finally assessed by this reflex. If the brainstem is functionally intact, injection of cold water into the ear, while head is supported in 30° elevation, stimulates movements of the eyeball. No response of the eyeballs to this denotes a very grave sign, and if it persists for more than an hour, death is certain
- *Analysis of motor response to command and stimuli:* Obeying commands is a good prognostic sign. Flexion response, and attempt at avoiding painful stimuli indicate good prognosis. On the other hand, extensor responses and/or assumption of *decerebrate posture* have a grave prognosis

  Even in noncomatose patients, the motor responses are more informative than sensory charting.

  In subarachnoid haemorrhage, the meningeal irritation leads to neck rigidity
- *Post-traumatic amnesia* (Return of continuous memory after head injury): It is the best guide for assessing the ultimate prognosis. If it exists less than 24 hours, the prognosis is good. Its extension beyond 24 hours is not a good prognostic sign
- Due to loose attachment and pliability of the epicranial aponeurosis, the external wound may not overlie the underlying fracture in a compound injury
- *Cardiac arrhythmias* (atrioventricular nodal and ventricular arrhythmias) are frequently associated with severe brain injuries
- *Assessment of level of consciousness:* Though not universally accepted, *Glasgow Coma Scale* has been observed to be reliable, and on the whole satisfactory to prognosticate the ultimate outcome of a head injury. Though it is fallacious when there are associated orbital injuries, diseases, speech problems, and pre-existing mental conditions, these can be out-weighed by its overall simplicity and practicability, since it gives an actual description of the patient's condition, rather than expressing in terms of coma, semicoma, and stupor.

  Three parameters (E, M, V) are mainly observed to assess the depth of the coma.

  By adding the scores of each component, the total Glasgow Coma Scale **(Table 19.1)** is determined. If the total score is 15 (E 4 + M 6 + V 5), the patient's level of consciousness is completely normal. A patient in deep coma will score only three. The *higher the score, better is the prognosis.*

TABLE 19.1: Glasgow Coma Scale.

E = Eye opening		M = Best motor response		V = Verbal response	
Spontaneous	—4	Obeys	—6	Oriented	—5
To speech	—3	Localises pain	—5	Confused conversation	—4
To pain	—2	Withdraws (flexion)	—4	Inappropriate words	—3
Nil	—1	Decorticate (flexion) rigidity	—3	Incomprehensible sound	—2
		Decerebrate (extension) rigidity	—2		—1
		Nil	—1	Nil	

The seriousness of cerebral dysfunction assessed using the Glasgow Coma Scale can be classified as: Mild (scores 13 through 15); Moderate (score 9 through 12); and Severe (scores 3 through 8 points). Patient with score less than 8 are in coma (Booth CM et al).

An alternative scoring system has been suggested as the FOUR Score coma scale. (**F**ull **O**utline of **U**n**R**esponsiveness) at the Mayo clinic (Wolf CA, et al. and Further Validation of the FOUR score scale by intensive care nurses. Mayo Clin Proc. 2007;82:435-438).

TABLE 19.2: Four score coma scale.

	Points				
Response	0	1	2	3	4
Eyes	Eyelids open, tracking and blinking on command	Eyelids open, but not tracking	Eyelids closed but open to loud voice	Eyelids closed but open to pain	Eyelids remain closed to pain
Motor	Thumbs up, fist or peace sign to command	Localising to pain	Flexion response to pain	Extensor posturing to pain	No response to pain or generalised myoclonus; status epilepticus

Contd...

Contd...

Response	Points				
	0	1	2	3	4
Brainstem reflexes	Pupillary and corneal reflexes present	One pupil wide and fixed	Pupillary or corneal reflexes absent	Pupillary and corneal reflexes absent	Absent pupillary, corneal and cough reflexes
Respiration	Not intubated regular breathing	Not intubated, Cheyne-Stokes pattern of breathing	Not intubated, irregular breathing pattern	Breathing above ventilator rate	Breathing at ventilator rate or apnoea

Source: Adapted from Demaerschalk BM, Meschia JF, et al. Advantages of the Mayo clinic FOUR Coma Score over the Glasgow Coma Scale in the intensive care unit, Mayo clinic Neurosciences update. As written on pages 747 of De Gowin's Diagnostic Examins 9th Ed. Vol 2-by Leblond RF, Degowin RL, Brown DD. Tata McGraw Hill Education Private limited' New Delhi-2011.

■ INVESTIGATIONS

- In any patient of head injury (specially unconscious ones)
  - Examination of vomitus—if it is there
  - Routine examination of urine—specially for sugar
  - Breath—analysis for alcohol, etc.
  - Blood urea and serum creatinine
- X-ray (in addition to the skull, the neck should be included, **Figs. 19.1 to 19.3**) whenever possible, but not at the cost of management of the head injury. Two real indications for an emergency X-ray are: depressed

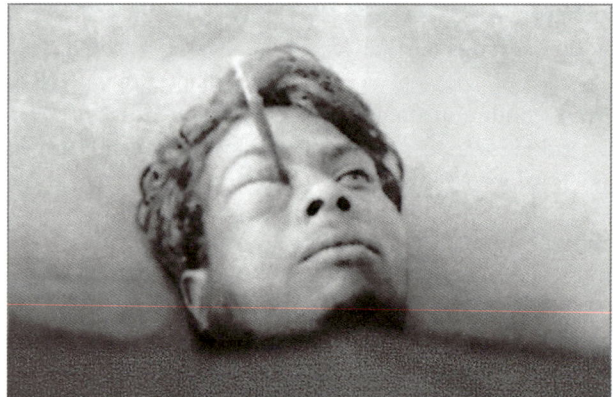

Fig. 19.1: An unusual arrow injury—piercing through the inner canthus of right eye.

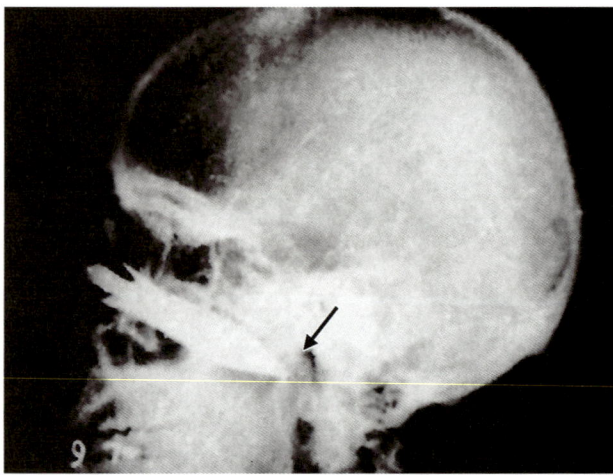

Fig. 19.2: The arrow tip almost to touch the medulla oblongata region.

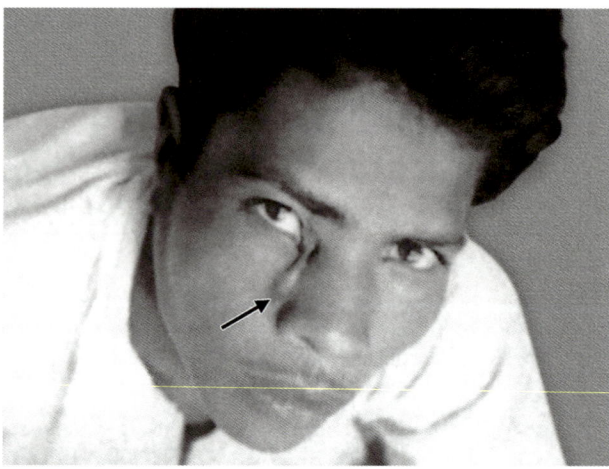

Fig. 19.3: After cautious removal of the arrow, the patient recovered fully except for the scar which can also be much reduced by proper plastic surgery.

TABLE 19.3: Features of fracture of base of the skull*.

Anterior cranial fossa	Middle cranial fossa	Posterior cranial fossa
Compounding through paranasal sinuses; bleeding and/or CSF or brain matter leak through nose; may be damage of 1, 2, 3, 4, 5, 6 cranial nerves; subconjunctival haemorrhage *Clinical difference* between subconjunctival haemorrhage following fracture of anterior cranial fossa and black eye (direct injury over face/eye)	• May be internal compounding through auditory meatus; blood and/or CSF through nose or mouth; may vomit swallowed blood; may be affection of 7th and 8th cranial nerves • By 48 hours following injury, bruising appearing at the mastoid process almost confirms fracture of middle cranial fossa (Battle's sign)	May cause serious haemorrhage due to rupture of the venous sinuses; may produce lesion of brainstem which may prove fatal; blood extravasates posterior to mastoid process; may be nystagmus and ataxia; 9th, 10th and 11th cranial nerves may be affected

Subconjunctival haemorrhage	*Black eye* **(Fig. 19.4)**
• Ecchymosis develops gradually (usually after 24 hours)	• Ecchymosis develops soon after injury
• Ecchymosis is circular, limited by attachment of orbital fascia to orbital margin	• Ecchymosis spreads even to the cheek and forehead
• Colour is usually purple-blue	• Reddish-purple colour
• Haemorrhage is subconjunctival and cannot be moved with conjunctiva, and its posterior limit cannot be seen	• Haemorrhage is conjunctival and moves along with conjunctiva, also posterior limit can be seen
• Eyeball may protrude due to retrobulbar collection	• Eyeball not protruded
• Conjunctiva may be swollen	• Eyelid swollen

* Bilateral symmetrical black eye is suggestive of fracture of the anterior cranial fossa **(Fig. 19.5)**

TABLE 19.4: Brain injuries.

	Cerebral concussion	*Cerebral irritation*	*Cerebral compression*
1. Effect of head injury	Mild	Mild to moderate	Severe
2. Onset	Immediate	Delayed	Immediate or delayed
3. Cause	Shock of brain	Irritation due to cerebral oedema, contusion of brain	Usually due to cerebral haemorrhage (clot), bony fragment, foreign body or laceration of brain
4. Consciousness	Initial unconsciousness for a short period	May be history of initial unconsciousness, remains drowsy and irritable, avoids light and keeps eyes closed, preferring darkness	Concussion may continue in deep unconsciousness • Initial restlessness, ending in deep unconsciousness • Concussion—lucid interval—deep unconsciousness
5. Attitude	While unconscious, the patient may be completely flaccid but recovers soon	Assumes attitude of flexion and lies curled up on the side	• May be flaccid in the beginning • One side may be paralysed, while the other shows incoordinated contractions and may later on become paralysed

Contd...

Contd...

	Cerebral concussion	**Cerebral irritation**	**Cerebral compression**
6. Pulse	Rapid with low volume	Initially rapid, gradually settles	• Initially rapid, gradually becomes slow and bounding, may again become rapid in terminal stage
7. Blood pressure	Falls	Initially falls, later on maintained	Falls initially, then gradually rises to maintain the cerebral circulation and again falls in the terminal stage
8. Respiration	Slow, shallow and rapid	Almost normal	• Initially slow, shallow and rapid; gradually becomes slow and deep suggestive of Cheyne-Stokes breathing • Stertorous breathing may develop (Cheeks puffing in and out with snoring noise) indicating onset of bulbar compression
9. Temperature	Subnormal	May be slightly higher	• Initially subnormal, then moderate pyrexia. Intracranial haematoma/secondary infections may lead to higher temperature • Extremely high temperature (40°-42° C) indicates pontine haemorrhage
10. Eye (pupil)	Slightly dilated, equal and reactive	Equal, reactive, remains slightly dilated but instantaneously constricts on testing	Hutchinson's pupil— *Normal side* • Initially normal reactive • Later on contracted • Last stage dilated and fixed • In pontine haemorrhage pinpoint fixed pupils *Affected side* • Contracted reactive • Dilated, may be fixed • Dilated and fixed
11. Reflexes	Absent, but recover	Irritable jerks	Paralysed side flaccid (jerks absent)
12. Residual effects	• May recover fully • May be followed by stage of irritation • May be followed by compression features either in continuity or with lucid interval	• May recover completely • May be residual headache, irritability, forget fullness, lack of concentration, abnormal psychic behaviour	• May end fatally If recovery—usually incomplete. Residual paresis, speech defects. Abnormal psychic behaviour. Lack of concentration, insomnia. Intracranial abscess, Jacksonian fits

TABLE 19.5: Injuries of intracranial blood vessels.

	Extradural (middle meningeal haemorrhage)	**Subdural haemorrhage**	**Intracerebral haemorrhage**	**Subarachnoid haemorrhage**
Incidence	Not common	Common	Common	Not common
Onset	Delayed manifestation (1–2 days)	Quite early manifestation	Early manifestation	Early manifestation
Site of injury on skull	• Temporal injuries—fracture skull with rupture of branches of middle meningeal artery (rarely anterior meningeal) • Haematoma on temporal region	Injury anywhere on the skull, even without fracture. Usually rupture of large cortical veins and/or laceration of the cortex	• Injury anywhere on the skull • With any type of brain injury	

Contd...

Contd...

	Extradural (middle meningeal haemorrhage)	**Subdural haemorrhage**	**Intracerebral haemorrhage**	**Subarachnoid haemorrhage**
Stages of manifestation	• Initially in a state of confusion or irritation, or concussion features—recover—after a variable period (few hours to days—lucid interval) again gradually becomes drowsy, and comatose • Gradually accumulating haematoma/clot presses the cerebral cortex from below upwards—producing facial, then upper limb, then lower limb paralysis	• No lucid interval Patient remains unconscious • Develops paralysis from the beginning (not in an orderly fashion) • Rapid deterioration	• No lucid interval • Patient unconscious • Develops paralysis from the beginning (not in an orderly fashion)	• Soon after injury rapid pulse, pyrexia, neck rigidity, severe headache, restlessness, positive Kernig's sign. After few hours lumbar discomfort with bilateral plantar response upgoing
Lumbar puncture	No blood in CSF	Blood in CSF	Blood in CSF	Blood in CSF

1. **Lateralisation of the lesion in extradural haemorrhage:** (i) Swelling and bruises in the temporal region—usually opposite to the side of paralysis (except in countre-coupe injury), (ii) Observation of Hutchinson's pupils, (iii) Temperature is higher on the paralysed side, (iv) Babinski positive (plantar up-going) on the side opposite to the haematoma pressing side, (v) Speech will be affected in case of left-sided injury of a right-handed person, (vi) Fracture of the skull usually denotes the underlying brain tissue damage—paralysis on the opposite side
2. **Severe complication of head injury:** Vasogenic Brain Oedema—Increased intracranial pressure occurs due to injury to the blood-brain barrier which results in leakage of protein and water into the intracellular spaces. This vasogenic brain oedema is preceded by a phase of brain swelling caused by the release of various substances, e.g. bradykinin, free radicals, lactate, CA++, prostaglandins, and neuropeptides—which have deleterious effects at cell level, mainly the cell membrane

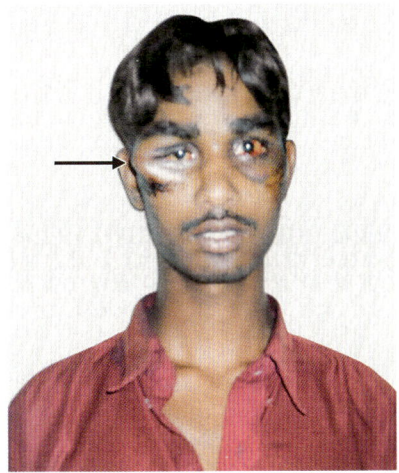

Fig. 19.4: Black eye due to orbital/external injury.

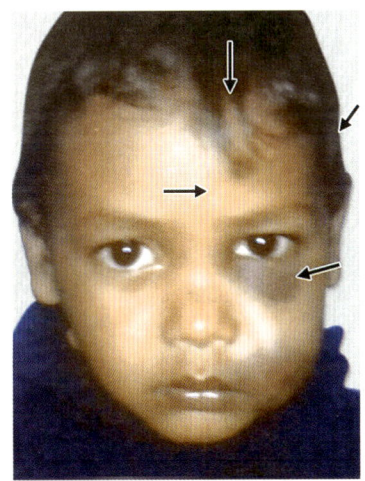

Fig. 19.5: Black eye like picture due to injury in left frontal and maxillary region.
Courtesy: Mrs Sabana, Ms Mileta, Ms Sarita

fracture and intracranial foreign body. This is also important from medicolegal point of view
- Lumbar puncture—(Usually not to be done in acute head injury), very cautiously (to avoid formation of pressure cone—which may be fatal) to see tension of CSF, any blood in CSF
- Cerebral/carotid angiography
- EEG—Not of much significance in acute head injury, but may be useful later on
- CAT scanning
- Stereoscopic studies
- NMR (MRI)
- Ultrasonogram
- Inspection burr holes in the skull.

■ BIBLIOGRAPHY

1. Iversen LD, Swiontkowski MF. The diagnosis and management of musculoskeletal trauma. In: Iversen LD, Swiontkowski MF (Eds): Manual of Acute Orthopaedic Therapeutics (4th ed), Boston: Little Brown and Company; 1995.1-19.
2. Pandey S, Sinha SN, Jha B, et al. An unusual arrow injury. Int Surg. 1972;57-589.

CHAPTER 20

Gross Assessment of Chest Injuries

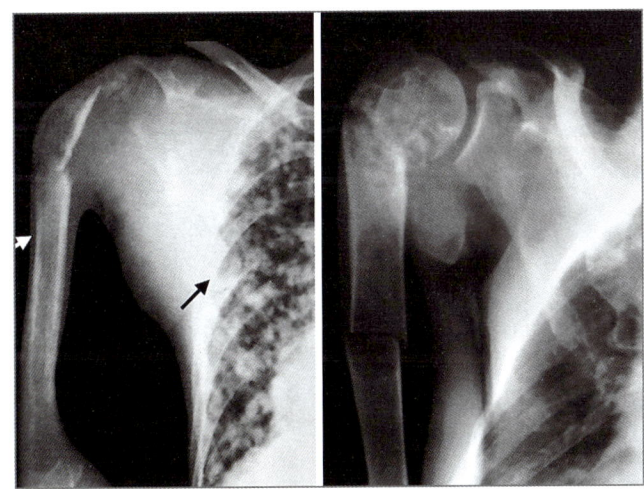

"The more you share your knowledge, the more you shine."
—*PP Wangchuk*

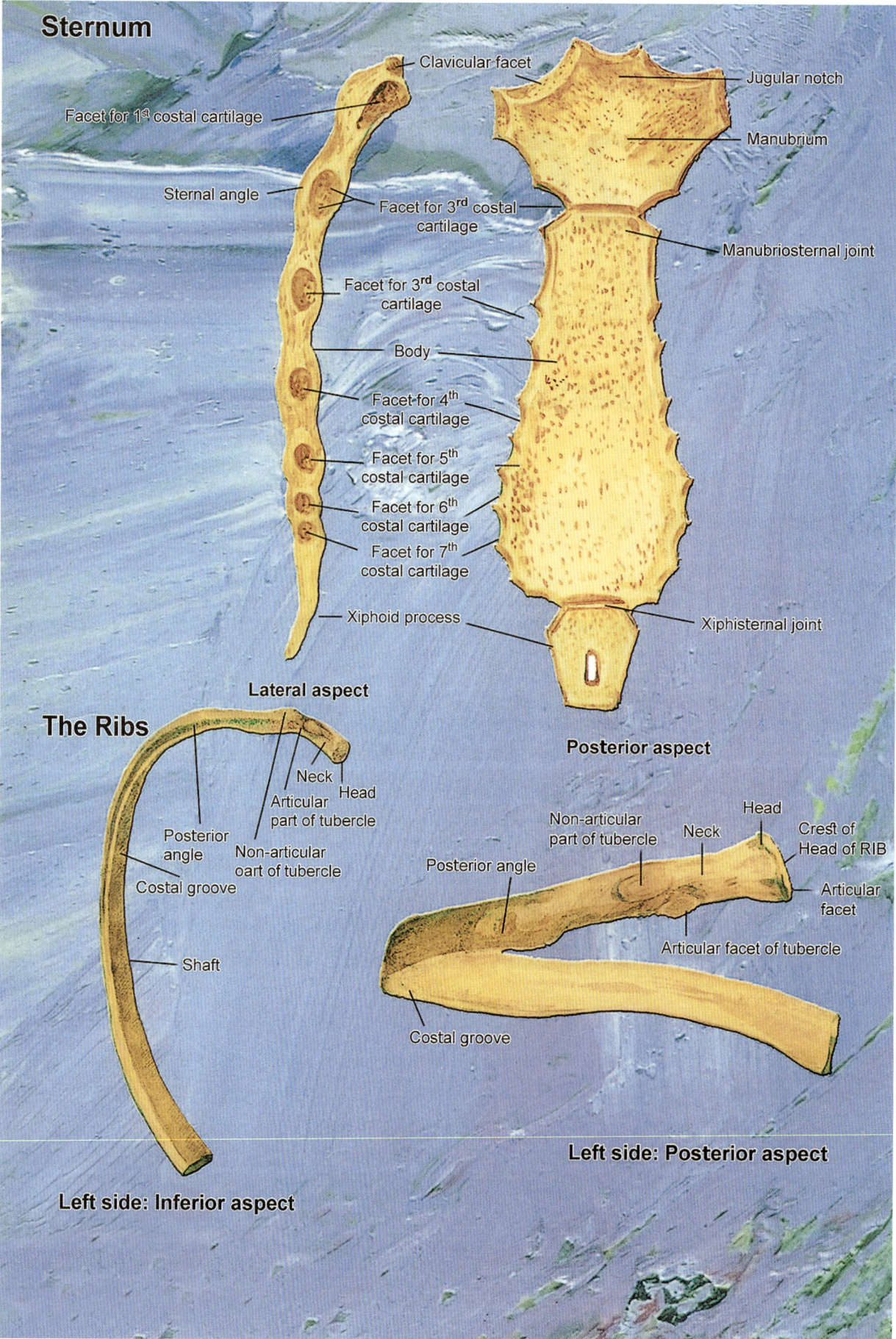

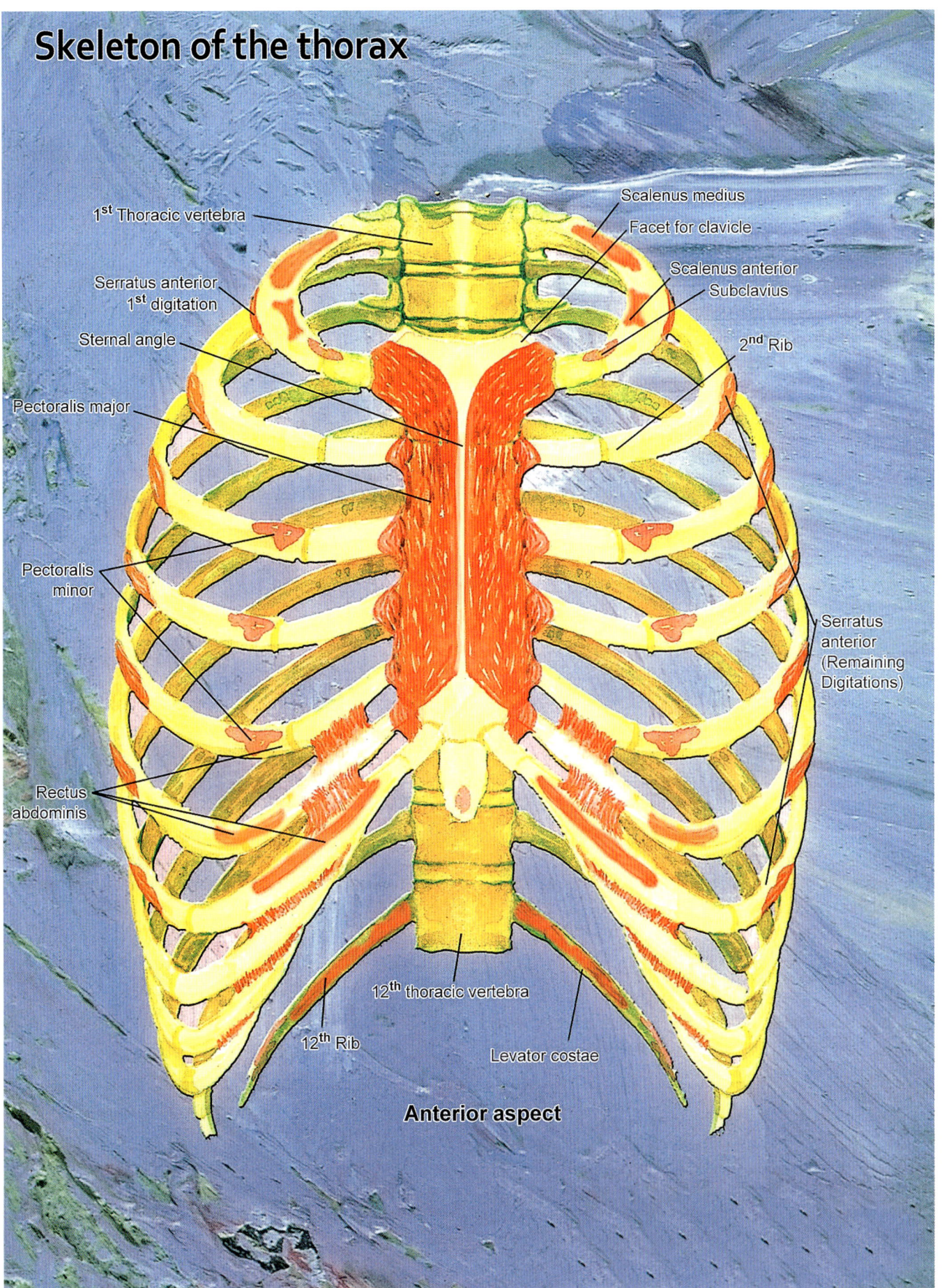

INTRODUCTION

Chest injuries cause approximately 25% of the deaths occurring due to war and allied injuries. Hence, their accurate diagnosis and prompt treatment is of great importance. In civil practice, causes of chest injuries include road traffic accidents; increasing criminal violence, (stab injuries, gunshot/missile injuries) and sports injuries. The main importance of chest injuries is in their effects on the vital organs of the chest, like lungs, heart and major blood vessels, giving rise to traumatic pneumothorax, haemothorax, mediastinal flutter, stove-in-chest, rupture of aorta and other catastrophies.

According to mode of violence, chest injuries can be: (i) non-penetrating (blunt trauma to thoracic cage), which usually produce contusion to lung, haemorrhage and oedema in alveoli and interstitial tissue, but rarely, even transection of trachea and/or bronchus leading to emphysema, pneumothorax and respiratory distress, (ii) penetrating injuries (minor pleural puncture to catastrophic heart, aortic and lung injuries).

Chest injuries may be classified as follows:

Group I
- Those peculiar to the chest wall:
- Subcutaneous emphysema
- Flail chest (paradoxical respiration)
- Open pneumothorax.

Group II
Those peculiar to the inner region of the chest:
- Closed pneumothorax
- Haemothorax
- Obstruction of lower airways due to secretions, leading to "*wet lung*" and aspiration pneumonitis.

Group III
Those peculiar to the inner most region of chest:
- Mediastinal emphysema and injury
- Cardiac tamponade
- Traumatic diaphragmatic hernia.

The mortality rate due to injuries of heart and great vessels and pulmonary insufficiency is still high.

Regardless of the classification, it is important to detect whether the thoracic cage was penetrated by a pointed object.

Chest Wall

Fracture of single or multiple ribs is not alarming, if the lung parenchyma or pleura has not been pierced. However, the patient feels pain even in regular breathing. The fracture can be best localised by asking the patient to point out the site of 'catch' due to pain while taking a deep breath. Palpation with the finger tip along the suspected rib will elicit maximum tenderness at the fracture site. One may feel crepitus as well.

Chest compression test should be avoided as far as possible, except in doubtful cases.

Compression Test

While sitting on a stool, the patient elevates his arms over the head. The base of one hand is placed over the sternum and the base of the other over the spine at the same level. The thorax is then gently compressed anteroposteriorly. When a rib has been fractured, this manoeuvre causes pain at the site of lesion.

Side-to-side compression may also be done if the fracture is located more anteriorly or in the sternum.

In multiple fractures of the ribs, though there may not be immediate complications, injury to the underlying pleura and lungs, later on, is a possibility. The pain in such case is of greater magnitude with limited excursion of that side of the chest, leading to post-traumatic atelectasis of the lung.

Injury of Lungs

There are two early features:
- *Haemoptysis:* In every case of chest injury, an early enquiry about coughing out of blood should be made
- *Surgical emphysema:* Due to traumatic rupture of pulmonary tissue, air percolates from beneath the visceral pleura to enter the hilum of the lung and via the mediastinum it appears in the neck. However, air may directly enter the subcutaneous tissue after rupture of both the layers of pleura.

EXAMINATION OF INJURIES OF THE CHEST (TABLE 20.1)

Usual complaints are: Swelling, pain, fever, difficulty in breathing, cough, haemoptysis. Enquire about the nature of violence and history of any previous chest disease.

General and systemic examinations: See whether the patient is in shock, restless, cyanosed, dyspnoeic or gasping. Pulse, temperature and blood pressure should be recorded. Also, look for any associated injury.

Attitude of the Patient

Fracture of sternum: The attitude is characteristic. The body is bent forward with the shoulders rotated inwards, the head is held downwards and forward.

Respiration: Note the type of the breathing patterns. The respiration may be:
- Abdominothoracic or abdominal or thoraco-abdominal or only thoracic

TABLE 20.1: Acute traumatic conditions of chest.

Type of injury	History	Clinical feature	Radiology	Other investigations	Complication	Treatment	Prognosis
1	2	3	4	5	6	7	8
1. Single rib fracture	• Injury • Heavy coughing • Closed cardiac massage • In asthmatics and osteoporosis even mild to moderate coughing/sneezing	Pain at the site of fracture (aggravated by deep breathing and coughing). Local tenderness; may be crepitus; compression test indicates sight of fracture. Fractures of lower ribs may involve underlying abdominal viscera	Fracture may not be shown in X-ray	—	Surgical emphysema • Felt as crepitus on gentle palpation	• May be ignored • Analgesics • Prophylactic antibiotics • Local infiltration of long acting local anaesthetic agent • Encourage normal respiratory pattern • Effective coughing after pressing the injured portion of chest • Ambulation (not bed rest) • Strapping of chest (not being preferred as regular procedure) • In case of massive surgical emphysema putting a wide bore needle or tube in subcutaneous tissue is needed	Good
2. Multiple rib fractures (on one side)	• Severe injury • Chest compression against hard object • Closed cardiac massage	• Marked pain at the site of fracture even on normal breathing; breathing is shallow. • Local tenderness ++, crepitus, (compression test should be avoided lest it may produce complications)	Fractures visible usually with overlap	—	• Surgical emphysema • Pneumothorax • Haemopneumothorax • Contusion of lungs	• Hospitalise the patient (some may require positive pressure ventilation) • Strapping of chest • Long-acting local anaesthetic infiltration after antiseptic preparation • Analgesics • Chest binder (Elastic corset) with pressure pads over injured area. In certain conditions, fixation of fractures by stainless steel wire/intramedullary rush pin/Judet clips, may be required	Fairly good
3. Fracture sternum	Severe direct injury from the front, e.g. impact of steering wheel (getting less) due to protective balloon incorporated in stem axis of steering; deceleration on to seat belts; closed cardiac massage	Pain in the sternal zone, tenderness at the fracture site, irregularity usually in a transverse line due to slight overlapping tendency of the fragments	Lateral and oblique views must be taken to exactly localise the site of fracture and displacement	• ECG (for any concomitant myocardial injury) • X-ray of dorsal spine (for any concomitant vertebral fracture	Myocardial injury, Vertebral injury, Mediastinal emphysema may be due to ruptured bronchus. Air may enter peribronchial space. Emphysema first appearing over suprasternal notch spreads, to neck, face, chest, abdomen and scrotum (Some are associated with multiple segmental rib fractures leading to flail chest and severe pulmonary insufficiency) rupture of aorta	• May be ignored • Analgesics • Rarely reduction by hooking the fragment, if markedly displaced • Management of associated serious injuries (e.g. myocardial injury, unstable chest injury, paradoxical movement of flail chest, etc.)	Fairly good

Contd...

Type of injury	History	Clinical feature	Radiology	Other investigations	Complication	Treatment	Prognosis
1	2	3	4	5	6	7	8
4. Multiple rib fractures at two sites (flail chest, stove-in chest) Flail—when ribs are fractured at two sites, usually anteriorly and posteriorly)	Severe injury, usually traffic accidents	Severe pain, respiratory distress, cyanosis, features of shock, paradoxical breathing (the portions of the ribs intervening the fracture sites forms a flail segment). With every inspiration, due to negative pressure in pleural cavity, this flail segment is sucked in and in expiration the flail segment is blown out and air comes from the opposite lung along the carina	• Affected lung space is collapsed to varying extent. • Fractured fragment obvious—usually with overlap	Screening to confirm the paradoxical breathing	Shock, cyanosis, traumatic wet lung (lung secretions fill in bronchi) May be lethal	First aid is by padded pressure over the flail segment • Endotracheal intubation and suction and cleaning of trachea and bronchial tree • Positive pressure ventilation • Towel-clip-traction of the flail fragment and stabilisation with a crammer wire circular frame • Internal fixation of the fractured ribs	If managed well • fairly good • may be lethal
5. Haemothorax (Blood in pleural cavity) Haemothorax is one of the most common manifestations after a blunt or penetrating chest trauma	• Laceration of lung parenchyma • Rupture of intercostal or internal mammary vessel	Pain chest. Respiratory distress. Cyanosis in severe cases. Tendency of silent chest. Dullness on percussion from below upwards. Muffled or absent breath sounds. Impaired vocal resonance	Radiopaque shadow filling the costophrenic and cardiophrenic angles and proceeding upwards	Aspiration (frank blood in pleural cavity)	May lead to clotting (clotting is rare due to churning). Pyothorax or Empyema	• Aspiration • Antibiotics • Respiratory exercises • Catheter drainage through 8th intercostal space in mid axillary line connected to water seal drainage	Fairly good
6. Haemopneumothorax (blood and air in pleural cavity) During the siege of the capital of the Mallians, Alexander the Great was *seriously wounded by an arrow in the chest. His faithful General Ptolemy said – "His breath as well as his blood spouted from the wound"*	Rupture of lung parenchyma or entry of air from outside	As above, hyperresonance and vocal fremitus, above the level of dullness. The line of dullness is horizontal when examined in the sitting position	Radiopaque shadow at the bottom of the lung field having a horizontal level, over which there is air in the pleural cavity	Aspiration (frank blood in pleural cavity)	• May lead to clotting (clotting rare due to churning) • Pyothorax or Empyema • Respiratory distress may increase • Pyopneumothorax	• Aspiration • Antibiotics • Respiratory exercises • Catheter drainage through 8th intercostal space • If needed, a 2nd catheter drainage in 2nd intercostal space anteriorly and connected to water seal drainage	Fair

Contd...

Type of injury	History	Clinical feature	Radiology	Other investigations	Complication	Treatment	Prognosis
1	2	3	4	5	6	7	8
7. Pyothorax (Empyema)—pus in the pleural cavity.	• Rupture of lung abscess in pleural cavity • Infection of haemothorax • Penetrating injury of chest	• Constitutional features of infection (febrile attacks and feature of toxaemia) • Findings of haemothorax exaggerated	Findings of haemothorax exaggerated	Aspiration of pleural cavity—pus	• Fever • Toxaemia, may even lead to lethal stage • Secondary lung abscess • May end in bronchopleural fistula or break subcutaneously (Empyema necessitans—impulse on coughing) or may even lead to sinus to exterior	• Repeated aspiration • Catheter drainage through 8th inter-costal space in mid axillary line connected to water seal system • Antibiotics • General restorative measures • Surgery—Evacuation of pus. Excision and/or decortication	Fair
8. Traumatic asphyxia	• Sudden compression of chest (crush injury) • Sudden retropulsion of blood into the bigger veins of chest, neck and head—leads to extravasation of blood into loose sub-conjunctival and subcutaneous tissues of face	• Marked subconjunctival congestion • Bleeding from nose and ears • Congested skin at face and neck • Petechial haemorrhage	Shock	— —	May be lethal unless and until attended very promptly	• Management of shock • Hyperbaric oxygen	Poor
9. Injury to lung parenchyma (contusion or laceration)	Closed or open chest injury	Haemoptysis, pain chest, surgical emphysema, respiratory distress, restricted chest movement, weak breath sounds	Features of localised consolidation of lung	—	• Pneumonia • Lung abscess	• Symptomatic • Antibiotics • Other expectant line of treatment	Fair

Contd...

Gross Assessment of Chest Injuries

Contd...

Type of injury	History	Clinical feature	Radiology	Other investigations	Complication	Treatment	Prognosis
1	2	3	4	5	6	7	8
10. Cardiac injury (usually haemopericardium)	Closed or open chest injury	• Typical triad of cardiac tamponade—increased area of cardiac dullness, muffled/inaudible heart sounds, gradual increasing of venous, and falling of arterial blood pressure. (rise in diastolic and fall in systolic blood pressure) • Features of shock	Increased cardiac shadow	Aspiration through left anterior 4th intercostal space—diagnostic (as blood comes out) and therapeutic, (as symptoms and signs improve)	Respiratory distress, cardiac shock—may be lethal	• Aspiration (may be repeated) through 4th intercostal space • Antibiotics • Specialised treatment	Fair
11. Thoracic major vessels injury (specially aorta)	Severe chest injury (specially penetrating injury) rapid deceleration, e.g. in car crash or fall from a great height	• Fever • Shock • Features of cardiopulmonary failure	In presence of minor leaks • Widening of mediastinum	—	Usually lethal	• Prompt treatment by specialised cardiothoracic team may save the patient	Poor
12. Injury to diaphragm (rupture of diaphragm) occurs in about 4 to 5% of chest injuries	Closed crush injuries • Penetrating abdominothoracic/thoraco abdominal injuries	• Features of shock • Features of peritonitis • Respiratory distress • Basal dullness • Muffled/inaudible breath sound	Radiopaque shadow in continuity with diaphragm (as if raised diaphragm) akin to haemothorax. On left side—herniated stomach may show gas. (cf. haemothorax)	Barium meal reveals position of stomach inside the chest Aspiration at lower chest does not reveal blood	• Cardiopulmonary compression features, profound shock (haemorrhagic) • Peritonitis	Thorough repair of rupture through thoraco-abdominal approach	Poor to fair

NB: The ***fracture of first rib*** is potentially serious chest injury, since it is well protected and requires a severe force to fracture, which may also lead to injuries to big vessels, head, neck, and abdomen. Mortality rate with fracture of first rib may be about 30%

NB: The **major life threatening problems** are tension pneumothorax, massive haemothorax, flail chest, thoracic major blood vessels injuries, open cardiac injury and traumatic asphyxia.
A tension pneumothorax is diagnosed by the signs of massive pneumothorax along with positive pressure in the intrapleural hemispace, causing mediastinal shift and decreasing venous return—which leads to a rapidly deteriorating respiratory and cardiovascular condition. Urgent aspiration of air relieve symptoms.
In flail chest patient can ventilate, but dyspnoea and cynosis persist. There is dissociated (discordinated) movements of the chest wall.
Besides definitive management, patient should be given immediate oxygen and put on ventilator

- Paradoxical breathing, i.e. indrawing of chest wall during inspiration and expansion during expiration.

Also note whether respiration is easy or laboured.

Local Examination

Inspection

Inspect the chest wall from all around (the clothes must be removed or cut open to see clearly) for any wound especially penetrating (whether it has penetrated the pleura) or sucking chest (suck-in chest) wound or for a paradoxical movement of a flail chest wall.

In case of penetrating wound, air and blood passes in and out of the wound with a loud sucking noise.

In late cases, it may be calcified showing whorl-like pattern. Ultrasonographically, it shows echogenic shadow with acoustic shadow. On CT scan, there is hypodense mass with thick peripheral rim. In MRI, a well-defined mass showing intermediate signal intensity at T1-weighted imaging and higher signal intensity at T2-weighted imaging. Histologically, foreign body granuloma is seen. Management consists of total excision.

It is interesting to know that Alexander the Great sustained an arrow injury in his chest during the siege of the capital of Mallians (modern Multan in Pakistan) producing the "sucking chest injury"—aptly complained as "his breath as well as his blood spouted from the wound". His surgeon Kritodemos of Kos treated him by extracting the arrow and covering the wound.

Look for any swelling on the chest. Surgical emphysema gives rise to a diffuse swelling.
- Presence of ecchymosis on the chest wall
- Presence of petechial haemorrhage in supraclavicular region at the side of the neck (traumatic asphyxia).

Examination of sputum: If sputum is blood-stained, it indicates injury to the lung.

Palpation

Palpate the ribs, besides the tenderness, which will be present in all injuries, crepitus [if present, indicates rib fractures (cf. crepitus in subcutaneous emphysema)], sternum, thoracic vertebrae, and any swelling if present. Ascertain the position of apex beat of heart. Feel for the vocal fremitus.

In the fractures of lower ribs, there is possibility of injury to abdominal organs, e.g. liver, spleen, etc.

Percussion: Undue resonance over the chest is suggestive of pneumothorax; normal cardiac dullness may be obliterated. Haemothorax and haemopericardium will be dull on percussion.

Auscultation: Auscultate for any crepitus.
- Diminution or absence of breath sounds indicates haemo/pneumothorax.

Heart: Muffled heart sounds with low pulse pressure and high diastolic pressure occur in haemopericardium.

A rapid thready pulse, falling blood pressure, distended neck veins, and distant muffled heart sounds indicate the development of cardiac tamponade.

If on inspection the patient appears to be in great respiratory distress, immediate management must be started.

■ BLUNT CHEST INJURY

Rib fractures are most common injuries in blunt chest trauma. The sensitivity of chest X-rays in showing the fractures of rib is limited, particularly in those involving the cartilage part of the rib. However, *ultrasonography using 7.5 MHz linear transducer is useful for detecting such fractures (which are often missed in plane X-rays).*

In blunt chest injury, there may be chest wall or intrathoracic injury. *The patient's prognosis is less favourable: when several ribs are broken* (mortality becomes higher if at least four ribs are broken) and when there are severe intrathoracic lesions, such as pneumothorax—mainly the tension pneumothorax; when there is tamponade of the pericardium;
- When there is rupture of diaphragm
- When there is contusion of lung
- When there is massive bleeding.

About 20–25% of patients with multiple rib fractures go in shock. Correct diagnosis and immediate management of above mentioned serious conditions are mandatory.

The *first sign of pulmonary insufficiency* is tachypnoea. The arterial oxygen tension is the most important parameter and may indicate loss of pulmonary capacity immediately after trauma, before the chest X-ray shows any pathology.

Intrapulmonary shunting increases considerably (from normal below 8% to 50% or more), soon after injury, except in patients with cardiac contusion (may occur in two-thirds of patients of blunt chest injury); heart failure or increased pulmonary vascular resistance (PVR). One of the most important development after blunt chest trauma is the rapid increase in pulmonary vascular resistance (PVR), which may remain elevated for even 3 weeks. PVR has been found to be the best haemodynamic predictor of survival.

Besides direct lung damage, pulmonary microembolic and margination of white cells in lung capillaries are important factors in the development of lung insufficiency.

Management of Pulmonary Insufficiency

Adequate oxygenation, fluid volume replacement and supportive care are the mainstay of management. Plasma expanders, plasma and blood and crystalloid should be administered according to the urinary output and CVP. Mechanical ventilation with volume-controlled ventilators is required for the patients who cannot maintain sufficient ventilation and oxygenation despite vigorous treatment with oxygen, physiotherapy and pain-relief (by even intravenous morphine, intercostal block or epidural anaesthesia).

In certain patients of blunt chest trauma, thoracotomy has to be done, e.g. in massive intrathoracic bleeding, acute cardiac tamponade, rupture of thoracic aorta or its large branches, rupture of trachea/main bronchus, rupture of diaphragm or oesophagus.

Intercostal tube drainage should be liberally used in blunt chest trauma.

Bolus doses of corticosteroids—methylprednisolone (30 mgm/kg)—in all chest trauma patients with several rib fractures and flail chest or lung contusion provides important beneficial effects. It helps in reduction in pulmonary vascular resistance and thereby reduction in right heart load, in reduction of the number of multiple organ failure, in lessening the complications, such as bronchial infection, septicaemia, fat embolism and disseminated intravascular coagulation. Further methyl prednisolone prevents chaotic activation of the complement cascade.

Complications in blunt chest trauma, especially in polytraumatised patient can be severe, such as adult respiratory distress, renal failure, hepatic failure, coagulation disorders, gastrointestinal bleeding, severe sepsis, etc.

The overall management of polytraumatised patients can be summarised as follows: Adequate oxygenation, proper fluid replacement, timely surgical intervention, adequate nutritional calorie, and substrate supplementation, management of septic complications.

In flail chest with failure to wean acute pain, with instability and chest wall defect, fractured ribs should be fixed. Latest method is to fix by minimally invasive absorbable plates and screws.

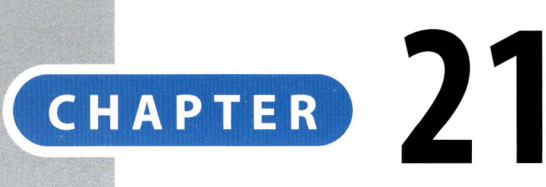

Gross Examination of Abdomen

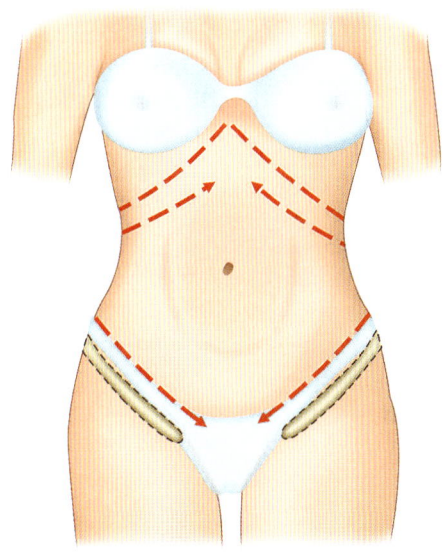

"Never ruin an apology with an excuse."
—**Benjamin Franklin**

No branch of medicine is independent, and inter-disciplinary basic knowledge is essential for examination of any patient. After all we are examining a patient, not just a system.

Anatomically 'abdomen' includes the area extending from the diaphragm to the pelvic floor; however, for practical purposes, abdominal area extends from the nipple line (representing highest point of dome of diaphragm) to the inguinopubic level.

Abdomen is not protected by any bony cage; hence is quite vulnerable to trauma.

In orthopaedic practice, examination of the abdomen is *required mainly after an accident*, since it is the third most commonly injured region of the body. In an accident service, the orthopaedic surgeon, being the chief of the team, has an obligation to ensure that the patient has no other vital injuries. In severe accidents, the abdomen may be involved both as closed or as open injuries.

Open injuries are usually obvious and they must get the attention of an abdominal surgeon at the earliest, because though it may look small on the surface, it might have grievously damaged in the deep. In closed injuries, one must be on the lookout to detect any visceral damage or internal haemorrhage. In managing abdominal injury one should never forget the dictum that *'it is always better to open and see the abdomen than to wait and repent'.*

■ HISTORY

In case of injury, enquire in detail regarding the nature of blow/hurt/or crush over the lower chest or abdomen. Note the site, character, progression and reference of pain; distention, *borborygmi*; and passing of urine, flatus, and stool. Enquire about the colour of urine, stool and vomitus.

Pain in the shoulder region during inspiration usually suggest subdiaphragmatic irritation due to blood or leaked gastrointestinal content [(in case of penetrating injury or rupture) of abdominal organ or viscera] or inflammatory lesion in that region.

Abdominal trauma occurs due to:
- Blunt trauma
- Penetrating trauma
- Iatrogenic injury
- Blast injury.

Blunt abdominal trauma (e.g. severe blow, hurt by or fall on blunt hard object) may produce severe intra or retroperitoneal injuries with relatively few clinical signs.

Repeated examination is essential regarding:
- General condition of the patient
- Local condition of the abdomen.

General Condition of the Patient

Look for facial expression; pulse—rate, regularity and volume, respiration (type of respiration), blood pressure, temperature, features of internal haemorrhage (i.e. increasing restlessness, increasing pallor, feeble to imperceptible pulse, gradual fall of blood pressure, sweating, air hunger, drowsiness, collapse).

In case of injury, *a rising pulse rate combined with falling blood pressure is highly suggestive of intra-abdominal injury.*

A quick systemic examination should be done to rule out any other vital injury.

Local Condition of the Abdomen

Certain helpful criteria while examining the abdomen:
- Patient should lie supine on a flat bed, *preferably* with flexed lower limbs
- Ask him to breath through the mouth, to relax the abdomen
- Now proceed by gently starting from the non-affected side to overcome the possible resistance offered by an apprehensive patient
- Always examine in supine position for abdominal complaints.

Inspection

Inspect from all sides, including the back. Look for skin condition, any prominence of veins, umbilicus, protuberance of abdomen, tattoo marks and any localised bulging on straining. In case of injury—look for bruising, abrasion, wound (site, number, entry/exit, protruding structure, discharge), abdominal distention, localised discolouration of skin.

Any lacerated wound or eviscerated bowel should be covered with a large sterile pack soaked in warm saline, at the earliest.

Palpation

Palpate from all sides. Be very gentle in abdominal palpation.
- *Abdominal wall:* For guarding, tenderness, herniation, and crepitus (surgical emphysema due to colonic injury, sternal fracture)
- *Abdominal cavity:* For viscera (liver, spleen, gallbladder, kidney, urinary bladder) any distention, and evidence of fluid in the abdomen, any palpable lump (note its characters in detail) **(Fig. 21.1)**.

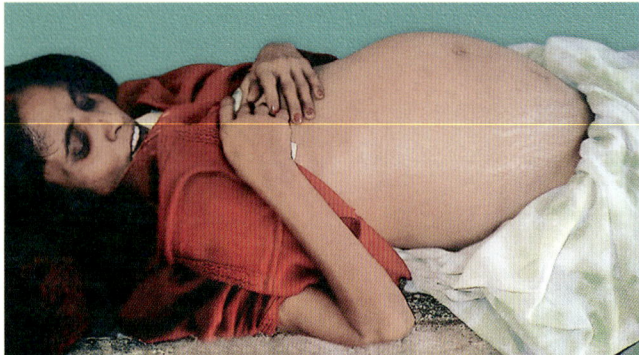

Fig. 21.1: Secondary deposits in liver with malignant ascitis—Primary in pelvis region affecting bones. Patient has cachectic look.

Percussion

Obliteration of liver dullness indicates *perforation of hollow viscus*. *Shifting dullness* indicates fluid in the peritoneal cavity. *Suprapubic dullness* signifies distension of urinary bladder. *With dullness in iliac fossa, suspect iliac abscess.*

Auscultation

Auscultation of all quadrants is mandatory. The continuous presence of normal bowel sounds in all quadrants is against the diagnosis of intra-abdominal injury (complete absence of bowel sounds indicates paralytic ileus or serious abdominal injury). Muffled and interrupted bowel sounds may be heard in mild intra-abdominal injury, mild paralytic ileus or early intra-abdominal bleeding. Increased bowel sounds indicate early intestinal obstruction (which may later turn into paralytic ileus). Note for any adventitious sound (arterial bruit).

Measurements

Repeated measurement of the *girth of abdomen* at the umbilicus should be done in cases of injury. *Gradual increase, coupled with clinical deterioration, is an important evidence of intraperitoneal bleeding.*

Per Rectal/Per Vaginal Examination

Tenderness and soft swelling in the rectovesical pouch, may indicate intraperitoneal haemorrhage or rupture of bladder.

■ INVESTIGATION

- *X-ray:* In plain X-ray of abdomen in sitting posture, *air (gas) shadow under diaphragm,* indicates perforation of hollow viscus. Distended intestinal loop shadows signify distention (obstruction). *Multiple horizontal fluid levels,* indicate paralytic ileus/obstruction.
- *Paracentesis and peritoneal lavage:* Aspiration of blood from sub-umbilical midline region helps in establishing the diagnosis of abdominal injuries.
  Diagnostic peritoneal lavage is particularly useful in comatose or semicomatose patients due to associated head injuries, alcoholic intoxication or drug ingestion.
- *Ultrasound:* In case of injury, increase in visceral shadow indicates perivisceral haematoma. Repeated ultrasonography, may be prognostic regarding increasing or regressing perivisceral haematoma.
- *CT scan:* It may help in diagnosing and localising the retroperitoneal haematoma.
- *Magnetic resonance imaging (MRI):* It helps in localisation of the pathology/injury more clearly.
- *Exploratory laparotomy:* Even diagnostic laparotomy may prove more rewarding, especially in case of unresolved suspicion, and may provide a chance of therapeutic surgical measures.

Key Diagnostic Points

Rupture Liver

Due to direct injury on right lower thorax and right upper abdomen (e.g. steering wheel injury).

- General features of extreme shock
- Tenderness and rigidity, more in right hypochondrium and lower right intercostal spaces
- Increased area of liver dullness
- Shifting dullness
- May be associated with fracture of right lower ribs.

Splenic Rupture

- Due to crush injury over left lower chest/left upper abdomen
- Usually with overlying fracture of left lower ribs
- Local tenderness and rigidity, more in left hypochondrium
- Hyperaesthesia and pain in left shoulder, referred from the left sub-diaphragmatic area (**Kehr's sign**)
- Persistent dullness mainly in left upper abdomen, and left flank, but shifting dullness in the right flank (**Ballance's sign**)
- Pointed finger tip pressure in between sternomastoid and scalenus medius in supraclavicular region initiates severe pain (**Saegessar's splenic point**).

Renal Injury

- Usually due to injuries in lumbar region (blow or fall or runover)
- Tenderness in and around the renal angle
- Varying swelling and dullness over the renal angle
- Passing of blood in urine
- All the samples of urine should be preserved to look for presence of blood in the urine. Haematuria may occur even after three weeks due to dislodgement of clot
- Abdominal distention may develop due to irritation of splanchnic nerves by retroperitoneal haematoma.

Urinary Bladder Injury

- Intraperitoneal rupture of bladder (20%)—follows injury while bladder is full and it leads to peritonitis
- Extraperitoneal rupture (80%)—follows pelvic injuries (*see* Chapter Pelvic Injury)—suprapubic tenderness, little dullness in hypogastrium, blood/clot in urine
- Severe injuries of most of the abdominal viscera produce profound shock
- Rupture of hollow abdominal viscera leads to severe peritonitis (abdominal pain, features of shock, rigid abdomen, muffled or absent bowel sounds)
- Rupture of major blood vessels is usually fatal.

In spinal injuries or following surgery on the spine, or a peritoneal lavage, the features of paralytic ileus commonly develop (distended abdomen and with tinkling bowel sounds). In these cases, or even after applying plaster jacket/

spica a very severe complication—*acute dilatation of the stomach*—may occur (acute distention of upper abdomen, very weak/absent bowel sounds, left diaphragm pushed up in chest which develops increased resonance, persistent vomiting, profound shock, unless managed very promptly—mainly by maintaining fluid and electrolyte balance and aspiration of stomach even by stomach tube, rather than Ryle's tube—this condition is fatal).

Among non-traumatic conditions, the abdomen and allied zones require examination for:
- Any referred pain (e.g. caries spine, spinal injury)
- Search for a cold/hot abscess (e.g. in abdominal wall; in pelvis—psoas abscess, iliac abscess)
- Palpating lower abdomen for vertebral prominence (e.g. in spondylolisthesis).

Iliac Abscess
- It is commonly confused with hip pathology
- Patient can be of any age—from a young child to an adult.
- Constitutional features—fever ranging up to 38.5°C or even more. Patient may be toxic
- Keeps the hip flexed and slightly externally rotated **(Fig. 21.2)**
- Resistant, firm tender mass felt in iliac fossa (which should be normally empty).
  (cf.) In *psoas abscess* resistant firm tender mass is felt by the side of the vertebrae. While palpating psoas abscess support the flank from behind by one hand and palpate by tips of four fingers of opposite hand against the sides of the lumbar vertebrae. The psoas abscess may sometimes extend beneath the inguinal ligament as a conical mass/swelling, which has a continuity with the psoas abscess in the iliac fossa

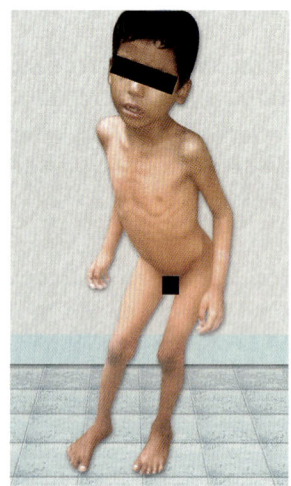

Fig. 21.2: Boy with right iliac abscess looking ill and keeping his right lower limb flexed slightly abducted and externally rotated at hip.

- Iliac fossa dull on percussion (compare with the other side)
- Take the patient in confidence, further flex the hip and demonstrate the free rotational movements of the hip (this rules out any hip pathology)
- Aspiration of pus is confirmatory.

Psoas bursitis: It is a painless effusion in the psoas bursa which presents as tense, nonfluctuant, immobile oblong or conical swelling beneath and below the inguinal ligament. However, there is no mass/swelling in the iliac fosse which distinguishes psoas bursitis from psoas abscess. It should also be differentiated from femoral hernia, in which impulse will be felt on coughing.

CHAPTER 22

How to Read X-ray Plate

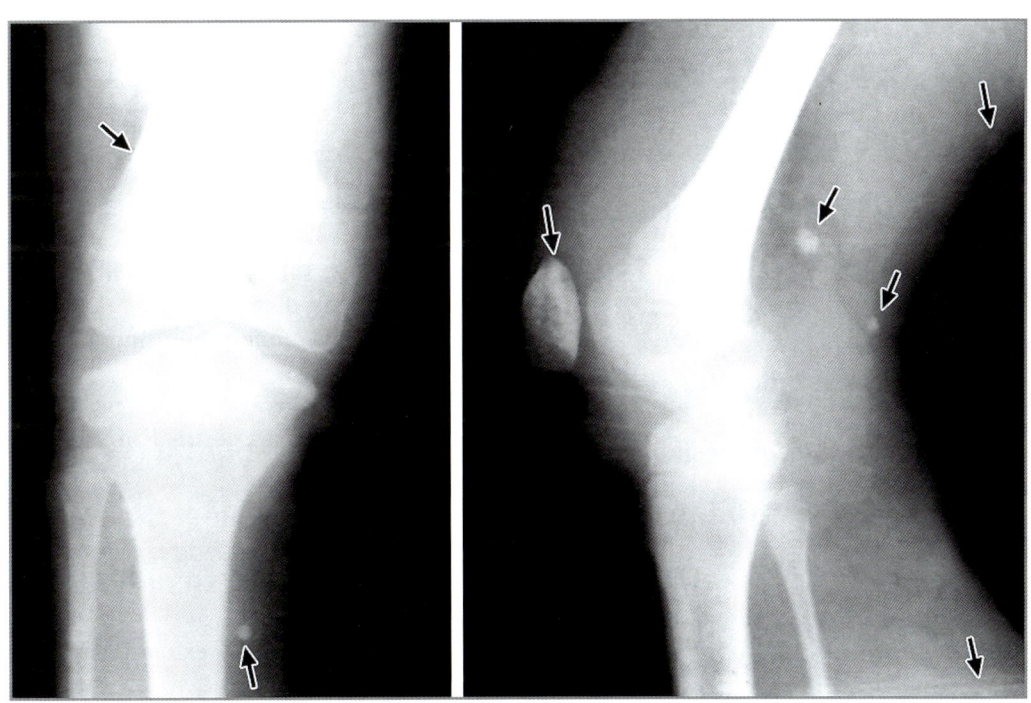

"The most disadvantageous peace is better than the most just war."
—*Desiderius*

READING AN X-RAY

For proper diagnosis, the quality of X-ray must be of good standard, i.e. adequately positioned, exposed, developed (so as to show all gradations of the grey scale by which fine differences of skin, subcutaneous tissues, muscle mass, intervening fascial planes, bone and joint details can be delineated), properly washed, nicely dried up and should be free from artifact.

While exposing for the bone and joint pathologies following general principles should be observed:
- It is always helpful to expose the desired portions both sides of the limbs for proper comparison
- Full length of the limb bone should be exposed if possible
- X-ray plate should be long enough to include the zones beyond the suspected length, and should include at least one joint above and one below the affected or even suspected site of lesion/injury. If that is not possible it should include at least one joint nearer to the pathology. In case of a joint, at least 1/3rd to 1/2 of the adjoining bones on either side must be included.
- All soft tissues from all around the bone/joint should be included
- X-ray must be taken in at least two planes—anteroposterior and lateral and preferably the oblique view should always be taken
- Special views are required for special visualisation whenever needed
- Stress views are required in suspected instability of any joint or suspected nonunion of a fracture
- In significant (more than 1 cm) leg length discrepancy, special leg-length films are the only way to discern and document the shortening and in case of the growing child follow the shortening through the growth period.

Inspect a plate against a bright light. Proceed in the following order—Confirm the name of the patient; type of X-ray (plain, contrast, tomogram, etc.) view taken, part exposed, extent of inclusion and side of the limb or part. Then read systematically:

Soft Tissue Shadow

Increased (generalised or localised), normal, decreased; texture, i.e. clear delineation of different layers; ground glass appearance (homogenous), etc. Any abnormal content, like shadow in soft tissue zone, e.g.
- Radiopaque shadow, e.g. metallic foreign body, bony piece (e.g. sequestrum, calcified spots parasites **(Figs. 22.1A and B)**, cysticerci, guinea worm, new bone forming tumours, calcified blood vessel wall, phleboliths, calcification in ligaments, faecolith (in case of pelvis, lumbar, sacral and coccygeal region of spine), myositic mass.
- Entrapped translucent area, e.g. air in sinus tract, gas in muscle planes (gas gangrene), surgical emphysema.

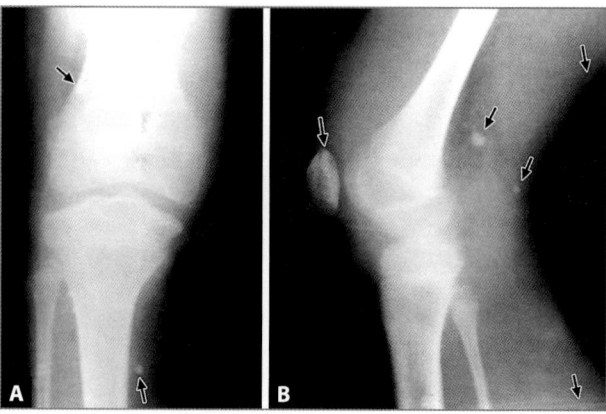

Figs. 22.1A and B: Haemangioma in thigh, and popliteal region. Note the calcified spots.

Joint

Joint space—(Radiological joint space = anatomical joint space + area occupied by articular cartilage)
- Periarticular tissues
- Clear, fuzzy
- Increased, normal, decreased
- Regular, uniform
- Any radiopaque shadow in the joint space
- Any bony trabeculation across the joint.

Articulating Bones

- Interrelation between the articulating bones (always compare with opposite side if possible) for congruity—normal, subluxated (partial dissociation), dislocated (complete dissociation)
- Margins—uniform, erosion, destruction, osteophytes, collapse
- Subchondral area—condensations, rarefaction, cysts/cyst like spaces, destruction, sequestrum

In X-ray picture of a long bone look for
- Overall alignment
- Average bone age, and sex (if possible)
- Different areas—articular ends, metaphyseal areas, diaphyseal area
- Cortical shadow—texture—normal, thickened, thinned, destruction, any dent on the cortex, breach in the continuity—pseudo or real fractures, reactionary bone laying—its type, pattern, extent, any associated lesions (subperiosteal longitudinal, onion peel or sunburst bone laying)
- Medullary shadow—mainly in the diaphyseal area—any cystic area, texture, any abnormal content, expansion of medulla, trabecular pattern
- Corticomedullary delineation
- Condition of growth plate shadow (in case of infants, children and adolescents)—uniformity, widening, destruction, premature fusion, irregular fusion, any other abnormal finding.

Bone-age Radiograph Atlas

The atlas of Greulich and Pyle for skeletal maturity and epiphyseal closure is widely used in many countries to assess skeletal age and to plan orthopaedic surgery. Compiling the data collected from institutional American children in 1950s. Greulich and Pyle produced an atlas comprising of a large series of standard anteroposterior radiographs of hand.

Each radiograph is assigned to a specific age in years and months and the patient's skeletal age is determined by comparing his/her radiograph with the standard in the atlas for the appropriate gender. However, such atlas should be a broad-guideline, and for more appropriate conclusion, such bone-age atlas should be prepared in each country, even then clear medicolegal statements about age cannot be made from X-rays alone.

Further care should be taken while using such atlas to predict years of remaining growth, when it concerns orthopaedic surgery as in leg lengthening or epiphyseal closure surgery.

■ BIBLIOGRAPHY

1. Greulich WW, Pyle SI. A radiograph atlas of skeletal development of the hand and wrist, 2nd ed. 1959.

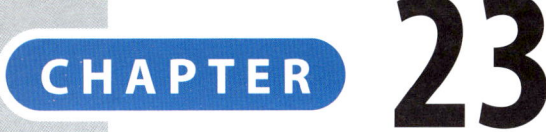

Advanced Diagnostic Imaging

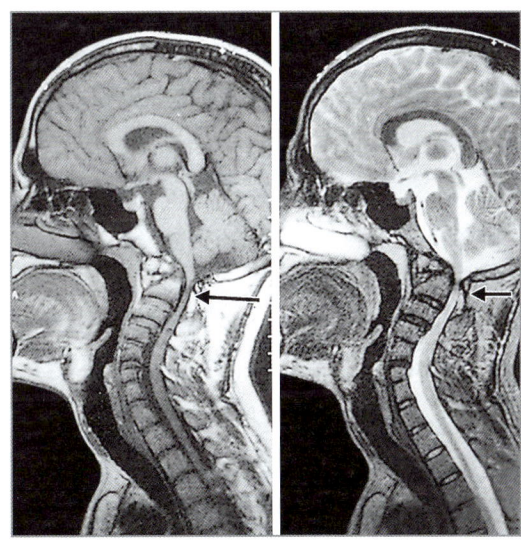

*"We can easily forgive a child who is afraid of the dark;
the real tragedy of life is when men are afraid of the light."*
—*Plato*

"Self-belief and Resilience are the key to sustaining growth"
—*Naik AM*

World's biggest radiotelescope launched in Netherlands (The Hague)
Scientists in the Netherlands have unveiled the largest radiotelescope in the world which is based near the northeastern town of Assen, but the antennas are spread out across the rest of the Netherlands and also in Germany, Sweden, France and Britain. Femke Boekhorst of the Netherlands Radio Astronomy Institute said—The LOFAR (Low-Frequency Array) consists of 25,000 small antennas measuring between 50 centimetres and 2 meters across, instead of a traditional large dish. When all antennas are combined, a giant telescope is produced with a diameter of about 1000 kilometres. The data gathered by the telescope will be dealt with by a supercomputer at the university of Groningen and transmitted to the institute. The observations over the data will allow to learn more about the origin of the universe, back to the moment right after the "Big Bang".

Technology has become the symbol of today's life and also of the modern medicine. After the discovery of X-rays by physicist Wilhelm Conrad Röentgen (1845–1922), this has become the most useful method of diagnostic imaging. *The advanced techniques of imaging are more or less 'developed and modified' forms of X-ray technology.* The goal of any imaging study is to define accurately the pathomorphological changes in any specific tissue, organ or part of body.

Conventional radiology is still the cornerstone of medical imaging and it constitutes the major bulk of investigations in any imaging establishment. Recent introduction of *'digital X-ray'* has improved the quality of image and provided the much avoided flexibility in acquisition and processing of images. The exposure radiation has also reduced by about 20–30%.

The introduction of rotograph plus panoramic dental X-ray is proving much useful in delineating the topography and health of the teeth and the jaw bones *(refer Fig. 18.3)*.

In computerised radiography (CR), any structure of a given region can be seen just by changing of window, such as a single exposure of chest X-ray done by CR system shows lung parenchyma, ribs, spine, heart by changing of window (cf. in conventional X-ray it will require three exposures).

Earlier radiographic imaging studies, e.g. *plain radiography*, *computed tomography* and *radionuclide studies* played major role in evaluation of musculoskeletal disorders. However, they focussed mainly on detection of osseous abnormalities. With the development of MRI, it is now possible to evaluate non-invasively the soft tissue structures as well.

To study the pattern, patency and possible pathology of blood vessels the peripheral angiography is fairly useful **(Fig. 23.1)**. The last decade has seen marked improvement in imaging techniques in terms of the agents available for use, the technology to provide the images and the computing software to analyse and display them.

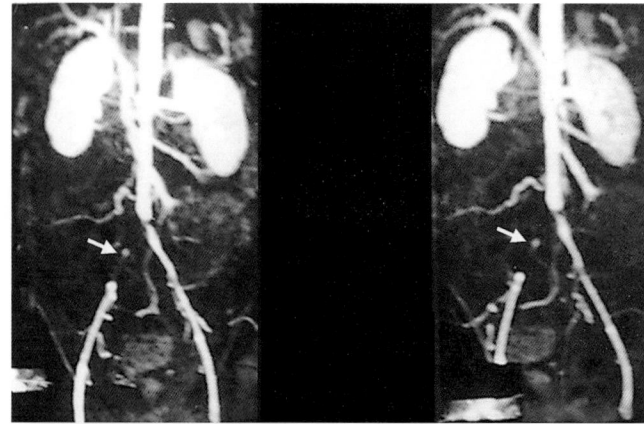
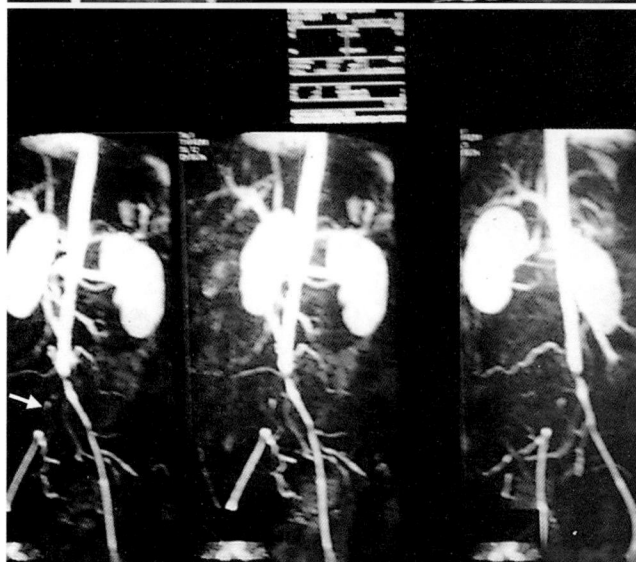

Fig. 23.1: Peripheral angiography showing complete block in the proximal segment of right common iliac, and intermittent block in left common iliac artery.

The use of LASER (L = Light; A = Amplification; S = Stimulation; E = Emission; R = Radiation) can further enhance the values of the imaging techniques (and also the therapeutic modalities).

Contrast media (air, gas, or iodine-based liquids) is used with X-rays for delineating the tract, cavities or spaces for knowing their size, patency, direction and occupancy. The contrast material is introduced (injected) into blood vessels, body fluids, cavities, tracts, and organs. This leads to a marked differences in the coefficient of absorption of the X-rays by the adjacent structures which provides diagnostic contrast between the tissues.

Usually contrast media are of following types as given in **Flowchart 23.1**.

Iodine-based liquids can be ionic, water soluble, or oily. The former two are less irritant, less toxic, miscible, and get rapidly absorbed and excreted. The latter is more irritant, more toxic, non-miscible and very slowly absorbable. Of the iodides, metrizamide—a non-ionic and least toxic and least irritant—is most commonly used. Contrast media is usually used for following investigations **(Table 23.1)**.

Flowchart 23.1: Contrast media (usually used with X-ray).

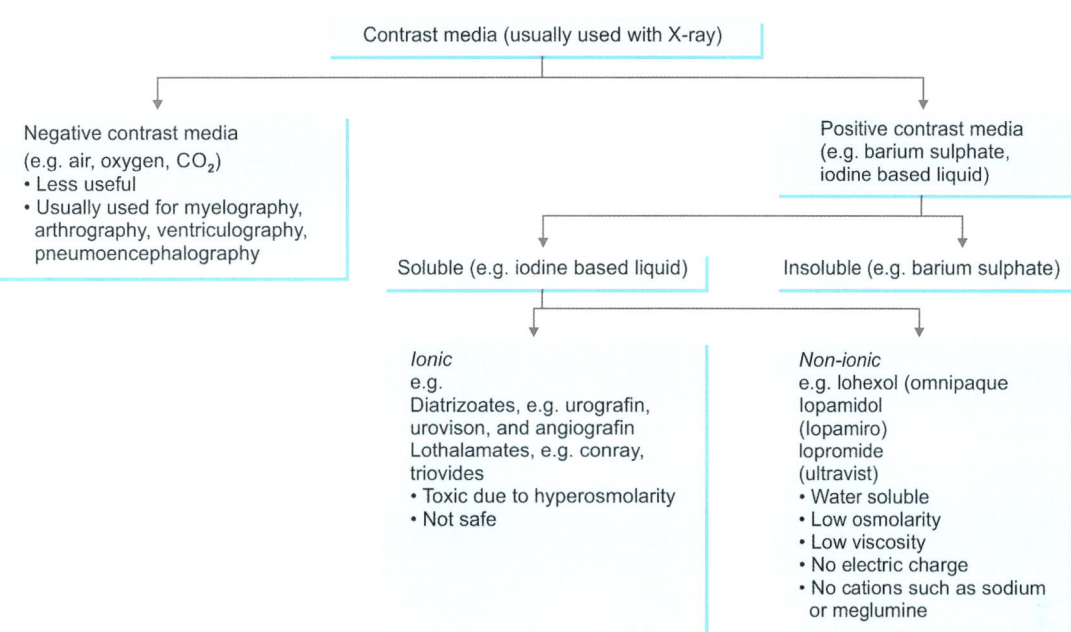

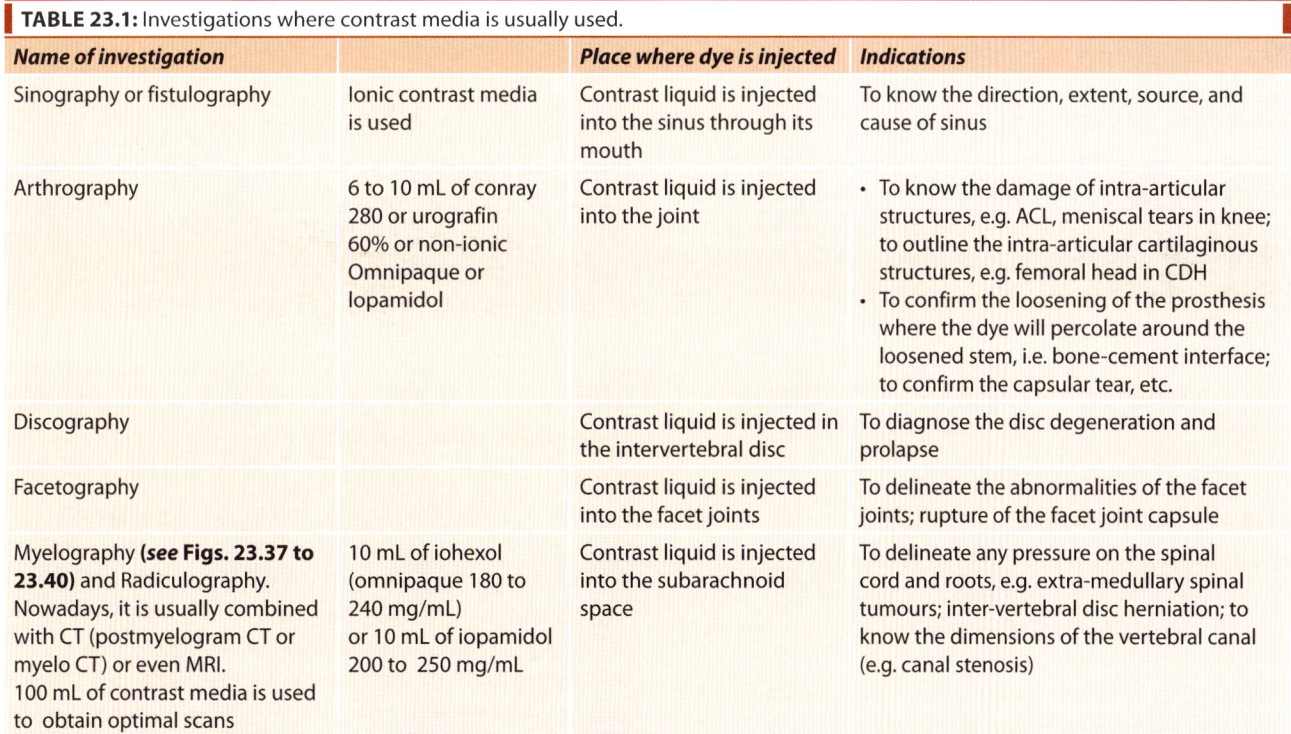

TABLE 23.1: Investigations where contrast media is usually used.

Name of investigation		Place where dye is injected	Indications
Sinography or fistulography	Ionic contrast media is used	Contrast liquid is injected into the sinus through its mouth	To know the direction, extent, source, and cause of sinus
Arthrography	6 to 10 mL of conray 280 or urografin 60% or non-ionic Omnipaque or Iopamidol	Contrast liquid is injected into the joint	• To know the damage of intra-articular structures, e.g. ACL, meniscal tears in knee; to outline the intra-articular cartilaginous structures, e.g. femoral head in CDH • To confirm the loosening of the prosthesis where the dye will percolate around the loosened stem, i.e. bone-cement interface; to confirm the capsular tear, etc.
Discography		Contrast liquid is injected in the intervertebral disc	To diagnose the disc degeneration and prolapse
Facetography		Contrast liquid is injected into the facet joints	To delineate the abnormalities of the facet joints; rupture of the facet joint capsule
Myelography (*see* Figs. 23.37 to 23.40) and Radiculography. Nowadays, it is usually combined with CT (postmyelogram CT or myelo CT) or even MRI. 100 mL of contrast media is used to obtain optimal scans	10 mL of iohexol (omnipaque 180 to 240 mg/mL) or 10 mL of iopamidol 200 to 250 mg/mL	Contrast liquid is injected into the subarachnoid space	To delineate any pressure on the spinal cord and roots, e.g. extra-medullary spinal tumours; inter-vertebral disc herniation; to know the dimensions of the vertebral canal (e.g. canal stenosis)

Note: After lumbar myelography, patients (more in young women) may develop headache (beginning within three days and lasting for three to five days)—spinal headache

In the past few years significant technological advances have been seen in the field of imaging of which those usefully concern the orthopaedic field are: (1) the increasing availability of 3 Tesla (3T) MRI scanning (2) newer modalities of positron emission tomography computed tomography (PET-CT) and PET-MRI.

■ MRI

Paramagnetic contrast agents are used to delineate the lesion in better way. They decrease the T_1 and T_2 of adjacent protons and act as proton relaxation enhancers. The contrast media dimeglumine gadopentetate (Magnevist) is commonly used.

Non-invasive diagnostic aids, such as *tomography, xeroradiography, ultrasonography, scintigraphy, computed axial tomography,* and *magnetic resonance imaging have definitely improved the accuracy of diagnosis without many of the attendant risks.* However, certain disadvantages of these diagnostic aids, as noted below, prevent them from being ordered as a routine procedure.

Disadvantages
- Most of them are too expensive
- The findings are too difficult for interpretation by average clinicians, except in too obvious pathologies, most of which can be fairly and accurately diagnosed by much less cheap good quality X-rays
- One has to mostly rely on the radiologist's report which is usually written without interaction with the clinicians and the patients. Hence at times, the reports confuse the clinical diagnosis
- Unless two or more of the above aids are combined, there is lack of specificity and accuracy in diagnosis.
- CT contains ionizing radiation; hence cannot be used in pregnant women AND should be used very judiciously in children.

■ TOMOGRAPHY

Tomography is the X-ray image focused on a desired plane. The word tomogram is derived from the word 'tomos' (= cut or section). By rotating the tube and the X-ray film in opposite directions on any imaginary pivot, the pictures produced on either side of the pivotal plane are blurred out. The object under study is demonstrated in a succession of different layers of the object cut into a number of sections or slices. Pictures obtained on different plane-cuts, reveal the lesions which are obscured on plane X-rays.

Its disadvantage is relatively high dose of radiation to the patient. The advent of CT and MRI has outdated the tomography.

Uses of Tomography
- Tomography can be helpful in clarifying the vague and obscured findings of plane X-rays, and occult injuries. It can assist in further assessment of a known fracture or fracture-dislocation
- It reveals the deep-seated lesions, e.g. osteoid osteoma, brodies abscess, infective focus, etc.
- It may help to identify a less obvious sequestrum or subchondral bony plate destruction in septic arthritis and thus distinguish it from periarticular osteoporosis, where the subchondral plate remains intact
- In spinal region, tomography is very useful for identifying the facet fractures and the obscured defects in the pars interarticularis
- It was earlier used to demonstrate the tuberculous infiltrations and cavities in the lung.

Orientation of Cone-Beam Computed Tomography

Standardization of head orientation is crucial in treatment planning and evaluation of treatment effects in patients with skeletal deformities. Natural head position (NHP) is recommended for two-dimensional (2D) and three-dimensional (3D) imaging/photography. NHP is the natural position of the head in which subject rests their head habitually. NHP also represents the true aesthetic and functional anatomic form of the face. Three-dimensional cone-beam computed tomography (CBCT) is considered to be a modern state-of-the-art imaging. It allows a smooth digital workflow from diagnosis to treatment planning and execution by integration with other digital technologies like digital models and 3D stereophotogrammetry. (Balachandran R 2019)

■ XERORADIOGRAPHY

'Xero' means 'dry'. The xeroradiography is dry procedure in which the wet process of developing and fixing the films are not used.

Routine X-ray exposures are also used in Xeroradiography. An aluminium plate is coated with the thin layer of selenium and charged electrically. Selenium plate has photoconductive behaviour. The X-ray beam is passed through the part of body, to be studied, to reach the plate. Here the response is registered as an electrically charged density pattern on the recording plate as the latent image, which is developed by blowing a thin powder (Toner) over selenium-coated plate on which the powder adheres in the proportion of the charge present over there. Then it is reproduced in the form of positive images on a plastic-coated paper which becomes the permanent record. The photoelectrical process involved here, is mainly sensitive to variations in the tissue density.

Uses of Xeroradiography

Xeroradiography produces a very high grade of soft tissue contrast, which is not obtained on routine radiography.

Vague, obscured and fuzzy lesions, e.g. subperiosteal erosions (e.g. in early osteomyelitis), early soft tissue calcification (e.g. in myositis ossificans), early cartilaginous calcification (e.g. in chondrocalcinosis, foreign bodies of low density), etc. can be displayed not only more easily but also earlier than by the use of plane X-rays. It is widely used for mammography.

Disadvantage of xeroradiography is that, for exposing the deeper and thicker part, a high dose of radiation is required.

■ ENDOSCOPY

The endoscopic oriented visualisation of inner part of a hollow viscera and tracts (like GI tract, urinary bladder, ureters, joints, etc.) has remained the primary tool for detecting the early signs of diseases including the cancers.

Advancements in this field have been tremendous. It includes the provision to view the live tissue inside the body at a cellular level in real time during an endoscopic investigation. It comprises a probe-based confocal laser endomicroscopy (pCLE) technique. It operates through a tiny microscope threaded through a single use endoscope and eliminates the time required for any biopsy.

■ ULTRASONOGRAPHY

Sounds of frequency higher than 20,000 Hz are called *'ultrasonics.'* Sounds of frequency lower than 20 Hz are called infrasonics or subsonics. We cannot hear the ultrasonic and infrasonic sounds. They travel with same speed as the audible sound.

Thus ultrasound is acoustic pressure wave at frequencies above the audible range of human hearing.

Ultrasonography can be utilised for diagnostic (ultrasonography) and therapeutic purposes. *Diagnostic ultrasonography employs a transducer that functions as a transmitter and a receiver of acoustic energy.* The *principle of ultrasonography* is based on the recording of reflection of sound waves from the resistances of different densities. High frequency sound waves produced by a transducer can penetrate several centimetres through the soft tissues. While passing through the tissue-interfaces, few of these sound waves are reflected back as echoes to the transducer. As the echoes are received as electrical signals, these can be registered as images on a screen or a plate with the help of various equipments. The tissues of different densities can be reproduced as images in gradations of grey, which can reasonably delineate the anatomical outline.

According to the structural character of the tissues, their echogenicity vary. They can be *highly echogenic (mostly solid, e.g. fat), mildly echogenic (e.g. semisolids) or echofree (e.g. fluid-filled cysts).*

As such ultrasound is a form of mechanical energy which is transmitted through and into biological tissues as an acoustic pressure wave at frequencies above the limit of human hearing. It is widely used in medicine as diagnostic, therapeutic and operative tool. For therapy and operative purposes, ultrasound of high intensities (1 to 2 $W/C\ m^2$) is used, which can cause considerable heating in living tissues. To take full advantage of this energy absorption such levels of ultrasound is used acutely to reduce pain and muscle spasm, to improve muscle movements and to decrease joint stiffness.

To use *ultrasound as a surgical instrument even higher levels of intensity (5 to 300W cm^2) is used* and sharp parts of energy are used to fragment calculi, to induce healing of non-unions, to ablate diseased tissues (e.g. in cataract) and even to remove methyl methacrylate cement during revision arthroplasty.

On the other hand, the *ultrasound intensity of lower magnitudes up to 50 mW/cm^2 are used to drive diagnostic devices*, which non-invasively image vital organs, foetal development, peripheral blood flow, metabolic bone diseases, such as osteoporosis, and also to evaluate fracture callus during healing. The intensity level used for imaging is five orders of magnitude below that used for surgery, and this intensity is non-thermal and non-destructive but still has potential to influence bone mass and morphology through strong sensitivity of bone tissue to physical stimuli.

Uses of Ultrasonography

The diagnostic range of ultrasonography has increased by leaps and bounds from obstetrics to imaging of almost all parts of body, especially with the introduction of high resolution real-time USG and Volusion 3D and 4D imaging systems. High frequency probes are available today.

- Ultrasonography has obvious advantage of easy availability, portability (can be used as bedside imaging), noninvasive nature, cost effectiveness. AND is of great help for evaluating muscle, tendon and joint due to its ability for dynamic evaluation and multiplanar capability.
- Due to contrast echogenicity of solid and cystic masses, ultrasonography is mainly useful in diagnosing the deep-seated cystic lesions, e.g. abscesses, haematomas, cysts, aneurysms, intra-articular fluids, etc; in differentiating between cellulitis, abscess, osteomyelitis.

  It is good at detecting abnormalities of superficial structures. Its resolution is 1 mm compared with 3 mm for MRI. It is also much cheaper than MRI
- It is almost routinely used to *screen the neonates for the developmental dysplasia (DDH) of hip.* The use of ultrasonography to examine the neonatal hip was introduced and developed by Graf R in 1980. Ultrasonography could provide images of soft tissue components of the infant hip, e.g. cartilaginous components of the femoral head and the acetabulum, the joint capsule and the acetabular labrum. Ultrasonography can well demarcate the relation between acetabular labrum and cartilaginous femoral head epiphysis. Without any risk of radiation or invasive procedure ultrasound offers a good visualisation of the position of the femoral head before ossification takes place.

Two methods of ultrasonography are used to delineate the developmental dysplasia of the hip (subluxation, dislocation, instability of hip and abnormalities of acetabular development):

- The static technique of Graf R (1980), which emphasised morphology and classifies the status of hip on the basis of angular measurement of the acetabulum.
- The dynamic method, described by Harcke HT et al. (1984) consists of a multipositional evaluation which resembles the physical examination.
- Ultrasonography can be helpful in diagnosing the rotator cuff injuries of the shoulder; internal derangements of the knee; in Perthes' disease of hip; growth and development in bony and cartilaginous portions of the femoral head; early changes like irregularity and fissuring and late

changes like flattening and fragmentation. However, the interpretation may be difficult and even inaccurate
- *Study of extent and nature of soft tissue masses;* muscle pathologies (e.g. rupture, inflammation, haematoma, myositis ossifans); tendon pathologies (e.g. tendinitis, tears, tumours); bursal pathologies (bursitis, chronic degenerative changes, etc.).

To confirm the clinical suspicion of fracture of clavicle in the neonate (in whom exposure to irradiation during the X-ray should be avoided) ultrasound can be safely done in which a small 7.5 MHz linear array transducer should be used. The sonographic picture presents interruption of the hyperechogenic zone of bone steps, axial deviation and visible periosteal lesions (as in other fractures). *Haematoma is indirect sign of fracture.*

- Sonography can detect *greenstick fractures* and is a very good method to assess the *formation of callus*
- Rib fractures are the most common injuries resulting from blunt trauma. The sensitivity of chest X-ray in showing the fractures is limited particularly in those involving the cartilage part of rib. Ultrasonography performed with a 7.5 MHz linear transducer *is useful in detecting such rib fractures*
- Calcaneal quantitative ultrasound offers a promising approach *to screen for osteoporosis* and may be applied to exclude osteoporosis-associated high risk fractures
- Low intensity pulsed ultrasound therapy can be used *to accelerate the fracture healing* in the fractures prone to delayed union (e.g. scaphoid), established delayed union or even non-union. Ultrasound signal composed of a burst width of 200 microseconds containing 1.5 megahertz sine waves with a repetition rate of 1 kilohertz and an intensity of 30 milliwatts per square centimeter, is used 20 minutes daily for a total period of 20 weeks or until the fracture unites well. The exact mechanism of its working is not known, however, through a variety of mechanisms (some biological and some physical) the processes of fracture healing are accelerated and augmented
- The ultrasonic instruments can be used *to remove the bone cements* during revision hip replacement, of course it is costly and it may cause bone necrosis.
- Ultrasound can be used for evaluation of peripheral nerves as most of them are easily assessable to ultrasound.
- Colour-Doppler is routinely used to delineate the patency, variations and diagnosis of vascular diseases. It is useful in assessment of the vascularity of any tumour. It is helpful in differentiating vessels from adjacent tissues.
- Interventional procedures like soft tissue biopsies and aspiration of joints are better done under ultrasound guidance.
- Advanced techniques such as harmonic imaging, panoramic imaging and alikes are proving to be extremely useful in the field of ultrasonography of musculoskeletal system.

Pitfalls of Ultrasonography

Acoustic shadowing caused by calcification, bone or air produces limitations of ultrasound and makes the assessment of deeper structures impossible.

When lower frequency probes are used to study deeper structures, as a large muscle groups, the resolution drops.

The ultrasound technology is highly operator-dependent, and meticulous technique is required to avoid pitfalls in the results.

The reflectivity of muscles and tendons can be erroneously interpreted, if correct angle is not maintained, which should be perpendicular to the structure being examined.

The role of ultrasound in musculoskeletal problems, even though, is now well established, it remains complementary to other modalities like, X-ray, CT, MRI, Scintigraphy.

SCINTIGRAPHY (RADIOACTIVE ISOTOPE OR RADIONUCLIDES STUDIES OR NUCLEAR IMAGING)

Nuclear imaging utilizes the physiology of the concerned organ to obtain its image distinct from anatomical imaging technologies. Nuclear medicine uses radioisotopes for diagnosis and treatment of diseases.

In the disease process, functional abnormalities always precede structural change. Scintigraphy is most sensitive modality to detect abnormality at the earliest **(Fig. 23.2)** hence it has been also termed as "functional imaging".

Different tissues take up radioactive isotopes (radionuclides) according to their activities, and emit photons, which can be recorded by simple rectilinear scanner or a gamma camera to produce an image. Radiotracers are injected intravenously and their passage through organs and parts being studied, is seen with gamma camera.

In orthopaedic practice, radioactive isotopes commonly used are technetium 99m phosphate (99mTc to study vascularity and osteoblastic activity), gallium 67 citrate (67 Ga to study macrophage uptake for diagnosing inflammation and infection), technetium-labelled sulphur colloid (99m Tc-Sc), and indium-111-labelled leucocytes to assess leucocyte concentration, e.g. in infections; Indium chloride is used to diagnose loosening of prosthesis. Of these isotopes, *technetium 99m has been found to be ideal for radionuclide imaging and it emits gamma rays*. It has a short half-life (6 hours) and appropriate energy characters for recording by gamma camera. It is excreted rapidly by the kidney into the urine. Combined with bone seeking phosphate compound, it is selectively concentrated in bony structures. The low background activity indicates clear visibility of any increased uptake.

Of recently, the *radioactive technetium-labelled hydroxymethylene diphosphonate (99m Tc-HDP) is being used intravenously and the uptake activities are recorded in three phases.*

Advanced Diagnostic Imaging

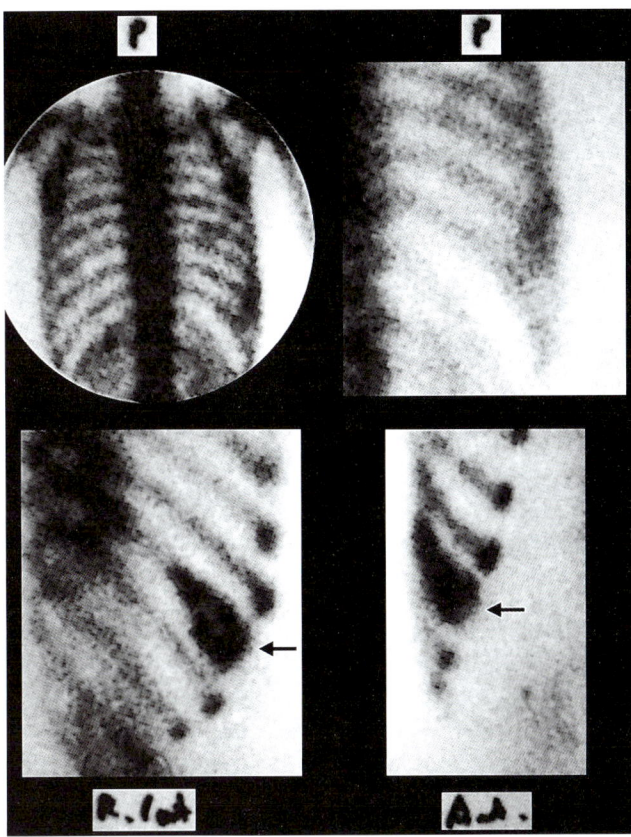

Fig. 23.2: Bone scintigraphy using technetium, showing increased uptake in right 8th rib (neoplasm) against the normal low background activity in rest of bones.

- *The flow phase:* It is akin to radionuclide angiogram demonstrating the blood flow.
- *Immediate* or perfusion or equilibrium or *blood-pool phase:* Immediately after the injection, the image shows relative vascular flow and distribution of radioisotope in the perivascular and extracellular space
- *Delayed or bone phase:* Two to four hours after the injection, when most of the isotope has been excreted, except that taken up in the bone by its osteoblastic activities.

Normally in the equilibrium phase, the periarticular vascular tissues take up the isotope most actively and produce darkest images, which gradually fade away.

Two to four hours later in the 'delayed phase', the uptake is more in the metaphyseal cancellous area showing more activity, and the outlines of bones are shown more clearly.

A negative three phase scan is good evidence of no significant underlying pathology, i.e. *"a nuclear medicine sedimentation rate".*

Abnormal recordings of the uptake are significant when it is sharply localised or obviously asymmetrical. *Broadly the abnormal recordings can be of four types:*

- *Increased uptake (activity) in the 'equilibrium' or 'perfusion' phase:* It *indicates increased vascularity of the soft tissues*, e.g. in acute (or even chronic) inflammatory changes

- *Decreased uptake (activity) in 'equilibrium' phase:* It indicates decreased vascularity of the soft tissues. It is an unusual finding
- *Increased uptake (activity) in 'delayed' phase:* It *indicates increased activities in the extracellular fluid* or *more enthusiastic cellular activities in the process of new bone formation* in fracture healing, inflammation of bone, bone tumours **(Fig. 23.2)**, revascularisation in osteonecrosis, myositic activities and heterotopic bone formation.

  Osteomyelitis focus usually presents as an area of increased tracer uptake (hot area), but in infants, due to oedematous occlusion of the intramedullary vessels, there is decreased delivery of the isotope leading to decreased tracer uptake (cold area).

  The tracer (technetium 99m) uptake will be more in the active bone tumours, bone involvements in malignant soft tissue tumours and occult bone metastasis
- *Decreased uptake (activity) in 'delayed' phase:* It indicates decreased vascularity of the bone, e.g. in avascular necrosis of femoral head, fibrotic replacement of bony tissues, etc.

Uses of Scintigraphy

- *Enthesopathy* (disease activities at the sites of tendon and ligament attachment to the bone), e.g. inflammatory, degenerative, metabolic, traumatic disorders affecting the pelvis, trochanter, humeral tuberosity, patella, osteitis pubis, etc.
- *Early detection and localisation of inflammatory changes,* e.g. acute osteomyelitis focus, bone abscess.

  Clinically, it becomes difficult to differentiate cellulitis from actual joint pathology. Hence, a 3-phase bone scan can be helpful as follows:

	Cellulitis	**Synovitis**	**Osteomyelitis**
First phase	+	+	+
Second phase	+	+	+
Third phase	–	+	+

  In synovitis, uptake will be on both sides of joint. While in osteomyelitis, bony uptake will be on one side
- *Early detection of bony metastasis*—On the whole scintigraphy has a high sensitivity but a low specificity for skeletal metastasis
- *Detection and localisation of avascular necrosis of bone* (e.g. *in* Perthes' disease, idiopathic osteonecrosis, avascular necrosis following fractures, etc.). *In Perthes' disease, it can be used to evaluate early stages of pathological process.* In the very early stage, uptake of technetium 99m is decreased, and it remains variable or is increased when the symptoms appear.

  Early diagnosis of *avascular necrosis is difficult* because the radiological changes appear late and artefacts are seen on MRI when metal is present. However, in a bone scan even the earliest changes of avascular necrosis can be detected as the *"bull's eye" sign* of decreased uptake in the centre of femoral head with diffuse uptake in the intertrochanteric region. In difficult cases, a bone marrow scan presents asymmetrical picture (against normal symmetrical picture) representing destruction (necrotic zone) in head of femur. However, one should be little cautious because early bone scans may suggest a more severe condition than really exists

- Detection of *infection in prosthetic replacement*
- *Early detection of stress fracture*—Indications of bone scanning in acute trauma is rare (e.g. in stress fractures in athletes prior to an important game, occult hip fractures in elderly, medicolegal cases), however, most of the bone scanning is performed in subacute conditions, e.g. occult fractures, avascular necrosis, reflex sympathetic dystrophic syndrome, etc.
- Detection of *degenerative joint diseases*
- *Studies of joint pathologies,* e.g. activity in rheumatoid arthritis, ankylosing spondylitis, osteoarthritis
- *Bone graft viability,* uptake, etc.

Conventional angiography can assess the *patency of graft vascular* supply which does not necessarily indicate graft viability at the cellular level. However, 3-phase bone scintigraphy with ^{99m}Tc-MDP is dependent both on vascular supply and the viable osteoblasts. The bone scintigraphy should be done 4–8 weeks after bone-grafting. Increased uptake of tracer at the graft site indicates intact graft vascularity and viability.

After acute injury to the scaphoid immediate bone scanning can be done and may be read as early as one hour after the injection of diphosphonate with effective result.

Early stress fractures are not visible on plane X-ray, however, the bone scan will show uptake on both the early blood pool and on the late images.

Pathological fractures scan may present characteristic appearance which may suggest the underlying pathology, e.g. in *osteoporosis* linear uptake in the vertebrae may be associated with fractures of the ribs. The site of uptake in a vertebral body determined by *single-photon emission-controlled tomography (SPECT)* may be more in keeping with malignancy and the planar bone can allow a rapid confirmation and assessment of the whole body to detect other metastatic lesions.

Setting-in of non-union is difficult to diagnose clinically and radiologically. However, the bone scan may be helpful since reduced uptake at the site of the fracture usually confirms an atrophic non-union.

In *early stages of reflux sympathetic dystrophy (RSD),* when radiological changes are hardly seen, the 3 phase hot bone scan showing increased vascularity along with diffuse uptake in the affected zone and intense periarticular uptake will be diagnostic.

Soft-tissue Injuries: Bone scanning is much helpful in diagnosing *avulsion and tendon injuries*, e.g. avulsion of hamstring attachment in the pelvis; avulsion of tibialis posterior tendon. In sports injuries, anterior and posterior impingement syndrome in the ankle can be well demonstrated.

Infection: Gallium has been the optional agent to locate infection in the body. However, though demanding (labour, facility and costwise), patient's own leucocyte may be labelled with either an indium or technetium-based products. Fluorodeoxyglucose (FDG)-*Positron emission tomography (PET) is used for localising infection in bone with about 100% accuracy.*

In localising infection in early stage in long bone (where radiograph shows initial changes by 10–14 days), the use of 3 phase bone scan is highly effective, and when combined with labelled leucocyte imaging it can also locate the pockets of infection in the bone, as early as the second day of infection. The first two phases of scan (blood flow and blood pool) will be abnormal in cellulitis and also in osteomyelitis, while the third phase or late images will show increased uptake in the bone in osteomyelitis. However, sometimes as a fallacy under the age of 6 months, bone scan may be normal or have reduced uptake.

FDG-PET can demonstrate increased uptake at the bone-prosthesis interface in the presence of infection. It can detect both loosening and infection and can help to differentiate between them in both hip and knee prosthesis, of course it is more useful in hip.

For spinal infections MRI is the optional investigation.

Tumours: Bones scanning with conventional disphosphonate is still mainly utilized to identify both primary and secondary bone tumours. It is also taken up by soft tissue metastasis from primary bone tumours, e.g. osteosarcoma.

Bone scanning cannot definitely differentiate benign from malignant tumours, however, any lesion with no uptake is most likely benign in nature, except osteoid osteoma. In osteoid osteoma, even if plane X-ray looks normal, scanning will show a highly localised area of markedly increased uptake. Scanning proves to be much useful to locate the lesion at operation and use of an intraoperative probe can demonstrate the site and later confirm the successful removal of the tumour.

Bone scan cannot always prove to be diagnostic in malignant lesions of bone, but three phases are always hot in malignant tumours.

Intramedullary skip metastases can be missed by both bone scan and MRI, however, bone marrow scintigraphy is more useful in defining the extent of tumour and intramedullary metastasis in both Ewing's sarcoma and osteogenic sarcoma. Soft-tissue metastases from osteo-sarcoma (but not from Ewing's sarcoma) can take up the scan. But for detecting soft-tissue metastases from Ewing's sarcoma gallium scanning is better. FDG-PET is useful for detecting the grade of primary tumour, distant metastases and for monitoring the treatment. FDG-PET with delayed imaging is useful in assessing the transformation of benign to malignant tumours, e.g. neurofibroma to neurofibrosarcoma.

Coregistration Imaging

To localise the pathology more accurately selective use of coregistration scanning can be a useful technique (e.g. for investigating patients with pain in foot, ankle or wrist, etc.)

Coregistration Processing

The X-ray is processed and digitised on a UMAX vist 58 flat bed scanner at 75 dpi. The co-ordinates of the position of the equivalent markers in the two images are identified. From the sets of pairs of markers, a transformation matrix is devised, which coregisters the radiograph and isotope scan so that these images can be superimposed on each other (Robinson et al. 1998).

■ IMMUNOSCINTIGRAPHY

Whereas X-ray, including CT, sonography, and MRI all visualise tumours by reason of the morphologic differences between the neoplasm and the surrounding healthy tissue, the nuclear medicine (scintigraphy) makes use of specific actions or reactions or special surface structure of tumour cells to demonstrate neoplastic tissue. In immunoscintigraphy, the radioactive labelled antibodies, directed against tumour-associated surface antigens, are injected intravenously and the site of the antigen-antibody reaction is located and imaged by recording the emitted gamma rays with a gamma camera. The development of *monoclonal antibodies and the possibilities of labelling them with short-lived technetium has significantly increased the use of immunoscintigraphy in clinical practice.*

Attempts are being made to use the antibodies for therapeutic purposes after labelling them with the substances, which emit alpha and beta rays rather than the gamma rays.

Presently, immunoscintigraphy is being utilised for making specific diagnosis of recurrence and metastasis in colorectal cancer and other tumours producing carcinoembryonic antigen (CEA), ovarian carcinomas, lymphomas and melanomas. This technique is rarely a meaningful method for primary tumour diagnosis (Weib, ML 1993).

■ NUCLEAR MEDICINE THERAPIES

Use of *Nuclear Medicine for therapies* is based on the principle of use of open sources of radioisotopes for selective delivery of radiation to the lesions/target organ. The differential uptake and lodging of radioisotope in the tumour, compared to normal bone forms the basis of nuclear medicine therapy.

For *pain palliation* (which may vary from 2 months to even 1.5 years) radioisotopes (like strontium-89, Samarium-153, Phosphorus-32, and Rhenium-186) are injected which gets localized in metastatic lesion and irradiate for much longer period. The pain relief is not by killing the tumour cells, rather by interruption of process that are maintained by humoral pain mediators in the tumour, like killing of peritumoral cytokine secreting cells. However, it should not be used for pain secondary to spinal cord or nerve invasion by metastasis.

Radiosynoviorthesis

In certain arthropathies, not responding to medical management nor indicated for surgery, nuclear medicine therapy can be used. High energy beta emitting radioisotopes (such as Yttrium-90, Rhenium-186, Phosphorus-32, Erbium-169, Holmium-166, Samarium-153- to be used according to the size of the target joint), when injected into the joint cavity in a colloid form are selectively taken up by the macrophages in the inflamed synovial lining which are destroyed giving relief in pain. This forms the main mode of management of the painful haemophilic arthritis, pigmented villonodular synovitis, Willebrand's disease, psoriatic arthritis, ankylosing spondylitis, collagenosis, rheumatoid arthritis, osteoarthritis. However, absolute contraindications are pregnancy, lactation, and relative contraindications are pre-existing severe myelosuppression, a recent fracture, history of recent arthroscopy.

■ CT/CAT SCAN

In 1974, Douglas Hounsfeld discovered the computerised axial tomography (CAT) scan machine, which opened the vistas of human anatomy with great precision and most of the time help patients get rid of an eager scalpel.

Computed Tomography (CT) produces transaxial cutting images through selected tissue planes, by which the anatomical planes, not delineable by plane X-rays, can be visualised. In CT scanning also, the X-ray is utilised. The X-ray emits from a X-ray tube installed inside a machine known as 'gantry'. The part to be CT scanned is kept in the round portion of the 'gantry'.

At first, a *'survey view' of the region* should be taken in which the affected area is selected and through it a series of cross-sectional images are obtained. Cutting slices are usually 5–10 mm apart, when done through the bigger joints or the tissues. However, much thinner slices are cut in case of small joints, intervertebral disc or smaller tissues.

CT relies on the same principles of physics as conventional X-rays, in which structures are distinguished from one another by their ability to absorb energy from X-rays. The X-ray tube emits a narrow beam of radiation as it passes in a series of scanning movements through an arc of 180° around the given part. The X-ray having passed through the part is also collected by a X-ray detector. The computer collects the information and processes them and displays as constructed picture on a television like screen.

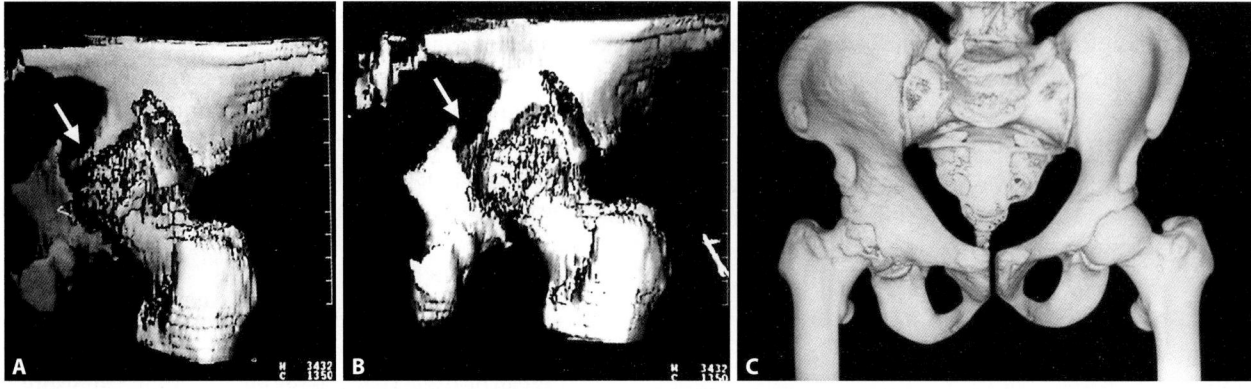

Figs. 23.3A to C: 3D reconstruction of central fracture dislocation of hip.

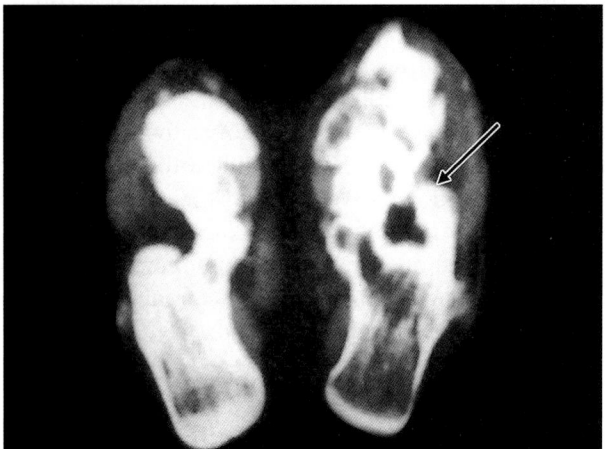

Fig. 23.4: CT of both hindfeet showing a cystic destruction in right talus (giant cell tumour).

Fig. 23.5: Enlarged view of right talus showing large areas of destruction in the neck, head and part of body of talus (giant cell tumour).

The value of CT is further increased when with the help of special equipment, different transaxial cut images are reconstructed in coronal or sagittal or even three dimensional (3D) images of bones with complicated shape, e.g. vertebrae, pelvic bone **(Figs. 23.3A to C)**.

CT displays the bony structures clearly but does not define accurately the soft tissues **(Figs. 23.4 and 23.5)**. CT delineates the bony anatomy architecture like cortical integrity more clearly. It helps in assessing ossification and calcification more accurately.

CT is based on the principle of X-ray attenuation, therefore, radio-opaque structures (such as bone, calcium) are dense on CT and look white and radiolucent structures (such as air, fat) look dark, and soft tissues appear gray.

Advantages of CT Scan

- Cross-sectional images
- No hinderances by overlying soft tissues
- Superior contrast resolution
- Detection of even early calcification
- Detection of soft tissue involvement in neoplasms
- Visualisation of joint details—cartilages and ligaments are better visualised. However, in CT scan of joints with prosthesis replacement, the prosthesis casts dense artefacts causing suboptimal evaluation of joint **(see Fig. 23.15A)**
- Various tissue characteristics can be delineated by measuring the Housefield units, especially in differentiating fat from other soft tissue and bones
- Contrast enhancement is possible by intravenous injection of iodine-based contrast medium.

The *main recent advances* in CT scanning are:
- Three-dimensional CT (3D)
- Real-time Multiplanar Reconstructions
- High-resolution CT
- Dynamic CT
- Dental CT
- Spiral CT
- Multidetector CT (MDCT)
- The limitation of scanning only in transverse (axial) sections has now been largely overcome in the new generation scanners with excellent reconstruction in any plane due to isometric "voxel" scanning providing unparalleled z-axis resolution i.e. the resolution in the reconstructed image is similar to original transverse image (Patil JK).

- CT scan is even superior to MRI in active trauma (fracture or dislocation); tarsal coalition; sterno-clavicular joint arthritis; sacroiliac joint erosion; intra-articular osteo-cartilaginous loose bodies; crowned dens syndrome—CPPD at C_2 dens.

Positron Emission Tomography (PET) (Figs. 23.6 to 23.12)

PET-CT imaging is a hybrid imaging. Both PET and CT are in the same gantry: PET component provides functional status, while CT component provides accurate localization of abnormal function.

Thus PET provides functional and metabolic status of body tissue and organ. PET is a unique imaging technology which provides in vivo noninvasive visualization/characterization/quantification of biologically and chemical process at cellular and subcellular level inside a living body. It has the ability to image: perfusion, metabolizing, abnormal protein deposits, respecter imaging, enzymes and transporters, infection and inflammation. In any disease process the functional and metabolic changes in cells appear much earlier than structural changes. Hence the disease site can be identified by PET imaging in the early stage.

- PET picks up metabolic activity and has tremendous potential in oncology both in initial evaluation and in monitoring response to treatment as well as infections. Combining the images of 'form', i.e. the anatomical structure provided by CT and MRI and those of function, i.e. metabolic or biochemical activity, provided by PET can be precisely aligned and correlated. PET combined with MRI reduces the radiation exposure when compared to a CT.

MRI is modality of choice for assessing the local extent of a primary lesion for surgical planning, however, PET has a limited role, albeit it may allow the noninvasive estimation of histologic grade of tumours.

The main disadvantage concerning PET is the difficulty and cost of producing and transporting the radiopharmaceuticals used for PET imaging, which are extremely short lived. The half-life of radioactive fluorine, used to trace glucose metabolism (using fluorodeoxyglucose FDG) is 2 hours only. Its production require a very expensive cyclotron and a production line for the radiopharmaceuticals. PET investigation is not all proof and can provide false negative or positive results.

The use of FDG-PET or PET/CT can lead to treatment optimization in the initial staging mainly in during sarcoma patients due to its superiority in detecting bone and lymph node metastases.

The integrated PET/CT machines can help in diagnosing the pulmonary nodules using the CT component.

- The first oncological application of PET was in the assessment of brain tumours. PET/CT is an important molecular imaging technique for the assessment of neurological disorders.
- The use of 2-fluoro-2-deoxy-D-glucose (FDG) and non-FDG novel PET radiopharmaceuticals facilitates the early diagnosis, delineation of extent, prognostication and monitoring of therapeutic response in several neuropathological states.
- Normally used radioisotopes for PET-CT are: 18F-FDG, 18F-PSMA, 18F-DOPA, 18F-Sodium fluoride etc. (By the help of Dr Ambuj Shrivastav 2023).

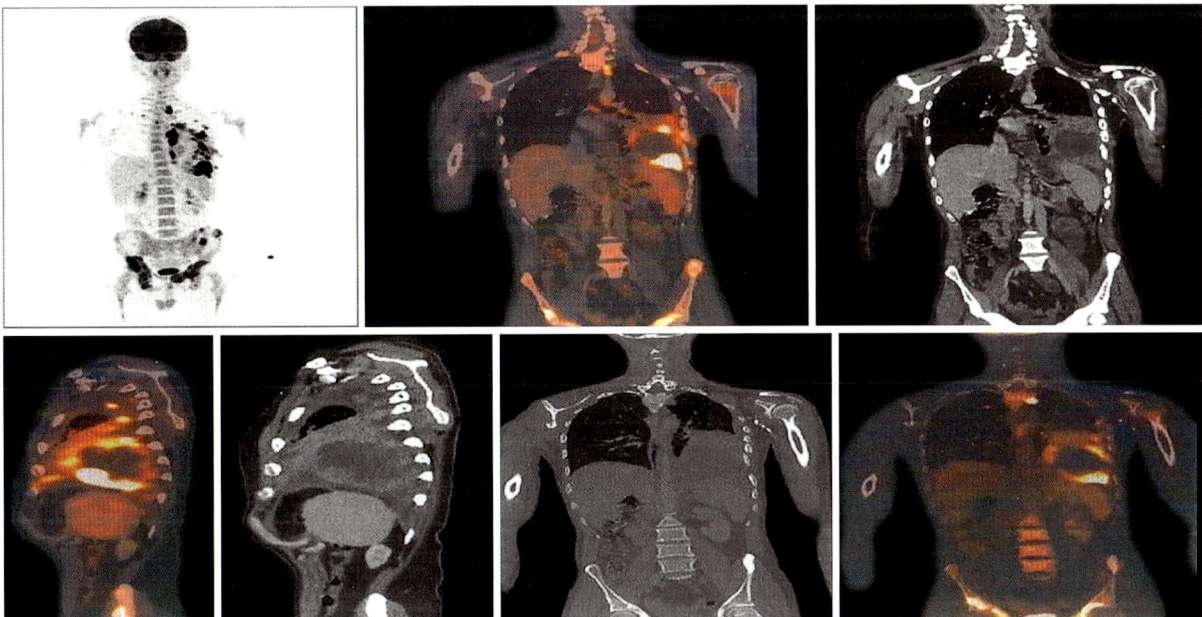

Fig. 23.6: *Brief clinical history:* Known case of adenocarcinoma of left lung with brain and bone metes. Post-chemotherapy status. (Completed 6th cycle of CT).

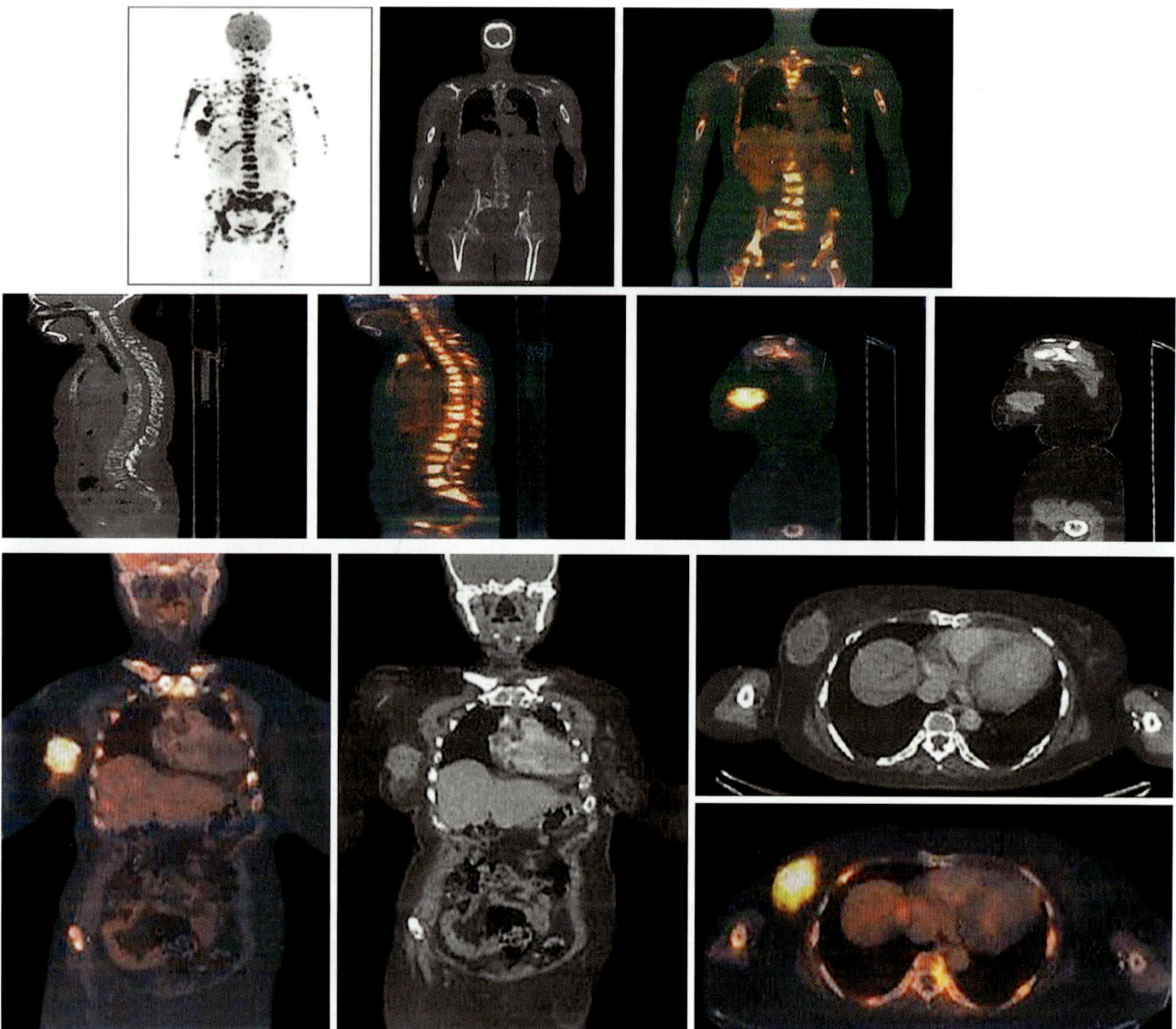

Fig. 23.7: *Brief clinical history:* A case of right breast lump (investigation). Initial diagnosis. Multiple metastatic mediastinal lymph nodes and extensive bone metes.

Uses of CT

CT has proved to be a very useful diagnostic aid in assessing the anatomical dimension of spinal canal, spinal trauma and diseases.

Canal Stenosis

Standard CT in cross-sectional mode can suggest foraminal narrowing. CT is useful in defining the lateral recess stenosis and foraminal stenosis, which is hardly possible in myelography.

CT is helpful in assessing the degree of encroachment of spinal canal by a fractured fragment, herniated intervertebral disc or any other space occupying lesion. The best way of confirming the diagnosis is by metrizamide or iohexol myelography combined with a reformatted computed tomography scan of the suspected segment. Combined with MRI, postmyelogram contrast CT can suggest 96–97% accurate diagnosis.

Radiation exposure of 4.8–7 rads, and the need for an invasive procedure for injecting the dye are disadvantages of contrast CT.

Spinal Trauma

Fractures of cervicothoracic and thoracic or thoracolumbar regions may be missed on plane X-rays. Injuries to osseous, ligamentous, and neurological structures can be evaluated with a high degree of accuracy through the sophisticated imaging technique like tomography, contrast myelography, postmyelogram CT with sagittal reconstruction, and MRI.

CT is helpful in assessing the degree of compromise of the spinal canal.

Advanced Diagnostic Imaging

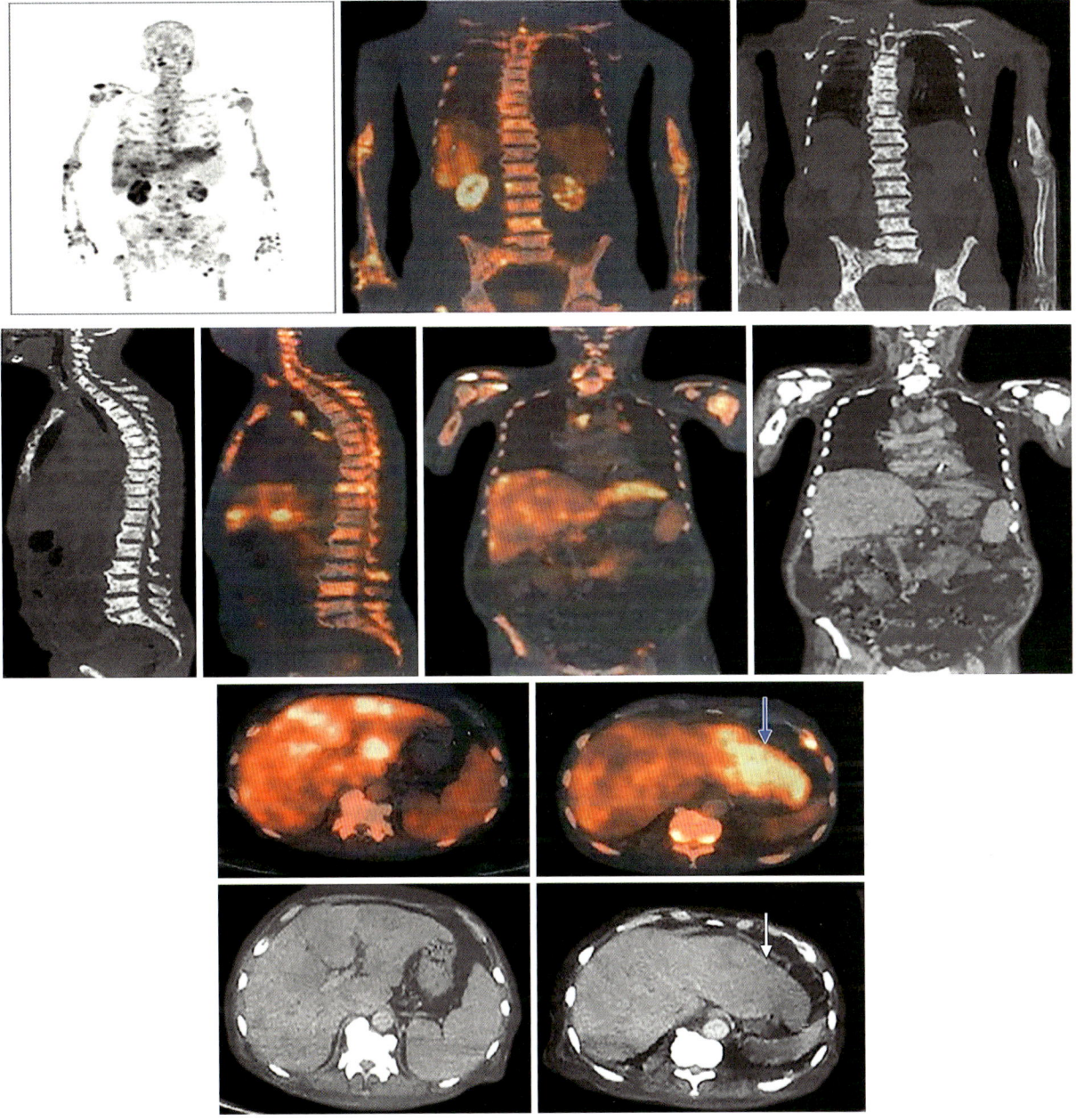

Fig. 23.8: *Brief clinical history:* Known case of adenocarcinoma prostate with multiple bone metes, Post-CT status. (Completed 8th cycle of CT) GS score – 5 + 5 = 10. Bilateral orchidectomy status. As a follow up case for further evaluation of the disease or bone metes.

Reformatted CT scans of the cervical spine usually present less distinct picture than in the lumbar spine.

Infections of Spine

Broad findings of the CT scan are more or less similar to those of plane X-rays including the lytic lesions in the subchondral zones, destruction of the end plate, sclerosed margin of the lytic lesions, lesser density and flattening of the disc, disruption of bone in the paradiscal and peridiscal regions, soft tissue shadows in epidural, paravertebral and paraspinal areas, and abscesses.

Postmyelogram CT clearly defines the compression of the spinal cord and other neural elements by abscess or sequestrum or bone or other materials.

Spinal Tumours

CT is of much use in assessment of the size, shape and infiltration of the tumours. Postmyelogram CT (myelo CT) clearly defines the space occupying growths in vertebral canal.

CT cannot demonstrate intraspinal tumours (unlike MRI) and arachnoiditis. It also cannot differentiate between old scars and new disc herniation.

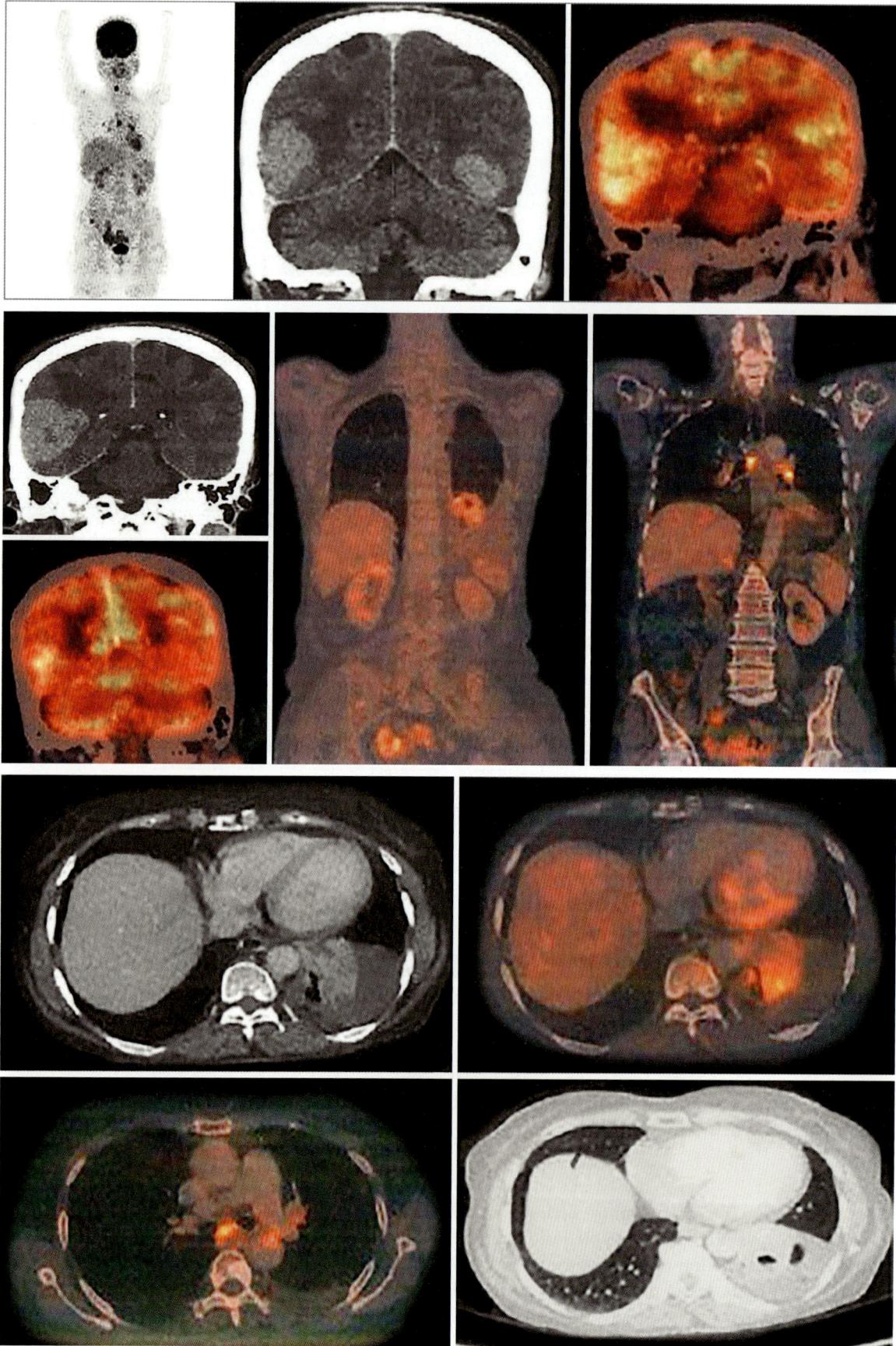

Fig. 23.9: *Brief clinical history:* Known case of carcinoma left lung with multiple bone, brain and liver metes. Post-CT status. Indication: For further evaluation of the disease.

Advanced Diagnostic Imaging

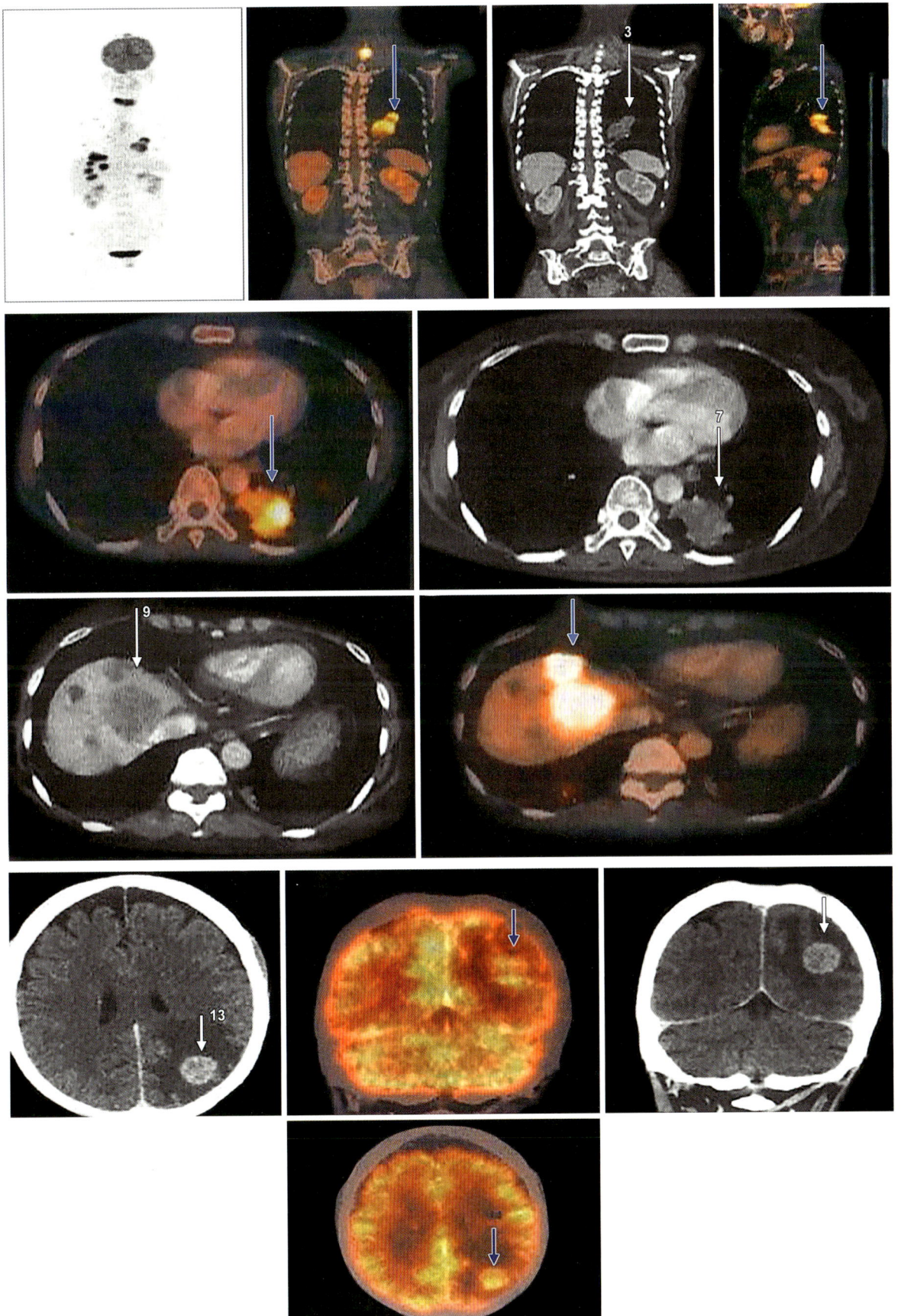

Fig. 23.10: *Brief clinical history:* Known case of carcinoma rectosigmoid colon with postoperative and post-CT, RT status. Now brain metes (evaluation). Indication: As a follow up case for further evaluation or brain metes evaluation.

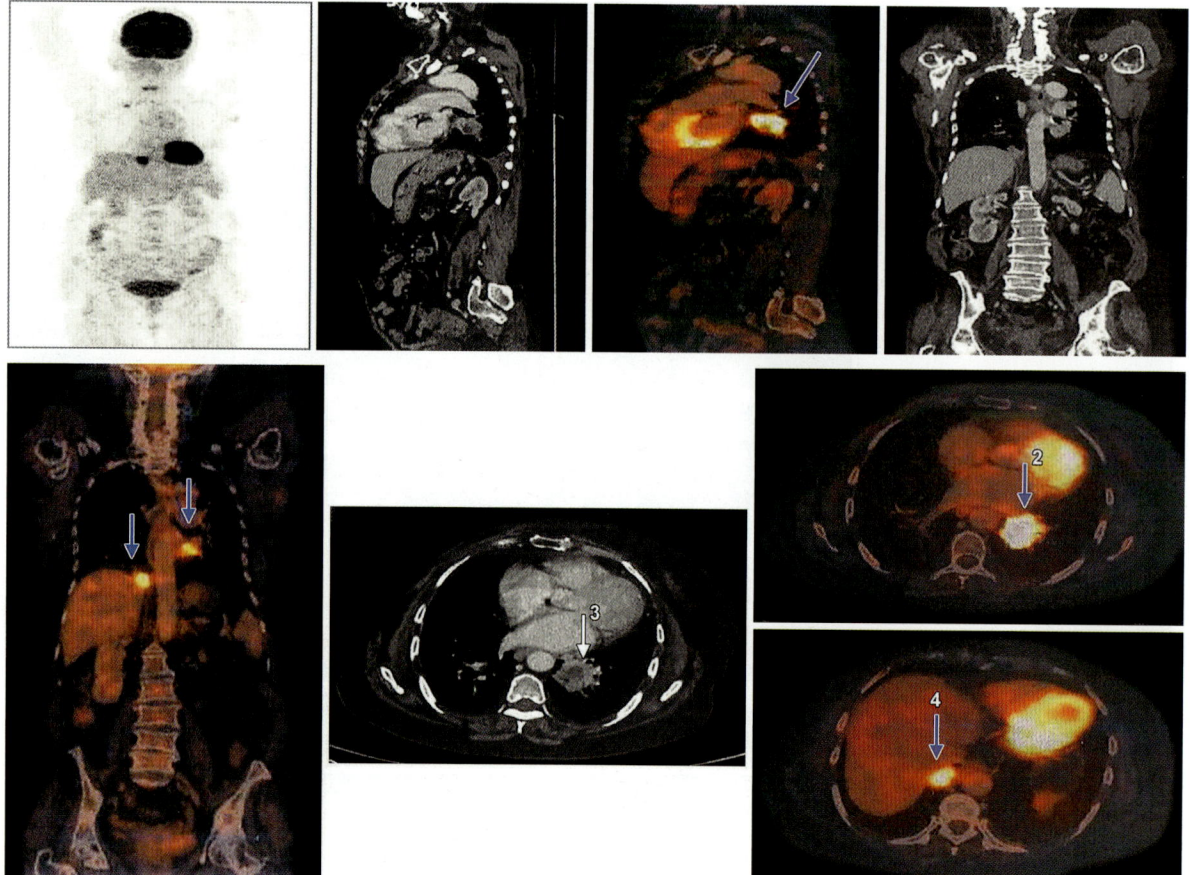

Fig. 23.11: *Brief clinical history:* Known case of carcinoma right breast with post-MRM status. Post-CT/RT status. Now lung metes evaluation. After MRM shows multiple lung and bone metes.

CT is a very sensitive investigation for detecting pulmonary metastases in malignant tumours.

Myelography combined with multiplanar CT scans can be of much use in assessing the intraspinal and extraspinal effects of spondylolisthesis including the evaluation of disc degeneration.

Other places, beside spine, where CT can be helpful:
Fractures not clearly delineable in plane X-ray, can be displayed by CT, e.g. carpal, tarsal (mainly calcaneal fractures and osteochondral fractures of talus), tibial condylar, and pelvic fractures (including the injuries and pathologies of sacroiliac joints); hairline fractures.

High resolution computed tomography has been found to be very useful in studying the meniscal tears, cruciate ligament tears, disorders of complicated joints, e.g. sacroiliac, sternoclavicular, etc.

CT can be useful in assessing the patellofemoral joint, synovial cysts and soft tissue tumours in and around the knee.

MAGNETIC RESONANCE IMAGING (MRI)

Magnetic resonance imaging (MRI) is a non-invasive scanning procedure which uses magnetism and radio waves to produce clear picture of the human anatomy. It forms pictures of the anatomy and physiological processes of the body in both healthy and diseased tissues.

The Nobel laureate Felix Bloch and EM Purcell discovered the physical phenomenon of Magnetic Resonance Imaging (MRI) in 1930/1946, based upon assessment of radiofrequency emissions from atoms and molecules in tissues, exposed to an external magnetic field.

The medical application of NMR (Nuclear Magnetic Resonance) was pioneered by Odebald and Lindstorm in 1955, while Damadian and Hinslow were the first to produce the NMR images on 3rd June, 1977. In the same year, Damadian completed construction of the first whole body scanner.

Paul C Lauterbur (of America) and Peter Mansfield (of Britain) were selected for Nobel prize in 2003 for introducing three-dimensional MRI.

The images recorded in MRI are more or less similar to those of CT scans, but have more clarity and tissue contrast. It gives detailed images of both bones and different soft tissues. The sectional images can be produced in any plane, and reconstituted to project three dimensional (3D) pictures. MRI is a non-invasive procedure and allows to visualise the structures directly in all orthogonal planes. Its resolution is 3 mm (compared with 1 mm for ultrasound).

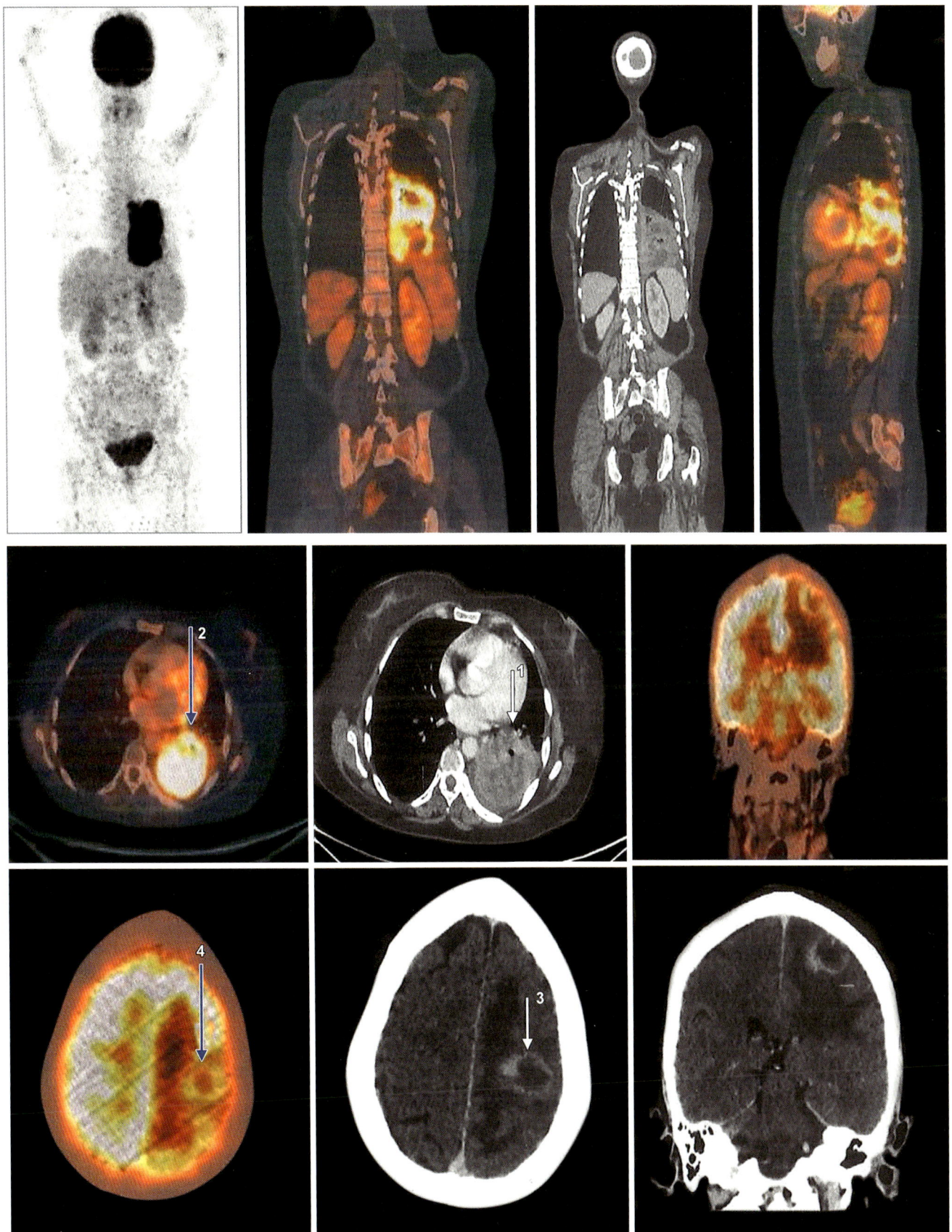

Fig. 23.12: *Brief clinical history:* A case of carcinoma left lung with brain metes. Fresh case. Initial diagnosis.

In this technique, there is interaction of nuclei of a selected atom with an external oscillating electromagnetic field, which is changing at a fraction of time at a particular frequency. Even though all atoms with odd number of protons have property of magnetic resonance, the hydrogen nucleus, because of its abundance in tissues and easy detectability, is used in the current technique of MRI. The technique of MRI uses the magnetic properties of hydrogen nucleus excited by radiofrequency radiation transmitted by a coil surrounding the part. The signal emitted from the excited hydrogen nuclei is detected as induced electric currents in a receiver coil.

The intensity of MR signals depends upon the concentration of hydrogen nuclei in the tissues underscanning and their spinning character and relaxation rates following proton excitation. The physical phenomenon of relaxation is expressed by two independent tissue constants T1 and T2, producing two signals simultaneously. While the images are produced, the tissue character can be 'weighted' or enhanced to provide complementary informations. The T1-weighted images are sharp, well-defined and almost anatomical in appearance. The T2-weighted images project more of the pathological characters of the tissues.

T1 or T2 weighting typically refers to the spin echo MR sequence. TR is the repetition time or time between 90° radiofrequency pulses, whereas TE is the echotime or time between the 90° pulse and the time the signal is received. *T1-weighted images* are short TR (300-1000 ms) and short TE (10-30 ms) and *provide excellent anatomic details, and fat as a high bright signal.* In contrast, *T2-weighted images* are long TR (1800-2500 ms) and long TE (40-90 ms) sensitive *for detecting oedema,* and shows water as a bright signal. An additional signal is obtained by suppressing the fat signal which is called short tau inversion recovery (STIR). It cannot be used to differentiate fluid collections (e.g. abscess) from localised soft tissue oedema.

A proton density sequence combines T1 and T2 weighting by having a long TR (> T1) and short TE (< T2). *This technique can be used to separate cartilage from bone.*

Appearances of various tissues on T1, and T2-weighted MR images appear high (white on MRI) or low (black on MRI). The brightness on MRI is compared with muscle. Different tissues appear as follows as T1, and T2-weighted MR images.

Structure	T1 Intensity	T2 Intensity
Fat, Fatty marrow	High	Lower
Hyaline cartilage	Intermediate	Intermediate
Muscle	Intermediate	Intermediate
Fluid or oedema	Low	High
Neoplasm	Low	High
Cortical bone	Very low	Very low
Tendon, ligaments	Very low	Very low

Tissues with maximum concentration of hydrogen nuclei emit high intensity signals producing the brightest images (e.g. fat, bone marrow, cancellous bone, etc.); those with little concentration of hydrogen emit low intensity signals projected as black (e.g. ligaments, bony cortex, tendons, air, etc.); and those with intermediate concentration are produced in the grey scale (e.g. cartilage, muscle, spinal canal, etc.).

Other frequently used pulse sequences are proton density and short tau inversion recovery (STIR), which has the property to suppress the signals from fat and increase the contrast for water containing tissues. These images greatly aid in detection of marrow and soft tissue disease, e.g. in muscle tears, osteomyelitis, bone marrow oedema or tumour involvement.

Various tissues and organs can be imaged clearly by properly adjusting the anatomical plane, type of coil, thickness of cut slice, and sequence of pulse and magnification.

With ever advancing technology, a wide variety of MRI imaging systems are now available. Scanners are determined and grouped by their field strength. High-field scanners, with superconducting magnets, possess field strengths more than 1.0 Tesla. Low-field scanner work at field strengths of 0.3–0.7 Tesla. New ultra low-field scanners work at less than 0.1 Tesla. Now more powerful systems (3 Tesla) are available for neuroimaging and cardiac imaging, which have the advantage of better resolution. Newer modalities of positron emission tomography-computed tomography (PET-CT) and (PET-MRI) are available.

On the whole, smaller and more specialised coils provide higher resolution and smaller fields of view, and at the same time maintain satisfactory image signal-to-noise ratios.

LAVA Flex is an excellent 3D diagnostic tool for visualising various abdominal conditions with uniform fat suppression. This 3D SPGR technique acquires an out-of-phase and in-phase echo within the same TR to synthesise water and fat images. It is frequently used for abdominal imaging with patients who are suspected to struggle with extended breath-hold times to maintain 20-22 seconds breath-hold (which is helpful in obtaining high-quality images due to breathing artifacts). The gadolinium-enhanced T1-weighted images, used to assess the bowel wall, allow better visualisation of the surrounding vasculature and tissues. The LAVA Flex gives excellent high resolution images with uniform fat suppression within fast scan time (<15 seconds).

Uses of MRI

MRI is marginally superior to spine myelo-CT in identifying the spinal lesions **(Figs. 23.25 to 23.35)**. It can suitably examine the entire spine, identify the degenerated disc, delineate the cord and root impingement **(Figs. 23.13 and 23.14)**, demonstrate the intra-spinal tumours **(Figs. 23.15 to 23.18)**, and evaluate the thecal spaces and tissues in the foramen **(Figs. 23.19A and B)**. If combined with postmyelogram CT, the accuracy of diagnosis may be up to 95%, and even non-symptomatic lesions can be identified **(Fig. 23.20)**.

- Spinal infections **(Figs. 23.17 and 23.21 to 23.24)** can be identified quickly and more or less accurately, and the

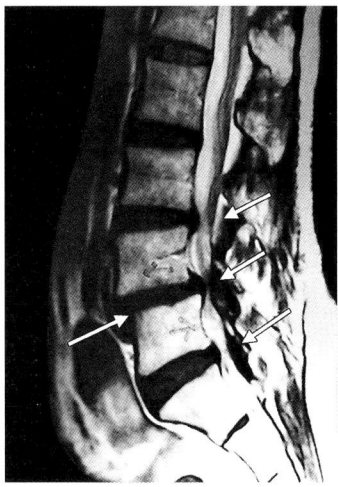

Fig. 23.13: MRI of lumbosacral spine showing lumbar canal stenosis and posterior herniation of degenerated discs pressing upon the cauda equina in L4-5 spondylolisthesis seen in mid-sagittal T1- and T2-weighted images.

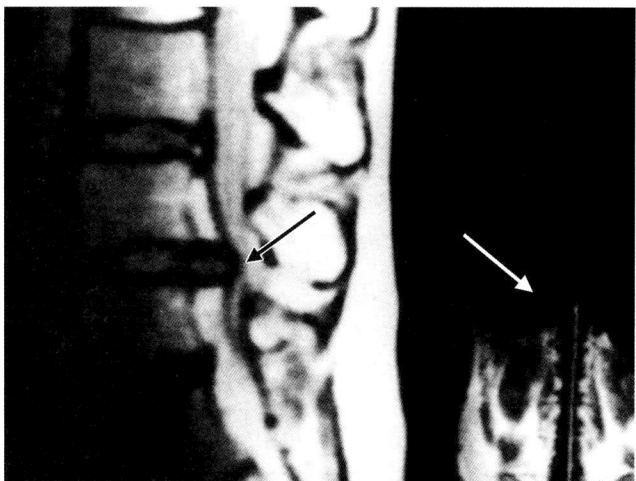

Fig. 23.14: MRI of lumbar region showing compression by L4-5 disc herniation.

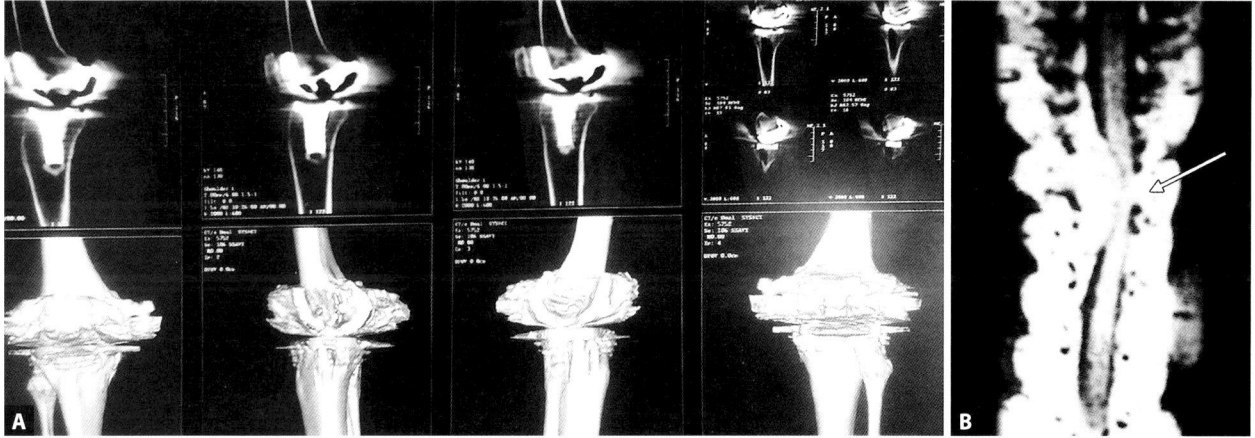

Figs. 23.15A and B: (A) CT in total knee joint replacement done in both sides of knee. Prosthesis casts dense artefacts causing suboptimal evaluation of joint. (B) MRI of dorsal spine T1-weighted image showing isointense extramedullary dumb-bell shaped spinal tumour, which looks hyperintense on T2-weighted image. The possibility is of neurofibroma.

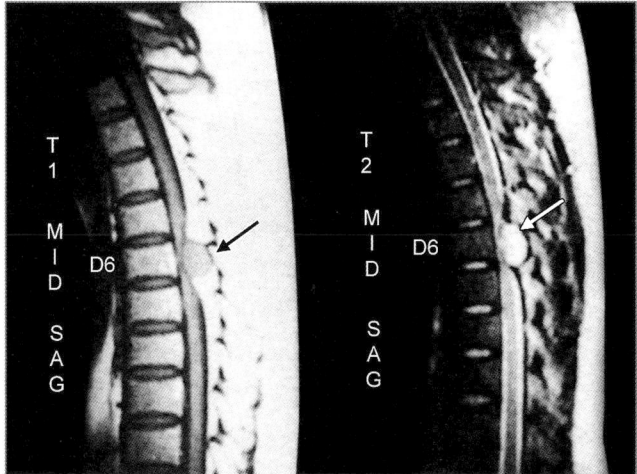

Fig. 23.16: MRI showing compression of the spinal cord by an oval extradural mass (neurofibroma).

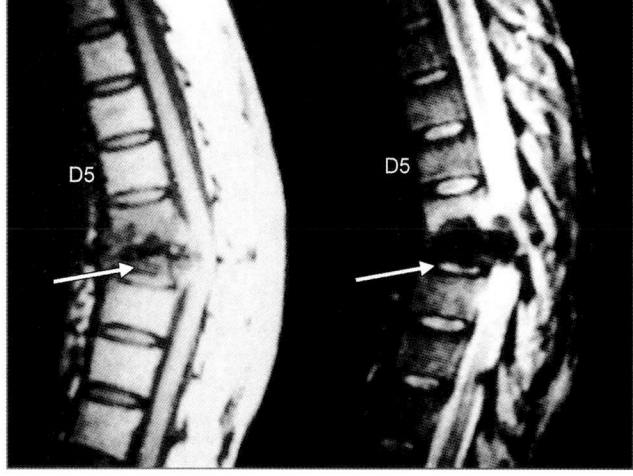

Fig. 23.17: T1- and T2-weighted midsagittal images showing extradural compression by a space occupying lesion (neoplasm or abscess).

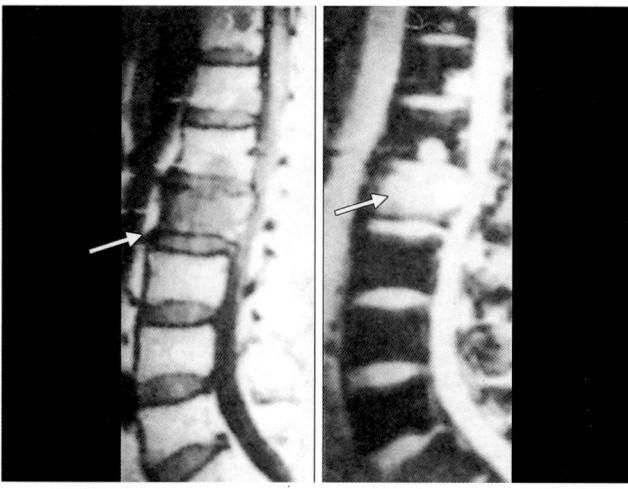

Fig. 23.18: MRI of lumbar and lumbosacral sagittal section showing multifocal hypointense areas in L2 vertebral body on T1-weighted image. Wedging of L2 vertebra, and impingement of the spinal cord by the posteriorly displaced portion of vertebral body (due to secondary metastasis).

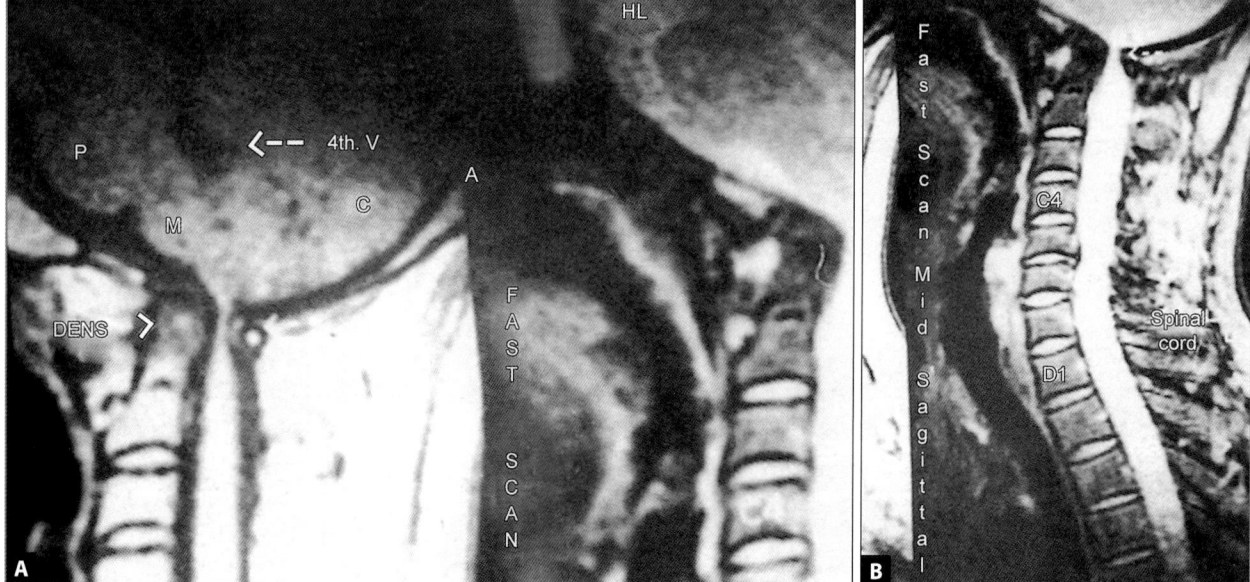

Figs. 23.19A and B: MRI of craniovertebral region. Mid-sagittal T1-weighted image shows the odontoid process lying above the plane of foramen magnum, causing marked reduction in the space and pressure over the spinal cord platybasia with basilar impression in craniovertebral junctional congenital anomaly.

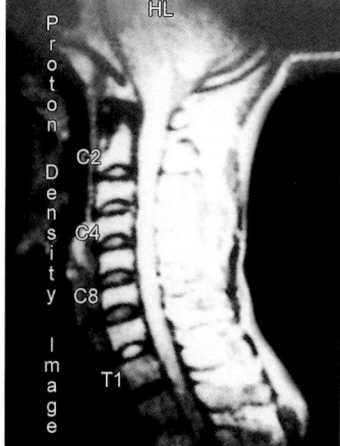

Fig. 23.20: MRI of cervical spine: Proton density and T2-weighted image shows a focal hyperintense area within the spinal cord at C3-C4 level suggestive of traumatic cord contusion.

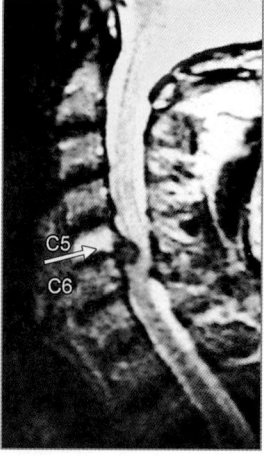

Fig. 23.21: T1-weighted mid-sagittal image showing compression at C5-6 levels due to tuberculous abscess.

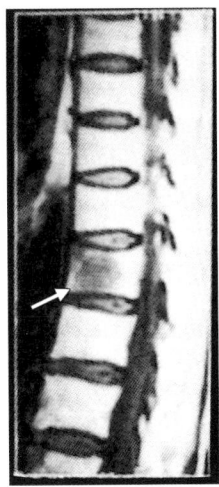

Fig. 23.22: MRI of dorsal spine showing focal hypointense area on T1 weighted image (which appears as hyperintense area on T2 weighted image) in D12 vertebral body—suggestive of tuberculous focus.

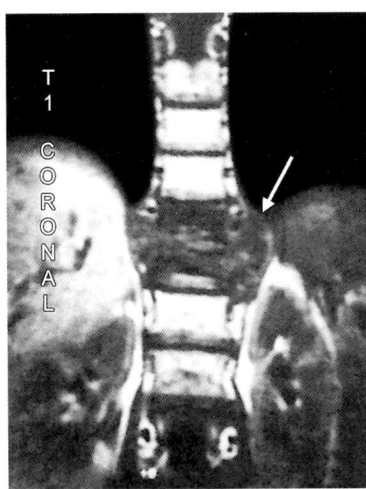

Fig. 23.23: Coronal section showing paravertebral abscess due to tuberculous infection.

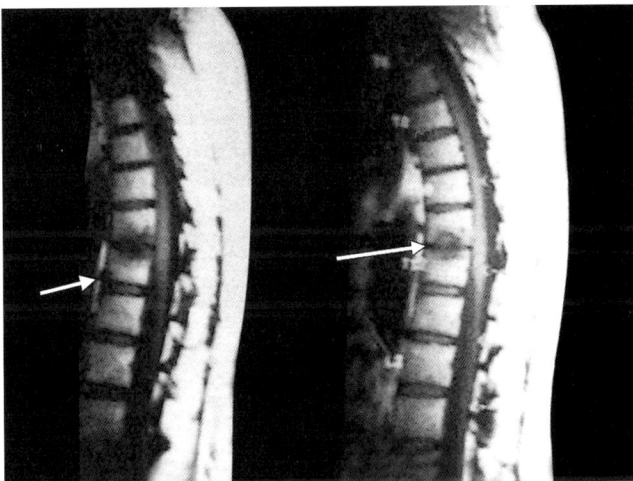

Fig. 23.24: T1-weighted mid-sagittal image showing almost kissing lesions of D10-11 and destruction of the intervertebral disc due to tuberculous infection.

extent of normal and infected tissues can be delineated in high quality MRI. To detect infection, T1-intermediate and T2-weighted views should be obtained in sagittal plane.

The MRI sequences typically used to evaluate the musculoskeletal system are the spin-echo, gradient echo, and STIR sequences. They provide excellent contrast and spatial resolution for the evaluation of normal anatomical structures and pathological changes within the body. Spin-echo T1-weighted sequences (a short relaxation time and a short echo time) are optimum to delineate tissues containing fat or blood and provide excellent anatomical detail. Spin-echo proton density-weighted sequences (a long relaxation time and a short-echo time) are also used to assess soft tissue and bone anatomy. Spin-echo T2-weighted sequences (a long relaxation time and a long echo time) are used to delineate tissue containing fluid or oedema. STIR and spin-echo fat-saturated T2-weighted sequences are particularly sensitive to fluid or oedema in soft tissues and osseous structures.

The high-signal intensity in cancellous bone on T1- weighted sequence: If the abnormal process contains increased free water (as with an inflammatory lesion or malignant cells), there is increased signal intensity in the cancellous bone on spin-echo T2-weighted and STIR sequence. If the pathology replacing the marrow fat contains fibrous tissue or additional mineralisation, there is low-signal intensity on all of the magnetic resonance images.

With MRI it is now possible to follow non-invasively the evolution of injury, repair and remodelling of tissue and the changes of tissue-aging.

Recent advances in MRI, including faster imaging sequences and improved surface coil design have markedly increased the amount of information provided by these images.

"*Kinematic MRI* refers to imaging a joint through a range of motion to examine the interactions between the soft tissue and osseous anatomy that comprise the joint" (Frank G Shellock & Christopher M. Powers 2001)

Elastography is a newer technique of MRI and ultra-sonography, which is used to assess tissue elasticity and stiffness.

1.5 Tesla MR unit, equipped with advanced MR technique, such as diffusion and perfusion imaging, spectroscopy, diffusion tensor imaging, contrast enhanced MR angiography functional MRI, etc. is quite useful.

MRI cannot differentiate between the pyogenic and non-pyogenic infections. The calcified areas of tuberculous abscesses, so well demonstrable in plane X-ray are not identified in MRI.

In infections, the patients usually remain in pain and agony, due to which they face a lot of difficulty in remaining still in a particular position for long periods. Hence, motion-induced degradation of the findings and artefact are common and misleading.

To increase the accuracy of early detection of infection and to monitor its various pathological processes, the contrast material *gadolinium-labelled diethylenetriamine penta-acetic acid (Gd-DTPA)* is being used in MRI. Gadolinium (non-allergic and non-radioactive) is a paramagnetic element used as a contrast agent in MRI. On T1-weighted images, gadolinium is distributed to areas of increased flow, hence it is a good marker of vascularity of tumours or of inflammation. Initial imaging technique must simplify the diagnostic work-up. In this respect, gadolinium-enhanced MRI is generally considered superior to all other imaging techniques. It is useful in detection of even doubtful infection and also enhances the sharp appearances of epidural and spinal infections, however, the added risk, expenses, and time have put reservations on its regular use.

Spinal Injuries

The *role of MRI in spinal trauma* is still evolving. MRI helps in patients with suspected spinal cord injury, epidural haematoma, traumatic disc herniation or ligamentous tear in the acute stage. It presents superior images of the lesions in the craniocervical and cervicothoracic regions. Its role in determining the prognosis for neurological recovery in traumatic quadriplegia or paraplegia, is being favourably reported.

In *investigating the low back pain,* the MRI has provided clinicians a non-invasive mechanism for viewing lumbar anatomy in great detail, however, MRI must be better related to the clinical features. Clinical findings correlate well with MRI findings but all MRI abnormalities do not necessarily have clinical symptoms or significance. The presence of

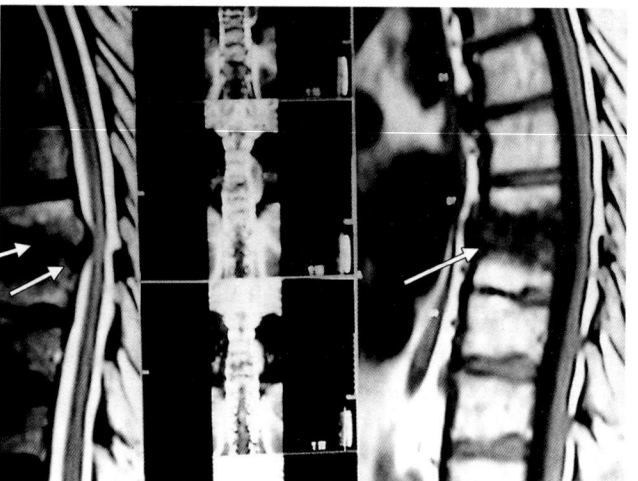

Fig. 23.25: Tuberculous collapse of adjacent vertebral bodies pressing on the spinal cord.

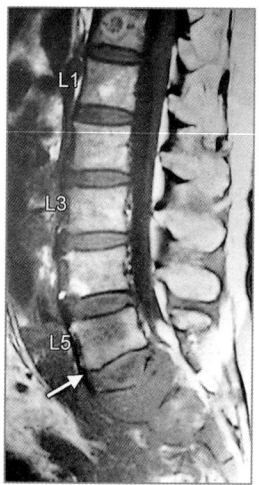

Fig. 23.27: Chordoma of sacrum.

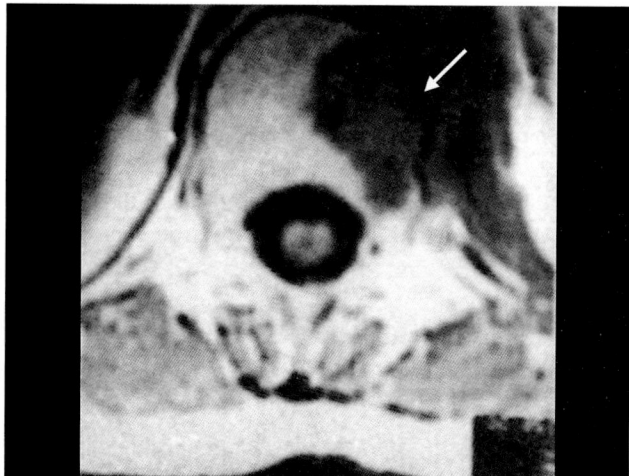

Fig. 23.26: Coronal weighted image of L3 vertebra reveals involvement of large area of soft tissues and destruction of right pedicle.

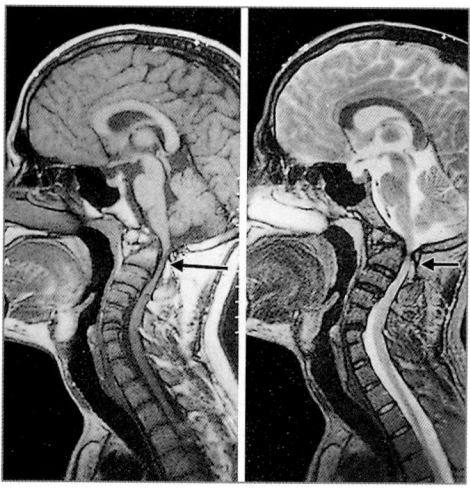

Fig. 23.28: MRI of brain and cervical region showing upper cervical canal stenosis producing constriction of the upper end of spinal cord.

Advanced Diagnostic Imaging

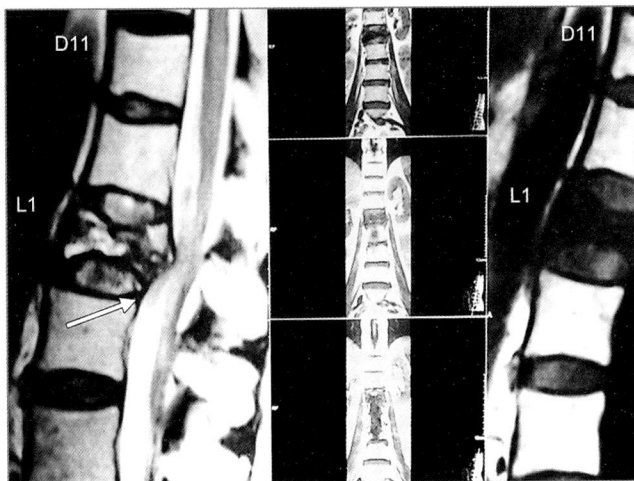

Fig. 23.29: Comminuted fracture of L1 body. The displaced fragment is pressing over the spinal cord.

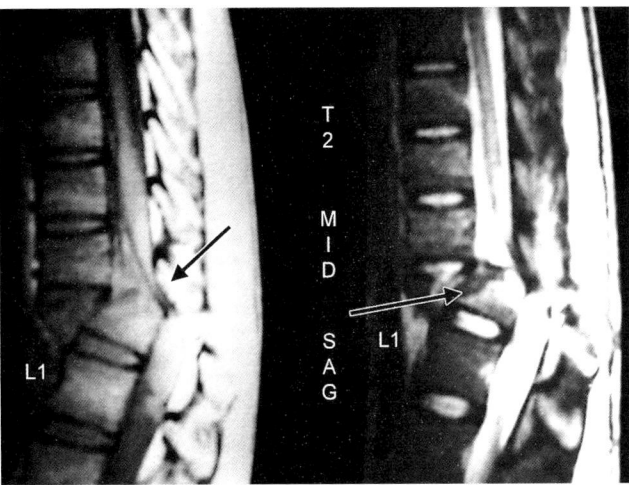

Fig. 23.31: T2-weighted mid-sagittal image showing complete transection of spinal cord in fracture dislocation of D_{12} vertebrae.

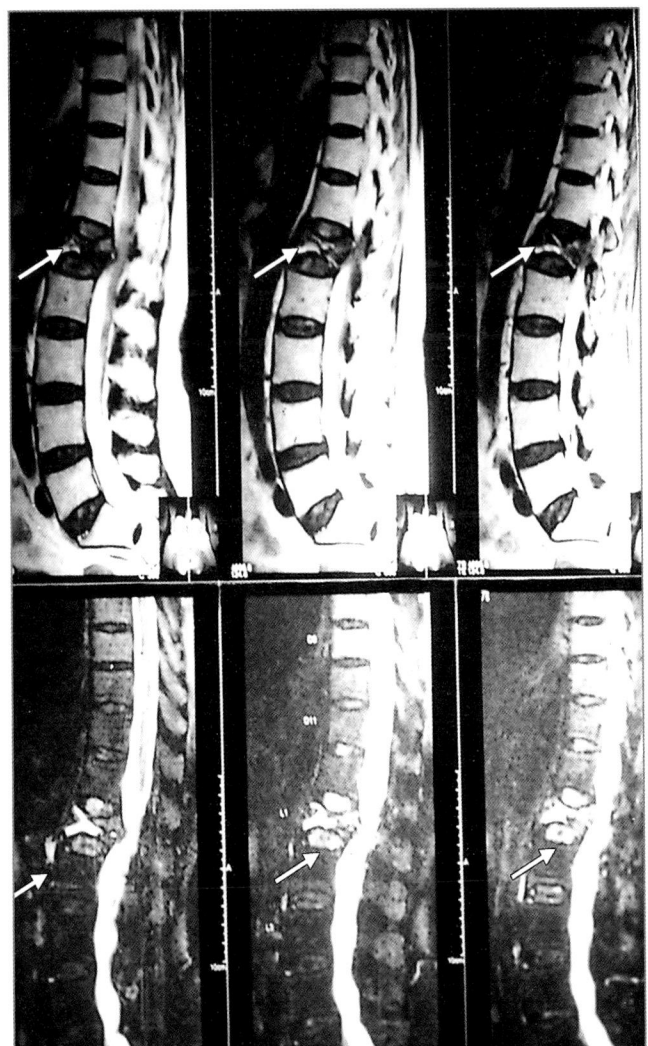

Fig. 23.30: Comminuted fracture of D12 vertebra producing marked pressure and damage of the spinal cord.

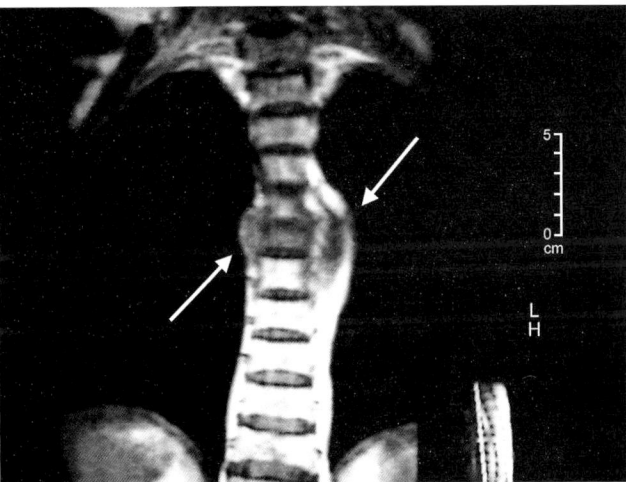

Fig. 23.32: Coronal section showing paravertebral abscess due to tuberculous infection.

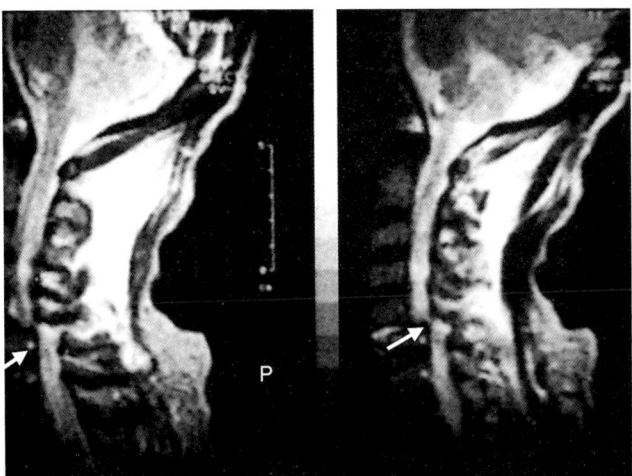

Fig. 23.33: T2-weighted image showing complete transection of cord at C6-7 levels.

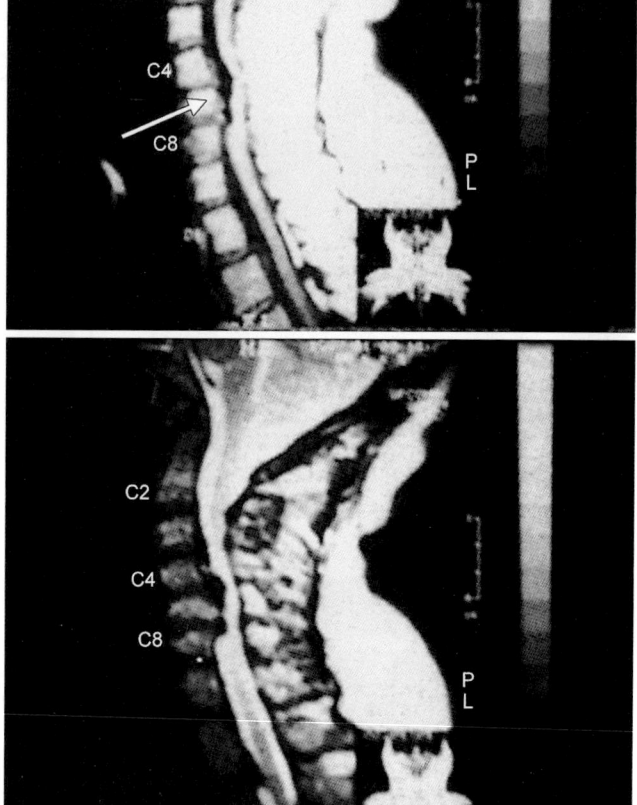

Fig. 23.34: T2-weighted image in mid-sagittal section showing epidural compression at C4-5-6 level probably due to calcification of posterior longitudinal ligament or thickened ligamentum flavum.

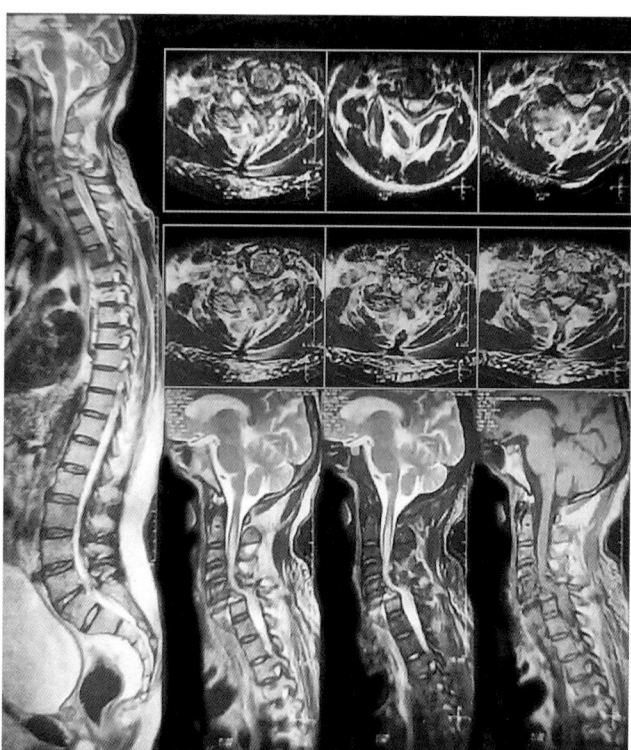

Fig. 23.35B: Comminuted fracture dislocation in upper cervical region

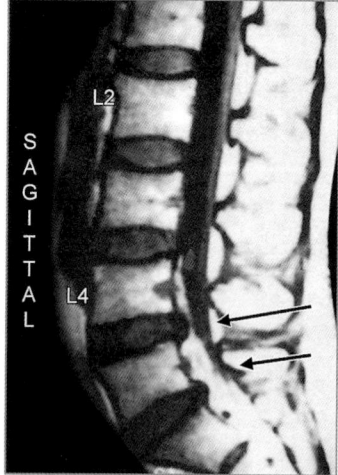

Fig. 23.36: T1-weighted mid-sagittal images showing intervertebral disc herniation pressing on cauda equina.

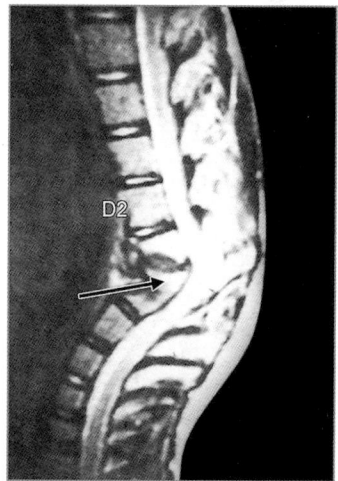

Fig. 23.35A: T2-weighted mid-sagittal section showing destruction at D3,4,5 with compression of cord due to internal gibbus.

centrolateral protrusion or extrusion with gross foramen compromise correlates with clinical signs and symptoms very well, but central bulges and disc protrusions correlate poorly with clinical signs and symptoms. The presence of neural foramen compromise is more important in determining the clinical signs and symptoms, but the type of disc herniation (bulge, protrusion or extrusion) correlates poorly with clinical signs and symptoms. The recent development of MRI scanning in the erect posture may well reveal biomechanical defects and spinal pathology, which are unrecognisable when the patient is supine.

The most common indication of MRI of spine is for evaluation of intervertebral disc disease. After disc surgery, MRI findings focus on early postoperative changes related

Advanced Diagnostic Imaging

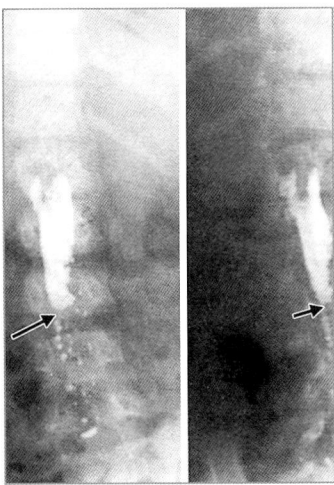

Fig. 23.37: Descending myelogram showing complete block at lower border of L4—cauda equina lesion due to massive intervertebral disc herniation.

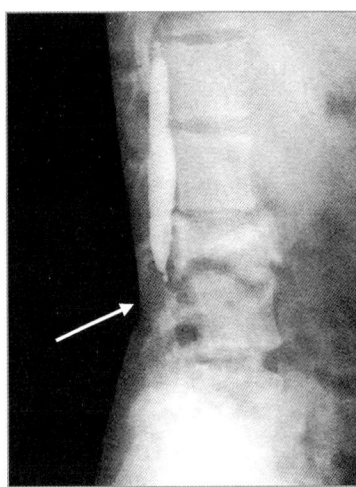

Fig. 23.39: Descending myelogram showing tapering block at the lower border of L3 vertebra due to unusual tuberculous concentrina collapse of L3.

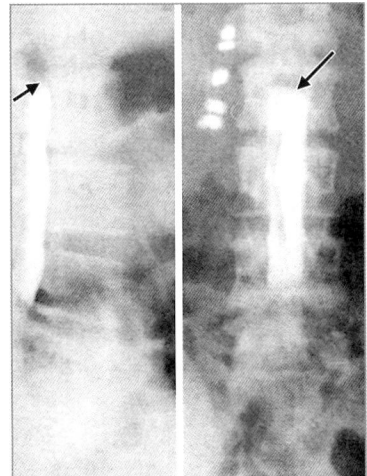

Fig. 23.38: Ascending myelogram showing block at L1 level due to meningioma.

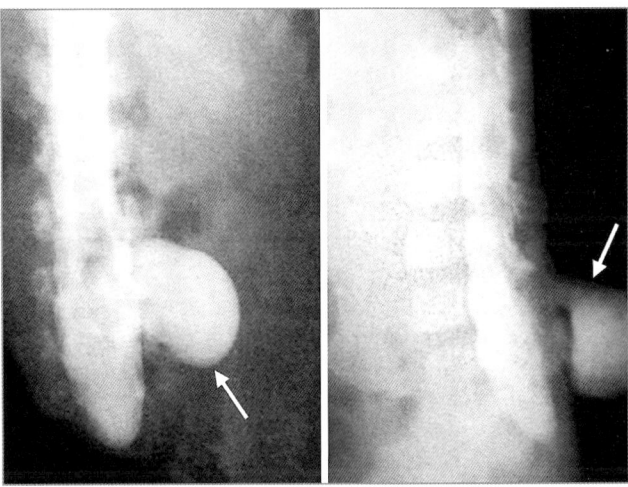

Fig. 23.40: Myelogram showing dye in pouch of meningocele.

to surgery, however, extensive soft-tissue changes present in the immediate postoperative period severely limits the usefulness of MRI. The recent development of magnetic resonance myelography (MRM) in MRI has the advantages in the visualisation of the thecal margins, nerve roots and nerve root sheaths. MRM is non-invasive, efficient and reliable tool in confirming postoperative decompression in lumbar discectomy, especially when the required expertise to analyse a complex and confusing postoperative MRI is not available. However, with fair numbers of false-positive and false-negative examinations, the diagnostic accuracy of MRM is insufficient to justify its use as an independent diagnostic tool.

Since MRI delineates the bone marrow excellently, it helps in early detection of both primary and secondary spinal tumours with high sensitivity on T1-weighted sequences.

In general bone and joint infections, MRI is not much helpful. In osteomyelitis, the marrow fat is replaced by oedematous fluid and cellular infiltrates. Hence in MRI, there is a decrease in normally present high marrow signals on T1-weighted images and a normal or increased signal on T2-weighted images.

MRI has a definite role (about 75% positive) *in early detection of the avascular necrosis of femoral head,* but its regular use for clinical decision making is still being developed. Accurate estimation of the extent of osteonecrosis of the femoral head and to calculate the volume and surface area of the osteonecrosis, MR images can be used but at the present time this method is too complicated for clinical application.

In Knee injuries/pathologies carefully performed clinical examination can give equal or even better diagnostic support in comparison with MRI scan, of course in several instances arthroscopy proves to be the gold standard especially in knee injuries. In internal derangements of knee, MRI appears to be useful non-invasive aid with high diagnostic accuracy, sensitivity, and negative predictive value.

In carpal tunnel syndrome, the synovial diseases, narrowing of the tunnel, and median nerve compression can be well delineated in MRI.

MRI appears to be a very accurate investigation for *assessing the extent of bone and soft tissue involvement by the tumour.* There is also possibility of assessing the actual nature of the tissues which can help in the pathological diagnosis besides anatomical delineation.

MRI of the *shoulder* is an exquisite modality for the proper *evaluation of various lesions and abnormalities,* e.g. rotator cuff tears, impingement, labral abnormalities and instability. Ultrasound though a good modality for rotator cuff degeneration and full thickness tears, is not a sensitive modality for partial thickness tears and is unable to visualise the labrum.

The proper mode for *evaluation of labrum abnormali-ties is MRI arthrography* with sensitivity up to 95% especi-ally in patients with shoulder instability, including recurrent anterior dislocations. For labral pathologies 20 mL of saline and diluted intra-articular gadolinium is injected under fluoroscopic control just as in routine shoulder arthrograms through anterior approach. Confirming the injection under radiograph, MRI is done after 20 minutes, obtaining T_1W and T_2W sequences in multiple planes.

In the elbow region, MRI is used to assess the tear and pathology of biceps and triceps tendons. In the wrist region, most common indication for MRI is to evaluate intrinsic carpal ligaments.

Diagnosis of damaged or disrupted interosseous membrane of the forearm is extremely difficult. However, the intact and disrupted interosseous membrane can be evaluated by the MRI. Axial T2-weighted fast spin-echo images with fat suppression provide the most accurate information. The use of fat suppression more clearly delineates the areas of oedema and injury in the trauma patients.

High resolution images of the inner ear structures give excellent detail of normal anatomy, *congenital anomalies and pathological changes of the inner ear.*

Advantages of MRI

- It is a non-invasive, versatile, and sensitive technique with fairly high degree of specificity and accuracy, and with no risk of ionizing radiation
- It does not require frequent repositioning as in myelography
- It produces clear and high soft tissue contrast differentiating the bone and soft tissues
- MRI scan is superior to CT scan in: cervical spine disease or instability; spinal stenosis or disc disease; internal derangement of knee; rotator cuff tears and tendinitis; tumour; skeletal muscle pathology; pigmented villonodular synovitis; sacroiliitis (inflammatory); tenosynovitis; synovitis;
- MRI is the only modality, that allows direct visualization of the marrow

MRI is complementary to CT scan and bone scintigraphy while evaluating bone tumours. However, as on today *PET (Positron emission tomography) Scanner* appears to be ultimate imaging modality in cancer management.

Disadvantages of MRI

Besides those enumerated in the beginning of the chapter, other noticeable disadvantages of MRI are:

- It is a costly investigation
- It requires the patient to lie still in a particular position, which can become painful and annoying
- The fear of remaining in a closed container for a long period *(claustrophobia)* may create a problem, affecting the final result of MRI. However, open gantry MR is quiet and powerful with non-claustrophobic-spacious patient opening and also provides excellent image quality (with multiplanar acquisitions, better soft tissue details, superior and prolonged contrast enhancement, selective enhance-ment—fluid/fat suppression, angiograms without contrast media, etc).

Contraindications for MRI

If patient is with resuscitation equipment (such as airway, metallic tube, tracheostomy tube) MRI will not accept such case (MRI is likely to destabilize the equipment).

Absolute contraindications for MRI, as on today, are intracerebral aneurysmal clips, automatic defibrillators, internal hearing aids (cochlear implants) and metallic ocular foreign bodies. Except for recently developed MRI-friendly cardiac pace makers, others are contraindicated.

Relative contraindications for MRI are first-trimester of pregnancy, recently placed (within 6 weeks) intravascular stents; patients fitted with metal external fixators; few types of infusion pumps, bone or nerve stimulators.

Now most of the orthopaedic implants, internal fixators and hardware can be safely scanned, however, stainless steel-made implants (especially the bigger ones) are likely to produce variable artefacts obscuring the clear vision of the adjacent tissues, and these can be hardly (or not) eliminated by adjustments of scan parameters.

Injudiceous and commercial use of MRI is proving harmful to both—patients [who mostly press for the treatment of MRI finding (±)], and doctors (who are forgetting the clinical examination, loosing the clinical acumen, and depend more upon the MRI findings, which can be misleading. Without clinical findings MRI should not be overrated.) Refer MRI syndrome on Page 649.

Redundant and unnecessary MRI must be eliminated to control the spiraling costs of health care.

MRI can be used in pregnancy; however it should be avoided in 1st trimester.

FUSION IMAGING

Scintigraphy (Nuclear imaging) provides excellent functional information while CT and MRI give finer anatomical details of an organ/part. Both are essential to obtain comprehensive and complete information about the organ, which can be possible when anatomic details and functional informations are fused together—by Fusion imaging. In this process, the image obtained from Gamma Camera is blended with a CT or MRI image and all are then obtained from a single picture.

SWAN*

SWAN is an excellent diagnostic technique for various brain pathologies and helps in their early detection.

The SWAN technique combines a unique 3D T2-based multi-echo acquisition with a special reconstruction algorithm. Several echoes are read out at different TE times and then combined as a weighted average, compiling magnetic signature of a whole range of tissues with varying degrees of T2 contrast. At the end, it provides a clear sub-millimeter-resolution 3D with significantly enhanced susceptibility information and greatly increased signal-to-noise ratio (SNR) on both 1.5 T and 3-0T field strength systems. One can visualise major vessels and large vascular structures using SWAN. It can accurately delineate small vessels and microbleeds. It also helps in early detection of brain calcification, venous angiomas, iron and calcium deposition in tissues, etc. Using this technique, the whole brain can be imaged in 3D high-resolution in 3–4 minutes.

The *radiologists* are playing notable roles in *interventional orthopaedics* such as radiofrequency ablation of osteoid osteoma, metastasis; image-guided procedures like ultrasound guided aspiration/injections /; catheter-guided angiographic procedures to select patients with vascular malformations, preoperative tumour embolization Frank GS & Christopher P Kinematic MRI of the joints 2019 by CRC Press.

BIBLIOGRAPHY

1. Armstrong P, Keevil SF. Magnetic resonance imaging-1: basic principles of image production. BMJ. 1991;303:35-40.
2. Balachandran R. Kharbanda OP, Sennimalai K, Neelapu BC. Orientation of Cone-Beam Computed Tomography Image: Persuit of perfect orientation plane in three dimensions - A retrospective cross-sectional study. Ann Natl Acad Med Sci. (India) 2019;55-4:202-9.
3. Bloch F, Hanson W, Packard ME. Nuclear induction. Physical Review 1946;69:127.
4. Damadian R. Tumour detection by nuclear magnetic resonance. Science. 1971;171:1151-53.
5. Hasin SF, O'Doherty MJ, Smith MA. Functional imaging and the Orthopaedic Surgeon. J Bone Joint Surg (Br). 2002; 84-B:315-21.
6. Herzog RJ. Magnetic resonance imaging of the shoulder. An instructional course lecture. J Bone Joint Surg. 1997;79-A: 934-51.
7. Kayser R, Mahlfeld K, Hyde C, et al. ultrasonographic imaging of fractures of the clavicle in newborn infants J Bone Joint Surg. 2003;85-B:115-6.
8. Kundu ZS. Classification imaging, biopsy and staging of osteosarcoma. Indian J Orthop. 2014;48:238-46.
9. Mansfield P. Multiplanner image formation using NMR spin echoes. J Physical Chem. 1977;10:55-8.
10. Patel PR, Dave BR, Deliwala UH, Krishnan A. Magnetic resonance myelography in early postoperative lumbar discectomy: An efficient and cost effective modality. Indian Jorthop. 2010;44:257-62.
11. Purcell EM, Torrey HC, Pound RV. Resonance absorption by nuclear magnetic moments in a solid. Physical Review. 1946; 69:37-8.
12. Robinson Ahn, Bird N, Screaton N, et al. Coregistration imaging of the foot. J Bone Joint Surg. 1998;80-B:777-80.
13. Rubin C, Bolander M, Ryaby JP, Hadjiargyrou M. The use of low-intensity ultrasound to accelerate the healing of fractures. J Bone Joint Surg (Am). 2001;832-A:259-70.
14. Ullrich Sprect (Ed). X-ray Contras Media. Berlin: Springer Verlag, 1989.
15. Weib ML. Nuclear medicine methods in oncology. Medical Focus International. 1993;XI.5:16.
16. Wentroub S, Grill F. Ultrasonography in developmental dysplasia of the hip. J Bone Joint Surg. 2000;82-A:1004-18.
17. Young-Min Kim, Ahn JH, Kang HS, et al. Estimation of the extent of osteonecrosis of the femoral head using MRI. J Bone Joint Surg. 1998;80-B:954-58.

Source: GE Healthcare leaflet.

CHAPTER 24

Syndromes Related to Orthopaedics and Traumatology

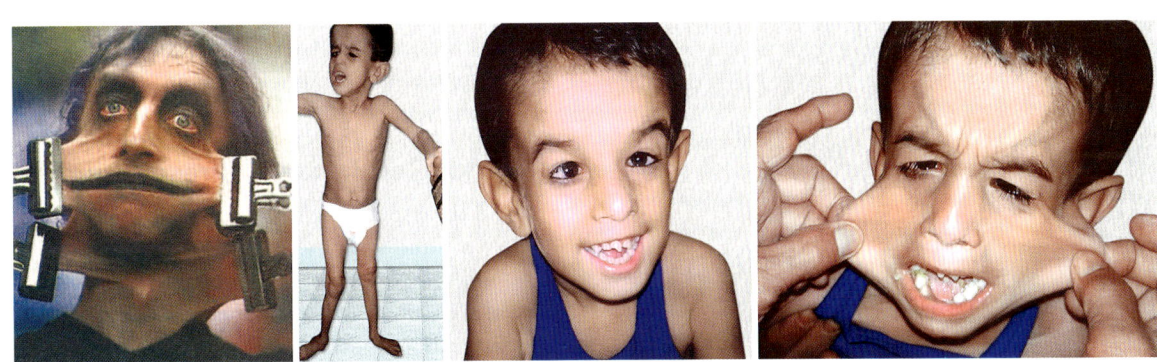

"Lonliness gives you an opportunity to discover yourself."
—*PP Wangchuk*

Acromegaly Syndrome

Hyperpituitarism (due to excessive production of growth hormone by pituitary gland e.g. in adenoma) if manifests after closure of growth plate it leads to the syndrome of Acromegaly and if it happens before closure of growth plate it is gigantism.

In acromegaly there is generalised thickening of skin, and enlargement of hands, feet, ears, nose and lips. There is expansion of skull, frontal bossing, prognathism (protrusion of lower jaw), macroglossia (enlargement of tongue) spacing between teeth). Hypertrichosis; hyperhidrosis; hyperpigmentation; soft tissue swelling. Complications, like – renal failure, cardiac failure, diabetes mellitus, carpal tunnel syndrome may develop.

Georg Mcist, a chemist at the university of Cambridge, lead author suggested that toxic protein clusters thought responsible for the cognitive decline associated with Alzheimer's disease reach different regions of the brain early then accumulate over the course of decades – this inference was drawn over the studies (reported as landmark research) carried out over 400 post-mortem brain samples from Alzheimer's and 100 positron emission tomography scans from people living with the disease to track the aggregation of tau, one of two key proteins implicated in the condition

Alzheimer Disease (Fig. 24.1)

Alzheimer Disease (described by German psychiatrist Alzheimer Alois in 1907) affects usually the elderly (about 44 mm people globally) (7th or 8th decade) who gradually loose their memory and orientation and get depressed with vacant look, and personality change. Early dementia is easily missed if not specifically sought. The disease is characterised by accumulation of amyloid deposits in the brain. The plaque is composed of neurotoxic beta-amyloid peptide. These peptides are cut out from a protein called the amyloid precursor protein and bind together to form plaques in the brain. The cause is partly genetic and perhaps partly environmental.

A different protease called cathepsin B is claimed to be elevated in brains of Alzheimer patients.

Gilles Guillemin (New South Wales) and his research team have demonstrated the involvement of a neuro-transmitter—a chemical called 'quinolinic acid' in producing Alzheimer's disease and few other brain diseases like autism, schizophrenia, etc. It is hoped that in future, it would be possible to stop the production of quinolinic acid by using specific enzyme inhibitors to block its production.

Scientists of Indian Science Institute Bengaluru have prepared a florogenic examination kit which can detect enzyme especially attached to Alzheimer disease. (Prabhat Khabar dated 15.6.2023) Frequent fasting at certain regular intervals may play some preventive role against Alzheimer disease.

Adams-Oliver Syndrome

Congenital scalp defects, occasionally ulceration. Sometimes with osseous skull defects, terminal reduction of one or more extremities with aphalangia, adactylia, acheiria, transverse hemimelia.

Adult Respiratory Distress Syndrome

Adult respiratory distress syndrome (ARDS) is a clinical syndrome which *commonly develop after severe trauma, multiple fractures, lung contusion, and fat embolism.* It can also occur after septicaemia, prolonged hypotension, gastric aspiration, massive blood transfusion, overdoses of certain drugs.

It manifests as:
- *Severe hypoxaemia,* resistant to supplemented oxygen therapy. The partial pressure of oxygen (PO_2) is less than 75 in patient receiving more than 50% oxygen
- *Diffuse fluffy pulmonary infiltrates* which involve both the lungs
- *Absence of increased pulmonary capillary hydrostatic pressure* probably due to cardiogenic cause. The pulmonary wedge pressure is less than 18
- No other explanation for the above findings. Lungs develop diffuse alveolar damage and become stiff.

Management of ARDS is primarily the treatment of its cause. Acute cases may need mechanical ventilation. Complication should be apprehended and prevented as far as possible.

Anterior Cord Syndrome

In this syndrome, there is *loss of neural functions* of the *anterior two-thirds of the spinal cord* (e.g. in spinal injury, space occupying lesions, etc.). Patient has *complete loss of*

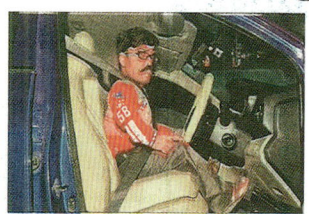

Fig. 24.1: Hindustan Times December 06, 2021.
Source: Rittman University of Cambridge shows an MRI image of a healthy brain (left) and an Alzhei brain with large black gaps where brain has shrunk.

motor functions below the level of lesion (cortico-spinal tracts) and *pain, touch and temperature sensations* (spino-thalamic tracts), but has sensations of vibration, proprioception, position and light touch due to intact posterior column. These preserved sensations help in improving the rehabilitation processes and overall prognosis.

Anterior Impingement Syndrome

It is an inflammatory process in which the *anterior capsule of the ankle joint is repeatedly impinged* with dorsiflexion in running and jumping sports. It leads to the formation of a bony spur at the anterior distal tibia and chronic pain in the ankle. It should be managed by ice *fomentation*, *NSAID* and *heel raise* in the footwear. The persistent problems can be relieved by arthroscopic debridement and removal of bony spur.

Anterior Interosseous Syndrome

Palsy of anterior interosseous nerve was first described by Tinel J in 1918 as 'Dissociated paralysis of median nerve'.

It is the *compression neuropathy of anterior interosseous nerve* (a branch of median nerve emerging at about 5 to 8 cm below the lateral epicondyle and it contains only the motor fibres for supplying the flexor pollicis longus, flexor digitorum profundus (to the index and middle fingers) and pronator quadratus muscles. Though this nerve contains only motor fibres, *pain in the forearm is the common complain* in this syndrome, which is *exacerbated by exercises and relieved by rest*. There is no significant sensory problems, except unexplained pain.

The Kilon-Neven sign is positive. The typical symptom is the inability to form 'O' with the thumb and index finger. Due to paralysis of flexor pollicis longus and flexor digitorum longus, the patient is not able to flex at distal interphalangeal joint of index finger and interphalangeal joint of thumb.

Several causes have been found to be responsible for this compression, such as tight musculotendinous arch of flexor digitorum origin; band from pronator teres origin; Lacertus fibrosus tightness; an aberrant or thrombosed blood vessels.

Main treatment is exploration and decompression of the nerve. If motor function does not recover, tendon transfers should be done: brachioradialis to restore flexion of the interphalangeal joint of thumb; flexor digitorum profundus of ring or middle finger to be transferred to restore flexion of DIP of index finger.

Anterior Tarsal Tunnel Syndrome

Marinacci AA (1968) described it as the entrapment neuropathy involving deep peroneal nerve beneath the inferior extensor retinaculum. It is usually produced by pressure of the dorsal strap of high heeled shoes. The patient complains of pain on the dorsum of the foot and usually dysesthesias or sensory loss in the first web space. Electromyography reveals the increased distal potency of the deep peroneal nerve with chronic denervation of the extensor digitorum brevis. Treatment consists of avoidance of irritant (dorsal strap of shoe-pressure) and decompression of the inferior extensor retinaculum and sometime also of extensor digitorum brevis.

Anterolateral Soft Tissue Impingement Syndrome

Following an ankle injury, localised area of fibrosis or *synovitis develops in the anterolateral region of the ankle*. Patients complain of persistent pain, swelling and catching sensation in the anterolateral region of the ankle joint. Treatment is by conservative measures like rest, immobilisation and NSAID. In failed cases, arthroscopic or open surgical resection of the impingement lesion may be required.

Antley-Bixler Syndrome

There are camptodactyly, long hands and fingers, multiple joint contractures, fusion of certain joints especially humerus with radius with carpus in continuity associated with brachycephaly, prominent forehead, proptosis, mid-face hypoplasia, deep nasal bridge and dysplasia of ears.

Apert's Syndrome

In 1906, Eugene Apert described such a group of children. It is a major genetic disorder with dominant inheritance with an incidence of about one in one lac born babies. It is one of a group of rare deformities known as acrocephalosyndactyly syndromes. There is deformity of skull due to disrupted bone growth and premature closure of coronal sutures which may lead to increased intracranial pressure and mental deficiencies with the syndactyly of fingers and toes. The syndactyly is of type I variety of Blauth's classification (*see* **Fig. 15.5**). There is extensive syndactyly with complete spoon-like deformity of hands and soft syndactyly of all toes. Common nail may be shared by all toes. There may be acrocephaly, strabismus, maxillary hypoplasia, high prominent forehead, flat occiput, flat or concave face, exophthalmos, (**Fig. 24.2**) high-arched perforated palate, hole in heart, etc. The hand in Apert's syndrome should be reconstructed as far as possible. Also ***see*** **Figs. 15.6** in Chapter 15.

Arnold-Chiari Syndrome

Also See Page 268.

In this congenital anomaly, there is downward displacement of the cerebellum through the foramen magnum of skull and by similar caudal elongation of the medullae. It has two major types:

Infantile type: Commonly associated with other midline defects such as spina bifida, meningocele, hydrocephalus, etc. Usually, the infant is brought with hydrocephalus, spina bifida or paraparesis resulting from myelomeningocele. It is usually managed by a ventricular shunting procedure for

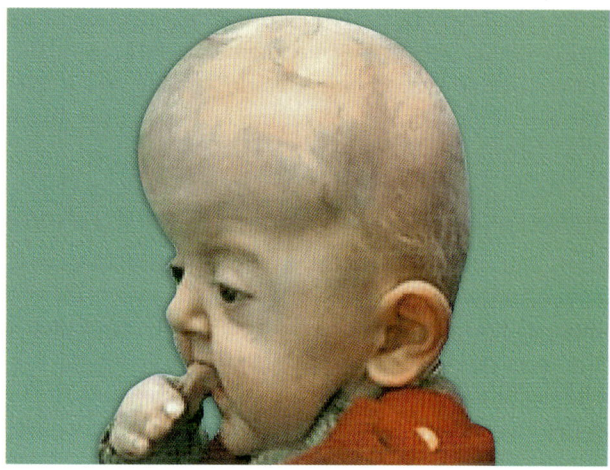

Fig. 24.2: Apert's syndrome.

hydrocephalus and repair of meningomyelocele. Prognosis, on the whole, is not good.

Adult type: Remains asymptomatic till adult life, when the patient may present with features of damage to the cerebellum, lower cranial nerves, pyramidal tracts and posterior columns; variable hydrocephalus; features of syringomyelia, fusion of cervical vertebrae, etc. Surgical enlargement of foramen magnum and decompression of cervicomedullary junction may help.

Baller-Gerold Syndrome

Premature craniosynostosis, radial ray defects, and occasionally other hand and forearm anomalies.

Battered Child Syndrome (Kempe CH 1962)

The infant remains neglected, malnourished, with retarded growth and development, and poor skin hygiene with bizarre skeletal (mainly the long bones) affections (effects of various old injuries in the infants' bones). The typical X-ray findings are symmetrical metaphyseal periosteal new bone formation as happens in periosteal avulsion and subperiosteal haemorrhage (Akbarnia 1976).

Battered Baby Syndrome (Child Abuse)

The recognition of this condition was emphasised when J Caffey in 1946 first drew attention to the association of *multiple fractures* of long bones of infants suffering from chronic subdural haematoma. It includes those *infants and young children* (usually below 2 years of age who are unable to protect themselves or narrate the history of injury) who sustain *repeated multiple deliberately inflicted injuries* (sometimes serious) at the hands of their parents (who do not want the children) or other adults (who are probably perverted or criminals or mentally ill). The injuries are bruises, abrasions, burns, fractures of long bones (usually in epiphyseal or epiphyseo-metaphyseal regions), ribs, etc., subdural haematoma with or without fractures of skull.

Parents usually give cautious, suspectable and bizarre history of injury. The alert clinician with a high index of suspicion must go in detail family and social history. The X-rays usually reveal evidences of healed earlier fractures.

Rathod (2016) has described a battered child as one who is a victim of deliberate nonaccidental physical trauma which has been inflicted by a person or persons responsible for his/her care. The concept of child abuse has now also includes physical and emotional neglect, physical abuse, psychological and sexual abuse. Child abuse may take place at homes, orphanages, schools, streets and juvenile prisons.

Battered Buttock Syndrome

A direct blow over the trochanter may cause a central dislocation of the hip and in the same process split the trochanteric fat capsule with displacement of the fat pad inferiorly. This is often mistaken for an unresolved haematoma. The clue to injury is the severe bruising which occurs initially.

Benign Hypermobility Syndrome

In this syndrome, which is more common in females, there are increased joint mobility, loose joints, daytime pain and night-time awakening with discomfort especially after exercises. In children and young adults, it is an important cause of musculoskeletal pain.

Bone Cement Implant Syndrome

It is a well-recognised complication of cemented arthroplasty. It is characterised by systemic hypotension, hypoxia, and pulmonary hypertension. Though it can be alarming, if appropriate therapy can maintain haemodynamic stability, even elderly critically ill patients will survive. The hazards of this syndrome can be reduced with use of certain anaesthetic and surgical prophylaxis. Use of TEE should be seriously considered during the use of bone cement, especially in arthroplasties.

Bone Marrow Oedema Syndrome

The term is based on early magnetic resonance imaging (MRI) finding. This syndrome can present in variable pattern like Transient Osteoporosis of Hip (TOH); Regional migration transient osteoporosis where features migrate from one joint to other; Partial transient osteoporosis in which a portion of foot or a portion of knee is involved. In 1959, Curtiss and Kincoid described a peculiar pattern of regional osteoporosis in women in 3rd trimester of pregnancy. Osteopenia appears as a late finding in plain X-ray (4–6 weeks after onset of symptoms). CT shows similar features as in X-ray. MRI shows diagnostic bone marrow oedema. Bone biopsy also reveals marrow oedema without evidence of ischaemic changes. Scintigraphy is sensitive but not specific.

Aetiology is unknown. Disease is self-limiting and does not need any intervention.

Management: Mainly consists of wait and watch, protected weight bearing, assurances, and symptomatic (analgesic, NSAID, traction). High level of suspicion and MRI are helpful in diagnosis. In TOH, MRI T1-weighted images reveal low signal intensity, while T2-weighted images reveal matching high signal intensity in bone marrow.

Differential diagnosis: Infective arthritis, rheumatoid arthritis, RSD, Villonodular synovitis, AVN of femoral head, etc.

Clinically in TOH, there is abrupt onset of pain in hip joint which exaggerates on weight bearing and relieves with rest. Disease passes through three phases: In first phase (lasting 1-2 months), there is rapid aggravation of pain and functional disability; in 2nd phase (lasting for 4-6 months) pain reaches a plateau of intensity; third phase lasts for 6-9 months and in it symptoms regress and hip joint becomes normal.

Brown-Sequard Syndrome

In hemicord dysfunction (hemisection of spinal cord)—frequently seen with extradural tumours, in penetrating injury or unilateral facet dislocation—the clinical features are *ipsilateral posterior column sensory loss and contralateral pain* and *temperature sensations loss, below the level of the lesion*. There will be *ipsilateral upper motor neuron lesion* below the involved segment and an *ipsilateral lower motor neuron lesion* at the level of damaged cord. However, there is not much functional deficit as some fibres cross over.

Caput Ulna Syndrome

Destructive changes following synovitis of the *distal radioulnar joint* especially in rheumatoid arthritis is called caput ulna syndrome. Clinically, there are soft (synovial) swelling over the distal part of ulna; *dorsal prominence and instability of distal end of ulna*, which is also tender; rotational movements of the distal radioulnar joint and dorsiflexion of the wrist are grossly restricted; weakness at wrist; less or loss of normal action of extensor carpi ulnaris and rarely of the extensors of little, ring and middle fingers due to pathological rupture of the tendons.

Carpal Tunnel Syndrome

It is the *most common compressive neuropathy* of upper extremity in which the *median nerve is compressed in the carpal tunnel* at the wrist. Sir James Paget described this condition in 1863 and Moersch coined the name of the syndrome (*see* Page 173).

Catel-Manzke Syndrome

There are mandibular hypoplasia, retroglossia, cleft palate, rudimentary phalanx and metacarpal, clinodactyly associated with congenital cardiac anomalies.

Cauda Equina Syndrome

It occurs due to *pressure on the roots of cauda equina* due to various causes, mostly the midline (central) herniated intervertebral disc, producing lower motor neuron type of lesion (*see* Page 269).

Cenani-Lenz Syndactyly Syndrome

There is almost complete (occasionally partial) syndactyly of all fingers, dysphalangism of toes, synostosis of metacarpals/radioulnar joint, and occasionally syndactylism.

Central Cord Syndrome

It is caused by *cervical hyperextension injuries* resulting in hematomyelia, contusion, cord swelling, and ischaemia of cervical spinal cord. The anterior horn cells may be damaged at the level of injury. There is *incomplete tetraparesis* and ill-defined patchy sensory loss.

The patient has *disproportionate greater weakness in the upper extremities as compared to the lower;* variable sensory dysfunctions and urinary bladder problems.

Management mainly concerns immobilisation of the cervical region and medicines to reduce the cervical oedema. Usually, the signs of neurological damage disappear in reverse order of their appearance. Overall prognosis is not bad but unpredictable, unless recovery starts early and rapidly.

Charcot-Marie-Tooth Syndrome (Peroneal Muscular Atrophy Disease)

The French neurologist Marie Pierre (1853-1940) of Paris was the first to describe this condition.

Charcot-Marie-Tooth disease (syndrome) is a hetero-geneous group of disorders which can result from genetic defects in many proteins of myelin sheath of the peripheral nerve.

In this autosomal dominant disease (syndrome), there is *peripheral neuropathy* associated with *weakness or loss of power of the intrinsic muscles* of the foot resulting in clawing of the toes. It is more common in males, but more severe in females. Details of family history and course of disease must be enquired. Type I of this disease (myelin sheath disease), starting 20 to 40 years is less severe. Type II starts in 5–15 years (axonal abnormality) of age and has severe motor and sensory deficit. Management is usually by surgery, however joint-sparing procedures should be tried first—failing which arthrodesis is indicated.

Chronic Compartment Syndrome

Few athletes have tendency to develop the symptoms of compartment syndrome after each exercise session. *Usually they have raised intracompartmental pressure even at rest (10–15 mm Hg* as against normal pressure of 0-4 mm Hg). After exercise, the pressure rises high (20–70 mm Hg) and it remains so even for 5–10 minutes after stopping the exercises.

Recurrent pain, temporary paraesthesia and *numbness* are the presenting features.

Changing the pattern and amount of exercises and limiting the physical activities (likely to aggravate the intracompartmental pressure) should help, otherwise surgical decompression is the only permanent solution.

Chronic Regional Pain Syndrome—Type I (Reflex Sympathetic Dystrophy, Algodystrophy)

Initially it is diagnosed clinically, and radiological changes occur after the condition is well established. In the early stage, the three phase 'hot' bone scan showing increased vascularity combined with diffuse uptake in the affected area and intense periarticular uptake will be diagnostic.

Clenched Fist Syndrome

(Psychoflexed hand-Birman and Lee 2012)
Two typical postures of the hand are acquired in psychiatric disorders:
- *Psychoflexed hand:* Here the ulnar three digits are severely flexed and contracted almost digging into the palm interfering with the hygiene and thereafter emits offensive odour.
  Clenched fist syndrome: In which the entire fist is clenched, however, the ulnar three digits are more severely involved.
- *Psychoextended hand:* In this condition the ulnar three digits are held in rigid hyperextension at the proximal interphalangeal joints and in flexion at the metacarpophalangeal joints. The index metacarpophalangeal joint remains in flexion, however, active flexion and extension is possible at the proximal interphalangeal joint, by which opposition to the thumb pulp remains possible. These problems are hardly cured/corrected. The psychiatric disorders should by managed along with possible stretching or casting or needed operation to improve the function of hand as far as possible.

Clinical Syndrome of Dementia

According to international criteria, the clinical diagnosis of Alzheimer's disease (*Also see* Page 634) (A degenerative progressive ailment of insidious onset characterised by deposits of amyloid plaque substances and several other inflammatory proteins in the brain. The plaque is composed of neurotoxic beta amyloid peptide. These peptides are cut out from a protein called the amyloid precursor protein and bind together to form plaques in brain. A different protease called Cathepsin B is claimed to be elevated in brains of Alzheimer patients) can only be made with a certainty in the persons suffering from clinical syndrome of dementia defined by:
- The existence of associated memory disturbances
- An impairment of at least one other higher function (language, executive function, performance of gestures, recognition of objects)
- These impairments should be severe enough to restrain the independence of the individual in daily life.

Alzheimer disease usually affects the elderly persons who gradually loose their memory and orientation and get depressed with vacant look.

■ COMPARTMENT SYNDROME

Compartment syndrome is a condition in which *increased pressure* (usually due to fracture haematoma) *within the osteo-musculo-fascial space* compromises the circulation of the contents of that space and thereby causes damage to the tissues in the compartment. It mainly occurs in the forearm and leg (*see* the Chapter on Compartment syndrome).

Compartment Syndromes of Leg

Anterior Tibial Syndrome or Anterior Compartment Syndrome

Increased pressure in the anterior compartment of leg (bounded by interosseous membrane posteriorly, the tibia medially, crural fascia anteriorly, and fibula laterally) on its contents (mainly the anterior tibial nerve and vessels), usually due to unaccustomed vigorous exercises by nonacclimatised athletes leads to ischaemic changes on the muscles and nerves. Athlete feels *sudden onset of severe continuous pain in the anterior part of leg, gradual hypoesthesia* and *paresis* (later on paralysis) of anterior group of muscles (i.e. tibialis anterior, extensor hallucis longus, extensor digitorum longus, peroneus tertius).

Prompt investigation (mainly measurement of intracompartmental pressure studies) and surgical decompression can avert the irreversible damage.

Lateral Compartment Syndrome (Peroneal Compartment Syndrome)

This rare condition may occur due to unaccustomed strenuous activities by the young persons leading to *increased pressure* in the *peroneal compartment* containing the peroneus longus and brevis muscles and superficial peroneal nerve. This syndrome may occur after rupture of peroneus longus tendon.

Posterior Compartment Syndrome

It may manifest as: (a) Superficial posterior compartment syndrome, and (b) Deep posterior compartment syndrome.

Superficial posterior compartment syndrome: This compartment contains the soleus, gastrocnemius and plantaris muscles and sural nerve (innervating the dorsolateral aspect of the ankle and foot), is rarely affected by increased pressure.

Deep posterior compartment syndrome: This compartment is separated from the superficial one by the transverse intermuscular septum and contains the tibialis posterior, flexor digitorum longus and flexor hallucis longus muscles and posterior tibial nerve and vessels. It is commonly affected by increased pressure leading to ischaemic effects on the muscles and nerves *(akin to Volkmann's ischaemic contracture in the forearm)*. Clinical features are almost the same as in forearm mainly being the pain on stretching the toes and paraesthesia in the early stage and later on hypoesthesia in sole and equinus deformity and clawing of the toes. Calf remains tense and tender in the early stage.

Prompt investigations and decompression (better by fibulectomy, which can decompress all the compartments of the leg) can avert the irreversible damage.

Complex Regional Pain Syndrome (CRPS)

Complex regional pain syndrome (CRPS) type 1 term was promoted by International Association for the Study of Pain (IASP) in 1994. It is defined as a syndrome which usually develops after an inciting noxious event and results in pain and tenderness which are disproportionate to the injury and is not limited to the territory of a single peripheral nerve.

Complex regional pain syndrome (CRPS) formerly known as reflex sympathetic dystrophy (RSD) and causalgia, has not only been dynamic but also controversial issue. It has been known over 125 years in history of medicine as pain emanating from or related to sympathetic nervous system under different names: Causalgia (1872); RSD (1943); Sympathetic maintained pain (1986); Sympathetically dependant pain (1997) and CRPS (1995); Exact cause or proper explanation of this condition is not known. Nomenclature like RSD is controversial, as it is neither reflex, nor sympathetic nor dystrophy. Patient's symptoms or pain are associated with sensory, motor or vasomotor dysfunction. It has also been labeled as a psychiatric disease, conversion/somatisation disorder, Munchausen syndrome or malingering associated with migraine or Raynauds disease. Women are more affected. Peak age incidence is 3rd and 4th decade.

Causalgia (Greek word "Klaus" = fire + "Algos" = Pair) described by Silas Weill Mitchell – father of modern neurology). *Diagnosis and management* are contentious and controversial. CRPS is a clinical diagnosis and there is no single diagnostic test. The typical case is obvious and mostly is as direct effects of trauma, fracture, cellulitis, arthritis and malignancy. There are no specific scientifically tenable treatment, but nevertheless there are numerous modalities of management, such as—sympathetic ganglion block; intravenous regional blocks; regional anaesthesia or analgesia, physical therapy, behavioural interventions, surgical intervention, etc. Manchikanti (2001) has suggested that radiofrequency neurolysis is a safe and effective modality of managing CRPS, especially due to developments and advances of radiofrequency neurolysis using the pulsed mode.

In CRPS, pain is typically out of proportion to that expected, and clinical features of vasomotor instability are the main complaints and findings. The vasomotor changes in CRPS I usually present three phases.

Phase I—The early vasomotor response of swelling and vasodilatation, usually occurring within three months of precipitating episode.

Phase II—The dystrophic phase with predominant vasoconstriction containing oedema and cold skin alongwith increasing stiffness, usually coming after 3 months.

Phase III—The atrophic phase with increasing atrophy of skin, muscle and soft tissues with fibrosis and contracture. Diffuse bony changes also occur as demineralisation in early stage, patchy osteoporosis, joint space remains almost normal. The typical sites involved are hand and foot, however, knee, elbow, shoulder and even hip (in pregnancy) may be affected.

A triphasic isotope bone scan is useful in aiding the diagnosis of CRPS, however, it is not diagnostic.

■ COVID TOE SYNDROME

Covid-19 can affect not only the lungs, but can lead to multiorgan disorders. Foot disorders are associated with Covid-19 present in the form of skin, vascular or neuromuscular manifestations. Skin lesions are dominated by chilblain. At the vascular level, there are severe manifestation including peripheral ischaemia that leads to necrosis and gangrene, which can lead to amputation. Neuromuscular workups may reveal painful foot, paretic foot, foot gait and balance disorders. (Millani A, Cherid H, Rachedi 2021).

Computer Syndrome

Prolonged sitting over the computer in a closed, crowded and isolated spaces and that too in a semicrouch or crouch position **(Fig. 10.1 on Page 286)** gradually leads to various physical problems, such as feeling of self-confinement, problems of posture, low backache, wrist-hand-finger problems, watering of eyes and other eye problems, frontal/occipit headache, repetitive stress disorders, psychological aberrations and other bizarre manifestations. Several such problems gradually improve with modification of job, sitting arrangements, adjustment of chairs and the screen, correcting the posture, using of ophthalmic glasses, certain exercises, etc. However, with very fast emerging use of computer, it is mandatory to look into the problem-creating aspects in the use of computer and improve accordingly.

Congenital Short Femur Syndrome (Proximal Focal Femoral Deficiency) (*see* Figs. 2.26 to 2.31)

The femoral deficiency consists of osseous defects and thereby produced various deformities. The spectrum of defective development of femur may vary from simple congenital short femur to complete absence of femur. There may be various associated dysplasias, instability, stiffness and deformities at hip, knee and pelvis.

According to portion and severity of deficiency, congenital short femur syndrome has been variously classified (AM Pappas has classified it into nine types—Pediatric Orthop 1983; 3: 45).

Treatment mainly consists of: (1) correction of deformities and reconstruction of hip, femur and knee by various osteotomies and lengthening of the femur; (2)

Orthotic/prosthetic fitment with or without reconstructive surgery or amputation.

Craniodiaphyseal Dysplasia (CDD) Syndrome

Craniodiaphyseal dysplasia is a rare sclerosing bone disease, the severity of which depends on its phenotypic expression. Hyperostosis can cause progressive foraminal stenosis leading to palsy of cranial nerves, epilepsy and mental retardation. Although the syndrome is rare, its pathophysiological and therapeutic considerations may be applicable to the management of stenosis of the spinal canal in other hyperostotic bone disorders.

Crush Syndrome (Traumatic Rhabdomyolysis)

This clinical entity occurs due to *prolonged continuous pressure on the muscles,* e.g. entrapment in disasters due to earthquake, mines (coal mines), multistoried building collapse; autocompression by the drug addicters.

Once the pressure is released from the muscles, the accumulated metabolites get released into circulation, in which there are large amount of intracellular potassium, phosphorus, lactic acid and myoglobin—this process has been named as 'reperfusion'. It produces *shock and renal failure* resulting in metabolic acidosis. The basic defect is impairment of sarcolemmic sodium-potassium-adenosine triphosphate activity (Knochel-1981).

Management should urgently aim at *prevention of renal failure*. It can be achieved by prompt and continuous intravenous infusion of saline and mannitol till myoglobin is no longer detected in urine. Continuous effective mannitol-alkaline diuresis washes off the metabolites released in reperfusion and also removes the oxygen-free radicals. Allopurinol is also used which limits the reperfusion injury by inhibiting xanthine oxidase activities. It also checks the hyperuricemia, often seen in this syndrome.

Meyer Betz (1910) observed after Sicily earthquake in 1909 and reported "rhabdomyolysis with the triple symptoms of myalgia, loss of muscle power and dark brown urine" Bywaters first used the english term "Crush syndrome in 1941 and for this entity Japanese used the term "atsuza".

Cryptophthalmos-Syndactyly Syndrome

Cryptophthalmos-syndactyly syndrome is a rare congenital abnormality due to failure of separation of eyelids during the 4th to 6th week of intrauterine life. The lid folds are absent; instead a continuous sheet of skin extends from the eyebrows over the eyes to the cheeks. It is usually bilateral and symmetrical, and is typically sporadic, however, occasionally it may be recessive or autosomal dominantly inherited. Syndactyly of fingers and/or toes may be associated with this condition (Sugar HS—The cryptophthalmos-syndactyly syndrome. Am J Ophthalmol 1968;66:897-9).

Cubital Tunnel Syndrome

It is the *entrapment neuropathy of ulnar nerve in the cubital tunnel*. This tunnel is a fibro-osseous ring formed by the back of medial epicondyle and the proximal part of ulna and bridged by a fascial sheet (Osborne's fascia). Cubital tunnel syndrome is the second most common compressive neuropathy of the upper limb.

Patient complains of pain, tingling and numbness with forced flexion of elbow (elbow flexion test is positive—forceful flexion of elbow initiates pain and tingling in ulnar nerve distribution), decreased sensation in forearm and hand, weakness in hand grip strength, and atrophy of first dorsal interosseous muscle.

Tinel's sign is positive at cubital tunnel.

In EMG, nerve conduction velocity may show slowing of conduction across the elbow.

There may be several causes. Patients in and after anaesthesia, keeping the flexed elbow on the bed or chest for prolonged period may develop compression in the cubital tunnel, since in the flexed position the ulnar nerve is stretched tightly within the cubital tunnel.

Mild form usually respond to nonoperative treatment (= avoiding acute/forceful flexion of elbow; local corticoid infiltration, etc). Refractory cases need surgery (= decompression; anterior transposition of ulnar nerve; medial epicondylectomy; subcutaneous transposition of ulnar nerve alongwith stabilisation in anterior position with a fasciodermal sling followed by immediate range of motion exercises provides reliable results with high patient's satisfaction).

Cushing's Syndrome (Fig. 24.3A)

Harvey Cushing, Professor of Surgery of Harvard University, Boston, USA (1869–1939) described this condition in 1932. It is produced by the *excessive production of corticotrophin from pituitary gland*. It mostly occurs in *females*; is

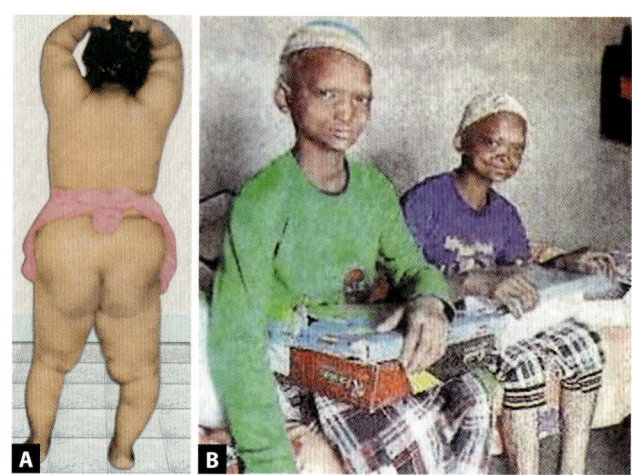

Figs. 24.3A and B: (A) Cushing syndrome; (B) Hypohidrotic ectodermal dysplasia (HED).
Source: Hindustan Times

characterised by *accumulation of fat on the trunk, neck, face*, which becomes *reddened and bloated*. The skin becomes thin and atrophic with striae developing in it mainly over the abdomen.

Systemic complications like *hypertension* and *glycosuria* develop. *Removal of secretary tissue* (pituitary lesion) may help.

Dead Leg or Chorley Horse Syndrome

The external violence (like a *direct heavy blow by any blunt object over the quadriceps muscle*) causes 'dead leg' or 'Chorley horse' syndrome due to local muscular bleeding. Patient has local pain, swelling, tenderness and difficulty in walking.

Management should be on the expectant lines.

Diabetic Foot Syndrome

The classical triopathy of the diabetic foot syndrome is angiopathy, neuropathy and infection either presenting alone or in combination. Neuropathy and infection underlie several foot problems, however, the vascular affections produce the most destructive changes. The diabetic vasculopathy is a progressive disease. The diabetic foot syndrome usually forms a part of generalised disorder, and is oftenly associated with retinopathy, nephropathy and cardiovascular affections. Overall, the prognosis of these patients depends upon an efficient health care system with specialised diabetic foot clinics and multidisciplinary services.

Diabetic Muscle Infarct (DMI) Syndrome

Diabetic muscle infarct was first described by Angervall and Stener and was termed 'tumoriform focal muscular degeneration' in 1965.

In diabetes mellitus, a painful mass may develop in thigh mimicking a sarcoma. On histological examination, it shows areas of haemorrhagic necrosis surrounded by muscle which present regressive changes and evidence of regeneration, pathological changes in blood vessels and intraneural diabetic microangiopathy.

In most of the cases, symptoms resolve spontaneously, however, the treatment of 'DMI' is mainly by analgesics and physiotherapy. In resistant cases, surgical resection of the involved muscle, decreases the pain and improves the function.

Diabetic Nerve Compression Syndrome

The peripheral nerves of the diabetic patients are very susceptible to compression and traction injuries, from the latent diffuse neuropathy of metabolic, ischaemic or mixed pathologies (Mulders et al. 1961). The posterior tibial nerve in tarsal tunnel; the peroneal nerve in fibular tunnel; the ulnar nerve in cubital tunnel; and the median nerve in carpal tunnel are at high risk in compressive neuropathies in diabetics.

Diffuse Idiopathic Skeletal Hyperostosis (DISH) Syndrome (Forestier's Disease)

Diffuse idiopathic skeletal hyperostosis is a *benign spinal disorder* characterised by bony proliferations. It may have familial predisposition. It is common in diabetics over the age of 50 years. Scheuermann's disease in adolescent age may be a predisposing factor.

The term 'diffuse idiopathic skeletal hyperostosis' (DISH) was coined by Resnick and Niwayama in 1976.

Its clear etiology is not known, however certain factors may be considered as contributing factors, such as mechanical irritation (like position of aorta leading to formation of bony bridges), genetic factors (HLA genes), biochemical factors (like fluoride, vitamin A) drugs (etretinate, isotretinoin, vitamin A derivatives); pathologic calcification of anterior longitudinal ligament of spine. (After Chadha R 2016)

Patient complains of *mild to moderate dorsal or lumbar backache with variable stiffness*. There may be associated pain in big joints and also in the heels.

Bone deposition occurs in paraspinal connective tissues, peripheral portion of the intervertebral disc and anterior spinal longitudinal ligaments, with horizontally oriented osteophytes (cf. ankylosing spondylitis where there are longitudinally oriented syndesmophytes), thick bridges and spurs. There is no squaring of vertebrae and no involvement of sacroiliac and apophyseal joints (cf. ankylosing spondylitis).

Non-operative management (reassurances, physiotherapy, NSAIDs and postural adjustments) is usually helpful.

Disseminated Intravascular Coagulation Syndrome

This syndrome is characterized by the systemic activation of blood coagulation.

The process generates intravascular thrombin and fibrin, which may result in the thrombosis of small to medium-sized vessels and ultimately organ dysfunction and severe bleeding. The exact cause is not known, and it may result as complication of infections, trauma, malignancy, toxic reactions etc. There is no single diagnostic laboratory test to confirm it. Dynamic assessment of coagulation parameters like global coagulation tests, prothrombin time, fibrinogen-platelet count and fibrinogen related markers should be repeatedly done.

Its management consist of treating the underlying cause and correct the initiating factor of excessive coagulation.

Double Crush Syndrome

Though electromyography experts suggest about this syndrome but it is still controversial. This syndrome may exist when carpal tunnel syndrome occurs in association with degenerative cervical spine disease. Proximal nerve entrapment may occur at cervical root level causing a disruption in axoplasmic flow in both afferent and efferent directions. The second entrapment is distally in the carpal tunnel, which causes second physiological insult along the course of the axon.

Down Syndrome

Down syndrome was discovered by Lejeune, Gauthier and Turpin (1959) and Jacob, Baikie, Court Brown and Strong (1959). It is *mostly caused by trisomy 21*. The chances of non-dysfunction of chromosome 21 increases with the maternal age. The syndrome is characterised by: *mongoloid face, mental retardation, general hypotonia, short stubby hands,* a *single palmar crease, incurving of little fingers,* wide space between great and second toes, outer flare of iliac wings, ligamentous hyperlaxity, atlantoaxial instability, dislocation of patella and hip, genu valgum, and flexible pes planovalgus. There may also be congenital heart disease (mainly the septal defects), congenital alimentary tract anomaly (typically duodenal atresia, Hirschsprung's disease).

In Down's syndrome, the incidence of subluxation of C1 to C2 is about 2%, and it can be seen at any age.

A simple maternal blood test can identify Down's syndrome with ACCURACY eliminating the need for invasive tests like amniocentesis that carry a risk of miscarriage. Babies with Down syndrome have an extra copy of chromosome 21, causing physical and intellectual (mental) impairment. A mother's blood may contain traces of her baby genetic codes and blood test can denote this extra code.

Economy Class Syndrome or Cheap Class Syndrome

Deep vein thrombosis (DVT) can develop when blood pools in a victim's legs due to long periods of immobility, such as on a prolonged aeroplane flight especially in economy class with crowded leg space, causing blood clots. The Thrombosis Research Institute in London has put the incidence of DVT in the passengers on long flight as one in 12,000 on an average. Heathrow in London receives at least two passengers developing DVT while on long flight. The conditions that raise one's risk (e.g. obesity, smoking, coronary artery disease, varicose veins, cancer, pregnancy, etc.) can act as a catalytic agent. Cheap class syndrome has killed 25 passengers at Narita airport in 8 years.

Prevention: (1) Walking up and down the cabin at least once in an hour; (2) Booking seats at the asle, exit rows, or near a bulkhead to increase leg room; (3) While seating often clenching of the toes which stimulates blood flow; (4) Avoid alcohol; (5) Drink enough of water; (6) Wearing of travel socks; (7) Taking aspirin tablet before flying which helps in thinning the blood.

EEC Syndrome (Ectrodactyly Ectodermal Dysplasia Clefting syndrome)

There is variable severe anomalies of midportion of the hands and feet along with cleft lip, cleft palate or both, sparse thin hair, sparse eyebrows and eye lashes, light dry hyperkeratotic skin, other eye defects, dysdontiasis (small carious teeth, hypoplastic teeth) and sometimes xerostomia.

Edward's Syndrome (Trisomy 18)

Due to *chromosomal aberrations*, the child usually have short radius, diminutive thumb ray, flexion deformities of the fingers of hands.

Ehlers-Danlos Syndrome (Figs. 24.4A and B)

Ehlers-Danlos syndrome is a group of syndromes caused by defective collagen metabolism. There are *skin changes of hyperextensibility, fragility, and bruisability* with resultant 'cigarette paper' scarring, marked *ligamentous laxity* of the joints and *bone fragility* with osteopenia. Virtually, it has no treatment. Also see benign hyermobility syndrome discussed earlier.

Garry Turner from UK holds the Guinness World Record for the Guinness World Record for the stretchiest skin thanks to the fact that he can extend the skin on his stomach 15.8 centimeters.

Ellis-van Creveld Syndrome

Ellis-van creveld syndrome is a *congenital anomaly of the foot* in which polydactyly (accessory digits) may be associated with chondroectodermal dysplasia, where there are chondrodysplasia, ectodermal dysplasia, polydactyly, congenital heart disease.

Extensor Retinaculum Syndrome of the Ankle

This syndrome consists of severe pain and swelling of the ankle; hyperaesthesia or anaesthesia in the web space of great toe; weakness of extensor hallucis longus and extensor digitorum communis; and pain on passive flexion of toes, especially the big toe.

It is usually produced in injury of the distal tibia physis. With fractures at this level, anterior displacement of the distal tibia compresses the contents of the tunnel roofed by the superior extensor retinaculum (like injury in the carpal tunnel). The pressure beneath the superior extensor retinaculum is raised to ischaemic level. The treatment consists of the release of the superior extensor retinaculum, and reduction and stabilisation of the fracture. In untreated cases, there may be residual sensory deficit in the first web space and paresis of extensor digitorum brevis which limits hyperextension of the toes.

Factitious Hand Syndromes

(From Campbell's Operative orthopaedics, 12th edition, Elsevier-Mosby; 2013:3491)

Three types of factitious hand syndromes have been identified by Grunert et al. depending on the physical presentation as: (1) self-mutilation and wound mutilation,

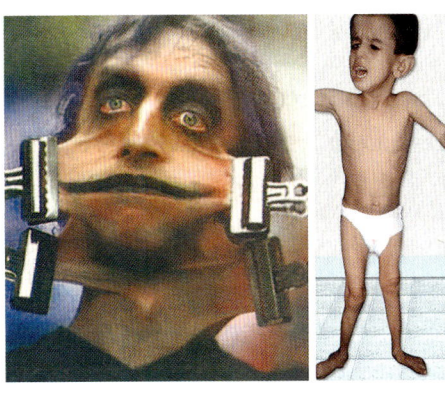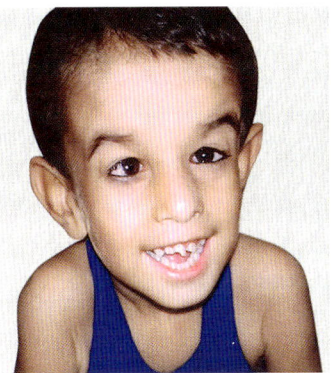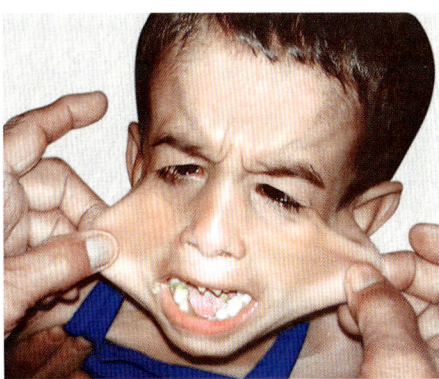

Fig. 24.4A: Ehlers-Danlos syndrome.

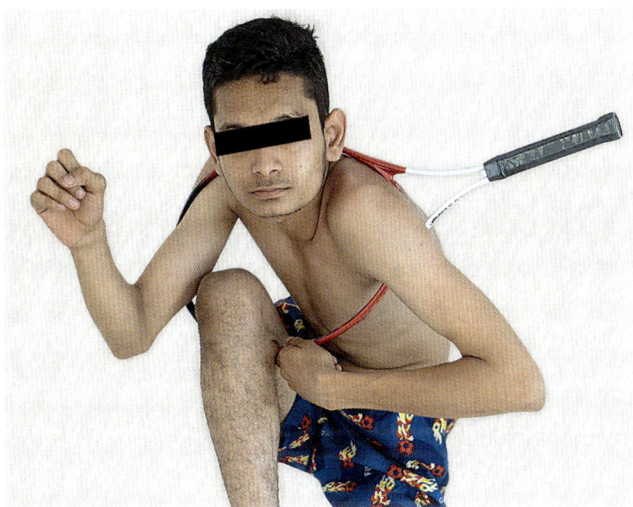

Fig. 24.4B: The rubber boy–He dislocates his arms to crawl through an unstrung tennis racquet, performs contortion, handstands and unique acrobatics.
Source: Newspaper

(2) oedema and (3) finger and hand deformities. These patients have clear psychological disorder. However, it is essential to rule out any organic cause for the presented conditions.

Failed Back Surgery Syndrome (FBSS) (After Kalbag, Ramani)

The *problems persisting even after the spinal surgery* may be named as FBSS. There may be several causes like ill-chosen patient, wrong level surgery, improper fixation, persistent instability of spine, malingerer patient, settlement of claims, etc. Reoperation may also not satisfy the patient, however in genuine cases, proper spinal stabilisation should help. More sophisticated technology has allowed the implanters to successfully address several cases of failed back syndrome by spinal cord stimulation.

There is alarming prevalence to this syndrome. Perhaps most common cause is numerous back surgeries which are being done without appropriately applying conservative measures, such as physical therapy, injection therapy, chiropractic, minimally invasive surgical techniques, etc. However, back surgery has a place in properly indicated patients.

Analysing critically the FBSS is a misnomer, since it is not a syndrome rather a symptom complex consisting of persistent or new onset of pain in back or leg or both, which the patients complain after variable period following back surgery.

Fanconi Syndrome

Fanconi syndrome is an autosomal recessive genetic disorder characterised by glucosuria, aminoaciduria, and hyperphosphaturia.

Fanconi anaemia is an autosomal recessive disorder in which all marrow elements are affected. There are pigmentation in the skin, heart and kidney malformations, radial club hand and thumb deformities. There is pronounced growth deficiency alongwith hypoplasia/aplasia of thumbs, triphalangism, patchy dirty brown skin pigmentation, unusual facies, microphthalmos, nystagmus, coloboma, microcephaly, pancytopaenia, aplastic anaemia, decreased foetal haemoglobin, hypoplasia of male genitalia, ear deformities, deafness.

Fat Emboli Syndrome

Fat emboli syndrome first described by Zenker in 1861 in association with long bone fractures is a self limited pulmonary disease, which usually *occurs within 3 days of fracture*. It is an important cause of acute respiratory distress syndrome.

It occurs due to the *entry of neutral fat into the vascular system*. It usually develops *24–48 hours after the traumatic fractures of long bones*, mostly after *multiple fractures*; *prolonged orthopaedic procedures* including the handling of long bones; trauma to fat laden tissues, e.g. fatty liver. Main manifestations are respiratory failure, cerebral dysfunction and petechiae.

Clinical manifestations are *mental aberrations, disturbances of consciousness* (confusion, delirium), which may progress to delirium and coma. There may be high *fever, tachycardia, marked dyspnoea, hypovolemic shock, petechial haemorrhages* over thorax and upper extremities. On auscultation, fine rales are found all over the chest. *X-ray chest* shows diffuse alveolar filling of both lung fields and *patchy pulmonary infiltrates.*

Arterial blood gas analysis reveal *hypoxemia* and *hypocapnia*. Haematocrit count is decreased and there may be thrombocytopenia. A *platelet count of less than 150,000* and PaO_2 *of less than 60 mmHg* is most useful diagnostic test. Oxygen saturation of less than 96% by pulse oximetry is highly suggestive. Fat in urine is rare. Management is mainly the meticulous supportive therapy.

Respiratory support is the cornerstone of prevention and treatment. Ethanol infusion, heparin and corticosteroids though used frequently, but have doubtful role. Shock is managed on its merit.

Felty's Syndrome

Felty's syndrome is rheumatoid arthritis with splenomegaly and leukopenia generally a neutropenia ($<2000/mm^3$) or thrombocytopenia. Felty syndrome occurs in 19% of RA patients with RF positive, articular manifestation and more extra-articular manifestation. Complications may be bacterial infections chronic non-healing ulcers and risk of developing non-Hodgkin's lymphoma. Treatment is same as for RA patients.

Fibular Tunnel Syndrome (Peroneal Nerve Entrapment)

See Pages 486 and 502 in Peripheral Nerve Injuries Chapter.

Fibromyalgia Syndrome (FM Syndrome; Fibrositis Syndrome)

Fibromyalgia syndrome is a problematic syndrome for both general practitioners and rheumatologist. It is a common syndrome of *musculoskeletal pain and fatigue*, which occurs *mostly among middle-aged women.* Its basic existence remained controversial, however, majority of researchers feel that FM is the result of a complex interaction between predisposing, precipitating and perpetuating factors and it should be regarded as a *"chronic wide-spread pain disorders".* During the months of development of this syndrome emotions, cognitions and behaviour changes may be seen. Manifestations are diffuse pain, fatigue, sleep disturbances, morning stiffness, headaches, irritable bowel—symptoms being modulated by weather conditions, stress and activities—these all adversely affect the quality of life to an extent comparable to other chronic diseases, such as rheumatoid arthritis, osteoarthritis, diabetes, etc. Different theories have been proposed to explain the pathogenesis of FM, however, management of FM has focussed on two pathophysiological aspects of the disease: (1) the altered serotonergic mechanism and (2) sleep disturbances.

First Ray Insufficiency Syndrome or First Metatarsal Insufficient Syndrome (Anatomically or Functionally or Both)

Generally, metatarsal length abnormalities lead to instability at their adjacent joints with geometrical deviations of the bone, loss of function, loss of the balanced forefoot architecture and loss of load distribution with overload on the adjacent rays. Several metatarsal osteotomies have been advocated to manage it. Of course footwear modifications and orthotic treatment should be tried first.

Frantic Life Syndrome (FLS)

The new technology coupled with a *demanding career and the pressure of household work* of a nuclear family, the globalisation bandwagon heralded by superfast and easily accessible technologies (like mobile phone and e-mail) have left *working women feeling under greater pressure to juggle work and home commitment* leaving less time for themselves. These all have made their lives more hectic than ever. They *feel exhausted and burnt out.* They may develop chronic backache and may become irritable. This condition has been dubbed as *"frantic life syndrome"* which is becoming more common, especially in bigger cities.

Freeman-Sheldon Syndrome

Freeman-Sheldon syndrome consists of *complex deformities* in which there are *whistling facies, epicanthus of eyes, small nose* with hypoplastic alae, small tongue, high palate, ulnar deviation of hands, thickened skin over proximal phalanges, equinovarus deformity of foot.

Froin's Syndrome

In lumbar puncture in spinal tumour (or due to any block), the CS fluid is often discoloured *yellow and has high protein content.* In 'Froin's syndrome', a pronounced yellow colour (xanthocromia) of CSF, is associated with high protein content and formation of coagulation. The viscosity of the fluid is markedly increased. On the whole, this is rare syndrome.

Frozen Shoulder Syndrome

Due to various non-traumatic (e.g. subacromial bursitis, bicepital tendinitis, capsulitis) or traumatic, the movements of the shoulder (especially internal rotation, external rotation, abduction) gradually get limited to *almost no movement at the glenohumeral joint,* i.e. the proper shoulder joint becomes frozen. However, the flexion and extension movements of shoulder are fully preserved.

Patient complains of pain in and around the shoulder, especially in the night. Muscles around the shoulder gradually atrophy. Joint line and periarticular zones are tendor. There is *no active or passive movement at the shoulder (except flexion or extension,* which are possible to fair extent).

X-ray shows osteoporosis of the bones around the joint, subchondral irregular cysts, and reduction of joint space. Diabetics are more susceptible. This syndrome may be self-limited.

Management mainly consists of *physical therapy, NSAIDs,* subacromial or intra-articular *corticosteroid injections.* If there is no satisfactory improvement, *manipulation* of the shoulder joint under general anaesthesia, arthroscopic debridement or decompression may be needed.

Gardner's Syndrome

It is an *autosomal Mendelian dominant hereditary disorder* characterised by:
- Multiple or solitary osteomas (mostly on frontal bone followed by maxilla, mandible, temporal bones, femur, fibula, etc.)
- Intestinal polyps (both of small and large bowel)
- Fibromas, including desmoid tumours, skin fibroma
- Sebaceous cyst
- Dentigerous cyst, and other dental abnormalities
- Associated malignant conditions [e.g. fibrosarcoma, malignant polyps (carcinomas), carcinomas of thyroid] have also been reported. Bony growths usually precede other lesions and their malignant transformation has not been reported.

Goltz-Gorlin Syndrome

Goltz-Gorlin syndrome is an autosomal dominant disorder with high degree of penetrance and variable expressivity (uncommon genetic condition), equal prevalence from 1/57,000 to 1/256,000 – in both sexes. It is characterized by the presence of multiple odontogenic keratocysts of jaws along with several other abnormal cutaneous, ophthalmic, and osseous displays. This syndrome is also known as "nevoid basal cell carcinoma syndrome'; jaw cyst; bifid rib syndrome. Since various systemic disorders are involved in this syndrome, its management involves multidisciplinary approach.

There are lentil-sized areas of dermal atrophy—irregular net-like, worm-like or stripped distribution, telangiectasis, hernias of adipose tissue and papillomas. Associated skeletal anomalies are syndactyly, hypoplasia or aplasia of digits.

Gorham-Stout Syndrome

(Gorham's Massive osteolysis; Gorham's diseases; disappearing bone disease; essential osteolysis; progressive atrophy of bone; idiopathic osteolysis; spontaneous absorption of bone; phantom bone; haemangiomatosis/lymphangiomatosis of bone; progressive osteolysis) (**See Figs. 17.87 to 17.89**)

Gorham-Stout syndrome is a rare condition, in which spontaneous progressive resorption of bone occurs.

'Idiopathic osteolysis' was first described by Jackson in 1872. Its aetiology is not well understood, however it may be due to increased number of paracrine-or autocrine-stimulated hyperactive osteoclasts (Moller *et al.* 1999). The resorbed bone is replaced by a markedly vascularised fibrous tissue.

Early potent *antiresorptive therapy* (e.g. with calcitonin or bisphosphonates) may prevent local progressive osteolysis.

Guillain–Barré Syndrome

Key Facts
- Guillain-Barré syndrome (GBS) is a rare condition in which a person's immune system attacks the peripheral nerves.
- People of all ages can be affected, but it is more common in adults and in males.
- Most people recover fully from even the most severe cases of Guillain-Barré syndrome.
- Severe cases of Guillain-Barré syndrome are rare but can result in near-total paralysis and problems breathing.
- Guillain-Barré syndrome is potentially life-threatening. People with Guillain-Barré syndrome should be treated and monitored as quickly as possible; some may need intensive care. Treatment includes supportive care and some immunological therapies.

Overview

In Guillain-Barré syndrome, the body's immune system attacks part of the peripheral nervous system. The syndrome can affect the nerves that control muscle movement as well as those that transmit pain, temperature and touch sensations. This can result in muscle weakness, loss of sensation in the legs and/or arms, and problems swallowing or breathing.

It is a rare condition, and while it is more common in adults and in males, people of all ages can be affected.

Symptoms

Symptoms typically last a few weeks, with most individuals recovering without long-term, severe neurological complications.

The first symptoms of Guillain-Barré syndrome include weakness or tingling sensations. They usually start in the legs and can spread to the arms and face.

For some people, these symptoms can lead to paralysis of the legs, arms, or muscles in the face. In approximately one third of people, the chest muscles are affected, making it hard to breathe.

The ability to speak and swallow may become affected in severe cases of Guillain-Barré syndrome. These cases are considered life-threatening, and affected individuals should be treated in intensive-care units.

Most people recover fully from even the most severe cases of Guillain-Barré syndrome, although some continue to experience weakness.

Even in the best of settings, a small number of Guillain-Barré syndrome patients die from complications, which can include paralysis of the muscles that control breathing, blood infection, lung clots, or cardiac arrest.

Causes

Guillain-Barré syndrome (GBS) is rare. The cause of it is not fully understood, but most cases follow an infection with a virus or bacteria. This leads the immune system to attack the body itself. Infection with the bacteria *Campylobacter jejuni*, which causes gastroenteritis (including symptoms of nausea, vomiting and diarrhoea), is one of the most common risk factors for GBS. People can also develop GBS after having the flu or other viral infections including cytomegalovirus, Epstein-Barr virus, and the Zika virus.

In rare instances, vaccinations may increase the risk of people getting GBS, but the chance of this occurring is extremely low. Studies show that people are much more likely to get GBS from infections such as the flu than from the vaccine given to prevent the infection, in this case the flu vaccine. Occasionally, surgery can trigger GBS.

Diagnosis

Diagnosis is based on symptoms and findings on neurological examination including diminished or loss of deep-tendon reflexes. A lumbar puncture or Electromyography (EMG) may be done for supportive information, though should not delay treatment. Other tests, such as blood tests, to identify the underlying trigger are not required to make the diagnosis of GBS and should not delay treatment. Anyone who is considered to possibly have GBS should be closely monitored for respiratory difficulty.

Treatment and Care

The following are recommendations for treatment and care of people with Guillain-Barré syndrome:
- Guillain-Barré syndrome is potentially life-threatening. GBS patients should be hospitalized so that they can be monitored closely.
- Supportive care includes monitoring of breathing, heartbeat and blood pressure. In cases where a person's ability to breathe is impaired, he or she is usually put on a ventilator. All GBS patients should be monitored for complications, which can include abnormal heart beat, infections, blood clots, and high or low blood pressure.
- There is no known cure for GBS, but treatments can help improve symptoms of GBS and shorten its duration.
- Given the autoimmune nature of the disease, its acute phase is typically treated with immunotherapy, such as plasma exchange to remove antibodies from the blood or intravenous immunoglobulin. It is most often beneficial when initiated 7 to 14 days after symptoms appear.
- In cases where muscle weakness persists after the acute phase of the illness, patients may require rehabilitation services to strengthen their muscles and restore movement.

WHO Response

WHO is supporting countries to manage GBS by:
- Enhancing surveillance of causative agents such as *Campylobacter jejuni* or Zika virus;
- Providing guidelines for the assessment and management of GBS;
- Supporting countries to implement guidelines and strengthen health systems to improve the management of GBS cases; and
- Defining the research agenda for GBS.

WHO's Intersectoral global action plan on epilepsy and other neurological disorders aims to address the challenges and gaps in providing care and services for people with neurological conditions such as GBS and ensure a comprehensive, coordinated response across sectors.

Hair-thread Tourniquet Syndrome/Hair Tourniquet Syndrome

(Ischaemic hair syndrome; Toe Tourniquet syndrome)

Hair tourniquet syndrome occurs when a piece of hair wraps around a small appendage of your baby's body. A thread from a blanket or a piece of clothing can also cause the condition. Hair tourniquets most commonly coil around your baby's toes, fingers or penis.

Hip Spine Syndrome

See as on Page 225.

Holt-Oram Syndrome

Holt-oram syndrome symmetrical or asymmetrical malformations of extremities like triphalangism, hypoplasia/aplasia of thumb, dysplasia/aplasia of radius and dysplasia of upper arm. Associated heart defects like septal defects (atrial septa) or other cardiac malformations.

Horner's Syndrome (*see* Page 507)

Peripheral Nerve Inj Chapter Brachial Plexus Inj

Hypohidrotic Ectodermal Dysplasia (Fig. 1B)

Hypohidrotic ectodermal dysplasia is a genetic disease in which the patient feels excessive heat. The HED patients usually present with few pointy teeth, hair peppered with grey, flat nose, dark and cracked skin, thin and reedy voice, and peculiar facial appearance. Management is mostly symptomatic (*Source:* Hindustan Times).

Idiopathic Ulnar Impaction Syndrome

See Ulnar Impaction Syndrome on Page 658.

Iliotibial Band Syndrome

This syndrome is caused by *friction between iliotibial band and the femoral condyle*. It is usually seen in runners. Normally, the iliotibial band stabilises the knee while running. The ground reaction force occurs medial to the knee joint during single-limb support in any activity. This ground reaction force produces an external varus movement. The role of iliotibial band is important in this situation where it stabilises the knee against the external force by generating an internal valgus movement, which helps to maintain an upright position.

At the maximum stance phase, in flexion of knee (at about 45%) there is a high valgus movement, when the iliotibial band lies directly over the lateral femoral condyle, making it most susceptible to a friction injury (augmented in runners, especially when the knee is aligned in neutral or varus position).

Pain and tenderness on the outer side of knee in the distal region of iliotibial band are the most common, presenting symptoms. Avoiding the irritating fits, practices and postures relieve the situation.

Impingement Syndrome of Shoulder (Swimmer's Shoulder)

In this condition, the *musculotendinous structures of the rotator cuff are repeatedly impinged* between the humeral head and the anatomical arch made up by the anterior portion of the acromion, the acromioclavicular joint and the coracoacromial ligament. This impingement is probably due to occult instability of shoulder.

Impingement syndrome is one of the most common causes of shoulder pain and dysfunction. It is typically *caused by mechanical encroachment of the bursal surface of the rotator cuff resulting from a narrowed coracoacromial arch*. Three progressive stages of subacromial impingement have been described: Stage I—oedema and haemorrhage in patients younger than 25 years; Stage II—fibrositis and tendinitis in patients 25–40 years; Stage III—Osteophytes and tendon rupture—patients often report having difficulty with those activities that require reaching overhead or behind the back. There may be tenderness along anterior acromion or supraspinatus insertion and pain with provocative impingement manoeuvres.

Management should be by restriction/avoiding of the triggering activities, NSAID, modification of the sports activities, physiotherapy, etc.

Inflammatory Syndrome

Inflammatory syndrome is *part of painful rheumatological syndromes*. It comprises of fatigue, anorexia, and possibly weight loss and fever. ESR is raised and sometimes there is inflammatory anaemia (microcytic, low serum iron, but low total iron-binding capacity).

Infrapatellar Contracture Syndrome (IPCS)

Paulos et al. (1987), coined the term *'Infrapatellar Contracture Syndrome* (an unrecognised cause of knee stiffness with patella entrapment and patella infera) for a group of patients with knee stiffness resulting from injury to knee or after surgery. There is loss of both flexion and extension and is variant of arthrofibrosis where there is an abnormal fibrosclerotic healing response in the anterior structures of knee including the fat pad, patellar retinaculum and patellar tendon.

Clinically, the key to diagnosis is *reduced patellar mobility*. A zero or negative passive patellar tilt or superior or inferior glide of less than 2 cm confirms the diagnosis. The problem may be suprapatellar entrapment with adhesions in the suprapatellar pouch (which usually responds to arthroscopic release) or infra- and peripatellar (gentle—not vigorous—exercises with NSAIDs may help, failing which surgical release of adhesions, release of the patellar tendon and a lateral retinacular release followed by graduated physiotherapy on CPM usually help).

Intersection Syndrome

Tenosynovitis of the second dorsal compartment over the wrist is called intersection syndrome. It is usually due to repetitive use of the wrist.

Patient complains of pain, and tender swelling at about 3–4 cm above the wrist where the abductor pollicis longus and extensor pollicis brevis cross or intersect the extensor carpi longus and brevis tendons. In advanced cases, local crepitus may be heard and felt.

Management consists of *rest to the part for three weeks, job modification* and *NSAID*. Local corticosteroid infiltration may help early recovery. In the resistant cases, second osteofascial compartment may need surgical release.

Intervertebral Disc Syndrome

These are very potent cause of mechanical low back pain. These include: (i) *disc herniation*, (ii) *degenerative disc disease* (*See* chapter on low backache).

Ischiofemoral Impingement Syndrome

In Ischiofemoral impingement syndrome (IFIS) there is pain in the hip region occurring due to trapping of quadratus femoris muscle in a decreased ischiofemoral space (IFS) or an abnormal quadratus femoris muscle infringing a normal ischiofemoral space. Such problem can be treated by excision of the lessor trochanter, of course when IFS is normal and quadratus femoris muscle is grossly malformed.

Jaccoud's Syndrome

Jaccoud's syndrome consists of *typical rheumatoid arthritis like deformities* of fingers (flexion deformities and ulnar deviation of metacarpophalangeal joints and swan-neck deformities of the digits) due to *nonerosive synovitis of systemic lupus erythematosus (SLE)*. Deformities develop due to soft tissue attenuation leading to ligamentous laxity. The main affections are the radial portion of the dorsal capsular hood of the metacarpophalangeal joints with ulnar subluxation of the extensor digitorum communis tendons and hyperextension of the proximal interphalangeal joint. In X-ray, there may be rarefaction, but the joint spaces are not reduced (cf. rheumatoid arthritis).

Kaposi Sarcoma Inflammatory Cytokine Syndrome (KICS)

Polizzotto, Uldrick and colleagues introduced the diagnosis of Kaposi sarcoma inflammatory cytokine syndrome (KICS) in 2012, showing how the disease mimics sepsis and may even require respiratory support. KICS can produce fevers, cachexia, pancytopenia and raised c-reactive protein (CRP) levels. KICS is a rare and fatal malignancy that is challenging to treat. The syndrome develops in individuals who are both human immunodeficiency virus (HIV) and human herpesvirus 8 positive. The diagnosis of disease is challenging. It mimics sepsis and has high mortality rate. A bone marrow biopsy is necessary for definitive diagnosis.

Klinefelter Syndrome – Key Syndrome

Klinefelter syndrome is due to *sex chromosome anomalies*, in which there is *an additional 'X' chromosome (XXY)*. Thus there are 47 chromosomes with the cell, containing two 'X' and 'Y' chromosome. The patients are male in character, with tall legs but the testes are atrophied with azoospermia, eunuchoid body habitus with gynaecomastia and female distribution of hairs; increase in sole to os-pubis length and mental retardation. They are subfertile.

Klippel-Feil Syndrome (Page 259, Figs. 8.77A to D)

Klippel-Feil syndrome is due to *congenitally fused vertebrae* (brevicollis), *usually in pairs, usually from C2 to C7*, either in multiple levels or single level.

The classic clinical findings are a *short neck* (fusion leads to reduced number of vertebrae), *a low posterior hairline* (headline) and *restricted neck movements*. However, only 50% of the patients show all the three elements.

About 50% the patients have deafness (as first described by Jalladeau in 1936).

Scoliosis, kyphosis or kyphoscoliosis and/or torticollis is also present in about 50% of patients. Platybasia may be associated.

Neurogenic phenomenon may be present, e.g. features of nerve root pressure—neuralgia with various manifestations; or spinal cord pressure—upper motor neuron lesion in lower limbs. Neurogenic complains require treatment: cervical traction and/or cervical support for root pressure features; but for resistant cases and spinal cord pressure, by surgical decompression.

Klippel-Trenaunay Syndrome (KTS)

This syndrome is characterised by *capillary malformations and venous anomalies with bony soft-tissue* hypertrophy on one or more limbs. Lymphatic malformation is often associated with this condition.

Knee-Spine Syndrome

See on Page 225.

Larsen Syndrome

Larsen syndrome is a rare disorder where there may have vertebral anomalies like spina bifida, hypoplastic vertebrae, cervical kyphosis and anteroposterior dissociation. Persistent and increasing cervical kyphosis itself may lead to the serious complication of anteroposterior dissociation with potential risk of paralysis and are difficult to treat. For mild and flexible cervical kyphosis Sakaura has recommended posterior spinal fusion, and for severe kyphotic deformity or in patients with neurological problems—anterior decompression and circumferential arthrodesis.

Larsen-Johansson Syndrome (Disease)

Probably occurring due to transition tendinitis at the lower pole of patella, the patient (in late childhood age) complains of pain and tenderness at the inferior pole of patella. In X-ray, there may be ossicle formation or apparent fragmentation. Ultrasonography may help in diagnosis. Treatment is symptomatic.

Ledderhose Syndrome (Plantar Fibromatosis)

Ledderhose syndrome is the plantar fibromatosis in which there is proliferative fibroplasia of the plantar aponeurosis like Dupuytren's contracture in the hand. The patient presents with nodular thickening in the aponeurosis mostly on the medial non-weight bearing areas. Management usually consists of shoe-modifications. But if the painful symptoms persist, wide surgical resection of the involved segment of fascia should be done. However, the recurrence rate is high.

Lesch-Nyhan Syndrome

It is a rare X-linked recessive disorder associated with virtually complete deficiency of HGPRT. It mostly occurs in males and its prevalence is 1 in 380,000. It has three major clinical manifestations:
- Over production of uric acid
- Behavioural problems
- Neurological disability

The enzyme HGPRT deficiency leads to increased levels of PRPP and decreased levels of IMP and GMP causing increased de novo purine synthesis which results in over production of uric acid, leading to gout like swelling in few joints.

One important feature of this syndrome is self-destructive behaviour like chewing of lips and fingertips. The patient develops cognitive dysfunction, aggressiveness and impulsive behavior. Treatment is symptomatic and to control increased uric level.

Linear Sebaceous Naevus Syndrome

Linear sebaceous naevus syndrome (LSNS), also known as epidermal naevus syndrome (ENS), is characterised by congenital anomalies affecting multiple systems in the body, including the skin, skeleton and central nervous system. The 'sebaceous naevus' was first recognised in 1895, when Jadasson described smooth yellow or brown verrucous skin lesions, free from hair follicles, and distributed in a localised, linear or generalised pattern. The naevi are symmetrical, tend to be more extensive on one side of body and follow a morphological pattern. There may be associated precocious puberty.

'Ligamentous Postural' Syndrome

In this syndrome, pain is particularly increased by maintenance of a particular posture, altering the position relieves the pain. Again the maintenance of the same position for longer period increases the intensity of pain.

Lofgren's Syndrome

Acute self-limiting arthropathy occurring in patients of sarcoidosis is known as Lofgren's syndrome. Patients present with erythema nodosum, symmetric migratory polyarthritis (affecting mainly the ankles, knees, wrists, hands) and hilar lymphadenopathy. The features resolve of their own in 2–3 months. However, reassurances and NSAIDs are helpful.

Low Testosterone Syndrome

(Synonyms: Male menopause; Andropause; Male climacteric; Veropause)

A more appropriate name of this condition should be ADAM—*Androgen decline in the aging male*. It is not related to hormonal changes only, but few people also develop psychological problem.

Contrarily to menopause in women, andropause is not an obligatory event in men, and when it does occur, its pathogenesis and hormonal aspects are very variable.

Clinical manifestations of ADAM consist of anxiety, depression, irritability, insomnia, reduced muscle and bone-mass, pain in bones and muscles, weakness, diminished libido, impotency, poor memory, diminished sexual body hair.

It is reasonable to treat androgen deficiency in early or late aging, provided a cautious urological check up has been carried out before treatment. Elderly men with symptoms of hypogonadism and a total testosterone level < 300 ng/dL should be started on testosterone replacement.

Maffucci's Syndrome

A Maffucci described this condition in 1881.

This syndrome consists of dyschondroplasia, *multiple enchondromas* with multiple cavernous *haemangiomas*, and phlebitis in the soft tissues.

Marfan's Syndrome

Bernard J A Marfan, a French paediatrician described this condition in 1896 as "dolichostenomelia", meaning there-by "long thin limbs".

It is a congenital disease mostly inherited as an autosomal dominant, however, sporadic cases do occur. The long slender phalanges and spider fingers have given this disease the name of arachnodactyly.

It is characterised by long and narrow skull, high arched palate, *disproportionally long elongated thin limbs (and thus finger-to-finger span with the outstretched upper limbs exceeds the height of the body), generalised joint laxity, spider fingers, achondroplasia, trident hand, short stubby equal fingers* (equal in length), *dislocation of lenses*, myopia, retinal detachment, blue sclerae, aneurysmal dilatation of aorta or pulmonary artery, *dissecting aortic aneurysm, prolapsed cardiac valves*, increased prevalence of hernias. The ears may be long and pointed. Thorax may be deformed as pectus excavatum (funnel breast) or pectus carinatum (pigeon breast). In spinal column, there may be fused vertebrae or spina bifida or kyphoscoliosis.

Perhaps Abraham Lincoln was suffering with Marfan's syndrome (as guessed by photographs).

Maroteaux-Lamy Syndrome

Maroteaux-Lamy syndrome is an autosomal recessive genetic disorder, characterised by *osseous and corneal changes without mental retardation*. Chondroitin sulphate B can be detected in urine.

McCune Albright Syndrome (Endocrinopathic Fibrous Dysplasia or Osteodystrophia Fibrosa)

This syndrome is characterised by *osteitis fibrosa disseminata, areas of pathological pigmentation* and *endocrine dysfunction* with *precocious puberty*, and *hyperthyroidism*.

Its management is difficult.

Fibrous dysplasia is a sporadic development skeletal disorder (monostotic or polyostotic) with medullary fibro-osseous lesions containing fibroblast-like spindle cells and immature woven bone. Fibrous dysplasia are following types:
- Monostotic
- *Polyostotic:* Monomelic form Polymelic form

- *Polyostotic with endocrinopathy:* McCune – Albright syndrome Mazabraud's syndrome
- Osteofibrous dysplasia

Medial Tibial Stress Syndrome (Medial Tibial Syndrome)

Medial tibial stress syndrome is not a compartment syndrome rather a *non-specific inflammatory condition* or stress *reaction of the bone affecting the periosteum of the deep posterior compartment of leg.* Patient complains of pain on the posteromedial aspect of leg after exercises which is usually relieved after rest, but it may persist for hours or days even with rest.

Posteromedial margin of distal third of tibia is tender. There may be marked pronation of the foot. X-ray is usually normal. Rest, hot moist fomentations, guarded gentle under warm-water exercises (to maintain the tone and flexibility of the muscles) usually relieve the condition. However, recurrence oftenly occurs.

Menkes Syndrome

It was first described in 1962 as a neurodegenerative disease, probably caused by copper deficiency and is characterized by psychomotor retardation, seizures and failure to thrive. The affected children have lesser strength in bone and are liable to sustain multiple fractures of long bone, including the birth fractures. However, the first fracture usually occurs by the age of 2–3 months. The X-ray picture is almost similar to those sustained in battered baby syndrome. (Danks et al. (1972).

Munchausen Syndrome By Proxy

Children, who are regularly brought by parents for examination of vague illness and with a history of undergoing multiple diagnostic or therapeutic procedures without any clear outcome, are at risk of undergoing child abuse, are included in the group of Munchausen syndrome by proxy. The biologic mother is almost always the culprit for inflicting the abuse on the child. (After Rathod C 2016).

Morquio's Syndrome

Morquio's syndrome is an autosomal recessive dysplasia caused by a deficiency in the enzyme N-acetylgalactosamine-6-sulfadase, which is essential for the degradation of keratin sulphate and chondroitin-6-sulphate. The gene for this lysosomal enzyme is located on chromosome 16. The diagnosis of Morquio's syndrome is made with a positive test for urinary keratan sulphate. Patients usually appear normal at birth but gradually show growth failure and spondyloepiphyseal dysplasia and develop abnormal appearance by 18 months of age. Thoracolumbar kyphosis, genu valgum and wrist instability usually develop.

Odontoid hypoplasia and upper cervical instability are most common in this syndrome—leading to cervical myelopathy. Atlantoaxial instability may lead to life-threatening dislocation. Prophylactic fusion of the upper cervical spine can prevent the development of myelopathy.

MRI Syndrome

Injudicious and commercial use of MRI is proving to be variably harmful both for patients and doctors. Several patients, especially the elite dash, governmental and industrial employees (whose medical bills are reimbursed) take the MRI as status symbol and ask from their doctors to prescribe MRI, where even it is not indicated nor necessary. Few doctors, yield to their pressure and prescribe unindicated MRI even without thorough clinical examination. Such patients keep on carrying MRI plates from doctor to doctor and ultimately get confused due to different opinions (due to various indications). Even few doctors proceed for treatment only on MRI report as if they have to treat the MRI and hardly the patient.

It is worthwhile noting that 20–70% of lumbar disc abnormalities has been detected in asymptomatic individuals by MRI (Boden et al. 1990, Jensen 1994, Boos et al. 1995).

Nagar Syndrome

The syndrome consists of *clubfoot in combination with acrofacial dysostoses.*

Acrofacial dysostoses are characterised by micrognathia, malar hypoplasia and upper limb abnormalities. The patients coming under this syndrome can be classified into two groups:
1. The *Nagar* Syndrome is characterised by *preaxial* limb defects.
2. The *Genee-Wiedemann* (Miller) Syndrome is characterised by *Postaxial* defects.

Nail-Patella Syndrome

Nail-patella syndrome is a major genetic disorder with *dominant inheritance dysplasia of nails, absent or small patellae* (which lead to recurrent dislocation), *iliac horns, and sometimes dislocation of the radial head.* It is linked to ABO blood group.

It is a peculiar autosomal dominant inherited condition in which the common findings are:
- Hypoplasia of the nail
- Hypoplastic or absent patella
- Hypoplasia of the capitellum
- Subluxation of the radial head
- A bony spur on the ilium.

Numb Chin Syndrome

Due to pressure on or infiltration of the (inferior alveolar nerve or mental nerve) branches of IX cranial nerve by (usually) malignant tissues (e.g. aggressive lymphoma), the patient (usually a young adult) complains of numbness in lower lip and chin. MRI and scintigraphy should be done for assessing the problem and managed accordingly.

Olecranon Impingement Syndrome (Hyperextension Overload Syndrome or Boxer's Elbow)

Olecranon impingement syndrome is *an overuse syndrome* caused by repetitive valgus extension overload of the elbow, e.g. *in throwing motions* which cause the olecranon process to impinge against the medial wall of the olecranon fossa. Athletes usually complain of local pain during the extension phase of throwing and catching or locking in or near extension.

There may be *swelling and tenderness on the posterior aspect of elbow*. Full extension of elbow may be limited. There may be palpable loose bodies. Forced valgus strain in full extension causes pain.

On X-ray, there may be *spur or evidence of old fracture* or *hypertrophy of the olecranon* tip or loose bodies in that region. Arthroscopic or open *removal of loose bodies or spurs* may be required to cure the condition.

Oral-Acral Malformation Complex (Syndrome)

There are microglossia, cleft lip, cleft palate, adhesion of tongue to upper jaw, fibrous bands between upper and lower jaws, micrognathia, transverse reduction, anomalies of the extremities, syndactyly, symbrachydactyly.

Overlap Syndromes

Overlap syndromes occur when patients meet criteria for the diagnosis of more than one connective tissue disease (e.g. patients with CLE may develop a positive rheumatoid factor and as erosive arthritis in a distribution similar to RA; the overlap of SLE and RA is known as RUPUS). About 25% of patients with one connective tissue disease will develop an overlap syndrome. Although the features of both diseases may occur concurrently, usually one syndrome gradually takes on the features of another.

Painful Hypertrophic Peroneal Tubercle Syndrome: (Y Tanaka et al.1995)

The peroneal tubercle lies at the lateral aspect of the calcaneus and functions as a fulcrum for the peroneus longus tendon. Since the report of Hyrtl [(cited by Francellon in 180 (cited by Tanaka et al. 1995), painful conditions caused by a hypertrophic peroneal tubercle have been recognized. The symptoms are caused by skin damage from shoe pressure, stenosing tenosynovitis of the peroneus longus tendon or the peroneus previs tendon, (Tanaka et al. cited several publications), entrapment neuropathy of lateral dorsal cutaneous nerve, which is the distal trunk of sural nerve and runs directly above the tubercle. Most of these problems have to be treated surgically.

Pancoast Syndrome (Superior Sulcus Syndrome)

Pancoast Henry Khurnath (1875-1939), Professor of Radiology, Philadelphia, USA described this condition. The apical cancer of lung usually invades the pleura at the thoracic apex, thoracic muscles in that region, the neurovascular bundles including the brachial plexus and cervical sympathetic chain. Besides pain in the local region there may be severe pain in neck, shoulder and axilla. Pain and paraesthesia may also be referred along the involved nerve, mainly along the arm or even down.

There may associated Horner's syndrome (unilateral miosis, ptosis, enophthalmos, absence of sweating on the ipsilateral face and neck).

Paraneoplastic Syndromes

Paraneoplastic syndromes include conditions like Hypertrophic Pulmonary Osteo Arthropathy (HPOA), which is a metabolic bone disease, occurring mostly in older patients having high risk for carcinoma lung (history of smoking, tobacco use, etc.). Usually patients complain of generalised bone pains, swelling of joints, chest pain, clubbing of fingers with inconclusive findings on other diagnostic modality. Bone scan should be done. CT of thorax may reveal a mass in the lung, for which CT-guided FNAC is recommended which may reveal lung cancer. HPOA may be associated with other malignancies like mesothelioma, lymphoma, pulmonary metastasis from osteogenic sarcoma, melanoma, renal cell carcinoma, etc.

Parkes-Weber Syndrome

Parkes-Weber syndrome (PWS) has almost the same characteristics as Klippel-Trenaunay syndrome (KTS) except that there are arteriovenous malformations (high flow lesions) instead of venous anomalies.

Patello-Femoral Syndrome/Excessive Lateral Pressure Syndrome/Patellar Pain Syndrome

It *may be taken as modern terminology for chondromalacia patellae*. Patient, usually adolescent girl complains of gradual onset of dull non-specific pain in the anterior knee (medial, lateral or superior to patella) or in retropatellar region. The symptoms aggravate with climbing or descending stairs and also in night. Clicking or crepitus may be felt. As situation advances, there may be a sense of giving way at knee, especially in descending stairs. Pathologically, there is inflammation of peripatellar soft tissues, drying out and later on breaking up of patello-femoral cartilage due to repetitive stressing in high flexion activities (e.g. in skiing, jumping and squatting). Management consists of exercises mainly to build up medial quadriceps and hamstrings.

Pierre Robin Syndrome

Symmetrically underdeveloped chin can be associated with cleft palate and breathing problems.

Piriformis Syndrome

This syndrome is the result of entrapment of sciatic nerve by the piriformis muscle as it passes through the sciatic notch (*see* Page 240 in the chapter on Spine).

Poems Syndrome

Poems syndrome—a multisystem disorder—is an acronym for polyneuropathy, organomegaly (enlargement of an organ), endocrinopathy, M protein (monoclonal immunoglobulin—a type of antibody), and skin changes (e.g. hyperpigmentation). Its exact cause is not known. In several cases, primary adrenocortical deficiency is revealed by systematic screening with a rapid ACTH test.

Poland Syndrome

There is aplasia of pectoralis major alongwith ipsilateral anomalies of the upper extremity mainly symbrachydactyly, absence of rays, hypoplasia of forearm, etc.

Postconcussive Syndrome

Postconcussive syndrome may be defined as the continuation of at least three of the following symptoms after minor head injury: headache, irritability, dizziness, impaired memory and concentration, fatigue, insomnia, and decreased tolerance for noise and light. The initial neurological examination and CT may be completely normal. However, neurological and neuropsychological assessments and scans detecting organicity (e.g. CT, MRI, and SPECT) may reveal impairment associated with postconcussive syndrome.

Posterior Compartment Syndrome

See Page 656.

Postphlebitic Syndrome

Postphlebitic syndrome occurs due to earlier occlusion of the deep veins, which remained unrecanalised, or due to destruction of the valves with persistent venous incompetence. The leg remains swollen with pitting oedema. Patient feels heaviness and dull ache in leg with prolonged sitting with legs down on floor or standing. There may be skin problems due to chronic stasis. Early management is essential to avoid long-term disabilities.

Post-traumatic Stress Syndrome/Disorder (PTSD)

Post-traumatic stress syndrome/disorder is a debilitating condition that follows a terrifying event. One thought it to be shell-shock or battle fatigue, was first brought to public attention by war veterans, but it can result from several physical and/or mental incidents, e.g. serious accidents (car, train wreck, plane crash, etc.), natural disasters (e.g. earthquake, floods, tsunami, etc.), violent attacks, e.g. mugging, rape, torture, being held captive, etc.), kidnapping, threatening to kill the person or his/her close one, witnessing of any mass-destruction, etc.

People with PTSD have persistent frightening thoughts, horror and memories of their ordeal. They feel emotionally numb. Children develop disorganised behaviour. About 5% of population are likely to develop PTSD. Women are directly vulnerable. PTSD may be acute (when symptoms last for about one month or chronic (symptoms continue for more than 3 months) or it may be delayed PTSD manifestation.

Management mainly consists of psychotherapy and allied medication.

Pronator Teres Syndrome

Pronator teres syndrome (Anterior Elbow Pain) also called median nerve compression syndrome at elbow—described by Kepell and Thompson.

It is *entrapment of median nerve due to compression by the pronator teres muscle, lacertus fibrosus, ligament of Struthers,* flexor digitorum superficialis, producing essentially the features of neuropathy of *high carpal tunnel syndrome*. There may be numbness and paraesthesia in the median nerve innervated digits, weakness in the thenar muscles, and pain in the wrist and forearm.

Tinel's sign is negative at the wrist.

The nerve conduction studies of the median nerve may be delayed, but delay is not at the wrist (cf. carpal tunnel syndrome).

Radial Tunnel Syndrome (Resistant Tennis Elbow)

Radial tunnel syndrome is the *entrapment (or compression) neuropathy of the posterior interosseous nerve* in the lateral aspect of proximal forearm. Patient may have weakness in the forearm muscles innervated by the posterior interosseous nerve or pain in the lateral aspect of the elbow region or both. Since the problematic site is nearer to the lateral epicondyle, it can be confused with lateral epicondylitis or tennis elbow.

Symptoms include fatigue or a dull aching pain at the top of forearm. It is mainly a clinical diagnosis, as the nerve conduction studies are often normal. Dynamic ultrasonography – a new diagnostic method and helps in identifying the site of compression. In radial tunnel syndrome arcade of Frohse has been identified as the most common site of compression once confirmed by dynamic ultrasonography, surgical decompression is the best treatment.

Reiter's Syndrome

As originally described in 1916, Reiter's syndrome is the clinical triad of urethritis, conjunctivitis and arthritis following an infectious dysentery or diarrheal illnesses. Now it is considered to be a form of radiation arthritis (a sterile inflammatory synovitis following an infection by organism which infect mucosal surface).

It is a variant of *inflammatory polyarthropathies*, affecting the sexually active males. They complain of asymmetric pain and swelling in the joints mainly of lower extremities or back and loss of weight. On examination, *evidences of urethritis, iritis, conjunctivitis and painless ulcerative lesions in mucous membrane* are seen. X-ray may reveal asymmetric sacroiliitis and isolated involvement of spine. Two cutaneous lesions—circinate balanitis serpiginous ulcer on glans penis and keratoderma blennorrhagicum—psoriasis form lesion on the plantar surface of heel and metatarsal heads are characteristics of Reiter's syndrome.

Laboratory findings are:
- HLA-B27 is oftenly positive
- C/H50 is increased in serum
- Joint fluid contain cells—5000 to 30,000 leucocytes/mm and Reiter's cell (macrophages containing 3 to 5 phagocytosed polymorphs).

It responds to NSAIDs to variable extent.

Reperfusion Syndrome

Reperfusion syndrome occurs in the synovial membrane after intraoperative distension (e.g. in arthroscopy with saline solution irrigation) in which there is alteration in synovial metabolism and local blood flow (compression of synovial blood vessels) after operation. There is increase in the local production of lactate, consumption of glucose in the synovial membrane and elevation in the levels of pyruvate. These findings may be of importance for the understanding of the pathological process leading to post-traumatic degeneration of articular cartilage, i.e. osteoarthritis.

Restless Legs Syndrome

Restless legs syndrome is a common (affecting 1 to 15% of adult population) curious sensorimotor disorder of unknown aetiology (though disorders like anaemia, iron deficiency and end-stage renal failure may be associated), first described by Ekbom in 1944. Legs are most frequently affected. There is motor restlessness with an urge to move due to uncomfortable sensations in affected limb. There is diurnal variation with worsening symptoms at night. There is usually periodic limb movements in sleep, which occur during non-rapid eye movement, and sleep. The most characteristic movements are a flexion jerk at the hip, knee and ankle. There is no specific treatment. Physiotherapy, transcutaneous electrical nerve stimulation (TENS), certain drugs (such as dopaminergics, benzodiazepines, opioids, anticonvulsants, etc.) may be helpful.

[Earley CJ. Restless legs syndrome. N Eng J Med. 2003; 348:2103-19].

Rett syndrome

Neuromuscular scoliosis is the most common orthopaedic condition seen in children with Rett syndrome. In this syndrome scoliosis develops in 75% of children by 13 years of age. C - or S-shaped curves can be seen with poorer function and walking ability with a deficit in the brain. There is no consensus that bracing is beneficial in reducing the progression of scoliosis in children with this syndrome.

Posterior spinal fusion is considered when a curve reaches 40° to 50°.

The survival of children of Rett syndrome who undergo spinal fusion for severe scoliosis has been shown to be better than those who were managed nonsurgically. This observation was more marked for children with early onset scoliosis in whom surgery could have a protective effect on respiratory function.

Pelvic fixation is usually needed to correct pelvic obliquity and restore sitting balance

Robert's Syndrome

Tetraphocomelia, cleft lip, cleft palate and mental retardation are usually seen in the patients suffering from this syndrome.

RS3PE Syndrome

RS3PE syndrome is characterised by acute severe onset of symmetrical synovitis of small joints of hand, wrists and flexor tendon sheath along with pitting oedema of dorsum of hand ('boxing glove' hand). Elderly white men are mostly affected. Symptoms respond well to low-dose prednisone and hydroxychloroquine.

Sanfilippo's Syndrome (Type V)

It is autosomal recessive, like Hurler's Disease, but the somatic manifestations are less severe whilst mental impairment is earlier and more severe. Corneal opacity is absent. Excessive heparitin sulphate is present in the urine. Deformities are moderate, and some hepato-splenomegaly is usually present.

Scheie Syndrome

Scheie syndrome is an autosomal recessive genetic disorder characterised by stiff joints, clouding of cornea, and chondroitin sulphate B in urine. There is no mental retardation. Chondroitin sulphate B is the defective mucopolysaccharide.

Seasonal Affective Disorder (SAD)

Seasonal affective disorder was first identified in 1984 with the typical seasonal mood swings associated with short days and long nights. Characteristically, the predominant symptoms are depression, bodyache, anxiety, irritability, low energy levels, carbohydrate craving, increased appetite and weight, increased need for sleep (which is disturbed) and impairment to work and socialise. Bright artificial light is the treatment of choice. The light treatment should be given between 7 AM and 9 AM every morning and response usually starts in first 4 days.

Severe Acute Respiratory Syndrome (SARS)

This new clinical syndrome said to be due to unidentified virus was first identified at Guangdong province of South China in November 2002, from where it spreaded to adjacent Hong Kong in February 2003—thence to Canada, Singapore, Vietnam, Thailand. It is characterised by cough, fever, respiratory distress leading to respiratory failure and death. It spreads through fomites and is rapidly fatal. Preventive measures (avoiding respiratory contamination by use of mask, immediate segregation of identified cases, etc.) must be taken with supportive measures. It may be self-limiting.

Sinus Tarsi Syndrome

Damage to proprioceptive system of foot (proprioceptive subtalar centre—interosseous ligament) in the adults due to various causes (traumatic, inflammatory, degenerative or idiopathic) is represented by 'Sinus tarsi syndrome' (O'Connor 1956; Hauser 1972). Patient may ascribe the problem to the few months earlier history of sprain. Manifestation may be acute (severe pain in front of lateral malleolus aggravated by active or passive flexion and inversion; tendor swelling in the region of mouth of sinus tarsi; negative X-ray, or chronic [no pain while at rest or walking on the level and smooth ground but may be in going up and down the stairs, jumping, running, etc. due to activation of the receptors (which are not stimulated while at rest or walking on level ground)]. In most of the cases, histological examination reveals it to be degenerative in origin. Treatment remains mostly operative—emptying the sinus tarsi and/or triple arthrodesis.

Sjogren Syndrome

Sjogren syndrome described by Henrich Sjogren of Stockholm in 1933 refers to a systemic disease manifested by dry eyes, dry mouth and arthritis. Typically affecting middle-aged female, its manifestations are due to lymphocytic infiltration of glandular and non-glandular organs. It may be primary or secondary (when there is accompanying evidence of another connective tissue disease—mostly rheumatoid arthritis).

Smashed Heel Syndrome

In fractures of calcaneum, the most common site of persistent pain, in unsatisfactorily treated patients is the heel pad. Prolonged period of non-weight bearing further adds to the heel pad dystrophy and pain.

Management mainly consists of exercises of the foot, gentle massage of the heel, and special footwear (gradually raised, softly padded heel top, and padded and well adapted heel counter). Local infiltration of corticoids may help in few cases.

Stickler's Syndrome

Stickler's syndrome is *an autosomal dominant disorder* characterised by irregularity in the development of epiphysis, late appearance and/or mottling of the ossification centres, knobby joints, stubby digits, severe progressive myopia with retinal detachment and blindness. There may be associated cleft palate, conductive deafness and spinal deformities (e.g. dorsal kyphosis similar to Scheuermann's disease).

Streeter's Syndrome (Congenital Ring Syndrome)

Streeter's syndrome is basically a *congenital constriction band (Streeter's band) syndrome* or amniotic band syndrome affecting the limbs/digits. Exact cause is not known, but suggestions have been the possibilities of constriction by the amniotic band, developmental failure of subcutaneous mesodermal mass, germ plasm defects, etc. **(Figs. 24.5 to 24.10)**.

Torpin (1965) enunciated the theory that rupture of amnion permits the foetus from entering the chorionic cavity

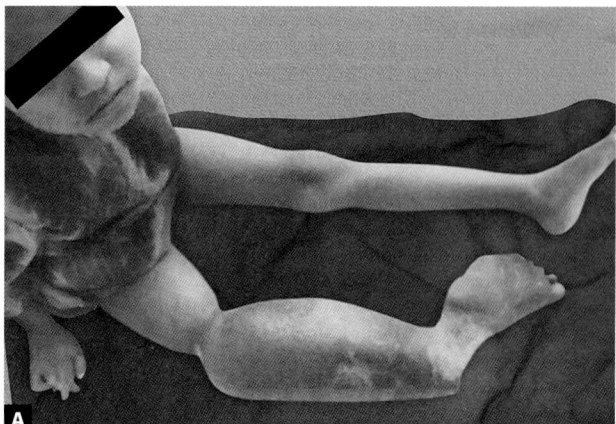
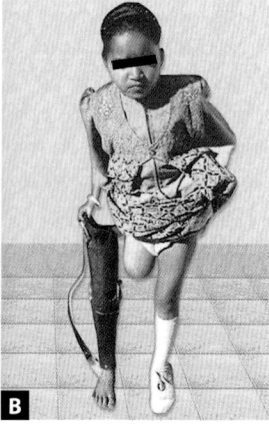

Figs. 24.5A and B: Neglected congenital constriction rings through thigh and leg leading to infected threatened gangrene of the leg and foot—amputated and fitted with above knee prosthesis.

Syndromes Related to Orthopaedics and Traumatology

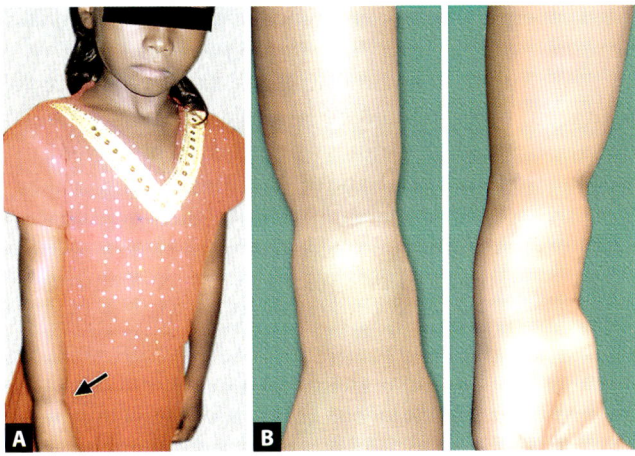

Figs. 24.6A and B: The only treatment of such condition (**Figs. 24.5A and B** patient) is the amputation just above the constriction ring in thigh and fitting with prosthesis. (A and B) Congenital constriction band in lower forearm. Management of such cases—wait and watch. Usually they remain as such, except for some swelling in the portion distal to the constricting band.

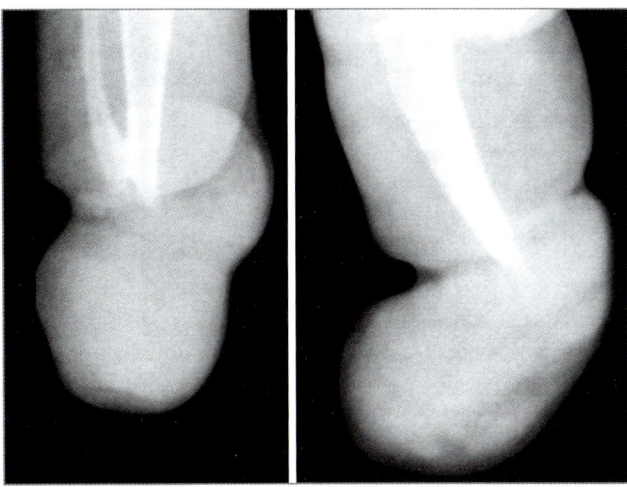

Fig. 24.9: X-ray of the leg and foot of same patient (**Fig. 24.9**).

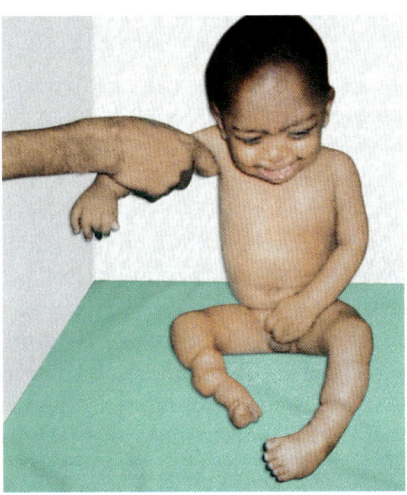

Fig. 24.7: Multiple congenital constriction rings in the legs with ill-developed right foot and associated clubfoot on left side.

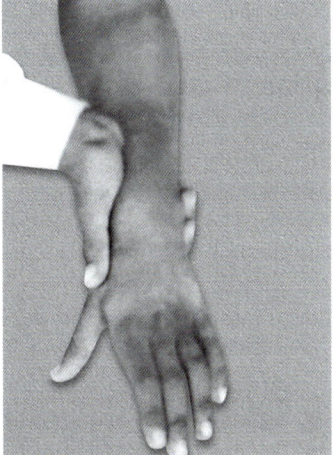

Fig. 24.10: Aquired constricting flat fibrous band following trauma (devitalised skin and subcutaneous tissue in a fan-belt injury). Varying swelling may appear in the distal (to flat constriction) part.

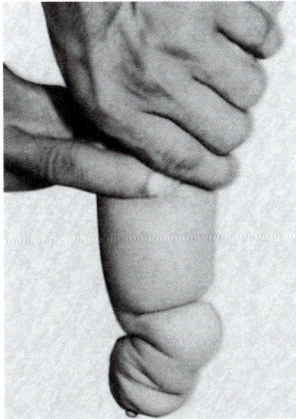

Fig. 24.8: Congenital constricting grooves in the lower leg with distorted development of leg and the foot is represented by only fibro-fatty soft tissue mass.

with tethering of extremities and resulting oligohydramnios produce clubfeet and other positional anomalies. Ruptured amnion acts as a band around the limb leading to constriction band in the limb or amputation in uterus.

The *depth of constricting ring varies from subcutaneous to bone* deep. Hennigan and Kuo classified the constricting bands into four grades according to severity; grade 1 band involves only the subcutaneous tissues; grade 2 band extends to fascia; grade 3 involves full thickness of fascia and requires release; grade 4 is almost congenital amputation. There may be *associated other congenital malformations* in other parts of the body or even distal to the ring, e.g. clubfoot, club hand, syndactyly, brachydactyly, symphalangism, hypoplastic or absent nails, rudimentary toes or fingers, etc. Due to obstruction in lymphatic and/or venous flow, there is usually ballooning of the distal part. Circulatory impediment of the distal part may necessitate amputation. The portion of the limb or digit proximal to the ring is usually normal.

Management: The shallow benign grooves may be ignored. The *deeper grooves need full depth excision and reconstruction by 'Z' plasty transposition flaps in stages.* No more than 50% of the circumference of the limb or digit should be *excised and reconstructed in one stage.* Complete groove (in circumference) should not be excised and reconstructed in one stage, lest gangrene may occur.

However, Greene and Hill (1993) have advocated one stage release of congenital constriction band. Since (circulation to skin flaps) blood supply to the skin is primarily from the musculocutaneous arteries that directly penetrate the subcutaneous and cutaneous tissue from underlying muscles, the single stage contracture release is feasible, which avoids repeat surgery, saves time and reduces the financial burden.

Subacromial Syndromes (Impingement Syndrome, Shoulder Impingement Syndrome)

These syndromes include *rotator cuff tears, tendinitis* Calcifying tendinitis of rotator cuff, and *impingements in the subacromial region.* There are several causes which can produce these problems, e.g. deformed acromion process (forward sloping, hooked or curved acromion); os acromiale; repetitive overhead use; faulty overhead sports; shoulder instabilities; shoulder injuries; impingements; degenerative changes; collagen arthropathy, etc.

Neer and Poppen (1987) described the supraspinatus outlet—consisting of the space between the acromion, coracoacromial ligament, coracoid acromioclavicular joint and glenoid—through which supraspinatus muscle passes. They considered the narrowing of the outlet as the main cause of shoulder impingement syndrome.

Patients complain of *pain in shoulder usually after some exertion*, especially in certain position. *Subacromial region* is tender. Presence of *impingement sign*: while the examiner stabilises the scapula, the patient is asked to elevate the arm forward, there will be pain—*primary impingement* sign. Then patient is asked to actively abduct the internally rotated arm, there will be pain—*Secondary impingement* sign.

The features may be confused with cervicobrachial neuralgia, thoracic outlet syndrome, acromioclavicular degenerative arthritis; suprascapular nerve entrapment.

Management consists of avoiding the overhead-activities; NSAIDs; fomentations; ice-therapy; subacromial corticosteroids injections; physiotherapy from very beginning; arthroscopic/surgical decompression with repair of rotator cuff tears. Ideally decompression of the coracoacromial arch in patients with shoulder impingement syndrome should be done only at the site of impingement. Simultaneous arthroscopic resection of the acromioclavicular joint and subacromial decompression can also produce good results in acromioclavicular pathology and concomitant subacromial impingement.

Extracorporeal shock wave therapy has been suggested for calcific tendinitis as an alternative to surgery.

Syndromes of Mucopolysaccharidoses (After DV Chavda) (Table 24.1)

Mucopolysaccharidoses are the biggest group of lysosomal storage diseases. In these disorders, there is deficiency of specific enzyme involved in breakdown of glycosaminoglycan. Lysosomes are the enzymes which degrade intracellular micromolecules into smaller units for cellular metabolism and utilisation. Defect in any enzymic activities leads to blockage in the breakdown process and intracellular accumulation of semidegraded compounds.

The mucopolysaccharidoses are divided into six major categories (I-VI) according to the substance that accumulates. All these come under one common group of mucopolysaccharides storage disorders. In these lesions, there is generalised skeletal abnormalities affecting the spine and limbs leading to dwarfism and visceral abnormalities. Skeletal manifestations vary in each type of MPS, but the common features are short stature, thickened bones with defective remodelling and abnormalities of joints.

TABLE 24.1: Types of mucopolysaccharidoses.

Type	Name of syndrome	Enzyme defect/deficiency	INCR urinary excretory	Prognosis
I	Herler syndrome: Gertrude described it in 1919. Ellis et al. named it Gargoylism	Alpha-L-iduronidase	• Dermatan sulfate ++ • Heparin sulfate +	Progressive disease; death by 10 years of age
II	Hunter syndrome: C Hunter described it in 1917	Sulfoidioconate sulfatase	• Heparin sulfate ++ • Dermatan sulfate +	Survival till about 3rd decade of life
III	Sanfilippo syndrome: SJ Sanfilippo et al. described it 1963	N-heparan sulfatase or alpha-acetylglucosaminidase cosaminidase	• Heparin sulfate ++	Survival till 3rd to 4th decade of life
IV	Morquio syndrome: L Morquio and JL Brailsford described it in 1929	N-Ac-Gal-6 sulfate sulfatase	• Keratin sulfate ++	Normal longevity
V	Scheie syndrome: HG Scheie et al. described it in 1962	Alpha-L-iduronidase	• Heparin sulfate + • Dermatan sulfate ++	Normal longevity
VI	Maroteaux-Lamy syndrome: Maroteaux-Lamy et al. described it in 1965	N-Ac-Gel-4 sulfate	• Dermatan sulfate ++	Guarded prognosis; death from cardiovascular causes

Tabatznik Syndrome (Heart/Hand Syndrome)

Tabatznik syndrome is a major genetic disorder with dominant inheritance. There is cardiac arrhythmia and malformation of upper extremities particularly 'stub thumb'.

Tarsal Tunnel Syndrome (Posterior Tibial Nerve Compression)

KECH described this syndrome (an entrapment neuropathy) in 1962, which is characterised by *compression of the posterior tibial nerve or its branches* (the calcaneal branch, lateral and medial plantar nerve) *in the tarsal tunnel* (a fibro-osseous tunnel formed by the medial wall of calcaneum and talus and medial malleolus, and roofed by the flexor retinaculum or laciniate ligament. It contains the posterior tibial nerve and its branches, posterior tibial artery and vein, tendons of tibialis posterior, flexor digitorum longus, and flexor hallucis longus). Posterior tibial nerve may be pressed from without or within the tunnel. Compression may be due to engorged veins, growths (like lipoma), fracture callus, ganglion from tendon sheath, exostosis, excessive valgus deformity of hind foot, etc.

Patients complain of burning, tingling, pain, paraesthesia, hypoesthesia, hyperesthesia, muscle cramps or numbness affecting the heel and/or sole of the foot and the symptoms may spread to the toes. Symptoms are usually unilateral and rarely bilateral, and they mainly occur while walking, during exercise, at night when the patient is at rest, and with positions of dorsiflexion and eversion of foot. Usually the symptoms (Lopez-de-Celis et al. 2020) increases with activities and overuse and gets relieved with rest. Occasionally, the pain may radiate along the posterior tibial nerve and/or its branches. Paresis/paralysis of some small muscles of foot may occur.

Diagnosis is based on clinical findings, positive Tinel's sign, nerve conduction studies and EMG studies.

Management consists of NSAID, shoe-modification, treatment of identified cause, corticosteroid injection, and surgical decompression especially in resistant cases.

Thigh Compartment Syndrome

As in the leg, compartment syndrome can occur in thigh as well due to blunt injury to thigh with prolonged compression by any heavy object or even body weight, with or without fracture of femur. It can occur *in any of the three compartments* of thigh (i.e. quadriceps, hamstring, adductor) but *quadriceps compartment* is *mostly involved*.

Thoracic Inlet Syndrome

See Page 236 in the chapter on Spine.

Thoracic Outlet Syndrome (Adson's Sign) (Fig. 24.11)

In a vice-like action, the axillary artery and brachial *plexus coursing over the first rib, may be compressed by the cervical rib* (rib, or rudimentary rib with fibrous band originating from the 7th cervical vertebra and inserting onto the 1st rib) producing various symptoms, e.g. burning, tingling, numbness in palm and/or finger tips. The lower trunk of the brachial plexus (mainly T1) is usually compressed leading to wasting of the interossei. Axillary artery compression may gradually lead to the post-stenotic dilatation with thrombus formation and embolism. First rib stress fracture, usually found in adolescent overhead throwing athletes (complaining of posterior shoulder pain while swinging the bat or pitching the ball), If not healed in 7 to 8 months with conservative treatment may have symptoms consistent with thoracic outlet syndrome (Funakoshi et al. 2019). Persistent symptoms can be only relieved by decompression (removal of cervical rib and/or fibrous band).

Thrombocytopaenia Absent Radius (TAR) Syndrome

There is bilateral aplasia of radius alongwith thrombocytopaenia. There may be frequent life-threatening episodes of bleeding or bleeding tendency.

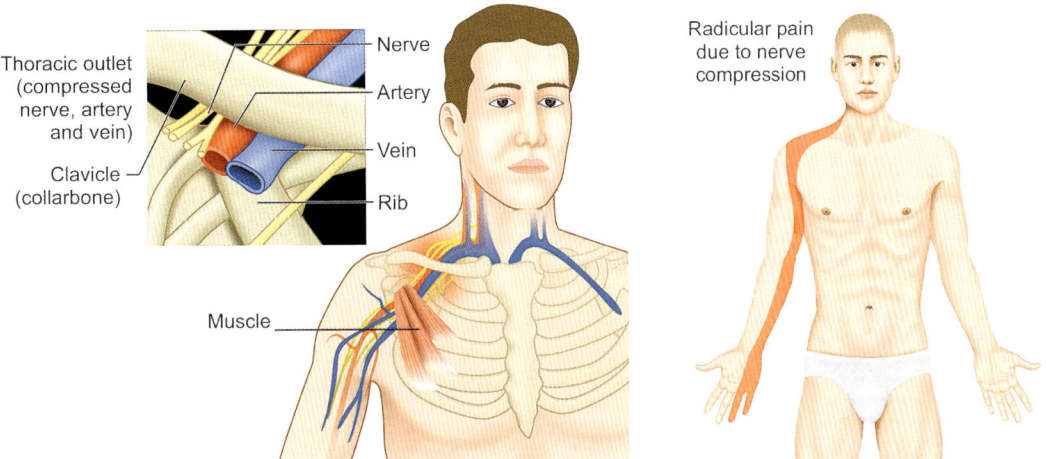

Fig. 24.11: Thoracic outlet syndrome.

Tietze's Syndrome

Tietze's syndrome is idiopathic self-limiting *costochondritis* occurring at the *costosternal junctional regions* usually in the age group 25 to 50 years characterised by painful tender enlargement of one or *more ribs (4th to 7th)*. The pain increases on deep breathing, coughing, sneezing, local deep pressure and chest compression. Reassurance and NSAID usually help. In resistant cases, local infiltration of corticosteroids is indicated.

Tethered Cord Syndrome

The filum terminale and lower end of spinal cord/or roots may get tethered to the vestigial remnants of spina bifida, which in due course may lead to various neurogenic disorders and deformities especially in ankle and foot region.

Touraine-Solente-Gole Syndrome (Pachydermoperiostosis)

Touraine-Solente-Gole syndrome is a rare type of hypertrophic osteoarthropathy. It has been found to be inherited by a Mendelian dominant or sex-linked trait affecting males (Fischer et al. 1964, Rimon 1965). Painful swelling around the knees, wrists and ankles are associated with periostitis, clubbing and skin and scalp thickening (pachydermis). Ankle swelling is due to periostitis.

Bone marrow failure may occur (Metz and Dowell 1965). The problems usually start at the age of puberty and progress for about 5 years.

Tourette Syndrome

Tourette syndrome is a neurodevelopmental disorder appearing in childhood and characterised by a complex array of vocal and facial tics, echolalia and coprolalia which often spoils the social function. Patient may reduce or even suppress the tics with much effort. There may be associated obsessive-compulsive disorder, attention-deficit disorder or hyperactive (manifestations) disorders.

Tourniquet Paralysis Syndrome

Due to *abnormal prolonged pressure by the tourniquet*, the *neurovascular tissues suffer resulting in paralysis.*

It is common in upper limb, in which all the nerves are affected leading to motor and sensory paralysis. Once paralysis occurs, the management is more or less on only expectant lines. The recovery should usually occur by three months.

In the upper limb, the pneumatic tourniquet should be applied at the upper arm with *a pressure of systolic +50 mmHg for the maximum of 1 to 1¼ hours.*

In the lower limb, it should be applied in the mid-thigh region with a pressure of *twice the systolic pressure for maximum of 1¼ to 1¾ hours.*

Turner Syndrome

Turner syndrome was described by Henry Turner in 1938 in seven girls who displayed the same phenotype.

It is due to sex chromosomal anomalies, in which *one 'X' chromosome is missing (XO)*. Nearly two-thirds of these patients have an 'XO' karyotype, the remainder are mosaics (XO/XX) or have partial deletion of the 'X' chromosome. Thus, there are only 45 chromosomes. The person is female in character with short stature, webbing of neck, broad chest with widely spaced nipples, low posterior hair line, peripheral lymphoedema, cubitus valgus. They have primary amenorrhoea and are infertile with rudimentary ovaries. They may have coarctation of aorta and pigmented naevi. They are usually active and asymptomatic with a low incidence of mental retardation and a normal life expectancy. Leg lengthening should be avoided in such patients.

Ulnar Impaction Syndrome

Ulnar impaction syndrome may be defined as a degenerative condition characterised by ulnar wrist pain, swelling, and limitation of movements related to excessive loading across the ulnar aspect of wrist. It is usually seen in patients with positive ulnar variance. Usual acquired predisposing conditions for this syndrome are malunion of distal radial fracture, premature physeal arrest of the distal part of radius, previous radial head resection, an Essex-Lopresti injury, etc. However, "Idiopathic ulnar impaction syndrome" occur in patients who have congenital or dynamic positive ulnar variance with wrist pronation and forceful grip without any history of fracture or premature physeal arrest.

Usually, there is subluxation of distal radioulnar joint in X-ray besides dissociation in relation between distal ends of radius and ulna (displacement of ulnar head from the distal aspect of the radius to be measured on lateral view X-ray of wrist with forearm in neutral rotation as radioulnar distance) usually there is degenerative cystic change in ulnar carpal bone.

Ulnar shortening osteotomy improves wrist function in patients with idiopathic ulnar impaction syndrome and reduces the subluxation of distal radioulnar joint.

Management

Symptomatic relief may be obtained by restriction of hurting efforts, NSAIDs, local analgesic application, corticoid infiltration, etc. Surgical measure such as ulnar shortening osteotomy improves the functions of wrist, reduces the subluxation of distal radioulnar joint and also leads to resolution of the cystic changes of the ulnar carpal bone.

Ulnar Tunnel Syndrome

Ulnar tunnel syndrome results from compression of the ulnar nerve in a tight triangular fibro-osseous tunnel (about

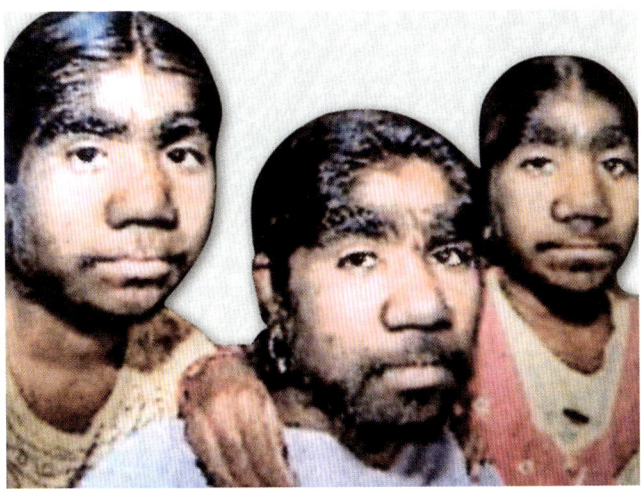

Fig. 24.12: Werewolf syndrome.
Source: Newspaper Hindustan Times.

1.5 cm long) situated in the wrist region. The tunnel is bounded by superficial transverse carpal ligament anteriorly, the deep transverse carpal ligament posteriorly, and pisiform bone and pisohamate ligament medially. The incidence of ulnar tunnel syndrome is much less as compared to carpal tunnel syndrome. The symptoms due to compression of ulnar nerve may be motor or sensory or both depending upon the site of compression. In compression, just distal to the ulnar tunnel, the deep branch of ulnar nerve which supplies the intrinsic muscles of hand, is affected. Compression may be caused by any space occupying lesion, such as any tumour, ganglion, ulnar artery aneurysm, fracture of hamate, arterial thrombosis, rheumatoid arthritis. The clinical features may be confused with cervicobrachial neuralgia, peripheral neuropathy, thoracic outlet syndrome, etc. Treatment mainly consists of decompression of tunnel and neurolysis of the compressed nerve. If the ulnar artery is occluded for several millimetres, in this zone, the features of Raynaud syndrome (phenomenon) may be observed in ulnar three digits, because the sympathetic nerve fibres for these digits pass along the ulnar artery. If it is so, the segmental resection of artery followed by vein graft should help.

Valgus Extension Overload Syndrome

It is uncommon entity seen in throwing athletes, like baseball players or pitchers. Patient complains of pain in posterior elbow region, due to repetitive stress, which leads to excessive shear forces on medial aspect of olecranon tip and olecranon fossa. This leads to lateral to lateral radiocapitellar compression and posterior extension overload with tension on medial collateral ligament. Chondrolysis, osteophyte formation and loose bodies develops.

Patient, complains of pain in posteromedial region of elbow during the active sports activities. Posteromedial region of olecranon becomes tender. Crepitus can be felt. Pain develops/increases with forced elbow full extension with a valgus stress. Recurrent symptoms can be managed by removal of bony spurs, even arthroscopically.

Werewolf Syndrome

Werewolf syndrome is an extremely rare genetic condition (incidence of about one in 1000 million) in which hairs are grown in disorganised fashion from head to foot with vague pain (may be psychological) in body. The face looks peculiar and dreadful. Though costly, the possible management is only the laser surgery **(Fig. 24.12)** (Source: HT)

■ BIBLIOGRAPHY

1. Akbarnia BA, Akbarnia NO. The role of orthopedist in child abuse and neglect. Orthop Clin North Am. 1976;7:733-41:
2. Baek GH, Chung MS, Lee YH, et al. Ulnar shortening osteotomy in idiopathic ulnar impaction syndrome. J Bone Joint Surg (B). 2005;2649 (Downloaded from www.ejbjs.org)
3. Birman MV, Lee DH. Factitious disorders of the upper extremity. J Am Acad Orthop Surgs. 2012;20:78. Quoted in Campbell's-Operative Orthopaedics, 12th edition vol four, Elsevier-Mosby 2013;3490.
4. Danks DM, Campbell PE, Stevens BJ et al. Menkes' kinky hair syndrome—an inherited defect in copper absorption with widespread effects. Pediatrics. 1972;50:188-201.
5. Das SP, Sahoo PK, Mohanty RN, Das SK. One stage release of congenital constriction band in lower limb from new born to 3 years. Ind J Orthop. 2010;44:198-201.
6. Funakoshi T, Furushima K, Kusano H et al. First-rib stress fracture in overhead throwing athletes. J Bone Joint Surg Am. 2019; 101:896-903.
7. Greene WB, Hill C. One stage release of congenital circumferential constriction bands. J Bone Joint Sug (AM). 1993;75: 650-5.
8. Kempe CH, Silverman FN, Steele BF et al. The battered child syndrome. JAMA. 1962-181:17-24.
9. Lopez-de-celis, Polo SC, Gonzalez-Rueda V et al. Dimensional changes of the tarsal tunnel during foot and ankle positions: anatomical study. J Foot Ankle Surg. 2020;59:763-7.
10. Miliani A, Chevid H, Rachedi M. Pathologies du pied associées a la covid-19-foot disorders associated with covid-19. Med Chir Pied. 2021;37:66-71.
11. Rathod C. The Battered Baby Syndrome (Child Abuse). Chapter 331, pp 3008, of textbook of orthopaedic and trauma, JAYPEE 3rd ed. 2016.
12. Sadaksharana J, Annapoorni AV. Gorlin-Goltz syndrome with multidisciplinary approach of treatment annals of the national academy of medical sciences (India). 2019;55-4:213-7.
13. Sakaura H, Matsuoka T, Iwasaki M, et al. Surgical treatment of cervical kyphosis in Larsen syndrome: report of 3 cases and review of the literature. Spine 3:E39,2007.
14. Sponseller P, Abousamra O. Neuromuscular spine deformity. Let's discuss spine deformity AAOS 2018 American Academy of Orthopaedic Surgeons: 39-58.
15. Tanaka Y, Takakura Y, Akiyama et al. Painful hypertrophic peroneal tubercle syndrome. Foot Diseases. 1995:11(1):29-33.
16. Torpin R. Amniochorionic mesoblastic fibrous strings and amniotic bands: Associated constricting fetal malformations or fetal death. Am J Obstet Gynaecol. 1965;91:65-75.

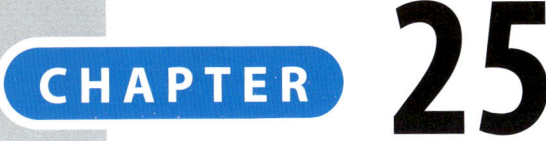

CHAPTER 25

Leg Ulcers

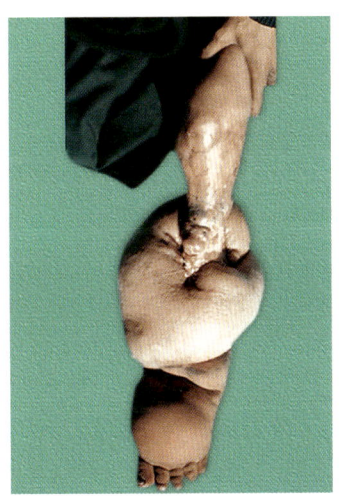

"The weak can never forgive, forgiveness is the attribute of the strong."
—*Mahatma Gandhi*

Ulcers of the leg pose a challenging task in terms of their morbidity and chronicity.

Leg is the common site for the ulcers due to various underlying causes. The *ulcers of the leg are always the sequelae and never the disease 'sui generis'.* The incidence of leg ulcers is about 1.5% in general, however in low socioeconomic group of persons and in tropics as a whole this incidence is about 15%.

■ CAUSES OF LEG ULCERS

On overall consideration, about 70% of these ulcers are due to vascular disorders, peculiarity interacting with skin and subcutaneous tissue.

The causes of leg ulcers can be broadly grouped under following headings:

- *Congenital ulcers:* The ulcer is not present at birth, but can develop due to underlying congenital causes, e.g. lymphoedema **(Fig. 25.1)**, arteriovenous fistulae.

- *Traumatic* **(Figs. 25.2 to 25.4, 25.23 and 25.25)**: It can be primary, e.g. in open injury with persistent skin loss or secondary, e.g. (i) after infection of underlying haematoma and its breaking down, (ii) rolled injuries (underwheel rolled injury or fan-belt injury) in which the devitalised skin and subcutaneous tissues get necrosed and break down.

- *Iatrogenic:*
  • Postoperative gaping of the wound
  • Breaking down of skin over the infected and/or projecting screw or plate or nail-head or pressing from underneath to sloughing (e.g. in subcutaneously placed plates).

- *Infective:*
  • Pyogenic—sequelae to acute/subacute/chronic osteomyelitis **(Fig. 25.22)**
  • Tuberculous ulcer **(Figs. 25.5, 15.110B)**
  • Pyoderma gangrenosum

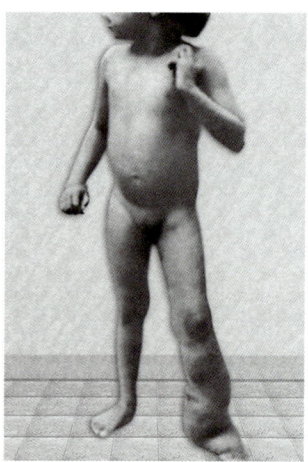

Fig. 25.1: Congenital lymphoedema in left leg with an ulcer on the medial aspect of leg (cf. filarial lymphoedema **Figures 2.54A to D**).

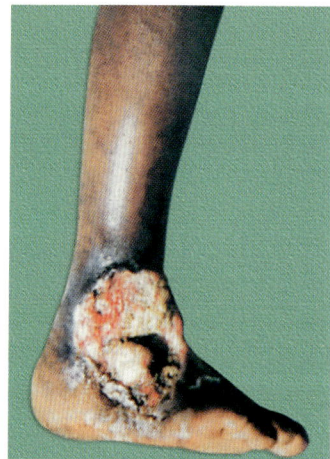

Fig. 25.3: Post-traumatic extensive resistant ulcers on the leg, ankle and foot.

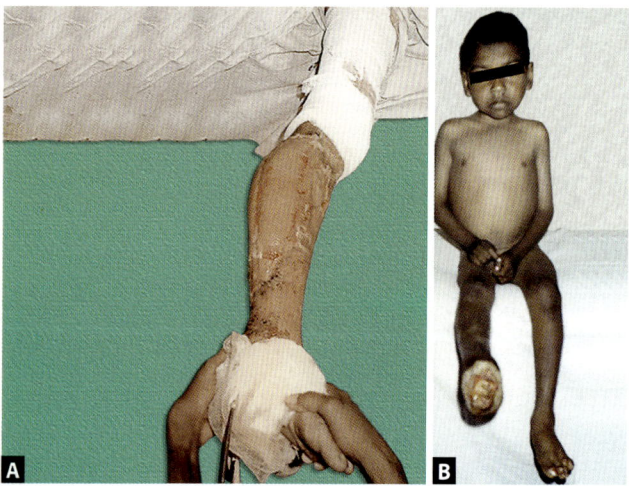

Figs. 25.2A and B: (A) Post-traumatic persistent ulcer; (B) 2½ years old persistent ulcer on lower leg and ankle following gangrenous fall out after snake bite.

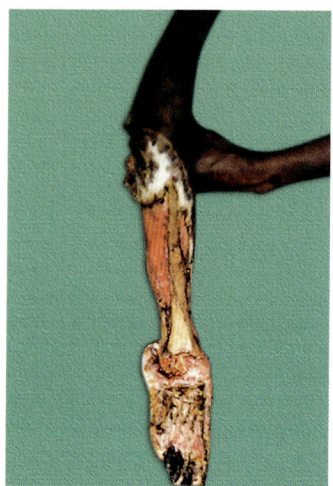

Fig. 25.4: 7 weeks old extensively damaged and devitalized wound (ulcer) on leg and foot due to road traffic accident—such limb has disarticulated from knee or and followed by suitable artificial limb.

- Syphilis or yaws **(Fig. 25.6)**—tertiary stage
- Hansen's disease (usually spreads up from the malleolar region **(Figs. 25.7, 25.8; and 15.102A)**
- Mycotic infection **(Fig. 15.112A)**
- Guinea worm ulcer **(Fig. 25.9)**.

■ *Tropical diseases:*
- Ulcers developing over the filarial elephantiasis **(Refer Figs. 2.55A to C)**
- Ulcer due to Leishmaniasis **(Fig. 25.10)**
- Aleppo boil
- Tularaemia.

■ *Tropical ulcer* **(Figs. 25.11 and 25.12)**:
- Predominantly seen in lower third of the leg
- Common in *equatorial and also in tropical zones*, especially in poor, unhygienic, malnutritioned people with intercurrent illness

- It is rather a clinical syndrome of no definite known aetiology. However, bacteriology reveals 'Fusobacterium ulcerans' (which has direct cytotoxic effects) along with other secondary invaders, e.g. *Borrelia vincentii, Pseudomonas, Staphylococcus, Streptococcus, Pneumococcus*, etc.

With history of minor trauma, scratch or prick, erythematous zone develops, over which vesicles and thence bullae containing serous or serosanguinous fluid appear. They rupture to result in painful dirty foul smelling ulcer with filthy purulent friable greenish/ yellowish/whitish grey/whitish slough and indurated margin. Ulcer spreads rapidly. Underlying fascia, muscles and tendons slough out, and bone gets affected. It may persist for more than 2 to 3 months as chronic ulcer with slow fibrotic healing. Histology of

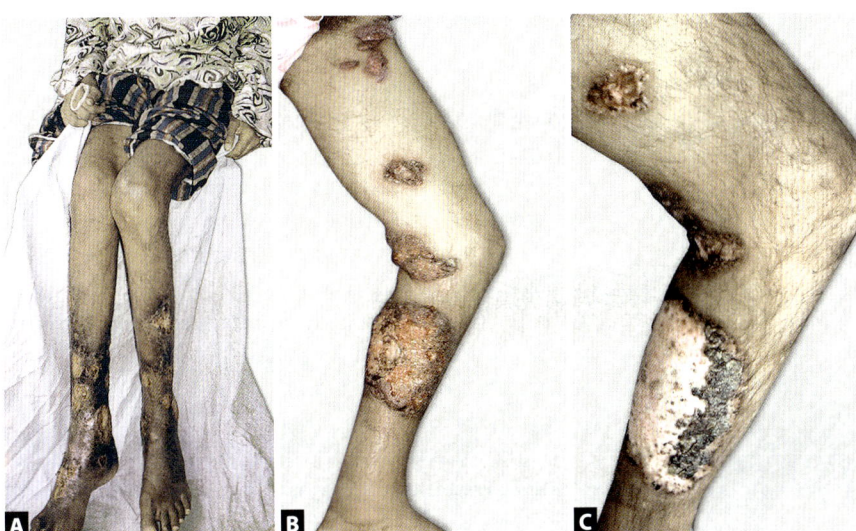

Figs. 25.5A to C: Tuberculous ulcer on thigh, legs and foot.

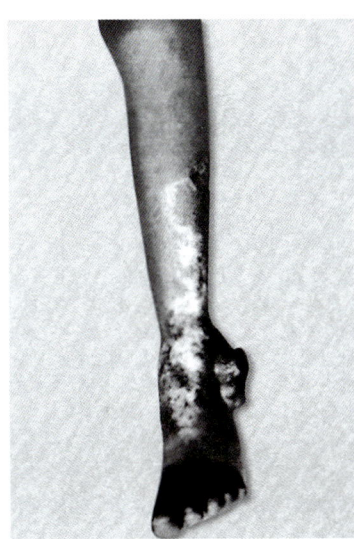

Fig. 25.6: Late yaws—gummatous framboesides.

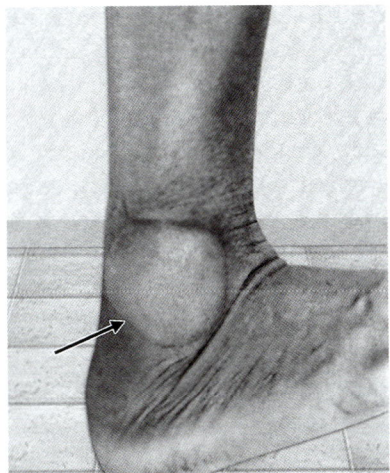

Fig. 25.7: Prior to break down bulla developed on the constant pressure point.

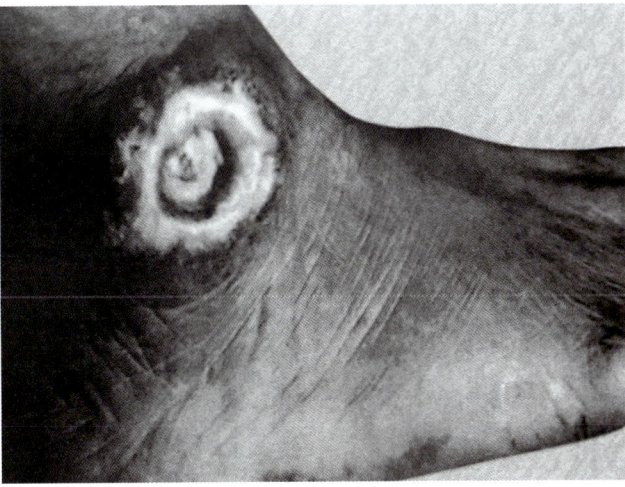

Fig. 25.8: Hansen's disease producing pressure necrosis ulcer on the lateral malleolus (professionally patient has to sit crossed-leg for hours together).

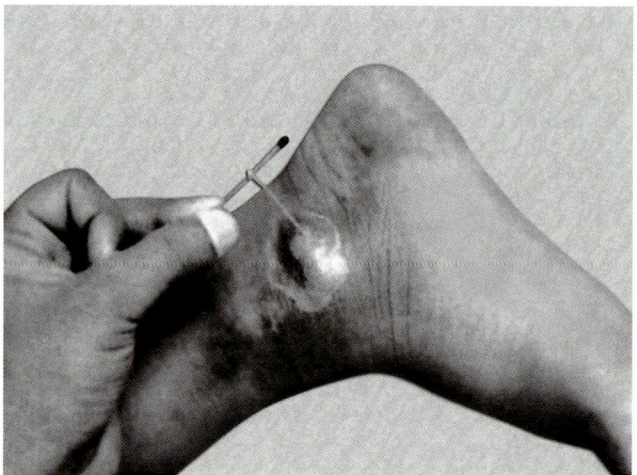

Fig. 25.9: Multiple ulcers on the medial aspect of lower leg and ankle due to guinea worm. Note the traditional way of removing the worm by coiling on a match stick.

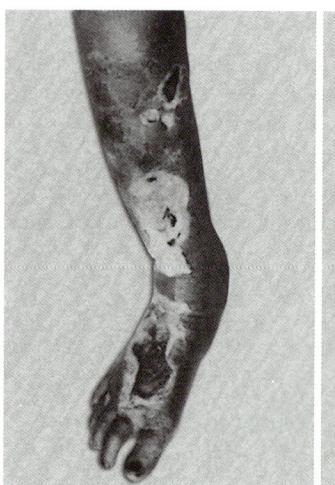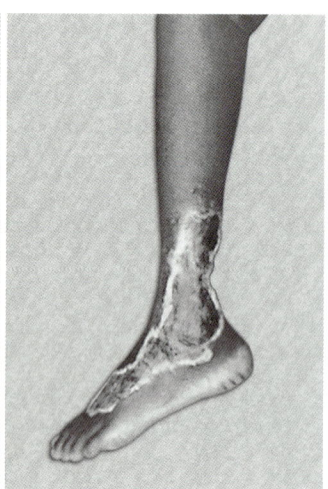

Fig. 25.12: Tropical ulcers. Note the extensive necrosis over the leg and foot with whitish purulent slough, developed following a minor injury by a wooden conical end.

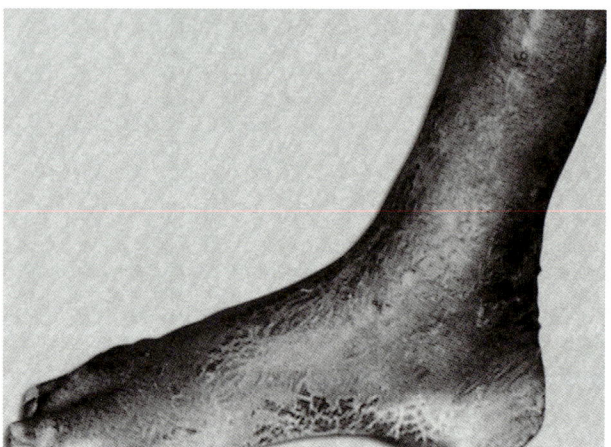

Fig. 25.10: Leishmaniasis ulcer.

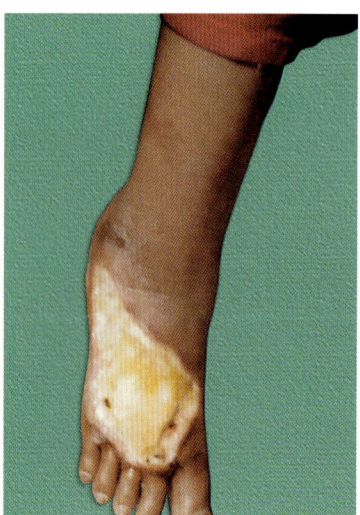

Fig. 25.11: Tropical ulcer in initial stage.

the edge of the ulcer usually shows epitheliomatous hyperplasia.

Even after healing recurrence may occur with marked fibrosis. Ulcer may turn to malignancy as differentiated squamous cell carcinoma.

- *Burn ulcers:* Leg is a common site of burn leading to persistent ulcers, e.g. in accidental fire, electric burn, chemical burn **(Figs. 25.13 to 25.17)**.
- Cold-Fire-Burn ulcer of heel-leg **(Fig. 15.125)**
- Ulcers related to vascular origin
  - *Venous diseases:* Venous stasis ulcers – defined as the persistent ambulatory venous hypertension of the lower extremities (Eberhardt RT et al. 2014) – are the most common type of ulceration seen on the lower extremities mostly in the elderly people (beyond 60 year of age). Most of the ulcers have delayed healing in alkaline pH environment. *Varicose ulcer* **(Figs. 25.17 and 25.18)***:* Chronic superficial or deep or both venous insufficiency leads to ambulatory hypertension which results in seepage of blood components into the pericapillary space. Unhealthy ischaemic tissue in such venous disease breaks down to persistent ulcer even with mild trauma.

    Patient complains of swelling and dull ache *in the lower leg*, more so after prolonged standing or keeping the leg dependant. *Hyperpigmentation, woody induration of skin, dermatitis* and *eczematous changes* pre or co-exist the ulcer. There may be history of bleeding.
  - *Arterial diseases*: Arterial insufficiency (e.g. in atherosclerosis, thromboangiitis obliterans, arterial thrombosis, arterial embolism, peri/polyarteritis nodosa, hypertensive ulcer (Martorell's ulcer), panangiitis (Erythema nodosum), frost bite (cold

Leg Ulcers

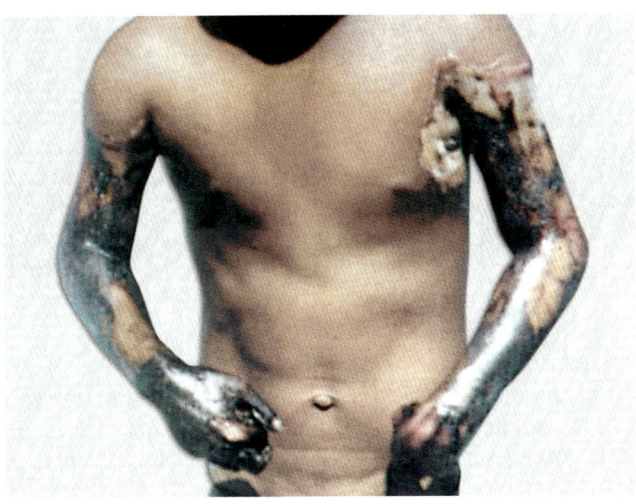

Fig. 25.13: Typical electrical burn of both upper limbs.

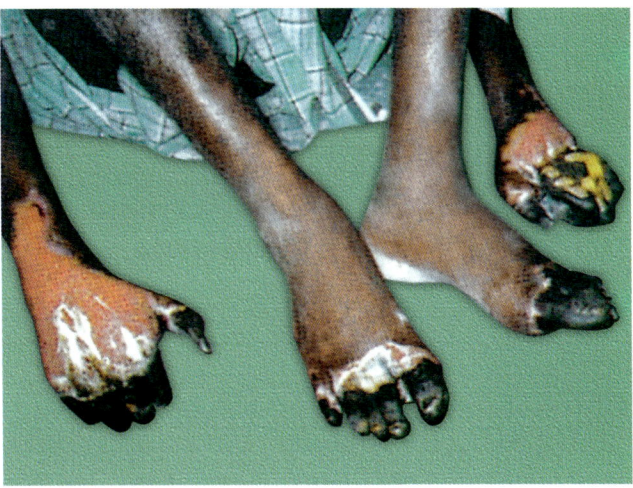

Fig. 25.16: Bilateral almost symmetrical gangrene of both hands and feet due to toxicity of an indigenous medicine.

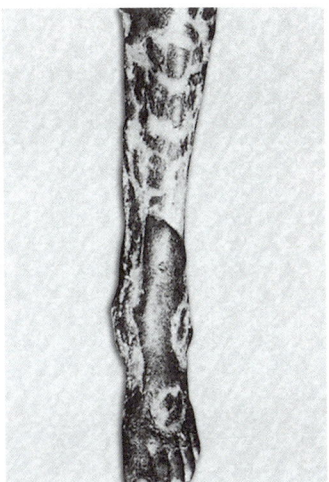

Fig. 25.14: Extensive post-accidental healed burn ulcers with patchy partial thickness skin cover.

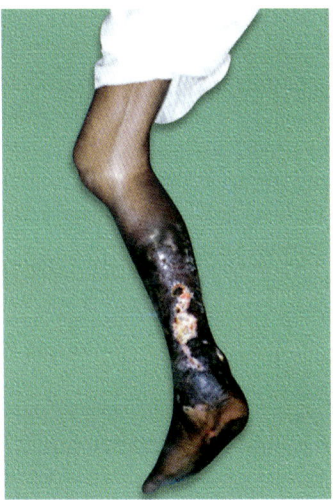

Fig. 25.17: Silencer-pipe burn ulcer in motorcycle accident.

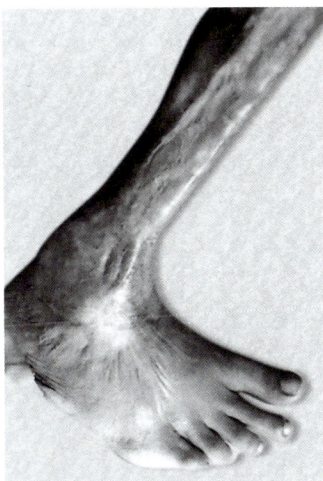

Fig. 25.15: 2-year-old post burn persistent ulcer with variable healing by second intention and contracture in ankle and leg.

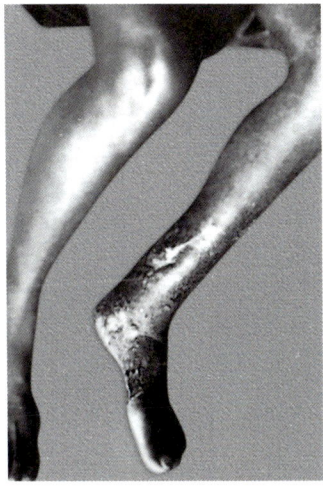

Fig. 25.18: Varicose ulcers on the medial aspect of ankle and lower leg.

injuries) produce ischaemic ulcers more on the foot (toes, interdigital clefts, heel, bony prominences) than the leg.

The patient complains of *intermittent claudication, tingling, numbness in toes, rest pain in night, changes in skin colour,* etc. The pain aggravates after walking, exposure to cold and elevation of leg. The peripheral pulse is less felt or absent. Ulcer develops rapidly destroying the deeper tissues.

- *Lymphatic diseases*: Lymphatic obstruction (congenital or infective—like filariasis) gradually leads to *lymphoedema* (painless pitting oedema of leg and foot), *chronic inflammatory changes* and fibrosis which lead to *elephantiasis* with *multiple furrows* and *fissures*, over which *ulcers* develop **[(Refer Figs. 2.55 and 25.19A and B)]**.
- *Arteriovenous fistulae* can also lead to chronic ulcers more or less due to same pathogenesis as due to venous insufficiency.
- *Vasculitis* can cause ulcers, e.g. SLE, polyarteritis, etc.
- *Erythrocyanosis frigida*: Ulcers of the leg associated with chillblain are more common in women. It starts with a bluish red infiltration and appearance of small vesicle, which breaks down to produce painful ulcer. There is loss of hair on the atrophied skin of leg and ankle becomes swollen.

■ *Dermatological disorders:* Ulcerations are seen in various skin conditions, e.g. allergic dermatitis; JUCCUYA (ulcer due to Leishmaniasis).

■ *Neoplasms:*
  - *Haemangioma*—ulcer may develop on haemangioma, which may bleed **(Figs. 25.20A and B)**.
    ◆ *Squamous cell carcinoma* **(Fig. 25.21)** usually develop over chronic ulcers due to other several causes. However, they may develop as primary carcinomatous ulcer as well
    ◆ *Basal cell carcinoma:* Leg is the second most common site after the face.
    ◆ *Marjolin's ulcer* **(Fig. 25.24)**; A slow growing carcinomatous (mostly squamous cell carcinoma) ulcer which may develop on the old scars (mostly on the post-burn scar) after a latent period of 1 to 30 years or even more
    ◆ *Melanoma:* Though melanoma develops more in the foot region, it can occur in the leg as well
    ◆ *Kaposi's sarcoma*
    ◆ *Non-Hodgkin's lymphoma.*

■ *Miscellaneous* **(see Figs. 25.13 to 25.16):**
  - *In battered babies*, the ulcer develop following repeated cutting or burning on the leg
  - *In mentally derailed persons*, persistent self-inflicted ulcers can be seen on the legs
  - *Beggars produce self-inflicted chronic ulcers* on the leg to attract the passerby with pity

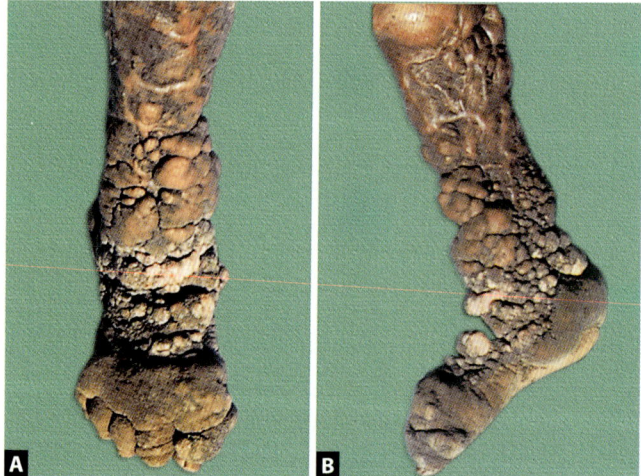

Figs. 25.20A and B: Advanced filarial elephantiasis with numerous fissurings, nodulations, keratinizations, ulcerations, etc. One attempt of surgical excision and skin grafting has been done with failure.

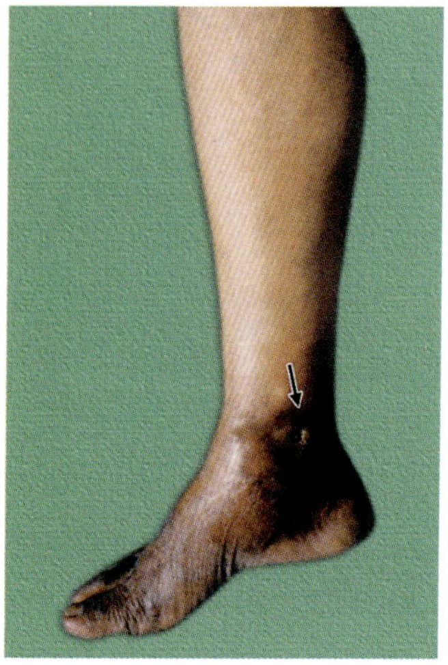

Fig. 25.19: Varicose ulcer.

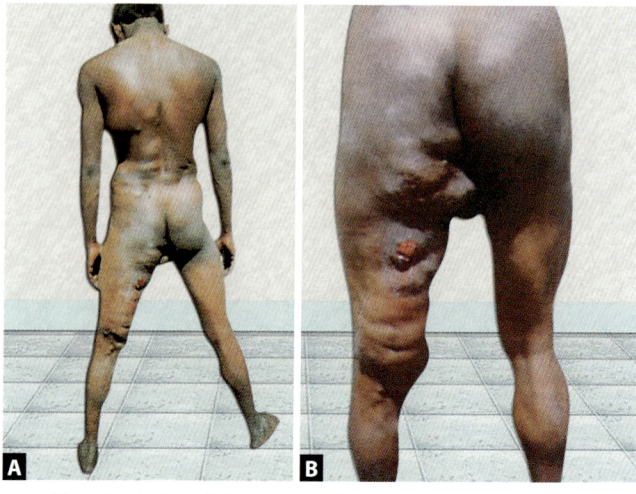

Figs. 25.21A and B: Extensive large vessel haemangioma with ulcers at several places.

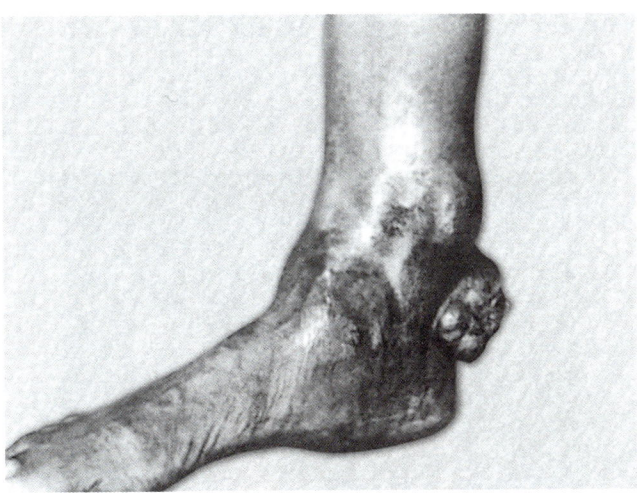

Fig. 25.22: Primary epitheliomatous ulcer on the lower medial aspect of leg and ankle Squamous cell carcinoma may complicate chronic neglected wounds specially in diabetic.

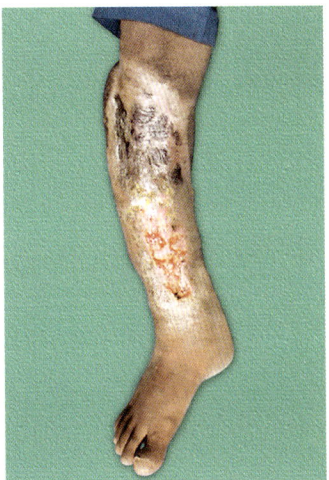

Fig. 25.23: 'K' nailing done for extensive compound fracture of leg bones. Partial thickness skin graft over the resistant portion of ulcer.

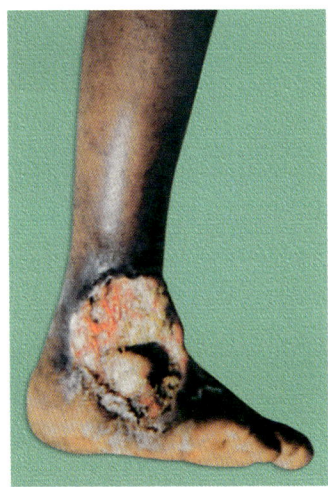

Fig. 25.25: Marjolin's ulcer developed over the post-traumatic scar.

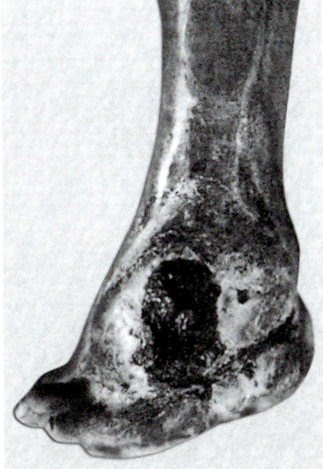

Fig. 25.24: Chronic post-traumatic persistent extensive ulcer on leg.

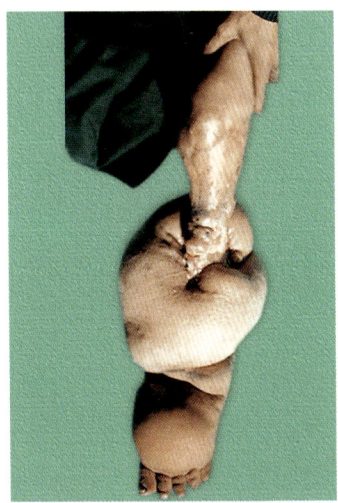

Fig. 25.26: Post-traumatic lymphoedema, elephantiasis and ulcer on the leg.

- Rarely ulcer may develop on the leg *in ulcerative colitis* and metabolic diseases
- Ulcer following snakebite **(Fig. 25.2B)**

■ BIBLIOGRAPHY

1. Eberhardt RT, Raffetto JD. Chronic venous insufficiency. Circulation. 2014;130:333-46.

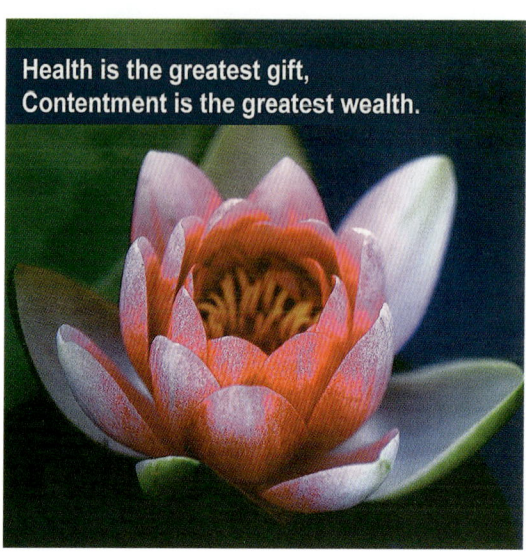

Index

Page numbers followed by *f* refer to figure, *fc* refer to flowchart, and *t* refer to table.

A

Abdomen
    distended 599
    girth of 599
    gross examination of 597
    local condition of 598
    quadrants of 275
    right upper 599
Abdominal muscle 261*f*
    weakness of 311
Abdominal wall 598, 600
Abdominis, external oblique 299
Abducent nerve 499
Abduct shoulder 506*f*
Abduction 327, 334, 338, 461*f*
Abductor digiti minimi 511
Abductor pollicis
    brevis muscle 510*f*
    longus 157*f*
        stress tests for 173
Abscess 609, 622, 623*f*
    axillary 104*f*
    bilateral paravertebral 229*f*
Acetabular development,
    abnormalities of 609
Acetabulum 60
Acheiria 38, 634
Acheriopodia 38
Achilles tendinitis 425, 470*f*
Achilles tendon 424
Achiria 38
Achondroplasia 68*f*, 69, 649
Achromia 81*f*
Acidosis 366*f*
Acoustic pressure wave 609
Acrofacial dysostoses 650
Acromegalic jaw 570
Acromegaly syndrome 634
Acromioclavicular degenerative arthritis 656
Acromioclavicular joint 101
    dislocation of 116
    sternoclavicular to 106
Acromion, angle of 106, 109
Actinomycetoma 477*f*
Acute respiratory distress syndrome 67
Adactylia 634
Adamantinoma 575
Adamkiewcz great spinal artery 212
Adams-Oliver syndrome 634
Adduction 327, 334, 338, 461*f*
Adductor muscles, contracture of 308*f*
Adductor tightness, autocorrection of 308*f*

Adenocarcinoma 615*f*
    prostate 617*f*
Adenoma 634
Adhesive capsulitis 120, 121
Adipose tissue 524
Adson's sign 657
Adson's test 237
Adult respiratory distress syndrome 634
Aerobic respiration 3
Agenesis 38
Agnathia 571
Ainhum 475
Air contrast radiography 258
Aitken's four-part classification 60
Akinesia 254
Albers-Schonberg disease 10*f*
Alcoholism, chronic 82
Algodystrophy 638
Alkaptonuria 292*f*
    musculoskeletal manifestation of 292*f*
Allergic dermatitis 666
Allis' test 348*f*
Allodynia 19
    spatial summation of 19
Allopurinol 90
Alpha-fetoprotein measurements 260
Alveoli 590
Alzheimer's disease 41, 634, 638
Amelia 38
    totalis 38
Ameloblastoma 575
Amnesia, post-traumatic 581
Amputation 38
Amyloid
    arthropathy 83
    precursor protein 638
    substances, deposits of 41
Anaemia 13*f*, 366*f*
    disease 366*f*
    aplastic 643
Anal canal 273
Anal reflexes 270
Analgesia 15
Analgia 18
Anconeus triangle 129
Andropause 649
Aneurysm 609
    aortic 269, 649
Angiography 531
    peripheral 606, 606*f*
Angular kyphosis 223, 223*f*
Anhidrosis 18

Ankle 649
    anteroposterior stress test of 423, 485
    arthrodesis of 422*f*
    attitude of 419
    clonus 252*f*
    common affections of 427
    congenital contracture of 8*f*
    extensor retinaculum syndrome of 642
    fracture dislocation of 428*f*
    jerk 251*f*, 270
    joint 415
        integrity of 417
        synovial reflection of 417
    lateral collapse of 422
    mortice 417
    movements of 461*f*
    neuropathic arthropathy of 431
    osteoarthritis of 431
    pathology 427
        effects of 418
    sprain of 428
    tuberculosis of 408, 427*f*
    villonodular synovitis of 430*f*
    zero axis of 461
Ankylosing spondylitis 223, 223*f*, 263, 264*f*, 269, 280, 281, 282*f*, 290, 358, 364*f*, 365*f*, 469, 613, 641
    advanced 265*f*
    secondary 263
Ankylosis 30, 136, 569
    acquired 571, 572
    causes of 96*t*
    congenital 571, 572
    types of 30, 96*t*
Annular grooves, congenital 181
Anoxia 366*f*
Anserine tendinopathy 385
Antagonists 31
Anterior compartment syndrome 638
Anterior cord syndrome 634
Anterior cruciate ligament 373
    injury 401*f*
Anterior impingement syndrome 429, 635
Anterior interosseous nerve 635
    compression syndrome 502
Anterior tibial
    artery 417, 418, 418*f*, 420*f*
    nerve 417, 501*f*
    syndrome 638
    tendon, insertional tendinosis of 445
    vein 417
Anterolateral soft tissue impingement
    syndrome 635

Anteversion, degree of 349*f*
Anticonvulsants 73, 653
Antigen, calcaneus 613
Antiresorptive therapy 645
Antley-Bixler syndrome 635
Anulus fibrosus 287
Aorta 594
Apert's syndrome 437, 437*f*, 635, 636*f*
Aphalangia 38, 634
Aplasia, bilateral 657
Aplastic anaemia 643
Apley's test 401, 402*f*
Apodia 38
Apprehension sign 111, 394, 402
Apprehension test 111, 402
Apraxia 253
Arachnodactyly 181
Arachnoid mater 212
Arachnoiditis 617
Arbeitsgemeinschaft für ostesynthese fragen 7
Arch
    anterior 435
    longitudinal 435
    transverse 435
Arm-drop-sign 111
Arnold-Chiari syndrome 260, 635
Arrhythmias, cardiac 581
Arterial blood gas analysis 644
Arterial diseases 664
Arterial insufficiency 481*f*, 664
Arteriography 35, 403, 404
Arteriovenous fistula 662, 666
Artery 144*f*
Arthritis 12*f*, 80, 92, 654
    chronic 80
    degenerative 93, 292*f*
    post-variolar 95*f*
    presentation of 80
    reactive 87, 88
    secondary 12*f*
    true 80, 80*t*
Arthrocentesis 34
Arthrodesis 136*f*, 140*f*, 422*f*, 507
    circumferential 648
    modified triple 306*f*, 442*f*
    triple 439*f*, 654
Arthrodial joint 371
Arthrofibrosis 389
Arthrography 35, 113, 349, 403, 404
Arthrogryposis 355*f*
    multiplex congenita 8*f*, 9*f*, 455*f*, 466
Arthrokinematics 80
Arthrolysis 147*f*
Arthroplasty, replacement 132*f*
Arthropodae 78
Arthroscopy 34, 113, 349, 403, 404, 411, 427, 465
Arthrosis 463
    degenerative 291, 358, 410, 410*f*
Arthrotomy 92, 113, 403
Articular cartilage 44, 44*f*, 602
    sliced fracture of 396
Articular facets 213
Articular ligaments 573
Articular surfaces, palpation of 385
Ashworth scale 322
    modified 322

Asphyxia, traumatic 593
Aspiration 349
    biopsy 34, 349
Aspirin 86
Astereognosis 254
Asthma 378*f*
Asynergid 253
Ataxia 247, 253
Athetosis 247
Atlantoaxial instability 642
Atlanto-axial
    joint 227
    subluxation 269
Atlanto-occipital joint 227
Atonic bladder 217
Atresia, duodenal 642
Atrioventricular nodal arrhythmias 581
Attention deficit hyperactivity disorder 314, 316
Attitude 103, 130, 158, 301, 329, 375, 457, 569, 583, 590
Auricular nerve, posterior 513*f*
Auscultation 29, 51, 235, 275, 403, 426, 464, 530, 595, 599
Autism 314, 316
    five types of 39*f*
    spectrum 39
    spectrum disorder 39*f*
Autoimmune disorders 314
Autosomal dominant 10*f*
    disease 637
    disorder 654
Autosomal mendelian dominant hereditary disorder 645
Autosomal recessive 10*f*
Avascular necrosis 349, 364*f*, 368, 479*f*
    bilateral 365*f*, 366*f*
Avulsion 396
Axial rotation stress test 276
Axillary folds, measurement of 109*f*
Axillary nerve 102
    test for integrity of 110
Axonotmesis 504

B

Back muscle exercise 293
Backache 287, 292
    chronic 290*f*
    clinical examination of 292
    compensation 291
    referred 292
    usual causes of 287
Backbreaking stresses, reduce 287
Baclofen 308*f*
Bacteria
    filamentous 477*f*
    gram-negative 486
Baker's cyst 384
Balance disorders 639
Ball joints 80
Ballance's sign 599
Baller-Gerold syndrome 636
Ballismus 247
Bamboo spine 263, 264
Barber's pilonidal sinus 196
Barlow's test 345, 345*f*
Barton's fracture 164*f*, 171

Basal cell carcinoma 666
Baseballer's elbow 133
Bathyanaesthesia 254
Batson's plexus 212
Battered baby syndrome 66, 636, 650
Battered buttock syndrome 636
Baumann's angle 130
Beggars produce 666
Behavioural therapy 294
Bell's palsy 499
Benediction attitude 190
Benzodiazepines 653
Bertolotti syndrome 287, 288
Biceps
    brachii 299
    bursa 388
    jerk 252*f*
Bicipital tendinitis 110, 121, 644
Bicipital tenosynovitis, tests for 110
Biopsy 34, 519, 531
    excisional 34
Birth defects, high prevalence of 37
Bisphosphonate treatment 11*f*
Bladder 255, 273
    automatic 217
    consists, nerve supply of 217
    intraperitoneal rupture of 599
Blast injury 598
Blastomycosis 185*f*
Blauth's classification 635
Bleeding, massive 595
Blood 312, 595
    culture 91
    flow 612
    pool 612
        phase 611
    pressure 584, 598
    vessels, major 590
Blount disease 382
Blowing out 419
Blue sclerae 11*f*
Blunt trauma 590, 598
    abdominal 598
Body
    anterolateral surface of 418
    immune system 645
    mass index 26
        high 26
Bone 96, 373, 614
    abscess 611
    age radiograph atlas 603
    anatomy 625
    around knee, ossification of 373*t*
    articulating surfaces of 79
    avascular necrosis of 68, 611
    cement 610
        implant syndrome 636
    densitometers 35
    deposition 641
    destruction, areas of 409
    disease 645
    expansion of 28
    formation 409
    girth of 28
    graft viability 612
    infections 629
    joint pains 366*f*
    lymphangiomatosis of 645

marrow 622
    failure 10*f*
    oedema syndrome 636
mineral density 72
nonhereditary dysplasia of 10*f*
ossification of 178*f*
pains 651
progressive atrophy of 645
prosthesis interface 612
resorption 203*f*
sarcomas 533*t*
scanning 612
scintigraphy 611*f*
spontaneous absorption of 645
tissue, microarchitectural
        deterioration of 72
tuberculosis 22
tuberculous infection of 184*f*
tumour 521, 522, 536*t*
    benign 525*t*, 532
    classification of 523
    primary malignant 536, 536*t*, 537-547
    secondary 522
    staging systems for malignant 533
    treatment of 533
turnover markers 74
typical long 44
Bony ankylosis 362*f*
Bony components 163, 417
Bony cortex 622
Bony growths, benign 409
Bony lesions 396-398
Bony loose bodies 396
Bony metastasis, early detection of 611
Bony palpation 385
Bony prominences 371
Bony sequestrum 28
Borborygmi 598
Borrelia vincentii 663
Botulinum-A toxin 308*f*
Bound foot deformity 481*f*, 485
Boutonniere deformity 188, 189*f*
Bow knee 379*f*, 382*f*
Bow leg 381, 382
Bowel control 255
Bowel sounds, complete absence of 599
Bowler's thumb 194
Bowstring test 237, 239
Boxer's elbow 651
Brachial artery 129
Brachial plexus 505, 507, 508
    test for integrity of 110
Brachial roots 236
Brachioradialis 635
Brachydactylism 181
Brachydactyly 655
Brachymetacarpia 181
Brachymetatarsia 437, 448
Brain 634
    injuries 583*t*
    MRI of 626*f*
Brainstem reflexes 582
Breast lump 616*f*
Brittle bone disease 11*f*
Brodie's abscess 59, 69*f*, 608
Broom test 140
Brown tumors 203*f*
Brown-Séquard syndrome 215, 254, 637

Bryant's sign 110
Bryant's triangle 342*f*
    fallacies of 342
    quantitative measurement of 342
Buccal cavity 570
Buccal mucosa 570
Buerger's disease 21, 475
Buerger's phenomenon 9, 19
Bull's eye sign 612
Bunionette 453
Bunnell test 188
Burn
    contracture 13*f*
    ulcers 664
Bursa
    anserinus 388
    around knee 388
    pathologies 610
Bursitis 610

C

Cachexia 648
Calcaneal apophysis, posterior 470*f*
Calcaneal apophysitis 470*f*, 483*f*
Calcaneal branch, medial 501*f*, 503
Calcaneal decompression 471
Calcaneal fasciitis 471*f*
Calcaneal fat pad 436
Calcaneal fractures 620
Calcaneal spur 471
    resection 471
    syndrome 471*f*
Calcaneal stress fracture 470*f*
Calcaneocavovalgus deformity 459*f*, 460*f*
Calcaneocavus foot 443*f*
Calcaneocuboid joint degenerative 463
Calcaneoplasty, endoscopic 470*f*
Calcaneovalgus foot 459*f*
    footprint of 460*f*
Calcaneum
    advanced malignant melanoma of 483*f*
    giant cell tumour of 475, 483*f*
    osteomyelitis of 483*f*
    tuberculosis of 470*f*
Calcaneus deformity, measurement of 464
Calcaneus foot 440
Calcar femorale 327
Calcium 406*f*, 614
    carbonate 74
    oxide 74
    pyrophosphate
        crystal inflammatory arthritis,
            chronic 90
        dehydrate, crystals of 398*f*
        deposition 90
        dihydrate crystal deposition disease 90
    silicate 74
    sulphate 74
Callaway's test 109
Callosity, types of 469, 469*t*
Callus, formation of 610
Caloric reflex 581
Campylobacter jejuni 646
Canal stenosis 616
Cancellous bone 622, 625
Cancer
    care 522

chemotherapy 367
    treatment of 535
Candle bone disease 10*f*
Capital epiphysis 362*f*
    fragmentation of 365*f*
Capital femoral epiphysis 364*f*
Capsular irritation sign 121
Capsular tear
    avulsion, posterior 412*f*
    haematoma 351, 352
Capsulectomy 140*f*
Capsulitis 80, 644
Capsulotomy 383*f*
Caput ulna syndrome 637
Carcinoma 523, 575, 621*f*, 645
    jaw 281*f*, 576*f*, 645
Carcinomatosis, secondary 281
Carcinomatous epulis 576*f*
Card test 462*f*, 511*f*
Cardiac failure 634
Cardiac tamponade 590
Cardiac valves, prolapsed 649
Cardiovascular disease 74
Cardiovascular system 26
Caries
    spine 261, 270, 600
    teeth 572
Carotid angiography 585
Carpal bones 179
Carpal dislocations 171
Carpal instability 172
Carpal tunnel 173*f*, 501*f*
Carpal tunnel syndrome 22, 173, 175, 509, 630, 634, 637, 641
    causes of 175
    stages of 174*t*
Carpometacarpal arthritis 22
Carpometacarpal joint 179, 197
    tuberculosis of 204*f*
Carpopedal spasm 247
Cartilage 622
Cartilaginous components 609
Cartilaginous surface 101
Catastrophic heart 590
Catel-Manzke syndrome 637
Cathepsin B 634
Cauda equina 214*f*, 269, 623*f*, 628*f*
    lesion 256, 629*f*
    roots of 637
Cauda equina syndrome 269, 637
    causes of 270
Caudal regression syndrome 261
Causalgia 16, 639
Cavernous lymphangioma 61
Cavity, abdominal 598
Cavovarus deformity 454*f*
Cell
    count 79
    of origin 523-525
Cellulitis 53, 481*f*, 611
Cementoma 575
Cenani-Lenz syndactyly syndrome 637
Central cord syndrome 637
Central fracture dislocation 351, 352, 614*f*
Central nervous system 26
Central spinal canal 261
Cephalothoracopagus 8*f*
Cerebellar tremor 22

Cerebellum 217
Cerebral compression 583
Cerebral concussion 583
Cerebral cortex 188
Cerebral irritation 583
Cerebral palsy 14*f*, 193*f*, 244, 303, 303, 304, 307*f*-309*f*, 314, 315, 321, 466
  aspects of 303
  incidence of 303
  typical 307*f*
Cervical
  compression test 236, 236*f*
  disc prolapse 236
  hyperextension injuries 637
  lymph nodes, different groups of 569
  movement, passive testing of 232
  roots stretch test 236
  spondylosis 236, 258, 269
  vertebrae 259*f*, 268*f*, 636
Cervical rib
  removal of 657
  syndrome 502
Cervical spine 158, 212*f*, 231, 232*f*, 233*f*, 569
  congenital lordosis of 225*f*
  disease 630
  lateral stretching of 236
  MRI of 624*f*
  test for active movement of 232
Cervicobrachial neuralgia 659
Chair test 140
Charcot's arthropathy 153*f*, 365*f*, 391*f*, 392*f*, 423
Charcot's gait 246
Charcot's joint 50
Charcot's neuroarthropathy 365*f*, 391
Charcot-Marie-tooth
  disease 466
  syndrome 637
Charley horse' syndrome 393, 641
Chauffeur's fracture 170, 170*f*
Cheap class syndrome 642
Chemotherapy 533
  anteroposterior 152*f*, 408*f*, 427*f*
Chest
  acute traumatic conditions of 591*t*
  barrel-shaped 46
  compression test 590
  expansion, measurement of 235
  injury of 590
  trauma, penetrating 592
  vital organs of 590
Chest injuries 590, 594
  blunt 595
  gross assessment of 587
Chest wall 590, 595
  indrawing of 595
Chiene's test 342, 342*f*
Chikungunya 95
Child abuse 636
Childress Duck-Waddle test 402
Chinese foot binding 481*f*
Chin-on-chest deformity 223*f*
Chlamydia trachomatis 88
Cholesterolaemia 13*f*
Chondroblasts 523
Chondrocalcinosis 397, 398*f*, 608
Chondroitin sulphate B 653

Chondromalacia 394
  patellae 397, 413
Chondrosarcoma 280, 527, 536*t*
Chorea 247
Christian priest 388
Chronic exertional compartment syndrome 138
Chronic regional pain syndrome 638
Chronic tension stress injuries 151
  manifestation of 133
Chvostek's sign 247
Ciliospinal reflex 580
Cine-radiography 35, 257, 403, 404, 465
Circulus vasculosus 44*f*
Circumduction 167, 339
Claudication 19
Claustrophobia 630
Clavicle
  dislocated sternal end of 117*f*
  fracture outer end of 119*f*
  sternal end of 118*f*
  subserves 101
Claw foot 448
Claw hand 190
Claw toe 448, 448*f*
Cleft feet 182*f*, 437
Cleft hand 181, 182*f*
  bilateral 182*f*
  typical 182*f*
Cleft lip 642, 651, 653
  congenital 8*f*
Cleft palate 637, 642, 651, 653
  congenital 8*f*
Clench teeth 570
Clenched fist syndrome 638
Clergyman's knee 388, 389*f*
Clinodactyly 202*f*
Club hand
  bilateral 160*f*
  congenital 159*f*
Clubfoot 454, 455*f*, 458*f*, 465-467, 476*f*, 655
  camp 454*f*
  deformities 466
  early 467
  grades of 467, 468
  late onset 467
  mild 456*f*
  moderate 457*f*
  severe 442*f*, 457*f*
  very late-onset 467
Clubhand 655
Clutton's joint 50
Coagulation defects 366
Coagulopathy 367
Cobb's angle 257
Cobb's method 257, 257*f*
Coccygodynia 283
Cochlear implants 630
Cockup deformity 453, 453*f*
Cockup splint 513
Codman's triangle formation 409
Colchicine 90
Cold abscess 119*f*, 153*f*, 164*f*, 204*f*, 228*t*, 229*f*, 281*f*, 331*f*, 332
  presence of 261
  sites of 227
  tracking of 229*f*-231*f*

Cold-fire burn 475
  ulcer 664
Collagen
  arthropathy 80, 269, 280, 407, 572
  diseases 379, 503
Collagenosis 613
Collapse, progressive 368
Collateral ligament 395
  medial 385
  test for integrity of 400
Colles fracture 65, 158, 165*f*, 169, 170*f*, 190*f*
  reverse 163, 170*f*
Coloboma 643
Comminuted fracture 627*f*
  dislocation 628*f*
Compartment syndrome 68, 138, 466, 638
  chronic 637
Complete brachial plexus palsy 506*f*
Complex regional pain syndrome 18, 19, 639
Compound palmar ganglion 161*f*, 163, 176
Compression sciatic neuropathy 502
Compression stress test 234, 276, 276*f*
Compression test 590
Computer syndrome 639
Computerised axial tomography 531
Concurrent therapy 535
Condylar fracture 396, 412
Condylar joint 79
Condyles, fracture of 572
Condylomata 275*f*
Cone-beam computed tomography, orientation of 608
Congenital constriction band syndrome 654
Congenital convex pes valgus 438, 441*f*, 446, 482*f*
Congenital ring syndrome 181*f*, 654
Connective tissue 11*f*
  disease, mixed 87
Consciousness 583
  disturbances of 643
  level of 581
Contractures 252
  assessment of 310
  grading of 310*t*
Contrast radiography 34, 258
Conus medullaris 214
Coprolalia 658
Coracoid process, tip of 106
Coracoiditis, test for detecting 112
Cord
  bladder 217
  contusion, traumatic 624*f*
  level 248, 250, 251
  total damage of 256
Core biopsy 34
Core needle biopsy 531
Corns 468
Corona radiata 215*f*
Cortex 44*f*
  expansion of 409
Corticoids, local infiltration of 654
Corticomedullary delineation 409, 602
Corticospinal system 217
  lesions of 249
Corticospinal tracts 635
Corticosteroids 85
  bolus doses of 596
  injection of 414
  injections 645

Cothymia 40
Cough 318
Cover up test 382
COVID-19 639
   toe syndrome 639
Coxa plana 349
Coxa vara 358
Cozen's test 140, 141*f*, 151
Craig's test 347
Cramps 19, 20
Cranial fossa
   anterior 583
   posterior 583
Cranial nerves 240, 313, 499, 500
   broad assessment of 499*t*
   examination of 569
   integrity of 499
Craniodiaphyseal dysplasia syndrome 640
Craniomandibular joints 573
Craniopagus 7*f*
Craniotabes 46
C-reactive protein 33
   raised 648
Crepitus 165, 173
Crossed-straight-leg-raising test 237
Cruciate integrity
   test for posterior 395
   tests for anterior 400
Cruciate ligament
   avulsion 395
   tears 620
Crude functions 178
Crush syndrome 67, 640
Cryptophthalmos-syndactyly syndrome 640
Crystal arthritis 80, 83, 430
Crystal synovitis 89
   arthritis 89
Crystalloid 595
Cubital fossa 147*f*
Cubital tunnel syndrome 511, 640
   test for 141
Cubitus recurvatum 135*f*
Cubitus valgus 130*f*, 658
   deformity 150*f*
   measurement of 137
Cubitus varus 130*f*, 137
   deformity 131*f*, 137
   measurement of 137
Curly toes 437, 452
Cursory regional examination 45
Cushing's syndrome 640, 640*f*
Cyanosis 255
Cycle-spoke injury 428
Cyst 385, 609
   dentigerous 575, 576*f*
   intraosseous keratinous 201
Cystic hygroma 61
Cystic swellings around knee 388
Cystography 35
Cytokines 94
Cytotoxicity 366

D

Darwinius masillae 3
de Quervain's disease 22, 162*f*, 163, 165, 165*f*, 172
   test for 165

Dead leg syndrome 393
Deafness 259
Decubitus complications 68
Deep infections 486
Deep infrapatellar bursa 388
Deep palpation 28, 50, 131, 162, 195, 275, 330, 385, 420, 459, 530, 570
Deep peroneal nerve 501*f*
Deep posterior compartment syndrome 638
Deep pressure tenderness 330
Deep reflexes 250*t*, 253
Deep thrust tenderness 227, 265
Deep vein thrombosis 642
Defibrillators, automatic 630
Deformity 12*f*, 19, 189*f*, 287, 647
Degenerative disc disease 647
Dehydration 366*f*
Dejerine-Sottas disease 176
Deltoid muscle 124*f*
   bilateral congenital contracture of 123*f*
   contracture of 103
Dementia, clinical syndrome of 638
Dental cyst 574, 576*f*
Denticulate ligaments 213
Depression 572
Dermatitis 664
Dermatological disorders 666
Dermatome 266
Dermatomyositis 87, 148*f*
Destructive cystic lesions 81*f*
Diabetes mellitus 74, 82, 365*f*, 634, 641
   end-stage complication of 365*f*
Diabetic foot 485
   infection 485*f*
   syndrome 641
   ulcers 485, 486
      classification of 486
Diabetic hand 189
Diabetic muscle infarct syndrome 641
Diabetic nerve compression syndrome 641
Diabetic neuropathy 365*f*, 482*f*
Diaphragm 599
   dome of 598
   injury of 594
   rupture of 594, 595
Diaphragmatic hernia, traumatic 590
Diaphyseal aclasis 159*f*
Diaphysis 44, 44*f*
Diarrhoea, symptoms of 646
Diastematomyelia 466
Diclofenac 308*f*
Diffuse idiopathic skeletal hyperostosis syndrome 641
Digestive problems 316
Digitless hand 181*f*
Digitus quintus varus 452, 453*f*
   super Inductus 453*f*
Direct pyramidal tract 218*f*
Disability 19
Disasters, natural 652
Disc
   disorders, region for 287
   herniation 647
      type of 628
   prolapse 237
      diagnosis of 289

   protrusions 237, 628
   surgery 628
Discitis 263
Discodural interaction 293
Discography 258
Disease modifying anti-rheumatic drugs 85
Dislocation 573
Dislocation
   anterior 330, 351, 352, 355*f*-357*f*
   elbow 143
   posterior 351, 352
   pure posterior 330
   traumatic 113
Disseminated intravascular coagulation syndrome 641
Distal epiphyses, osteochondritis of 472
Distal intercondylar line 101
Distal interphalangeal joint 94, 200*f*, 448
Distal radioulnar joint 637, 658
   ballottement of 163
   instability of 163
   stability of 172
Distraction stress test 234, 276, 276*f*
Doll's eye phenomenon 581
Dolorimeter 18
Dopaminergics 653
Doppler flowmetry 35
Doppler ultrasonography 35
Dorsal bunion 452
Dorsal interossei muscles 203*f*
Dorsal kyphosis 69*f*
Dorsal spinal muscles 318
Dorsal spine 212*f*, 233
   MRI of 625*f*
Dorsal spinocerebral tract 218*f*
Dorsalis pedis artery 420*f*
Dorsiflexion 422, 461*f*
Dorsolumbar caries spine 219*f*
Double crush syndrome 641
Dowager's hump 73, 223
Down's syndrome 642
Dragging gait 244
Drawer sign, anterior 423
Drawer test 399*f*
   anterior 399
Drive diagnostic devices 609
Drop thumb deformity 190*f*
Drummer's palsy 190*f*
Drunkers gait 245
Duchenne muscular dystrophy 316, 317
Duck gait 244
Duga's test 110, 110*f*
Duplication toes 452
Dupuytren's contracture 120, 191, 192*f*
Dupuytren's disease 22, 191
Durkan compression test 175
Dynamic structural deformity 443
Dyschondroplasia 61*f*, 377, 649
Dyschromia 81*f*
Dysdiadochokinesia 253
Dysenteric arthropathy 96
Dyskinesia 247
Dysphagia 315
Dysplasia 345
   developmental 330, 358, 609
   fibrous 122, 123*f*, 367*f*
Dyspnoea, marked 644
Dystonia 247

E

Echinococcus granulosus 269
Echolalia 658
Economy class syndrome 642
Ectrocheiria 38
Ectrodactyly 38
    ectodermal dysplasia clefting
        syndrome 642
Ectromelia 38
Ectrophalangia 38
Ectropodia 38
Edward's syndrome 642
Egawa's test 511
Egg-shell crackling 163
Egyptian foot 460*f*
Ehlers-Danlos syndrome 642, 643*f*
Eichhoff test 173
Elastography 625
Elbow 133
    affections of 142
    bilateral unreduced posterior
        dislocation of 147*f*
    Charcot's arthropathy of 153*f*, 365*f*
    chronic septic arthritis of 153*f*
    congenital
        dislocation of 154*f*
            flexion contracture of 132*f*
    controls flexion of 255
    excisional arthroplasty of 136*f*
    flexor of 131
    forced flexion of 640
    fracture dislocation of 144
    joint 127, 129, 132*f*
        posterolateral dislocation of 147*f*
    movements of 135*f*
    pathology 142, 143
    post-burn contracture of 14*f*, 153*f*
    septic arthritis of 152
    tuberculosis of 152
    ulnar nerve compression at 511
    villonodular synovitis of 133*f*
Electrodiagnosis 518
Electromyography 518
Elephantiasis 45, 70*f*, 479*f*
    post-traumatic 72*f*
Ellipsoid joints 79
Ellis-van Creveld syndrome 642
Ely's test 347
Emphysema 590
    surgical 590, 602
Empyema 593
Encephalitis, autoimmune 314
Enchondroma 184*f*, 185*f*
    multiple 649
Endocarditis, bacterial 83
Endocrinal functions 26
Endocrinopathic fibrous dysplasia 649
Endocrinopathy 650
Endoneurium 501
Endoscopy 608
Enneking's classification 532
Enneking's system 533
Enteropathic arthritis 88
Enthesopathy 611
Enzyme
    defect 656
    deficiency 656

Enzyme-linked immunosorbent assay 34
Epicondylar fracture, medial 148
Epicondylar region, palpation of 133
Epicondylar tips, localisation of 133*f*
Epicondyle, medial 148*f*
Epicondylectomy, medial 640
Epicondylitis
    lateral 139
    medial 141*f*, 151
    test for lateral 139, 141
Epidermal naevus syndrome 649
Epilepsy 314
Epineurium 501
Epiphyseal fracture 396
Epiphyseal growth plate 44, 314*f*
Epiphyseal injury 161*f*
Epiphyseo-metaphyseal regions 636
Epiphysis 44
Episodes 366*f*
Epithelial odontomes 574
Epithelial surface, discontinuity of 27*t*
Epstein-Barr virus 646
Equilibrium reactions 253
Equinocavovarus deformity 476*f*
    severe 476*f*
Equinocavovarus foot, severe 442*f*
Equinovarus deformity 466, 476*f*
    acquired 466*t*
Equinus deformity 438
    measurement of 464
Equinus foot 438, 439*f*
Erb's palsy 110, 505*f*, 506*f*, 508
Erichson's sign 348
Erythema nodosum 664
Erythrocyanosis frigida 666
Erythrocyte sedimentation rate 33
Essex-Lopresti injury 658
Etretinate 641
Eumycetoma 477*f*
Eupraxia 253
Evan's classification 353*fc*
Eve's disease 575
Eversion sprain 429
Everted foot 440, 443*f*
Ewing's sarcoma 268, 475, 479*f*, 536-547, 612
Excessive lateral pressure syndrome 651
Exophthalmos 635
Exoskeleton 476
Exostosis 151
    familial 528*f*
    multiple 23*f*, 528*f*
Extensive multiple neurofibromatosis
    neurofibroma 513*f*
Extensor carpi
    radialis longus 157*f*
    ulnaris 157*f*, 299
Extensor digiti minimi 157*f*
Extensor digitorum 157*f*, 167, 167*f*, 299
    longus 420*f*
        tendon 172*f*, 417
Extensor hallucis longus 420*f*, 638
    tendon of 417
Extensor indicis 157*f*
Extensor pollicis
    brevis 157*f*
    longus 157*f*, 167, 167*f*, 299, 513*f*
        tendon, rupture of 190*f*

Extensor retinaculum, superior 642
External rotation 327, 334, 338
External vertebral venous plexus 212
Extracorporeal shockwave lithotripsy 121
Extraperitoneal rupture 599
Extrapyramidal system 217
Extrinsic vascular pressure 366
Eye 584
    epicanthus of 644
    opening 581
    problems 639

F

Fabella 398
Faber manoeuvre 239*f*, 347
Facet joint injections 294
Facetal arthropathy 267
Facial expression 598
Facial muscles 318
Facial nerve 499
    palsy 499
Factitious hand syndromes 642
Faecal matter 278
Failed back syndrome 643
Fajersztajn test 237, 238, 238*f*
Fallacies 233, 248, 250, 251, 337
Fanatic life syndrome 292
Fan-belt injury 662
Fanconi anaemia 643
Fanconi syndrome 643
Fan-shaped deltoid ligament 417
Fascicles 298
Fasciculation 106
Fat 622
    accumulation of 641
    emboli syndrome 643
    embolism 67, 634
    pad inferiorly 636
Fatigue 644
Febuxostat 90
Feet 434
    congenital malformation of 436
Felty's syndrome 644
Femoral capital epiphysis 364*f*
Femoral condyles 385, 386*f*, 647
Femoral deficiency 639
    severe congenital 60
Femoral head 60, 349
    avascular necrosis of 629
    bilateral avascular necrosis of 366*f*
    painful avascular necrosis of 366*f*
    vascular supply of 353*f*
Femoral neck 60
    anteversion of 347*f*, 381, 382
Femoral nerve 516, 517
    stretch test 237, 239, 239*f*
Femoral root stretch 266
Femoral shaft, multiple fractures of 67*f*
Femoral supracondylar osteotomy 376*f*
Femorotibial compartments 371
Femur
    congenital acute bowing of 72*f*
    congenital anterolateral bowing of 69*f*
    congenital pseudoarthrosis of 49*f*
    fracture of neck of 366
    Garden type fracture of neck of 353*f*
    osteomyelitis of 54*f*
    reconstruction of 639

Ferguson's method 257, 257f
Festinant gait 245
Fever 644
    enteric 572
Fibrillation potential 519
Fibrocartilaginous structure, circumferential rim of 101
Fibrodysplasia ossificans progressiva 148
Fibro-fatty soft tissue mass 655f
Fibromyalgia syndrome 644
Fibro-osseous tunnel 657
    triangular 658
Fibroproliferative disease, benign 191
Fibrosarcoma 645
Fibrosclerotic healing response, abnormal 647
Fibrositis syndrome 644
Fibrous
    band 657
    sheath 179
    tissue 186f, 524
Fibula
    articulates, head of 371
    congenital
        absence of 60f
        pseudoarthrosis of 52
    overgrowth of 57f
Fibular tunnel syndrome 503, 644
Figure of 4 test 239, 239f
Filarial elephantiasis 71f, 475f, 479f
Filarial lymphoedema 70f, 662f
Filum terminale 214
Fine needle aspiration cytology 34, 531
Fingers
    abduction of 200f
    adduction of 200f
    deformity of 189f, 647
    flexion contracture of 205f
    flexor sheath of 195f
    normal movements of 198t
    post-burn contracture of 136f
Finger-to-finger contact 166
Finkelstein's test 165
Fire arm injury 506
First ray insufficiency syndrome 644
Fissures 470f
Five fingers quadriceps 245, 301
Fixators 31
Fixed abduction deformity, angle of 337f
Fixed deformity, correction of 307
Fixed flexion deformity 335, 391
Fixed kyphosis 223
Flabby skin 46
Flaccid flat feet 445
Flail chest 590, 592, 596
    wall 595
Flail joints 310
Flat foot 441f, 444
    anterior 435, 472
Flexible cervical kyphosis 648
Flexible flat foot 445
    test for 444
Flexible hind foot valgus 463
Flexion 337
    deformity 190f, 374, 647
    extension 333
Flexor carpi
    radialis 174f

ulnaris 168, 174f, 511
    calcific tendinitis of 172
Flexor digitorum
    longus 420f
        tendon of 417
    profundus 200f, 299
    sublimis 299
        tendon 201
Flexor hallucis longus 421f
    tendon of 417
Flexor tendons, synovial sheaths of 179, 180f
Flexor tenosynovectomy 176
Floating patella 387
Fluid
    collections 622
    filled cysts 609
    in joint 28, 134
        tests for 386
    levels, multiple horizontal 599
    presence of 349
    quantity of 386
Fluoride 50, 641
Fluorodeoxyglucose 615
Fluoronavigation 6
Fluorosis 50, 50f
Focal femoral deficiency, proximal 639
Foetal surveillance techniques 465
Folic acid 366f
Foot 433
    ailments 434
    angle 241
    applied anatomy of 435
    attitude of 419
    bones, ossification of 436
    broad divisions of 436t
    calcaneovalgus deformity of 59f
    callosity of 469t
    circumferential measurement of 464f
    congenital
        anomaly of 642
        contracture of 8f
    deformities 377f, 438
        compensation 454
        typical attitudes of 302
    dorsum of 476f
    evolution of 434
    flat 241f
    gait 639
    haemangiosarcoma of 475, 479f
    hyperplasia of 475, 478f
    hyperpronation of 443
    involvement 485
    length of 435
    longitudinal measurement of 463f
    movements of 461f
    multiple problematic deformities of 13f
    pathology 464
    post-burn contracture of 484f
    rectangular 455
    side car deformity of 446
    spread 453, 453f
    square 455
    to ankle, relation of 420
    tuberculosis of 475
    X-ray of 24f
    zero axis of 461
Foot-drop gait 244
Footprints 34, 246, 441f, 465
    electrical recording of 465

Footwear
    examination of 457, 460f, 461f, 464
    wrinkling of 464
Foramen magnum 624f
Forearm 638
    bones 46f
    movements of 165
    rotational movements of 136f
    supinator of 131
    X-ray of 61f
Forefoot 436, 454, 472
    abduction 447, 447f, 462
        movements of 462f
    adduction 447, 447f, 462
        movements of 462f
    Egyptian type of 455
    types of 455
Forestier's disease 641
Four score coma scale 581t
Fracture 10, 62
    acetabulum 280f
    around shoulder 115
    calcaneum 470f
    classification of 63t, 353fc
    clavicle 116, 119f, 508
    complicated status of 65t
    complications of 67
    displacements of 64
    fixation of 406f
    forearm 201f
    healing 64t, 610
    high risk of 52
    indirect sign of 610
    leg bones, congenital 48f
    neck femur 351, 352
        classification of 352t
    open reduction of 406f
    patella 393, 393f, 412
        types of 393f
    pelvis 351, 352
    scaphoid 171
    sternum 591
    transverse 151f, 393f
    trochanter 351, 352, 354f, 355f
    ununited 65
Fragilis ossium 11f
Frantic life syndrome 644
Freeman-Sheldon syndrome 644
Freezing shoulder 120
Freiberg's disease 472, 472f
Fresh Smith's fracture 170f
Friction test 402
Froin's syndrome 644
Froment's sign 511f
Frost bite 664
Frozen shoulder syndrome 120, 644

G

Gadolinium-labelled diethylenetriamine penta-acetic acid 626
Gaenslen's test 276
Gait 218, 240, 301, 304f, 305
    abnormal 241
    analysis 246
    antalgic 245
    ataxic 245

calcaneus 245
cerebellar 246
circumduction 244, 246
crouch 244
cycle 241*f*
equinus 244
festinating 245
hemiplegic 244
hysterical 246
in-toeing 244
lathyriatic 244
painful 245
recognised patterns of 243
Galeazzi's fracture 149*f*
Galeazzi's sign 347, 348*f*
Gallbladder 598
Ganglion around wrist 173
Gangrene 478*f*
tissue 486
Gardner's syndrome 645
Gas gangrene 602
acute 67*f*
Gastrocnemius 423
tear 423
tendinitis of 411
Gastrocsoleus 299
contraction of 251*f*
Gaucher's disease 367, 368
Gauvain's sign 346
Genee-Wiedemann syndrome 650
Genitourinary system 26
Genome, study of 36
Genu recurvatum 383*f*, 384*f*, 406*f*
bilateral 384*f*
congenital 383*f*
congenital 383*f*
deformity 383
gait 245
unilateral 384*f*
Genu valgum 69*f*, 375*f*-378*f*, 380
bilateral 49*f*, 366*f*
idiopathic 366*f*
causes of 377
dislocation of 642
idiopathic 379
idiopathic bilateral 378*f*
incidence of 377
measurement of 392
Genu varum 376, 376*f*, 380, 381*f*
fallacies of 381
idiopathic 380*f*
bilateral 379*f*
measurement of 392
Geographical topography 300
Giant cell tumour 162*f*, 163, 173, 409, 475, 483*f*, 536-547, 614*f*
Gibbus, acute 223*f*
Gigantism 39, 634
Ginglymi 79
Glandular organs 654
Glasgow Coma Scale 24, 581, 581*t*
Glenohumeral articulation 101
Glenohumeral joint 101, 644
Glenoid fossa, articular surface of 102
Glenoid labrum 101
Glide test 394
Glomus tumour 195, 484
Glossopharyngeal nerve 500

Glucocorticoids 73
Gluteal bulge 331*f*
Gluteal fold 331*f*
abnormal 346
Gluteal lurch 301
Gluteal region 332
Gluteus maximus 299, 371*f*
contracture 331*f*, 332*f*
bilateral 331*f*
gait 245
Gluteus medius gait 245, 299
Glycoprotein lubricin 79
Glycosuria 641
Goldthwaite's sign 276, 277, 277*f*
Golfer's elbow 133, 151
Goltz-Gorlin syndrome 645
Gomphosis 78
Gonococcal arthritis 83, 88
Goniometer 30
Goose foot 388
Gordon's sign 249*f*
Gorham's diseases 82, 645
Gorham-Stout syndrome 645
Gout 89
pathogenesis of 89
Gouty arthritis 82*f*, 474
Gower's sign 317
Graft vascular supply, patency of 612
Granulocyte scintigraphy 35
Greater trochanter 331*f*, 342*f*
palpation of 347*f*
Greater tuberosity 106
Grecian foot 455, 460*f*
Green stick fracture 62
Green-Anderson's chart 51
Grinding test 401, 402*f*
Gross spinal cord deformity 261
Growth epiphysis 66*f*, 378*f*
Growth factors 94
Growth plate 44*f*, 314*f*
Guillain-Barré
paralysis 466
syndrome 313, 645, 646
Guinea worm 602
ulcer 663
Gunshot injuries 590
Guthrie test 34
Guttman's test 255, 518
Guyon's canal 158, 501*f*
pressure in 511
Gyrus, posterior central 215*f*

H

Haemangioma 268, 280, 602*f*, 649, 666
Haemangiomatosis 645
Haemangiomatous mass 124*f*
Haematoma 609, 610
Haemopericardium 594
Haemophilia 407
Haemophilic arthritis 80
Haemophilus influenzae 91
Haemopneumothorax 592
Haemoptysis 590
Haemorrhage 67, 590
extradural 585
intracerebral 584
middle meningeal 584

petechial 644
subarachnoid 584
subdural 584
subperiosteal 636
Haemorrhagic disease 378
Haemothorax 590, 592
Haenslen's test 277*f*
Haglund's deformity 470*f*
Haglund's syndrome 470*f*
Haglund's triad 470*f*
Hair
follicles 649
tourniquet syndrome 646
Hallux dolorosus 452
Hallux fluxus 452
Hallux limitus 452
Hallux rigidus 452
Hallux valgus 450, 450*f*
bilateral 450*f*
congenital 451*f*
bunion 450
Hallux varus 451, 451*f*, 452*f*
bilateral 446*f*, 452*f*
deformity 452*f*
Hamilton ruler test 109, 109*f*
Hammer-toe deformity 449, 449*f*
Hamstrings
contracture of 384
testing for flexibility in 348
Hand 177, 649
bones 179, 203
deformity of 188
functions, gross assessment of 180
gangrene of 201*f*
grotesque deformity of 14*f*
infections of 195
movements of 196
multiple problematic deformities of 13*f*
on head sign 236, 258
print 201
spaces of 179
supporting head sign 236
syndrome 657
to knee gait 245, 301
tuberculosis of 204*f*
typical garden spade deformity of 170*f*
Hand-hygiene, routine 10
Hand-Schüller-Christian disease 13*f*
Hansen's claw hand deformity 203*f*
Hansen's cold abscess 515*f*
Hansen's disease 474, 474*f*, 476*f*, 503, 513*f*, 515*f*, 663
Hansen's neuropathy 510, 511*f*
Harris hip
function scale 350, 350*t*
score 349
Harrison's groove 378*f*
Harrison's sulcus 47*f*, 378*f*
Hart's sign 348
Haversian canals 203*f*
Hawkin's test 121
Head injury 580
assessment of 580
gross examination of 579
severe complication of 585
Headaches 644
Hearing 10
aids, internal 630

Heart 595
    disease, congenital 642
    failure 595
    syndrome 657
Heat therapy 289
Heberden's node 186*f*
Heel 439
    pad 436
        pain 471
    pain, posterior 470*f*
    painful 469, 470*f*
    strike 241*f*
    thrust test 332
    walking 32
Helicopod gait 244
Hemihypertrophy, congenital 9*f*
Hemimelia, transverse 634
Hemimilia 38
Hemiplegia 194*f*
Heparin 73
Heparitin sulphate, excessive 653
Hepatic failure 22
Hereditary familial disorder 23*f*
Herler syndrome 656
Hernia, femoral 331*f*, 600
Herniated disc compression nerve 269*f*
Herniation, true 265
Heterotopic calcification 147
Heterotopic ossification 147
    causes of 148
Higamentum flavum, hypertrophied 267
Hill-Sachs lesion 113*f*
Hindfoot 436, 465*f*
    oblique view for 464
    valgus, severe 463
Hinge joint 79, 129
Hip 94, 325
    abduction, limitation of 346
    abductor mechanism of 344
    affections, non-traumatic 358*t*
    bilateral
        congenital dislocation of 357*f*
        septic arthritis of 362*f*
    central fracture dislocation of 614*f*
    Charcot's disease of 365*f*
    congenital
        contracture of 8*f*
        dislocation of 358
    controls flexion of 256
    developmental dysplasia of 330, 358, 609
    dislocation of 345, 642
    disorders of 345
    fixed abduction deformity of 336
    fixed adduction deformity of 337
    fixed deformities of 334
    fixed flexion deformity of 335
    fixed rotational deformities of 337
    functions, broad assessment of 349
    in flexion, measuring abduction of 346
    instability of 60, 344
    intra-articular pathology 328
    knee-ankle-foot orthoses 405*f*
    normal movements of 333*t*, 337
    oblique projection of 349
    osteoarthritis 94
    pain of 328
    pathology 351
    reconstruction of 639
    region, involvement of 309
    septic arthritis of 54*f*, 357*f*, 358, 362*f*
    spine syndrome 225, 646
    tests for 343
    transient osteoporosis of 636
    traumatic 351*t*
    tuberculous arthritis of 363*f*
Hip joint 60, 273, 327, 365*f*
    advanced tuberculous arthritis of 363*f*
    anterior dislocation of 355*f*-357*f*
    bilateral idiopathic avascular
        necrosis of 365*f*
    central-fracture dislocation of 356*f*
    dislocation of 354*t*
    inspection of 330*t*
    pathological dislocation of 362*f*
    posterior dislocation of 355*f*
    space 328
    synovitis of 330
    tenderness of 330
Hirschsprung's disease 642
Histoplasmosis 185*f*
Hitchhiker's sign 173
Hodgkin's deposits 270
Hollow foot 458*f*
Holmium-166 613
Holt-Oram syndrome 646
Homan's sign 422
Homogentisic acid 292*f*
Hooding deformity 189
Horner's syndrome 646, 651
Horse's tail 269
Hot swollen joint, evaluation of 91*fc*
Housemaid's knee 388, 389*f*
Howship's lacunae 203*f*
Human hearing, audible range of 609
Human immunodeficiency virus 33, 97, 648
    infection, spread of 22
Hume's fracture 149*f*
Humeral head
    avascular necrosis of 117*f*
    plays, vascular supply of 101
Humerus
    congenital pseudoarthrosis of 49*f*
    fracture of lateral condyle of 149
    head of 106
    lower articular end of 129
    open fracture of 512*f*
    proximal end of 101
    supracondylar osteotomy of 131*f*
    surgical neck of 117*f*
Hunter syndrome 656
Hurler's disease 653
Hyaline cartilage, layer of 79
Hydrocephalus 635
Hydrops knee 410*f*
Hydroxychloroquine 90
Hyperalgesia 15, 19
Hypercalcaemia 184*f*, 203*f*
Hypercalciuria 184*f*, 203*f*
Hypercallus 508
Hypercholesterolemia 186*f*
Hyperesthesia 657
Hyperextensibility, skin changes of 642
Hyperextension 200*f*
    overload syndrome 651
Hyperhidrosis 21, 634
Hyperkeratosis 478*f*
Hyperlipidaemias 367
Hypermobile 310
Hypermobility syndrome, benign 636
Hyperostotic bone disorders 640
Hyperparathyroidism 184*f*, 203, 203*f*
    primary 184*f*, 203*f*
Hyperpathia 19
Hyperphosphatemia 203*f*
Hyperphosphaturia 184*f*
Hyperpigmentation 634, 664
Hyperpituitarism 570, 634
Hyperplasia 182*f*, 446*f*, 571
    angiofibroblastic 151
    X-ray of 478*f*
Hypertension 641
Hyperthyroidism 649
    clinical features of 15
Hypertonia 249
Hypertrichosis 634
Hypoaesthesia 516
Hypoalgesia 15
Hypocapnia 644
Hypochromia 81*f*
Hypoesthesia 638
Hypogastric ganglion 218*f*
Hypoglossal nerve 500
Hypohidrotic ectodermal dysplasia 646, 640*f*
Hypophalangia 38
Hypophosphataemia 184*f*, 203*f*
Hypoplasia 569, 571, 643
    femoral 60
Hypoproteinaemia, prolonged 67
Hypothalamus 218*f*
Hypothenar eminence 186
Hypothyroidism, clinical features of 15
Hypotonia 249
Hypoxaemia 644
    severe 634
Hypoxia 636
Hysterical tremor 22

I

Idiopathic clubfoot 467, 467*f*
    clinical grades of 467*t*
Idiopathic ulnar impaction
        syndrome 646, 658
Iliac abscess 600
    suspect 599
Iliac crest 234, 331*f*
Iliac fossa 331*f*, 599, 600
Iliac plate, pyogenic infection of 281
Iliac spine
    anterior superior 331*f*, 337*f*, 338*f*, 340, 342*f*
    posterior superior 331*f*
Iliac vessels 273
Ilio-costal distance 234
Iliofemoral ligament 327
Ilio-occipital distance 235
Iliopsoas 299
Iliotibial band
    attaches 372
    contracture 311
    syndrome 647
Iliotibial tract 371*f*
    testing for tightness of 301
Ilizarov apparatus 47*f*
    advantages of 47

Ilizarov distraction 72f
Ilizarov method 384f
Immobilization 47
Immune system modulation 501
Immunity
    cell-mediated 54
    humoral 54
Immunoscintigraphy 613
Impingement sign, secondary 656
Impingement syndrome 647, 656
Impingement tests 346
Index finger, sensory loss in 129
Indomethacin 90, 398f
Infection 612
    acute 477
    bacterial 263
    burns 47
    chronic 82
    epidural 626
    traumatic 72f
Inflammation 610
Inflammatory bowel disease, peripheral arthritis of 83
Inflammatory lesions, acute 44
Inflammatory polyarthritic conditions 83
Inflammatory syndrome 647
Infraclavicular fossae 106
Infraclavicular nerve 229f
Infradian rhythm 16
Infrapatellar bursa, superficial 388
Infrapatellar bursitis 389f
Infrapatellar contracture syndrome 647
Infrapatellar fossae 387f
Ingrowing nail 477, 480f, 481f
Inguinal ligament 331f
Injury 22, 288
    abdominal 599
    aortic 590
    bizarre history of 636
    cardiac 594
    external 585f
    iatrogenic 598
    modes of 22
    on skull, site of 584
    penetrating 590
    severe 278
    type of 591, 592-594
Inner ear 630
Instability, assessment of 163, 312
Intensity, higher levels of 609
Intercalary bone 485
Intercalary defects 38
Internal capsule 215f
Internal rotation 327, 334, 338
    gait 244
Internal snapping hip 328
Internal vertebral venous plexus 212
International Osteoporosis Foundation one-minute osteoporosis risk test 74
Interosseous nerve, posterior 151, 501f, 502, 512, 517, 652
Intersection syndrome 647
Interstitial tissue 590
Intervertebral disc
    bulge of 214
    disease 213, 628
    extrusion of 214
    herniation, massive 629f
    pathology 288
    prolapse 264, 269
    protrusion of 214
    sequestration of 214
    structure of 214
    syndrome 647
    unit of 287
Intestinal obstruction 599
Intra-abdominal bleeding 599
Intra-articular
    fluids 609
    fractures 66
    ligaments 371, 391f
    structures, function of 395
Intracerebral aneurysmal clips 630
Intracompartmental pressure 638
Intracranial blood vessels, injury of 584t
Intractable plantar fasciitis 471
Intradiscal electrothermal therapy 294
Intradiscal injections 289
Intramuscular injections 317
Intrathoracic bleeding, massive 596
Intrauterine moulding 222
Intrinsic minus hand 187f
Intrinsic muscles 637
    test for 462f
Intrinsic occlusion 366
Intrinsic plus
    hand 188f
        test for 188
    test, reverse 188
Inversion sprain 428
Inverted foot 440, 442f
Involuntary movement 246, 254
Iodine-based liquids 606
Ipsilateral fibula 57f
    tibialization of 57f
Ipsilateral lower motor neuron lesion 637
Ipsilateral posterior column sensory loss 637
Iridocyclitis 291
Irritability 32
Irritable bowel 644
Ischaemic hair syndrome 646
Ischaemic muscle 519
Ischial tuberosity 331f
Ischiofemoral impingement syndrome 647
Ischiofemoral space 647
Isotretinoin 641
Isthmic spondylolisthesis 266, 267

J

Jaccoud's syndrome 647
Jack test 445
Jamshidi needle 531
Janeway spots 196
Jaundice 13f
Javelin Thrower's elbow 133, 151, 152
Jaw
    advanced carcinoma of 576f, 577f
    ankylosis of 571, 573f
    movements, pain on 569
    swelling of 574t, 577
    typical locking of 14f
Jebsen-Taylor hand function test 180
Jersey finger 194
Jersey thumb 194f
Jiggers infection 475, 479f
Jobe test 112
Joint 77, 602, 608
    active movement of 31
    affections of 7
    ankylosis of 69f, 96, 569
    aspiration of 85, 91, 113
    Charcot's disease of 391f
    classification of 78fc
    collapse 428
    deep palpation of 28
    diseases, degenerative 612
    exposed 371
    infections 629
    inflammation, miscellaneous 91
    interphalangeal 204f
    laxity 649
    line 28
        palpation of 133, 385
        tenderness 428
    osteoarthritis 93
    paralysed 31
    pathologies 612
    several 83
    space 602, 639
    stiffness of 30, 68, 389
        types of 30, 30t
    stress, reduction of 86
    swelling of 651
    tuberculosis 22
Jone's triple tendon transfer 514
Jug test 140, 140f, 151
Jumper's knee 385
Juxta-articular fractures 66

K

Kaposi's sarcoma 666
    inflammatory cytokine syndrome 648
Kernig's sign 238
Kidney 598
Kienbock's disease 164f, 171, 172
Kiloh-Nevin sign 510
Kinesthetic sensation 254
Klinefelter syndrome 648
Klippel-Feil syndrome 104, 104f, 105f, 234, 259f, 648
Klippel-Trenaunay syndrome 648
Klumpke's paralysis 188, 507, 508
Knee 369, 371, 389, 649
    anterior
        dislocation of 406f
        translation of 373
    arthrodesis 314f, 410f
    articular surface of 371
    bilateral congenital posterolateral dislocation of 405f
    Charcot's arthropathy of 365f, 392f
    chronic septic arthritis of 408f
    congenital
        contracture of 8f
        dislocation of 383f
        unilateral posterior dislocation of 405f
    controls extension of 256
    degenerative arthrosis of 410f
    flexion
        contracture of 375f
        deformity of 374
    gait 304f

hyperextension of 52, 60*f*
inflamed 374
instability of 60, 399
jerk 251*f*, 270, 371
movements, normal 390*t*
ossification around 373*f*
osteoarthritis of 94, 382*f*, 411
osteoarthrosis of 382*f*
pathology 403, 404
posterior fracture dislocation of 406*f*
reconstruction of 639
spine syndrome 225, 648
stiffness of 390
transepiphyseal arthrodesis of 306*f*, 314*f*
triple deformity of 375, 375*f*
tuberculosis of 408*f*
varus valgus collapse of 410
Knee joint 402
    bilateral flexion contracture of 8*f*
    flexed attitude of 375
    internal derangements of 395, 396*t*, 630
    triple deformity of 375*f*
Knobby joints 654
Knock flat foot 454
Knock knee gait 245
Kothari's angle 337*f*
Krause's end bulb 254
Kryptos 481
Kyphoscoliosis 221*f*, 287, 648
Kyphosis 648
    congenital 224
    presence of 261
Kyphotic deformity 223

L

Labile kyphosis 223
Labrum abnormalities, evaluation of 630
Lachman Drawer manoeuvre 473
Lachman's sign 400
Lachman's test 400, 400*f*
Lag sign 121
    presence of 121
Laquer's sign 276, 277, 277*f*
Large glandular enlargements 570
Larsen syndrome 648
Larsen-Johansson
    disease 648
    syndrome 648
Lasegue's sign 237
Lasegue's test 237, 238, 238*f*
Laser Doppler flowmetry 35
Lateral antebrachial cutaneous nerve, compression of 503
Lateral condylar fracture, degree of 149
Lateral meniscus, cyst of 388
Lateral popliteal nerve 385, 501*f*, 502, 514, 515*f*, 517
Lateral stretch test 236
Latissimus dorsi 299
Ledderhose syndrome 648
Leg
    and foot lies, neurovascular bundle of 372
    anterior part of 638
    compartment syndromes of 638
    component, observe alignment of 376
    congenital
        angular deformities of 52
        shortening of 60*f*

pain of 290
    anterior 425
shortening of 66*f*
ulcers 661
    causes of 662
unilateral radicular type of 290
Legg-Calve-Perthes' disease 349, 363*f*, 364*f*, 367
Lenses, dislocation of 649
Leprosy 153*f*, 475*f*, 509
Lesch-Nyhan syndrome 648
Lesions 396-398, 511
    clinical localisation of 255
    inflammatory 572
    tumour like 523, 524
Lesser toe deformities 448
Lever arm disease 306
Ligamentous postural syndrome 292, 649
Ligaments 622, 641
    controlling group of 423
    postpartum relaxation of 281
Ligamentum
    denticulatum 212
    flavum 628*f*
    patellae 385, 393
        avulsion of 393*f*, 395
        rupture of 395
Limb
    deformity of 50
    lengthening 47
    malformations, congenital 37
    paralysed 310
Linear measurement 29, 108, 168, 234, 310, 339, 392, 426
Linear sebaceous naevus syndrome 60*f*, 649
Lipoma 275*f*, 657
Lipomeningocele 261
Lissauer's tract 218*f*
Little disease 315
Little equinus 438
Little league elbow syndrome 133, 151
Little toe, congenital elevation of 437
Liver 598
    cirrhosis 73
    disease, chronic 74, 391*f*
    dullness, obliteration of 599
Lobstein's disease 11*f*
Lobster-claw hand 182*f*
Locomotor system 178
Lofgren's syndrome 649
Long bones
    blood supply of 44
    congenital deficiencies of 52
    examination of 43, 146
    fracture of 62
Long saphenous vein 420
Long thoracic nerve 508
Loose bodies 401
    causes of 402
Lordosis 224, 225
Low back pain 269*f*, 286, 287*t*, 626
    management of 293
    non-specific 287
Low backache 285, 290*f*
    chronic 286, 290*f*
    prevention of 294
Low serum iron 647
Low testosterone syndrome 649

Lower back muscles 265
Lower extremity, congenital anomalies of 51
Lower femoral growth, physeal injuries of 378
Lower humeral epiphysis, fracture separation of 142
Lower jaw
    absence of 571
    protrusion of 634
Lower limb 29, 253, 505, 517, 600, 658
    compensate shortening of 60*f*
Lower lumbar sciatic compressive radiculopathy 239
Lower motor neuron 217, 269
Lower radial epiphysis, fracture separation of 169
Lumbar canal stenosis 290, 623*f*
Lumbar disc prolapse 237
Lumbar discectomy 629
Lumbar lordosis 211, 224*f*, 335*f*
Lumbar puncture 585
Lumbar spine 212*f*, 233, 273
    canal stenosis, diagnosis of 290
    muscles 318
Lumbar spondylosis 289, 289*f*
Lumbar vertebrae, sacralisation of 288*f*
Lumbo-pelvic joint complex 273
Lumbosacral belt 289, 293
Lumbosacral spine, MRI of 623*f*
Lunate
    dislocation 171
    malacia 171
Lung
    contusion of 595, 634
    injury of 590
    insufficiency, development of 595
    parenchyma 590, 593
Luxatio erecta 103
Lymph glands 81*f*, 333, 410*f*
    examination of 419
Lymph nodes 26
Lymphadenopathy 109
Lymphangiography 35
Lymphangioma 61
    congenital cavernous 61*f*
    over ankle 431*f*
Lymphatic diseases 666
Lymphatic malformation 648
Lymphatic obstruction 666
Lymphatic system, congenital malformation of 61
Lymphoedema 61*f*, 662, 666
    congenital 9*f*, 70*f*, 123*f*, 662*f*
    peripheral 658
    post-traumatic 72*f*
Lymphomas 613

M

Macrodactylism 181, 182*f*, 183*f*
Macrodactyly 437, 439*f*
Macroglossia 634
Madelung's deformity 160*f*, 176
    bilateral congenital 160*f*
Madelung's wrist 160*f*
Madura foot 477*f*
    advanced 477*f*
    ulcers 477*f*

Index

Madura hand 185f
Maduromycosis coccidioidomycosis 185f
Maffucci's syndrome 649
Magnetic belt 293
Magnetic resonance imaging syndrome 650
Magnuson pointing test 240
Malformation, congenital 81f, 268
Malignancy 67
Malingerer's backache 291
Malleolar tip, medial 340
Malleoli, interrelation of 420
Mallet finger 193, 193f
Mallet thumb 193, 193f
    deformity 190f
Mallet toe 449
Malunited fractures 11f
Malunited supracondylar fracture 131f
Mandible 567
    fracture of 573
    hyperplasia of 569
    ossification of 569
    ramus of 572
Mandibular hypoplasia 637
Mannitol-alkaline diuresis 640
Marble bone disease 10f
March fracture 472
Marfan's syndrome 649
Marie-Strumpell's disease 290
Marjolin's ulcer 666
Maroteaux-Lamy syndrome 649, 656
Marrow hypertrophy 366
Marrow replacement 366
Martorell's ulcer 664
Massage 293
Mastication, muscles of 569
Masticatory muscles 573
Mastoiditis 572
Maxillary hypoplasia 635
McCune Albright syndrome 649
McMurray's osteotomy 94
McMurray's test 401, 401f
Measles 572
Mechanical stress 281
Medial longitudinal arch 435
    collapse of 444
Medial meniscus
    cyst of 388
    tear 412
Medial tibial stress syndrome 650
Median nerve 129, 502, 509
    complete surgical decompression of 175
    compression 175
        syndrome 652
    damage of 505
    injury 510f
Mediastinal emphysema 590
Mediastinal injury 590
Medical education 6
Medulla 44f
Medullary shadow 602
Medullary tumours 523
Megalodactylism 181, 182f
Melanoma 470f, 575, 613, 666
Melorheostosis 10f
Meningioma 290f, 629f
Meningocele 260
    pouch of 629f

Meniscal tears 620
Meniscus 372
    test for 401
Menkes syndrome 650
Menopausal symptoms 74
Menopause, male 469
Mental aberrations 643
Mental retardation 14f, 649
Mental stress 90
Meralgia paraesthetica 501f
Mercurial poisoning 22
Merkel's disc 254
Metabolic disease 503
Metacarpal bones 179
Metacarpophalangeal joint 179, 204f, 513f
    tuberculosis of 184f
Metallic foreign body 602
Metaphyseal artery 44f
Metaphyseal system 44, 45
Metaphysis 44, 44f
Metaphysitis, multiple 13f
Metastasis 533
Metastatic carcinoma 575
Metastatic lesions, symptoms to 528
Metastatic mediastinal lymph nodes,
    multiple 616f
Metastatic tumours 536-547
    soft tissue sarcomas 536t
Metatarsal bones 436
Metatarsal cuneiform joint 452f
Metatarsal insufficient syndrome 644
Metatarsal rise sign 463
Metatarsal stress fracture 473
Metatarsalgia 472
Metatarsals adducted 447
Metatarsophalangeal joint 82f, 448, 452f, 472f
Metatarsus adductus 447, 447f
    bilateral 482f
    congenital 437, 439f, 447
Metatarsus primus
    elevates 452
    varus 452f
Meterecom 35
Methicillin resistant *Staphylococcus aureus* 486
Methotrexate osteopathy 73
Methyl salicylate 86
Methylprednisolone 596
Microcephaly 643
Microembolisation 366
Microfractures 367
Microglossia 651
Micrognathia 569, 571
Microphthalmos 643
Middle column 213
Middle cranial fossa 583
Middle radioulnar union 165
Midfoot 436
Migratory pattern 83
Migratory polyarthritis 87
Mill's manoeuvre 140, 141f, 151
Miller syndrome 650
Miner's elbow 154
Minimally invasive
    absorbable plates and screws 596
    surgery 451
Miserable malalignment 394
Missile injuries 590

Modern imaging techniques 258
Monoarticular affections 407
Monoarticular arthritis 82, 82t
Monoclonal immunoglobulin 652
Monosodium urate monohydrate crystals 90
Monteggia fracture 149f
    dislocation 148, 149, 149f, 149t
Monteggia lesions, classification of 149t
Moon-walk 242
Morning stiffness 83, 95, 290, 644
Morquio's syndrome 650, 656
Morrant Baker's cyst 385, 389
Morris's bitrochanteric test 342, 342f
Morton's metatarsalgia 472, 501f, 503
Motor cortex 215f
Motor dysfunction 246, 639
Motor function 240, 247
Motor nerve conduction test 518
Motor neuron 519
    disease 317
Motor system 214
    applied anatomy of 214, 217t
Motor unit 298
Movement
    abnormal 391, 423
    axis of 390
    coordination of 253
    development of 303
    method of assessing 134
    muscles involved in 572
    normal range of 333
    passive 31
Move-Theater sign 394
Mucopolysaccharidoses 656
    syndromes of 656
    types of 656t
Mucous membrane 653
Muffled heart sounds 595
Multifocal chronic pyogenic osteomyelitis 58f
Multifocal osteoarticular tuberculosis 202f
Multifocal pyogenic arthritis 81f
Multifocal tuberculosis 184f, 478f
Multiplanar reconstruction 35
Multiple congenital constriction rings 655f
Multiple deformities 11f
Multiple epiphysitis, typical X-ray of 9f
Multiple fractures 10f, 634
Multiple injuries 66f
Multiple myeloma 268, 536-547
    sternal puncture in 531
    suspect 268
Mumps 572
Munchausen syndrome 650
Muscle 96, 317, 385, 622
    abdominal 261f
    accessory 390
    action 31
    anterior abdominal 225
    assessment chart 310
    bulk of 247, 309
    cells, striated 524
    condition 27
    cramps 657
    crush injury 317
    curve 518
    fibres 519
        groups of 22
    function of 299

hypertrophy of 303f
imbalance lead 449
name of 318
pathologies 610
power of 252
  assessment of 517
  controlling 31
  grading of 31t, 310
  record of 318
spasm of 261
tears 622
tone of 247, 309, 322
wasting of 95
weakness of 32
  proximal 87
Muscular contraction 298
Muscular dystrophy 314, 316
  congenital 316
Muscular fasciculations 22
Muscular tenderness 87
Muscular torticollis, congenital 220
Musculoskeletal manifestations 97
Musculoskeletal neoplasms, staging system for 533
Musculoskeletal oncology 532
Musculoskeletal pain 644
Musculoskeletal system, components of 78
Musculoskeletal tumours, malignant 533, 533t
Musculotendinous contractures 306
Muslim's callus 470f
Mycetoma 185f, 477f
Mycobacterium
  bovis 92
  leprae 475f
  tuberculosis 92
Mycotic infection 663
Myelocele 261
Myelogram 629f
Myelographic study 258
Myelomatosis, multiple 280
Myelomatous 574
Myelomeningocele 260, 635
Myelosuppression, severe 613
Myerding graded spondylolisthesis 267
Myofibrosarcoma 529f
Myopathic gait 244
Myopathy 24f, 203f, 316, 316f, 466
  diagnostic of 317
Myositic mass 147f
  around hip 367f
Myositis 147f
  ossifans 610
  ossicans 68, 146, 148, 608
    progressiva 148
Myotonia, congenital 303f
Myriad postures 178

N

Nagar syndrome 650
Nail 518
  fold 518
Nail-patella syndrome 650
Narath's sign 347
Nausea, symptoms of 646
Navigation
  role of 532
  system, disadvantages of 532

Neck 26
  anteroinferior surface of 418
  extensors 318
  inferolateral surface of 418
  short 648
  superior surface of 418
Neck-shaft angle, development of 327
Necrotic zone 612
Necrotising fasciitis 67
Needle biopsy 34, 258
Neer's impingement test 111
Neighbouring joint mildly swollen 54
Nelaton's line 342, 342f
Neoadjuvant therapy 535
Neoplasm 280, 431, 623f, 666
Neoplastic conditions 291, 409, 575
Neoplastic nature 522
Nerve 45, 144f, 502
  accessory 500
  action potential recording 518
  affection 68
  affections of 515
  conduction 504
    monitor 518
  fibre groups 217
  hourglass deformity of 176
  injury
    test for median 509f
    types of 504t
  neurolysis of 515f
  repair 507
  root supply 318
  stimulation 518
  supply 134, 166, 231, 333, 334, 390, 572
  tissue 524
Nervi erigentes 218f
Nervous system, peripheral 475f
Neural complications 265
Neuralgia 648
Neuro developmental disorders 314
Neurofibroma 514f, 623f
Neurofibromatosis 46f
  congenital 10f
  syndrome of 513f
Neurogenic claudication 20, 20t
  bilateral 290
Neurogenic pain 16, 16f
Neurolemma sheath 501
Neurological examination 240, 312
Neurolysis 471, 507
Neuroma, interdigital 472
Neuromuscular disorders 82, 314
Neuromuscular junction 519
Neuromuscular scoliosis 653
Neuropathic ankle and feet 423
Neuropathic arthropathy 80
Neuropathic pain 16
Neuropathy 641
  entrapment 501f, 657
  peripheral 637, 659
  stages of 16, 17f
Neuropraxia 504
Neurosensory testing 35, 459
Neurosyphilitic ulcer 475
Neurotmesis 504
Neurotomy 471
Neurotoxic beta amyloid peptide 634, 638
Neurotrophic tyrosine kinage 18

Neurovascular examination 277
Neurovascular tissues 658
Neutral zero position 30
Neutrophil response 54
New disc herniation 617
Noble compression test 347
Nociceptive pain 16
Nociceptors 15
Nocturnal stiffness 290
Nodules, examination of 29
Non-glandular organs 654
Non-Hodgkin's lymphoma 644, 666
Non-inflamed infrapatellar bursa 389f
Non-nodal non-erosive degenerative joint disease 93
Non-steroidal anti-inflammatory drugs 85, 86, 289
Non-symptomatic lesions 622
Nonsynovial joints 78
Non-synovial joints, variants of 78
Non-traumatic conditions 600
Non-verbal pain scale 17, 18t
Nuclear imaging 35, 404, 631
Nuclear medicine 610, 613
  for therapies, use of 613
  therapies 613
Nucleus
  gracilis 215f
  pulposus 214, 287
Numb chin syndrome 650
Nutrient artery 44f
Nutrient system 44
Nutritional status 13
Nystagmus 643

O

O'brien test 122
O'brien's needle test 424
Ober's test 301
Obesity 469
  paradox 26
Obeying commands 581
Oblique ligament 395
Obstetrical brachial plexus lesion 506
Obstetrical palsy 506
Obturator nerve 516
Occipito-atlanto-axial region, tuberculous infection of 261
Occiput-to-wall test 233
Occupational therapy 140f
Ochronosis 292f
Ochronotic arthritis 292f
Ocular torticollis 220
Oculocephalic reflex 581
Oculomotor nerve 499
Oculovestibular reflex 581
Odontoid hypoplasia 650
Odontomes 575
Oedema 590
  around ankle 419
Olecranon
  bursitis 132f, 154
  fracture of 150, 151f
  impingement syndrome 651
Olfactory nerve 499
Oligospinal tract 218f
Omphalopagus 8f

Onychocryptosis 477
Onychogryphosis 484
Open biopsy 531, 532
Open fish-mouth appearance 411*f*
Open fontanelles 46
Open injuries 598
Open pneumothorax 590
Open reduction internal fixation 144*f*
Open surgery, moderately 6
Open-wedge valgus distal tibial osteotomy, medial 423
Opioids 652
Oppenheim's sign 249*f*
Optic nerve 499
Oral-acral malformation complex 651
Orthopaedic
   practice 610
     surgery, computer-assisted 6
     symbol of 4*f*
Orthotomography 51
Ortolani's sign 344, 345*f*
Os accessorium supracalcaneum 485
Os calcaneus secundarius 485
Os infranaviculare 485
Os intercuneiform 485
Os intermetatarseum 485
Os peroneum 485
Os subcalcis 485
Os subfibulare 485
Os subtentaculi 485
Os supranaviculare 485
Os trigonum 485
Os vesalianum 485
Oschner's clasp test 509*f*
Osgood-Schlatter's disease 397, 412, 413, 413*f*
   reverse 398
Osler's nodes 196
Osseous
   and corneal changes 649
   focus 409
   heteroplasia, progressive 147
   odontomes 575
Ossicles, accessory 484
Ossification 274
   around elbow 130*f*
     joint 129
Osteitis
   deformans 70
   fibrosa cystica 184*f*, 203*f*
   pubis 282*f*, 283
Osteoarthritis 10, 80, 93, 95, 95*t*, 197, 382*f*, 410, 613
   primary 410
Osteoarthropathy, hypertrophic pulmonary 651
Osteoarthros 410
Osteoarthrosis 93
Osteoblast 525
Osteoblastic activity 610
Osteoblastoma 525-527
Osteoblasts 523
Osteochondritis 470*f*
   dessicans 397, 398*f*, 399*f*, 402
Osteochondrodysplasia, form of 69
Osteochondroma 160*f*, 280, 283, 525-527
   multiple 528*f*
Osteochondromatosis 398*f*
Osteoclastoma 268, 409

Osteoclasts 523
Osteodystrophia fibrosa 649
Osteogenesis
   imperfecta 10*f*-12*f*, 23*f*, 67, 67*f*, 377
     congenita 67
     tarda 67
Osteoid osteoma 280, 525-527, 608
Osteokinematics 80
Osteoligamentous vertebral canal, narrowing of 289
Osteolysis
   essential 645
   idiopathic 645
   progressive 645
Osteoma 525-527
Osteomalacia 45, 67, 223, 280, 280*f*, 282*f*, 291, 469
   congenital 11*f*
Osteomusculofascial space 638
Osteomyelitic calcaneum 483*f*
Osteomyelitis 9*f*, 10, 47, 53, 54, 58*f*, 62, 66*f*, 72*f*, 81*f*, 119*f*, 153*f*, 184*f*, 204*f*, 378*f*, 381*f*, 572, 608, 611, 612
   acute 378, 611, 662
     haematogenous 54, 54*f*
   characteristics of 53*t*
   chronic 56, 56*f*-59*f*, 66*f*, 378*f*, 473*f*, 575*f*, 662
   extensive 66*f*
   post-traumatic 54
   primary subacute 56
   sets 54
   subacute 55, 56*f*, 119*f*, 575*f*, 662
Osteomyetis 125*f*
Osteonecrosis 160*f*, 172, 349, 365*f*, 629
   idiopathic 611
Osteopathia condensans disseminata 12*f*
Osteopenia 11*f*, 74, 367
Osteopetrosis 10*f*
Osteopoikilosis 10*f*, 12*f*
Osteoporosis 67, 69*f*, 72-74, 223, 612
   age-related 73
   primary 73
   screen for 610
   secondary 73
   severe 74
Osteoporotic compression fractures 291
Osteopsathyrosis 11*f*
Osteosarcoma 268, 409, 528*f*, 536*t*, 612
   primary 536-547
Osteosarcopenia 74
   concept of 74
Osteosynthesis 132*f*
Osteotomy 136*f*
Otitis media 572
Out-toeing gait 244
Ovarian carcinomas 613
Overlap syndromes 651
Overriding toes 452
Ozonucleolysis 289

P

Pachydermoperiostosis 658
Paget's disease 67, 68*f*, 70, 71, 223, 269, 280
   bone 71
Pain 15, 18, 32, 94, 102, 350
   abdominal 599

   causes of 469, 471, 472
   characteristics of 19*t*
   contralateral 637
   early morning 293
   palliation 613
   pathophysiology of 16
   perception, loss of 505
   recurrent 637
     episodes of 94
   severe 120, 654
   site of origin of 16
   types of 5
Painful arc syndrome 111, 111*f*, 121
Painful hypertrophic peroneal tubercle syndrome 651
Painful limp 428
Pale mucosal fibrosis 570, 572
Palm and figures, skin creases on 178
Palmar aspect 161
Palmar dorsiflexion 166
Palmar fascia 179
Palmar flexion 166, 167*f*
Palmaris longus 167, 168*f*, 174*f*
Palpate lymph glands 419
Palpating dorsalis pedis 459
Palpating joint 571
Palpating styloid processes, method of 162
Palpation 28, 50, 106, 162, 195, 226, 309, 330, 384, 420, 459, 517, 530, 570, 595, 598
   superficial 50, 131, 162, 195, 226, 274, 330, 384, 420, 459, 530, 570
Panangiitis 664
Pancoast syndrome 651
Pancoast tumour 508
Pancytopaenia 643, 648
Pandey's calcaneal sling sliding osteotomy 305*f*, 460*f*
Pandey's test 345, 345*f*, 346*f*
Pantalar arthrodesis 313*f*, 314*f*
Paper chromatography 532
Paper pull-out test 473
Paracentesis 599
Paradoxical breathing 595
Paradoxical respiration 590
Paraesthesia 255, 638, 657
   temporary 637
Paralysis 299, 585
   depth of 504
   period of 301
   type of 299, 301
Paralytic ankle and feet 423
Paralytic diseases 312
Paralytic hip 358
Paralytic ileus 599
Paralytic kyphoscoliosis 221*f*
Paralytic subluxation 107*f*
   diagnostic of 106
Paralytic supinated foot 442*f*
Paralytic valgus collapse 482*f*
Paramagnetic contrast agents 607
Paraneoplastic syndromes 651
Paraparesis 635
Paraplegia 262
Paraspinal connective tissues 641
Paraspinal muscles 219*f*
   tone of 227
Parathyroid
   function tests 74

Index

gland 203*f*
hormone 184*f*, 203*f*
Paresis 638
Paretic foot 639
Parkes-Weber syndrome 651
Parkinsonian tremor 21
Paronychia 195*f*, 196, 484
    acute 480*f*, 481*f*
    mild chronic 480*f*
    severe acute 480*f*
Paronychium 518
Parotid stones 572
Parotitis 572
Paroxysmal trepidant ataxia 244
Pars interarticularis 213
Patchy osteoporosis 639
Patchy pulmonary infiltrates 644
Patella 385
    anomalies of 393
    bilateral recurrent dislocation of 413*f*
    blood supply of 372
    chronic dislocation of 395
    congenital dislocation of 52
    dislocation of 398, 642
    fracture of 395
    habitual dislocation of 395
    importance of 372
    lateral dislocation of 413*f*
    lower pole of 648
    recurrent dislocation of 394, 412
    slipping 412
Patellar ballottement 387
Patellar clonus 252*f*
Patellar jerk 251*f*
Patellar malalignment 413
    dynamic evaluation of 394
    physical examination for 394
Patellar mobility, reduced 647
Patellar pain 394
    syndrome 651
Patellar tap 387, 387*f*
Patellar tendinitis 385
Patellofemoral articulation 403*f*
Patellofemoral compartment 371
Patellofemoral compression test 388, 410
Patellofemoral joint 387
Patellofemoral syndrome 397, 651
Pathological fracture 12*f*, 66, 66*f*, 69*f*, 123*f*, 162*f*, 203*f*, 612
Pathological rupture 637
Patrick's test 239*f*, 277, 347
Pectoralis major 299
Pectus
    carinatum 46, 377*f*
    excavatum 46, 377*f*
Peculiar swelling 190*f*
Pellegrini-Sticda's disease 385, 397
Pelvic affections 278
Pelvic bone 283
    metastasis 281*f*
Pelvic examination 277
Pelvic fixation 653
Pelvic fractures 620
    classification of 278
Pelvic injury 273, 516
Pelvic pathology 278
Pelvic peritoneum 273

Pelvic ring
    normal 279*f*
    stable fracture of 279*f*
    unstable fractures of 279*f*
Pelvic tilt 337*f*
Pelvic traction 289
Pelvis 271, 273, 334, 337
    compression stress test of 276*f*
    injury of 278*t*
    ipsilateral triple dislocation of 279*f*
    skeletal framework of 273
    trefoil shape of 282*f*
Pendulum test 239
Percussion tenderness 227
Percussion test 175
Percutaneous interstitial laser photocoagulation 527
Percutaneous vertebroplasty 291
Perianal saddle anaesthesia 254
Periapical abscess 575*f*
Periarthritis 120
Periarticular rarefaction 281
Periarticular tissues 602
Pericardium, tamponade of 595
Perineum, widening of 329*f*, 345
Perineurium 501
Periodic limb movements 653
Perionychium 518
Periosteal artery 44*f*
Periosteal system 44, 45
Periosteum 44*f*
Peripheral nerve 32, 188, 348, 501, 513*f*
    injury 497, 505, 517
        assessment of 505
        causes of 503
    integrity of 168
Peritoneal lavage 599
Peritumoral cytokine secreting cells, killing of 613
Perivisceral haematoma 599
Peromelia 38
Peroneal artery 418, 418*f*
Peroneal compartment 638
    syndrome 638
Peroneal muscular atrophy disease 637
Peroneal nerve 501*f*, 514
    entrapment 503, 644
Peroneal spasm 470*f*
    test for 425, 425*f*
Peroneal tendinitis, clinical findings of 446
Peroneal tendon
    disorders 445
    recurrent subluxation of 429
    sheath, chronic stenosing tenosynovitis of 445
Peroneal tubercle lies 651
Peroneus brevis 299
Peroneus longus 299
Peroneus tertius 299, 638
    tendon of 417
Persistent ulcer, post-traumatic 662*f*
Perthes' disease 358, 364*f*, 609, 611
Perthes' hip 358
Pes abductus 447, 448*f*
Pes anserine 388
Pes cavus 443, 443*f*
Pes planus 50*f*, 441*f*, 444, 444*f*, 454
Pes transversus 453, 453*f*
Pes valgus 440*f*, 441*f*, 482*f*

Phalanges 179, 436
    congenital absence of 181*f*
Phalanx, proximal 183*f*
Phalen's test 175
Phantom
    bone 645
    limb pain 16
    sciatica 218
Phenylbutazone 398*f*
Phenytoin 73
Phocomelia 38
Phosphorus-32 613
Photopodogram 465
Physeal fracture 62*f*
Physical therapy 645
Physiological genu
    valgum 377
    varum 377
Physiomechanics 572
Pia mater 212
Pierre Robin syndrome 569, 651
Pigeon
    breast 649
    chest 46
Pigmented villonodular synovitis 430
Pill-rolling tremor 21
Pincer nails 481*f*
Pins and needles 255
    sensation 293
Piriformis syndrome 240, 502, 652
Pisa syndrome 9, 14*f*
Pisiform-hamate tunnel 511
Pitcher's elbow 133, 151
Pituitary lesion 641
Pivot joint 79
Pivot shift test 400, 401*f*
Plane joints 79
Plantar fasciitis 469, 470, 470*f*, 471
Plantar fasciotomy 471
Plantar fibromatosis 648
Plantar flex ankle joint 421
Plantar flexion 422, 422*f*
Plantar plate 473
    pathology 473
Plantar reflex 249*f*
Plantarflexion 461*f*
Plantigrade foot 439*f*
Plasma 595
    expanders 595
Plaster disease 68
Plastic surgery 104*f*
Plathysmography 35
Pleura 590
    penetrated 595
Pleural cavity 592, 593
Pleural puncture, minor 590
Plexus
    anterior 212
    posterior 212
Pneumothorax, closed 590
Pobble foot 437, 437*f*
Podoscopy 465
POEMS syndrome 652
Poland syndrome 652
Policeman receiving tip 103
Poliomyelitic deformities 298*f*
Poliomyelitis 299, 312, 377, 430, 466
Polio-paralysis 313*f*-315*f*, 384*f*, 406*f*

muscles
    affected in 299
    escaping 299
Polyarteritis nodosa 87
Polyarthralgia denotes pain 82
Polyarthritis 82
Polyarthropathies
    chronic inflammatory 73
    inflammatory 652
Polyarticular arthritis 82, 82t
Polydactylism 181
Polydactyly 437, 437f
Polymyalgia rheumatica 83, 89
Polymyositis 87
Polyneuritis 317
Polyps, malignant 645
Polytraumatised, management of 596
Poncet's disease 96
Poor skin hygiene 636
Popeye muscle 132f
Popeye sign 132f
Popliteal aneurysm 389
Popliteal angle, measurement of 373f
Popliteal fossa 419
Popliteal nerve, medial 515
Positive ankle impingement sign 426
Post-Achilles
    bursitis 470f
    pathology 425f
        test for 425
Post-burn
    contractural adduction deformity 123f
    contracture 139f, 570
Postconcussive syndrome 652
Posterior compartment syndrome 638, 652
Posterior cruciate
    avulsion 412, 412f
    ligament 395
    tear 395
Posterior tibial nerve 417, 501f, 503, 514f
    compression 516, 657
Post-irradiation neoplasms 523
Postmenopausal osteoporosis 73
Postphlebitic syndrome 652
Postural abnormalities 9
Posture, maintenance of 211
Post-viral arthritis 154
Potential elements 19
Pott's disease 261
Pott's fracture 428, 428f
Pott's paraplegia 262t
Pott's puffy tumour 9f
Preacher's hand 190
Pre-Achilles
    bursitis 420, 470f
    pathology 425f
        test for 425
Preaxial radial hemimelia 183
Preiser's disease 171
Prepatellar bursa 388
Prepatellar bursitis 389f
Presacral nerve 218f
Pressure sore, search for 255
Pretendinitis 463
Primary bone tumour 522, 612
    classification of 523t
Primitive reflexes 323
Prognathism 569, 571, 634

Prominent parietal region 46
Pronator teres 299
    syndrome 652
Prone hip-extension test 336
Proprioceptive sensation, absence of 391
Prostate, carcinoma of 281f
Prosthetic replacement 612
Protein
    content 79
    inflammatory 638
Proton beam therapy 535
Proton therapy 535
Protrusio acetabuli 280, 280f
    bilateral 280f
Protrusion 572
Proximal femoral
    focal deficiency 60
    metaphysis 364f
Proximal synovial uniaxial pivot radioulnar joint 165
Pseudoarthrosis 46f, 48f, 60, 65, 132f
    congenital 46f, 48f
Pseudoganglion 157f
Pseudogout 90
Pseudolipoma 106f
Pseudomuscular hypertrophy 303f, 317
Pseudoparesis 13
Pseudosciatica 227
Pseudoseptic arthritis 92
Pseudotumours 522
Psoas
    abscess 600
    bursitis 600
Psoriatic arthritis 83, 88, 613
Psychoextended hand 638
Psychoflexed hand 638
Psychological disturbance 16
Psychological pain 16
Pubic bones 10f
Pubic rami 282f
Pubic symphysis 273, 279
Pubic tubercle 328, 331f
Pudendal nerve 218f
Pulmonary bed 522
Pulmonary capillary hydrostatic pressure 634
Pulmonary hypertension 636
Pulmonary insufficiency
    management of 595
    sign of 595
Pulmonary tuberculosis 261
Pulmonary vascular resistance 595
Pulse 584
Pump handle test 276, 277f
Pupil 580, 584
Pyoderma gangrenosum 662
Pyogenic abscess 204f
Pyogenic arthritis 81f, 116, 204f
Pyogenic chronic osteomyelitis 57f
Pyogenic dactylitis 184f
Pyogenic osteomyelitis 204f, 263
    calcaneum, chronic 477f
Pyothorax 593
Pyramidal affection 249
Pyramidal cells 215f
Pyramidal fibres 215f
Pyrophosphate arthropathy 398f

Q

Q angle 402
Quadriceps active test 399
Quadriceps apparatus 392
    injuries 393f
    integrity of 392
    lesions 395
Quadriceps avoidance gait 245
Quadriceps contracture
    bilateral congenital 383f
    causes of 390
    congenital 383f
Quadriceps expansion 385, 395
Quadriceps femoris 299
Quadriceps gait 245
Quadriceps lag 391
Quadriceps muscle 641
Quadriceps tear
    compensation 393, 393f
    incomplete 393, 393f
Quadriceps tendon rupture 395
Quadriceps tightness 390
Quantitative ultrasound 74
Quinizarin powder turns purple 518
Quinolinic acid 634

R

Rachitic bilateral
    bow leg 49f
    genu valgum 50f, 366f, 377f
Rachitic dwarfism 46
Rachitic genu valgum, bilateral 377f
Rachitic genu varum 381f
    bilateral 379f, 380f
Rachitic rosary 46, 47f
Rachitic windswept deformity 406f
    X-ray of 406f
Radial and ulnar deviation 166
Radial bursa 196
    infection 195f
Radial club hand, bilateral 183f
Radial nerve 110, 129, 178, 501f, 502, 512, 517
    damage of 505
    injury 513f
Radial styloid process, fracture of 170, 170f
Radial tunnel syndrome 652
Radiation
    exposure 616
    therapy 367
Radicular odontomes 575
Radiculopathy 289f
Radioactive isotope 610
Radioactive isotope studies 35
Radioactive scanning 258
Radioactive technetium-labelled hydroxymethylene diphosphonate 610
Radio-capitellar articular disease 151
Radiofrequency denervation 294
Radioisotope scanning 51
Radionuclide studies 35
Radioscintigraphy 403
Radiosynoviorthesis 613
Radioulnar arthritis, post-traumatic
    inferior 171

Radioulnar joints 165
Radius, congenital absence of 159*f*
Raffinis end bulbi 254
Range of motion 134
Range of movement 166, 231, 333, 334, 390
Raynaud's phenomenon 21, 87
Raynaud's syndrome 659
Reading X-ray 602
Reconstructive surgery 203*f*
Record muscle power, proforma to 318
Rectal examination 275, 348
Rectum 273
Rectus abdominis 318
Rectus femoris contracture test 347
Recurvatum, congenital 52
Reeling gait 245
Reflex 240, 248, 250, 251, 253, 584
    elicitation of 518
    name of 308
    superficial 248*t*, 253
    sympathetic dystrophy 638, 639
Reflux sympathetic dystrophy, early
        stages of 612
Regional lymph gland enlargement 522
Rehabilitation 86
    procedures 300*f*
Reiter's cell 653
Reiter's syndrome 83, 87-89, 652, 653
Relaxation occurs 298
Relocation test 111
Renal angle 227
Renal failure 634, 640
    prevention of 640
Renal function tests 532
Renal impairment 73
Renal injury 599
Renal rickets 367*f*
    X-ray of 46*f*
Reperfusion syndrome 653
Repetitive stimulation 518
Residual effects 584
Resistant tennis elbow 652
Respiration 582, 584, 590
    type of 598
Respiratory disease, chronic 378*f*
Respiratory distress 590, 595
Respiratory support 644
Respiratory system 26
Restless legs syndrome 653
Reticuloendothelial cells 54
Reticulospinal tract 218*f*
Retinaculum, tightness of 394
Retraction 572
Retrocalcaneal bursitis 420, 470*f*
Retroglossia 637
Retropulsion 245
Rett syndrome 653
Rhabdomyolysis, traumatic 640
Rhenium-186 613
Rheumatic fever 83, 87, 572
Rheumatoid arthritis 73, 74, 83, 85, 86, 95,
        95*t*, 152, 163, 172, 188, 189*f*, 190*f*,
        269, 280, 291, 391*f*, 407, 430, 451,
        469, 485, 613, 648
    affecting elbow 152
    juvenile 83, 87, 88*f*
    pathogenic stages of 85

Rheumatoid factor 87
Rheumatoid hand 190*f*, 203*f*
Rheumatoid hip 358
Rheumatoid nodules 84
Rheumatoid spondylitis 290
Rheumatological syndromes, part of
        painful 647
Rib fracture
    multiple 591, 592
    single 591
Rib hump 221
Rickets 280, 405
    stigmata of 45
Rigid flat foot, congenital 446
Rigid hind foot valgus 463
Rigidity 249
Risus sardonicus 14*f*
Road traffic accidents 590
Robert's syndrome 653
Robotic gait 246
Robotic surgery 6
    use of 6
Rocker-Bottom flat foot 446
Rocking horse gait 245
Roentgen-stereophotogrammetric
        analysis 35
Rolling-pin test 140
Romberg's sign 253
Roseta stone 286
Rotational movements 135
Rotational stress test 401, 401*f*
Rotator cuff 101, 111, 647, 656
    function of 110
    tears 630, 656
    tendinitis of 111
Rotatory movements 572
RS3PE syndrome 653
Rubro spinal tract 218*f*
Rudimentary foot 438
Rudimentary limbs 8*f*
Rupture 610
    liver 599
    tendon, rounded ends of 424
Rust sign 236

S

Sabre tibia 45, 49*f*
Sacral spine 212*f*
Sacroiliac arthritis 281
Sacroiliac joint 234, 273, 278, 279*f*, 281, 281*f*,
        282*f*, 365*f*
    CT scan of 282*f*
    fusion 264
    MRI of 282*f*
    pathology of 237, 620
    tenderness 291
    tuberculosis of 281
Sacroiliac strain 281
Sacroiliitis 282*f*, 288*f*, 290, 630
Sacrospinalis 299
Sacrum
    chordoma of 626*f*
    congenital absence of 280*f*
Saddle anaesthesia 289
Saddle joints 80
Saegessar's splenic point 599

Salmonella 89, 96
    typhimurium 88
Salter-Harris classification 62*f*
Samarium-153 613
Sandwich vertebrae 10*f*
Sanfilippo's syndrome 653, 656
Sarcoidosis 367
Sarcoma 523, 529*f*, 575
Sarcomatous 574
Sarcopenia 74
Scalene syndrome 502
Scalp
    defects, congenital 634
    oedema of 9*f*
Scanogram 257
Scaphoid 366, 610
    shift test 165, 172
    osteonecrosis of 171
Scapula
    congenital elevation of 104
    to humerus 102
    typical bilateral winging of 508*f*
    winging of 508
Scapular muscles, gross wasting of 316*f*
Scapulothoracic gliding 101
Scarlet fever 572
Scarpa's triangle 331*f*
    base of 332
Scheie syndrome 653, 656
Scheuermann's disease 223
Scheuermann's kyphosis 287
Schindylesis 78
Schober test 234
Schoemaker's line 342, 342*f*
Schwann's cell sheath 501
Sciatic nerve 237, 273, 502, 505, 514, 517
    entrapment of 240
Sciatic neuropathy 239
Sciatic notch 240
Sciatic radiculitis 239*f*
Sciatic scoliosis 265
Sciatic stretch test 238, 238*f*, 346
    alternative method of 239*f*
Sciatica 218, 269*f*
Scintigraphy 35, 71, 404, 531, 610, 631
    uses of 611
Scissor-gait 243, 305
Sclerae 292*f*
Scleroderma 86
Sclerosis 282*f*
    multiple 22
Scoliosis 10, 220, 222, 257*f*, 648
    angle of 257*f*
    computer-aided assessment of 258
    congenital 220*f*, 221*f*, 222
    degenerative 222
    etiological classification of 222*t*
    etiology of 221
    hysterical 223
    idiopathic 222
    infantile idiopathic 222
    management of 223
    severe 268
Scoliotic curves, methods of measuring 257
Scurvy 377, 405, 407*f*
    X-ray of 407*f*
Seasonal affective disorder 653
Sebaceous naevi 60*f*

Secretary tissue, removal of 641
Segmental instability, role of 287
Sellar joints 80
Semilunar cartilage 395
Semimembranosus bursa 389
Senile
    kyphosis 223
    osteoporosis 291
    spine, curvature of 212f
    tremors 21
    type osteoporosis 73
Sensorial organ 434
Sensory
    area 506-512, 514-516
    assessments 240
    dysfunctions 637
    functions 254
    pathways 215f
    system 215
        applied anatomy of 214
Septal defects 642
Septic arthritis 81f, 141f, 153f, 163, 362f, 378, 381f, 572
    acute 81f, 91, 408
    bacterial 91
    chronic 125f, 153f, 408, 408f
Sequestrum 602
Seronegative spondyloarthropathies 89
Serratus anterior paralysis, traumatic 508f
Serum
    acid phosphatase 532
    alkaline phosphatase 532
    biochemistry 33
    creatinine phosphokinase 317
    enzyme 312
Sesamoid bones 435
Sever's disease 470f, 483f
Severe acute respiratory syndrome 654
Sex chromosome anomalies 648
Sexually active males 652
Shenton's arc, continuity of 349
Shigella 96
    flexneri 88
Shin splints 425
Shiny corners 264
Shock 67, 640
    absorber 434
    extracorporeal 656
    hypovolemic 644
Short femur syndrome, congenital 639
Short limb gait 245
Short shuffling gait 245
Short stubby equal fingers 649
Short tau inversion recovery 622
Short-echo time 625
Short-leg gait 245
Shoulder 123f, 131
    affections 103, 113
    anterior dislocation of 103, 103f
    arthrodesis of 507
    chronic septic arthritis of 125f
    common affections of 113t
    congenital dislocation of 124f
    dislocation of 115f, 124f
        classification of 114fc
    fixed abduction
        contracture of 125f
        deformity of 103f, 104f, 124f
    fracture dislocation of 117f
    girdle 158
        congenital malformation of 104
    habitual dislocation of 115f
    impingement syndrome 121, 647, 656
    instability, test for anterior 111
    MRI of 630
    muscles 506f
    pain, posterior 657
    pathology 112
    posterior dislocation of 117f
    preglenoid dislocation of 116f
    primary septic arthritis of 119f
    septic arthritis of 119f, 125f
    short rotators of 299
    subcoracoid dislocation of 116f
    upward subluxation of 117f
Shoulder joint 99, 109
    injury of 102
    manipulation of 645
    recurrent dislocation of 113
    tenderness of 106
    tuberculosis of 119f
Sickle cell
    anaemia 366f
    disease 366f
    haemoglobin 366f
        C disease 366f
    hemoglobinopathy 366f
    thalassemia 366f
    trait 366f
Sickle foot 447
Side bending 233
Side car deformity 446
Side-to-side compression 590
Signal-to-noise ratio 631
Simmond's test 424
Sinding-Larsen-Johansson's disease 398
Single palmar crease 642
Single-photon emission-controlled tomography 612
Sinography 35
Sinus 92
    multiple 275f
    persistence of 28
    tarsi 418f, 654
        syndrome 654
    track denoted 59
    tract 602
Sitting ability 305
Sitting root test 237, 239
Sitting status 320
Sjogren syndrome 654
Skeletal changes 69
Skeletal deformities 220f
Skeletal limb deficiencies, congenital 37
Skeletal muscle 298
    pathology 630
Skeletal system 211
Skeleton, heritable disorders of 10f
Skew foot 453
Skin 27, 518
    chronic infective disease of 477f
    woody induration of 664
Skull, deformity of 635
Sleep disturbances 644
Slipped capital
    epiphysis, bilateral 364f
    femoral epiphysis 358
Slocum test 399
Small disk protrusions 237
Small nose 644
Smashed heel syndrome 654
Smith's fracture 163, 165f, 169, 170f
Snapping elbow 135
Snuffbox, palpation of 163
Societal limitation 298
Socket joint 80, 327
Soft corns 468
Soft tissue 96, 630, 648
    calcification 608
    components 417
    disease 622
    growths
        benign 409
        malignant 409
    injury 429f, 612
    lesions 396-398
    masses 610
    palpation of 385
    region 330
    shadow 409, 602
    swelling 634
Sole
    of footwear, study of 464
    skin of 436
Soleus tear 423
Space of Parona 179
Spastic diplegia 244, 318
Spastic flat foot 444f
Spastic gait 244
Spastic pes valgus, bilateral 445f
Spasticity 249
Speed's test 110
Sphincter
    external oblique 218f
    internal 218f
Spider fingers 649
Spina bifida 259, 261f, 466, 467, 467t, 476f, 635
    incidence of 260
    manifesta 227, 260, 261f, 476f
    occulta 260, 260f, 476
Spina ventosa 183f
Spinal artery
    anterior 212
    embolism 269
    posterior 212
Spinal canal 622
    anatomical dimension of 616
    stenosis 267, 270, 289
Spinal column 213
    line of 236
Spinal cord 188, 211, 213, 255, 624f, 626f, 627f, 634
    arteries of 212
    blood vessels of 212
    complete transection of 627f
    compression of 623f
        paraplegia of 268
    hemisection of 215, 254
    lower end of 214f
    meninges of 212
    monitoring 35
    platybasia 624f
    section of 215f
    segment 255, 255t

stimulation 643
  tracts of 217
  transverse section of 218*f*
  veins of 213
Spinal deformity 69*f*
  typical 14*f*
Spinal disorder, benign 641
Spinal excursion anteroposterior 235*f*
Spinal infections 612, 622, 626
Spinal injuries 599, 600, 626, 634
Spinal instability 263
Spinal longitudinal ligaments, anterior 641
Spinal movements 233
Spinal nerve
  posterior division of 230*f*
  typical mixed 501
Spinal pain 218
  acute 218
  chronic 218
  subacute 218
Spinal pathology 256, 258, 628
Spinal processes, congenital fusion of 259*f*
Spinal region 227, 608
Spinal roots 188, 211
Spinal stability 213
Spinal stenosis 289, 630
Spinal stenotic syndrome 19, 289
Spinal surgery 643
Spinal tenderness 227*f*
Spinal trauma 616, 626
  anatomical dimension of 616
Spinal tuberculosis 261, 263
Spinal tumours 268, 268*fc*, 270, 617
  primary 629
  secondary 629
Spinal zones 257
Spindle cells 186*f*
Spine 207, 211, 255, 268
  anterior column of 287
  curvature of 211, 212*f*, 220
  degenerative arthrosis of 291
  depends, stability of 213
  development of 211
  infections of 617
  lateral flexion test of 237, 238
  ligament of 641
  linear measurement of 235*f*
  measurements of 234
  night pain in 218
  posterior column of 287
  stress test of 235
  tumours of 268
  with cord level, relation of 255
Spin-echo T1-weighted sequences 625
Spinotectal tract 218*f*
Spinothalamic tract, lateral 218*f*
Spino-thalamic tracts 635
Spleen 598
Splenectomy 368
Splenic rupture 599
Spondyloarthropathy 87
Spondylolisthesis 225*f*, 226*f*, 257, 266, 289, 623*f*
  classification of 267
  degenerative 267
Spondylolysis 257, 267, 267*f*, 289
Spool-shaped trochlea 129
Sporotrichosis 185*f*

Sports injuries 590
Sprengel's shoulder 104, 105*f*, 259
Sputum, examination of 595
Squamous cell carcinoma 666
Squat test 402
Squeezing 51
Stab injury 506, 590
Stamping gait 245
Staphylococcus 196
  aureus 56, 91, 263, 486
  epidermids 56
Starch iodine test 255
State-of-the-art imaging 608
Static clawfoot 448
Static problems 306
Stato-acoustic nerve 500
Stature disturbances 38
Steering wheel injury 599
Steindler's fasciectomy 439*f*
Stenosing tenosynovitis, chronic 165, 445
Stenosis
  causes of 289
  primary 289
  secondary 289
Step sign 163
Stereognosis 254
Sternoclavicular dislocation 116
Sternoclavicular joints 292*f*
Sternoclavicular tuberculosis 122
Sternocleidomastoid 318
Sternum, fracture of 590
Stickler's syndrome 654
Stiff hind foot valgus 463
Stiff hip gait 245
Stiff knee gait 245
Still's disease 88
Stir-fry test 141
Stove-in chest 592
Strabismus 635
Straight-leg-raising 237
  test 234, 237, 276, 343, 343*f*
  reverse 237
Strain
  injury, repetitive 23
  traumatic 281
Streeter's band 654
  syndrome 654
Streeter's syndrome 52, 654
Streptococcus 91
  pneumoniae 91
Stress
  fracture 612
    early detection of 612
  injuries 470*f*
  radiology 427
  syndrome, post-traumatic 652
  test 276, 395, 400*f*, 423, 462
    types of 276
  X-ray 403
Stressful life 287
Stride length 241
Strontium-89 613
Structural dorsolumbar scoliosis 220*f*
Student's elbow 131*f*, 154
Subacromial bursa 122*f*
Subacromial bursitis 121, 644
Subacromial impingement, test for detecting 111

Subacromial syndromes 656
Subarachnoid space 212
Subchondral area 602
Subclavian artery, aneurysms of 508
Subcutaneous emphysema 590
Subcutaneous tissue 477*f*
Subdiaphragmatic irritation 598
Subluxated sternoclavicular joint 118*f*
Subluxatio erecta 117*f*
Submental cyst 577*f*
Subperiosteal cysts 187*f*
Subperiosteal erosions 608
Subperiosteal haematoma 407*f*
Subperiosteal swelling 9*f*
Subscapularis 299
  musculotendinous units of 102
Sub-talar arthritis 470*f*
Sub-talar degenerative arthritis 463
Sudden rapid growth 522
Sudden sciatic stretch test 238, 239*f*
Sudeck's osteoneurodystrophy 68
Sui generis 662
Sunray spicules 409
Superficial posterior compartment syndrome 638
Superior sulcus syndrome 651
Superiosteal cysts 203*f*
Suppurative paronychia, acute 480*f*
Supraclavicular region 158
Supracondylar femoral osteotomy 377*f*
Supracondylar fracture 142, 143, 144*f*
Supracondylar region 158
Supracondylar ridges 133*f*
  palpation of 132
Suprapatellar bursa 388
Suprapatellar infrapatellar fossae 387*f*
Suprapatellar pouch 387*f*, 647
Suprapubic dullness 599
Suprascapular nerve entrapment 503, 656
Supraspinatus
  tendinitis 121
  test for complete rupture of 110
Supratrochanteric depression 331*f*
Supratrochanteric measurement 341
Supratrochanteric region 332
Sural nerve entrapment 499, 501*f*
Sutures 78
Swan-neck deformity 188, 189*f*, 648
Swayback 225
Sweat test 518
Sweating, excessive 21
Swelling 19, 83, 585
  anterolateral 421*f*
  anteromedial 421*f*
  around shoulder 106
  atypical neurofibromatous 275*f*
  diffuse 163
  inflammatory 574
  posterolateral 421*f*
  posteromedial 421*f*
  spindle-shaped 185
  type of 574
Swimmer's shoulder 647
Swollen hands 87
Sympathetic nervous system 639
Sympathetic trunk 218*f*
Symphalangism 181, 202*f*, 655
Symphysis 78

Synchondroses 78
Syndactylism 70*f*, 205*f*
Syndactyly 437, 437*f*, 655
Syndesmophytes 264
    bilateral 264
Syndesmosis 78
Synergists 31
Synovectomy 133*f*, 427*f*
Synovial blood vessels, compression of 653
Synovial chondromatosis 398*f*
Synovial fluid 79, 90
Synovial hypertrophy, test to diagnose 426
Synovial impingement sign 426
Synovial joint 78, 79
    compensation 371
Synovial membrane 79
    villi of 398*f*
Synovial osteochondromatosis 398*f*
Synovial swelling 133*f*, 421, 427*f*
    features of 386
Synovial thickening 28, 385
Synovial xanthomatosis 186*f*
Synovioma 409
Synovitis 80, 80*t*, 398*f*, 611, 630
    develops 635
Synovium 524
Syphilis 49*f*
    congenital 13*f*, 81*f*, 410*f*
    stigmata of 13*f*, 49
Syringomyelia 254, 391*f*
Syringomyelocele 261
Systemic hypotension 636
Systemic lupus erythematosus 86
    nonerosive synovitis of 648
Systremma 20

T

T1-weighted sequence 625
Tabatznik syndrome 657
Tabes dorsalis 391*f*
Tabetic arthropathy 391*f*
    neuropathic joint 391*f*
Tachycardia 644
Tachypnoea 595
Tackling spasticity 306
Tailor's ankle 430
Tailor's bunion 453
Talepes equinus deformity 438
Talipes equinovarus, congenital 437
Talus
    blood supply of 418, 418*f*
    Ewing's sarcoma of 475, 479*f*
    foot 454
    osteochondral fractures of 620
Tardy median nerve palsy 173
Tardy ulnar nerve palsy 511
Targeted therapy 535
Tarsal coalition 437
Tarsal tunnel 657
    syndrome 501*f*, 503, 516, 657
Tarso-metatarsal joints 470*f*
Tear 610
    full thickness 630
    of rotator cuff, test for complete 110
Technetium 99m 611
Technetium-labelled sulphur colloid 610
Tectorial membrane 213

Tectospinal tract 218*f*
Teeth, pressure of 577
Telescopic test 343, 343*f*
Temperature 254, 584, 598
    sensations loss 637
Temporomandibular joint 265*f*, 567, 569, 570, 572
    anatomical landmark of 569
    ankylosis, unilateral 572*f*
    congenital bilateral ankylosis of 569
    dislocation 577*f*
    dislocation of 573
    movements of 572*t*
    palpation of 571*f*
    subluxation of 573
Tenderness 32, 471
Tendinitis 610, 630, 656
Tendinopathy 172
Tendinosis 470*f*
Tendo-Achilles 420, 424
    complete rupture of 424*f*
    lengthening 442*f*
    rupture of 424, 431*f*, 460*f*
        partial 424*f*, 470*f*
        test for 424
    testing for tightness of 311
    tightness 439
Tendon 96, 136, 385
    anterior group of 420
    discontinuity of 463
    giant cell tumour of 186*f*
    low degeneration of 463
    pathologies 610
    sheath, fibroma of 524
    transfer 507
Tendovaginitis 425*f*
    test for 425
Tennis elbow 139, 150
    tests to 140
Tenosynovitis 630, 647
Tension pneumothorax 595
Tension tests 237
Tensor fascia femoris 299, 314*f*, 371*f*
    complex deformity 301, 301*f*, 302*f*
        assessment of 311
    contracture 302*f*
    deformities complex 301
Terminal flexion, limitation of 391
Tetanus 572
    early stage of 14*f*
Tetany 247
Tethered cord syndrome 658
Tetracycline staining studies 532
Tetraphocomelia 653
Textiloma 522
Thalamus 215*f*
Thalidomide tragedy 37
Theatre cocktail party syndrome 292
Thenar eminence 186
Thermal fibres 215*f*
Thigh
    compartment syndrome 657
    lateral cutaneous nerve of 516, 517
Thomas test 335*f*
Thompson's test 424, 424*f*
Thoracic cage 590
Thoracic inlet narrowing 223
Thoracic inlet syndrome 237*f*, 502, 657
    test for 110, 236

Thoracic outlet syndrome 237, 656, 657, 657*f*, 659
Thoracolumbar kyphosis 650
Thoracopagus 7*f*
Thoracotomy 596
Thorax 228
    right lower 599
Thorn prick ulcer 474
Thromboangiitis obliterans 21
Thrombocytopaenia absent radius syndrome 657
Thromboembolism 67
Thrombosis 269, 366
Thumb 197
    abduction of 168, 197*f*
    acute paronychia of 480*f*
    adduction of 197*f*
    aplasia of 643
    Felon of 196*f*
    flexion deformity of 190*f*
    loss of opposition of 509
    movements of 196
    nail test 385
    normal movements of 197*t*
    post-burn contracture of 136*f*
    whitlow of 204*f*
    zero position of 200
Thumb-in-palm deformity 194
Thyroid, carcinoma of 645
Thyrotoxicosis 22
Tibia 57*f*, 413*f*
    anterior surface of 388
    bilateral pseudoarthrosis of 46*f*
    chronic osteomyelitis of 70*f*
    congenital pseudoarthrosis of 47*f*, 48*f*, 52
    pseudoarthrosis of 52
    side-to-side flattening of 49*f*
    vara 382
Tibial artery, posterior 417, 418, 418*f*, 420*f*, 657
Tibial condylar 386, 620
    accessible articular surface of 386*f*
Tibial diaphysis, destruction of 57*f*
Tibial hemimelia 53
Tibial nerve 515
Tibial spine fracture 396, 411*f*
Tibial tendon dysfunction, posterior 420, 440*f*
Tibial tubercle apophysitis 413
Tibial tuberosity, avulsion of 393*f*, 394
Tibialis anterior 299
    tendon of 417
Tibialis posterior 299
    muscle-tendon, function of 462
    tendon 417, 425, 425*f*
        dysfunction 445, 462
Tibiofibular syndesmosis comprises 417
Tibiofibular torsion 418
Tics 247
Tietze's syndrome 658
Tinel's sign 175, 640
    method of 517
Tinkling bowel sounds 599
Tissues 622
Toe
    cockup deformity of 453
    movements of 462
    sign 463
    tourniquet syndrome 646
    windswept deformities of 446*f*, 451

Toe-heel gait 245
Toenail, disorders of 476
Toe-walking 32, 244
Tomography 35
　uses of 608
Tongue
　adhesion of 651
　enlargement of 634
　sign 316*f*, 317
Topallenesthesia 254
Tophi 89
Torticollis 220, 247
　acquired 220
　congenital 220*f*
Tortoise foot 475, 479*f*
Total knee
　joint replacement 623*f*
　replacement 382*f*, 410*f*
Touch
　superficial 254
　tenderness 330
Touraine-Solente-Gole syndrome 658
Tourette syndrome 658
Tourniquet paralysis syndrome 658
Tourniquet test 175
Trachea, rupture of 596
Tract of Burdach 215*f*, 218*f*
Traction injury 506
Transillumination 387
　test, method of 388*f*
Transitional lumbosacral anatomy 287
Transitional vertebra syndrome 288
Transmitted movement 29
Trapezius 299, 507
Trauma
　abdominal 598
　penetrating 598
　severe 634
Trefoil pelvis 280, 282*f*
Tremor 21, 22, 247
Trendelenburg's gait 244, 344, 344*f*
Triangular fibrocartilage, inferior surface of 157
Triceps jerk 252*f*
Triceps muscle 136
Trident hand 649
Trigeminal nerve 499
Trigger finger 193
　management of 194
Trigger point 28
Triponema pallidum bacteria 13*f*
Trisomy 18 642
Trochanter, fibrous dysplasia of 367*f*
Trochanteric bursitis 330
Trochanteric fracture 330
Trochlear nerve 499
Trochlear notch 129
Trochoid joint 79
Trophic ulcer 260*f*, 474, 474*f*, 476*f*
　pre-ulcerative appearance of 474*f*
Tropical diseases 663
Trousseau's sign 247
Tru-cut needle-biopsy system 531
True prolapse 265
Trunk 231
　movements of 233
Tubercle, posterior 418
Tubercular rheumatism 96

Tuberculosis 163, 202*f*
　spine 261
Tuberculous abscess 624*f*
Tuberculous arthritis 81*f*, 116, 152*f*
　advanced 152*f*, 363*f*
Tuberculous caeca 81*f*
Tuberculous dactylitis 183*f*, 184*f*
Tuberculous hip 358
Tuberculous infection 238*f*, 625*f*, 627*f*
Tuberculous synovial thickening 81*f*
Tuberculous synovitis 92, 362*f*
Tuberculous tenosynovitis 176
Tuberculous ulcer 662
Tumoral calcinosis 97
Tumour 466, 522, 610, 612
　benign 522, 532
　diagnosis, primary 613
　grades of primary 612
　intra-spinal 622
　lymph nodes metastasis 533
　malignant 523
　primary 522
　secondary 522
　vascularity of 626
Tunga penetrans 479*f*
Tunnel view 403
Turner syndrome 658
Twist tenderness 227
Typical cubitus valgus deformity 137*f*
Typical gouty tophi 474*f*
Typical rheumatoid
　arthritis 647
　hand 189*f*
Tyrosine metabolism, hereditary disorder of 292*f*

U

Ulcer 27*t*, 662
　arteriosclerotic 475
　causes of 474
　chronic 666
　condylomatous 275*f*
　congenital 662
　depth 486
　hypertensive 664
　malignant 27
　non-healing 644
　non-specific 27
　specific 27
　tropical 663
Ulcerative lesions, painless 653
Ulna, distal end of 637
Ulnar bursa infection 195*f*, 196
Ulnar claw hand 510
Ulnar dominance 511
Ulnar impaction syndrome 658
Ulnar nerve 129, 153*f*, 501*f*, 502, 510, 517, 640, 641
　anterior transposition of 640
　damage of 505, 512*f*
　entrapment neuropathy of 640
　injury 511*f*
　paralysis 187*f*, 190
Ulnar palsy, high 511
Ulnar paradox 511
Ulnar shortening osteotomy 658
Ulnar side 162

Ulnar styloid processes 163*f*
Ulnar tunnel syndrome 658
　incidence of 659
Ulnar-median nerves paralysis 187*f*
Ultrasonography
　pitfalls of 610
　uses of 609
Unicameral bone cyst 123*f*
Untradian rhythm 16
Unusual facies syndrome 60
Upper limb 29, 253, 299
　disorder, work-related 23
　muscles, hypertrophy of 313*f*
　peripheral nerves of 129
Upper motor neuron 217
Upper radioulnar synostosis, congenital 136*f*
Uraemia 22
Urate crystals 474*f*
Ureters 608
Urethra 273
Urethritis, evidences of 653
Uric acid 89
　production of 649
Urinary bladder 218*f*, 598, 608
　injury 599
　innervation of 217, 218*f*
　problems 637
Urine
　chemistry 312
　routine examination of 582
Uterus 273

V

Vacuum disc sign 266
Vagina 273
Vague 91
　low backache and stiffness 290
　nerve 500
Valgus collapse 423*f*
　at ankle 422
Valgus extension overload syndrome 659
Valgus foot 440, 440*f*
Vanishing bone disease 82
Varicose
　ulcer 664
　veins, congenital 72*f*
Varicosities 419
Varus deformities 452*f*
Varus foot 440, 440*f*
Varus recurvatum gait 246
Vascular affections 188
Vascular claudication 20, 20*t*
Vascular malformations 69, 269, 270
　osseous involvement in 68
Vascular origin, ulcers of 475
Vascular tumours 524
Vasculitis 366
Vasogenic brain oedema 585
Vasomotor
　assessment 518
　changes 255
　dysfunction 639
　effect 506-510, 512, 514-516
　functions 240
　swelling 255
Vehicular accidents 506
Veins 45, 212, 417

Venography 35
  epidural 258
Venous diseases 664
Venous stasis ulcers 664
Ventral spinocerebellar tract 218*f*
Ventral spinothalamic tract 218*f*
Ventricular arrhythmias 581
Verbal response 581
Veropause 649
Vertebra 211
  arterial supply of 212
  artery, branches of 212
  body 258
  column 213
    weight transmission along 214
  end plates 287
  localisation of 255*t*
  osteomyelitis 55
  spine 255
  superior end 257
Vertebral bodies, squared anterior 264
Vertical measurement 464
Vertical talus
  bilateral congenital 438*f*
  congenital 438, 438*f*, 441*f*, 446
Vessels 96, 348
Vestibular nerve 500
Vestibulospinal tract 218*f*
Vestigial synovial folds 372
Villonodular synovitis 80, 613, 630
Violence, mode of 590
Viral arthritis 83, 95
Viscera 598
Visceral assessment 255
Visceral functions 240
Viscosity, measurement of 79
Visual loss 10
Vitamin A 641
  derivatives 641
Vitamin D 376*f*, 406*f*
  deficiency 405
Vitiligo 81*f*
Vocal and facial tics 658

Volkmann's ischaemia 66, 129, 139*f*
  acute 68
  contracture 9, 14*f*, 138, 139*f*, 140*f*, 145*t*, 466, 638
  management, severe 139*f*
Volume-controlled ventilators 595
Vomiting
  examination of 582
  symptoms of 646
von Bechterew's disease 290
von Recklinghausen's disease 203*f*
Vrolik's disease 11*f*

W

Waddling gait 244
Wagner-Meggitt classification 485
Walking ability 305
Walking like robot 246
Walking status 320
Warm tender swollen joint 92
Wart 469, 469*t*
Washerman's reaction 33
Washerwoman's strain 22
Weakness 32
Web infection 195*f*
Webbed neck, congenital 104
Weight bearing position 403
Well leg raising test 237
Werewolf syndrome 659, 659*f*
Whistling facies 644
Wide-spread pain disorders, chronic 16, 644
Willebrand's disease 613
Wilson's test 402
World's oldest cancer 522
Wringing test 140, 140*f*
Wrist 649
  arthrodesis of 140*f*
  controls extension of 255
  dorsum of 162
  grotesque deformity of 14*f*
  pain, post-traumatic chronic 172
  pathology 168, 169
  post-burn contracture of 136*f*, 159*f*
  radial deviation of 168
  septic arthritis of 162*f*
  stenosing tenosynovitis 172
  synovial reflections of 157
  three prominent flexors of 174*f*
  tuberculosis of 172
  typical garden spade deformity of 170
  ulnar nerve compression at 511
Wrist drop 190
  splintage for 513
Wrist joint 155, 157
  line, localisation of 162*f*
  movements of 167*f*
  swellings around 163
  tuberculosis of 164*f*
Wry neck 220

X

X chromosome 317, 658
Xanthine oxidase inhibitor 90
Xanthocromia 644
Xanthoma 186*f*, 470*f*
  multiple 186*f*
Xanthomatosis 475
  multiple 186*f*
Xanthomatous swellings, multiple 478*f*
Xeroradiography 34, 608
  disadvantage of 608
  uses of 608

Y

Yergason's manoeuvre 110
Yersinia arthritic infection 89
Yttrium-90 613

Z

Zig-zag deformity 47
Zika virus 646